NUTRITION

IN HEALTH AND DISEASE

Helen S. Mitchell

A.B., PH.D., SC.D., *Research Consultant, Harvard School of Public Health; Nutrition Consultant, Head Start Program, O.E.O.; Dean Emeritus of the School of Home Economics and formerly Research Professor of Nutrition, University of Massachusetts, Amherst; Exchange Professor Hokkaido University, Sapporo, Japan; Formerly Principal Nutritionist, Office of Defense, Health and Welfare; Professor of Physiology and Nutrition, Battle Creek College.*

Henderika J. Rynbergen

B.S., M.S., *Professor of Science, Emeritus, Cornell University-New York Hospital School of Nursing. Formerly Director of Dietetics, American University Hospital, Beirut, Lebanon; Food Clinic Dietitian, Vanderbilt Clinic, Presbyterian Hospital, New York; Food Clinic Dietitian, Barnes Hospital, St. Louis; and Nutritionist, Community Health Association, Boston*

Linnea Anderson

M.P.H., *Associate Professor, Public Health Nutrition, University of Michigan; formerly Nutrition Consultant, Michigan Department of Public Health*

Marjorie V. Dibble

B.S., M.S., *Chairman, Department of Nutrition and Food Science, College of Home Economics, Syracuse University*

COOPER'S
NUTRITION
in HEALTH
and DISEASE

Fifteenth Edition

Mitchell

Rynbergen

Anderson

Dibble

J. B. LIPPINCOTT COMPANY

Philadelphia   **Toronto**

FIFTEENTH EDITION

Copyright © 1968, by J. B. Lippincott Company

Copyright, 1928, 1929, 1930, 1931, 1933, 1935,
1938, 1941, 1943, 1947, 1950, 1953, 1958, 1963
by J. B. Lippincott Company

This book is fully protected by copyright and, with the exception of brief extracts for review, no part of it may be reproduced in any form, by print, photoprint, microfilm, or any other means, without the written permission of the publishers.

Distributed in Great Britain by
Pitman Medical Publishing Co., Limited, London

Library of Congress Catalog Card Number 68-20822

Printed in the United States of America

Preface

As in previous editions this text presents a comprehensive review of the principles of nutrition as they apply to the needs of normal persons of all ages and to the more specific dietary needs of individuals suffering from certain pathological conditions.

Part One, in a completely revised first chapter, introduces the student to the scope of the science of nutrition and its application, including the role of the nurse, the dietitian and the nutritionist in promoting good nutrition through the proper use of food. A brief discussion of federal, state and local agencies involved in food and nutrition services is followed by a discussion of world food problems confronting the United Nations and other international agencies.

The chapters concerned with specific nutrients (Chapters 2 through 8), their chemical composition, functions in the body and the food sources of these nutrients have been revised extensively. Since students entering educational programs in nursing come to their professional courses with more background in chemistry and the life sciences than previously, these chapters include more details in nutritional science than earlier editions. For example, special attention has been given to present concepts of fat metabolism, including our understanding of the role of saturated and unsaturated fats and cholesterol in the American diet.

An entirely new chapter on digestion, absorption and metabolism (Chapter 9) has been added to clarify the interrelationships among these processes. The mechanisms involved in the transport of nutrients across the intestinal mucosa, and the role of enzymes in the metabolism of nutrients in the tissues are included in this chapter.

The discussion of regional, cultural and religious influences on food habits in Chapter 11 has been expanded to include pertinent material from the Overseas Supplement to the 14th edition. Good nutrition is possible using a wide variety of different food patterns, but a knowledge of food values is necessary to accomplish this goal even when foods are plentiful. This is even more true when food is scarce and of limited variety. This chapter should be useful to professional persons working with special groups in the U. S. and in other countries.

Chapter 16 is devoted to the world-wide problem of malnutrition. Special emphasis is given to protein-calorie malnutrition as it affects primarly the preschool child, resulting in marasmus or kwashiorkor. Whereas, in earlier decades, emphasis was placed on the high death rates in the age group 1–4, the concern now is with the possible effect of malnutrition on mental development of those who survive early deficiencies and seem to recover physically. At the same time, food research has made it possible to use indigenous foods to supply adequate protein and other nutrients in the form of food mixtures suitable for children as well as for adults. This chapter also includes discussions of vitamin and mineral deficiencies which still occur around the world in spite of current knowledge of causes, cures and prevention.

Chapter 17, Safeguarding Our Food Supply, has been completely rewritten. Although most foodborne diseases are on the decrease in the U.S. outbreaks of foodborne salmonella infections have increased significantly in the past decade. At the same time there is considerable public concern about the control of food additives, pesticide residues and other food contaminants. Food faddists are apt to exaggerate these problems. The increasingly active role of the federal agencies in the public health protection of our food supply is a source of reassurance.

v

As in past editions other chapters in Part One discuss the Recommended Dietary Allowances; the nutritional needs during pregnancy and lactation; current practices in infant feeding; the special nutritional needs of growing children and the teenager during the adolescent growth spurt, and the needs of adults as they grow older.

Part Two, Therapeutic Nutrition, presents the principles of diet modification in the treatment of disease. The Introduction and Chapter 18 focus on the patient and the roles of the nurse, the dietitian and the physician in the dietary phase of patient care. Many of the chapters in this section have been extensively revised. Atherosclerosis, arteriosclerosis and various forms of heart disease are discussed in line with present and rapidly advancing knowledge in regard to advisable diets for these conditions. New approaches in the treatment of obesity are featured in the chapter on weight control.

Chapter 25, dealing with diseases of the kidney, includes a discussion of the dietary care of patients on hemodialysis, and of the very low protein diet for patients with oliguria for whom dialysis is not available.

Where possible, Exchange Systems, used widely since 1950 for calculating pattern dietaries for patients with diabetes, have been modified for use when other nutrients or caloric requirements are involved. For example, exchange lists are included for diets restricted in sodium, for protein, sodium and potassium restriction, and for fat-controlled diets.

Suggestions for the more liberal dietary treatment of peptic ulcer are included in Chapter 26, Diseases of the Stomach and Esophagus. The malabsorption syndromes, including disaccharidase deficiencies and defective monosaccharide absorption, gluten-induced enteropathy, cystic fibrosis and tropical sprue, and the use of medium-chain triglycerides in the treatment of some of these disorders have been added to other discussions of the dietary treatment of Diseases of the Intestines, Chapter 27.

The low-taurine diet, recently reported as successful in the treatment of psoriasis, has been included in Chapter 30, Allergy and Diseases of the Skin. A discussion of favism has been added to Chapter 31, Diseases of the Blood.

Chapter 34, Diseases of Children, has been extensively revised. It includes directions for the ketogenic diet, recently again proved valuable in the treatment of epilepsy in children not responding to drug therapy. The section dealing with inborn errors of metabolism has been greatly expanded and includes discussion of the metabolic enzymes involved. The most recent findings on phenylketonuria and newly revised Exchange Lists for phenylalanine-controlled diets are included. A discussion of several other errors of metabolism and their dietary treatment has been added.

Part Three includes the basic principles of food selection and preparation, and selected recipes for modifying food preparation for therapeutic diets. These include recipes for increasing caloric and protein content, and for control of calorie, carbohydrate, sodium, and fatty acid intake. Recipes for gluten-restricted and allergy diets are also given.

Part Four, as previously, includes various reference tables, extensive bibliographies and a glossary of terms used. Table 1 is the general food value table. Table 2 is the Food Composition Table for Short Method of Dietary Analysis (3rd revision) which is convenient for quick estimates in dietary surveys. Table 3, Fatty Acid and Cholesterol Content of Foods, has been added for use in planning fat-controlled diets. Table 4, Essential Amino Acid Content of Foods, is also new. Physical Growth Standards for children ages 2 to 18 have been added in Table 11. Also the new height and weight tables for adults, adapted from Sargent, have been included in an attempt to assist individuals to relate body weight to body type as well as to age and height.

An extensive and current bibliography, classified by subjects, will be of special help to instructors and others wishing to pursue certain subjects in greater depth than is possible in a text. The Glossary of terms used has also been expanded and brought up to date.

THE AUTHORS

Acknowledgments

The authors wish to express their deep appreciation to their many friends and colleagues for generous help given them during the preparation of the 15th edition of *Nutrition in Health and Disease*. One of the compensations for the arduous work involved in such a revision is the contact with and the courtesy extended by investigators, associates and other authors for permission to use material from their work and research.

Special thanks are due to Miss Mary Egan, Chief of the Nutrition Section, Division of Health Services, Children's Bureau, Department of Health, Education and Welfare, for specific suggestions given in the preparation of Chapters 12, 13, 14 and 34 dealing with the nutrition of mothers and children; to several members of the staff of the Consumer and Food Economics Research Division of the Department of Agriculture for conference time and supplying information and illustrative materials, especially tabular material for Part Four; to Dr. L. J. Tepley, Chief of Applied Nutrition, UNICEF, United Nations, for a file of pictures and information regarding malnutrition in many countries; to Dr. Moises Behar, Director of the Institute for Nutrition for Central America and Panama, Guatemala, for photographs and information regarding malnutrition in Central America; to Dr. Eugene H. Stevenson, Assistant to the Director, Division of Nutrition, Food and Drug Administration, for advice on up-to-date regulations on food protection discussed in Chapter 17; to Olin Mathieson Chemical Co. for permission to use the picture of healthy children of many nationalities in Chapter 11; to Mrs. Alice Stewart for revision of the pattern diet of Southeastern U.S.A. used in Chapter 10; to Dr. Franz J. Ingelfinger, Editor of the New England Journal of Medicine, for permission to use the graph of the intestinal epithelial cell in Chapter 9, and to Dr. Eva Donaldson Wilson, Department of Home Economics, Ohio State University, for permission to use the revised Food Composition Table for Short Method of Dietary Analysis in Part Four.

Also to Mrs. Marjorie Zukel, Nutrition Consultant, Heart Disease Control Program, Public Health Service, Department of Health, Education and Welfare, for help in preparing the tables of fat-controlled diets; to Dr. George L. Bailey and to the dietary staff of the Peter Bent Brigham Hospital, Boston, for help with Chapter 25, Diseases of the Kidney; to Dr. Marvin H. Sleisenger of the Department of Medicine, Cornell Medical Center, who made available the photographs of the mucosa of the jejunum in celiac disease before and after treatment; to Dr. Daphne A. Roe of the Graduate School of Nutrition, Cornell University, for permission to use the low taurine diet and for help in preparing the text material relating to it; to Miss Geraldine Getty of the Arkansas Children's Hospital, for obtaining the photograph of hospitalized children eating together at table used in Chapter 34; and to Miss Helen E. Walsh, Chief, Bureau of Public Health Nutrition, Department of Public Health, State of California, for permission to use Tables of Phenylalanine Content of Food in Chapter 34.

Lastly, the authors wish to acknowledge the patience and skill of their editors, David T. Miller, J. Stuart Freeman, Jr. and Naomi Coplin, in converting the manuscript into a book.

To all these, mentioned and unmentioned, the authors express gratitude, while recognizing that any errors which may inadvertently appear in the text are solely their own responsibility.

Contents

Part One: PRINCIPLES OF NUTRITION

Part Two: DIET IN DISEASE

Contents

Part Three: MODIFICATION OF FOOD FOR THERAPEUTIC DIETS

Part Four: TABULAR MATERIAL AND BIBLIOGRAPHY

PART ONE
Principles of Nutrition

CHAPTER 1

Growth of the Science of Nutrition and Its Application

Nutritional Status U.S.A. • *Role of the Nurse, Dietitian and Nutritionist in Promoting Good Nutrition in the Community* • *U. S. Agencies Engaged in Nutrition Activities* • *Nutrition—A National and International Issue*

FOOD—MAN'S FIRST CONCERN

Food, the sustainer of life itself for all living creatures, has of necessity been the concern of man down through the ages. Just as most wild animals are today, for thousands of years man was a hunter and gatherer. About 6,000 years ago when the earliest civilizations were established, he became a food producer, the better to alleviate his hunger. For less than 70 years, however, man has gradually accumulated the knowledge necessary to provide food not only to satisfy hunger, but also to nourish his body so that he may realize its full potential. In the 20th century man has developed the science of nutrition and has learned how specific nutrients in foods support growth and maintain life.

To provide food for the millions of individuals in today's world is a complex problem involving not only nutrition science but many other disciplines: agriculture, marketing, microbiology, food technology, economics, education, psychology, anthropology, medicine, sociology and perhaps others.

Evolution of Nutrition Research

Early in the 20th century research workers in food chemistry and in physiology in Europe, America and Japan demonstrated the need of good-quality protein for the growth of animals. Later the concept of the number and the kinds of minerals needed for growth came to include trace elements, as well as those present in larger amounts. At the same time, other workers showed the presence and the need for certain "accessory food factors," later called vitamins. Then followed in rapid succession studies of amino acids, essential fatty acids, hormones, enzymes, chemical regulators and intermediary products of digestion and metabolism.

Research methods and scientific tools have kept pace with changing concepts. First, the chemist analyzed foods for protein, fat, total ash and moisture, and assumed the balance to be carbohydrate in nature. Then he analyzed the ash for its specific mineral constituents. Later, animal-feeding experiments supplemented the chemist's data by showing that hitherto unrecognized food factors were necessary for growth and that the rate of growth could be used to measure the presence of such substances. This method is known as bio-assay. Now microorganisms are being used, and the method is called microbiologic assay.

Nutrition research today encompasses more and more facets requiring teams of scientists from several disciplines. Survey teams conducting nutritional status studies may require a physician, a nutritionist, a nurse, a biochemist, an anthropologist and a laboratory technician. The study of food values and how to improve them demands the skills of chemists, physicists and food technologists as well as the nutrition scientist. New methods and tools for research have permitted progress from the earlier and, sometimes, crude animal experiments to more accurate observations on humans. The use of radioactive isotopes and tagged elements have led to a better understanding of metabolic pathways of specific nutrients. And the science of genetics has shown us how DNA and RNA control protein synthesis (See Chap. 9). Such studies have in turn opened new vistas on the abnormalities related to certain metabolic diseases and to their possible prevention and treatment.

Nutrition and Dietetics Defined

Nutrition may be defined as the combination of processes by which the living organism receives and utilizes the nutrients from food for the maintenance of its functions and for the growth of tissues. Malnutrition results when the organism fails to receive or cannot utilize the essential nutrients.

Dietetics is the application of the science of nutrition and food management to the feeding of individuals or groups. The dietitian is particularly aware of the variation in nutrient needs determined by the sex, age, activity, and physical condition of the individual or group. Psychology as well as socioeconomic factors play an important role in the functions of the dietitian.

NUTRITIONAL STATUS U.S.A.

In the United States we have used two methods to determine what people are con-

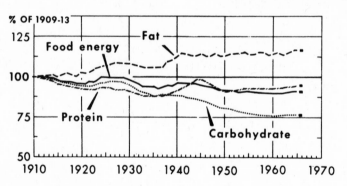

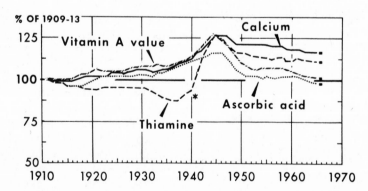

Fig. 1-1. Trends in per capita consumption of nutrients in the United States, 1910–1966. (*Top*) Food energy, protein, fat and carbohydrates. (*Bottom*) Calcium, vitamin A, thiamine and ascorbic acid. * Enrichment initiated. ▬ 1966 preliminary. (U.S.D.A. Agricultural Research Service, 1966)

suming and one method to determine nutritional status. The first two methods are (1) household food consumption surveys, and (2) statistics on the disappearance of food from our markets.

Household Consumption Surveys. A nationwide survey was made in the United States in 1965-66. Earlier surveys were made in 1936, 1942, 1948, and 1955. In 1965-66, data of household usage of foods were collected from 15,000 homes during the four seasons of the year and in different sections of the country. Although data from this last survey are not completely summarized as yet, the findings from this and the earlier surveys show changing trends both in food selection and in the nutritional quality of American diets.

Findings from such surveys help to focus attention on areas where improvement in nutrition is needed. This may be accomplished by popular education or by a concerted attempt to improve the food supply. For instance, the data from one of the earlier surveys were responsible for the initiation of bread and flour enrichment (See Chap. 10). Information from later surveys will undoubtedly be put to use by industry and through educational channels to benefit the consumer.

Market Disappearance Statistics. Figure 1–1 shows the trends in U. S. consumption of nutrients from 1910 to 1966. These trends are derived by the Agricultural Research Service of the U. S. Department of Agriculture from the statistics available to them on the quantities of foods that disappear from the retail markets each year. It is interesting to note the decrease in the consumption of carbohydrate and the increase in fat. The decrease in carbohydrate is due primarily to a decrease in the consumption of bread and potatoes.

Nutritional Status Surveys. Surveys of the nutritional status of a large number of individuals, which include medical inspection, biochemical analysis of blood and urine, and dietary histories, have not been done recently in the U. S. The Public Health Service conducted such surveys in the late 1940's in various parts of the country. From 1947 to 1958 studies were sponsored by the Cooperative State Agricultural Experiment Stations and the Agricultural Research Service of the U.S.D.A. A digest of the latter survey was published in 1959 by Agnes Fay Morgan and is the most comprehensive statement to date on this subject.[1]

At present it appears that the population as a whole consumes a diet adequate in essential nutrients and is free from frank deficiency symptoms, but from a variety of research there are indications that all age groups do not fare equally well. There are signs that we need to be especially concerned with the nutritional status of pregnant women, infants and preschool children and adolescent girls. For pregnant women, infants and preschool children socioeconomic factors may be affecting food intake. At the same time we are faced with a problem of overnutrition: obesity and, possibly, certain chronic diseases are the results of too much food.

EVIDENCE THAT BETTER DIETS CAN BENEFIT NUTRITIONAL STATUS

In wartime it was demonstrated that "improvement of the diet of workmen whose diet was not previously up to the standard for health was followed by increased output without any conscious increased effort and also by a reduction in the number of accidents."[2] In the United States the importance attached to proper feeding of industrial workers has come to be appreciated to the extent that provision of adequate food for employees has continued to be emphasized where there is progressive plant management. The feeding of men in the armed forces is constantly under study to improve both palatability and nutritive quality of the food because authorities appreciate the importance of the right food for health, morale and general stamina of the men.

Among the postwar studies, those in Newfoundland and in the Philippines are notable examples of measured accomplishment. In Newfoundland, many fisherfolk

---

[1] Morgan, A. F.: Nutritional Status, U.S.A. Cal. Agr. Exp. Station Bull. 769. Berkeley, Oct., 1959.

[2] Orr, J. B.: Brit. Med. J., *1*:73, 1941.

live in isolated coastal villages shut off from outside supplies except for about 2 months in the summer. One of the authors made a survey in several of the northern outposts 15 years prior to the study begun in 1944 in some of the southern village outposts. The conditions in 1944 were depressingly similar to those found earlier. The signs and the symptoms found on clinical examination and biologic tests in 1944 were indicative of a multiple vitamin deficiency. The enrichment of margarine with vitamins A and D and of all white flour with three B vitamins plus iron and calcium became effective in June, 1944. A follow-up survey in 1948 found a striking improvement in health, particularly in those symptoms which might have been expected to respond to the nutritional factors provided in the enrichment program. Beriberi, which had been widespread prior to 1944, was practically nonexistent in 1948, and tuberculosis deaths were reduced by half in 8 years.[3] The policy of flour enrichment in Newfoundland has been maintained since her union with Canada in 1949, and there is enthusiastic support for it as a consequence of the health improvement.

Beriberi has long been associated with the eating of polished rice, the form preferred by most oriental peoples. Few countries have adequate statistics to give a true picture of the incidence of beriberi, but the Philippines have kept records since 1920. On the peninsula of Bataan, deaths from beriberi had ranged from 150 to 300 a year, and as many as 12,000 persons gave evidence of health continually impaired by beriberi symptoms. Since the initiation of the rice-enrichment program in 1949, inspired and directed by Dr. R. R. Williams, the incidence of beriberi has been reduced about 90 per cent, and not a single death from beriberi occurred during the next 2 years.[4] Even though education may have stimulated some improvement in food habits and in methods of milling rice over a long period of time, it is unlikely that any such accomplishment as that reported above ever could have been realized from education alone, even within the lifetime of children.

Other studies on smaller groups in this country in institutions where diet could be controlled and nutritional status studied have shown good results. Food providing essential nutrients not only can cure deficiencies and allow for optimal growth of children but also make the difference between mediocre and buoyant health.

ROLE OF THE NURSE, DIETITIAN AND NUTRITIONIST IN PROMOTING GOOD NUTRITION IN THE COMMUNITY

The Nurse in the Hospital may be of great assistance in helping a patient understand and carry out the doctor's diet order, whether normal or therapeutic. She may also consult with the dietitian in planning a menu which the patient will accept. In assisting the patient with his diet she may also influence his family's food plan and, thereby, improve the food selection for the whole family.

In the out-patient clinic the nurse, by using an educational approach which the patient understands and accepts, can help in the selection of an adequate and appropriate diet. To change food habits is usually a slow process. Thus, at each clinic visit, the nurse has the opportunity to help the patient gradually to make the necessary adjustments.

In the obstetrics unit of the hospital, the nurse has a unique opportunity to discuss with the mother her own diet as well as that of her family, during her prenatal visits to the doctor. After the birth of the baby, new mothers particularly will have many questions on feeding the baby which the nurse can answer (See Chap. 13).

The public health nurse may be in a position to observe community nutrition problems more closely than any other person. Her function may be largely educational or it may involve giving some bedside care or directing the home health aide or housekeeper. She has an opportunity to carry practical nutrition into many homes untouched by other services. Her evaluation of family, or individual, food habits may

[3] Medical survey and resurvey in Newfoundland, 1944 and 1948. Canad. M.A.J., 52:227, 1945; 60: 329, 1949.

[4] Williams, R. R.: Am. J. Nursing, 52:447, 1952.

disclose nutrition problems that might be improved by instruction in food preparation. When such instruction is carried out in the home, suggestions should be made in line with the cooking facilities available.

When money for food is limited it is particularly important to be able to guide the homemaker in the selection of low-cost foods that will provide adequate nutrition for all members of the household.

The school nurse has intimate contact with the children, is usually respected by them and sometimes may be more successful than the child's mother in influencing food habits. She may be able to help the mother when a child needs guidance or has eating problems. At school the nurse may be consulted about the school lunch menus, or, in cases where the school lunch does not provide for the best nutrition, she may help to improve the program. She often plans or assists with the educational program for the improvement of nutrition either in the classroom or the lunch room.

Where communities or schools employ "nurse-teachers" with broad responsibilities in school health programs, nurses are often called on to serve on school health committees. They must be prepared to help to coordinate health programs, including nutrition education. They are often the most logical link between the school, the home and the community services.

The dietitian and public health nutritionist, both specialists in foods and nutrition, are ready to help the nurse in solving nutrition problems either in the hospital or the community. The public health nutritionist, available in larger communities, functions primarily as an educator, sometimes working with the school nurse, sometimes with the public health nurses caring for families in their homes. In any situation the specialist in foods and nutrition is ready to assist the nurse, or in complex problems, assume the responsibility for working directly with the family.

U. S. AGENCIES ENGAGED IN NUTRITION ACTIVITIES

Numerous federal, state and local government agencies, private agencies, and industrial and educational institutions are engaged in various phases of nutrition research and education. Their publications are generally available to nurses and nutritionists and many of them are valuable aids to professional education, or for use

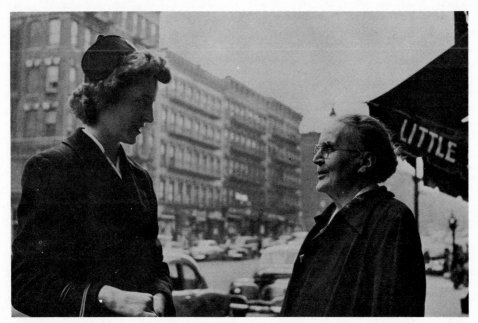

FIG. 1-2. A public health nurse discusses a problem with one of her patients. (Photo from The New York Hospital, New York, N. Y.)

in educational programs with the lay public. A few of the groups from which reliable information can be obtained are listed in the following paragraphs.

Official Agencies. *The U. S. Department of Agriculture* (U.S.D.A.) has many divisions concerned with food and nutrition. Of particular interest are two sections of the Agricultural Research Service: the Consumer and Food Economics Research Division and the Human Nutrition Research Division. They conduct research and surveys, such as those referred to earlier in this chapter, and also publish numerous bulletins which serve as references for everyone working in the field. For example, the Consumer and Food Economics Research Division publishes Agriculture Handbook #8, "Composition of Foods: Raw, Processed, Prepared," which is widely used as a reference. Table 1, Part IV in this book was compiled primarily from this reference. The Department of Agriculture, through the state educational agencies, also administers the school lunch program which may feed as many as 19 million children in a school day.[5]

The Department of Health, Education, and Welfare (HEW) has several units involved in nutrition research or service. The Children's Bureau (CB) is concerned with health services to mothers and children, including the nutritional needs of pregnant women, infants and children. The Food and Drug Administration (FDA) through its regulations is involved in protecting the safety of our food and drugs. The Public Health Service (PHS) is involved both in nutrition research and service. It carries on and supports research through the National Institutes of Health, and, through state and local health agencies, is involved in service programs.

The Office of Economic Opportunity (OEO) in the Executive Office of the President is vitally concerned not only with the welfare of the economically deprived part of our population but also with the health of this group. The Head Start Program for preschool children is one example of their activities.

[5] Leverton, R. M.: The world's biggest lunch counter. Food and Nutrition News, 38, March, 1967.

The nutrition activities of these and other agencies are coordinated at the federal level by the Interagency Committee on Nutrition Education. Their *Nutrition Committee News* is a valuable source of information for nurses and dietitians.

Other Agencies, Professional Societies and Institutions. The Food and Nutrition Board of the National Academy of Sciences —National Research Council was established in 1940 to consider questions pertaining to nutrition measures necessary during World War II. The Academy is a quasi-governmental agency. The Food and Nutrition Board has taken the leadership in promoting nutrition research and its application to health. The Recommended Dietary Allowances, the yardstick to good nutrition, was one of their first accomplishments and has been revised at 5-year intervals since it was first published in 1941.

The American Institute of Nutrition (AIN) is a professional society for nutrition scientists and publishes the Journal of Nutrition. The American Society of Clinical Nutrition, a division of the AIN, publishes the American Journal of Clinical Nutrition.

The Nutrition Foundation, Inc., established in 1941 by the food and allied industries, "seeks to make essential contributions to the advancement of nutrition knowledge and its effective application, and thus serve the health and welfare of the public." Since 1942 the Foundation has published Nutrition Reviews—abstracts of current scientific literature in nutrition. Throughout the years the Foundation has also published semipopular brochures on nutrition topics of current interest.

The American Dietetic Association (ADA), the professional society for dietitians, was founded in 1917 during World War I by pioneers in the then emerging profession of dietetics. The Association began publication of the *Journal of the American Dietetic Association* in 1925, and continues to report research and studies in food and nutrition and in the administration of food service. In addition, the Association publishes educational materials which are as useful to nurses, doctors, teachers and others in related professions as to dietitians.

Unreliable Organizations. In recent years several widely advertised organizations, which were deliberately given names similar to those of organizations mentioned above, have issued unreliable publications in the field of nutrition and dietetics. They have even led some professionally trained people to accept fads and false ideas about food requirements, vitamin and mineral supplements, and the "dangers" of commercial fertilizers and food additives.

NUTRITION—A NATIONAL AND INTERNATIONAL ISSUE

Ever since World War II scientists in technically advanced countries have become increasingly aware of world food problems. Surveys have been made in many of the developing countries in an effort to understand their specific problems of food production, distribution, conservation, and nutrient content of the local food supply. The public press has repeatedly commented that the world food supply is not keeping pace with the population explosion. It requires a more scientific analysis of the world situation, however, to know where to start in solving the dilemma.

It is generally agreed that the realistic approach is to give the kind of aid that will help the developing countries to help themselves. The Agricultural Extension Service in the U. S. worked with rural families during the 1920's and '30's, to improve food production by better agricultural procedures. The program, which is still continuing, is so successful that today we are exporting our surplus farm produce to other countries. The lessons learned from extension methods in this country are now being applied in modified form among rural and village people in many underdeveloped countries.

Dr. Philip R. Lee, Assistant Secretary of the U. S. Department of H.E.W., comments:

An effective program to fight malnutrition must consider many interlocking causes. The daily diet of men is conditioned by what they grow, by what they can buy, and by what the food practices of their parents and grandparents have been. One factor is common to all: tradition. To accelerate dietary improvements among malnourished peoples, it is best to begin with food resources they are accustomed to. Introduction of new habits must be presented patiently and tactfully.[6]

For many years the U. S. Government has been concerned with "freedom from hunger" campaigns. The Foreign Aid Program and the Food For Freedom Program initiated in 1966 included combating malnutrition as a major objective. The Agency for International Development (AID) began in 1966 to add vitamins A and D to the nonfat dry milk which was being sent to developing countries to improve the diets of millions of children.

Dr. Lee continues:

These new programs to combat malnutrition are being combined with expanded United States efforts to aid agricultural production and food technology, to improve health services, to make family planning services available to those who wish them and to increase educational opportunities.[6]

These efforts are closely coordinated with international organizations such as FAO, WHO, UNICEF and UNESCO, described in the next paragraphs.

Prevalence of Poor Nutrition in the World

In any survey nutritional status must be measured by medical examination of individuals and by statistical data which distinguish between the prevalence of subnormal nutrition and frank deficiencies. Even though dietary surveys may show diets to be faulty and even seriously inadequate according to our standards, physical evidence of malnutrition may not be conspicuous. However, habitual malnutrition predisposes people to physical ills and defects, and early malnutrition may affect ability to learn. Thus a careful distinction should be made between the extent to which diets seem to be inadequate, as shown by dietary surveys, and the prevalence of actual deficiency conditions in a population group.

The first World Food Survey, made in 1946, was based on somewhat inadequate

---

6 Lee, P. R.: Nutrition and world health. Nutrition News, 29:9, 1966.

data from 70 countries with some 90 per cent of the world's population. The later surveys, reported in 1952 and 1963, were even more inclusive. The last one, based on more reliable data from over 80 countries, covered about 95 per cent of the world population.[7] The people in less developed countries were found to have an average intake of just over 2,100 calories compared with over 3,000 calories for people in developed countries. More serious was the finding that "the intake of animal protein in these countries and regions is only one fifth of that in the more developed areas."[7] The food intakes in the less developed countries are considerably short of the requirements, and, in fact, it is estimated that at least 20 per cent of the

[7] FAO Basic Study No. 11. Third World Food Survey, Rome, Italy, 1963.

population in these areas are undernourished and 60 per cent are malnourished. Even looking only to the needs of the development decade 1965 to 1975, the world food supplies will have to be increased by more than 35 per cent merely "to sustain the world's population at its present unsatisfactory level of diet."[7]

Such world surveys do not tell the true extent of malnutrition in each country or the areas or seasons in which conditions are the worst; however, they do focus attention upon countries or areas where further nutritional status studies should be made. A world map on page 216 shows the extent and distribution of calorie-protein malnutrition among young children (See Chap. 16). Some of the deficiency diseases discussed in Chapter 16 seldom occur in the United States today but all are found in the world today.

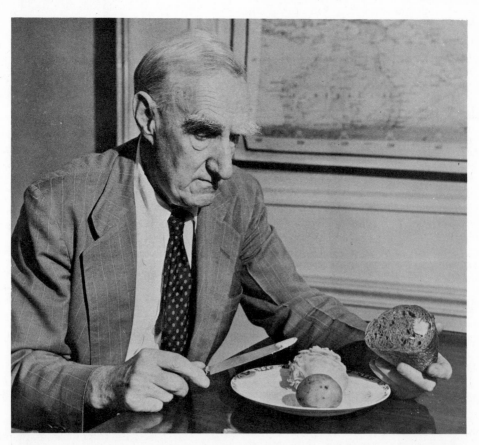

Fɪɢ. 1-3. Lord John Boyd Orr, first Director General of the Food and Agricultural Organization of the United Nations. (Science Service, Inc., Washington, D. C.)

Not all subnormal nutrition should be designated malnutrition, but the problem demands attention, as indicated by this comment by W. H. Griffith, a veteran in the field:

The prevalence of subnormal nutrition and frank malnutrition in the world today, despite amazing advances in knowledge during the past fifty years, is troubling. Even in the United States there is sufficient evidence of faulty food practices to suggest that we have not succeeded in doing an effective and persuasive job of education about nutrition. Physicians and clinical investigators have a large stake in this problem and the role of medicine in nutrition is increasing in extent and importance.[8]

World Approach to Solving Nutritional Problems

Implementation of ideas to improve the world situation has become a function of a number of UN agencies, set up for specific purposes and staffed by experts from many countries. Those agencies concerned with health and nutrition will be mentioned briefly.

The Food and Agriculture Organization (FAO) was the first of the permanent United Nations agencies to start planning for a better fed world. FAO became a full-fledged international organization in Quebec, Canada, in 1945 under the leadership of Lord John Boyd Orr, a world leader in the field of nutrition. He was the 1949 recipient of a Nobel Peace Prize in recognition of his leadership in this work.

The FAO is today one of the largest UN agencies, with headquarters in Rome and with 120 or more countries participating in its work. FAO publications are directed principally to administrators, technicians and other specialists in the broad fields of agriculture and nutrition who are making an effort to raise standards of living.

The World Health Organization (WHO), with headquarters in Geneva, Switzerland, came into being in 1948, with 120 countries now collaborating in an effort to achieve the highest possible level of health.

Such a goal demands cooperation of several countries in matters such as control of communicable diseases and the setting up of international standards for drugs, pesticides and other biological substances and for exchange of scientific knowledge. WHO publishes technical and semitechnical bulletins in several languages and a monthly WHO Chronicle which provides news of health activities in various countries.

Joint FAO/WHO technical committees work together on food and agriculture problems and organize and conduct meetings with experts from specific areas concerning health problems in those areas. These meetings and reports are concerned, first, with finding out specific needs and how they can best be met and then following up with plans for educational programs. A joint FAO/UNICEF/WHO program for the development of protein-rich foods has been in progress for years and some results of this project are most encouraging.

The United Nations Educational, Scientific and Cultural Organization (UNESCO) is also concerned with improving the living standards of the world's people. To that end UNESCO has been attempting to provide, through its Fundamental Education Program and through active cooperation with government agencies in respective countries, means whereby more people may have at least an elementary education. UNESCO aims to promote collaboration among nations through education, science and culture in order to further human rights and freedoms without discrimination as to race, sex, language or religion.

The United Nations Children's Fund (originally United Nations International Children's Emergency Fund) (UNICEF) was founded in 1946 as an outgrowth of World War II to meet the emergency needs of children in war-ravaged countries. UNICEF is currently assisting in over 500 long-range programs in more than 100 countries, where they are especially concerned about the welfare of mothers and children. The U. S. donates surplus milk through UNICEF after the needs of the U. S. school feeding programs have been

[8] Griffith, W. H.: Food as a regulator of metabolism. Am. J. Clin. Nutr., *17*:391, 1965.

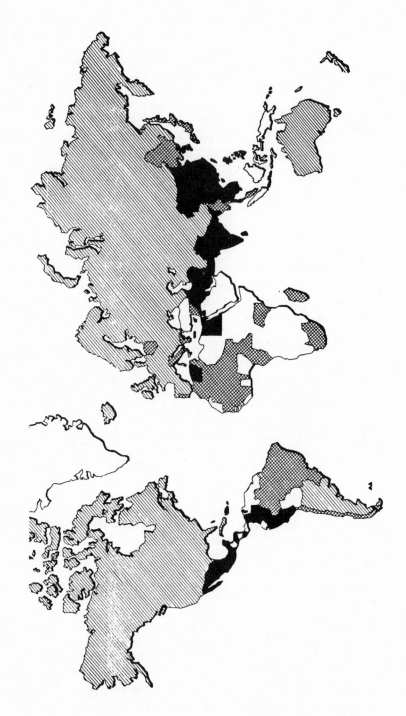

FIG. 1-4. A difference in calories. ■ Poor: below 2,250 calories per person. ▨ Medium: 2,250-2,750 calories per person. ▨ Good: over 2,750 calories per person. (Kihss, Peter: U.N. Sets the Table. Food and People Series No. 2, a UNESCO project. New York, Manhattan Publishing Co.)

met. UNICEF Christmas cards and the "Trick or Treat" program at Halloween (sponsored by UNICEF) have become symbols of concern and are a means of giving tangible aid.

Many other member countries of the UN besides the United States contribute generously to these UN agencies and also have international projects of their own. A Round-table Conference, sponsored by UNICEF and held at Bellagio, Italy, in 1964, was entitled "Planning for the Needs of Children in Developing Countries" and involved many cooperating agencies. The International Nutrition Congresses and other regional conferences held in recent years were all concerned with working out more specific guide lines for each country or area to meet the needs of children in those areas. No two countries have exactly the same problems.

This chapter has presented just a brief sketch of the evolution of the science of nutrition and of the many opportunities for its application in today's world. Scientists have been aware of some of the problems for decades and have been studying how to solve them. The public has now become aroused to support action. Results of national and international efforts toward a better-fed world will be worth watching in the decades to come.

STUDY QUESTIONS AND ACTIVITIES

1. How old is the science of nutrition?
2. Define the words *nutrition* and *dietetics*.
3. What groups in the population of the United States are still in need of some concern in terms of their nutritional status?
4. Which of the three major food groups has shown increased consumption in the past 50 years? Which has decreased? What foods are responsible for the decrease?
5. Give scientific evidence that improvement of nutritional status is possible as a result of food enrichment.

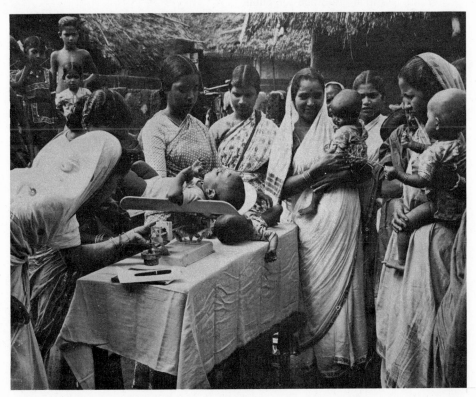

Fig. 1-5. Indian mothers crowd around the scales to learn about good nutrition for their children and hygienic habits. (UNICEF photo by Jack Ling)

6. What role does the nurse have in the promotion of good nutrition?

7. Name some of the U. S. Government agencies involved in research and service programs in nutrition. Have you used any of their publications or seen them in the school library?

8. What are some of the professional organizations in the field of nutrition? Have you used any of their publications?

9. What are the most pressing nutrition problems in the world? (Class project: Collect clippings from newspapers and magazines on world nutrition during the next month. Post on bulletin board.)

10. Who is Lord John Boyd Orr?

11. Name some of the United Nations agencies concerned with nutrition and food production. What popular method is used by UNICEF to aid in financing its program?

SUPPLEMENTARY READING ON THE APPLICATION OF NUTRITION

Ase, K., *et al.*: Nutrition education for public health nurses. Am. J. Publ. Health, 56:938, 1966.

Beeuwkes, A.: Nutrition education in schools of public health. Am. J. Publ. Health, 56: 926, 1966.

King, C. G.: Trends in international nutrition programs. J. Am. Dietet. A., 48:297, 1966.

Methods of Planning and Evaluation in Applied Nutrition Programs. WHO Technical Report Series, No. 340, 1966.

Sipple, H. L.: The Nutrition Foundation's first twenty-five years; a quarter century of nutrition science progress. Nutr. Rev., 24:353, 1966.

Stiebeling, H. K.: How far have we come? J. Home Econ., 59:341, 1967.

Todhunter, E. N.: The story of nutrition. Chap. 2, Food. Yearbook of Agriculture. U.S.D.A., Washington, D. C., 1959.

Vaughan, M. E.: Nutrition consultation for public health nurses. J. Am. Dietet. A., 49: 505, 1966.

For further references see Bibliography in Part Four.

CHAPTER **2**

Carbohydrates

*Man's Major Source of "Fuel" · Photosynthesis · Simple Sugars ·
Complex Carbohydrates · Plant Sources of Carbohydrates · Animal Sources of Carbohydrates*

MAN'S MAJOR SOURCE OF "FUEL"

Carbohydrates, chiefly in the form of cereal grains and root vegetables, are the major sources of energy for most peoples of the world. They provide from 45 to 50 per cent of the calories of the American diet and a far higher percentage for many other peoples. They are the cheapest and the most easily digested form of fuel for human and animal energy. The protein-sparing function of carbohydrates whereby they supply the energy needs and "spare" protein for other purposes is an important consideration if the supply of protein is limited. "Carbohydrate, the fuel of life" applies to more people than does the more common phrase, "Bread, the staff of life."

The proportion of total calories derived from common carbohydrate foods around the world throws light on the respective standards of living in various countries. Most of the peoples of Asia and the middle eastern countries, Africa and Latin America derive over 80 per cent of their calories from grains and potatoes or other root vegetables. As economic standards have gone up, especially in the United States and Great Britain, the amount of sugar in the diet has increased while the amount of starch has decreased proportionately (Table 2–1). The grains and other carbohydrate foods used typically in different countries will be mentioned as the food sources are discussed.

Carbohydrates are the chief form in which plants store potential energy. They are compounds of carbon, hydrogen and oxygen and are synthesized from the water of the soil and the carbon dioxide of the air by the green chlorophyll in the leaves which makes use of solar energy. This process is known as photosynthesis. The reaction is so complex that man has yet to understand fully and duplicate the chemical laboratory of the green leaf. Only in 1960, after years of painstaking research, did chemists learn how to synthesize a chlorophyll-like compound—and it required 55 separate and complicated steps. One cannot help but wonder how many steps

TABLE 2–1. Changes in the Pattern of Carbohydrate Consumption*

	Total Calories from Carbohydrate		Calories from Sugars and Syrups	
	United Kingdom	United States	United Kingdom	United States
1910	56%	48%	13%	11%
1962	57%	47%	18%	16%

*Greaves, J. P., and Hollingsworth, D. F.: Proc. Nutr. Soc., 23:136, 1964.

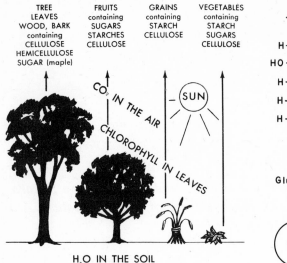

TREE LEAVES WOOD, BARK containing CELLULOSE HEMICELLULOSE SUGAR (maple)

FRUITS containing SUGARS STARCHES CELLULOSE

GRAINS containing STARCH CELLULOSE

VEGETABLES containing STARCH SUGARS CELLULOSE

CO_2 IN THE AIR

CHLOROPHYLL IN LEAVES

SUN

H₂O IN THE SOIL

FIG. 2-1. Synthesis of carbohydrates in plants.

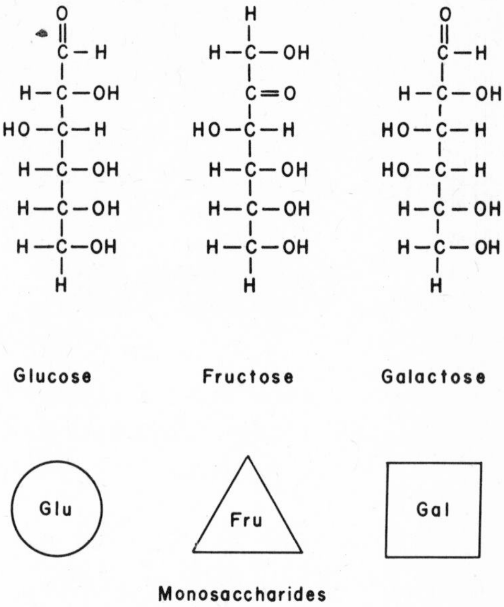

Glucose   Fructose   Galactose

Glu   Fru   Gal

Monosaccharides

FIG. 2-2. Diagram shows chemical structure of the monosaccharides glucose, fructose, and galactose. Each of these sugars is a hexose containing 6 carbon atoms, 12 hydrogen atoms and 6 oxygen atoms.

Nature takes for the entire process of photosynthesis of the sugar molecule.

The largest proportion of the sun's energy which is transformed into potential energy by plants appears in some form of carbohydrate. The single sugars (monosaccharides) probably are synthesized first, and then small molecules are combined to form the larger and more complex molecules called polysaccharides (See Fig. 2–1). Small amounts of fats and proteins also are synthesized by plants.

SIMPLE SUGARS

Monosaccharides (Fig. 2–2) are the simplest carbohydrate units and are classified according to the number of carbons in the molecule. Hexoses, sugars containing 6 carbon atoms, are the nutritionally significant sugars found in foods although others, particularly pentoses, which contain 5 carbon atoms, are produced in the metabolism of foodstuffs. The single hexoses, glucose, fructose and galactose, require no digestion and are readily absorbed from the intestine directly into the blood stream (See Chap. 9).

Glucose, also called dextrose, is abundant in fruits and vegetables. It is the form of carbohydrate to which all other carbohydrates are converted eventually for transport in the blood and for utilization by the tissues of the body.

Fructose, also called levulose or fruit sugar, is found associated with glucose in many fruits and vegetables, and especially in honey.

Galactose is not found free in nature but is derived from the disaccharide lactose, found in milk, by hydrolysis.

Sugar alcohols, sorbitol and mannitol, have a sweetening effect similar to glucose. Sorbitol, which is found in many fruits and vegetables, is very slowly absorbed into the blood stream and can apparently be metabolized without insulin. It has the same caloric value as glucose, the sugar from which it is derived. Mannitol, found in pineapples, olives, asparagus, and carrots, may also be added as a drying agent to other foods. Since it is poorly absorbed, mannitol supplies about one half the caloric value of glucose.

The disaccharides (Fig. 2–3)—sugars containing two hexose units—that are commonly encountered in foods are sucrose

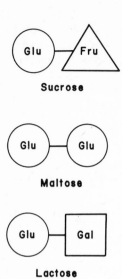

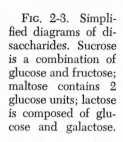

Fig. 2-3. Simplified diagrams of disaccharides. Sucrose is a combination of glucose and fructose; maltose contains 2 glucose units; lactose is composed of glucose and galactose.

Sucrose

Maltose

Lactose

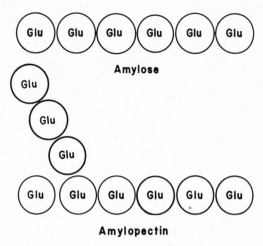

Amylose

Amylopectin

Forms of Starch

Fig. 2-4. Simplified diagrams of amylose and amyolpectin, the two forms of starch found in foods. Amylose molecules consist of 250 to 300 units of glucose in a straight chain. Amylopectin, in addition to containing the straight chain units of amylose, also has branched chains and is composed of over a thousand glucose units.

Disaccharides

(cane or beet sugar), maltose (malt sugar) and lactose (milk sugar). Disaccharides are split by specific enzymes in the digestive tract into monosaccharides, or by acid hydrolysis commercially. Each of the three disaccharides has distinct characteristics of interest in human nutrition.

Sucrose—ordinary granulated, powdered or brown sugar—is one of the sweetest forms of sugar and costs the least. On hydrolysis sucrose yields equal amounts of fructose and glucose, or invert sugar, as this mixture is commonly called.

Maltose, or malt sugar, does not occur free in nature but is manufactured from starch by enzyme or acid hydrolysis. Maltose, easily utilized by the body, is often used in combination with dextrin in infant formulas where it is desirable to have a soluble form of carbohydrate which does not readily ferment in the digestive tract. Two molecules of glucose are formed by the hydrolysis of maltose.

Lactose, or milk sugar, is the only one of the common sugars not found in plants. It is formed only in the mammary glands of lactating mothers, animal or human. It is less soluble and more slowly digested than the other two disaccharides. Lactose is only about ⅙ as sweet as sucrose and hence is responsible for the blandness of

milk. When hydrolyzed, a molecule of glucose and a molecule of galactose are formed.

COMPLEX CARBOHYDRATES

For more stable and efficient storage of potential energy, the plant and animal world packs its fuel in units larger than the sugars—i.e., dextrin, starch, cellulose, and glycogen. All of these are polysaccharides, the molecules of which may contain several hundred times as many glucose units as those of the sugars. Consequently they are much less soluble and more stable but differ markedly among themselves as to digestibility and resistance to spoilage. Since there is so much moisture in all growing plants, one essential characteristic of a storage material is insolubility. To be suitable for human food, however, a carbohydrate must be subject to digestion by the enzymes of the digestive tract. Starches and dextrins fall into this category, but celluloses and hemicelluloses which occur in food are more or less resistant to digestion.

Dextrins occur mostly as intermediate products in the partial hydrolysis of starch by enzymatic action or in cooking. They are made up of many glucose units joined together with the same linkage as maltose and the straight chains of starch. The individual molecules are smaller than starch and they do not have the thickening property of starch.

Starch, the chief form of carbohydrate in the diet, occurs in two forms: (1) amylose, a straight chain polysaccharide of glucose, and (2) amylopectin, the branched chain polysaccharide of glucose (Fig. 2–4). Starch is found in cereal grains, vegetables and other plants. The starch of the grain is mostly in the endosperm (See Fig. 2–5), encased in a protective covering of cellulose (the bran or the husk). The starch granule in the endosperm consists of tiny particles of starch usually arranged in concentric layers in a pattern of characteristic shape and appearance. The starch granules in turn may be enclosed in cells of larger size. This storage of starch in plants may be compared to warehouse storing of small packages of prepared cereal in cartons, with the cartons in turn packed in larger containers for ease in handling.

Cellulose, found in the framework of plants, is also a polysaccharide of glucose but with a different type linkage between the glucose molecules. It is the chief constituent of wood, stalks and leaves of all plants and of the outer coverings of seeds and cereals. Cellulose forms the more or less porous walls of cells in which water, starch, minerals and other substances are stored in the plant much as honey is held in the comb.

No known enzyme secreted in the human intestine can digest cellulose because it cannot break the linkage between the glucose units, but bacterial fermentation or disintegration may play a role in dissolving the substances that bind together the cellulose fibers or particles. Thus the cellulose of tender shoots may disappear completely from the intestinal tract.

The indigestibility of cellulose is its major asset, since the undigested fiber furnishes the bulk necessary for efficient and normal peristaltic action (muscular contraction) of the intestines. Research has demonstrated that the normal colon performs better when a reasonable amount (4-7 Gm.) of bulk or residue is present.

Glycogen, or "animal starch," is the form in which the animal stores its carbohydrate. It is a polysaccharide similar to amylopectin but with more branched chains and higher molecular weight. When more glucose than can be immediately metabolized enters the blood stream, the normal individual can combine many glucose molecules (up to 30,000) to form glycogen. By the same token, when glucose is needed, glycogen can be broken down and glucose becomes quickly available (See Chap. 9). In the living mammal both the liver and muscle can store glycogen. The liver glycogen is the more quickly available for replenishing blood sugar. The muscle glycogen is used primarily as fuel for the muscles. In muscle meat as purchased little glycogen is present because it disappears during rigor mortis.

Other polysaccharides, such as the pectic substances, agar, alginates and carrageenens (Irish moss), cannot be digested but are used in various foods because of their colloidal property—i.e., the ability to absorb water and form a gel. Commercial pectin, prepared from cull apple peels and cores or the albedo of lemons and available as liquid or powder, is used primarily for

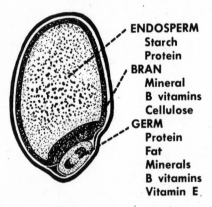

ENDOSPERM
Starch
Protein
BRAN
Mineral
B vitamins
Cellulose
GERM
Protein
Fat
Minerals
B vitamins
Vitamin E

FIG. 2-5. A grain of wheat has three parts. All are used in whole-wheat flour but only the endosperm in white flour. Note what a small part of the grain is germ. (Wellman Food Plannings, Lippincott)

making fruit jellies. Agar is used as a thickening agent in candy manufacturing and in processing meats; the alginates and carrageenens are used in the manufacture of ice cream to give body and smooth consistency; they are also used as stabilizing agents in other food processing.

PLANT SOURCES OF CARBOHYDRATES
Cereal Grains

The ancient Romans called Demeter, the Greek goddess of the grains and harvests, Ceres, and from her name the word cereal is derived. Because of their wide cultivation, their good keeping qualities, bland flavor and the great variety of products that can be manufactured from them, cereals have continued to be the staple of the human diet from prehistoric times to the present. Most of them belong to the botanic family of grasses, with the exception of buckwheat. Each of the cereals has characteristic properties and uses.

Rice has the widest use of any cereal in the world. It is the staple food for Asia, the Near East, some Latin American and African countries and is widely used elsewhere. It provides as much as 70 to 80 per cent of the calories for the larger part of the population of these areas.

About 80 per cent of the billion and a half Asians are involved in the production and distribution of rice. To meet the ever increasing demand for rice, the International Rice Research Institute in the Philippine Islands directs work on improving rice production and has recently announced a new strain with improved yield and drastically reduced growing time, an important feature for colder climates.

Rice is usually milled as white rice, the form preferred by most people, although much of the vitamin and mineral content is lost in the milling. When the ancient home milling process, which involves parboiling or steaming before polishing, is used, some of the vitamins are forced into the center of the kernel and thus are conserved. Converted rice, now available in the United States, is commercially processed by a similar method and has a somewhat higher vitamin content than ordinary white rice. Rice enrichment, by the addition of a high vitamin "premix," is being practiced in Japan, the Philippine Islands and parts of the United States. The "premix," which is heavily fortified with certain B vitamins, is applied to the white rice together with a protective coating that is highly resistant to cooking losses.

Unpolished brown rice and "wild rice," both of which contain more of the original minerals and vitamins than does white rice, have limited use because of their different flavor, poor keeping quality and high price. Rice-eating countries do not use rice for bread making but use it in place of bread. Rice flour is used in making a wide variety of delectable snack foods in some of the oriental countries.

Wheat is the next most common cereal used throughout the world and the most widely used in the Americas and Europe. It can be milled for a variety of uses—as breakfast cereals, as flour for bread, cakes, pastries, crackers and for macaroni products. It lends itself to bread making better than other grains because of its high gluten content, which is necessary for yeast breads that demand kneading. Wheat is equally good for baking-powder breads, cakes and cookies. Certain varieties of wheat are preferred for bread flour, others for cake flour, but for both the flour is manufactured by roller- or impact-milling—complicated processes designed to produce a pure white flour containing none of the bran or the germ. The final product represents 70 per cent or less of the wheat kernel. The outer coatings and the germ, which contain the bulk of the minerals and vitamins, are sold mostly as stock feed. A small amount of pure wheat germ is processed for human consumption. Some bran is also processed for use as high-roughage breakfast cereals.

A small proportion of our wheat crop in the United States is milled as whole-wheat or Graham flour and some as whole-wheat breakfast cereal. Hard winter wheat is milled as semolina for the manufacture of macaroni, spaghetti, vermicelli and noodles. A wide variety of these products are used in Italy and elsewhere in Europe as well as in the Americas and the Orient.

Corn (or *maize*) is used for human food in many countries in a variety of forms:

cornmeal, white and yellow; hominy grits; samp, or hulled corn; popcorn; cornflakes or similar ready-to-eat cereals; and as a source of cornstarch, corn syrup and corn oil. All of these products are processed from several varieties of mature field corn. Yellow or white cornmeal is cooked as mush or grits and is used in griddle cakes or in cornmeal breads, corn pone, muffins, johnnycakes and, in Central and South America, for tamales and tortillas. Cornstarch is sold commercially as a thickening agent in cooking. Corn sugar and syrup are made by hydrolyzing the starch in the corn, i.e., breaking it down into dextrins, maltose and glucose. Corn oil is extracted from the corn germ by a carefully controlled commercial process. The special properties of corn oil will be discussed in Chapter 3.

Oats are used chiefly in the form of rolled oats or oatmeal in the United States and western Europe. In recent years some ready-to-eat cereals have been processed from oats. Oat products carry more of the original kernel than do most other processed cereals, and, thus, oats lose fewer nutrients between the field and table.

Rye is similar to wheat in many respects; rye flour may be used with wheat or by itself for bread making. Rye breads such as pumpernickel or Swedish rye are used in northern and central Europe and in Russia more commonly than in the United States.

Barley is used mostly as "pearled" barley, which is the kernel left after the bran and the germ have been removed. Barley flour is made by grinding the "pearls." In the United States pearl barley has limited use in soups and in the making of gruels for invalid diets. In some other countries such as Korea and Japan barley is raised and used as a low-cost substitute for rice by the poorer people.

Buckwheat is not a true cereal botanically, i.e., it does not belong to the grasses as do the other cereals, but it serves the same purpose for human food. The bran, or the husk, is removed and the rest of the kernel is rolled and bolted to produce buckwheat flour. In the United States its most common use is in buckwheat griddle cakes and waffles; in Japan buckwheat noodles are relished. In Europe buckwheat is used in making heavy breads, gruels, puddings, cakes and beer.

Millet is a staple food for millions of people in India, Russia, China and Africa but is little known in the United States. It can be raised where land is too poor and the climate too dry to grow wheat, rice, corn or most other grains. Millet is used in eastern Europe for making flat bread or porridge. Russian "kasha" (cereal), often made from millet, may also be made from wheat or buckwheat.

Milling of Grains. Natural grains carry not only the store of carbohydrates already mentioned but also protein and certain minerals and vitamins essential for good nutrition. The vitamin-B-complex factors present in the natural whole grains are usually sufficient in amount to help form the enzymes necessary for the metabolism of the carbohydrate of the grain. The balance of nature is upset when we find it desirable to modify natural grains by milling them to produce a whiter, more easily digested flour with better keeping qualities when stored. In so doing some of the minerals and vitamins are lost or discarded in the millings. It is interesting to note that the latter find excellent use as animal feed. Attempts to educate people accustomed to white-flour products to return to the use of whole-grain products have never been successful. Consequently, the expedient of enrichment of bread and flour was initiated in the United States during World War II, with other cereal products of various types added to the list later. Thiamine, riboflavin, niacin and iron are the factors added (See Chap. 10). Bread and flour enrichment is of first importance because bread constitutes one of the main sources of calories in the American diet.

Fruits

Fruits and vegetables constitute a less concentrated source of carbohydrates than do the cereals because of their high water content. In fruits the carbohydrate is mostly in the form of the monosaccharides glucose and fructose. The disaccharide, sucrose, may be found in a few fresh fruits, and most canned fruits contain added sucrose or glucose unless specifically labeled "canned without added sugar." The soluble sugars along with the fruits' acids and traces of volatile oils give fruits their appetite appeal and odor, which is further enhanced by color and texture.

The sugar content of fresh fruits may vary from 6 to 20 per cent, those of canteloupe and watermelon being the lowest and that of banana one of the highest. Of course, dried fruits such as prunes, apricots, raisins, dates and figs have a much higher sugar content (near 70%) due to their low moisture content. The caloric value of fruits—fresh, canned or frozen— is determined largely by their sugar content.

Although most fruits are considered highly desirable raw, plantains, which are related to the banana except for being larger, are not palatable unless cooked. Because of their high starch content these fruits are an important source of carbohydrates in many tropical countries and when boiled, baked or fried are frequently used in the main course of the meal.

The avocado pear and the olive are different from all other fruits because of their high fat content, which gives them a comparatively high caloric value in spite of their low carbohydrate content.

Most fresh fruits also contain some cellulose or hemicellulose. This type of bulk, along with the fruit acids, seems to serve as a stimulant to intestinal motility for many people.

Vegetables

Under the term *vegetables* are grouped foods representing practically every part of the plant—leaves, stems, seeds, seed pods, flowers, fruits, roots and tubers. They vary as widely in composition as they do in function in the plant and may contain anywhere from 3 to 35 per cent of carbohydrate in the forms of starch, sugars, cellulose and hemicellulose.

Obviously, the caloric value of vegetables varies with the per cent of carbohydrate present, but, in general, the high water and cellulose content of leaf, flower and stem vegetables puts them in the low-calorie

TABLE 2–2. Carbohydrates in Common Starchy Foods and Sweets

STARCHY FOODS	Per Cent
Barley, pearled	79
Breads, all types	52-58
Cassava, meal and flour	85
Cornmeal and grits	74-78
Crackers	71-74
Macaroni, spaghetti and noodles	73-77
Oatmeal or oat cereals	70
Potatoes, cooked	19
Rice or rice cereals	79
Rye flour	68-78
Wheat flour	69-79
Wheat cereals	72-80

SWEETS	Per Cent
Cakes	56-62
Candies	56-99
Cookies	60-80
Dried fruits	75-88
Honey	80
Jams and jellies	65-71
Syrups	74
Cane or beet sugar	100

class. These include all the green leafy vegetables, plus celery, asparagus, cauliflower, broccoli and Brussels sprouts. The roots, the tubers and the seeds of plants have a higher starch and sugar content and less water and, therefore, provide more calories per unit of weight. These include all kinds of potatoes, beets, carrots, turnips, parsnips, peas, beans and lentils.

The cellulose and hemicellulose found typically in vegetables also varies in amount and digestibility. Some forms of cellulose such as that in certain leafy and stem vegetables and in sweet corn are so resistant even to bacterial digestion and so frequently irritating that they may not be tolerated by some adults or by young children.

Root vegetables often provide much of the carbohydrate in the diets of certain African, Latin American and Asian peoples. Since they are for the most part very poor in protein, their wide use creates certain nutrition problems, particularly in infant feeding where they may take the place of more nutritious foods. Cassava, also called manioc or yuca, has a long root which is

1 to 3 inches thick. It is frequently grated, dried and powdered as a "meal"—tapioca or arrowroot. Taro, which is also grown in tropical and subtropical countries, can be baked or boiled like a potato. The Hawaiians boil the eddoes (as the roots are called), then peel and grind them with water to make *poi*, the sticky pastelike food so popular in the Islands. Other roots and tubers such as sweet potatoes, yams, turnips, and Jerusalem artichokes may also be used as staple foods at certain times by various peoples.

Nuts

Nuts seldom are thought of as a source of carbohydrate because of their high content of fat and protein. However, because of their low moisture content, they contribute from 10 to 27 per cent total carbohydrate. They also contain from 1 to 2 per cent of fiber. Peanuts, which are really legumes, are usually classed with the nuts because of their composition and common usage.

Because of the high fat content, nuts digest slowly. Chopping or grinding improves digestibility. In the form of nut butter and combined with other foods, there is usually no digestive difficulty. Peanut butter may be used in sandwiches or as an ingredient of a dish.

Other Plant Sources of Carbohydrates

Common table sugar—the refined white granulated or powdered sugar or brown sugar—is processed from either sugar cane or sugar beets.

Sucrose is the chief source of sweetening used in most desserts, ice creams, candies and soft drinks. The average per-capita consumption of sugar in the United States is estimated at approximately two pounds per week. This means, of course, that some persons use much more than this, and others consume far less. Since sugar is 99.9 per cent carbohydrate and furnishes almost 4 calories to the gram, those who use the average amount or more are getting more than 3,500 empty calories per week. Sugar is concentrated fuel but furnishes no other nutrients. Furthermore, candies and other sweets are reputed to aggravate dental

caries, a major health problem. Sugar consumption in the form of candies, soft drinks and rich desserts is certainly a contributing factor to the great American problem of obesity (Chap. 21).

Molasses is a by-product of sugar refining and carries more of the mineral content of the original plant than do the refined sugars.

Maple syrup and sugar are made by boiling down the sap from sugar maples. This was one of the kinds of sugar used earliest in America—its source known to the Indians and taught to the early settlers by them. Regardless of flavor or color, which are due to traces of other factors, the sugar in all of the above products is the disaccharide sucrose.

Corn syrup, made from field corn by hydrolysis of the starch, is mostly glucose and maltose.

Honey, made by bees from flower nectars, contains a mixture of the two monosaccharides, glucose and fructose. The fructose in honey makes it taste sweeter than corn syrup because fructose has a sweeter taste then either glucose or maltose.

Sorghum syrup is made from the sweet juice of the sorghum stem, and its use is confined largely to the southeastern and south central states. Grain sorghums are also used for food in parts of India, China and Africa.

Other forms of plant life not usually classed as vegetables are the seaweeds used for food in many countries, notably Japan. Certain varieties of seaweed are sources of *agar* and *alginates*.

Change of Form

Interchanges among the different forms of carbohydrate in the plant world are interesting and significant factors in food quality and keeping properties. As growth proceeds, there is constant exchange from one form to another. In fruits such as the banana the carbohydrate is in the form of starch in the maturing fruit, but some of it is changed to sugar as the fruit ripens. In some vegetables sugar synthesized by the leaves is stored as starch, as in potatoes and in mature beans, peas and corn. People like fresh green corn and green peas because the carbohydrate is still partly sugar. Connoisseurs of fresh garden vegetables are aware of how quickly the sugar of corn and green peas disappears after harvesting, and how much more delicious they are when used immediately after picking. This change is due to the enzymes that are present in the vegetables, and the change is stopped as soon as the enzymes are destroyed by heating. Thus, frozen vegetables that have been blanched promptly after harvesting and before freezing may have better flavor than do so-called fresh vegetables that have been shipped long distances and stored before appearing at market.

ANIMAL SOURCES OF CARBOHYDRATES

Most animal foods, such as meats, poultry and fish, contain only traces of carbohydrate in the form of *glycogen* used for muscle contraction. Eggs also contain only traces of carbohydrate. Only liver contains an appreciable amount, and this in the form of glycogen. In all animals the liver serves as a temporary storehouse for quickly available fuel for the body, and it may contain from 2 to 6 per cent of glycogen. Another source of glycogen in foods is the seafood, scallops, which are the muscles of shellfish and contain about 3 per cent of glycogen.

Fresh milk contains about 5 per cent of carbohydrate in the form of *lactose*, a disaccharide. When consumed in amounts greater than those ordinarily present in milk, some lactose may not be digested. An undigested residue of lactose in the large intestine has a laxative action which may be desirable in certain instances but in excess causes diarrhea. Lactose is an excellent medium for the growth of certain useful acid-tolerant bacteria and has been used therapeutically to increase this type of bacterial flora in the large intestines. Lactose also seems to increase the absorption or utilization of calcium, and often this finding is cited as the reason for the efficient utilization of calcium from milk. Sometimes lactose is given as an accompaniment of calcium salts prescribed for

persons who have an allergy to milk and must obtain their calcium in another form.

A summary of the types and amounts of carbohydrates found in various foods was recently compiled by Hardinge *et al.*[1]

STUDY QUESTIONS AND ACTIVITIES

1. From what compounds are carbohydrates synthesized by plants? What is the process called?

2. Name the monosaccharides and give some food sources of each.

3. What kind of sugar is made from cane or sugar beets? Where else may this same sugar be found in Nature?

4. In what way is the sugar of milk unique? How is it classified chemically?

5. Which carbohydrates are most common in fruits? In root vegetables?

6. What type of food provides the most common source of carbohydrate and calories for the world's people? What are some of the regional or national preferences?

7. What is another name for "animal starch"? Where is it found? Of what significance is it in animal nutrition?

8. Certain polysaccharides are not digested by intestinal enzymes. Which are they? In which foods do we find them? What is their function?

9. Compare the sweetness of the sugars. Why does honey taste sweeter than cane syrup?

10. List the carbohydrate foods you consumed in the past 24 hours. How wide a variety of plant sources is represented?

11. How does your sugar intake compare with that of other carbohydrate sources? If it seems high, how can you replace it with more nutritious but equally desirable foods?

12. Glance at the "ready to eat" cereal shelf in the local supermarket. How many cereal grains are represented? What added ingredients do some of them have? Do you consider this beneficial? What would you judge to be the difference in cost between a serving (1 ounce) of ready-to-eat cereal and a cooked cereal?

---

[1] Hardinge, M. G., *et al.*: J. Am. Dietet. A., *46*: 197, 1965.

SUPPLEMENTARY READING ON CARBOHYDRATES

Harper, A. E.: Carbohydrates. Chap. 8, Food. Yearbook of Agriculture, Washington, D. C., U.S.D.A., 1959.

Hodges, R. E.: Present knowledge of carbohydrates. Nutr. Rev., 24:65, 1966.

Macdonald, I.: Symposium on Dietary Carbohydrates in Man. Am. J. Clin. Nutr., 20:65, 1967.

For further references see Bibliography in Part Four.

CHAPTER 3

Fats and Other Lipids

Fats in the Human Diet • Kinds of Fats and Their Characteristics • Essential Fatty Acids • Animal Sources • Plant Sources • Other Lipids

FATS IN THE HUMAN DIET

Fats are a form of stored energy in animals as important as carbohydrates are in plants. Although there are wide differences among individuals and regions, surveys indicate that Americans as a group consume more than 40 per cent of their calories as fat (Table 3–1). Visible fats from such sources as butter, margarine, shortening, and salad and cooking oils account for about 40 per cent of the fat intake, whereas the fats of meats, eggs, milk, cheese, nuts and cereals, often referred to as invisible fats, contribute about 60 per cent of the total fat in the American diet. Data in Table 3–2 detail the actual contribution made by different foods to the total fat in the average diet.

Because people differ so widely in their patterns of food preparation and in their eating practices in regard to fat, reliable information as to the actual consumption of this nutrient is difficult to obtain. Some homemakers use considerable amounts of fat for frying and flavoring foods; others may use methods of preparation, especially in the cooking of meats and poultry, which markedly reduce the amount of fat in the cooked food. Habits vary in regard to the eating or discarding of fat on meat, the use of table fats on breads and cream on cereals and the use of salad dressings. People who are accustomed to a large amount of fat in their diet are unhappy when they are deprived of it. The psychological value of visible fat in the diet is far greater than that of the hidden or invisible fat, although physiologically the latter serves an identical purpose.

There is no physiological evidence that the human body needs as much fat as Americans consume, but neither is there proof that such amounts are harmful. Some experts recommend a moderate reduction whereby fat would provide 25 to 30 per cent of the total calories in the diet. Even this much fat is not a physiologic necessity for all people, as has been demonstrated by the extremely low-fat diets consumed by large population groups throughout the world. In many countries of the Orient, the Middle East and Africa the average diet provides less than 20 per cent of the total calories in the form of fat, as compared with twice that amount in the American diet.

TABLE 3–1. Trends in Fat Consumption During Selected Periods—U. S.*

Period	Calories Per Capita Per Day	Fat Per Capita Per Day (Grams)	Fat Calories (Per Cent)
1909-13	3490	125	32.2
1935-39	3270	133	36.6
1964	3170	147	41.4

*Figures adapted from Nutritive Value of Food for Consumption, United States, 1909–64, Friend, B., Agricultural Research Service 62-14, U.S.D.A., Washington, D. C., 1966.

TABLE 3–2. Food Consumption per Capita per Year and Percentage of Total Fat Contributed by Major Food Groups for Selected Periods*

Food Group	1909-13		1935-39		1964	
	Lbs.	Per Cent of Total Fat	Lbs.	Per Cent of Total Fat	Lbs.	Per Cent of Total Fat
Meat	141.4	34.6	120.1	27.6	155.7	32.2
Poultry	17.5	1.8	16.2	1.5	38.8	1.9
Fish	13.3	1.0	13.1	0.8	13.6	0.9
Eggs	37.4	3.8	36.4	3.5	39.9	3.4
Dairy products† excluding butter	177.0	14.9	202.0	15.8	236.0	14.4
Butter	17.6	14.1	17.0	12.9	6.8	4.6
Other fats and oils	23.0	22.6	32.3	29.6	43.8	35.4
Fruits	176.3	0.3	199.0	0.3	163.1	0.3
Vegetables	202.9	0.3	231.2	0.5	204.8	0.5
Potatoes‡	205.0	0.3	147.0	0.2	104.9	0.1
Dried beans, peas, nuts and soya products	16.3	1.9	18.9	3.3	16.5	3.4
Flour and cereal products	291.0	3.8	204.0	2.5	144.0	1.5
Sugar and other sweeteners	89.1	0.0	110.5	0.0	111.1	0.0
Coffee and cocoa	9.9	0.6	15.9	1.6	15.3	1.4

*Figures from Nutritive Value of Food Available for Consumption, United States, 1909–64, Friend, B., Agricultural Research Service 62-14, U.S.D.A., Washington, D. C., 1966.
†Milk equivalents given in quarts.
‡Includes sweet potatoes.

In recent years the American consumer has modified somewhat his selection of fats. For instance, there is an increase in the use of soybean, corn and cottonseed oil, in the consumption of poultry, in the substitution of margarine for butter and the use of nondairy "creamers" and toppings, instead of cream from milk. Table 3–2 shows the difference in per cent of total fat contributed by the major food groups during 1909-13, 1935-39 and in 1964. These changes have led to differences in the composition of total fat in the diet. Although the amount of saturated fat has not varied in the last thirty years, the per cent of polyunsaturated fat has increased from a ratio of polyunsaturated to saturated (P/S) (see p. 27) of 0.23 in 1936 to 0.33 in 1963. Of the 145 grams of fat available per person per day in 1963, saturated fatty acids contributed 37 per cent; oleic acid (monounsaturated), 40 per cent; linoleic acid (polyunsaturated), 12 per cent.[1]

[1] National Research Council Publication 1147. Dietary Fat and Human Health. Washington, D. C., 1966.

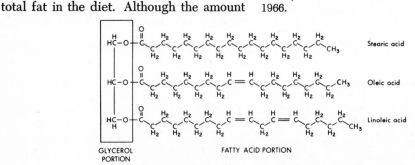

FIG. 3-1. Diagram shows the three fatty acids, stearic (saturated), oleic (monounsaturated), and linoleic (polyunsaturated), combined in ester linkage with glycerol to form a triglyceride or fat.

Fats serve multiple purposes in the diet. In addition to their high fuel value, some act as carriers of essential fatty acids and vitamins. That fat makes a meal more satisfying is due partially to its slow rate of digestion, its satiety value, and to the flavor it gives to other foods.

KINDS OF FATS AND THEIR CHARACTERISTICS

Fats, oils and fat-like substances, because of similar solubilities, are classified as lipids (Table 3–3). They are insoluble in water. Like carbohydrates, fats are composed of carbon, hydrogen and oxygen but in proportions that greatly increase their energy value. Fats that are fluid at room temperature are usually called oils, while those that are solid are called fats. Both are primarily mixtures of triglycerides, i.e., compounds of three fatty acid molecules attached to a glycerol molecule in the form of an ester (Fig. 3–1). They contain a variety of different fatty acids in varying proportions.

The type and configuration of the fatty acids in fats are responsible for differences in flavor, texture, melting points, absorption, essential fatty acid activity and other characteristics. Fatty acids vary in length from 2 carbons to more than 20 carbons and are referred to as short chain (2-6 carbons), medium chain (8-12 carbons) and long chain (more than 12 carbons). Reference may also be made to extra long chain fatty acids, or those over 20 carbons. Natural fats contain 16 and 18 carbon fatty acids in the largest quantities, although short chain fatty acids are found in butterfat and coconut oil. In addition to being present in relatively small amounts in natural fats, triglycerides containing medium chain fatty acids are commercially prepared from such fats as coconut oil. The ease with which such medium chain fatty acids are hydrolyzed, absorbed and transported have made them useful in treating patients with certain types of malabsorption syndromes (See Chap. 9, Fat Absorption and Chap. 27, Diseases of the Intestines).

Fatty acids are also classified as saturated or unsaturated, depending on the presence or absence of double bonds. A double bond occurs when two adjoining

TABLE 3–3. Classification of Lipids

I. Simple Lipids
   A. Mono-, di- and triglycerides—esters of fatty acids with glycerol
   B. Esters of fatty acids with high-molecular-weight alcohols
     Waxes
     Cholesterol esters
     Vitamin A and D esters

II. Compound Lipids
   A. Phospholipids—phosphorus-containing lipids
     Lecithins
     Cephalins
     Sphingomyelins
   B. Glycolipids—sugar-containing lipids
     Cerebrosides
     Gangliosides
   C. Lipoproteins

III. Derived Lipids
   A. Fatty acids
   B. Sterols
     Cholesterol
     Ergosterol
     Bile acids
     Steroid hormones
     Vitamin D
   C. Hydrocarbons
     Squalene
     Carotenoids
     Aliphatic hydrocarbons
   D. Fat-soluble vitamins
     Vitamin A
     Vitamin E
     Vitamin K

carbons each have one less hydrogen atom than they normally hold. Then a double bond between the two carbons satisfies the carbon valence of 4. Fatty acids such as oleic are called monounsaturated because they contain one double bond, while linoleic, linolenic and arachidonic acids, which contain 2, 3, and 4 double bonds respectively, are called polyunsaturated (Fig. 3–1.) The polyunsaturated fatty acids have been shown in certain instances to lower blood cholesterol level, whereas saturated fatty acids may actually tend to raise the serum cholesterol level. Table 3–4 shows the fatty acid composition of some common animal and vegetable fats. Saturated fatty acids, particularly the long chain fatty acids and their glycerides, have higher melting points and hence tend to be solid in form at room temperature. These fats

TABLE 3—4. Analyses of Major Fatty Acids Typical of Some Fats of Animal and Plant Origin*†

| | SATURATED | | | | MONOUNSATURATED | | POLYUNSATURATED | | | |
	Lauric 12:0	Myristic 14:0	Palmitic 16:0	Stearic 18:0	Palmitoleic 16:1	Oleic 18:1	Linoleic 18:2	Linolenic 18:3	Arachidonic 18:4	Other Polyenoic Acids
ANIMAL FATS										
Lard	..	1.5	27.0	13.5	3.0	43.5	10.5	0.5	..	..
Chicken	2.0	7.0	25.0	6.0	8.0	36.0	14.0	..	..	..
Egg	..	..	25.0	10.0	..	50.0	10.0	2.0	3.0	..
Beef	..	3.0	29.0	21.0	3.0	41.0	2.0	0.5	0.5	..
Butter	3.5	12.0	28.0	13.0	3.0	28.5	1.0	..	..	..
Human Milk	7.0	8.5	21.0	7.0	2.5	36.0	7.0	1.0	0.5	..
Menhaden (fish)	..	9.0	19.0	5.5	16.0	..	..	..	..	48.5
VEGETABLE OILS										
Corn	..	..	12.5	2.5	..	29.0	55.0	0.5	..	..
Peanut	..	..	11.5	3.0	..	53.0	26.0	..	..	..
Cottonseed	..	1.0	26.0	3.0	1.0	17.5	51.5	..	..	..
Soybean	..	..	11.5	4.0	..	24.5	53.0	7.0	..	..
Olive	..	..	13.0	2.5	1.0	74.0	9.0	0.5	..	..
Coconut	49.5	19.5	8.5	2.0	..	6.0	1.5	..	..	..

*Composition is given in weight percentages of the component fatty acids (rounded to nearest 0.5) as determined by gas chromatography. The number of carbon atoms: number of double bonds are indicated under the common name of the fatty acid. These data were derived from a variety of sources. They are representative determinations, rather than averages, and considerable variation is to be expected in individual samples from other sources.

†Adapted from Dietary Fat and Human Health, National Research Council Publication 1147, Washington, D. C., 1966.

are found in greater amounts in animal sources. Oils for the most part contain large amounts of unsaturated fatty acids, have lower melting points and are chiefly of vegetable origin. Coconut oil is a notable exception, however, since it is almost 90 per cent saturated but short and medium chain acids account for its being an oil. Animals, including man, are able metabolically to increase or decrease the chain length of fatty acids by the addition or removal of 2 carbon fragments and can convert the saturated fatty acid stearic to the monounsaturated fatty acid oleic by removal of 2 hydrogens. Man cannot, however synthesize the polyunsaturated fatty acid, linoleic; hence, this is considered to be an essential fatty acid (EFA).

In addition to the length of the fatty acid chain and the degree of saturation, the configuration of the fatty acid at the double bond as well as the position of the double bonds are factors which determine the role of fats in nutrition. The fatty acids in most natural fats are in the *cis* form, which means that at the double bond the molecule turns back on itself ⌐⌐. In processed fats such as margarine much of the fatty acid has been changed into the *trans* form whereby the chain is stretched out ⌐⌐⌐. This increases the melting point so that a desirable consistency for a table or cooking fat is accomplished with a low degree of saturation. Hydrogenation, the addition of hydrogen atoms, increases the degree of saturation and changes a liquid oil to a solid fat. These changes in the configuration of fats have been found not to affect their caloric value.

A clear distinction should be kept in mind between oils which are true fats and the hydrocarbons derived from petroleum, such as lubricating oil or purified mineral oil. The latter contain carbon and hydrogen but no oxygen. Mineral oil is completely indigestible in the animal body and cannot be classified as a food. Formerly, it was used in place of true fats in certain low-calorie diets. This procedure is generally discouraged because mineral oil tends to interfere with the absorption of the fat-soluble vitamins. It is particularly detrimental when used in a food such as salad dressing and when taken with meals. Vegetable gums are now frequently used in low-calorie salad dressings to achieve the desired consistency.

ESSENTIAL FATTY ACIDS (EFA)

An essential fatty acid is one which is necessary for normal nutrition and which cannot be synthesized by the body from other substances. Linoleic acid, the polyunsaturated fatty acid most abundant in nature, is the main essential fatty acid to be considered. Linolenic acid, which was at first classed as one of the essential fatty acids, is not active in relieving the dermatitis of essential fatty acid deficiency; arachidonic acid, which is effective in curing the deficiency, can be synthesized in the body from linoleic acid.

Demonstration of an essential fatty acid deficiency in animals requires the rigid exclusion of fat from the diet. Therefore, it is not surprising that evidence of essential fatty acid deficiencies in adult humans has not been recognized. However, Hansen, Wiese and associates[2,3] have demonstrated a fatty acid deficiency in infants, which proves beyond a doubt that essential fatty acids (EFA) are required by humans. After establishing normal blood levels for 2, 3 and 4 double bond fatty acids by surveying healthy infants and children,[4] the same serum levels in poorly nourished children were studied. In the latter group they found not only decreased blood levels of the fatty acids containing 2 and 4 double bonds—i.e., those with EFA activity—but also many cases of dermatitis similar to the symptoms of essential fatty acid deficiency seen in animals. Blood levels of fatty acids with three double bonds which are inactive physiologically were increased. More recently these investigators have been able to evaluate over 400 infants fed formulas containing varying amounts of linoleic acid. Again the dry and scaly skin of dermatitis was the most frequent finding among the infants receiving formulas low in linoleic acid. Infants also seemed to grow better

[2] Hansen, A. E., and Wiese, H. F.: J. Nutrition, 52:367, 1954.
[3] Hansen, A. E., et al.: Pediatrics, 31:171, 1963.
[4] Wiese, H. F., et al.: J. Nutrition, 52:355, 1954.

FAT

In Average Servings of Foods
Classified in the Four Food Groups

	Average serving grams	Grams of Fat in one serving
GROUP I: MILK and EQUIVALENTS		
Whole milk, 1 cup	244	10
Cheese, Cheddar or Blue mold, 1 oz.	30	9
Ice cream, 1/6 quart	60	8
Cream, Light, 2 tbsp.	30	6
GROUP II: MEAT, POULTRY, FISH, EGGS and NUTS		
Ham, cooked, 1 slice	60	17
Frankfurter, cooked, 1	50	14
Chicken, breast, fried, 3 oz.	90	14
Hamburg, cooked, market ground, 1 patty	50	10
Lamb chop, lean only, 1 chop	66	6
Egg, whole, one	50	6
Haddock, fried, 1 fillet	90	5
Pecans and walnuts, 1/2 oz.	15	10
Almonds and cashews, 1/2 oz.	15	8
Peanut butter, 1 tbsp.	16	8
GROUP III: VEGETABLES and FRUITS		
Avocado, ripe, 1/2 medium	100	16
Ripe olives, 5 large	33	10
Potato chips, 10 large	20	8
French fried potatoes, 10 pieces	50	7
GROUP IV: BREAD, CAKES and CEREALS		
Chocolate cake with fudge icing, 1 piece	120	14
Pie, apple or cherry, 1 section	135	13
Doughnut, one	33	6
Plain cake, 1 piece	50	4
FATS and OILS		
Salad oil, 1 tbsp.	14	14
Butter or margarine, 1 tbsp.	14	11

THERE ARE NO RECOMMENDED DIETARY ALLOWANCES FOR FAT

THIS LINE REPRESENTS APPROXIMATELY 1/4 THE FAT AVAILABLE FOR CONSUMPTION PER DAY PER CAPITA IN USA

FIGURE 3-2

and required fewer calories for growth when there was an adequate supply of EFA.

Although evaporated milk has proved satisfactory in infant feeding, Wiese et al.[5] suggest that the amount of linoleic acid supplied by evaporated milk formulas (1-2%

[5] Wiese, H. F., et al.: J. Nutrition, 66:345, 1958.

of total calories) may be considered minimal, whereas breast milk, which is 4 to 5 times higher in linoleic acid, contains optimal amounts of EFA. Attention was called by these authors to the infrequent incidence of eczema and other skin manifestations in breast-fed infants when compared with those on cow's milk. Analysis of the linoleic acid content of commercial infant formulas and precooked cereals indicates that these also make an important contribution of EFA to the infant diet.[6]

Although the adult human requirement of essential fatty acids is not known, the Food and Nutrition Board of the National Research Council states that, "Linoleic acid in the range of 1 to 3 per cent of total calories appears to meet the infant requirement and probably adult needs, which are presumably less than those of infants."[7] The exact function of linoleic acid and its derivatives in the body is not understood but such acids are known to be essential structural elements for synthesis of tissue lipids and hence should receive particular attention in infant feeding.[8]

ANIMAL SOURCES OF FATS
(See Fig. 3–2)

The body fat of each form of animal life is typical of the species but varies with function in the body and the temperature of the environment. The fat of cold-blooded animals—fish, for example—is a soft fat which remains plastic in the low-temperature environment in which the fish live. The fats of warm-blooded animals have higher melting points but are also plastic at the body temperature of each species. As a rule, the fat of herbivorous animals is harder than the fat of carnivorous animals. When adipose tissue of animals is subjected to heat, the fat liquefies and separates from the connective-tissue cells in which it was stored. Thus pork fat is "tried out" in the manufacture of lard. Sheep have the hardest body fat of any

domestic animal; when extracted, it is known as mutton tallow. Poultry fats are intermediate between meat and fish fats both in hardness and in the content of polyunsaturated fatty acids.

The fat of fish is always fluid at cold temperature and is therefore called an oil. Fish fats contain a higher proportion of polyunsaturated extra-long-chain fatty acids than do the meat or poultry fats (See Table 3–4). However, there is a great difference in the fat content of fish, which varies from less than 1 per cent to more than 12 per cent. Thus fish are classified either as low in fat or high in fat. The amount in all fish varies somewhat with the season of the year, with the time of spawning and with changes in feeding conditions. It may be noted that certain fish which have very little fat in the edible portion have a comparatively large amount in the liver. Fish liver oils are extracted and refined for use as rich sources of vitamins A and D.

Milk fat is in an unstable emulsion which breaks (i.e., separates) on standing and allows the cream to rise. Homogenization of milk produces a more stable emulsion with smaller fat globules, and, therefore, the cream does not separate. Butter is the milk fat plus some moisture and milk solids separated by churning; the finished product contains about 85 per cent of fat. Butter contains very little polyunsaturated fatty acid, as will be noted in Table 3–4. Butter is valued as a good source of vitamin A.

PLANT SOURCES OF FATS
(See Fig. 3–2)

All fats in the plant kingdom are oils at room temperature. Most vegetables and fruits contain less than 1 per cent of fat, with the exception of avocados and olives, as may be seen in Figure 3–2. The nuts and the seeds have a higher fat content. Seed oils are mostly extracted or expressed for use as pure oils for culinary and other purposes. Many of these have a high proportion of linoleic acid, as may be seen in Table 3–4.

Margarines and cooking fats are usually made from vegetable oils, cottonseed, soybean and corn oils by the process of hydro-

[6] Hughes, G., *et al.*: Clin. Pediat., 2:555, 1963.

[7] National Research Council Publication 1146. Recommended Dietary Allowances. Washington, D. C., 1964.

[8] Holman, R. T.: J.A.M.A., 178:930, 1961.

TABLE 3–5. Selected Fatty Acids in Margarines*

| Types of Margarine (first ingredient named on label) | Amount in 100 Grams | | | |
| | Total Fat (Grams) | Total Saturated Fatty Acids (Grams) | Unsaturated Fatty Acids | |
			Oleic (Grams)	Linoleic (Grams)
Hydrogenated or hardened fat	81	18	47	14
Liquid oil	81	19	31	29

*Figures from Composition of Foods: Raw, Processed and Prepared. Agricultural Handbook No. 8. U.S.D.A., Washington, D. C., 1963.

genation. This chemical process involves the introduction of hydrogen into the fat molecule under carefully controlled conditions to produce a fat with exactly the right melting point and other properties for culinary purposes. Hydrogenation also results in transforming part of the fat to the *trans* form to obtain the desired consistency. Fat thus formed is homogenized to form a creamy smooth product, but evidence of its being a mixture is given by the grainy texture of such a fat once it has been melted and allowed to harden again—the high and the low melting point ingredients are no longer evenly mixed.

The public demand for unsaturated fat has prompted margarine manufacturers to reduce the amount of hydrogenation to a minimum in order to retain as much of the unsaturated fatty acid as possible. Margarines are manufactured by either partially hydrogenating the total amount of vegetable oil to the desired consistency or by adding liquid vegetable oil to a more completely hydrogenated solid fat. The latter type contains approximately twice the amount of linoleic acid. The first ingredient named on the label of the margarine package tells the consumer which product he is selecting: "liquid corn oil plus hydrogenated corn oil" means that the margarine has been processed by the second method and hence would have a higher ratio of polyunsaturated to saturated fatty acids (Table 3–5). The fat thus prepared is churned with cultured milk and other ingredients to give the product the flavor of butter. All brands are now fortified with vitamin A to the equivalent of average butter, and some have vitamin D added. Therefore, margarine is nutritionally the equivalent of butter and sometimes is preferred because of the lower cost and the higher content of unsaturated fatty

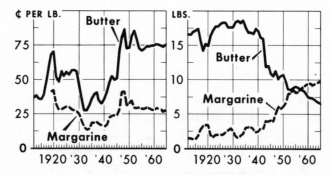

FIG. 3-3. Changes in the cost and consumption of butter and margarine in the United States from 1912 to 1965. (*Left*) Retail prices. (*Right*) Consumption per civilian. (U. S. Department of Agriculture, 1966)

acids. All states now permit the sale of margarine to which coloring has been added; Wisconsin in 1967 was the last state to legalize such sales. The change in the consumption of butter and margarine in the last 20 years is significant (See Fig. 3–3).

OTHER LIPIDS

Phospholipids

In addition to fats, the phospholipids play very important roles in metabolism. They are structural compounds in cell membranes, essential components of certain enzyme systems and most probably are involved in the transport of lipids in the body. Their chemical structure is similar to fats except that a phosphoric acid radical and a nitrogen-containing base have replaced one of the fatty acids. Lecithin, a water-soluble derivative of fats, is the most abundant of the phospholipids in both tissues and foods where, because of its emulsifying properties, it serves as a solubilizer and stabilizer. Other phospholipids, cephalin and sphingomyelin, are also present in most tissues, the latter primarily in brain and lung tissues as a constituent of the myelin sheaths. Foods which contribute phospholipids to the diet include liver, brains, heart and egg yolk. Lecithin may also be added as an emulsifier to margarine, cheese products and other processed foods.

Choline, a part of the lecithin molecule, is now known to be essential to the prevention of fat accumulation in the liver. Other substances, such as the essential amino acid methionine and its derivatives, also have the function of preventing fatty liver. Such substances are called lipotropic because they have the ability to move or mobilize fat.

Cholesterol and Other Sterols

The two most common sterols are ergosterol, found in plants, and cholesterol, found in animal tissues. Cholesterol, an essential constituent of many cells, especially nerve and glandular tissues, is found in high concentration in the liver, where it is synthesized and stored, and in the blood, where it serves in the transport of fat.

Egg yolks and brains are particularly rich sources of cholesterol in the diet. Other important food sources include butter, cream cheese, heart, kidneys, liver, sweetbreads, lobster, shrimp, crab and fish roe. For additional food sources, see Table 3, Part 4.

In normal individuals the body compensates for the level of cholesterol intake in the diet through changes in the synthesis, degradation and excretion of the compound. Cholesterol synthesis may vary from 0.5 Gm. to 2 Gm. per day. Conversion in the liver to bile acids is the chief method of degradation and excretion, but cholesterol as such may also leave the body through the feces by excretion into the bile. Although as much as 50 per cent of the cholesterol synthesized each day in the body may be secreted with the bile into the intestines, much of it may also be reabsorbed in the process of fat absorption.

The maintenance of a normal level of blood cholesterol is of great physiologic importance. It is a precursor of Vitamin D (see Chap. 7) and closely related to several hormones in the body. It should not therefore be considered an abnormal substance in the body but one that has vital functions to perform. The Food and Nutrition Board's Report on Dietary Fat and Human Health states:

Evidence to support the concept that increased plasma concentrations of cholesterol are atherogenic is considerable but not conclusive. The type and quantity of dietary fat and the amount of cholesterol eaten influence the cholesterol concentration in the blood. Fats high in saturated fatty acids support a somewhat higher plasma cholesterol concentration than do those rich in polyunsaturated fatty acids. Many, but not all, population studies indicate that diets high in fat, among other nutrients, are correlated with higher concentrations of plasma cholesterol and with increased prevalence of cardiovascular disease. However, proof of a causal relationship is lacking.[9]

Further discussion of the relationship of blood cholesterol levels to atherosclerotic disease is discussed in Chapter 23.

---

[9] National Research Council Publication 1147. Dietary Fat and Human Health. Washington, D. C., 1966.

Lipoproteins

Most of the lipids in the body are transported in the blood by combining with proteins. The lipoproteins are classified according to their density as chylomicrons (containing primarily triglycerides from dietary fat and very little protein), low-density lipoprotein, or LDL (containing triglycerides in transport from the liver to adipose tissue, and phospholipids, cholesterol and protein which assist the transport) and high-density lipoproteins, or HDL (which are higher in protein and lower in lipid than the LDL). The free fatty acids are transported in the plasma bound to the protein albumin.

STUDY QUESTIONS AND ACTIVITIES

1. What can be said about the human requirement for fat in the diet? How does American consumption compare with that of some other countries?

2. What changes have occurred in the consumption and selection of fats by American consumers in the last 50 years? Explain why there may be large differences in the amount of fat consumed by individual families?

3. What is meant by saturated and unsaturated fatty acids? Give illustrations of each.

4. Which of the polyunsaturated fatty acids is most widely distributed in foods? What types of foods contribute the most of this factor?

5. From what sources are margarine and some of the cooking fats manufactured and by what process?

6. Is there evidence that the level of fat in the diet of Americans may be a hazard to health? In what way?

7. Name the essential fatty acids. Why are they called essential? Can any of them be synthesized in the body?

8. Besides its use for energy, what other functions does fat perform in the body?

9. What are phospholipids? Sterols? Where are they found in the body? Which sterols may be converted to vitamin D?

10. What are the normal functions of cholesterol in the body? How is the excess excreted?

SUPPLEMENTARY READING ON FATS

Coons, C. M.: Fats and Fatty Acids. Chap. 7. Foods. Yearbook of Agriculture. U.S.D.A., Washington, D. C., 1959.

Holman, R. T.: Council on Foods and Nutrition. How essential are fatty acids? J.A.M.A., *178*:930, 1961.

Council on Foods and Nutrition: The regulation of dietary fat. J.A.M.A., *181*:411, 1962.

National Research Council Publication 1147. Dietary Fat and Human Health. Washington, D. C., 1966.

For further references see Bibliography in Part Four.

CHAPTER 4

Proteins

*Vital Importance and World Use · Composition and Synthesis ·
Amino Acids—Essential and Nonessential · Quality of Protein ·
Protein Requirements · Food Sources of Protein · Stability of
Proteins in Foods*

VITAL IMPORTANCE AND WORLD USE

Every animal, including man, must have an adequate source of protein in order to grow and maintain itself.

Proteins have long been recognized as the fundamental structural element of every cell of the body. More recently, specific proteins and protein derivatives have been identified as the functional elements in certain specialized cells, glandular secretions, enzymes, and hormones. In their role as enzymes, proteins control the breakdown of food for energy and the synthesis of new compounds for maintenance and repair of body tissues. When they are supplied in amounts greater than necessary for growth and maintenance, proteins contribute to the energy pool of the body and, similarily, if carbohydrates and fats are not sufficient to meet energy demands, protein will be diverted for this purpose. Thus, protein well deserves its name, which is of Greek derivation, meaning "of first importance." Since proteins are the principal constituents of the active tissues of the body and the body is, in turn, dependent upon food protein for these indispensable substances, the quality and the quantity in the daily diet are of prime importance.

In many parts of the world, the developing countries particularly, food sources of protein, especially proteins of good quality, are extremely scarce. There is some evidence that in countries where the quality and the quantity of protein and other nutrients are inadequate, the stature of whole groups of people may be affected. When height and weight growth curves of groups of preschool children in Mexico, Lebanon (Arab refugees), Hong Kong, and Thailand were compared with those of United States (Iowa) children, growth retardation was evident in the former groups. Children in Ethiopia, Jordan, and Vietnam were also shorter and weighed less than Iowa children between the ages of one and seventeen years.[1] The increased stature of Japanese youths has paralleled increases in the Japanese diet of both total protein and protein from animal sources[2] (See Chap. 14). Similarly, Japanese who have lived in the U. S. for a generation or more have shown a marked increase in stature—clear evidence that heredity was not the determining factor[3]; and Australians and New Zealanders, perhaps the heaviest meat-eaters on the globe, have large physiques.

The United States has ample sources of protein available (approximately 100 Gm. per capita per day), and more than two thirds of it comes from meat, fish, poultry,

---

[1] Pre-School Child Malnutrition–Primary Deterrant to Human Progress. NAS-NRC Publication No. 1282. Washington, D. C., 1966.

[2] Mitchell, H. S.: J. Am. Dietet. A., *40*:521, 1962.

[3] Gruelich, W. W.: Science, *127*:515, 1958.

eggs, and dairy products (Fig. 4–1). Although surveys indicate that most of the North American population consume an adequate amount, there are still people who, for economic or other reasons, may not get enough protein.

COMPOSITION AND SYNTHESIS

Proteins, like fats and carbohydrates, are composed of carbon, hydrogen and oxygen, and, in addition, they must contain nitrogen. Often sulfur and phosphorus and sometimes other elements such as iron (in hemoglobin) and iodine (in thyroxine) are incorporated into the protein molecule.

Plants can synthesize proteins from the nitrates and the ammonia in soil and decaying vegetable matter. Water and carbon dioxide from the air provide the necessary carbon, hydrogen and oxygen. Animals are dependent on plants for this synthesis because animal cells cannot utilize simpler forms of nitrogen, and animal metabolism of protein, in turn, eventually yields the forms of nitrogen which only plant life and microorganisms can utilize. This sequence of events is called the nitrogen cycle.

Proteins are made up of some 22 or more nitrogen-containing compounds known as animo acids. All the amino acids are organic acids containing at least one acid group (COOH) and one amino group (NH₂). Certain amino acids, however, have two acid groups (acidic), others have two amino groups (basic), and still others may contain ring structures (aromatic) or sulfur groups. These amino acids are joined together by chemical linkages called peptide bonds in which the acid group of the first amino acid is attached to the nitrogen group of the next amino acid (Fig. 4–2). Two amino acids so linked are called a dipeptide; three amino acids, tripeptides. Polypeptides are composed of 10 to 100 amino acids. Those molecules containing over 100—sometimes several thousand—amino acids are referred to as proteins. The order in which all these amino acids are arranged is determined by the genetic code—the DNA (deoxyribonucleic acid) found in the nucleus of every cell (see Chap. 9). Because protein molecules are so large, with molecular weights ranging from 10,000 to several million, they have certain properties in common with colloidal solutions; the fact that protein molecules are too large to pass through cell membranes is important in physiology. For example, plasma proteins, because they cannot penetrate the capillary membranes, remain in the blood vessels and have an important effect on regulating water balance in the body (see Chap. 6).

The first of the amino acids to be identified was discovered over 125 years ago; the last of the 22 listed in Table 4–1 was isolated and identified in 1935 by W. C. Rose. During the century between these discoveries much of the basic chemistry and

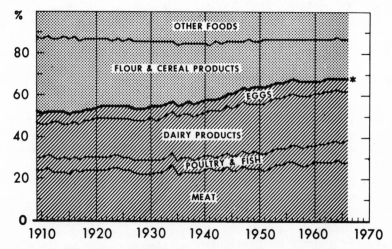

Fig. 4-1. Sources of protein in the diet of the U. S. population from 1910 to 1966. *–Total animal sources. (U.S.D.A. Agricultural Research Service, 1966)

physiologic significance of proteins came to be understood. With the realization that the constituent amino acids were important factors in determining the nutritive value of a protein, many investigations were conducted to find out which of them were indispensable and which could be excluded safely from the diet without interfering with normal growth and body function.

Amino Acids: Essential and Nonessential

Amino acids that the body cannot synthesize in adequate amounts are called essential or indispensable because they must be supplied by the diet in proper proportions and amounts to meet the requirements for maintenance and growth of tissue. Nonessential or dispensable amino acids are those the body can synthesize in sufficient amounts to meet its needs if the total amount of nitrogen supplied by protein is adequate (Table 4–1).

Nitrogen balance studies have been used to determine the amounts of essential amino acids required by various groups. An individual is in nitrogen equilibrium or balance when the nitrogen intake from protein is approximately equal to the nitrogen lost in the feces and urine. An adult consuming a diet that contains sufficient amounts of the essential amino acids will be in nitrogen equilibrium. If an essential amino acid is removed from the diet, negative nitrogen balance results. In this case more nitrogen is being lost than is consumed because tissues requiring the essential amino acid cannot be maintained and hence are broken down and their nitrogen excreted. Nitrogen equilibrium will again be attained when the lacking essential amino acid is supplied in amounts adequate to maintain tissues. Positive nitrogen balance, i.e., nitrogen intake

TABLE 4–1. Classification of Amino Acids with Respect to Their Need for Growth and Maintenance of Body Tissue

Essential	Nonessential
Isoleucine	Alanine
Leucine	Asparagine
Lysine	Aspartic acid
Methionine	Cysteine
Phenylalanine	Cystine
Threonine	Glutamic acid
Tryptophan	Glutamine
Valine	Glycine
Arginine*	Hydroxyproline
Histidine†	Proline
	Serine
	Tyrosine

*Arginine can be synthesized by the animal organism, but, since the rate of synthesis may be limited, a dietary supply may be necessary for maximum growth.

†Histidine is required for growth, but is not needed for maintenance by the adult human.

from protein greater than nitrogen loss in urine and feces, occurs only when new tissues are synthesized such as in growth and pregnancy.

According to Rose[4] eight amino acids are essential for maintenance of nitrogen equilibrium in man. The essential amino acid requirements for young men and women are given in Table 4–2. Men in an older age group who were studied by Tuttle and associates[5] appear to differ in their requirements; studies thus far indicate an increased need for methionine and lysine. Infants and children also appear to have proportionally greater demands for certain amino acids than the young adults.[6] In addition,

[4] Rose, W. C.: Nutr. Abstr. and Rev., 27:631, 1957.

[5] Tuttle, S. G., *et al.*: Am. J. Clin. Nutr., 16:225, 1965.

[6] Evaluation of Protein Quality. NAS-NRC Publication No. 1100. Washington, D. C., 1963.

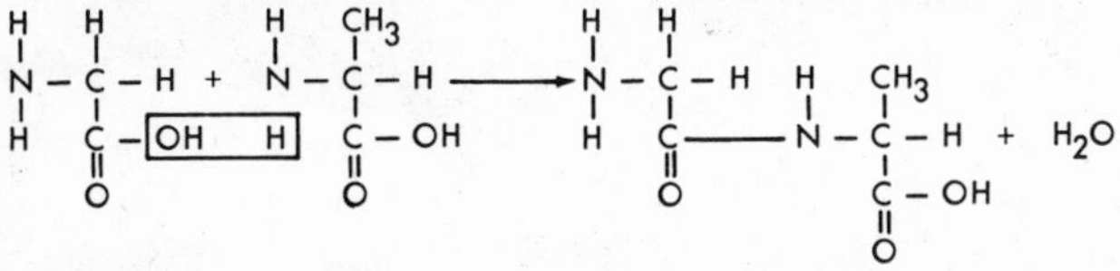

Glycine   Alanine   Glycylalanine

FIG. 4-2. Diagram shows amino acids glycine and alanine joined by peptide linkage to form the dipeptide glycylalanine.

TABLE 4-2. Minimum Requirements
of Essential Amino Acids*
(gm. per day)

Amino Acid	Young Men	Young Women
Leucine	1.10	0.62
Isoleucine	0.70	0.45
Lysine	0.80	0.50
Threonine	0.50	0.31
Tryptophan	0.25	0.16
Valine	0.80	0.65
Methionine	1.10	0.55†
Phenylalanine	1.10	1.12‡

*Figures from Rose, W. C., *et al.*: J. Biol. Chem., 217:987, 1955; Leverton, R. M., *et al.*: J. Nutr., 58:59, 83, 219, 341, 355; Swenseid, M. E., Williams, I., and Dunn, M. S.: J. Nutr., 58:495, 507, 1956; and Jones, E. M., *et al.*: J. Nutr., 60:549, 1956.
†Includes cystine.
‡Includes tyrosine.

infants probably require histidine as an essential amino acid.[7]

Factors in addition to the age, sex and physiologic condition of an individual influence the requirements for specific amino acids. If total protein intake is low, small surpluses of certain amino acids can increase the need for others. The nonessential amino acids in the protein also affect the quality of the protein. For example, the amount of the sulfur-containing essential amino acid methionine required may be somewhat reduced if cystine, a sulfur-containing nonessential amino acid is supplied in the diet. Likewise, the presence in the diet of tyrosine, a nonessential amino acid similar in structure to phenylalanine, may reduce the requirement for phenylalanine. Thus, much definitive work on amino acid

_____

[7] Holt, L. E., *et al.*: Protein and Amino Acid Requirements in Early Life. New York, New York University Press, 1960.

requirements has been accomplished, but many pieces of the puzzle are still missing.

Because of the identification of specific requirements for certain amino acids, it has become necessary to separate consideration of protein needs into two categories. One is the requirement for the essential amino acids, those the body cannot synthesize at a rate to meet its need. The other is the requirement for total protein—or total nitrogen, as it is sometimes called—which must be available to the body for the synthesis of the nonessential amino acids.

QUALITY OF PROTEIN

The effects of proteins on the maintenance or growth of animals are determined by the amounts of each of the eight to ten essential amino acids which are present in the specific protein. Osborne and Mendel in their pioneer work with rats showed that individual proteins differed in their ability to maintain life and support the growth of their animals. Casein (milk protein), when fed at a level of 18 per cent of the total calories, both maintained life and supported growth and hence was classified as a complete protein. Gliadin (wheat protein), since it maintained life but did not support growth, was called a partially incomplete protein. Incomplete proteins such as zein (corn protein) were those which could not even maintain life because they were lacking in one or more of the essential amino acids. Since casein was found to be only half as effective in supporting growth when fed at the 9 per cent level as it was at the 18 per cent level, it was recognized that quality and quantity were both important in determining the effectiveness of proteins.

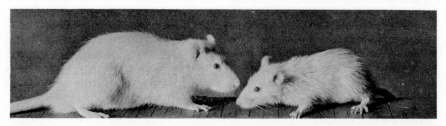

FIG. 4-3. Adequate and inadequate protein (18 per cent vs. 4 per cent). Rats of the same litter. This deficiency produces stunted growth but no deformities.

Animal proteins, such as meats, poultry, fish, eggs, milk and cheese, provide good quality protein in liberal amounts and are termed complete proteins. The exception to this is gelatin, the protein derived from animal connective tissue which, because of its lack of tryptophan, is classified as an incomplete protein. Proteins from plant sources are usually not of as good quality as those from animal sources because one or more of the following essential amino acids are in short supply: lysine, methionine, threonine and tryptophan. They are therefore incomplete or partially incomplete. The best quality plant proteins are found in legumes, such as beans, peas and peanuts, and in nuts. The protein in bread and cereals and in vegetables other than those mentioned and in fruit are all incomplete. These proteins are nevertheless an important part of the food intake, since their amino acids are a part of all tissue protein molecules. If they were not included in the diet, the body would need to synthesize them from the more important essential amino acids.

By comparing the proportions of essential amino acids present in a food protein of unknown quality with those in an ideal protein the deficiency of essential amino acids, if any, can be calculated. Egg protein contains a pattern of essential amino acids closely approximating the proportions determined as indispensable for humans, and was at first used as an ideal protein for comparison. Later, the Food and Agricultural Organization[8] proposed a desirable pattern of essential amino acids with which comparisons could be made; by using this "ideal pattern," the amino acid content of food combinations as well as individual foods could be appraised. Then, in 1965, a joint FAO/WHO committee recommended that the proteins of human milk or eggs again be used as the reference pattern[9] (Table 4–3).

The FAO committee also proposed a protein score based on the calculation of the most limiting amino acid in a given food or combination, i.e., the amino acid that falls farthest below the ideal pattern. If the most limiting amino acid is 80 per cent of the ideal, then the protein score is considered to be 80. A diet with a protein score above 70 is considered satisfactory if the amount of total protein is liberal. When the score is below 70, even an increase in the total amount of such a poor quality protein in the diet cannot supply a sufficient amount of the limiting amino acid. In these instances, another protein which can supply the limiting factor must be added to improve the protein quality of the diet.

---

[8] Protein Requirements. FAO Nutrition Studies, No. 16. Rome, Italy, 1957.

[9] Joint FAO/WHO Expert Group: Protein Requirements. Tech. Report 301, World Health Organization. Geneva, Switzerland, 1965.

TABLE 4–3. The FAO Pattern and the Proteins of Egg, Human Milk and Cow's Milk*
(Gm./100 Gm. of protein)

Essential Amino Acids	FAO Pattern	Egg	Human Milk	Cow's Milk
Arginine†	—	6.6	4.1	3.7
Histidine†	—	2.4	2.2	2.7
Lysine	4.2	6.6	6.6	7.9
Leucine	4.8	8.8	9.1	10.0
Isoleucine	4.2	6.6	5.5	6.5
Methionine	2.2	3.1	2.3	2.5
(Total sulfur amino acids)	4.2	5.4	4.3	3.4
Phenylalanine	2.8	5.8	4.4	4.9
(Total aromatic amino acids)	5.6	10.8	9.9	10.0
Threonine	2.8	5.0	4.5	4.7
Tryptophan	1.4	1.7	1.6	1.4
Valine	4.2	7.4	6.3	7.0

*Adapted from Evaluation of Protein Quality. NAS-NRC Publication No. 1100. Washington, D. C., 1963.
†See Table 4-1.

Fortunately, most of our foods contain a mixture of proteins, one of which often supplements another. More to the point, however, is the fact that we combine several different foods in a meal, the proteins of which tend to supplement one another because of their varying amino acid content. For instance, cereals which are low in lysine are usually eaten with milk, which provides a generous amount of this factor. Thus, cereal and milk or bread and cheese are good combinations. It is obvious that this type of complementary value among foods makes a varied diet more desirable than a restricted one.

The concept of protein supplementation has also been applied in areas where animal proteins are not readily available. Attempts to provide palatable low-cost foods with an adequate amino acid balance from inexpensive indigenous foods has resulted in combinations of various types of vegetable proteins. One such product is "Incaparina" developed by the Institute of Nutrition in Central America and Panama (INCAP). It consists of a mixture of ground maize, sorghum, cottonseed flour, torula yeast and vitamin A.[10] A number of other countries in Asia, the Near East and Africa have developed similar products to meet the protein needs of young infants. Small amounts of animal protein such as skim milk or fish meal have also been added to mixtures of vegetable proteins to improve their quality. Another example is seen in the enrichment of cereal grains with one or more of the amino acids which are the limiting factors, such as the addition of lysine to wheat. These mixtures provide a relatively good source of protein, particularly for the growing child, who suffers the most from poor quality and inadequate protein intake.

PROTEIN REQUIREMENTS

Any quantitative estimate of protein requirement must take into account the quality of the proteins involved. The Food and Nutrition Board recommends a daily intake of 1 Gm. of protein per Kg. of body weight for the adult. Hence the recommendation for the "reference man and woman" is 70

and 58 Gm. respectively (see Chap. 10). The Board recognized, however, that these were not minimum needs inasmuch as adults can be maintained in nitrogen balance on protein intakes of less than half the recommended dietary allowance when the protein is of high quality, i.e., Biological Value 100. If proteins of lower Biological Value are used, the minimum requirement increases proportionately. Biological value refers to the proportion of absorbed nitrogen which is retained by the subject. The recommended allowances for growing children are higher per unit of weight to meet the needs for growth. This is true also for the pregnant woman and the nursing mother, both of whom naturally need an extra supply to provide for the nourishment of two organisms.[11]

The trend at the present time is toward an increasingly liberal protein allowance for all ages, so as to provide for less obvious needs as well as for growth and maintenance. For example, antibody formation requires protein and hence resistance to infections is reduced when protein intake is inadequate.[12]

It is highly desirable that at least one third of the daily protein intake be derived from animal sources, which is usually the case in the average diet in the United States. It is also strongly recommended that some good quality protein be included in every meal, since the tissues must have all of the essential amino acids present at one time for tissue synthesis. If they are not, they may be metabolized and wasted. This rule applies particularly to breakfast and lunch, for these are the meals most likely to be sketchy, and often contain little if any protein. It is also worth noting that, since protein foods with high protein scores are the most expensive class of foods in the diet, there is a tendency among low-income groups to consume less than recommended amounts of proteins, both quantitatively and qualitatively.

10 Scrimshaw, N. S., and Bressani, R.: Fed. Proc., 20:80, 1961.

11 Recommended Dietary Allowances. 6th Ed. NAS-NRC Publication 1146. Washington, D. C., 1964.

12 Scrimshaw, N. S.: Borden's Rev. Nutr. Res., 26:17, 1965. (No. 2.)

PROTEIN

In Average Servings of Foods
Classified in the Four Food Groups

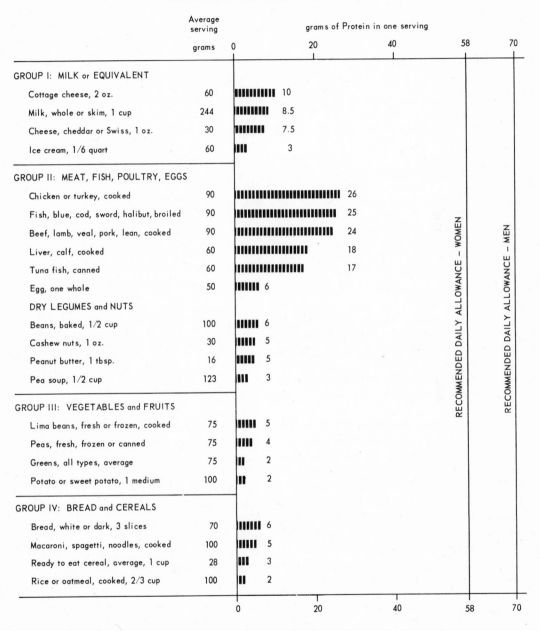

FIGURE 4-4

TABLE 4–4. Protein in Pattern Dietary for 1 Day*

Food Group	Amount in Gm.	Household Measure	Calories	Protein Gm.
Milk or equivalent	488	2 cups	320	17
Egg	50	1 medium	81	7
Meat, fish	120	4 ozs. cooked	376	30
Vegetables:				
Potato, cooked	100	1 medium	65	2
Green or yellow	75	1 serving	27	2
Other	75	1 serving	45	2
Fruits:				
Citrus	100	1 serving	43	1
Other	100	1 serving	85	—
Bread, white enriched	70	3 slices	189	6
Cereal, whole grain or enriched	30	1 oz. dry or		
	130	⅔ cup cooked	89	3
Butter or margarine	14	1 tbsp.	100	—
		Total	1,420	70

*For basis of calculation, see Pattern Dietary in Chapter 10.

A basic dietary pattern for a day (Chap. 10) is useful in planning menus. This dietary pattern (Table 4–4) of approximately 1,400 calories provides a liberal amount of protein, more than three fourths of which is derived from animal sources. Additional foods chosen to supply the extra calories would also provide more protein.

Protein requirement may be modified by certain pathologic conditions. During convalescence from debilitating diseases or surgery, extra protein will hasten recovery and rehabilitation. For this reason the earlier tendency to reduce protein intake in many diseases, with a few exceptions, has been reversed. The nurse should, however, recognize that certain diseases (see Chaps. 25, 28 and 34) may require limiting the total amount of protein or the amount of a specific amino acid in a patient's diet.

FOOD SOURCES OF PROTEIN

From the bar chart of average servings (Fig. 4–4), it is evident that the first two food groups supply the most protein per serving and are also the best quality proteins. Dry legumes and nuts are included as meat alternates in Group II because they contain the best quality of plant proteins.

Animal Sources of Protein

Group I. Milk and Milk Products. The foods listed in this group—milk, cheese and ice cream—all derive their protein from milk. The proteins of milk are casein and lactalbumin, both complete, i.e., they contain a good balance of amino acids. Milk is the protein food that Nature provides for the young of the species, and, around the world, milk from many different mammals is used for human food. Milk is almost essential for the infant; it is equally good as a source of protein for older children and adolescents during the growing years. Adults also should get some of their protein from milk and milk products. Nonfat dry milk, better known as dried skim milk, is an excellent source of milk protein and calcium at comparatively low cost. (See Chaps. 35 and 36 for ways of using dried skim milk.)

Cheese is the term applied to any product made from the concentrated curd of milk. Cheese is thought to have been the first manufactured food, the process for which was probably discovered accidentally when milk was stored in a bag made from the stomach of a cow, which contains rennin. The action of rennin on milk causes the curds to form and the whey to separate. Although a certain amount of the milk nutrients remains in the whey, the majority remains in the curd, which provides a large amount of the natural food value in milk in concentrated form. The curd in cottage cheese is formed by the development of or addition of lactic acid bacteria to skimmed milk.

Both food value and flavor of the many kinds of cheese that are available today depend on the composition and the methods of ripening which are used in production.

Group II. Meat, poultry and fish are all forms of animal tissue protein synthesized by each species to meet its specific needs for growth and maintenance. Such proteins are remarkably similar in amino acid content to the amino acid requirements of man. Meat, poultry and seafoods vary in protein content in inverse ratio to the moisture content: veal 28, beef 25, lamb 24, poultry 20 and fish 15 to 20 Gm. of protein per 100 Gm. of fresh product. Pork contains more fat than other meats, and the fat is embedded in the muscle in such a way that it is not easily removed.

Variety meats is a term applied to the organs and the glands of animals. They include tongue, liver, kidney, sweetbreads (thymus gland of calf or lamb), beef or calf heart and beef brains. The organ meats tend to be much richer in vitamins and minerals than muscle meats. Popular luncheon meats such as spiced ham, pressed meat loaves, liverwurst and various types of cold sausages such as bologna and frankfurters are sometimes classed as variety meats. They contain from 11 to 17 per cent of protein in a convenient form for quick lunches.

Poultry is a general term covering a variety of domestic birds including chicken, turkeys, geese and ducks. After roasting, the protein content of the lean meat of most poultry is about 30 per cent; after frying or broiling the proportion of the protein content is slightly less than it is after roasting, because less moisture is lost.

Fish, including shellfish, compare favorably with meats and poultry as good sources of protein and in many countries are the chief source of animal protein. In the United States an effort is being made to stimulate the use of more varieties of both salt and fresh water fish. In other countries such products as fish sausage, fish flour and meal and other processed fish foods of high protein value are being developed to improve the protein supply. Shellfish are low in fat and somewhat lower in protein ratio than fish because of their higher water content. For selection and preparation of meat, poultry and fish see Chapter 35.

Eggs are in a class by themselves, a protein food of high nutritive value. As mentioned previously, egg protein contains the essential amino acids in proportion so nearly like the theoretical ideal protein that it is often used experimentally as the reference standard in evaluating the protein of other foods (Table 4–3). Eggs contain 13 per cent of protein—less than meats, poultry or fish because of their higher water content. The egg white is one of the best examples of a pure colloidal solution of a protein (ovalbumin), containing 11 per cent of protein and 89 per cent of water. The protein of the yolk is more concentrated (16%) and much more complex. It contains lipoprotein, phosphoprotein, nucleoprotein and possibly others, all of which provide nourishment for the embryo chick and are equally valuable as human food.

Plant Sources of Protein

Group III. Vegetables are poor sources of protein; the only ones that provide more than 1 or 2 per cent are the legumes. These may run as high as 5 or 6 per cent when they are fresh and still higher in the dried form. For this reason, and because they provide one of the better quality of plant proteins, they are listed as meat alternates in the Four Food Group chart. Soybeans, which are the highest in protein content of the legumes, are not used much for human food in the United States, but they are important sources of protein in many countries where animal foods are scarce. Soybean milk, curd, cheese and flour are a few of the soybean products used by Orientals. In India, according to Patwardhan,[13] pulses (legumes) and beans could be produced and used more extensively than at present with great advantage because of their high nutritive value. They are especially important in a country where animal protein is scarce or the population is largely vegetarian.

Peanuts are really legumes although they are often classed as nuts. Roasted peanuts and peanut butter contain about 26 per cent of protein, although roasting reduces the availability or destroys about 10 per cent of three of the essential amino acids present. Peanuts—or groundnuts, as they are called in many countries—are often used without roasting or with much less heating than is common in this country.

Nuts in general are good sources of protein of fairly high quality. Because they are expensive they are seldom eaten in sufficient quantity to make an important contribution to the protein of the diet.

Group IV. Breads and cereals make an important contribution to the protein of the diet, not only because of their liberal consumption but also because many of their uses encourage or increase the consumption of animal proteins such as milk, eggs, meat and fish. The protein of uncooked grains ranges from 7 to 14 per cent. The grain proteins are low in one or more essential amino acids, e.g., wheat is low in lysine, corn in tryptophan, rice in tryptophan and the sulfur-containing amino acids, cystine and methionine. However, plant proteins may supplement each other in such a way that a combination may provide a better balance of amino acids than any one food alone.

STABILITY OF PROTEINS IN FOODS
Bacterial Spoilage

Chemically pure proteins are fairly stable, but in the moist state in which they generally are found in foods they decompose readily at room temperature, owing to bacterial action, and may form substances toxic to the body. In this respect, nitrogenous foods are more unstable and will decompose more readily than carbo-

---

[13] Patwardhan, V. N.: Am. J. Clin. Nutr., *11*:12, 1962.

hydrates and fats. Therefore, protein foods such as fresh meat, fish, milk and eggs should be kept in the refrigerator to prevent or delay their decomposition.

Effect of Heat on Protein Foods

Proteins are somewhat modified by heat, both in physical properties and in physiologic availability. In ordinary cooking, proteins such as those in egg, meat and fish are coagulated by heat, but the amino acid content is not changed.

STUDY QUESTIONS AND ACTIVITIES

1. Why is good-quality protein important for breakfast as well as for other meals?

2. For what specific purposes are proteins used in the body?

3. What is meant by the terms nitrogen equilibrium, limiting factor and polypeptide?

4. The structural components of proteins are amino acids. How many of these are known? Do tissues vary in the requirements for specific amino acids?

5. What is meant by "essential amino acids"? Are the same ones essential for maintenance as for growth?

6. Explain three ways that proteins may be supplemented to improve the quality of the diet. What is meant by protein score? Biological Value?

7. What theory is suggested as to why most Australians and New Zealanders are taller than people of similar racial strains living elsewhere?

8. What are the best food sources of complete proteins? Which food groups furnish the most protein? Compare the quality of protein from plant and animal foods.

9. What is the effect of heat on protein?

10. What are the National Research Council recommendations for protein? Which foods must be included in the daily dietary, and how much of each, in order to ensure good nutrition?

11. The high-protein foods listed in Figure 4–4 contain appreciable amounts of other food constituents. Look at the Pattern Dietary in Chapter 10 and see what each supplies.

SUPPLEMENTARY READING ON PROTEIN AND AMINO ACIDS

Brock, J. F.: Dietary protein in relation to man's health. Fed. Proc., *20*:61, 1961 (Fifth Int. Congress on Nutrition).

FAO: Nutrition Requirements. FAO Nutrition Studies No. 16. Rome, Italy, 1957.

Food and Nutrition Board: Evaluation of Protein Nutrition. National Research Council Pub. 711. Washington, D. C., 1959.

Food and Nutrition Board: Evaluation of Protein Quality. National Research Council Pub. 1100. Washington, D. C., 1963.

Joint FAO/WHO Expert Group: Protein Requirements. Tech. Report 301, World Health Organization, Geneva, Switzerland, 1965.

Leverton, R. M.: Proteins and Amino Acids. Chaps. 5 and 6, Food. Yearbook of Agriculture, U.S.D.A., Washington, D. C., 1959.

For further references see Bibliography in Part Four.

CHAPTER 5

Energy Metabolism

Energy and Heat • Measurement of Food Calories • Measure of Energy Expended • Basal Metabolism • Factors Influencing Total Energy Requirements

Atomic power may make the headlines, but solar energy is still the power that makes life on earth possible. However, of all the sun's energy that reaches the earth only a fraction of 1 per cent can be adapted or stored for future use. Even the most efficient man-made devices for harnessing some of the sun's energy are less efficient by far than plants. Here the amazing process known as *photosynthesis* (p. 15) uses the sun's light energy to manufacture carbohydrates from the carbon dioxide of the air and the water from the soil. No animal is capable of accomplishing this synthesis. Thus, the potential or stored energy of the plant world becomes the food of animals who, in turn, spend that energy in the form of heat and work or store the surplus as body fat (See Chap. 2, Fig. 2–1).

Metabolism may be used in a general sense to refer to all types of changes that occur in food nutrients after they have been absorbed from the gastrointestinal tract and to the cellular activity involved in utilizing these nutrients (See Chap. 9). Sometimes the word is used in a more specific sense, as in protein metabolism, to refer to the total picture of what happens to protein in the body. These changes, which result ultimately in the combustion of foodstuffs, with the release of heat or energy, constitute what is called energy metabolism.

ENERGY AND HEAT

Energy is expended whenever work is performed by the body in the completion of any function, small or large. It matters not whether the action is voluntary, such as walking, sitting and the various acts involved in the performance of one's daily work, or involuntary, such as in respiration, digestion, the circulation of the blood, and the maintenance of muscular tone.

The body must be supplied with food as a source of energy to maintain its temperature and perform its work. There is a direct relation between the amount of work performed, the heat produced by the body and the total food intake. One cannot perform more work than is provided for by the food intake unless one uses the reserve supply stored as adipose tissue. This latter is dramatically illustrated by the loss of body fat in starvation.

Heat in Relation to Metabolism. Heat is the result of combustion of fuels outside the body and also of the oxidation of foods in our bodies. Since heat is a by-product of all energy spent as work, heat can serve as a measure of energy metabolism. As it is necessary in scientific work to have measures of length (centimeter, inch) and measures of weight (gram, ounce), so is it necessary to have a measure of heat. A Calorie (kilo calorie) is the amount of heat required to raise the temperature of one kilogram of water one degree centigrade.

In our more common measures, it is approximately the amount of heat required to raise the temperature of four pounds of water one degree Fahrenheit. This is a large calorie and is 1,000 times the small calorie, the unit used by physicists.

MEASUREMENT OF FOOD CALORIES

A bomb calorimeter is a device for measuring calories, the stored fuel in foods. The apparatus shown in Figure 5–1 is carefully designed for measuring all the heat produced by the complete oxidation of an accurately measured amount of any food. The apparatus is insulated thoroughly against loss of heat, and the amount of heat produced is measured by the change in temperature of a measured amount of water.

Physiologic Calorie Values. The calorie value of nutrients determined by the bomb calorimeter must be modified to take account of losses in digestion and excretion. From a large number of determinations Atwater derived the well-known physiologic fuel values:

	Calories per Gm.
Protein	4
Fat	9
Carbohydrate	4

These values were approximate only, but they served reasonably well when applied to foods in the average American diet. This method of calculating the calorie value of individual foods had been used since 1900, although the inaccuracies were recognized. In the Agriculture Handbook No. 8 published by the U. S. Department of Agriculture in 1963,[1] calorie values are calculated by a modification of the procedure that had been in use for over 60 years. Instead of applying the general caloric factors 4,9,4 to the percentage composition of food, as had been done previously, more specific factors were used. These new factors take into consideration further research data on the fuel values of foods.

The new values for most foods approximate the old values, but they are more ac-

[1] Watt, B. K., and Merrill, A. L.: Composition of Foods: Raw, Processed, Prepared. Agricultural Handbook No. 8. U. S. Department of Agriculture, 1963.

curate for foods such as whole wheat, where there is a large indigestible fraction. For practical purposes, however, it is still possible to estimate the caloric value of most foods by applying the old physiologic fuel values to the percentage composition for protein, fat and carbohydrate.

The need for revising the U. S. method of calculating food values was emphasized during World War II, when international committees were concerned with the world's food supply. They could not talk the same nutrition language unless they could agree on methods of estimating the nutritional value of foods. As a result, the FAO Nutrition Division published its find-

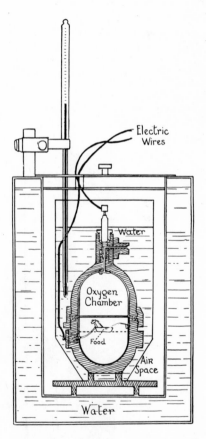

Fig. 5-1. Diagram of the parts of a bomb calorimeter. The water in the inner chamber changes in temperature when the food is burned. The water in the outer chamber acts with the intervening air space as insulation.

ings in 1947.[2] The policies and the data given in that publication became the basis of the present method of calculation. Table 1, in Part Four, Composition of Foods, is based on Handbook No. 8 and Bulletin 72.[3]

MEASURE OF ENERGY EXPENDED

The actual energy expended by the body throughout a given period may be determined by placing a human subject in a special calorimeter. The heat given off by the subject is absorbed by the water in the coils surrounding the well insulated chamber, where, by an accurate mechanism, the total heat may be measured. This procedure is known as direct calorimetry. As there are in existence only a few calorimeters large enough for making direct observations on human beings, and since they are exceedingly expensive, this method is used only for scientific research.

---

[2] FAO: Energy-Yielding Components of Food and Computation of Calorie Values. Washington, D.C., FAO, 1947.

[3] Nutritive Value of Foods. Home and Garden Bull. No. 72. Washington, D. C., U.S.D.A., 1964.

By another method, known as indirect calorimetry, the rate of metabolism is calculated from the oxygen intake or from the oxygen intake and carbon dioxide content of the expired air, as measured by a respiration apparatus. By determining either the oxygen consumed or the carbon dioxide exhaled in a given number of minutes, the caloric expenditure can be calculated. This principle may be applied to persons engaged in various types of activities or when lying at rest. If the subject is moving about, he has to carry his respirator with him (Fig. 5–2). Under basal conditions, or when work is performed in a stationary position, a tank-type apparatus is used.

BASAL METABOLISM

The energy expended under basal conditions includes the work of

1. Maintenance of muscle tone and body temperature
2. Circulation
3. Respiration
4. Other glandular and cellular activity.

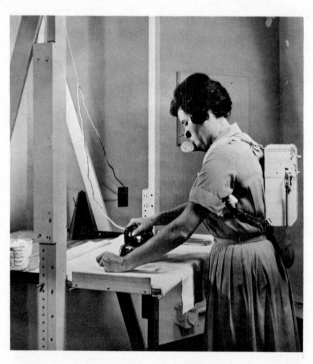

Fig. 5-2. Subject wearing respirometer to measure calorie expenditure while standing to iron at a work-surface level of 36 inches from the floor. (U.S.D.A. Office of Information)

In order that there may be some basis of comparison for tests, the rate of metabolism must be studied under standard basal conditions. Therefore, it is specified that the subject be lying down, awake and at complete rest, and that the test be taken at least 12 hours after the last meal and several hours after any vigorous exercise.

In the morning before breakfast is the most convenient time to comply with these conditions. The rate of metabolism as determined under these "standard" conditions is known as the basal metabolic rate (BMR). Marked variations in the basal rate of metabolism are an indication of disease.

Formerly, the basal metabolism test was used extensively as a means of diagnosis, particularly in cases of hyperthyroidism, hypothyroidism, myxedema and other endocrine disturbances which may alter the metabolic rate. Since the thyroid hormone, thyroxine, has the greatest effect on the metabolic rate, measurement of protein-bound iodine (PBI)—the combination of iodine-thyroxine with certain proteins in the blood—is a more accurate diagnostic test. It requires only a small sample of the patient's blood, and is easier for both the patient and the physician. The normal range for PBI is from 4 to 8 micrograms per 100 ml. of plasma.

Factors Determining Basal Metabolic Rate (BMR)

There are normal variations in basal metabolism, the causes of which lie within the body itself: the size, the shape and the composition of the body, the age of the individual and the activity of certain internal glands. It is generally accepted that a variation of from 10 to 15 per cent either way from the accepted metabolism rate (all variables considered) is within normal limits. Complete tables of average metabolic rates for men and women of different age, height and weight are used for comparison with the measured rate. The basal metabolism of an average man and woman would be about 1,650 and 1,350 calories, respectively.

The surface area of the body is used as a measure of size in these studies. The skin of the body is a radiating surface from which heat is given off continually. Therefore, the greater the skin area, the greater will be the amount of heat lost by the body and, in turn, the greater the necessary heat production by the individual. It has been found that a tall, slender person has a greater surface area than a shorter, stout person of the same weight; that is, surface area is proportional to height multiplied by weight.

The higher the proportion of active muscular tissue the higher the metabolic rate will be, because fatty tissue has a much lower rate. Thus, the athlete will tend to have a higher rate than a sedentary man of the same age and size.

Age and growth are responsible for normal variations in basal metabolism. The relative rate is highest during the first and the second years of life and decreases after that, although it is still relatively high through the ages of puberty, in both girls and boys. During adult life there is a steady decrease in rate, with a marked drop in old age, due undoubtedly to lower muscle tone resulting from diminishing muscular activity.

Sex probably has little effect on metabolism, although women in general have a lower metabolism than men. This may be accounted for by habitually less activity or by a difference in body composition, women usually having more fat and less muscular development than men.

Climate has little effect on the BMR of American subjects but has been shown to have an effect on Japanese. A variation of 17 per cent in the BMR of Japanese subjects is reported. The higher rates were recorded in the winter and the lower in the summer.[4] When Canadians living in Japan were compared to Japanese, the Canadian subjects did not show this seasonal change even though they were living under the same environmental conditions as the Japanese. Factors such as the size of the subject, composition of the diet and seasonal differences in energy expenditure probably influence the adaptation of basal metabolism to changes in climate.[5]

---

[4] Sasaki, T.: Fed. Proc., 25:1165, 1966.

[5] Yakiyashi, K.: Fed. Proc., 25:1169, 1966.

TABLE 5–1. Energy Expenditure for Everyday Activities*

	Cal./ Kg./Hr.	Cal./ Lb./Hr.
Asleep..........................	.9	.4
Bicycling, mod. speed.............	3.8	1.7
Cello playing....................	2.5	1.1
Dancing, foxtrot.................	5.2	2.4
Dancing, waltz..................	4.4	2.0
Dishwashing.....................	2.2	1.0
Dressing and undressing..........	1.9	.9
Driving an automobile............	2.1	1.0
Eating a meal	1.5	.7
Horseback riding, trot............	5.8	2.6
Ironing.........................	2.2	1.0
Laundry, light...................	2.5	1.1
Lying still and awake.............	1.2	.5
Painting furniture	2.8	1.3
Playing Ping-pong...............	5.9	2.7
Piano playing, moderate..........	2.6	1.2
Reading aloud...................	1.5	.7
Running........................	8.8	4.0
Sewing by hand.................	1.5	.7
Sewing, elec. mach..............	1.5	.7
Sitting quietly, watching TV........	1.4	.6
Skating........................	4.9	2.2
Standing, relaxed...............	1.7	.8
Sweeping, vacuum cleaner........	4.1	1.9
Swimming (2 mi./hr.).............	9.8	4.5
Tailoring.......................	2.1	1.0
Typing rapidly..................	2.2	1.0
Walking, 3 mph.................	3.3	1.5
Walking, 4 mph.................	4.9	2.2
Writing........................	1.5	.7

*Adapted from Taylor, MacLeod & Rose: Foundations of Nutrition. Ed. 5. New York, Macmillan, 1956. (Calculated by adding to original figures 1 cal./Kg./hr. for BMR plus 10 per cent for influence of food).

There is, however, a tendency for the basal metabolic rate of many individuals to decrease when they move from a temperate to a tropical climate. European women living in India had a lower BMR than women of similar body composition studied in the United States.[6]

Racial differences in metabolism have been noted, but it is not certain whether these differences relate directly to genetic factors or to environmental factors such as climate, dietary patterns and body size. In 1957 the Committee on Caloric Requirements of the Food and Agricultural Organization of the United Nations reported that "As far as present knowledge goes in-

dividuals of the same size, living in the same environment and having the same mode of living will have the same caloric requirements whatever their race. In other words race *per se* does not influence caloric requirements."[7] However, more recently a study of Indian and European women living in India showed that the Indian women had lower basal metabolic rates than the European women even when differences in height, weight and muscle mass were considered.[8]

The state of nutrition may effect the BMR. In order to conserve energy during severe starvation or prolonged undernutrition, the body adapts by decreasing its metabolic rate, possibly by as much as 50 per cent.

Diseases such as infections or fevers raise the BMR in proportion to the elevation of the body temperature, approximately 7 per cent for each degree Fahrenheit rise in temperature.

The secretions of certain endocrine glands, such as the thyroid, the adrenals and the pituitary affect metabolism. The secretion of the thyroid gland has the most marked effect. Hyperthyroidism is that condition in which the metabolism is accelerated by increased production of thyroxine, while hypothyroidism is characterized by a decrease resulting in subnormal metabolism. Adrenalin, a secretion of the adrenals, causes a temporary increase in the BMR. Those pituitary hormones which stimulate thyroid and adrenal secretions also affect the metabolic rate.

FACTORS INFLUENCING TOTAL ENERGY REQUIREMENTS

For all voluntary activities the energy needed is in direct relation to the intensity of the exercise. For instance, a moderate amount of energy is needed for walking, whereas for the heavy labor of digging a ditch or for the active exercise of tennis a much greater number of calories is needed.

Muscular work is the greatest factor influencing energy requirements. Mental work, strange as it may seem, does not af-

6 Mason, E. D., *et al.*: Human Biology, 36:374, 1964.

7 Calorie Requirements. Nutr. Studies, 15. FAO, Rome, 1957.

8 Mason, E. D., *et al.*: Op. cit.

TABLE 5–2. A Nurse's Activities for 1 Day—Calculation of Energy Expended

	Time Engaged in Activity in Hours	Calories per Pound	
		Per Hour	Total
Activity:			
Asleep....................................	8	0.4	3.2
Lying still, awake..........................	1	0.5	0.5
Dressing and undressing.....................	1	0.9	0.9
Sitting in class, eating meals, studying, watching TV..	6½	0.7	4.6
Clinical experience (6 hours):			
Walking................................	1	1.5	1.5
Standing...............................	1	.8	.8
Care of patient.........................	4	1.1	4.4
Walking to and from work..................	½	1.5	.7
Recreation:			
Playing piano..........................	½	1.2	.6
Dancing................................	½	2.0	1.0
	24		
		Total per lb.	18.2
		Weight in lbs.	130
	Total energy expended for the day		2,366

fect the total metabolism sufficiently to be detected easily. Investigators, working with very delicate apparatus, found that nerve tissue, when active, does expend some energy, but that the amount is minute compared with the total energy output of the body. In exceptional cases, physical work may be the means of increasing the metabolism by as much as 4,000 calories per day. In every case the food intake should equal in caloric value the heat units expended by the body (except, of course, in overweight individuals who find it necessary to reduce). A man doing sedentary work may require only 2,500 calories per day, while a man doing exceedingly hard manual labor may require as much as 5,000 calories. The calorie allowances given for different age and sex categories in the Recommended Daily Dietary Allowances apply to individuals engaged in moderate physical activity (see Chap. 10). For men, the range is from 2,900 down to 2,200; for women, from 2,100 to 1,600 calories, the lower figures being for the older age groups.

Table 5–1 gives the average energy expenditure per pound or per kilo per hour for several everyday activities. Obviously, not all types of activity have been measured but, in using this table to estimate energy expenditure, the data requiring similar exertion may be used for an activity for which no figure is given.

Individual variation in the amount of energy spent in performing a given task or activity may be considerable. One person may sit so relaxed that he spends no more energy than another may spend lying down. One person makes more motions in doing a job than another. Thus, in calculating the energy expenditure for a day from such a table one can expect only an approximate figure because of the many variables and the difficulty of estimating the exact length of time spent in each activity. Nevertheless, it is interesting to see how the energy intake calculated from food eaten compares with the calculated energy expenditure for the same day.

A student nurse weighing 130 pounds and in clinical practice for 6 hours a day may estimate her total energy expenditure for the 24 hours from the list of activities. The results of such a calculation are given in Table 5–2 as a sample. An office girl with less activity would expend considerably fewer calories, but a man weighing more and in sedentary occupation may expend about the same calories as the more active woman.

TABLE 5–3. Approximate Increase Above Basal Needs for Listed Activities

	Per Cent Above Basal
Bed rest (hospital patient)............	10
Sedentary activity, knitting...........	30
Light activity, tailor or nurse..........	50
Moderate activity, carpenter, painter...	75
Severe activity, lumberman, stone mason	100

A quick estimate of the energy needs of a moderately active person may be made as follows:

Basal needs = 1 cal./Kg./hr.

Weight in Kg. × 24 = BMR for 1 day

BMR plus 50% = total energy needs for light activity.

The increase above the basal is proportional to the degree of activity, as indicated in Table 5–3 for the rough estimation of energy needs.

Habitual muscular exercise not only increases the total energy metabolism but affects the basal rate, because energy is required to maintain muscle tone. On the

other hand, sleep lowers metabolism because the muscles are relaxed. A prolonged period of absolute rest in bed means loss of muscle tone and lowered metabolism.

A person who habitually consumes more calories than he expends for work plus body heat tends to store the extra food as body fat (adipose tissue). This is easy to do, especially when one's activities are less than they were previously. Frequently, eating habits are not adjusted to fit reduced activities. Therefore, it is not surprising that people tend to gain weight with age; it is more surprising that they do not gain more weight. A fuller discussion of weight control and the treatment of obesity is given in Chapter 21.

Age and body weight affect total energy requirement as well as the BMR. Of course, activity is the biggest variable, but, in general, activity decreases with age as does the metabolic activity of the tissues. Recognizing these changes, the National Research Council has listed caloric allowances for individuals of various body weights at different ages, assuming moderate physical activity (Table 5–4).

TABLE 5–4. Adjustment of Calorie Allowances for Adult Individuals of Various Body Weights and Ages*

(At a mean environmental temperature of 20° C. [68° F.] assuming average physical activity)

Desirable Weight			Calorie Allowance		
Kgs.	Pounds		25 Years	45 Years	65 Years
		Men	(1)	(2)	(3)
50	110		2,300	2,050	1,750
55	121		2,450	2,200	1,850
60	132		2,600	2,350	1,950
65	143		2,750	2,500	2,100
70	154		2,900	2,600	2,200
75	165		3,050	2,750	2,300
80	176		3,200	2,900	2,450
85	187		3,350	3,050	2,550
		Women	(4)	(5)	(6)
40	88		1,600	1,450	1,200
45	99		1,750	1,600	1,300
50	110		1,900	1,700	1,450
55	121		2,000	1,800	1,550
58	128		2,100	1,900	1,600
60	132		2,150	1,950	1,650
65	143		2,300	2,050	1,750
70	154		2,400	2,200	1,850

*National Research Council: Recommended Dietary Allowances. Pub. 1146. Washington, D. C., 1964.

The ingestion of food increases the metabolic rate. It was demonstrated that a fasting man had a metabolism averaging 9 per cent lower than that on the days when food was consumed. However, metabolism goes on during fasting, showing that the body must continue metabolizing even though the tissues are called on to make up the deficit. This explains the loss of weight and wasting in severe illness and starvation.

With prolonged fasting and subsequent loss of weight, the body tends to adjust itself by lowering the metabolic rate. This is comparable with setting back a thermostat so that the organism runs at a lower rate. This adjustment is true of adults, but children who are undernourished may have a higher rate, which makes undernutrition in children even more serious than in adults. So far there is no satisfactory explanation of this difference.

Specific Dynamic Action of Protein. Not all kinds of food are oxidized with an equal effect on metabolism. Protein stimulates metabolism, so that a greater amount of heat is produced in its metabolism than in that of similar quantities of fats and carbohyrates. This effect is commonly known as the specific dynamic action of protein. Carbohydrates and fats have a much less marked effect, but the slight stimulation that results from the intake of food of any type accounts for the fact that metabolism tests usually are taken before breakfast when no food has been eaten for at least 12 hours. For a person on an average diet the specific dynamic action of food may account for a rise of about 10 per cent above the basal.

Climate, season, housing and clothing affect metabolism, chiefly through their bearing upon the regulation of body temperature. The heat produced in the body by metabolic processes must be conserved or given off in such a way as to maintain the body temperature at a remarkably constant figure. If no heat were lost from the body during average daily activity, the temperature would rise about 2° F. an hour. In winter we purposely curtail our heat loss from the body by wearing heavier clothing and living in heated houses; in summer we wear thinner clothing to expedite greater losses. However, nature has provided for a carefully controlled loss of heat that may vary as climate and environment dictate. A thinly clothed person on a cold winter day may shiver. This process is a series of rapid muscular contractions set up involuntarily in the body to increase heat production in order to make up for the rapid heat loss. Evaporation of perspiration from the skin is a mechanism employed by the body to reduce temperature. Insensible perspiration is evaporating continuously with a slight loss of heat, but sensible perspiration means greater heat loss and affords a welcome cooling effect when the body is overheated in warm weather or after strenuous exercise.

As part of this mechanism for regulating body temperature the total metabolism may vary with the environmental temperature. FAO[9] recommends a 5 per cent decrease in calories for each 10° C. rise, and a 3 per cent increase for each 10° C. drop in environmental temperature from a mean of 10° C. One exception to the rule, reported by Consolazio *et al.*,[10] concerns men working in extreme heat, where the body temperature may rise. In these cases the energy expenditure for any given task was greater than at a moderate temperature.

Although essential nutrients should be considered in the selection of an adequate diet, it must be remembered that the caloric value is fundamentally one of the most important points. "No supplements of [amino acids], vitamins or mineral elements can alter the laws of the conservation of energy. Calories are still needed . . . to furnish energy for muscular work"[11] and maintain body functions.

When emergencies arise in war or famine, it is total calories which must be provided first to keep people alive and satisfied. The quality and the nature of the calories can be adjusted later to meet specific needs.

___

9 Calorie Requirements. Nutritional Studies, No. 15. FAO, Rome, 1957.

10 Consolazio, C. F., *et al.*: J. Nutrition, 73:126, 1961.

11 DuBois, E. F., and Chambers, W. H.: J.A.M.A., *119*:1183, 1942.

STUDY QUESTIONS

1. Explain the use of the word *metabolism* in the expressions "energy metabolism" and "protein metabolism."

2. What is the unit of measure for energy and how is food energy measured? Define it specifically.

3. What are the so-called physiologic fuel values? How can they be used to estimate food values?

4. Milk has the percentage composition of 3.5 Gm. of protein, 4 Gm. of fat and 5 Gm. of carbohydrate per 100 Gm. Calculate the caloric value of a glass of milk weighing 240 Gm.

5. What is measured in a basal metabolism test? Under what conditions must the test be performed? Name the factors that affect the basal metabolic needs of any given individual.

6. What is the largest single factor affecting the total energy requirements? List other factors that play a part in the total calories needed.

7. Calculate the energy requirement of a moderately active 60-Kg. (132 lb.) nurse by the quick method of allowing 24 calories per Kg. of body weight for basal needs plus 50 per cent for activity. Now use Table 5–1 and calculate her energy needs more carefully. Compare the figures. Is the quick method reasonably accurate?

8. How long will it take a nurse weighing 130 pounds to walk off (at 3 mph) a ¾ c. serving of ice cream (207 calories)?

9. The basal metabolism of a man of average size is about 1,650 calories per day; of a woman of average size, about 1,350 calories. If the measured basal metabolism for such a person were 12 per cent below average (−12), how many calories per day would each be expending under basal conditions?

10. When there are acute food shortages, which should relief agencies supplying a minimum of food to relieve starvation consider first—calories, protein or vitamins?

SUPPLEMENTARY READING ON CALORIE REQUIREMENTS AND ENERGY METABOLISM

Consolazio, C. F., *et al.*: Energy requirements of men in extreme heat. J. Nutrition, *73*: 126, 1961.

Konishi, F.: Food Energy Equivalents of Various activities. J. Am. Dietet. A., *46*:186, 1965.

Moore, M. E., Pond, J., and Korsluad, M. K.: Energy expenditure of pre-adolescent girls. J. Am. Dietet. A., *49*:409, 1966.

Review: Food intake and energy expenditure. Nutr. Rev., *14*:48, 1956.

———: Variability in Basal Metabolic Rate (book). Nutr. Rev., *25*:12, 1967.

———: Variability in caloric intakes. Nutr. Rev., *24*:39, 1966.

Whedon, G. D.: New research in human energy metabolism. J. Am. Dietet. A., *35*: 682, 1959.

For further references see Bibliography in Part Four.

CHAPTER 6

Water and Mineral Metabolism

Water in Relation to Body Function • Water Intake and Output • Electrolytes and Non-electrolytes • Acid-Base Balance • Vital Minerals and Their Distribution • Mineral Content of Foods • Calcium and Phosphorus • Iron • Sodium and other Mineral Elements • Trace Elements or Micronutrients

FLUIDS AND ELECTROLYTES

Water in Relation to Body Function

Water is more essential to life than is food, for a person may live weeks without food but only days without water. It is an essential component of blood, lymph, the secretions of the body (extracellular fluid) and of every cell in the body (intracellular). About half the adult weight is water, 60 per cent for men, 54 per cent for women. The internal environment of the body is bathed in fluids (which contain certain electrolytes) held in compartments of the body (extracellular and intracellular spaces) divided by semipermeable membranes. The extracellular compartment (the space outside the cell membrane) accounts for ⅓ of the body water and includes the fluid in plasma and in interstitial spaces; intracellular fluid contains ⅔ of the body water.

Fluid is necessary for the functioning of every organ in the body. It is the universal medium in which the various chemical changes of the body take place. As a carrier it aids in digestion, absorption, circulation and excretion; it is essential in the regulation of body temperature; it plays an important part in mechanical functions, such as the lubrication of joints and the movement of the viscera in the abdominal cavity. Waste products from the tissues are transferred to the blood in watery solutions; they are carried by the blood, which is about 80 per cent water; and they are excreted via the kidneys in the urine, which is about 97 per cent water (Fig. 6–1).

The same water is reused many times and for different purposes. Approximately 8 liters of digestive juices are produced and secreted by the glands in 24 hours (see Chap. 9). The water that carries the enzymes into the digestive tract is used during absorption to carry the digested nutrients into the blood and lymph. Over 4 liters of water are always circulating in the blood stream. Water is the carrier of nutrients throughout the body. It is estimated that some 50 liters of water cross cell membranes in a day. In the kidney large volumes of water carry the dissolved waste material through the capsule of the uriniferous tubules, but, in passing through the tubules, most of the water, with some of its useful dissolved material, is reabsorbed. The urine which is excreted is the concentrated aqueous solution of the waste products.

Water Intake and Output

Water normally is lost from the body by four routes: from the skin, as sensible and insensible perspiration; from the lungs, as water vapor in the expired air; from the kidneys, as urine; and from the intestines, in the feces. A minimum of 800 ml. of water is lost daily through the skin and lungs, and this amount may increase in hot, dry environments. The kidney eliminates approximately 1,000 to 1,500 ml. of water in the urine; fecal losses approximate 200 ml. daily but increase greatly when diarrhea occurs. Large water losses also result from excessive perspiration due to fever, vomiting, burns or hemorrhage (see Fig. 6–2).

Fluids are replaced by the ingestion of liquids and foods containing water. Although some water (14 ml. per 100 calories) is formed within the body as an end product of food metabolism, from 4 to 6 cups (1-1½ liters) of water or other liquids should be consumed daily in order to ensure a sufficient amount of water for body functions. Many foods contain a high percentage of water (Fig. 6–3) and may provide as much as 1 liter a day. Once ingested, water is absorbed rapidly from the digestive tract into the blood and lymph, although enough water is retained with food residues in the colon to produce a soft stool.

Homeostasis—Water Balance. Water balance is carefully regulated within the body and normally a balance between intake and output is maintained, provided that there is free access to water. Thus the weight of a man varies by approximately only ⅓ pound in a 24-hour period.

When water losses are increased owing to excessive sweating or diarrhea, for example, the kidneys conserve water by making less urine. This action of the kidneys is under the control of the pituitary antidiuretic hormone (ADH), which stimulates the renal tubules to increase the reabsorption of water.

Excessive loss of water results in sensations of extreme thirst. The mechanisms for stimulating thirst are located in the hypothalamus and are activated by an increase in the solute concentration in body fluid. Thirst is a sensation of dryness at the root of the tongue and the back part of the throat and is Nature's signal that liquid intake must be increased.

Dehydration. Dehydration may be fatal, a fact that further emphasizes the importance of water in the body. The German physiologist Rubner stated that we can lose all our reserve glycogen, all reserve fat and about one half of the body protein without great danger, but that a loss of 10 per cent of the body water is serious and from 20 to 22 per cent loss is fatal.

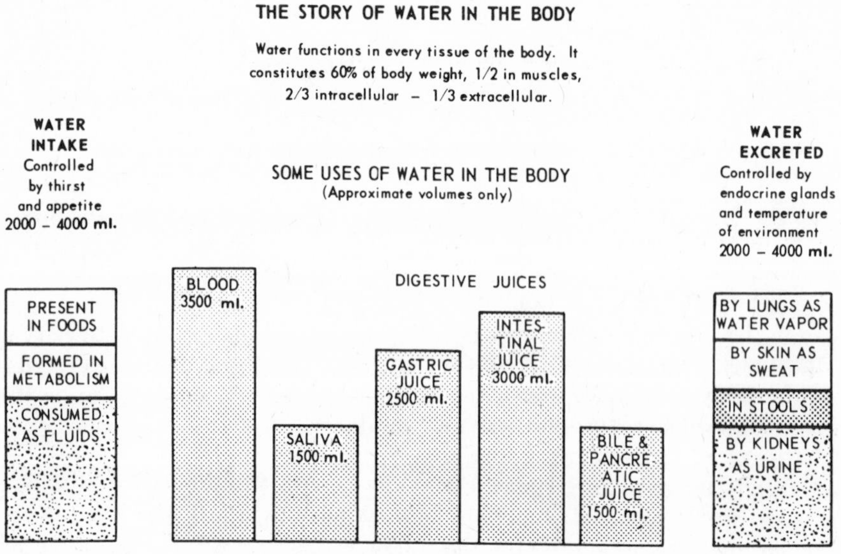

THE STORY OF WATER IN THE BODY

Water functions in every tissue of the body. It constitutes 60% of body weight, 1/2 in muscles, 2/3 intracellular – 1/3 extracellular.

WATER INTAKE
Controlled by thirst and appetite
2000 – 4000 ml.

SOME USES OF WATER IN THE BODY
(Approximate volumes only)

WATER EXCRETED
Controlled by endocrine glands and temperature of environment
2000 – 4000 ml.

PRESENT IN FOODS

FORMED IN METABOLISM

CONSUMED AS FLUIDS

BLOOD 3500 ml.

SALIVA 1500 ml.

GASTRIC JUICE 2500 ml.

DIGESTIVE JUICES

INTESTINAL JUICE 3000 ml.

BILE & PANCREATIC JUICE 1500 ml.

BY LUNGS AS WATER VAPOR

BY SKIN AS SWEAT

IN STOOLS

BY KIDNEYS AS URINE

FIGURE 6-1

The term dehydration implies more than change in water balance—there are always accompanying changes in electrolyte balance. When the water supply is restricted or when losses are excessive, the rate of water loss exceeds the rate of electrolyte loss. The extracellular fluid becomes concentrated, and osmotic pressure draws water from the cells into the extracellular fluid to compensate. This condition is called intracellular dehydration and is accompanied by extreme thirst and nausea. This is only one example of the 17 specific imbalances of the body fluids that are recognized at present, according to Snively.[1]

The tremendous nutritional and physiologic importance of water is easy to demonstrate.[2] To evaluate the relative effect of water and carbohydrate supplements on work performance, six dogs were run to exhaustion on a treadmill. When they ran without food or water supplement 17 hours after the last meal, they were able to expend an average of 1,190 calories. With a carbohydrate supplement without water they could expend 1,300 calories. When allowed to drink while running, each dog consumed 1.5 liters of water during the run and increased his endurance until he expended 2,140 calories. The reviewer also noted that Sir Edmund Hillary, the first

[1] Snively, W. D., Jr., Sea Within. p. 55. Philadelphia, Lippincott, 1960.

[2] Review: Nutr. Rev., *19*:23, 1961.

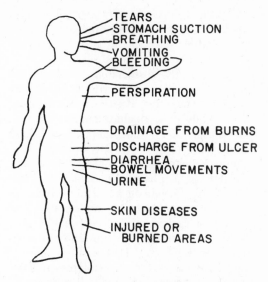

FIG. 6-2. Ways in which water and electrolytes may be lost. (Snively, W. D.: Sea Within. Philadelphia, J. B. Lippincott, 1960)

person to climb Mt. Everest, attributed the success of his expedition during the last few days of the ascent to an adequate supply of water which other expeditions had lacked.

Electrolytes and Non-electrolytes

Chemical compounds that dissociate in water, breaking up into separate particles called ions, are known as electrolytes, and the process is referred to as ionization.

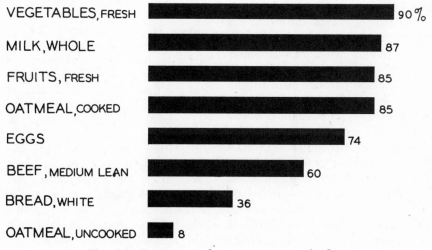

FIG. 6-3. Percentage of water in common foods.

Salts, acids and bases are electrolytes; compounds such as glucose, urea and protein are called non-electrolytes because they are molecules that do not ionize.

Each ion, the dissociated particle of an electrolyte, carries an electric charge, either positive or negative. Positive ions (cations) in the body fluids include sodium (Na^+), potassium (K^+), calcium (Ca^{++}), and magnesium (Mg^{++}). The negative ions (anions) include chloride (Cl^-), bicarbonate (HCO_3^-), phosphate (HPO_4^{--}), sulfate (SO_4^{--}), ions of inorganic acids such as lactate, pyruvate, aceto-acetate, and many protein derivatives. Electrical balance is always maintained in the fluid compartments of the body. To measure the total combining power of electrolytes in solution, a unit of measure related to the number of electrical charges carried by the ions present in solution must be used. This unit is referred to as milliequivalents (mEq.). The cations and anions in each fluid compartment of the body, as measured in milliequivalents, are equal.

Electrolyte Composition of the Body Fluids. Sodium is the major cation in plasma and interstitial fluid and chloride is the major anion. The major cation in intracellular fluid is potassium and the major anion is phosphate. Other ions are present in varying amounts in the different body fluids. Specific functions of these minerals will be discussed later in this chapter.

Osmotic Pressure. As previously stated, the fluid compartments of the body are separated by semipermeable membranes. These permit free exchange of water molecules but partially or completely prevent passage of dissolved particles such as glucose or electrolytes. If there is a solution containing a relatively large number of dissolved particles on one side of a semipermeable membrane and a solution containing a relatively small number of dissolved particles on the other, the force of osmosis is brought into play. Osmotic pressure causes water to pass across the semipermeable membrane from the less concentrated to the more concentrated solution, until the concentration of dissolved particles on both sides is equal.

Hence, exchanges of water between the various fluid compartments of the body occur as a result of osmotic pressure, which, in turn, is due chiefly to the concentration of electrolytes. Osmotic pressure in the cellular fluid is regulated mainly by the concentration of potassium and in the extracellular fluid by the concentration of sodium. If there is a loss or gain in either of these electrolytes in one compartment, the osmotic pressure is disturbed, and an increased amount of water will then be found in the compartment of greater osmotic pressure.

Plasma protein also plays an important role in maintaining osmotic equilibrium in the extracellular compartments. By remaining in the plasma it tends to prevent the leakage of water into the interstitial spaces, where an excess of extracellular fluid is known as edema.

Excess water losses may also result in excess loss of electrolytes. These are not always replaced through water intake, in which case serious problems may result. Moreover, as already noted, intracellular dehydration results when the rate of water loss from the body is greater than the rate of electrolyte loss.

Acid-Base Balance

Electrolytes play an important part in maintaining the acid-base balance in the blood and throughout the tissues. The maintenance of this balance is a function of normal metabolism. The reaction of the blood is slightly alkaline (pH 7.3-7.45), varying only within narrow limits, regardless of the amount of acid products formed in metabolism. This equilibrium is maintained by a series of buffers in the blood and the tissue fluids. These buffers, which have a tendency to resist changes in their pH when treated with strong acids or bases, contain a weak acid or base and a salt of this acid or base. They have been likened to a chemical sponge in that they can soak up or release anions or cations as needed to maintain the normal pH. The principal buffers in the regulation of acid-base balance are the bicarbonate-carbonic acid system, the phosphate system, the hemoglobin-oxyhemoglobin system and the proteins.

Acid products formed in metabolism are disposed of through either the lungs or the kidneys. The respiratory mechanism reacts quickly but the renal system adapts itself over longer periods of time. The respiratory system controls the removal from the blood of CO_2 and can either increase or decrease its loss by regulating the depth and rate of respiration. The kidneys, however, remove hydrogen ions from the body by excreting acids and, at the same time, return bicarbonate to the blood. This accounts for the urine having a more acid reaction (pH 5.5-6.6) than the plasma. The reaction of the urine may vary widely in a normal individual because the amount of acid or base end-products of metabolism will vary and the excess must be eliminated.

When the supply of buffer susbtances becomes depleted due to starvation or inability to metabolize food properly, a condition known as acidosis may result. Actually, the blood does not become acid, but the term *acidosis* is used to indicate the lowered alkaline reserve which results when the basic elements are used up faster than they are replenished. This may happen in severe diabetes, when the organic acids from faulty fat metabolism accumulate.

Alkalosis is the opposite of acidosis. This may occur when severe vomiting over a period of time causes a great loss of hydrochloric acid. The body quickly adjusts when the acute condition is relieved.

Acid-Base Reaction of Foods. Conclusive evidence is not as yet available in regard to the practical importance of the acid-base balance of foods in relation to health. Experience and scientific evidence indicate a wide range of adaptability on the part of the human body and do not support the "scare" propaganda with which certain food faddists promote the sale of "alkalizing" compounds to prevent acidosis.

The usual mixed diet contains a good balance of acid and basic factors. The basic elements, sodium, potassium, magnesium and calcium may occur as salts of inorganic acids, such as phosphates, sulfates, or chlorides, or organic acids. The mineral elements are sometimes referred to as "ash" because they do not "burn" up. When foods are metabolized in the body, the mineral elements are released to func-

tion in maintaining the acid-base balance; the organic acids are mostly oxidized to carbon dioxide and water. Foods are said to be acid or basic according to whether the acid or the basic elements in the ash predominate. Most fruits contain organic acids combined with basic inorganic elements. When such compounds are oxidized in the body, they leave an alkaline ash. Some other foods, such as cereals and meats, not at all acid in taste, yield end products that are strongly acid. Thus, by potential acidity or alkalinity of foods is meant the reaction that they will ultimately yield after being oxidized in the body.

Some workers have attempted to establish quantitative figures for the excess of acid or basic elements in foods, but the significance of these figures now is questioned; therefore, they have been omitted. A simple classification will be found in Table 8, Part Four.

MINERALS
Vital Minerals and Their Distribution

Although mineral elements constitute but a small proportion (4%) of the body tissue, they are essential both as structural components and in many vital processes. Some form hard tissues such as bones and teeth; some are in the fluids and soft tissues. For some functions it is the balance of mineral ions that is important—for example, in bone formation, the amount and the ratio of calcium and phosphorus; for normal muscular activity, the ratio between potassium and calcium in the extracellular fluid. Electrolytes, of which sodium and potassium salts are the most important, are the major factors in the osmotic control of water metabolism as discussed earlier in this chapter. Other minerals may act as catalysts, in enzyme systems, or as integral parts of organic compounds in the body, such as iron in hemoglobin, iodine in thyroxine, cobalt in vitamin B_{12}, zinc in insulin and sulfur in thiamine and biotin.

Plant life and animals, as well as bacteria and other one-celled organisms, all require proper concentrations of certain minerals to make life possible. In fact, changes in concentration of minerals, small in themselves, can be fatal to various forms of life.

TABLE 6–1. Mineral Composition of
an Adult Human Body

Element	Per Cent of Total Ash	Gm./70 Kg. Man
Calcium (Ca).............	39	1,160
Phosphorus (P)...........	22	670
Potassium (K)............	5	150
Sulfur (S)...............	4	112
Chlorine (Cl)............	3	85
Sodium (Na).............	2	63
Magnesium (Mg).........	0.7	21
Iron (Fe)................	.15	4.5
Iodine (I)...............	.0007	.02

Thus, common salt, which in dilute solution is necessary for most forms of animal life, becomes a preservative when foods are salted or kept in brine because the concentration kills bacteria. On the other hand, marine forms (fish and shellfish) quickly die when subjected to fresh water. In the human body also, the maintenance of a normal concentration of minerals in body fluids is essential.

The principal minerals which the body requires are calcium, phosphorus, potassium, chlorine, sodium, sulfur, magnesium, iron and iodine. These elements are present in the body in amounts as given in Table 6–1. Several minerals are used by animals in trace quantities and are sometimes called micronutrients; these are copper, manganese, cobalt, zinc, fluorine, molybdenum, selenium and chromium. Aluminum, arsenic, boron, cadmium and silicon also are present as trace elements in animal tissue, but their function is uncertain.

Mineral Content of Foods

In unrefined foods, minerals are present in various forms mixed or combined with proteins, fats and carbohydrates. Processed or refined foods, such as fats, oils, sugar and cornstarch, contain almost no minerals. The total mineral content of a food is determined by burning the organic or combustible part of a known amount of a food and weighing the resulting ash. The ash then is analyzed for individual mineral elements. Most foods have been analyzed for 10 or more mineral elements, but in dietary practice the figures most commonly used are those for calcium, phosphorus and iron and, for therapeutic purposes, sodium, potassium and magnesium (Tables 1 and 5, Part Four).

Minerals such as iodine, copper and other trace elements which are essential for life may be found abundantly in drinking water in certain areas or in foods grown in the soil of those areas, whereas in other parts of the country they are deficient in both soil and water. Still other mineral elements, such as sodium, potassium, chlorine, sulfur and magnesium—all necessary in human nutrition—are so universally present in foods that we recognize no need to worry about deficiencies.

The question of relative availability of mineral elements for physiologic processes continues to stimulate new investigations in this field. Fifty or more years ago, the opinion prevailed that the organic forms of minerals found in plant and animal foods were better utilized than the inorganic. However, modern research has disproved this theory. Today we are aware that many minerals occur in inorganic form in natural foods and, as such, are absorbed from the digestive tract without change.

Calcium and Phosphorus
Functions of Calcium and Phosphorus

Structures of Bones and Teeth. The adult human body contains approximately 2 per cent of calcium and 1 per cent of phosphorus. Ninety-nine per cent of the calcium and 75 per cent of the phosphorus in our bodies are found as constituents of bone and teeth, giving to them strength and rigidity.

Bone is made up of very small crystals, containing chiefly calcium phosphates and also small amounts of carbonates, magnesium, sodium and fluorine, which are set in the protein network or matrix. It contains blood and lymph vessels, nerves and bone marrow. The nutrients needed for bone metabolism pass from the blood vessels into the interstitial fluid that surrounds the crystals, so that exchanges between the tissues and the blood are easily accomplished.

Bone is constantly being synthesized and broken down. In children, bone synthesis —the formation of new bone—is greater than the destruction or resorption of bone; on the other hand, the skeletal changes frequently observed in old age occur when bone resorption dominates and there is a decrease in the absolute amount of bone (osteoporosis). In the normal adult the two processes are equally balanced, with both the mineralization (incorporation of calcium in bone) and the demineralization (resorption of calcium) being dependent on a normal functioning of the matrix cells.

Hormones control these processes. The parathyroid hormone controls the resorption of calcium from bone, and recently a thyroid hormone—thyrocalcitonin—that prohibits release of calcium from bone has been identified.

Bone, like other tissue, is in a state of dynamic equilibrium with the constituents of the plasma and other tissue. Calcium and phosphorus, when the food supply is abundant, can be stored in the trabeculae at the ends of the bones. From this storehouse these minerals are readily available to meet the needs of other tissues of the body when the dietary intake of calcium or

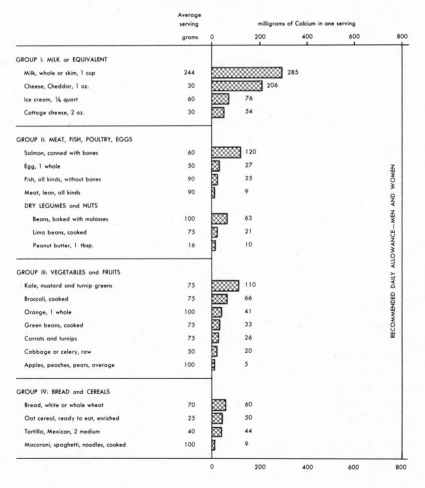

FIGURE 6-4

phosphorus is inadequate. However, if calcium has not been stored in the trabeculae, calcium will be withdrawn from bone structure itself. Prolonged removal of calcium from bone naturally results in bones more easily bent or broken. When calcium phosphate is removed from bone, the remaining tissue is as flexible as cartilage; in fact, it is essentially the same as cartilage. Cartilage precedes bone in the development of the fetus and the young animal, and normally the calcium phosphate is deposited in it as growth and strain demand. When nature's plan is thwarted by an inadequate supply of these minerals in food, or by an inability to utilize them, growth may be retarded, or, as more often happens, growth in size continues, but the new bone is abnormal in structure and poorly calcified. This may result in the bowed legs, enlarged ankles and wrists, prolapsed thorax and other bone deformities characteristic of rickets.

Tooth structures, particularly the dentine and enamel, are metabolically more stable than the bones. There is little turnover of calcium from the teeth.

Functions in Serum and Soft Tissues. When compared with the amounts in bones and teeth the concentrations of calcium and phosphorus in the blood are small, but their presence in normal amounts is essential for body function. Although they are often associated because they function together in the skeletal structures, elsewhere in the body their functions are quite distinct. A normal calcium level in the blood is necessary for blood clot formation, because it acts as a catalyst in the conversion of prothrombin to thrombin. Calcium has a vital role in maintaining muscle tone and irritability; it is required for normal nerve transmission; it is an activator of several enzymes; and it influences the permeability of cell membranes. The neuromuscular hyperirritability characteristic of tetany occurs when the blood calcium level falls below normal.

Phosphorus is a necessary constituent of every cell in the body. It is part of the nucleic acids DNA (deoxyribonucleic acid) and RNA (ribonucleic acid) which determine the genetic code (see Chap. 9).

Phosphorus is part of the ATP (adenosine triphosphate)-ADP (adenosine diphosphate) energy-transporting systems in the cells (see Chap. 9) and is also a component of the phospholipids which are involved in the emulsification and transport of fats and fatty acids. Phosphates, as previously mentioned, also assist in maintaining the acid-base balance of the blood.

Food Sources of Calcium and Phosphorus

It is apparent in Figure 6–4 that milk and milk products are the most important sources of calcium in readily available form. A few of the green, leafy vegetables used commonly in the Southern states are good sources of calcium, but others such as spinach, chard, beet greens and rhubarb contain sufficient oxalic acid to form insoluble calcium oxalate, thus rendering the calcium unavailable. In most sections of the country greens are not used regularly enough or in sufficient quantity to be relied upon to replace milk, but they are important when milk is scarce or unobtainable. Meats and poultry are poor sources of calcium. Cereal products contribute little, except where breads are enriched with calcium or are made with a high percentage of milk solids. The pattern dietary of 1,400 calories provides almost the recommended allowance of 800 mg. (0.8 Gm.), which will be supplemented by the calcium of the foods added to make up the needed calories (see Table 6–3 and Chap. 10).

Phosphorus is more widely distributed than calcium and less likely to be deficient in the average diet. Poultry, fish, meats, cereals, nuts and legumes, as well as milk and milk products, are all good sources. In the cooking of vegetables, there may be slight losses of calcium and phosphorus, especially if the cooking water is discarded.

Factors Affecting Absorption and Retention

All of the calcium and phosphorus in foods is not available to the body. Approximately 20 to 40 per cent of the calcium and 70 per cent of the phosphorus consumed by an individual is absorbed from the intestinal tract into the blood stream to become available. The amounts absorbed, however, may be greatly increased during periods of rapid growth when mineral needs are high. Individuals on limited intakes of calcium also are more efficient in their utilization than those on more liberal intakes. These factors help explain the following statement from the World Health Organization's report on Calcium Requirements. "In general, children and adults in most countries can grow normally and live healthily on a daily calcium intake between 300 mg. and 1000 mg. or, in the absence of nutritional disorders and if their vitamin D status is adequate, on even somewhat lower or higher intakes."[3]

Various factors, in addition to need, influence the efficiency of calcium and phosphorus absorption. Adequate amounts of vitamin D, an acid pH in the upper part of the intestinal tract, and a normal motility of the gastrointestinal tract enhance the absorption of these minerals. On the other hand, large amounts of fats, phytates (phosphorus compounds found in cereals) or oxalates which can form insoluble compounds with calcium may interfere with intestinal absorption.

In cases of parathyroid disturbances variations in calcium absorption and retention are even greater than under normal conditions. Hypercalcemia (high serum calcium) may occur in hyperparathyroidism, and hypocalcemia (serum calcium below normal) may result after operative removal of the parathyroid glands.

Dietary Requirements

The dietary requirements of calcium and phosphorus for children and adults have been investigated extensively. There is not, however, universal agreement among the experts on the interpretation of the findings.

The problem of balance studies to determine calcium and phosphorus requirements is complicated. As already mentioned, there are many factors which affect the amount of calcium absorbed and retained by the body. A person is said to be in equilibrium with respect to any nutrient if the intake approximately equals the output. The as-

TABLE 6–2. Bases for Calculating the Adult Recommended Dietary Allowance for Calcium*

Urinary calcium excretion	175 mg./day
Endogenous fecal calcium excretion	125 mg./day
Loss of calcium in sweat	20 mg./day
Total calcium losses	320 mg./day
Calcium absorbed from food	40 per cent

$$\frac{320}{x} \times \frac{100}{40} = 800 \text{ mg./day}$$

Recommended dietary allowance for adult	800 mg./day

*Figures from Recommended Dietary Allowances. National Academy of Sciences/National Research Council Publ. No. 1146. Washington, D. C., 1964.

sumption that end products of metabolism appear in the urine and unabsorbed material in the feces does not hold for calcium and phosphorus. Some metabolized (endogenous) calcium and phosphorus may be excreted via the intestinal tract. Moreover, the evidence that man can maintain calcium balance over a wide range of calcium intakes (the amount required to maintain this balance is largely determined by past dietary history) has caused one authority to question the use of balance studies to estimate calcium requirements.[4]

The Recommended Dietary Allowances (as revised in 1964) give 0.8 Gm. (800 mg.) per day as adequate for adults, with an additional 0.5 Gm. recommended for the second and third trimesters of pregnancy and during lactation. The bases for calculating the adult requirement are given in Table 6–2. The same allowance is recommended for women, despite their smaller average size, as for men, to ensure ample stores in preparation for maternity.

Special attention should be given to the calcuim intake of older people, especially women, because of their tendency commonly to decrease their intake when there may be even an increased need. For this group, a population at high risk for development of osteoporosis, the RDA of 800 mg. may allow little margin of safety. The occurrence of osteoporosis in elderly people is discused in Chapter 32.

[3] FAO/WHO Expert Committee on Calcium Requirements: WHO Chronicle, *16*:251, 1962.

[4] Hegsted, D. M.. J.A.M.A., *185*:588, 1963.

Some scientists consider that the Recommended Dietary Allowances for calcium are higher than necessary for health. Hegsted[5] comments that the allowances other than those for lactating women "appear to be far out of line with the evidence available and with everyday experience." More recently the FAO/WHO Expert Committee on Calcium Requirements[6] came to the conclusion, after evaluating surveys from several countries, that calcium deficiencies in man were not common and adults could adapt to a "suggested practical allowance" of 0.4 to 0.5 Gm. of calcium per day when necessary, but this level is not recommended as optimal.

The calcium and phosphorus requirements for growth have been investigated in children of different ages by observing the level of intake at which maximum retention of calcium and phosphorus is attained. Growth of bone requires the storage of new calcium and phosphorus as well as replacement. The growth requirement varies with age, being highest in relation to weight in the infant, lower and fairly constant after the first year and until puberty, when there is a rise again during the period of rapid growth. The recommended allowances of calcium for children take into account the different ages and sex needs. Calcium is the only nutrient listed for which the allowance per day for children of all ages is as great as it is for adults.

A careful selection of foodstuffs rich in calcium and phosphorus is necessary to meet these needs. For infants, the intake requirements may well be stated in terms of the amount of milk, since this is the chief food source. For older children, the requirements for calcium and phosphorus are most easily met by including a quart of milk a day or its equivalent in milk products. The calcium and the phosphorus content of milk is not only high but in good proportion, and these factors are more readily available from milk than from most other foods. During all periods of growth

vitamin D, or sunshine, is essential for the most efficient absorption and utilization of these two minerals. Compare this with the story of vitamin D in Chapter 7.

In the Recommended Dietary Allowances no figures are given for phosphorus because dietary deficiencies of phosphorus are uncommon when diets are adequate in calcium and protein. In general, the phosphorus allowance should be at least equal to the calcium allowance, especially for children and for women during the latter part of pregnancy and during lactation.

Iron

There is less than 5 Gm. of iron in the body of a normal healthy adult, but its importance to our well-being is strikingly out of proportion to the quantitative figure. Sixty to 70 per cent of the iron in the body is found in hemoglobin; iron stores in the liver, spleen, and bone marrow account for the next largest concentration of iron (30-35 per cent). Small but essential amounts of iron are found in muscle myoglobin; in transport form (bound to protein-transferrin) in the blood serum; and in every cell as a constituent of certain enzymes and chromatin (colored) materials.

Functions of Iron

Hemoglobin Synthesis. Iron is a necessary constituent of hemoglobin, the coloring matter of the red blood cells, and as such is vital to the processes of nutrition. Hemoglobin is a compound composed of the protein, globin, and the iron-containing pigment, heme. The heme is responsible for the characteristic color and oxygen-carrying capacity of blood. Hemoglobin combines with oxygen in the lung capillaries to form oxyhemoglobin, which travels in the blood stream to the tissues where the oxygen is released to take part in oxidative processes. Part of the carbon dioxide formed is carried back by the same hemoglobin, which drops its load in the lungs and starts out with a new supply of oxygen. Hemoglobin values below 12 to 14 Gm./100 ml. of blood are considered low.

The synthesis of hemoglobin proceeds concomitantly with the maturation of the red blood cell in the bone marrow, and lasts the

---

[5] Hegsted, D. M.: Nutr. Rev., *15*:257, 1957.

[6] FAO/WHO Expert Committee on Calcium Requirements: WHO Chronicle, *16*:251, 1962 (July).

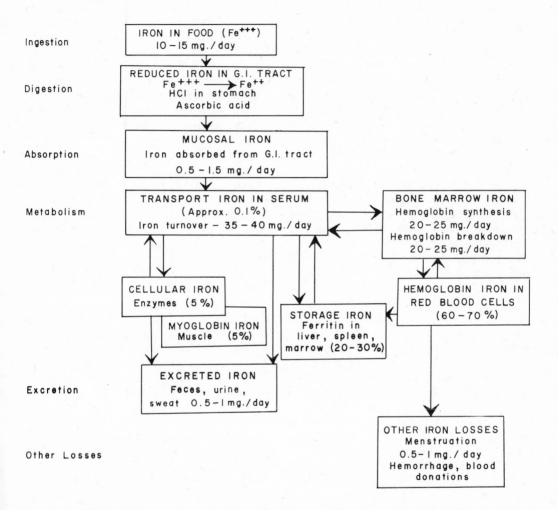

Fig. 6-5. Schematic diagram of iron pathways in the body. Figures in parentheses indicate approximate per cent of total body iron in each compartment. Average amounts of iron consumed, absorbed, turned over in the body and excreted per day are also included.

"lifetime" of the cell—120 days. When the cell is disintegrated, the hemoglobin molecule is again split into its components, the iron-compound heme undergoing certain changes which make the iron available for reuse. Hence, the iron of our bodies is used very efficiently and normally is not used up or destroyed but is conserved and utilized again and again. Small amounts of unabsorbed iron may be lost in the stools, a very small quantity is excreted in the urine, and traces may be lost through the skin in perspiration. Loss of blood due to hemorrhage, menstruation, or blood donations is responsible for the major losses of iron from the body.

Hemoglobin synthesis depends on the presence of copper. The discovery of the catalytic action of copper in the use of iron for elaboration of hemoglobin was dramatic because it was the first proof of the function of one inorganic element in the utilization of another; copper is not present in the hemoglobin molecule. Adequate protein must also be available for synthesis of the complex compound hemoglobin. Other dietary essentials, especially certain vitamins, seem to aid in this process, according to Leverton,[7] who demonstrated that young women could maintain their hemoglogin level on less iron if all the other essentials were present in the diet.

Myoglobin. Myoglobin, found only in the muscle tissue, is related to blood hemoglobin in both structure and function. It is an oxygen-carrier capable of supplying oxygen to the muscles and removing carbon dioxide.

Cellular Iron. As part of the various enzymes that catalyze oxidation-reduction processes in the cell, iron has an important role in tissue respiration.

Iron Transport and Storage

All of the iron in the plasma is transport iron. It is absorbed from the intestinal mucosa into the blood stream, where it is bound to transferrin, a protein compound, which transports iron to the bone marrow for hemoglobin synthesis, to the liver or spleen for storage or to other tissues for

[7] Leverton, R. M., and Marsh, A. G.: J. Nutrition, 23:229, 1942.

their use. Normally, two thirds of the transferrin (or iron-binding capacity of the blood) is bound to iron. In iron deficiency or when there are increased demands for iron (as in pregnancy), the iron-binding capacity increases in an attempt to trap more iron for the body. On the other hand, in hemochromatosis (abnormal amounts of iron deposited in tissue) the iron binding capacity is drastically reduced. Hence, the measurement of serum iron and the iron-binding capacity of the blood is another method used to determine the iron status of individuals.

Iron is stored as ferritin in the liver, spleen, intestinal mucosa, and in all reticulo-endothelial cells (connective tissue cells which ingest solid particles). When iron is deposited in abnormally large amounts, such as in iron-loading or excessive blood transfusions, hemosiderin, a compound similar to ferritin but containing more iron, is formed. The stores of iron, as well as the iron released from the disintegration of the red blood cells, are available to the body for hemoglobin synthesis. Hence, the iron actually used daily by an individual far exceeds that supplied by the dietary intake for the same period. Figure 6–5 illustrates the various pathways of iron in the body.

Food Sources of Iron

The best food sources of iron are found in the meat, fish, poultry and egg group. The green, leafy vegetables, potatoes, dried fruits and enriched bread and cereal products are the best plant sources. Milk and milk products are conspicuously low in iron (Fig. 6–6). Foods such as molasses and raisins, popularly featured as good sources of iron, are rich on a percentage basis, but small servings of these foods used infrequently do not constitute as important a source of food iron as some staple foods, such as whole-grain or enriched breads and cereals. The iron content of all common foods is given in Table 1, Part Four. Note that foods poor in iron have a noticeable lack of pigment, which is significant, since iron salts are all colored and usually lend color to a food rich in this element. Compare, for instance, egg yolk with egg white, molasses with white sugar, whole with milled grains, and spinach with celery. With a few exceptions, such as the potato and enriched white bread, it may be helpful to remember that white foods are not good builders of red blood.

The basic dietary of 1,400 calories provides 10.4 mg. of iron. Additional foods to supply extra calories would be necessary to bring this total up to the recommended level of 15 mg. for the adult female (See Table 6–3 and Chap. 10).

Factors Affecting Iron Absorption

As was the case with calcium and phosphorus, not all the iron present in foods is absorbed into the body. In fact, in the normal adult with adequate iron stores usually less than 10 per cent of the iron in food is absorbed; infants and young children absorb greater amounts of the iron from their food. The iron content of the intestinal epithelium plays an important role in regulating the iron equilibrium of the body. Iron from body pools can be concentrated in the mucosa of the small intestines, where it may act to regulate the entry of dietary iron to the cell. As iron is needed, it is transferred from mucosal cells into the body; excess iron is sloughed off with the mucosal cells into the gut and

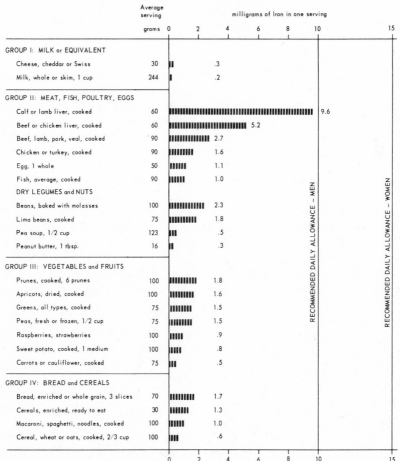

IRON

In Average Servings of Foods
Classified in the Four Food Groups

	Average serving grams	milligrams of Iron in one serving
GROUP I: MILK or EQUIVALENT		
Cheese, cheddar or Swiss	30	.3
Milk, whole or skim, 1 cup	244	.2
GROUP II: MEAT, FISH, POULTRY, EGGS		
Calf or lamb liver, cooked	60	9.6
Beef or chicken liver, cooked	60	5.2
Beef, lamb, pork, veal, cooked	90	2.7
Chicken or turkey, cooked	90	1.6
Egg, 1 whole	50	1.1
Fish, average, cooked	90	1.0
DRY LEGUMES and NUTS		
Beans, baked with molasses	100	2.3
Lima beans, cooked	75	1.8
Pea soup, 1/2 cup	123	.5
Peanut butter, 1 tbsp.	16	.3
GROUP III: VEGETABLES and FRUITS		
Prunes, cooked, 6 prunes	100	1.8
Apricots, dried, cooked	100	1.6
Greens, all types, cooked	75	1.5
Peas, fresh or frozen, 1/2 cup	75	1.5
Raspberries, strawberries	100	.9
Sweet potato, cooked, 1 medium	100	.8
Carrots or cauliflower, cooked	75	.5
GROUP IV: BREAD and CEREALS		
Bread, enriched or whole grain, 3 slices	70	1.7
Cereals, enriched, ready to eat	30	1.3
Macaroni, spaghetti, noodles, cooked	100	1.0
Cereal, wheat or oats, cooked, 2/3 cup	100	.6

RECOMMENDED DAILY ALLOWANCE – MEN

RECOMMENDED DAILY ALLOWANCE – WOMEN

FIGURE 6-6

TABLE 6–3. Calcium and Iron in Pattern Dietary for 1 Day*

Food Group	Amount in Gm.	Household Measure	Calories	Calcium Mg.	Iron Mg.
Milk or equivalent..........	488	2 cups	320	576	.2
Egg.....................	50	1 medium	81	27	1.2
Meat, fish, poultry..........	120	4 ozs. cooked	376	13	3.3
Vegetables:					
Potato, cooked..........	100	1 medium	65	6	.5
Green, leafy, and yellow..	75	1 serving	27	45	.8
Other.................	75	1 serving	45	18	.8
Fruits:					
Citrus.................	100	1 serving	43	11	.2
Other.................	100	1 serving	85	10	.8
Bread, white, enriched......	70	3 slices	189	59	1.7
Cereal, whole grain or enriched...............	30 130	1 oz. dry or ⅔ c. cooked	89	12	.9
Butter or margarine........	14	1 tbsp.	100	3	..
			1,420	780	10.4

*For basis of calculation, see Pattern Dietary in Chapter 10.

lost.[8] The mechanism for regulating iron absorption is not well understood at present but Moore and his associates[9] with the use of radioactive iron have shown that normal men and women absorb from 1 to 12 per cent of food iron whereas subjects with an iron deficiency absorbed 45 to 64 per cent when fed the same amounts of iron.

The form of the iron in food also affects its availability; ferrous (Fe^{++}) salts are absorbed more efficiently. Hence, since most food iron is in the form of ferric (Fe^{+++}) salts, they must be reduced for efficient absorption. Ascorbic acid and other reducing agents have been shown to enhance iron absorption. Iron from liver, muscle and enriched bread was absorbed better than that from eggs or various vegetables.[10,11,12]

Large amounts of fiber, or substances that form insoluble complexes with iron such as phytates and certain sulfur-containing compounds, reduce absorption. As might be expected, diarrhea also results in poor absorption.

Dietary Requirements for Iron

Adults. The recommended allowance for women is 15 mg. of iron per day, with an additional 5 mg. per day during the second and third trimesters of pregnancy and during lactation. These recommendations assume that at least 10 per cent of the iron will be absorbed from the diet. After menopause in women, when menstruation has ceased, the sex difference in the iron requirement no longer exists.

The 10 mg. of iron per day recommended for men may be more liberal than is necessary, because there is evidence that the male adult needs relatively little iron. Usually, this need is met if the diet is adequate in other respects. However, this figure has been retained until more data on the subject are available, because this level can be attained without difficulty, and a generous intake may be desirable for other reasons.

[8] Conrad, M. E., *et al.*: J. Clin. Invest., 43:963, 1964.
[9] Moore, C. V., and Duback, R.: J.A.M.A., 162: 197, 1956.
[10] Chodos, R. B., *et al.*: J. Clin. Invest., 36:314, 1957.
[11] Steinkamp, R., *et al.*: Arch. Int. Med., 95:181, 1955.
[12] Moore, C. V., and Duback, R.: Op. cit.

Children. During the period of rapid growth, when an increase in red cells and hemoglobin is taking place, provision for new material as well as replacement requires a more liberal supply of iron. The anemias of infancy and childhood are evidence of the shortage that frequently occurs, although nature seems to have made provision for the period of nursing. Milk is essentially low in iron, but a reserve of this mineral provided by the high hemoglobin level of the infant at birth is economically conserved for repeated utilization. The potential shortage of iron that may occur by the sixth or the seventh month may be forestalled by the early use of fortified cereals, egg yolks, vegetable purées, and other suitable sources of iron.

Adolescents. Few data are available for the requirements of this age group. The allowance of 15 mg. recommended was estimated on the assumption that needs are at least as much as for the adult female. Menstruation in adolescent girls means loss of hemoglobin and, consequently, an increased demand for all blood-building elements. Chlorosis or adolescent anemia in girls may be due to a low reserve of iron, or of other factors necessary for blood building, when menstruation begins. Languor and exhaustion result from the lack of an adequate oxygen supply to the tissues, in turn due to a lack of hemoglobin. Boys are growing rapidly at this age and also need iron for hemoglobin building, but even at an early age, before menstruation starts, girls seem to need more iron than boys of the same age.[13]

Sodium and Other Mineral Elements

Sodium is the most abundant cation in the extracellular fluid of the body. It acts with other electrolytes in the regulation of the osmotic pressure and the acid-base equilibrium. Sodium is a major factor in maintaining a proper water balance within the body and also functions in preserving the normal irritability of muscles. One milliequivalent of sodium weighs 23 mg.

The sodium intake of Americans has been estimated to be between 3 and 7 Gm. per day (equivalent to 7.5-18 Gm. of table salt/day), which is more than adequate for usual body needs. This amount may need to be reduced in certain diseases where water or electrolyte balance is disturbed. The sodium content of various foods is given in Table 5, Part Four, but it must be remembered that drinking water may also be an important consideration in determining sodium intake.[14,15]

Most of the salt consumed is excreted by the kidneys, with variable amounts lost through the skin and stools. In the normal individual, sodium is almost completely absorbed from the gastrointestinal tract but substantial losses may occur with vomiting and diarrhea. The skin losses may increase greatly when there is profuse perspiration from strenuous physical exertion in a hot environment. Under such circumstances salt depletion may be accompanied by heat exhaustion. Salt tablets taken with a liberal amount of water may be advised under these conditions.

Potassium is found principally in the intracellular fluid, where it plays an important role in cell metabolism, enzyme reactions and the synthesis of muscle protein from amino acids in the blood. Potassium ions maintain osmotic equilibrium with the sodium ions in the extracellular fluid. However, a small amount of potassium in the extracellular fluid is necessary for normal muscular activity. Thirty-nine mg. of potassium equals 1 milliequivalent.

Potassium requirements have not been established but an intake of 0.8 to 1.3 Gm./day is estimated as approximately the minimum need. Potassium is widely distributed in our foods, the average intake varying from 0.8 to 1.5 Gm. of potassium per 1,000 calories.[16] Although potassium deficiency is most unlikely in the healthy individual, medications such as certain diuretics and adrenal cortical hormones may cause potassium depletion if efforts are not made to replace potassium in the diet.[17] As with

[13] Johnston, F. A.: J. Am. Dietet. A., *29*:758, 1953.

[14] White, J. M., *et al.*: J. Am. Dietet. A., *50*:32, 1967.

[15] Cooper, G. R., and Heap, B.: J. Am. Dietet. A., *50*:37, 1967.

[16] Recommended Dietary Allowances. National Research Council Publ. No. 1146. 1964.

[17] Krehl, W. A.: Nutrition Today, *1*:20, 1966.

sodium, potassium losses may also be increased with vomiting and diarrhea. Meats, cereals, fruits, fruit juices and vegetables are good sources of potassium. Values for the potassium content of foods are given in Table 5, Part Four.

Chloride is the anion most commonly combined with sodium in the extracellular fluid and, to some extent, it is also found with potassium in the cells, but, unlike these bases, chlorine can pass freely between these two fluids through the cell membranes. The chlorides are among the electrolytes that help to maintain the osmotic pressure and acid-base equilibrium in the body. During digestion some of the chloride of the blood is used for the formation of hydrochloric acid in the gastric glands and is secreted into the stomach where it functions temporarily with the gastric enzymes and is then reabsorbed into the blood stream along with other nutrients. The approximate intake of 3 to 9 Gm. daily from foods and from added table salt easily meets the requirement. The only time when the body may be depleted of chloride is after the loss of gastric contents due to vomiting. Excess chloride is readily excreted by the kidneys and the skin, mostly as sodium chloride.

Magnesium in the body is divided between the bone and other tissue, about 70 per cent being combined with the calcium and the phophorus in the complex salt of the bone, the rest being unevenly distributed in the soft tissues and fluids. The highest concentrations occur in the muscles and the red blood corpuscles.

Magnesium functions as a cofactor in enzymatic reactions of carbohydrates, protein and energy metabolism. Seelig, in reviewing the published data on magnesium, has suggested that diets in western countries, which contain less magnesium (less than 5 mg./Kg./day) than do oriental diets (more than 6 mg./Kg./day), may be marginal in their magnesium content.[18] This may be a contributing factor in the magnesium deficiency found in chronic alcoholism (where there is an increased excre-

tion of magnesium[19]) and in the formation of renal calculi. In the latter instance, in rats it was found that magnesium was necessary to prevent calcium deposits, in amounts dependent on the level of phosphates in the diet.[20] However, recent balance studies on 18 normal and 7 obese adults indicate that magnesium intakes of 0.30–0.35 mEq./Kg. per day in normal subjects is adequate to maintain magnesium balance. Actually, magnesium requirements of obese subjects per kilogram of ideal weight were the same as those of the normal, non-obese subjects.[21]

Studies at the Harvard School of Public Health[22] on the interrelationship between dietary magnesium, quality and quantity of fats, hypercholesterolemia and lipidosis have demonstrated with rats that high dietary magnesium seemed to decrease lipid deposits in the blood vessels, although it did not decrease the blood cholesterol level. Further research on the functions of magnesium in metabolism may ultimately unravel some of the present biochemical puzzles.

Magnesium salts are both diuretic and laxative. The cathartic action is due to the slow absorption of magnesium from the intestines and the consequent drawing of water into the gut.

Magnesium is widely distributed in foods: it is a part of the chlorophyll molecule in green vegetables and is also found in nuts, cereal grains and seafood. Table 5, Part Four gives the magnesium content of various foods.

Sulfur is part of the protein in every cell of the body and occurs in most food proteins. Thus, the sulfur intake is usually sufficient if the protein is adequate. Sulfur occurs in a number of physiologically important organic compounds; in the amino acids methionine, cysteine and cystine; in insulin, glutathione, heparin, thiamine and biotin. Keratin (the protein of hair, fur,

---

[18] Seelig, M. S.: Am. J. Clin. Nutr., *14*:342, 1964.

[19] Sullivan, J. F., *et al.*: Am. J. Clin. Nutr., *13*: 297, 1963.

[20] Review: Nutr. Rev., *24*:43, 1966.

[21] Hellerstein, E. E., *et al.*: J. Nutrition, *71*:339, 1960.

[22] Jones, J. E., *et al.*: Am. J. Clin. Nutr., *20*:632, 1967.

nails and hoofs) is rich in sulfur; thus, the sulfur-containing amino acid requirement of hairy animals tends to be higher than that of humans.

Trace Elements or Micronutrients

Many inorganic elements occur in animal tissues in extremely small quantities and, in some instances, are detected only by spectrographic methods or by the use of radioactive elements. These are known as micronutrients or trace elements because they are found only in such minute quantities. However, this does not mean that they are unimportant, for it is now known that some of them are absolutely essential, usually in some enzyme system, although the functions of others are not well understood.

Essential Micronutrients

Iodine was one of the first micronutrients to be recognized as vital in nutrition, and it is still one of the most important.

Common goiter has been known since prehistoric times, but it was not recognized as a deficiency disease until the late 19th century. Baumann discovered iodine in the thyroid gland in 1895, and from then on iodine was used more or less as a preventive or curative treatment for endemic goiter. Before that time burnt sponge (a good source of iodine) had been a popular remedy.

Not until 20 years after Baumann's discovery was serious attention given to iodine as prophylaxis against goiter in large population groups. No doubt action was stimulated by the high incidence of goiter among draftees from certain states during World War I.

Function of Iodine and Thyroid Activity. Before surveys were made of the iodine content of soil, it had been noted that the disease of common goiter was unevenly distributed over the United States and that it seemed to be most prevalent in the very regions where there was the least iodine. This early suspicion was confirmed, and we now recognize that common goiter is primarily an iodine-deficiency disease.

As an essential constituent of the thyroid gland in man and in animals, sufficient iodine must be supplied if that gland is to synthesize enough of the hormones thyroxine (T_4) and triiodothyronine (T_3) to function normally.

Dietary iodine is absorbed from the gastrointestinal tract into the blood; about 30 per cent is removed by the thyroid gland for the synthesis of thyroid hormone and the rest is excreted by the kidneys. The amount of iodide present in the body of an adult is estimated to be about 25 mg., most of it concentrated in the thyroid, where it is stored in the form of thyroglobulin, a complex of protein and iodide. Proteolytic enzymes break down this compound, and thyroxine and small amounts of triiodothyronine are excreted into the circulating blood. When the amount of thyroid hormone in the serum is decreased, the pituitary gland releases a thyroid-stimulating hormone (TSH) which causes the thyroid gland to produce more cells and increase in size in an attempt to manufacture more hormone. This results in enlargement of the thyroid gland, or simple goiter.

Natural Food Sources of Iodine. The fact that goiter is not evenly distributed throughout the world or even in the United States indicates that some areas must provide natural protection through food or drinking water. People who live near the coasts and consume generous amounts of seafood probably get an adequate amount of iodine from these sources. In Japan, where seaweed as well as other seafoods in wide variety are popular, the iodine intake is estimated to be 0.5 to 1.0 mg. per day. The iodine requirement for health is probably between 0.1 and 0.2 mg. per day. The incidence of goiter in Japan is the lowest of any country in the world.

Since growing plants pick up iodine when it is present in the soil, plant foods vary widely in iodine content according to the soil in which they are grown. Thus, plant foods grown near sea coasts and in our southern states contain more iodine than those grown in the Great Lakes area or other regions where the surface soil is low in iodine. For this reason it is impossible to list the iodine content of foods in tables of food composition. Since our urban markets today abound in foods grown in many different regions there is less likely to be a severe iodine deficiency even in so-called goitrous regions. It is a very different situation where rural people confine their diet chiefly to home-grown products in mountainous regions where the soil is notably low in iodine.

In the early days, when crude salt was made by the evaporation of sea water and was used without purification, goiter was less common. This is an ironic touch, for the following sections describe the "introduction" of iodized salt in the 20th century for goiter prevention.

Goiter Prophylaxis. The suggestion was made by Marine and Kimball that iodine might be administered to children in goitrous regions as a preventive measure. Consequently, as an experiment, iodine was administered to school children in Akron, Ohio, with remarkably successful results. By a similar project, in three cantons in Switzerland the incidence of goiter was diminished during 3 years from 87 to 13 per cent. These demonstrations suffice to show that the body requirements for iodine, although they are exceedingly small, must be met in order to prevent goiter. Many sections of the country, notably the east coast and the southern states, as well as California on the west coast, need pay little attention to this factor because iodine is indigenous. However, in the goitrous regions this was a problem requiring attention, and Michigan led the way in its solution by promoting education in goiter therapy as a public-health measure.

Administration of iodine as a prophylactic measure against goiter had to be planned as a public-health activity so that it would reach all people in an area in safe but significant amounts. The use of tablets either at home or in school was impractical, and the adding of iodine to drinking water was too expensive. Common salt is used by nearly everyone in somewhat comparable amounts. Therefore, a small percentage of an iodine compound was added to table salt to be marketed in goitrous regions, and an educational campaign was conducted to inform people why they should buy and use iodized salt.

This plan was adopted by Michigan in 1924, and all salt manufacturers in the state put on the market a table salt containing 0.02 per cent of sodium iodide. Eleven years later the results of this plan adopted by the Michigan Department of Health far exceeded the hopes of those who instigated it. The incidence of endemic goiter or enlarged thyroid has been reduced almost to nil.[23] The decrease in the sale of iodized salt that has occurred since publicity on the subject has fallen off is paralleled by a slight increase in the number of goiters in school children. The discontinuance of iodized salt in one county in Michigan was followed by a marked rise in the incidence of goiter within 3 years.

In states where the use of iodized salt was not encouraged, the incidence of thyroid enlargement has remained fairly constant over the same period of years.

In 1941, the National Study Committee on Endemic Goiter resolved that the content of potassium iodide in table salt and in salt for domestic animals should be 0.01 per cent, provided that a suitable stabilizer was used. This amount was calculated from per capita consumption of salt to be sufficient for the prevention of endemic goiter and not great enough to cause harmful effects in other types of thyroid disorders. Iodized salt has since been continuously available in groceries in parts of the country where it is needed and at no increased cost to the consumer. However, education is still necessary if all people are to understand why it is desirable to choose iodized salt when shopping. Iodized salt is now being introduced into other countries where common goiter is endemic, probably as a result of its successful use in this country (See Chap. 16).

Goitrogens are substances that tend to produce goiters, and it has been demonstrated experimentally that such a substance is present in vegetables such as cabbage, Brussels sprouts, cauliflower, rutabagas and peanuts. Goitrogenic action is prevented by cooking, and an adequate supply of iodine inhibits or prevents it.

---

[23] McClure, R. D.: J.A.M.A., *109*:783, 1937.

Copper is essential for the utilization of iron in the synthesis of hemoglobin and as a constituent of many enzymes that function in tissue metabolism. Copper may function in the formation of bone and the maintenance of the myelin sheath in the nervous system. It is absorbed from the gastrointestinal tract and transported to the various tissues loosely bound to plasma proteins. Ceruloplasmin, a second and larger blood copper fraction, is assumed to be the serum copper enzyme. Copper compounds are also found in the liver, kidney, heart, brain and red blood cells. Cartwright and Wintrobe[24] have recently reviewed copper metabolism in man.

In some invertebrates, hemocyanin, a copper-containing protein in blood, functions as an oxygen carrier as hemoglobin does for vertebrates. The average American diet contains about 2.5 to 5.0 mg. of copper, and it has been estimated that the human requirement may be 2.0 mg. or less per day for adults. A copper deficiency has not been noted in humans, but certain domestic animals may show signs of copper deficiency and rats deprived of this element cannot bear normal young. Food sources of copper include liver, kidney, shellfish, nuts, cereals, cocoa and chocolate.

Manganese plays essential roles in both plant and animal nutrition. The human body contains about 10 to 20 mg., but little is known of its distribution. Manganese is absorbed rapidly and is also exchanged rapidly between the blood and tissue cells. It seems to function in blood formation and is found in high concentration in the mitochondria of the cells. Manganese is an important element in many enzyme systems. It is a normal part of the enzyme arginase, which is necessary for the formation of urea, and it functions as an activator of certain other enzymes as well. The manganese requirement of man is not known, but the average diet probably supplies enough. Blueberries and wheat bran are the richest known sources; nuts come next. The manganese content of plants is dependent on soil content.

Cobalt is a component of vitamin B_{12}, a nutritional factor necessary for the formation of red blood cells. An overdose of cobalt given to animals experimentally has been shown to produce polycythemia, i.e., red cells in excess of normal. There is ample cobalt present in the average diet, and there is no danger of an excess from natural foods.

Zinc occurs in animal and plant tissue in slightly smaller amounts than iron. Insulin is known to contain zinc, as does the enzyme carbonic anhydrase which plays an important role in the maintenance of equilibrium between carbon dioxide and carbonic acid. Recent studies in Egypt and Iran have indicated that zinc deficiency does occur in humans.[25,26] Although there are differences among the authorities[27,28] in interpreting these findings, dwarfism, hypogonadism, and iron-deficiency anemia were symptoms found in these populations where zinc intake was presumed inadequate. Zinc insufficiency may also result from chronic alcoholism where zinc excretion is greatly increased even when zinc levels in the serum are low.[29]

Studies at the University of Rochester have shown a relationship between zinc and wound healing.[30] When daily doses of zinc were given to a group of patients undergoing surgery, their wounds healed considerably faster than another group not receiving zinc supplements.

The average diet contains approximately 10 to 15 mg. of zinc, and excretion figures indicate that this amount is adequate to maintain positive balance except perhaps in tropical countries where sweat excretion may account for increased losses.[31]

[24] Cartwright, G. E., and Wintrobe, M. M.: Am. J. Clin. Nutr., *14*:224, 1964.

[25] Prasad, A. S., *et al.*: Am. J. Clin. Nutr., *12*:437, 1963.

[26] Reinhold, J. G., *et al.*: Am. J. Clin. Nutr., *18*: 294, 1966.

[27] Cable, Y. D., *et al.*: Am. J. Clin. Nutr., *18*:421, 1966.

[28] Prasad, A. S.: Am. J. Clin. Nutr., *20*:648, 1967.

[29] Sullivan, J. F., and Lankford, H. G.: Am. J. Clin. Nutr., *17*:57, 1965.

[30] Strain, W. H., *et al.*: Surg. Forum, *11*:291, 1960.

[31] Luecke, R. W.: Borden Rev. Nutr. Res., *26*:45, 1965.

Fluorine has long been recognized as a normal constituent of bones and teeth, the dental enamel being especially rich in this element. The fluorine content of surface soils and water supplies varies widely; this, naturally, influences the fluorine content of food grown in the region and, in turn, the level of human consumption.

Excess fluorine is now recognized as the cause of mottled enamel in the permanent teeth of children in certain areas of the world. This condition is endemic in limited areas—i.e., in the Texas Panhandle and adjacent areas—and is commonly known as dental fluorosis. The mottling occurs when fluorine is present in the drinking water in concentrations of 1.5 ppm. (parts per million) or more. In these same areas the low incidence of dental caries attracted comment. Subsequently, the relation of traces of fluorine in local water supplies to the low incidence of dental caries has been studied extensively.[32,33] The question of finding a level of fluorine in drinking water low enough to eliminate mottled enamel, but high enough to reduce the incidence of dental caries, had to be answered. It is now estimated that 1 ppm. is about the critical level, and if this amount is added to the water in a community, a reduction of 50 to 60 per cent in dental caries in children may be anticipated. Large-scale experiments now in progress in several communities point the way to effective use of fluorine prophylaxis. Mass control of dental caries in children is indeed a possibility in the future. (See further discussion of this subject in Chap. 16.)

While fluorine, says Hodge,[34] cannot "be listed literally as an element essential to life . . . it is now established beyond reasonable doubt that optimal quantities of fluorides are desirable and beneficial in improving tooth health."

There is also some evidence that fluoride is effective in the treatment of osteoporosis. Increased retention of calcium accompanied by a reduction in bone demineralization was observed in patients receiving fluoride salts.[35]

Molybdenum is an essential micronutrient associated with or functioning as a constituent of two or more oxidative enzymes. The few foods known to contain as much as 0.6 ppm. of molybdenum are legumes, cereals, organ meats and yeast. Molybdenum may be active metabolically in deriving energy from fats.

Selenium also has joined the ranks of essential micronutrients within the last decade. According to Schwarz[36] selenium is an integral part of an organic substance that protects rats against necrotic liver degeneration and prevents degenerative changes of other types in the liver and muscle in lambs, pigs, chicks, turkeys, calves, mice and mink. It also is closely associated with vitamin E in some of its curative action.

Chromium is the latest micronutrient that has been recognized as essential in animal nutrition and is associated with carbohydrate metabolism—the ability of the body to use glucose.

When low chromium diets were fed to rats, they developed, first, diabetes and then vascular lesions similar to atherosclerosis. Evidence that chromium levels are higher in human infants than in adults and that the concentration in human tissues varies greatly in different parts of the world (depending both on dietary habits and the amount of chromium in water supplies) raises many questions, which are currently under investigation, as to the role of chromium depletion in the incidence of chronic diseases such as diabetes and atherosclerosis in man.[37,38]

Chromium appears to function by increasing the effectiveness of insulin, thereby facilitating the transport of glucose into the cell.[39] See Chapter 22 for a discussion of the role of insulin and diabetes.

[32] McClure, F. J.: J.A.M.A., *139*:711, 1949.

[33] Ast, D. B., *et al.*: J. Am. Dent. A., *52*:291, 296, 307, 1956.

[34] Hodge, H. C.: J.A.M.A., *177*:313, 1961.

[35] Bernstein, D. S., *et al.*: J. Clin. Invest., *42*:916, 1963.

[36] Schwarz, K.: Nutr. Rev., *18*:193, 1960.

[37] Schroeder, H. A., *et al.*: J. Chron. Disease, *15*: 941, 1962.

[38] Mertz, W., *et al.*: J. Nutrition, *86*:107, 1965.

[39] Review: Nutr. Rev., *25*:50, 1967.

Toxicity and Tolerance of Higher Levels of Micronutrients

It is intriguing and worthy of note, says King, that eight of these trace elements "fit the pattern of discovery as an essential nutrient after several decades of biologic study that had been undertaken originally because in high concentrations [the element] had been dangerous" to some form of animal life. These findings of recent years "show how urgent the need is for the public as well as scientists to understand the concept that all nutrients are safe or useful to the body within a limited quantitative range."[40]

Trace Elements of Doubtful Significance

No one has yet been able to demonstrate that aluminum, arsenic, boron, cadmium and silicon are essential to animal life. However, all are found in traces, both in animal and in plant tissues.

Recent studies by Schroeder on trace metals implicates cadmium in the development of hypertension in the rat. This mineral is present in the kidneys in very small amounts at birth but gradually increases with age. High levels were found in patients with high blood pressure.[41] Proof of the relationship between cadmium and human hypertension must await further studies on both animals and humans. With the possible exception of cadmium, other trace metals appear to be harmless in the amounts and forms found in foods.

Contrary to an earlier popular misconception, traces of aluminum from cooking utensils or in baking powders are harmless.

Arsenic is found in seafoods and in the human body. It accumulates in hair and in nails, but its biologic function is not understood. It has been used therapeutically since the Middle Ages. Overdoses cause gastrointestinal disturbances, but there is no danger of an excess from natural foods.

---

40 King, C. G.: J. Am. Dietet. A., 38:223, 1961.
41 Schroeder, H. A.: J. Chron. Dis., 18:647, 1965.

STUDY QUESTIONS AND ACTIVITIES

1. If water in the body is not sufficient for metabolic needs, what makes a person aware of this particular need?

2. What happens in growth if calcium and phosphorus are inadequate in the dietary? Why are these 2 minerals usually discussed together?

3. Milk is the single best source of calcium in the diet. See if you can write a diet which meets the calcium requirement for the adult, allowing cheese but omitting milk. Repeat, omitting both cheese and milk.

4. What situation results when the iron intake of the diet is low? Name 4 good food sources of iron other than liver.

5. Give the reasons underlying the supposition that adult men may need very little, if any, iron in their intake. Why will adult women continue to need small amounts?

6. How does iodine function in the body? Where in the United States and in the world is iodine lacking in surface soil and water? What is being done to overcome such shortages?

7. Compare the calcium and iron supplied by the 1,400-calorie Pattern Dietary (Table 6–3) with the recommended allowances for these minerals.

8. Which minerals are most important in maintaining the electrolyte balance in the body? How is this accomplished?

9. Which of the micronutrients are known to be essential for animal life? Discuss the function of four of these nutrients.

10. For what tissues is fluoride important? How is this nutrient supplied to the body?

11. Are the blood and the tissues basic or acid in their reactions? How would you answer someone who said that she could not eat tomatoes "because they made her blood acid"? How does the body maintain its acid-base balance?

12. What nutrients are involved in the synthesis of hemoglobin?

13. How do water and electrolytes function together in blood and tissue metabolism?

SUMMARY OF MINERAL ELEMENTS IN NUTRITION
(The information summarized here is given in more detail in the text.)

Element	Rich Sources	Dietary Allowance for Adults	Function in the Body	Elimination
Calcium	Milk, cheese, some green vegetables	0.8 Gm. daily	Bone and tooth formation; coagulation of blood. Regulates muscle contractibility including heartbeat; activates enzymes; bone and tooth formation	Feces chiefly; some in urine and sweat
Phosphorus	Milk, poultry, fish, meats, cheese, nuts, cereals, legumes	Estimated—1.2 Gm.	Forms high-energy phosphate compounds for muscular and tissue cell activity, constituent of DNA, RNA, phospholipids and buffer system	Urine and feces
Iron	Liver, meat, legumes, whole or enriched grains, potatoes, egg yolk, green vegetables, dried fruits	Women, 15 mg.; men, 10 mg.	Constitutent of hemoglobin, myoglobin and tissue cells	Feces (mostly unabsorbed iron), small amounts in sweat
Iodine	Seafoods, water and plant life in nongoitrous regions; sodium iodide in iodized salt	Estimated—0.10-0.15 mg.	Necessary for formation of thyroxine, a hormone of the thyroid gland	Urine
Sodium	Common salt, seafoods, animal products	Estimated—about 0.5 Gm.	In extracellular fluid, regulates electrolyte and water balance, muscle irritability	Urine chiefly, and sweat
Potassium	Meats, cereals, vegetables, legumes, fruits	Estimated—0.8-1.3 Gm.	In intracellular fluid, regulates electrolyte and water balance and cell metabolism	Urine chiefly, and sweat
Magnesium	Nuts, cereals, legumes, green vegetables	Estimated—200-300 mg.	Constituent of bone; in soft tissue related to carbohydrate protein and lipid metabolism, regulates muscles and nerves	Feces chiefly; some in urine
Chlorine	Common salt, seafoods, animal products	Estimated about 0.5 Gm.	Forms acid in gastric juice; helps to regulate electrolyte and water balance	Urine chiefly, and sweat
Sulfur	Protein foods	Adequate if protein is adequate	Constituent of all body tissues—hair and nails especially and of specific organic compounds	Urine and feces
Micronutrients	Leafy foods, cereals, fruits, legumes, meats, seafoods	Minute traces	Enzyme, hormone or vitamin constituents; act as catalysts	Urine and feces
Copper	Liver, nuts, legumes	Estimated about 2.0 mg.	Aids in utilization of iron in hemoglobin synthesis; constituent of many enzymes	Feces chiefly

SUPPLEMENTARY READING ON WATER AND MINERALS

Baker, E. M., *et al.*: Water requirements of men as related to salt intake. Am. J. Clin. Nutr., *12*:394, 1963.

Brown, E. B.: The absorption of iron. Am. J. Clin. Nutr., *12*:205, 1963.

Cartwright, G. E., and Wintrobe, N. M.: Copper metabolism in normal subjects. Am. J. Clin. Nutr., *14*:224, 1964.

Council on Foods and Nutrition: Symposium on human calcium requirements. J.A.M.A., *185*:588, 1963.

Editorial: Iron overload. J.A.M.A., *191*:668, 1965.

Finch, C. A.: Iron balance in man. Nutr. Rev., *23*:129, 1967.

Knutson, J. W.: Fluoridation. Am. J. Nursing, *60*:196, 1960.

Krehl, W. A.: The potassium depletion syndrome. Nutrition Today, *1*:20, 1966.

Lowenstein, F. W.: Iodized salt in the prevention of endemic goiter: a world-wide survey of present programs. Am. J. Pub. Health, *57*:1815, 1967.

Luecke, R. V.: Significance of zinc in nutrition. Borden Rev. Nutr. Res., *26*:45, 1965.

Peden, J. C., Jr.: Present knowledge of iron and copper. Nutr. Rev., *25*:321, 1967.

Review: Salt supplementation during fasting in the cold. Nutr. Rev., *23*:45, 1965.

Seelig, M. S.: The requirement of magnesium by the normal adult. Am. J. Clin. Nutr., *14*:342, 1964.

Swanson, P. P.: Calcium in Nutrition. Pamphlet. Chicago, National Dairy Council, 1965.

For further references see Bibliography in Part Four.

CHAPTER 7

Fat-Soluble Vitamins

All Vitamins: Definitions • History • Vitamin Units and Assay Methods • Vitamin Content of Foods • The Fat-Soluble Group: Vitamin A • Vitamin D • Vitamin E • Vitamin K

GENERAL DISCUSSION OF ALL VITAMINS

The term *vitamine,* meaning a vital amine, was proposed by Funk in 1911 to designate a new food constituent necessary for life which he thought he had identified chemically. Other terminology was proposed as new factors were discovered, but the word *vitamin,* with the final "e" dropped to avoid any chemical significance, met with popular favor.

At first the individual vitamins were named by letter or according to their curative or preventive properties, but present opinion favors names descriptive of the substance. As the chemical structure of each vitamin is discovered, it is named appropriately, if it is not already a recognized compound. However, the lettered nomenclature may still be used to some extent, especially in popular discussions of the subject. From time to time new vitamins are postulated and are added to the accepted list after extensive research.

When a supposedly single vitamin proved to be more than one chemically and physiologically unrelated compound, the term *complex* was incorporated as additional identification, as in the B complex.

Sometimes it is convenient to group the vitamins according to solubility. Vitamins A, D, E, and K are fat soluble. Two water-soluble groups are recognized—those having vitamin C activity and the large group known as the vitamin B complex.

Definitions. *Vitamins* are potent organic compounds that occur in small concentrations in foods; they perform specific and vital functions in the cells and the tissues of the body. They cannot be synthesized by the organism and their absence or improper absorption results in specific deficiency diseases. They differ from each other in physiologic function, in chemical structure, and in distribution in food.

Vitamins may be classified according to their function as biological catalysts in the many and varied enzyme systems of the body or as constituents of body compounds such as the visual pigments. Olsen has recently suggested the possibility that certain fat-soluble vitamins may regulate the synthesis of protein at the genetic level.[1]

A brief review of *enzyme* terminology is appropriate before the specific functions of the various vitamins are discussed. Enzymes are said to contain at least two parts: the prosthetic group, or cofactor portion, and the protein portion. The specific amino acids which compose the protein part of the enzyme are determined by the genetic code (Chap. 9) and this portion is often referred to as the *apoenzyme.* Either mineral ions (such as Ca^{++}, Mg^{++}, Zn^{++}) or vitamins or, in many instances, both, make up the cofactor portion of the complete enzyme (holoenzyme). The vitamin portion of the enzyme is usually called the

[1] Olsen, R.: Am. J. Clin. Nutr., *20:604,* 1967.

78

coenzyme and the mineral the *activator*,[2] hence the term coenzyme as applied to certain vitamins.

There are also terms that apply to vitamins in general. A *provitamin,* or *precursor,* is a compound structurally related to a vitamin which the body can convert to a vitamin active compound. The word *avitaminosis* means literally without vitamins, although it is generally used with a letter following (e.g., avitaminosis A) to indicate a specific deficiency of that factor. The word *deficiency* may be used to indicate varying degrees of shortage: mild, moderate, severe or complete. The possibility of an excess intake of certain vitamins has been postulated, and in some instances a large excess has proved to be harmful; such a condition is termed *hypervitaminosis.* Early symptoms of vitamin deficiencies so vague that they are rarely noted except by a medical nutritionist are called *marginal.*

History. A few physicians early recognized the connection between food habits and the incidence of certain diseases. Beriberi was described in the 7th century and scurvy in the 13th, but it was centuries later that certain foods were recommended as protective. The first vitamins were discovered as "accessory factors" in foods which had proved to be curative for specific deficiency diseases. In other words, vitamins were first recognized by their absence rather than by their presence.

In the early years of the 20th century workers in Germany, the Netherlands, Great Britain and the United States were beginning to use animals for nutrition experiments. A number of investigators showed that purified rations containing only protein, fat, carbohydrate and minerals would not support growth. They observed that natural foods provided some substances other than the basal constituents which were essential for normal growth and well-being. These workers initiated the search for "accessory food factors," later called vitamins. Since then our knowledge of vitamins has grown rapidly.

---

[2] Wagner, A. F., and Folkers, K.: Vitamins and Coenzymes. p. 7. New York, John Wiley & Sons, 1964.

There are still, however, wide gaps in our understanding of the total vitamin story. For instance, although we can recognize a specific vitamin deficiency and cure it with appropriate amounts of the vitamin, the actual role of certain vitamins in metabolic processes still remains to be defined.

Vitamin Units and Assay Methods. Feeding tests on animals at first offered the only device for testing foods for their vitamin content. Procedures of this type, called the bio-assay method, are still the basis of comparison for the standardization of newer chemical or microbiologic methods of assay. After the chemists succeed in concentrating, identifying and synthesizing a vitamin, its content is expressed in metric weights of the pure crystalline substance.

The only vitamin values still given in International Units (I.U.) as originally defined by a League of Nations committee are vitamins A and D. All others are given in milligrams (mg.) or micrograms (mcg.), whichever is appropriate. The FAO/WHO Expert Committee on Vitamin Requirements has suggested that vitamin A values also be given in micrograms (mcg.).

Vitamin Content of Foods. Determination of the specific vitamin activity of natural foods becomes an increasingly difficult task as the number and the complexity of the vitamins increase. Tables 1 and 6, Part Four, give figures for many of the vitamins in foods. Vitamin losses in the cooking and the storage of food will be mentioned more specifically under each vitamin, but, in general, certain principles of vitamin conservation are worth noting. Fat-soluble vitamins (A, D, E, K) are not easily lost by ordinary cooking methods and they do not dissolve out in the cooking water. Water-soluble vitamins (B complex and C) are dissolved easily in cooking water and a portion of the vitamins actually may be destroyed by heating; therefore, cooking food only until tender in as little water as feasible is, in general, the best procedure. Vitamin losses due to storage of vegetables tend to parallel the degree of wilting; such losses are progressive in the long storage of fresh fruits and vegetables.

THE FAT-SOLUBLE GROUP

The 4 fat-soluble vitamins A, D, E, and K have nothing in common as to function or chemical structure except that they are all soluble in fat and fat solvents. Absorption from the intestinal tract follows the same path as the fats; thus, any condition that interferes with fat absorption may result in poor absorption of these vitamins. They can all be stored in the body to some extent, mostly in the liver, and as a consequence of storage manifestation of deficiencies is likely to be slower than for most of the water-soluble group. In several instances, vitamin activity is not confined to a single substance and several related substances produce a similar effect on the body.

Vitamin A

History. Vitamin A was the first of the fat-soluble vitamins to be recognized. This happened in 1913 when two groups of workers—McCollum and Davis, at the University of Wisconsin, and Osborne and Mendel, at Yale—demonstrated independently that rats fail to grow normally on diets lacking in natural fats. At about the time growth ceased the eyes became inflamed and apparently infected. This characteristic eye disease, known as xerophthalmia, was relieved in a few days by the addition to the diet of a little butter fat or cod-liver oil which contained the protective or curative factor known as vitamin A.

Nomenclature. Today we recognize a group of structurally related compounds that have vitamin A activity. Those found in animal products are colorless or only slightly pigmented and the most common of these *preformed vitamins* is vitamin A alcohol, or *retinol*. Other forms which have specific physiologic reactions include vitamin A aldehyde, or *retinal*, and vitamin A acid, or *retinoic acid*.

A number of forms of *provitamin* A are found in the yellow carotenoid plant pigments. *Beta-carotene* has the highest biological activity of the carotenes, yielding two molecules of vitamin A per molecule of beta-carotene.

Some animal products such as cream and butter may contain both preformed vitamin A and carotene, because some of the provitamin may remain unchanged.

Although vitamin A values in most food composition tables are given as International Units, the Report of the Joint FAO/WHO Expert Group on Requirements of Vitamin A, Thiamine, Riboflavine and Niacin, 1967, urges that this practice be changed and that units of weight be used.[3] This will necessitate that tables of food composition report separately the amount of retinol, beta-carotene and other mixed carotenoids in individual foods.

International Units can be converted to micrograms as follows:[4]

1 I.U. (or U.S.P. unit) of vitamin A
 = 0.3 mcg. retinol
 = 0.6 mcg. beta-carotene
 = 1.2 mcg. other mixed carotene with vitamin A activity.

---

[3] Requirements of Vitamin A, Thiamine, Riboflavine and Niacin. FAO Nutrition Report Series 41. Rome, 1967.
[4] Idem.

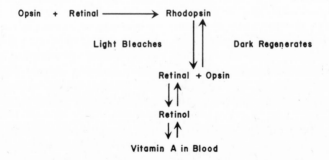

Fig. 7–1. Function of vitamin A in scotopic vision.

This approach to evaluating the vitamin A content of foods is recommended because, as will be discussed later, the vitamin A requirement depends on the proportion of vitamin A (retinol) to provitamin A (carotene) in the diet.

Functions of Vitamin A

Constituents of Visual Pigments. The best-defined function of vitamin A is its role in the visual process. Vitamin A aldehyde, retinal, combines with the protein opsin, to form rhodopsin, or visual purple, in the rods of the retina of the eye which are responsible for vision in dim light (scotopic vision). When light strikes the eye, the rhodopsin is bleached to yield the original protein opsin and retinal. The retinal is converted to retinol and, although most of it is reconverted to retinal to combine again with opsin, some is lost and must be replaced. Adaptation to dim light depends on the completion of the cycle. When bright light has caused excessive bleaching of the visual purple, the eyes' ability to regenerate it appears to be directly related to the amount of vitamin A available. The "dark adaptation" test which measures the eyes' ability to recover visual acuity in dim light has been used as a means of determining vitamin A status. Insufficient vitamin A for the synthesis of rhodopsin results in night blindness, or *nyctalopia*.

The cones of the retina which are responsible for vision in bright light (photopic vision) also contain a light-sensitive vitamin A–protein complex, iodopsin.

Maintenance of Epithelial Tissue. With the discovery that vitamin A acid participates in the synthesis of mucopolysaccharides, some metabolic explanation has been found for the role of vitamin A in maintaining normal epithelial membranes and the mucus-secreting activity of these cells. When vitamin A is deficient, the membranes lining the nose, the throat and other air passages, the gastrointestinal and the genitourinary tracts show changes in the epithelial cells known as keratinization. Rough, dry and scaly skin, especially on the arms and thighs, may also occur with vitamin A deficiency.

Whenever these tissue changes occur, the natural mechanism for protection against bacterial invasion is impaired and the tissue may easily become infected. Clinical observations show that normal mucous membranes lining nose, throat, sinuses and ear passages are the best defense against infections and that adequate vitamin A is an important factor in maintaining the normal functions of these membranes. Renal calculi may also be related to the keratinization of the urinary tract.

Damage to the epithelial layer of the eye is one of the most important clinical signs of vitamin A deficiency in humans, particularly children (see Chap. 16). There is a drying and thickening of the conjunctiva; the tear ducts fail to secrete; keratinization results, with the epithelial cells of the cornea becoming opaque and sloughing off. Infection and permanent blindness may follow if vitamin A is not administered.

Growth and Reproduction. Failure to grow occurs in vitamin A deficiency, as it does in many other nutrient deficiencies, before any other symptoms appear. Therefore, growth retardation indicates a problem which may be nutritional but, by itself, it does not indicate a specific cause.

Vitamin A is essential to normal reproduction in rats, pigs and other animals. Studies have shown that for successful reproduction and lactation the diet must furnish more vitamin A than is needed for good growth. Female rats on a minimal supply of vitamin A intake may show no outward signs of vitamin A deficiency, yet they are not able to bear or rear vigorous young. With an outright deficiency there is an interference with the normal estrus cycle in the female and a testicular degeneration in the male rat. Sows deprived of adequate vitamin A may give birth to litters of pigs with defective eyes or without eyeballs. This finding was one of the first evidences that prenatal malnutrition might cause abnormalities in the fetus.

Other Metabolic Processes. Animal studies indicate that vitamin A (alcohol or acid) functions in maintaining adrenal cortex cells, particularly those that produce the hormone cortisone which influences glycogen synthesis. In this case it has been stated that vitamin A deficiency results in a "chemical adrenalectomy."

Bones also depend on vitamin A for normal development. Vitamin A is required for the release of protein-splitting enzymes from the cell lysosomes to break down the cartilage structure, a process which is necessary for bone remodeling. Hence, control of bone deposition and resorption is not coordinated in a growing animal on a vitamin-A–deficient diet and structural defects in epiphyseal bone formation result. Tooth formation may similarly be impaired.

The nerve damage that frequently appears in vitamin A deficiency is thought to be related to the compression of the growing nervous tissue by a skeleton that ceases to grow.

Absorption, Transport and Storage of Vitamin A and Carotene

Vitamin A. Dietary vitamin A (i.e., retinyl esters) is hydrolyzed in the gastrointestinal tract to retinol and as such is absorbed across the mucosal cell membrane into the cell where it recombines with a fatty acid, usually palmitic. Vitamin A (retinyl) palmitate then travels in the chylomicrons by way of the lymphatic system and blood stream to the liver, where it is stored.

Liver stores of vitamin A (retinyl esters) are hydrolyzed by enzymes to free retinol which is transported by lipoproteins to the tissues of the body where a metabolic requirement exists. The liver stores can maintain the blood at relatively constant vitamin A levels even when the diet is deficient.[5] Hence, vitamin A deficiencies may not develop for long periods of time, depending on the reserve stores in the liver and the ability of the body to mobilize these reserves of vitamin A.

It is estimated that the liver may contain as much as 95 per cent of the vitamin A of the entire body, with small amounts in adipose tissue, lungs and kidneys. Infants and young animals probably have low reserves of vitamin A at birth but, if they are well fed, they store it rapidly. The liver gradually acquires, over a period of

years, an increasing reserve of vitamin A which normally reaches its peak in adult life. The advantage of this reserve is chiefly to take care of temporary shortages or increased requirements. Obviously, an intake above minimum requirement must be maintained most of the time if such a reserve is to be built up. Reserve stores of vitamin A are evident even in young animals.

Carotene. In the presence of fat and bile acids carotene is absorbed into the intestinal wall, where some is converted to vitamin A. The carotene that is not converted is absorbed into the lymph and carried to the blood stream. Some carotene is stored in adipose tissue. According to the recent report of the FAO/WHO committee on vitamin requirements approximately one third of the carotene in food is available to the body. Moreover, the amount of available carotene which is then converted to vitamin A varies considerably, but, in general, only about half is converted to vitamin A. Thus, in the human the utilization efficiency of carotene is ⅙; in other terms, 1 mcg. of beta-carotene would have the same biological activity as 0.167 mcg. of vitamin A alcohol, retinol.

Inadequate protein intakes decrease the absorption, transport and metabolism of both vitamin A and (to an even greater extent) carotene.

Dietary Requirements for Vitamin A

Human requirements for vitamin A are based on studies of two kinds: nutritional status studies on various population groups throughout the world and controlled depletion experiments carried out on man and other animals. Field studies have indicated that in countries where the vitamin A intake is 3,000 to 9,000 I.U. per person per day, vitamin A deficiency is rarely seen, whereas, in other countries, on intakes of 1,000 to 2,500 I.U. vitamin A deficiency is known to occur in the population. Depletion studies have examined the amount of vitamin A necessary to maintain normal dark adaptation in both humans and other animals.

The National Research Council's recommended allowance of 5,000 I.U. daily for

---

[5] Roels, O.: Nutr. Rev., *24*:131, 1966.

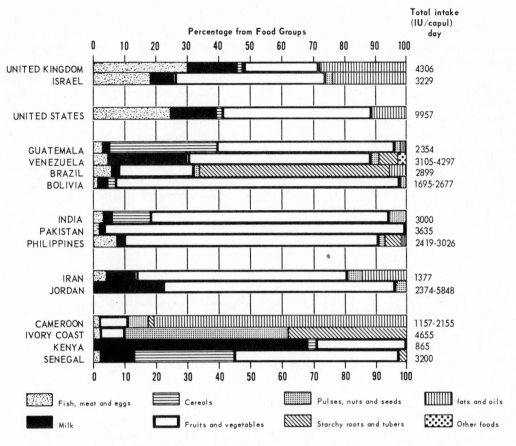

FIG. 7–2. Sources of vitamin A in the diets of population groups surveyed in some countries. (Report of a Joint FAO/WHO Expert Group: Requirements of Vitamin A, Thiamine, Riboflavine, and Niacin. FAO Nutrition Meetings Report Series No. 4. Rome, 1967.)

the average adult is approximately double the minimum requirement in depletion studies. The requirement assumes that the American diet provides at least ⅓ of the vitamin A as preformed vitamin A (retinol) and ⅔ or less from carotene. This implies that 4,000 I.U. of beta-carotene and 1,000 I.U. of retinol provide the allowance of 5,000 I.U. If the total amount were supplied from preformed vitamin A, 3,000 I.U. would be adequate.

To permit adequate stores of vitamin A and to meet the needs of growth, liberal allowances of vitamin A are recommended for infants and children, ranging from 1,500 I.U. in infancy to 5,000 I.U. during adolescence. In addition to the 5,000 I.U. for women, an extra 1,000 I.U. is recommended during pregnancy and an extra 3,000 I.U. during lactation.

The FAO/WHO committee on vitamin requirements adopted a recommended intake of 750 mcg. (2,500 I.U.) of retinol per day for the normal adult. No additional recommendation for pregnancy was made, provided that the usual diet supplied the recommended adult intake. To cover the vitamin A secreted in the milk, 1,200 mcg. (4,000 I.U.) of retinol was recommended during lactation. Recommendations for infants are based on the amount of vitamin A in breast milk. Suggested levels for children range from 300 mcg. (1,000 I.U.) for the 6-month-old to 750 mcg. (2,500 I.U.) for the older adolescent.

Since carotene, which is less efficiently utilized (⅙) than retinol, is often the major source of vitamin A activity in the diet, the recommended intake of vitamin A is modified depending on the per cent of vitamin A supplied by carotene. For instance, in diets containing 60 per cent of the vitamin A in the form of carotene (e.g., in the United States) the recommended amount of vitamin A is 1,500 mcg., or 5,000 I.U., which is the allowance set by the National Research Council for the United States. It is also of interest to note that, when carotene supplies all the vitamin A, the recommendation becomes 15,000 I.U. for vitamin A. Figure 7–2 illustrates the per cent of vitamin A supplied by various food groups in different countries throughout the world. (For complete table of vitamin A allowances for all age and sex categories see Chap. 10.)

Hypervitaminosis A. An overdose of vitamin A may cause serious injury to health. It is most likely to happen when children are given too much of a high potency supplement. The symptoms of hypervitaminosis A are loss of appetite, abnormal skin pigmentation, loss of hair, dry skin (with itching), pain in long bones and increased fragility of bones in general. Such symptoms have been observed in children who were given 50,000 to 75,000 I.U. of vitamin A daily for some time.

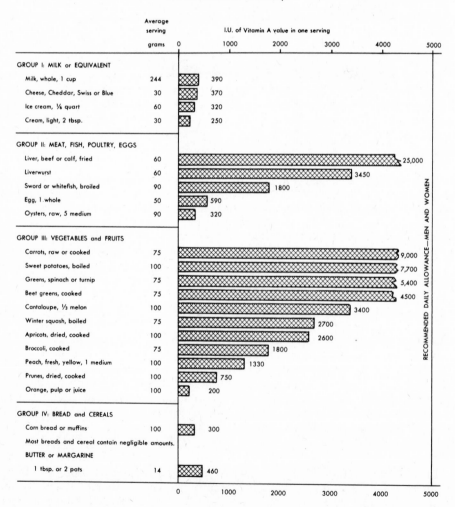

VITAMIN A VALUE

In Average Servings of Foods

Classified in the Four Food Groups

FIGURE 7–3

In three cases of adolescent girls reported by Morrice and Havener,[6] massive doses of 90,000 and 200,000 I.U. of vitamin A caused symptoms of brain tumor (pseudotumor cerebri), along with most of the syndrome described above.

Food Sources. The richest natural sources of vitamin A are the fish-liver oils, which usually are classed as food supplements rather than as foods. They vary according to species and season when caught, but commercial brands are well standardized for our convenience.

All animal livers are good sources of vitamin A, but they are not as rich as fish liver. All milk products that include milk fat, such as whole milk, butter, cream or full cream cheese, are rich in vitamin A. The milk of cows on green pasture is usually higher in vitamin A than is the milk of stall-fed animals.

Carotene is abundant in carrots, from which it derives its name, but it is also present in even higher concentration in certain green, leafy vegetables and grasses in which the color of the chlorophyll masks the yellow of the carotene. In certain species such as corn there is more carotene—hence, more vitamin-A activity—in yellow varieties than in white. In certain African countries red palm oil is used extensively and contributes greatly to the carotene intake.

Animal foods that contain mostly preformed vitamin A seem to be more efficient sources of this factor for humans than are the precursors found in plants. However, the ample supply of carotenes in plant foods may well contribute a large share of the vitamin A requirement. Cooking, puréeing or mashing of vegetables rupture the cell membranes and thereby make the carotene more available. Figure 7–3 shows the relative vitamin A values of some common foods in 4 food groups.

Vitamin D

History. Rickets has been known as a deficiency disease of infants for several centuries. Renaissance painters often depicted

children with rachitic deformities signs so common as to be considered normal. The history of rickets as a deficiency disease is much older than our knowledge of how to prevent it. In the early 19th century cod-liver oil was a well known folk remedy in Holland; somewhat later it was accepted as a therapeutic agent for rickets by physicians in Holland, France and Germany. During the latter part of the 19th century cod-liver oil lost favor with the medical profession because physicians could not explain its action. It was not used extensively then for many years until the period of World War I, when active research on the prevention and the treatment of rickets was inaugurated.

Early workers recognized that normal bone growth apparently was controlled by some substance in natural fats. This unknown factor was credited with some control over the metabolism of calcium and phosphorus.

Research on the chemical nature of vitamin D was initiated in 1924, when Steenbock and Hess demonstrated independently that antirachitic activity could be induced in foods containing certain fat-soluble substances by exposure to ultraviolet light. This discovery of the activation of fat-like substances by ultraviolet rays permitted the manufacture of a concentrated vitamin D preparation such as viosterol long before the pure crystalline vitamin D, calciferol, was isolated in 1935.

Nomenclature. Although about 10 compounds with vitamin-D activity have been identified, the two most important are vitamin D_2, or *ergocalciferol*, and vitamin D_3, *cholecalciferol*. As the names imply, these active vitamins are formed by the irradiation of two provitamins: ergosterol, found in lower forms of plants (such as yeast and fungi) and a form of cholesterol (7-dehydrocholesterol) found in the skin and other animal tissues. They appear to be equally effective in man.

Measurement of Vitamin D. The International Unit (I.U.) of vitamin D is the activity of 0.025 mcg. of pure crystalline vitamin D_3. One U.S.P. unit equals one I.U.

Criteria used for judging the severity of experimental rickets are roentgenograms

[6] Morrice, G., Jr., and Havener, W. H.: J.A.M.A., *173*:1802, 1960.

(X-rays) showing the total mineral content of bone and the calcification of the metaphyses (the growing portion) of the long bones. The last observation was used in developing a standardized line test on rats which was formerly employed for routine assays of vitamin D preparations. Rats were fed on a rickets-producing diet until a definite stage of early rickets occurred; the source of vitamin D (the product to be tested) was then fed and the animals were sacrificed on the 11th day. Longitudinal sections of certain bones were stained in silver-nitrate solution, which darkens only the calcified areas. Figure 7–4 shows the progressive degrees in recalcification, or healing, that take place in rachitic bone when graded doses of vitamin D are administered.

Other promising methods have been developed which shorten the time and the expense of vitamin D assays. In spite of these advances in the investigation of vitamin D —long recognized as necessary for the normal calcification of bones—many questions remain to be answered in regard to the mechanisms of action of this vitamin.

Functions. By increasing the amount of calcium and phosphorus that is absorbed from the lower end of the gastrointestinal

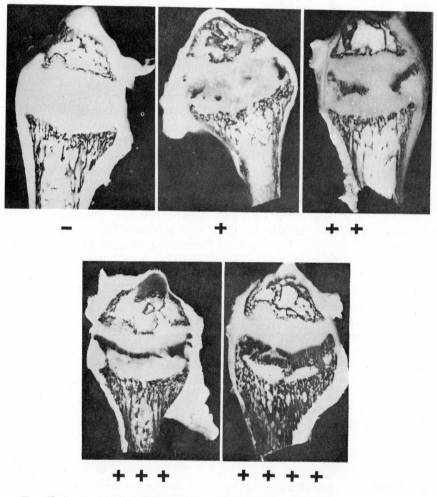

Fig. 7–4. Progressive degrees of recalcification or healing of rachitic bones due to graded doses of vitamin D. The increasing extent of the dark areas, where the white band appeared in the first photo, indicates mineral deposits. Photo marked ++++ represents one Steenbock or 2.7 U.S.P. units of vitamin D. (Wisconsin Alumni Research Foundation)

tract, vitamin D increases the availability of these nutrients, a particularly important function when dietary sources of calcium and phosphorus are limited. Bone calcification (see Chap. 6) requires both calcium and phosphorus. Hence, the role of vitamin D in expediting the utilization of phosphorus by increasing, first, its absorption and, then, the resorption of phosphates from the kidney and, finally, the conversion of organic phosphorus to inorganic phosphate, may prove to be the vitamin's primary function in maintaining normal bones. The relationship between vitamin D and citric acid metabolism is not well understood, but in vitamin D deficiency the serum citrate level drops as does the rate of bone calcification.

Further discussion of the role of vitamin D in the prevention of rickets and other deficiency diseases will be found in Chapter 16.

Absorption, Transport and Storage. Vitamin D is absorbed in the presence of bile primarily from the jejunum and is transported, like vitamin A, in the lymph chylomicrons to the blood stream. Reserves are found in the liver, skin, brain and bones, in all of which it is stored for future use.

Human Requirements. Since vitamin D may be supplied either by ingesting it in foods or supplements or by exposure to certain wavelengths of sunlight, its requirement has been difficult to determine.

There is good evidence that vitamin D is needed throughout the growth period. The recommended daily allowance of 400 I.U. permits maximum calcium retention during childhood and adolescence, and similar recommendations (400 I.U.) are made for both formula-fed and breast-fed infants. The premature infant who is growing rapidly and is usually not exposed to sunlight for a considerable length of time is more prone to develop rickets than the full-term infant and hence should be assured an adequate amount of vitamin D.

The adult requirement is not known but it is assumed to be so small that the average individual will receive sufficient vitamin D in the diet and by exposure to sunlight. During pregnancy and lactation, however, 400 I.U. daily are recommended, and small amounts of vitamin D may also

be desirable for others who get little exposure to sunlight.

Hypervitaminosis D. Vitamin D has been demonstrated to have specific toxicity when administered in overdosage. Usually toxicity is not manifest except after huge doses. Estimations are that 20 per cent of adults receiving a daily dose of 100,000 I.U. of vitamin D for several weeks or months would develop hypercalcemia. A comparable amount for infants based on weight would be 10,000 to 30,000 I.U. per day. Cases of vitamin D toxicity occur "because of unjustified and indiscriminate medical use of the vitamin, lack of appreciation of its toxicity and the self-administration of highly concentrated preparations."[7]

The maximum safe level of vitamin D for infants has yet to be precisely established, although intakes of 1,600 I.U.—four times the recommended dietary allowance—have not interfered with the rate of growth in either length or weight of infants.[8] However, evidence that certain infants may be more sensitive to the toxic effects of vitamin D and may develop hypercalcemia on intakes of 2,000 I.U. has caused considerable concern regarding the infant's total intake of this vitamin.[9] It is particularly important that the mother recognize the need for vitamin D but even more important that she be aware of the harmful effects of overdosage. This means, of course, that the physician and the mother should be aware of the sources of vitamin D in the diet as well as in supplements.

In adults, hypercalcemia has been accompanied by symptoms such as anorexia, nausea, weight loss, polyuria, constipation and azotemia. Similar symptoms are seen in infants, and, in certain rare severe forms, mental retardation also occurs.

Sources of Vitamin D

Sunshine. The low incidence of rickets in tropical climates suggested that sunshine might play a role in its prevention. Even after it had been demonstrated conclu-

---

[7] Fomon, S. J., *et al.*: J. Nutrition, 88:345, 1966.
[8] Review: Nutr. Rev., *19*:158, 1961.
[9] Report: Pediatrics, *31*:512, 1963.

sively that the ultraviolet light from sunshine aided in the healing of rickets, it was difficult to understand the connection between this effect of light and that of vitamin D from sources such as cod-liver oil. Eventually, the puzzle was solved when it was discovered that vitamin D activity could be produced by irradiation. In the skin a form of cholesterol is activated to vitamin D_3 when exposed to sunlight; by absorption into the circulation, this cholecalciferol (vitamin D_3) protects the body against rickets. The amount of ultraviolet light in sunlight varies with the season and the locality, as does the total amount of sunlight. These rays are also filtered out by fog, smoke and ordinary window glass. Thus, it is obvious that an adequate natural source of ultraviolet light is impossible in northern climates during the winter

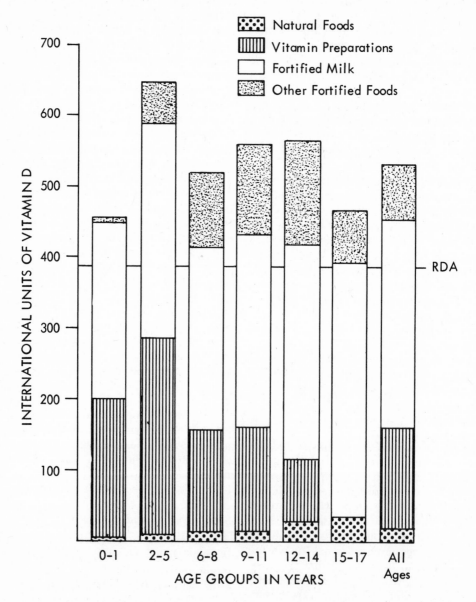

Fig. 7–5. Average daily intakes of vitamin D by age groups and sources. (Dale, A. E., and Lowenberg, M. E.: J. Pediat., 70:954, 1967)

months. Thus, some other source of vitamin D is needed.

Similarly, the pigments in the skin which protect against overproduction of vitamin D in the dark-skinned peoples living in the tropics also reduces the effectiveness of the smaller amount of irradiation in temperate climates. As a result, the incidence of rickets is higher in dark-skinned babies living in temperate zones than in either light-skinned babies in this zone or dark-skinned infants in the tropics.

Foods and Supplements. The natural distribution of vitamin D in common foods is limited to small, often insignificant, amounts in cream, butter, eggs and liver. Thus, we have come to depend upon fortified foods, fish-liver oil or concentrates for preventive and therapeutic use.

It was necessary to decide on one food, commonly used by children, to be fortified with a standard amount of vitamin D. Thus, the Council on Foods and Nutrition of the American Medical Association made the following decision:

"Of all the common foods available, milk is the most suitable as a carrier of added vitamin D. Vitamin D is concerned with the utilization of calcium and phosphorus, of which milk is an excellent source."[10]

Vitamin D milk now on the market is produced by adding a vitamin D concentrate to homogenized milk; the present standard of 400 I.U. per quart means that a quart of milk provides a day's requirement of vitamin D. All brands of evaporated milk also have vitamin D added, and strong recommendations to fortify nonfat milk solids with vitamins A and D have also been made by the American Medical Association.[11] Promiscuous fortification of a variety of other foods with vitamin D does not seem to be either necessary or desirable.

In the numerous fish-liver oils investigated there is a wide range of potency. This seems to vary with the season of the catch and the oil content of the livers.

The highest potency oil often is yielded from fish that give the lowest amount of oil. Concentrates are made from the natural fish-liver oils or by irradiating pure ergosterol and cholesterol. Such preparations are labeled with the exact units per dose or per capsule and are prescribed accordingly. A protective dose to meet the daily requirement is considerably less than what may be prescribed as a curative dose.

In a recent study of the consumption of vitamin D by children (birth to 18 years) the average daily intake for all age groups was above 400 I.U. Fortified milk supplied the largest amount of vitamin D, the percentage increasing with age. Vitamin preparations were more important in the infant and preschool groups than with the older children. Fortified foods contributed to intakes of vitamin D over the recommended dietary allowance, particularly in school age group (Fig. 7–5).[12]

Stability. Vitamin D in foods and in food concentrates is remarkably stable to heating, aging and storage. Vitamin D milk that is warmed for the baby is still a reliable source of this factor.

Vitamin E

History. The existence of a dietary factor essential for reproduction in the rat was recognized in the early 1920's by Evans; it was given the name vitamin E, or antisterility factor, by Sure in 1924. Much of the experimental work has been done on rats, the males and the females being affected differently. Vitamin E deficiency leads to destruction of germ cells in the testes of the male and thus to permanent sterility. In a female mated with a normal male, ovulation and implantation of the ovum may take place normally, but about halfway through the gestation period resorption of the developing fetus occurs and no young are born. With less severe vitamin E deficiency, which may permit the birth of a weakling litter, the chances of survival are poor because this same deficiency seems to interfere with lactation or later with growth of the young.

[10] Council on Foods and Nutrition A.M.A., Decision. J.A.M.A., *159*:1018, 1955.

[11] Council on Foods and Nutrition A.M.A., Statement. J.A.M.A., *197*:1107, 1966.

[12] Dale, A. E., and Lowenberg, M. E.: J. Pediatrics, *70*:954, 1967.

Earlier work on nutritional muscular dystrophy in rabbits has been repeated with other animals, and the nutritional deficiency factor has been identified as vitamin E. However, clinical evidence fails to indicate that vitamin E is a significant factor in human reproduction or muscular dystrophy. In fact, the role of vitamin E in human nutrition has not been well defined.

Nomenclature. Eight naturally occurring compounds have vitamin-E activity. They are fat-soluble alcohols of high molecular weight, closely related in structure. Alphatocopherol is the most active form. It deteriorates on exposure to light and decomposes upon irridation with ultraviolet light. Contact with lead and iron hastens destruction. Tocopherols, because they are readily oxidized themselves, have antioxidant properties and prevent deterioration of certain foods by oxidation. This same characteristic probably exerts a protective action upon vitamin A.

Functions and Physiologic Significance of Vitamin E in Humans. Vitamin E appears to function as an antioxidant in the body, protecting the unsaturated fatty acids from oxidation. Possibly as a result of this function, vitamin E helps maintain the structural integrity of cell membranes. Other antioxidants, including the mineral selenium, may replace or spare vitamin E in certain of its functions.[13]

Red blood cells from subjects on low vitamin E and high polyunsaturated fatty acid (PUFA) dietary intakes have less resistance to hemolysis in the presence of hydrogen peroxide than those from individuals on higher vitamin E and lower PUFA intakes. This test is one of the measurements used to determine the vitamin E status of individuals. Although vitamin E deficiencies in man are rare, considerable interest has been shown because of the relationship of vitamin E to PUFA and the present trend toward increasing the latter in the diets of certain individuals.

Formation of abnormally large red blood cells (macrocytes) in vitamin E deficiency is believed to be related to the role of

vitamin E in nucleic-acid formation. Macrocytic anemia in infants with kwashiorkor was greatly improved by administering vitamin E.[14] Premature babies tend to have very low levels of vitamin E, owing to limited transfer through the placenta. When such infants were fed formulas high in PUFA, Hussan and his associates reported the occurrence of a skin condition which also responded to vitamin E therapy.[15]

Human Requirement. The Food and Nutrition Board states that vitamin E requirement varies between 10 and 30 mg. per day for adults, depending on both the level of PUFA in the diet and the amount of other substances (such as selenium) which may spare vitamin E. For infants, a level similar to that found in human milk (0.5 mg./Kg.) is suggested. Horwitt[16] has reported extensive studies on men of the relationship of PUFA to vitamin E requirements.

Food Sources. Wheat germ and wheat-germ oil afford the richest source of this factor, but it is so widely distributed in common foods that it is actually difficult to obtain a food mixture for experimental purposes that is deficient in vitamin E.

Herting reported that, in individual vegetable oils and fats, the tocopherol levels varied according to source of the plant, time of harvest, stability after harvest, refining procedure and commercial hydrogenation procedures. When estimates of man's requirement for vitamin E as related to PUFA were compared with the amount of both substances in common edible oils high in polyunsaturated fatty acids (cottonseed, corn, safflower and soybean), only cottonseed supplied sufficient vitamin E to counterbalance the effect of its PUFA content.[17] Table 7–1 lists some common food sources of vitamin E.

---

[13] Roels, O. A.: Nutr. Rev., 25:33, 1967.

[14] Majaj, A. S.: Am. J. Clin. Nutr., *18*:362, 1966.
[15] Hussan, H., *et al.*: Am. J. Clin. Nutr., *19*:147, 1966.
[16] Horwitt, M. K.: J. Am. Dietet. A., *38*:231, 1961.
[17] Herting, D. C., and Drury, E.-J. E.: J. Nutrition, *81*:335, 1963.

TABLE 7–1. Food Sources of Vitamin E*

Food	Milligrams per 100 Gm.
Fats and Oils	
Corn oil	
Unhydrogenated	100
Hydrogenated	105
Cottonseed oil	
Unhydrogenated	91
Hydrogenated	80
Soybean oil	
Unhydrogenated	101
Hydrogenated	73
Coconut oil	8
Mayonnaise	50
Margarine (made with corn oil)	47
Butter	1
Fruits and Vegetables	
Tomatoes, fresh	0.85
Green peas, frozen	0.65
Banana	0.42
Carrots	0.21
Orange juice, fresh	0.20
Potatoes, baked	0.085
Cereal Grains	
Yellow cornmeal	3.4
Whole-wheat bread	2.2
Cornflakes	0.43
White bread	0.23
Meat, Fish, Poultry, and Eggs	
Beef liver, broiled	1.62
Egg	1.43
Fillet of haddock, broiled	1.20
Ground beef	0.63
Pork chops, pan-fried	0.60
Chicken breast	0.58

*From Bunnel, R. H., et al.: Am. J. Clin. Nutr., 17:1, 1965.

Vitamin K

History. In 1935 Dam recognized a severe deficiency disease in newly hatched chicks fed on a ration adequate in protein, minerals and all known vitamins. Hemorrhage apparently was due to a fall in prothrombin, the clotting agent in the blood; normal clotting time was restored by administering hog-liver fat or by feeding alfalfa. The antihemorrhagic factor found in these materials Dam called vitamin K—Koagulation Vitamin.

This discovery and the identification, the isolation and the synthesis of compounds with vitamin K activity have made possible extensive clinical use of this vitamin for the control and the prevention of hemorrhages due to vitamin K deficiency.

Nomenclature. Vitamin K is a yellowish crystalline substance. At least two forms (K_1, phylloquinone, and K_2, farnoquinone) occur naturally and a number of simpler substances with antihemorrhagic properties have been synthesized. Vitamin K_3, menadione, from which vitamin K_2 is synthesized, is the most potent and is also available in water-soluble analogues. The K vitamins are heat resistant but are destroyed by alkalis, strong acids and certain oxidizing agents. In the concentrated form vitamin K seems to be sensitive to light.

Vitamin K can be measured in micrograms of the pure synthetic compound, and the vitamin K activity of other substances can be expressed in similar terms. One method of assay uses young chicks and is based on the minimum dose that will maintain the normal coagulation time of the blood at the end of 1 month.

Function. Vitamin K is essential in blood coagulation for the maintenance of normal prothrombin time through its effect on prothrombin and factor VII (proconvertin). It may also be involved in the synthesis of other factors involved in blood coagulation. Prothrombin levels regulate the rate of blood coagulation; when they are low, the coagulation is depressed. Dicumarol, a vitamin K antagonist, is used in anticoagulation therapy.

Vitamin K may also have a role in the phosphorylation of glucose in the cell.

Human Requirement. For most people the vitamin K in the average diet plus that available from bacterial synthesis in the intestines is adequate, and no quantitative estimate of human requirement has been attempted.

Since a food deficiency of vitamin K is rare, the deficiency state is more likely caused by failure to absorb or utilize the vitamin. The absorption of vitamin K seems to be dependent on the presence of bile and the normal digestion and absorption of fats. The use of mineral oil in re-

FAT-SOLUBLE VITAMINS

	A	D	E	K
Active Chemical Forms	Retinol Retinal Retinoic acid Carotenes α, β, γ, etc.	Cholecalciferol Ergocalciferol	Tocopherols α, β, γ, etc.	Vitamin K_1 and K_2, menadione and other naphthoquinones
Important Food Sources	Liver Egg yolk Butter, cream Margarine Green and yellow vegetables Apricots Cantaloupe	Irradiated foods Small amounts in: Butter Egg yolk Liver Salmon Sardines Tuna fish	Wheat germ Leafy vegetables Vegetable oils Egg yolk Legumes Peanuts Margarine	Cabbage Cauliflower Spinach Other leafy vegetables Pork liver Soybean oil and other vegetable oils
Stability to Cooking, Drying, Light, etc.	Gradual destruction by exposure to air, heat and drying, more rapid at high temperatures	Stable to heating, aging and storage Destroyed by excess ultraviolet irradiation	Stable to methods of food processing Destroyed by rancidity and ultraviolet irradiation	Stable to heat, light and exposure to air Destroyed by strong acids, alkalis and oxidizing agents
Function	Maintains function of epithelial cells, skin, bone, mucous membranes, visual pigments	Calcium and phosphorus absorption and utilization in bone growth	Antioxidant in tissues, related to action of selenium	Necessary in formation of prothrombin, essential for clotting of blood
Deficiency: Signs and Symptoms	Night blindness Glare blindness Rough, dry skin Dry mucous membranes Xerophthalmia	Rickets Soft bones Bowed legs Poor teeth Skeletal deformities	Increased hemolysis of red blood cells. Macrocytic anemia and dermatitis in infants	Slow clotting time of blood Some hemorrhagic disease of newborn Lack of prothrombin
Adult Human Requirement	5000 I.U., when 1/3 from animal sources	Children and adolescents, 400 I.U.	Needed, but amount unknown	Unknown

ducing diets or as a laxative interferes seriously with the absorption of vitamin K as well as with the other fat-soluble vitamins. The prophylactic use of vitamin K in the prevention of hemorrhage in the newborn is practiced in some hospitals. A vitamin K preparation may be administered orally to the mother before delivery and a single dose of 0.5 to 1 mg. parenterally to the infant immediately after birth. If mothers have received anticoagulant therapy, their infants should be given 2 to 4 mg. of vitamin K immediately after birth.

From germ-free studies researchers suspect that excess doses of vitamin A may be antagonistic to vitamin K.[18]

Hypervitaminosis K. Vitamin K can be toxic if given in large doses over a prolonged period of time. Symptoms of vitamin K toxicity reported by Smith and Custer[19] are hypoprothrombinemia, petechial hemorrhages and renal tubule degeneration, and, in premature infants, hemolytic anemia.

In 1963 the Food and Drug Administration recommended the removal of menadione from all food supplements. Vitamins K_1 and K_2 are still permitted in carefully regulated amounts.

Food Sources. Vitamin K is fairly widely distributed in foods. It appears abundantly

[18] Review: Nutr. Rev., 24:125, 1966.

[19] Smith, A. M., Jr., and Custer, R. P.: J.A.M.A., 173:502, 1960.

in cauliflower, cabbage, spinach, pork liver and soybeans and, to a lesser extent, in wheat and oats. It can be synthesized in the lower gastrointestinal tract by the bacterial flora. However, since vitamin K is absorbed mainly from the upper section of the tract, only limited amounts are probably absorbed. Medication such as antibiotics which reduce intestinal flora decrease the synthesis of vitamin K.

Storage. Vitamin K is not stored easily in the body, but, according to clinical reports, whatever is stored is found in the liver.

STUDY QUESTIONS AND ACTIVITIES

1. How was the word *vitamin* derived? Can you define a vitamin as distinct from any other food nutrient?

2. Give some events and names of people of interest in the history of vitamin discoveries.

3. Describe the function of each of the fat-soluble vitamins and good food sources of each, if there are any.

4. Does the depth of yellow color in butter or egg yolks indicate the vitamin A potency? Why, or why not?

5. Since the supply of vitamin D is small in natural foods, what commercial process is used to produce vitamin D foods? Which foods are commonly fortified with vitamin D?

6. How does vitamin E function in animal nutrition? Is it essential for humans?

7. When is a deficiency of vitamin K most likely to occur and what prophylactic measures are sometimes recommended?

8. Are any of the fat-soluble vitamins toxic if used in too large quantities? For which one is special caution necessary when concentrates are administered to infants?

SUPPLEMENTARY READING ON FAT-SOLUBLE VITAMINS

Council on Foods and Nutrition: Fortification of nonfat milk solids with vitamins A and D. J.A.M.A., *197*:1107, 1966.

Dale, A. E., and Lowenberg, M. E.: Consumption of vitamin D in fortified and natural foods and in vitamin preparations. J. Pediat., *70*:952, 1967.

Herting, D. C.: Perspective on vitamin E. Am. J. Clin. Nutr., *19*:210, 1966.

Review: Vitamin A toxic reactions. Nutr. Rev., *22*:109, 1964.

Roels, O. A.: Present knowledge of vitamin A. Nutr. Rev., *24*:131, 1966.

———: Present knowledge of vitamin E. Nutr. Rev., *25*:33, 1967.

Wefring, K. W.: Hemorrhage in the newborn and vitamin K prophylaxis. J. Pediat., *63*:663, 1963.

For further references see Bibliography in Part Four.

CHAPTER 8

Water-Soluble Vitamins

Ascorbic Acid · The Vitamin B Complex · Thiamine · Riboflavin · Niacin · Vitamin B₆ · Pantothenic Acid · Vitamin B₁₂ · Folacin · Biotin · Vitamin Antagonists

ASCORBIC ACID

Introduction. The history of scurvy as a deficiency disease in man is discussed in Chapter 16. Experimental scurvy was first induced in guinea pigs in 1907 by Holst and Frolich in Norway; these animals, unlike the rat, the chicken, the dog and other domestic animals, develop characteristic hemorrhages around the joints, teeth and other bony structures very similar to the symptoms in man. Man, the primates and guinea pigs do not possess the ability to synthesize vitamin C when this vitamin is missing from their diets and must rely totally on the vitamin C ingested with their food.

Properties. By 1932 the isolation of vitamin C in pure crystalline form had been accomplished independently by two groups of workers. The chemical structure was identified and the product synthesized in physiologically active form soon afterwards, and in 1938 "ascorbic acid" was officially accepted as the chemical name of vitamin C. It occurs naturally in foods in two forms, the reduced form (usually designated as *ascorbic acid*) and the oxidized form, (*dehydroascorbic acid*). Both are physiologically active and both are found in body tissues. The ascorbic acid in fruits and vegetables and the synthetic form are equally well utilized.

Measurement. Measured by chemical titration, the potency of ascorbic acid is expressed in milligrams. It is an active reducing agent and bleaches certain dyes rapidly. This property is used in the quantitative determination in foods and tissues.

Guinea pigs always have been the preferred experimental animals for bioassay work because of their susceptibility to a deficiency of ascorbic acid, and they are still used for demonstration of such a deficiency and for comparative assays (Fig. 8–1).

Functions. Vitamin C has a variety of roles in the life processes, but to date the specific biochemical functions of ascorbic acid are not well understood. One of the most significant is its role in the formation of *collagen*, the protein substance that cements the cells together. Collagen contains the amino acids hydroxyproline and hydroxylysine, which are mainly formed in the body from the amino acids proline and lysine; ascorbic acid appears necessary for this conversion. Failure to synthesize collagen results in delayed healing of wounds. There is an actual increase in the amount of ascorbic acid present at the site of the wound during healing.

Because of failure of the osteoblasts to function properly in scurvy, bone disorganization results. Tooth dentin may also be adversely affected by vitamin C deficiency, although structural defects in the teeth rarely occur in man. Shortages of this vitamin also result in weakened capillary walls, which in turn leads to hemorrhages of varying degree.

Ascorbic acid functions in the metabolism of the amino acids phenylalanine and tyrosine. It is also necessary in the conversion of the inactive form of the vitamin, folic acid, to the active form, folinic acid, and in the regulation of the respiratory cycle in mitochondria and microsomes.

Ascorbic acid enhances the absorption of iron by reducing the ferric to the more readily absorbed ferrous form.

Clinical experience with a number of infections accompanied by fever shows a decreased blood level of ascorbic acid, indicating either increased need for this vitamin or increased destruction of it at this time. It appears, however, that a suboptimal intake of vitamin C is not a predisposing cause of any of these diseases. It has also been observed that the normally high concentration of ascorbic acid in the adrenal cortex is depleted whenever the gland is stimulated by hormones or certain toxins.

Administration of large doses of ascorbic acid appears to protect an individual exposed to very low environmental temperatures. Although there is not complete agreement regarding the relationship of ascorbic acid and stress, Baker in a recent review stated that he believed "there is definitely an increased requirement for ascorbic acid in all forms of stress; however, we do not, at this time, have sufficient knowledge to state an absolute or quantitative level of increased requirement."[1]

---

[1] Baker, E.: Am. J. Clin. Nutr., 20:583, 1967.

Absorption, Storage and Excretion. Absorption of ascorbic acid takes place in the upper part of the small intestines. It is circulated in the blood stream to the tissues of the body. The amount of ascorbic acid in different tissues varies; adrenal and pituitary tissue, brain, pancreas, kidney, liver and speen have relatively high concentrations; blood cells contain more than blood serum. When tissues have attained their maximum concentration of vitamin C, they have reached the state known as *saturation,* and excess ascorbic acid is excreted in the urine. It is generally believed that a habitual intake of vitamin C of between 80 and 100 mg. daily will keep a person in a state approaching saturation, which condition is probably more conducive to optimum health than one in which there is no reserve.

Human Requirement. Elaborate studies have been made to determine human requirements for ascorbic acid at different ages, under different conditions of environment, under physical exertion, in fevers and in infections. The amount necessary to prevent frank symptoms of scurvy in humans is far less than that recommended for an optimum state of health. Saturation tests after graded levels of intake and observations on blood ascorbic acid have been the chief techniques used for studying human requirements.

The National Research Council recommends 70 mg. daily for adults and 30 mg. extra during pregnancy and lactation. Growing children need relatively more than adults. (See Table 10–1, Chap. 10). During and following fevers and infections the

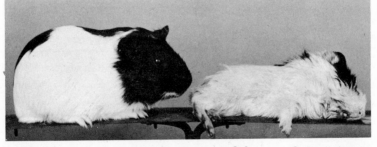

Fig. 8–1. Scurvy results from vitamin C deficiency. Guinea pigs are used for experiments in vitamin C because they need a food source of this factor, even as humans do. (*Left*) Normal guinea pig. (*Right*) Scorbutic guinea pig. (Nutrition Laboratory, Battle Creek Sanitarium)

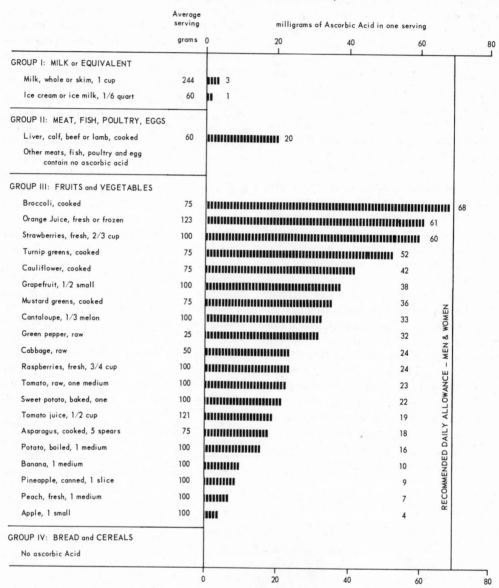

ASCORBIC ACID

In Average Servings of Foods
Classified in the Four Food Groups

	Average serving grams	milligrams of Ascorbic Acid in one serving
		0 20 40 60 80
GROUP I: MILK or EQUIVALENT		
Milk, whole or skim, 1 cup	244	3
Ice cream or ice milk, 1/6 quart	60	1
GROUP II: MEAT, FISH, POULTRY, EGGS		
Liver, calf, beef or lamb, cooked	60	20
Other meats, fish, poultry and egg contain no ascorbic acid		
GROUP III: FRUITS and VEGETABLES		
Broccoli, cooked	75	68
Orange Juice, fresh or frozen	123	61
Strawberries, fresh, 2/3 cup	100	60
Turnip greens, cooked	75	52
Cauliflower, cooked	75	42
Grapefruit, 1/2 small	100	38
Mustard greens, cooked	75	36
Cantaloupe, 1/3 melon	100	33
Green pepper, raw	25	32
Cabbage, raw	50	24
Raspberries, fresh, 3/4 cup	100	24
Tomato, raw, one medium	100	23
Sweet potato, baked, one	100	22
Tomato juice, 1/2 cup	121	19
Asparagus, cooked, 5 spears	75	18
Potato, boiled, 1 medium	100	16
Banana, 1 medium	100	10
Pineapple, canned, 1 slice	100	9
Peach, fresh, 1 medium	100	7
Apple, 1 small	100	4
GROUP IV: BREAD and CEREALS		
No ascorbic Acid		

RECOMMENDED DAILY ALLOWANCE – MEN & WOMEN

FIGURE 8–2

TABLE 8–1. Comparative Ascorbic Acid Dietary Standards for Male Adults in Selected Countries*

Country	Ascorbic Acid Mgs.
U.S.A.	70
Canada	30
Central America and Panama	50
Japan	65
Netherlands	50
Norway	30
The Philippines	75
South Africa	40
United Kingdom	20
U.S.S.R.	70

*Adapted from Recommended Dietary Allowances. National Academy of Sciences. National Research Council Publ. 1146, 1964.

demand for ascorbic acid seems to be increased, either because of rapid destruction or because of an increased need. A regular and adequate intake of ascorbic acid is emphasized because of the limited storage and constant need.

Opinions differ more widely as to what constitutes an adequate or optimal intake of ascorbic acid than for any other nutrient. The so-called standards from various countries given in Table 8–1 vary from minimal but adequate to optimal.

Food Sources. It is obvious from the bar chart (Fig. 8–2) that the commonly used fruits and vegetables of Group 3 are the richest sources of ascorbic acid, with citrus fruits, strawberries, cantaloupe and a number of raw, leafy vegetables topping the list. Canned or frozen citrus juice may be the cheapest source of vitamin C when fresh citrus fruit is scarce or expensive, and may even be cheaper than tomato juice, because it takes 3 times as much tomato as citrus juice to supply the same amounts of vitamin C.

Many factors affect the ascorbic acid content of fruits and vegetables; variety, maturity, length of storage, part of the plant, seasonal and geographical factors all have their influence. As plants mature they generally have less ascorbic acid; the sprouts of beans or grains, however, do contain vitamin C. Exposure to sunlight also tends to increase the plant's ascorbic

acid content. Food value tables give average representative amounts, whereas any individual food may vary considerably from this value.[2] From analyses of the ascorbic acid content of such foods as potatoes, cabbage and broccoli purchased during the winter in northern Vermont, the authors[3] conclude "that certain vegetables, as purchased during the winter months, provide dependable quantities of total ascorbic acid, even though they have been subjected to transportation, storage and handling."

In some countries indigenous fruits high in vitamin C are overlooked, even though they are readily available. For example, in Puerto Rico the acerola (*azarole,* or West Indian cherry) has the highest ascorbic acid content of any known food.[4] Only recently has attention been called to it, and the acerola has become popular. In Great Britain during World War II rosehip and black-currant syrups or jams served to supplement the meager supply of vitamin C from garden vegetables. Even before the war in northern Russia an extract of pine needles rich in vitamin C was being added to berry juice as a health beverage for school children. In another part of northern Europe raw turnip juice saved the lives of many infants who otherwise would have died of scurvy. Depending upon diet, mother's milk may contain more ascorbic acid than average cow's milk and considerably more than is found in pasteurized milk, thus affecting the amount and the timing of additional sources needed in an infant's diet.

Stability in Foods. Of all the vitamins, ascorbic acid is the most unstable to heat, oxidation, drying and storage, which makes it one of the most difficult nutrients to supply in adequate amounts to troops or civil populations in wartime. In World War II army rations included a lemon powder fortified with ascorbic acid; if men would not drink lemonade, as was frequently the case, their ration was deficient in vitamin C.

[2] Merrill, A. L.: J. Am. Dietet. A., *44*:264, 1964.
[3] Livak, J. K., and Morse, E. H.: J. Am. Dietet. A., *41*:111, 1962.
[4] del Campello, A., and Asenjo, C. F.: J. Agriculture, *61*:161, 1957.

Alkalinity, even in a slight degree, is distinctly destructive to this vitamin; therefore, soda should never be added to food in cooking. Acid fruits and vegetables lose much less ascorbic acid on heating than nonacid foods. Vitamin C is extremely soluble in water and dissolves out of some vegetables during the first few minutes in the process of cooking.

To reduce as much as possible the loss of ascorbic acid in cooking vegetables, the use of the least possible amount of cooking water, short cooking time (water should be boiling when vegetable is added) and little chopping or cutting is recommended. Studies have shown that baked, boiled or steamed potatoes retain a large proportion of their vitamin C if cooked whole. Fresh fruits and more especially vegetables lose vitamin C activity rapidly when stored at room temperature and somewhat less rapidly at refrigerator temperatures. Expert advice is not to shell peas, cut beans, or peel vegetables until ready to cook. Quick freezing of fruits and vegetables destroys little if any of this factor. To retain a maximum of the ascorbic acid, frozen fruits should be used promptly after thawing, and frozen vegetables should be plunged directly into boiling water for immediate cooking.

VITAMIN B COMPLEX

Introduction. As early as 1897, Eijkman, a Dutch physician stationed in Java, noticed that the poultry at the prison hospital showed symptoms similar to those of his patients suffering from beriberi. This malady developed in the chickens when they were fed on the polished-rice table scraps thrown out from one prison; recovery followed the feeding of brown rice from another prison. The results of the investigation were published in an obscure journal.

Years later great scientific significance was attached to the findings, for Eijkman had discovered that there was a deficiency in polished rice, although he had not realized its significance. Experimental work with rats, pigeons and dogs during the early part of this century led to the recognition of a hitherto unknown food essential that came to be known as vitamin B. Ani-

mals deprived of this factor lost appetite, ceased to grow and often developed characteristic symptoms of polyneuritis, a loss of muscular control and partial paralysis. Many of these symptoms in animals were similar to those of beriberi in man, particularly the effect on the nervous system.

Subdivision into Separate Factors. Numerous workers began to observe a complexity of symptoms due to deficiencies among peoples with different dietary patterns. These reports were confusing until the discrepancies in experimental findings and the diversity of physiologic properties ascribed to this so-called vitamin B led to the recognition of several factors instead of one. From then on the group was known as the vitamin B complex, and each fraction received separate designation—letter, descriptive name or chemical term—as research progressed to disclose the chemical nature of each.

At present some 12 fractions of the vitamin B complex are generally recognized, and others are postulated. Those discussed in this chapter are thiamine, riboflavin, niacin, vitamin B_6, vitamin B_{12}, folacin, pantothenic acid and biotin, with brief comments about several others.

Distribution and Properties. Certain properties, the solubility in water and the distribution in many common foods are similar for all members of the B complex. The very fact that several of the fractions occurred together in the same food gave rise to the early idea that there was only one substance. New factors identified are classified as belonging to the B complex if they are water-soluble and are abundant in liver and yeast; dry yeast is the richest natural source of the B complex.

Thiamine

Introduction. The polyneuritic symptoms similar to beriberi recognized by Eijkman in his chickens resulted from lack of the vitamin-B_1 fraction of the B complex. Beriberi is described in Chinese history, and some of the earliest attempts to treat it are reported from Japan and the Philippines. The recognition of its cause and of its possible cure by better diet is one of the landmarks in the history of nutrition. Takaki, a medical officer in the Japanese marines during the 1880's, was alarmed at the number of cases of beriberi—169 on one ship with 25 deaths. He proposed a theory that the food must be at fault and helped plan an experiment to prove it. A special training ship was sent out on a 287-day voyage; the revised ration included more vegetables, meat and "condensed milk," and less rice. There were only 14 cases of beriberi and no deaths on the trip; the 14 men who were sick had refused to eat the meat and the milk. According to the original report, Takaki attributed the improvement to an increase in nitrogen. The experiment, reinterpreted in view of modern knowledge, really demonstrated that foods containing more thiamine protected the men against the deficiency disease beriberi.

The pioneering work of Dr. Edward B. Vedder in the Philippines around 1910, when he cured babies dying of beriberi by feeding them a rice bran extract, and the subsequent long quest for the active principle in rice bran make a fascinating story. It is well told by Dr. R. R. Williams in his book entitled *Toward the Conquest of Beriberi*.[5] This account of Dr. Williams' own 26-year search for what proved to be a vitamin, of its identification and eventual synthesis is a classic in nutrition research.

Properties. Thiamine was synthesized by R. R. Williams in 1936 as a climax to his 26 years of interest in the subject. The pure vitamin, usually sold as thiamine hydrochloride, has a yeasty taste and odor and is water-soluble. The natural and synthetic products are identical in physiologic activity. In the dry state thiamine hydrochloride is stable and is not easily destroyed by heat or oxidation. In water solution it is less stable, but in an acid medium it is more stable than in a neutral or an alkaline medium.

Rice enrichment has been practiced for years in some of the rice-eating countries. The Rice Research Institute in the Philippines is working on the development of improved strains of rice and also on methods of enrichment, and much of the rice used in Japan is enriched.

Measurement. Thiamine content of foods may be expressed in milligrams or micrograms (1 mg. = 1,000 mcg.). Human requirements and potency of synthetic compounds or concentrates are expressed more often in milligrams.

Chemical and microbiologic methods of assay have largely replaced the older bioassay methods in which rats and pigeons were used as experimental animals. Now that these rapid methods of assay are available, extensive determinations of vitamin values of foods before and after storage and cooking are possible, and tables of food values include such figures.

Functions. Thiamine, as thiamine pyrophosphate (cocarboxylase), functions as a coenzyme in at least 24 enzyme systems. In carbohydrate metabolism (see Fig. 9–3) thiamine is necessary for the formation of acetyl coenzyme A from pyruvate and for the decarboxylation (removal of CO_2) of α-ketoglutarate in the Krebs' Cycle. In thiamine deficiency pyruvic and alpha-ketoglutaric acids tend to accumulate in the body and have been measured as a means of determining thiamine nutriture. It should be pointed out, however, that the accumulation of these two metabolites in the tissues is not necessarily the cause of the clinical symptoms of thiamine deficiency, but they represent a biochemical abnormality which is usually related to inadequate thiamine intakes.[6]

The enzyme transketolase also requires thiamine as a coenzyme. Present in red blood cells, liver, kidney and other tissue, transketolase is necessary for the synthesis in the body of the five-carbon sugars, such as ribose, found in DNA, RNA and other nucleotides. The transketolase activity of the red blood cell has also been determined as a means of measuring thiamine nutriture, since it is depressed when insufficient amounts of thiamine are present in the diet.[7]

Although there is no well defined relationship at the present time between the biochemical abnormalities and the clinical manifestations which result from thiamine

5 Williams, R. R.: Toward the Conquest of Beriberi. Cambridge, Harvard University Press, 1961.

6 Sauberlich, H. E.: Am. J. Clin. Nutr., *20*:528, 1967.

7 Brin, M.: J.A.M.A., *187*:762, 1964.

THIAMINE

In Average Servings of Foods
Classified in the Four Food Groups

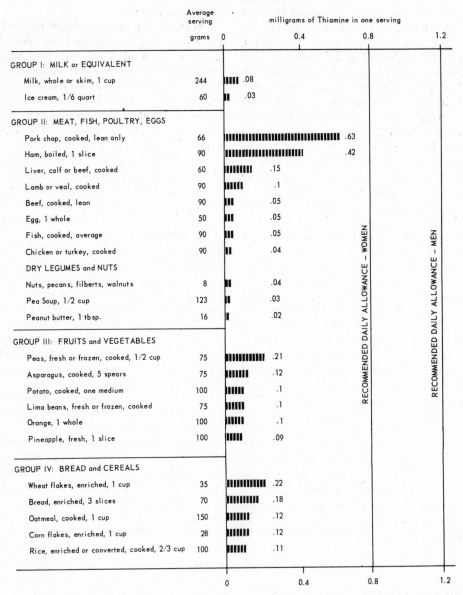

	Average serving grams	milligrams of Thiamine in one serving
GROUP I: MILK or EQUIVALENT		
Milk, whole or skim, 1 cup	244	.08
Ice cream, 1/6 quart	60	.03
GROUP II: MEAT, FISH, POULTRY, EGGS		
Pork chop, cooked, lean only	66	.63
Ham, boiled, 1 slice	90	.42
Liver, calf or beef, cooked	60	.15
Lamb or veal, cooked	90	.1
Beef, cooked, lean	90	.05
Egg, 1 whole	50	.05
Fish, cooked, average	90	.05
Chicken or turkey, cooked	90	.04
DRY LEGUMES and NUTS		
Nuts, pecans, filberts, walnuts	8	.04
Pea Soup, 1/2 cup	123	.03
Peanut butter, 1 tbsp.	16	.02
GROUP III: FRUITS and VEGETABLES		
Peas, fresh or frozen, cooked, 1/2 cup	75	.21
Asparagus, cooked, 5 spears	75	.12
Potato, cooked, one medium	100	.1
Lima beans, fresh or frozen, cooked	75	.1
Orange, 1 whole	100	.1
Pineapple, fresh, 1 slice	100	.09
GROUP IV: BREAD and CEREALS		
Wheat flakes, enriched, 1 cup	35	.22
Bread, enriched, 3 slices	70	.18
Oatmeal, cooked, 1 cup	150	.12
Corn flakes, enriched, 1 cup	28	.12
Rice, enriched or converted, cooked, 2/3 cup	100	.11

RECOMMENDED DAILY ALLOWANCE – WOMEN

RECOMMENDED DAILY ALLOWANCE – MEN

Figure 8–3

deficiency, several possibilities have been suggested[8]: failure to provide sufficient energy to the cell, failure to deliver a compound essential to the heart or nerves or accumulation of toxic substances.

Loss of appetite, constipation, irritability and fatigue are all symptoms that have been associated with low thiamine intakes. Changes in the central nervous system affecting peripheral nerves, eye-hand coordination and mental ability are found among chronic alcoholics who have inadequate intakes of thiamine. The various forms and symptoms of beriberi are discussed in Chapter 16.

Absorption, Storage, Excretion and Synthesis. Thiamine is absorbed from the small intestine and undergoes phosphorylation in the intestinal mucosa. It is found in cells as thiamine monophosphate or pyrophosphate. Thiamine cannot be stored to any extent in the animal body, although certain tissues—heart, brain, liver, and kidney—tend to have higher concentrations than others. These amounts decrease quickly when thiamine is not supplied, so an adequate daily intake is important. When excess thiamine is supplied, it is excreted in the urine, thus providing another measure of the adequacy of thiamine intake.

Although some thiamine may be synthesized by bacterial action in the large intestine of humans, very little is believed to be absorbed.

Human Requirement. Since thiamine functions primarily in terms of carbohydrate metabolism, the recommended allowances suggested by both the National Research Council's Food and Nutrition Board and the FAO/WHO Expert Committee are based on calorie levels. Since the minimum requirement is approximately 0.2 mg. per 1,000 calories, the recommended daily allowance was set at 0.4 mg. per 1,000 calories for males (1.2 mg. daily) and females (0.8 mg. daily). However, when calorie intake is less than 2,000 calories, 0.8 mg. is still recommended. Increased amounts are suggested by the Food and Nutrition Board for the last two trimesters of preg-

nancy and for lactation, 0.2 mg./day and 0.4 mg./day respectively, in addition to the allowance recommended for the non-pregnant woman. Recommendations for infants and children are the same as adults, 0.4 mg. of thiamine per 1,000 calories (see Chap. 10).

Food Sources. Thiamine is widely distributed in a large variety of animal and vegetable tissues, but there are few foods in which it occurs in abundance. This is strikingly emphasized in Figure 8–3, which shows the thiamine content of average servings of some common foods. Obviously, several servings of even the better sources of thiamine are needed to meet the recommended allowance. Therefore, enrichment of bread and cereals was instigated to make it easier for the average person to meet his requirement economically. Since bread constitutes about one fifth of the calories in the average American diet and since only a very small fraction of the bread consumed in this country is made from whole wheat, the enrichment of white flour and bread with thiamine, riboflavin, niacin and iron was a logical step. On the basis of the average per capita consumption of flour and bread in the United States, as much as 35 per cent of the daily thiamine requirement is now supplied by these foods. For more details about enriched flour and bread see Chapter 10.

Dry yeast and wheat germ are the richest natural sources of thiamine, but they are eaten only in relatively small amounts. Except for pork, which is outstanding, muscle meats contain less than the organs, such as liver, heart and kidney. Fruits in general are poor sources of this vitamin.

Stability in Foods. The losses of thiamine in cooking are dependent upon several factors, such as type of food, method of preparation, temperature, length of cooking and the acidity or alkalinity of the cooking medium. Research indicates that on the whole fresh vegetables retain thiamine well during cooking. From a trace to 15 per cent is dissolved in the cooking water, and up to 22 per cent may be destroyed by cooking. If the cooking water is discarded, thiamine losses may be from 20 to 35 per cent.

---

[8] Handlin, P.: Fed. Proc., *17*:31, 1958.

In acid foods this vitamin is quite stable, but its activity is destroyed rapidly by sulfite, a fact which may explain the loss of thiamine in dried fruits, such as apricots and peaches, treated with sulfur.

Thiamine is well retained in cereals, since they generally are cooked slowly and at a moderate temperature and the cooking water is used. Baked products lose about 15 per cent of their original thiamine. Generally, the losses in cooking meat are greater than in other foods, ranging from 25 to 50 per cent of the raw value.

Riboflavin

Introduction. The second member of the B complex—riboflavin—was recognized in the 1920's when it became evident that some growth-promoting properties of vitamin B were retained after heat had destroyed the antiberiberi properties. In 1932 the vitamin was identified as part of an enzyme and was synthesized in 1935.

Properties. Riboflavin in water solution has a yellow-green fluorescence. Although it is stable to heat, acid and oxidation, it is sensitive to alkali and in solution is easily destroyed by light. This vitamin always should be kept in dark bottles.

Measurement. The only reliable unit for riboflavin is the metric weight of the pure substance. Human requirements for this vitamin are expressed in milligrams and the amount in foods in milligrams or micrograms (1 mg. = 1,000 mcg.).

Physical-chemical and microbiologic methods of assay are used for determining the riboflavin content of foods, tissues, etc.

Functions. Riboflavin functions as a part of a group of enzymes called flavoproteins which are involved in the metabolism of carbohydrates, fats and proteins. Flavin mononucleotide (FMN) and flavin adenine dinucleotide (FAD) are two important riboflavin-containing enzymes which catalyze oxidation-reduction reactions in the cells. As hydrogen carriers these enzymes transfer hydrogen from the niacin-containing enzymes to the iron–cytochrome system, after which the hydrogen is combined with oxygen to form water. Thus riboflavin is essential for the release of energy within the cell (see Chap. 9).

Since riboflavin takes part in a number of chemical reactions within the body, it is essential for normal tissue maintenance. Deficiency of riboflavin causes damage to a variety of different types of tissues. It has been demonstrated that riboflavin deficiency in man may be characterized by pallor of the mucous membrane of the lips and splitting of the lips at the angles of the mouth, a condition known as cheilosis.

Riboflavin also plays an important role in relation to the eye. Ocular symptoms appear consistently on a low riboflavin diet and may precede all other manifestations. Eye-strain and fatigue, itching and burning, sensitivity to light and frontal headaches are the most frequent complaints. Cataracts have been observed in rats, mice, chickens and monkeys after prolonged deficiency of riboflavin. In man, riboflavin deficiency is apt to occur along with a deficiency of other members of the B complex.

Absorption, Storage and Excretion. Riboflavin is absorbed through the walls of the small intestines where it is phosphorlylated before entering the blood stream. It is carried to the tissues of the body and incorporated into cellular enzymes. There is no great storage capacity in the body for this vitamin. It has been suggested that under stress the body can conserve its store of riboflavin much better than it can conserve thiamine. The excess riboflavin is excreted in the urine and urinary levels of riboflavin are used to assess riboflavin status in the body.

Human Requirements. The Food and Nutrition Board of the National Research Council has set the recommended dietary allowance for riboflavin at 0.6 mg. per 1,000 calories or 1.7 mg. for the average 18- to 35-year-old male and 1.3 mg. for the average 18- to 35-year-old female. Since the minimum requirement is approximately 0.3 mg. per 1,000 calories, this permits a 100 per cent margin of safety. An increment of 0.3 mg./day for pregnancy and 0.6 mg./day for lactation is suggested. The recommended dietary allowance for infants and children is also 0.6 mg. per 1,000 calories. The actual recommendation for each age and sex group is given in Chapter 10.

RIBOFLAVIN

In Average Servings of Foods
Classified in the Four Food Groups

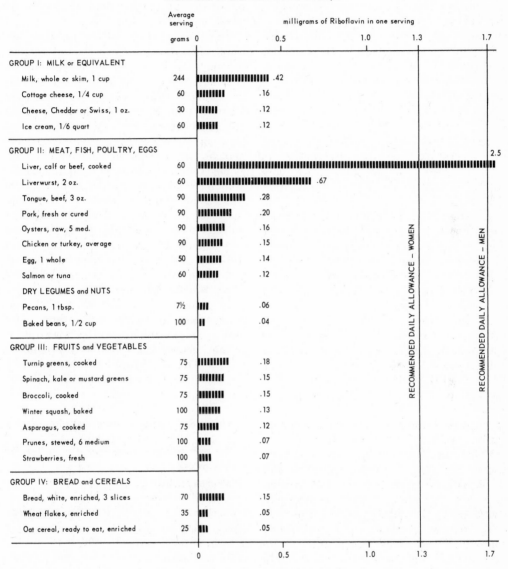

FIGURE 8–4

The FAO/WHO Expert Committee set the riboflavin recommendation at 0.55 mg. per 1,000 calories for all age groups.

Food Sources. Riboflavin is widely distributed in animal and in vegetable foods, but only in small amounts in most of them. Organ meats, milk and green leafy vegetables are the outstanding food sources.

This is strikingly emphasized in Figure 8–4, which shows the riboflavin content of average servings of some common foods and the contribution they make toward the day's requirement.

The average person is not apt to get an optimum amount of riboflavin unless he consumes a generous amount of milk. The addition of riboflavin in the enrichment of flour and bread has helped to raise the average intake.

Stability in Foods. Riboflavin is stable to ordinary cooking processes but unstable in alkaline solutions. It is stable in milk—an important source—if the milk is distributed in cartons or dark bottles or otherwise protected from light. One half or more of the riboflavin in milk may be lost in two hours if exposed to light.

Niacin

Introduction. When Elvehjem reported the spectacular cure of blacktongue in dogs by means of nicotinic acid, now known as niacin, the logical supposition was that a niacin deficiency might be the cause of pellagra in humans. Later, Spies and others demonstrated that most of the classic symptoms of pellagra were relieved by the administration of niacin. However, most persons suffering from pellagra have multiple deficiencies, and it has been found that certain symptoms formerly associated with the disease are not relieved until thiamine and riboflavin are supplied along with niacin. Earlier concepts of pellagra being related to a protein deficiency have been clarified by the discovery that one of the amino acids—tryptophan—is a precursor from which niacin may be synthesized in the animal body. Human pellagra is discussed fully in Chapter 16.

Properties. Nicotinic acid had long been known as a simple organic compound, but its physiologic properties were not realized until it was isolated from potent liver concentrates by Elvehjem and associates in 1937. In the dry state it is a very stable compound, and, unlike some other members of the B complex, it is even stable to alkali. Nicotinic acid is commonly called niacin to avoid confusion because it has none of the physiologic properties of nicotine found in tobacco.

Two forms of this vitamin—*nicotinic* acid and *niacinamide*—have antipellagra activity. Therapeutic doses of nicotinic acid may cause temporary flushing or hot flashes, but niacinamide does not produce this reaction.

Measurement. Niacin in foods and niacin requirement are both expressed in milligrams of the pure chemical substance.

Chemical and microbiologic methods for niacin assay are now used generally in place of animal assays. Dogs were the only animals with which early bio-assays could be made, and such tests were based on the blacktongue-preventing value.

Functions. Niacin, like thiamine and riboflavin, also functions as a coenzyme in energy metabolism. It is part of the enzymes NAD (nicotinamide adenine dinucleotide) and NADP (nicotinamide adenine dinucleotide phosphate), which are hydrogen carriers essential in the release of energy from carbohydrates, fats and protein. These niacin-containing enzymes transfer hydrogen from the oxidizable material (i.e., carbohydrate) to the riboflavin-containing enzymes (see Functions of Riboflavin). They are also involved in the synthesis of proteins and fats. Hence a variety of tissues, including the skin, gastrointestinal tract and nervous system, are affected by niacin deficiency. (See Pellagra, Chapter 16.)

Large doses of niacin (100 to 200 times the recommended allowance) administered orally have resulted in the lowering of serum cholesterol and beta-lipoprotein levels. The mechanism of this action is not understood, and only the acid form is effective, not the amide.

TABLE 8–2. Approximate Calculation of Niacin from Tryptophan

Dietary protein...........	60 grams
Tryptophan content 1% (approx.).............	0.01
Tryptophan.............	0.60 Gm. or 600 mg.
60 mg. of tryptophan = 1 mg. of niacin........	$600 \div 60 = 10$
Niacin equivalents from tryptophan...........	10 mg.

Relationship of Tryptophan to Niacin. The amino acid tryptophan can be converted to niacin in the body. Research studies have indicated that approximately 60 mg. of tryptophan are equivalent to 1 mg. of niacin. Animal and vegetable protein contain about 1.4 per cent and 1 per cent of tryptophan respectively. Table 8–2 illustrates how an approximate amount of niacin equivalents can be calculated from protein. Total niacin equivalents equal the preformed niacin plus the niacin equivalents available from protein.

Recommended Dietary Allowances. Both the Food and Nutrition Board and the FAO/WHO Expert Committee have established the recommended dietary allowance for niacin equivalents at 6.6 mg. per 1,000

calories for all age groups. Depending on calorie intake, the 1964 NRC-RDA for males is from 15 to 19 mg. of niacin equivalents daily and for females 13 to 14 mg. daily. An increase of 3 mg. and 7 mg. respectively above the allowance for the non-pregnant woman is recommended during pregnancy and lactation by the Food

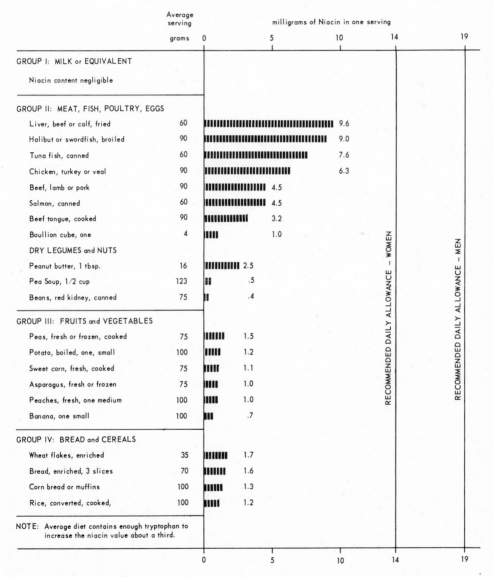

NIACIN

In Average Servings of Foods
Classified in the Four Food Groups

	Average serving grams	milligrams of Niacin in one serving
GROUP I: MILK or EQUIVALENT		
Niacin content negligible		
GROUP II: MEAT, FISH, POULTRY, EGGS		
Liver, beef or calf, fried	60	9.6
Halibut or swordfish, broiled	90	9.0
Tuna fish, canned	60	7.6
Chicken, turkey or veal	90	6.3
Beef, lamb or pork	90	4.5
Salmon, canned	60	4.5
Beef tongue, cooked	90	3.2
Boullion cube, one	4	1.0
DRY LEGUMES and NUTS		
Peanut butter, 1 tbsp.	16	2.5
Pea Soup, 1/2 cup	123	.5
Beans, red kidney, canned	75	.4
GROUP III: FRUITS and VEGETABLES		
Peas, fresh or frozen, cooked	75	1.5
Potato, boiled, one, small	100	1.2
Sweet corn, fresh, cooked	75	1.1
Asparagus, fresh or frozen	75	1.0
Peaches, fresh, one medium	100	1.0
Banana, one small	100	.7
GROUP IV: BREAD and CEREALS		
Wheat flakes, enriched	35	1.7
Bread, enriched, 3 slices	70	1.6
Corn bread or muffins	100	1.3
Rice, converted, cooked,	100	1.2

RECOMMENDED DAILY ALLOWANCE – WOMEN

RECOMMENDED DAILY ALLOWANCE – MEN

NOTE: Average diet contains enough tryptophan to increase the niacin value about a third.

Figure 8–5

TABLE 8–3. Vitamins in Pattern Dietary for 1 Day*

Food Group	Amount in Gm.	Household Measure	Calories	Vitamin A I.U.	Thiamine Mg.	Riboflavin Mg.	Niacin Mg.	Ascorbic Acid Mg.
Milk or equivalent.....	488	2 cups	320	700	.16	.84	.3	5
Egg...............	50	1 medium	81	590	.06	.15	..	..
Meat, fish, fowl.......	120	4 ozs. cooked	376	280	.14	.23	6.1	..
Vegetables:								
Potato...........	100	1 medium	65	..	.09	.03	1.2	16
Green or yellow....	75	1 serving	27	4,700	.05	.10	.5	25
Other...........	75	1 serving	45	300	.08	.06	.6	12
Fruits:								
Citrus...........	100	1 serving	43	140	.06	.02	.3	43
Other...........	100	1 serving	85	365	.03	.04	.5	4
Bread, white enriched.	70	3 slices	189	..	.17	.15	1.7	..
Cereal, whole grain or enriched........	30 130	1 oz. dry or ⅔ c. cooked	89	..	.08	.03	.7	..
Butter or margarine...	14	1 tbsp.	100	460	..	..	..	..
		Totals......	1,420	7,535	.92	1.65	11.9	105

*For basis of calculation, see Pattern Dietary in Chapter 10.

and Nutrition Board. Infants and children follow the same recommendations as adults.

Storage and Excretion. Little is known regarding the extent of storage of niacin in the body, but probably it is stored in the liver. It is eliminated in the urine largely as derivatives and, to a smaller extent, as free niacin. This diversity of end products has added to the difficulties of metabolic studies of niacin.

Food Sources. In general, meat, poultry and fish are better sources of niacin than plant products, as emphasized in Figure 8–5, showing average servings. The use of meat drippings is recommended, because niacin is easily dissolved out of foods in cooking. Whole grain and enriched products make an appreciable contribution. Fruits and vegetables other than mushrooms and legumes are insignificant sources of niacin. Milk and eggs are poor sources of preformed niacin but good sources of its precursor tryptophan.

Food values as given in Fig. 8–5 and in most food tables (Table I, Part Four) are not in *niacin equivalents* because such values are almost impossible to determine. Thus, when the listed niacin content of foods in a diet fails to meet the niacin equivalent recommendations, one may calculate the approximate amount available from tryptophan (Table 8–2). In the average diet in the United States, with adequate amounts of protein, the niacin value may be increased by one third or more.

Vitamins in Pattern Dietary for One Day

The contribution made by the Pattern Dietary (see also Chap. 10) to the 5 vitamins for which we have specific recommendations is given in the accompanying table. Since the pattern dietary provides only 1,400 calories, the foods chosen to supplement these will also provide additional vitamins to bring the totals up to the recommended allowances.

Vitamin B₆ Group

Introduction. Pyridoxine was identified in 1938 as a separate fraction of the B complex. Subsequently, vitamin B₆ proved to be a complex of 3 closely related chemical compounds—*pyridoxine, pyridoxal* and *pyridoxamine*—all of which are active physiologically. The need for this factor was first demonstrated in rats, but it is now established that it is needed by most animals. A deficiency is associated with a peculiar type of anemia in some species and extreme muscular weakness, dermatitis and nervous disorders in others. Vitamin B₆ can be synthesized by intestinal organisms in the rat, but whether or not this is true in humans has not been established.

The need for and the function of vitamin B₆ in humans has been demonstrated conclusively in both adults and infants. The accidental destruction of this factor in a canned-milk formula resulted in the occurrence of nervous irritability and convulsive seizures in young infants.[9] Rapid recovery followed injection of the vitamin, proving conclusively that the symptoms noted were a result of a deficiency.

Functions. The mechanism of the action of pyridoxine and its several analogues is associated closely with the synthesis and metabolism of amino acids. Pyridoxal phosphate (PALP), the coenzyme form of vitamin B₆, is necessary for transamination, the process by which the amino group (NH_2) from one amino acid is transferred to another to produce a different amino acid needed for protein synthesis. The transaminase activity (B₆-containing enzymes catalyzing transamination) of the blood can be measured as a means of assessing vitamin-B₆ status.[10]

PALP-containing enzymes are also involved in decarboxylation and desulfuration (removal of CO_2 and H_2S groups) of amino acids. The conversion of tryptophan to niacin requires vitamin B₆. If a large dose of tryptophan (Tryptophan Load Test) is administered to an individual with a pyridoxine deficiency, an intermediary product in the conversion—xanthurenic acid—accumulates and can be measured in the urine. When vitamin B₆ is present in adequate amounts, more nicotinic acid is formed and xanthurenic acid excretion is not increased. Folic acid metabolism is also dependent on pyridoxine-containing enzymes.

Coursin recently discussed several different aspects of vitamin-B₆ deficiency in man. He points out that in extreme cases of vitamin-B₆ deficiency there have been clear-cut symptoms of anemia, oxalate stone formation or central nervous system abnormalities. In addition, consideration must be given to what appear to be sub-optimal intakes by some people and increased needs of pregnant females and those taking certain birth control pills.[11]

A vitamin-B₆ Dependency Syndrome of genetic origin has been identified in which the patient requires large amounts of the vitamin to prevent convulsive seizures and mental retardation. Similiar deficiencies of other B₆-dependent enzymes have also been identified where only massive doses of the vitamin facilitated enzyme activity.[12] Much research work is focusing on this vitamin at the present time and we can expect soon to understand better its role in nutrition.

Human Requirements. Evidence available from animal experiments and human volunteers indicates that the daily intake of vitamin B₆ should be from 1.5 to 2 mg. when the daily protein intake is 100 Gm. or more. An allowance of 400 mcg./day for bottle-fed infants is suggested as adequate. High protein diets, pregnancy, and isoniazid therapy for tuberculosis are all believed to increase the need for vitamin B₆. Pyridoxine supplements during pregnancy may protect against dental caries.[13]

Food Sources. Of the animal foods, pork and the glandular meats are the richest, with lamb and veal relatively better than fish or beef muscle. Milk and eggs are only

9 Coursin, D. B.: J.A.M.A., *154*:406, 1954.

10 Linkswiler, H.: Am. J. Clin. Nutr., *20*:547, 1967.

11 Coursin, D. B.: Am. J. Clin. Nutr., *20*:558, 1967.

12 Review: Nutr. Rev., *25*:72, 1967.

13 Hillman, R. W., *et al.*: Am. J. Clin. Nutr., *10*:512, 1962.

fair sources. Of the plant foods, legumes, potatoes, oatmeal, wheat germ and bananas are the richest, with cabbages, carrots and other vegetables providing fair amounts. The B_6 content of foods is determined by a microbiologic method. (See Table 6 in Part Four.)

Pantothenic Acid

Introduction. Pantothenic acid is another of the vitamin B complex group first recognized as essential for rats, dogs, pigs, pigeons and chicks. The complete synthesis of pantothenic acid was accomplished in 1940. A deficiency has been reported to cause emaciation, loss of hair and graying of hair in dark animals, ulcers of the intestinal tract and damage to several internal organs.

Functions. Pantothenic acid is a part of coenzyme A which plays a basic role in metabolism—in the release of energy from carbohydrates, fats and proteins, and also in the synthesis of amino acids, fatty acids, sterols, and steroid hormones. It is also essential for the formation of porphyrin, the pigment portion of the hemoglobin molecule.

Human Requirement. A definite dietary requirement for pantothenic acid has not been established. In a survey by Chung, et al.[14] it was found that pantothenic acid activity of high-cost diets averaged 16.3 mg. per day and for the poorest diets 6.0 mg. per day. These workers estimate that the average American diet provides from 10 to 20 mg. per day, which is liberal in terms of the estimated need of 10 mg. per day.

Food Sources. The word *pantothenic*, meaning widespread, indicates that the distribution of this vitamin is extensive. Figures on the pantothenic acid content of foods are limited in number. Yeast, liver, kidney, heart, salmon and eggs are the best sources. Other good sources are broccoli, mushrooms, pork, beef tongue, peanuts, wheat, rye and soybean flour. About one half of the pantothenic acid is lost in the milling of grains, which constitute an

[14] Chung, A. S. M., *et al.*: Am. J. Clin. Nutr., 9:573, 1961.

important, if not a rich, source of this factor in the average diet. Fruits are relatively poor sources of this vitamin. (See Table 6 in Part Four.)

Vitamin B_{12}

Introduction. Ever since the discovery that liver was effective in the treatment of pernicious anemia research workers have been hunting for the active principle, or "extrinsic" factor, in liver. At first it seemed that folic acid was the answer, but it proved to be ineffective in relieving many of the symptoms of the disease. In 1948 a more active substance, B_{12}, isolated from liver, was found to be effective in microgram quantities in the therapy of pernicious anemia as well as in other types of macrocytic anemias. Thus, vitamin B_{12} is probably identical with Castle's "extrinsic" factor. Its oral effectiveness is enhanced by the "intrinsic" factor found in normal gastric juice, as was true of the active factor in liver extracts. The "intrinsic" factor is essential for the absorption of the vitamin B_{12}. Pernicious anemia is discussed further in Chapter 31.

The suggestion that vitamin B_{12} may act as a growth factor for children as it does for poultry, pigs and ruminants has not been well confirmed. The natural variation in the growth of children is so great that the relatively small effect of B_{12} is difficult to demonstrate. Furthermore, there is no evidence of a widespread deficiency of this factor among American children.

Properties. The structure of vitamin B_{12} was established by Todd in 1955 as an extremely complex nitrogenous compound containing 1 atom of cobalt (cyanocobalamine). Two of the active forms of this vitamin are cyanocobalamin (Vitamin B_{12}) and hydroxocobalamin (Vitamin B_{12a}). Vitamin B_{12} coenzymes are called cobamides. Cobalt, long known as a trace element essential for some animals, never before had been found in a natural organic compound.

Vitamin B_{12} is remarkably potent. It has a biologic activity 11,000 times that of a standard liver concentrate formerly used in the treatment of pernicious anemia.

Thus B_{12} appears to be one of the most potent biologically active substances known. It has been administered therapeutically in doses of from 6 to 150 mcg. Comparative effects with folic acid in other types of anemia require doses of from 20,000 to 50,000 mcg.

Functions. Vitamin B_{12} functions as a coenzyme in various chemical reactions in the cell. It is particularly important in the bone marrow where the red blood cells are formed and in nervous tissue. The synthesis of nucleic acids and, hence, of DNA depend on B_{12}-containing enzymes. Cobamides are also involved in folic acid metabolism.

A diagnostic test for the determination of vitamin-B_{12} deficiency depends on the role of B_{12} in the metabolism of certain fatty acids. Methylmalonic acid (MMA), which requires vitamin B_{12} for its breakdown to succinic acid, is excreted in the urine of individuals deficient in vitamin B_{12} and can be measured to assess B_{12} adequacy.[15]

Absorption, Transport and Storage. Since vitamin B_{12} has the largest and, probably, the most complicated molecule of any of the water-soluble nutrients, it is not surprising that its deficiency is caused more frequently by problems of absorption than by dietary inadequacy. Of equal interest is the fact that its absorption requires the presence in the gastric secretions of an even larger molecule, a mucoprotein called Castle's "intrinsic factor" (IF). The B_{12}-IF complex forms in the stomach, passes through the upper part of the small intestine to the ileum, where the IF attaches itself to the epithelial cells specific to this area of the gut and thereby facilitates the transfer of vitamin B_{12} into the ileal epithelium. Calcium is also necessary for this transfer. Three hours are required for the transport of B_{12}, whereas only seconds are required for most water-soluble compounds. Since the IF is not found in lymph or plasma, it must remain in the intestinal tract.[16]

When cobalamin is released into the bloodstream, it is attached to another protein and carried to the various tissues. Protein-bound vitamin B_{12} not immediately needed is stored in the liver, which is capable of storing relatively large amounts of this nutrient. As the quantity of the vitamin increases in the diet, the per cent absorbed decreases.

Although in some instances very large therapeutic doses of B_{12} given to pernicious anemia patients have caused some of the nutrient to be absorbed, in the absence of IF, vitamin B_{12} usually must be administered parenterally.

Human Requirement. The Food and Nutrition Board suggests that between 3 and 5 mcg. daily of vitamin B_{12} is adequate unless stores have been depleted, whereupon 15 mcg. per day will be necessary to replenish liver stores.

In pernicious anemia patients who have been treated to replenish their stores 1.5 mcg. daily given parenterally will meet the body needs; continuous treatment at predetermined intervals is indicated.

Food sources of vitamin B_{12} have not been widely investigated, but on present evidence the content of liver and kidney is high; of milk, muscle meats and fish, medium.

In surveys of typical diets the remarkable difference in the vitamin B_{12} content between the adequate and the poor diets emphasizes the importance of the contribution made by meats and other animal products to the B_{12} intake.

Folacin (Folic Acid)

Introduction. Folic acid was first recognized as a dietary essential for chicks in 1938 and later was shown to be a requirement of other animals. Folacin was first used clinically in 1945 by Spies, who showed it to be effective in the treatment of macrocytic anemias of pregnancy and tropical sprue, and these findings have since been confirmed.

Folic acid (pteroylglutamic acid, PGA) is transformed within the living organism to a biologically active form called folinic acid (N^5 formyl THFA) or "citrovorum factor."

15 Herbert, V.: Am. J. Clin. Nutr., 20:562, 1967.
16 Wilson, T. H.: Nutr. Rev., 23:33, 1965.

Functions. There are five known enzyme forms of folacin, and their major role is in the transfer of one-carbon units to various compounds in the synthesis of DNA, RNA, methionine and serine.[17]

The amino acid histidine requires folic acid for its complete utilization. When folic acid is not available, the intermediary product, formiminoglutamic acid (FIGLU), is excreted in the urine. FIGLU excretion levels can then be used to determine folic acid nutritional status.

Folic acid deficiency in man results in megaloblastic anemia, glossitis, and gastrointestinal disturbances. Because of the interdependence of vitamins B_{12}, B_6, ascorbic acid and folic acid the anemia found in these deficiency diseases may be similar and may respond to treatment with one or several of these nutrients. It should be pointed out, however, that even though the anemia in pernicious anemia may be relieved by folic acid, only vitamin B_{12} cures the neurologic symptoms (see Chap. 31).

Absorption, Excretion and Storage. Folic acid is readily absorbed by the gastrointestinal tract and carried by the blood to the tissues of the body. It is stored primarily in the liver, and excess is excreted in the urine.

The questions of both dietary folic acid deficiency[18] and secondary folic acid deficiency have been raised. In the case of the latter numerous possible causes have been cited: failure to absorb dietary folate; increased urinary excretion of folic acid; increased folate destruction; interference in the synthesis or activation of enzymes necessary for its utilization; and production of anti-folates.[19]

Human Requirements. Evidence that folacin and folinic acid are essential for humans is based on curative responses of patients with macrocytic anemias and on experimental work on primates deprived of these factors. Available information concerning requirements is also based on therapeutic responses of patients to daily doses of 200 to 500 mcg. of folacin. Chung *et al.*[20] found that high-cost and low-cost diets averaged 0.193 and 0.157 mg. of total folic acid activity respectively. A total folic acid content of 0.15 mg., which should supply at least 0.05 mg. of active folic acid, is considered adequate. There are probably increased needs during pregnancy and in patients with cirrhosis.

Since more than 0.1 mg. of folic acid per day may prevent anemia but not cure the neurologic symptoms of pernicious anemia, vitamin preparations which contain more than 0.1 mg. of folic acid cannot be sold without prescription.

Food Sources. The presence of this group of factors in green leaves was the basis for the name folacin (*folium,* meaning *leaf*). In addition to their presence in green leaves, these factors are found in liver, meats and fish, nuts, legumes and whole grains. (See Table 6 in Part Four.)

Many of the folates in food are easily destroyed by storing, cooking and other processing. Because of the destruction of folic acid activity in dried milk, it has been suggested that ascorbic acid be added as a preservative to the milk before processing.[21]

Biotin

Introduction. Biotin, another member of the vitamin B complex, was first isolated in 1936 as a growth essential for yeast cells. Previous to this date numerous workers had described factors called by various names but having similar antidermatitis properties. These several factors proved to be identical and are now known as biotin. Investigations have shown that a biotin deficiency can be produced in rats, rabbits and monkeys by feeding a substance called avidin found in raw egg white. Avidin inactivates biotin and is known as an antivitamin.

Biotin deficiency has been recognized in man only when diets have included large amounts of raw egg white. Intestinal synthesis of biotin is common in most animals and probably in man.

[17] Review: Nutr. Rev., *24*:289, 1966.
[18] Herbert, V.: Am. J. Clin. Nutr., *20*:562, 1967.
[19] Review: Nutr. Rev., *24*:289, 1966.

[20] Chung, *et al.*: op. cit. (ref. 14).
[21] Ghitis, J.: Am. J. Clin. Nutr., *18*:452, 1966.

TABLE 8–4. Water-Soluble Vitamins

Vitamin	C		Fractions of the Vitamin B Complex					
	Ascorbic Acid	Thiamine	Riboflavin	Niacin	Pantothenic Acid	Pyridoxine	Folacin Vitamin B12	Biotin
Important food sources	Citrus fruits Strawberries Cantaloupe Tomatoes Sweet peppers Cabbage Potatoes Kale, parsley Turnip greens	Pork Liver Organ meats Whole grains Enriched cereal products Nuts Legumes Potatoes	Liver, milk Meat, eggs Enriched cereal products Green, leafy vegetables	Liver, poultry Meat, fish Whole grains Enriched cereal products Legumes Mushrooms	Liver Organ meats Eggs, peanuts Legumes Mushrooms Salmon, whole grains	Pork Organ meats Legumes, seeds Grains Potatoes Bananas	Liver and other organ meats, milk, eggs Folacin in green leafy vegetables	Liver Organ meats Peanuts Mushrooms
Stability to cooking, drying, light, etc.	Unstable to heat and oxidation, except in acids Destroyed by drying and aging	Unstable to heat and oxidation	Stable to heat in cooking, to acids and oxidation Unstable to light	Stable to heat, light and oxidation, acid and alkali	Unstable to acid, alkali, heat and certain salts	Stable to heat, light and oxidation	Folacin unstable to heat and oxidation	
Function: Essential in	Formation of intercellular substance, cellular oxidation and reduction	Carbohydrate metabolism, coenzyme form cocarboxylase	Carbohydrate, fat and protein metabolism, coenzyme forms FMN and FAD	Carbohydrate, fat and protein metabolism, coenzyme forms NAD and NADP	Carbohydrate, fat and protein metabolism, coenzyme form coenzyme A	Metabolism of amino acids—coenzyme form PALP	Growth, blood formation, choline synthesis amino acid metabolism	Fatty acid synthesis, carboxylation reactions
Deficiency manifest as	Scurvy Sore mouth Sore and bleeding gums Weak-walled capillaries	Beriberi (man) Poor appetite Fatigue Constipation	Eye sensitivity Cheilosis (man)	Pellagra (man) Dermatitis Nervous depression Diarrhea		Convulsions Anemia Renal calculi	Macrocytic anemias, sprue and pernicious anemia	Lassitude Anorexia Depression Anemia
Adult human requirement	Men and women 70 mg.	Men and women 0.4 mg./1000 calories	Men and women 0.6 mg./1000 calories	Niacin equivalent men and women 6.6 mg./1000 calories	Probably 10 mg./day	Probably 1.2-2 mg.	Probably folacin, 0.15 mg. B12, 3-5 mcg.	Probably 150-300 mcg./day

Functions. Biotin plays an essential role as a coenzyme in CO_2 fixation; fatty acid synthesis, for instance, requires a biotin-containing enzyme to form malonyl coenzyme A from acetyl coenzyme A.

The role of biotin in protein and carbohydrate metabolism is less clear, and its relationship to the synthesis of transfer RNA (See Chap. 9) also needs further elucidation.

There is also some evidence that biotin is necessary for the utilization of vitamin B_{12} and that, like folic acid, it participates in one-carbon metabolism.[22]

Biotin deficiency results in lassitude, anorexia, depression, malaise, muscle pain, nausea, anemia, hypercholesterolemia and changes in the electrocardiograph.

Human Requirements. Most American diets contain 150 to 300 mcg. of biotin per day which is entirely adequate for good health.

Food Sources. Few foods have been analyzed for this factor. It is abundant in liver and other organs, in mushrooms and peanuts. Lesser amounts occur in milk, eggs and certain vegetables and fruits. (See Table 6 in Part Four.)

Other B-Complex Factors

Para-aminobenzoic acid (PABA) is a moiety of pteroylmonoglutamic acid (PGA), one of the forms of folic acid, and is no longer considered a vitamin.

Inositol was first considered to be a vitamin in 1940 but there is no evidence today that humans cannot synthesize all that is needed by the body.

Choline and Betaine. The classification of these 2 nitrogenous compounds as vitamins is questioned by some. They are structural components of body cells rather than catalysts. Choline occurs in foods as well as in the body in relatively large amounts and has never been associated with a deficiency disease in man. The body can make choline from methionine, an amino acid, with the aid of vitamin B_{12} and folacin. The action of choline, betaine or methionine in the prevention of "fatty livers" is known as lipotropic (fat moving). Choline

is distributed widely in plant and animal tissues, and a deficiency is not likely in the average diet. Betaine is formed by the oxidation of choline

ANTIVITAMINS OR VITAMIN ANTAGONISTS

Research in the chemical structure of vitamins has led logically to more understanding about their characteristic reactions. Some are destroyed by oxidation or light or are inactivated by reaction with other compounds. Any substance which prevents the absorption or metabolic functioning of a vitamin in the body is called an antivitamin or a vitamin antagonist; avidin is an antagonist to biotin.

One type of antagonist is a compound so similar in chemical structure that it starts to react like the true vitamin but cannot finish the reaction, thus blocking the space where the real vitamin could function. An interesting example of this type of reaction is a folic acid antagonist which has been used clinically in the treatment of malignant growths. The theory is that rapidly dividing cells may need more folic acid than normal cells, and therefore an antagonist might inhibit growth of the abnormal cells. Unfortunately, the folic acid antagonist inhibits growth in normal as well as abnormal cells.

Antibiotics and, possibly, some of the sulfa drugs used in the treatment of infections may be vitamin antagonists. Normally, bacteria in the intestinal tract have the ability to synthesize certain vitamins. When a sulfa drug or an antibiotic is given orally, it may make some of the intestinal bacteria incapable of vitamin synthesis, thus inhibiting growth. Conversely, in other animals antibiotics seem to stimulate growth by changing the balance of the intestinal microorganisms.

STUDY QUESTIONS AND ACTIVITIES

1. From a historical point of view, which deficiency diseases were first recognized as such?

2. List properties and food sources of ascorbic acid. Why is this factor the most difficult to supply in army rations or for arctic expeditions?

---

[22] Bridgers, W. F.: Nutr. Rev., 25:65, 1967.

3. How has the human need for ascorbic acid been studied? What is meant by a state of saturation?

4. How many fractions of the vitamin B complex are recognized today? Which ones are listed in the Recommended Dietary Allowances?

5. Which vitamins of the B complex group function in the release of energy from carbohydrates, fats and proteins? Name the coenzyme forms of each of these vitamins.

6. Name the scientist largely responsible for isolating and synthesizing thiamine.

7. What methods may be used to assess the nutritional status of a person with respect to thiamine?

8. What single food is the best source of riboflavin in the diet?

9. Is it easy to obtain sufficient quantity of thiamine in the diet? Which two common foods are good sources? Will these supply adequate amounts? (See Pattern Dietary in Chap 10.)

10. What is meant by the term "niacin equivalent"?

11. Which vitamins are likely to be reduced in foods under following treatment:

(A) Bottled milk exposed to sunlight
(B) Cabbage kept overnight after shredding
(C) Vegetables to which soda has been added in cooking
(D) Potatoes peeled and allowed to soak 2 to 3 hours before cooking?

12. Which group of vitamins are preventive and curative of macrocytic anemias? Which one is called the "extrinsic factor" and is the one most potent in pernicious anemia?

13. What is meant by an antivitamin, and how is the vitamin activity destroyed or prevented?

SUPPLEMENTARY READING ON WATER-SOLUBLE VITAMINS

Baker, E. M.: Vitamin B_6 requirement for adult men. Am. J. Clin. Nutr., 15:59, 1964.

Beaton, G. H., and McHenry, E. W.: Nutrition—A Comprehensive Treatise. Vol. II, Chaps. 2, 3, and 4. Academic Press, New York, 1964.

Bridgers, W. F.: Present knowledge of biotin. Nutr. Rev., 25:65, 1967.

Chung, A. S. M., et al.: Folic acid, pantothenic acid, and vitamin B_{12} in human dietaries. Am. J. Clin. Nutr., 9:573, 1961.

Food and Nutrition Board, National Research Council: Recommended Dietary Allowances. Publ. 1146, Washington, D. C., 1964.

Horwitt, M. K.: Nutritional Requirements of man, with special reference to riboflavin. Am. J. Clin. Nutr., 18:458, 1966.

Joint FAO/WHO Expert Group: Requirements of vitamin A, thiamine, riboflavine and niacin. FAO Report Series 41, Rome, 1967.

Review: Present knowledge of folacin. Nutr. Rev., 24:289, 1966.

Wilson, T. H.: Intrinsic factor and B_{12} absorption—a problem in cell physiology. Nutr. Rev., 23:33, 1965.

For further references see Bibliography in Part Four.

CHAPTER 9

Digestion, Absorption and Metabolism

Digestive-Absorptive Processes · Metabolism · Catabolism · Anabolism · Disposal of End Products

DIGESTIVE-ABSORPTIVE PROCESSES

Since the organs and the processes of digestion and absorption may have already been studied in anatomy, physiology and chemistry courses, this section will focus primarily on the nutrients which form the substrates, the specific enzymes involved in the hydrolysis reactions and the products that are formed by the digestive process. The mechanisms of absorption will also be discussed. One should remember, however, that foods are eaten in a variety of forms and combinations; cooking and other processing methods may, therefore, begin the breakdown of complex compounds such as starch and collagen (protein) before foods are ingested.

It has been only in recent years with the development of research techniques that the study of digestion, and particularly absorption, has entered a new and exciting phase. The use of the peroral biopsy and the intubation tube[1] to study absorption in humans, and the study of absorption mechanisms using small segments of intestines from animals have added greatly to our present knowledge of digestion and absorption.

Digestion

The two major and interrelated processes of digestion—i.e., the mechanical and the chemical—proceed simultaneously.

[1] Wilson, T. H.: Intestinal Absorption. Phila., W. B. Saunders, 1962.

In the first category are the muscular contractions of the walls of the gastrointestinal tract which move the food in solution (chyme), making contact possible between the food and the digestive enzymes. The second—chemical digestion—is the process of hydrolysis by which carbohydrates, fats and proteins are divided into simpler units which can be absorbed through the walls of the small intestine. Table 9–1 reviews briefly the chemical digestion of carbohydrates, fats and proteins. Each enzyme involved in the process is specific for the substrate, e.g., pepsin (gastric protease) acts only on proteins and is capable of breaking them down only as far as polypeptides.

In addition to the enzymes listed in Table 9–1 there are other chemical substances which affect digestion. The stomach secretes hydrochloric acid (HCl) which (1) activates the gastric protease pepsinogen to pepsin, (2) creates the proper acidity for the digestion of protein, (3) acts as a bacteriocidal agent, and (4) increases the solubility of certain minerals such as iron and calcium. Gastric secretions also contain *mucin* which protects the lining of the stomach from the HCl both by neutralizing the strongly acid contents and by forming a protective covering on the gastric epithelium.

Bile, excreted by the liver into the duodenum, emulsifies the fat, breaking it down into smaller globules to provide a larger surface area so that it can be acted upon more readily by the lipase. Bile,

TABLE 9–1. Digestion of Carbohydrates, Fats and Proteins

Source of Enzyme	Enzyme +	Substrate →	Products

Mouth
  Salivary glands
	Salivary amylase
	  ptyalin
		Starch	→ Dextrins and maltose

Stomach
  Gastric mucosa
	Gastric protease
	  pepsin
	  rennin
		Proteins
		Casein
			→ Polypeptides
			→ Paracasein (insoluble)

	Gastric lipase	Emulsified fat	→ Fatty acids and glycerol

Small Intestine
  Pancreas
	Pancreatic proteases
	  trypsin
	  chymotrypsin
	  carboxypeptidases
		Proteins and
		  Polypeptides
			→ Smaller polypeptides and
			  amino acids

	Pancreatic lipase
	  steapsin
		Fats	→ Mono and diglycerides
			  fatty acids and glycerol

	Pancreatic amylase amylopsin	Starch	→ Maltose

Intestinal mucosa
  Brush border
	Intestinal peptidases
	  aminopeptidase
	  dipeptidase
		Polypeptides
		Dipeptides
			→ Smaller polypeptides and
			  amino acids

	Intestinal disaccharidases
	  sucrase
	  maltase
	  lactase
		Sucrose
		Maltose
		Lactose
			→ Glucose and fructose
			→ Glucose (2 molecules)
			→ Glucose and galactose

TABLE 9–2. Hormones of the Gastrointestinal Tract

Hormone	Stimulus	Action

Gastric mucosa
  Gastrin..................
	Presence of protein derivatives
	  and mechanical distension in
	  the pyloric region.
		Stimulates secretion of HCl by the
		  gastric glands.

Small intestine mucosa
  Enterogastrone.............
	Presence of fats, or acid chyme
	  in the intestine.
		Inhibits gastric secretion and
		  motility.

Secretin...................	Presence of polypeptides and
	  acid chyme in the duodenum.
		Stimulates secretion of very alka-
		  line enzyme-poor fluid from the
		  pancreas.

Pancreozymin..............	Presence of polypeptides and
	  acid chyme in the duodenum.
		Stimulates pancreas to secrete
		  enzyme-rich fluid.

Cholecystokinin.............	Presence of fat in the duodenum.	Stimulates contractions of the gall-
		  bladder, with the expulsion of
		  bile into the duodenum.

Enterocrinin...............	Presence of acid chyme in the
	  duodenum.
		Stimulates secretion by glands in
		  small intestine.

which is slightly alkaline, also neutralizes the acidity of the chyme.

Hormones, which also affect the digestive process, are produced in the mucosa of the gastrointestinal tract. Table 9–2 lists the hormones, their stimuli and the action which they have on the secretion and motility of the gastrointestinal tract.

Absorption

Sites of Absorption

Absorption consists primarily of the transfer of nutrients from the lumen of the small intestine through the intestinal epithelium into the *lamina propria*, where the nutrients enter the blood and lymph ves-

TABLE 9–3. Sites of Absorption of Nutrients
from Gastrointestinal Tract

Nutrient	Site in Small Intestine
Glucose	Lower duodenum Upper jejunum
Amino Acids.........	Lower duodenum Jejunum
Fats...............	Lower duodenum Upper jejunum
Iron...............	Duodenum
Calcium.............	Duodenum
Sucrose.............	Lower jejunum Ileum
Lactose.............	Jejunum Upper ileum
Maltose.............	Jejunum Upper ileum
Vitamin D..........	(?) Ileum
Vitamin B₁₂	Ileum

sels. Although limited amounts of water, alcohol, simple salts and glucose are absorbed through the gastric mucosa, the small intestine is by far the more important organ for absorption.

Specifically, the most active absorptive area in the small intestine is the lower part of the duodenum and the first part of the jejunum.[2] (See Table 9–3.)

[2] Davenport, H. W.: Physiology of the Digestive Tract. Chicago, Year Book Publishers, 1961.

Structure of Intestinal Wall. The inner lining, or mucosa, of the small intestine is gathered up into folds and covered by a mass of fingerlike projections (villi) which increase its surface area tremendously (Fig. 9–1). With the development of the electron microscope and biopsy methods, the villi can now be studied in much greater detail. The epithelial cells which cover them have a so-called brush border consisting of thousands of tiny rodlets, or *microvilli,* which further increase the surface area available for absorption. A triple-layered membrane, made up of two layers of protein with a layer of fat in between, defines the outside edge of the microvilli. The single layer of epithelial cells lining the lumen rests on a connective tissue structure (lamina propria) which contains blood and lymph vessels. See schematic drawing, Figure 9–2.

For normal absorption to occur the substrate—for instance, glucose—must enter the intestinal epithelial cell and make its way across the cell where it sometimes undergoes a chemical change. Then the substrate, glucose in this case, not only must leave on the opposite side of the cell but must pass through two additional layers of tissue before it is finally within a blood vessel. If the substrate were a fat-soluble

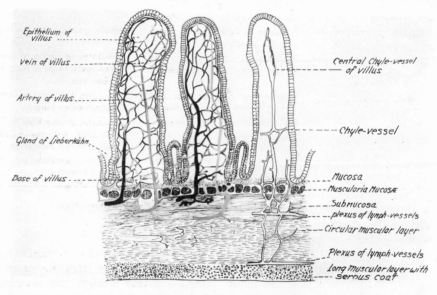

FIG. 9–1. Diagrammatic drawing (after F. P. Mall) showing the great extension of absorbing surface of the intestinal lining due to projecting villi.

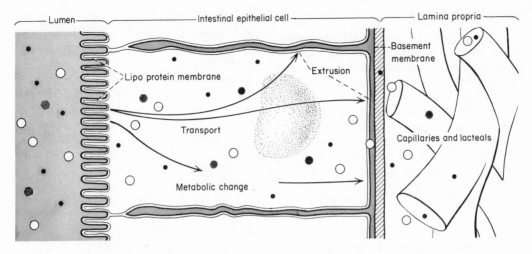

FIG. 9–2. Diagrammatic drawing, showing the process of absorption of nutrients from the lumen through the intestinal epithelial cell into the blood and lymph vessels of the lamina propria. (Ingelfinger, F. J.: Gastrointestinal Absorption. Nutrition Today, 2:3, 1967)

nutrient such as a long-chain monoglyceride, the process would be similar, except that it would enter a lacteal or lymph vessel rather than a blood capillary. Figure 9–2 schematically represents nutrients in the process of absorption.

Mechanisms of Absorption

Several current theories explain the various mechanisms used to accomplish the process of intestinal absorption.[3] Since the lipoprotein membrane of the microvilli makes the cell relatively impervious to water and water-soluble substances, there is a need to explain how large amounts of water constantly enter and leave the cell.

Pores. It is postulated that this bulk-flow of water is permitted by the presence of so-called pores, or channels, throughout the epithelium. These pores are just large enough to allow water, certain electrolytes and very small water-soluble molecules to enter the cell.

Carriers. Larger molecules are thought to enter the cell by the action of carriers. These carriers, located in the lipoprotein membrane, can attach themselves to a water-soluble compound and temporarily render it fat-soluble and, thereby, ferry it across the lipid layer of the membrane.

Some carriers may be involved with two types of compounds such as glucose and galactose. These sugars then compete for the available carriers. The number of carriers are also probably limited, and hence carrier transport will slow down or cease as vehicles become unavailable. This passive carrier-mediated diffusion continues only until there is a balance between the solutes in the cell and those in the lumen.

Pumps. In order to achieve continued absorption when there is a greater concentration in the cell or in the blood than in the lumen, a nutrient must be actively transported or pumped across the membrane barrier. These "pumps" require energy to operate but they do permit a very large and rapid transfer into the body of such nutrients as glucose, galactose, many amino acids, sodium and probably calcium, iron and vitamin B_{12}.

Pinocytosis, which is an amoebalike action of the epithelial cell membrane whereby a food particle or molecule is encompassed and thus brought into the cell, accounts for the absorption of large molecules such as those of a protein or a fat.

The roles which these mechanisms play in the absorption of monosaccharides, glycerides, fatty acids and amino acids will be briefly discussed.

[3] Ingelfinger, F. J.: Nutrition Today, 2:2, 1967.

Carbohydrates

Carbohydrates (disaccharides) are hydrolyzed to monosaccharides in the process of absorption by the disaccharidases in the brush border of the epithelial cell. The very large quantities of the three monosaccharides, glucose, galactose and fructose, which the body is able to absorb has called for an explanation over and above the fact that they are water-soluble. Since they are larger molecules than would be able to pass through the so-called pores, a carrier mechanism has been suggested for all three. In addition, glucose and galactose, which probably compete for the same carriers, may also be pumped across the intestinal barrier. Since the latter mechanism is active transport, which does not depend on the concentration of the sugar in the blood being less than in the intestines but actually permits the sugar to go from a lower to a higher concentration, it requires energy. This energy in turn is supplied by the metabolism of the glucose within the cell. The transfer of sodium and hence of fluid also depends on the metabolism of glucose. It is interesting to note that all the intestinal disaccharidases have reached their normal activity at the end of fetal life and hence the normal infant is able to absorb the various sugars.[4]

Glucose, galactose and fructose are transported from the capillaries to larger blood vessels and finally to the portal vein, which carries them to the liver where galactose and fructose are converted to glucose. From the liver glucose is transported to the tissues as needed or converted into glycogen for storage.

Fats

Fats are presented for absorption in the form of monoglycerides, fatty acids and glycerol. Bile salts and phospholipids aid in their passage into the intestinal membrane cell. Once inside the mucosal cell, the monoglycerides and long-chain fatty acids are recombined into triglycerides and then, with the assistance of beta-lipoprotein, the fat enters the lacteals. It is transported by the lymph vessels to the thoracic duct, which empties into the left subclavian vein. Here the triglycerides in the form of chylomicrons enter the blood stream slowly and are carried to the liver and adipose tissue for metabolism and storage. Very hard fats, those with completely saturated long-chain fatty acids, are absorbed less readily than softer fats. Other fat-soluble substances such as cholesterol and vitamins A, D, E, and K are absorbed with the triglycerides.[5]

Short-chain and medium-chain fatty acids (see Chap. 3) do not recombine as triglycerides but leave the mucosal cell as free fatty acids and glycerol. As such they are absorbed directly into the blood capillaries in the villi and carried by the portal vein to the liver. Here they may be metabolized or carried to the tissues for metabolism. Fats which have been specially processed to produce only the medium-chain fatty acids can be used for patients when normal fat absorption is impaired (see Chap. 27).

Proteins

Proteins are absorbed chiefly as amino acids by much the same route as monosaccharides are transported, primarily by specific carriers and by the so-called pump mechanisms. Some protein may also be absorbed as peptides[6] or even as polypeptides. The latter may account for certain allergic reactions to specific food proteins.[7] Although most amino acids enter the capillaries and are carried to the liver by the portal vein, some may remain in the epithelial cell to be used in the synthesis of intestinal enzymes and new cells. This endogenous protein from digestive enzymes and cells should be considered along with dietary protein when determining the total amount of amino acids available to the body at any given time. Endogenous protein when degraded in the gastrointestinal tract may contribute to maintaining a constant amino acid supply and, hence, temporarily delay a specific amino acid deficiency.[8]

[4] Mansford, K. R. L.: Proc. Nutr. Soc., *26*:27, 1967.

[5] Mead, J. F.: Nutr. Rev., *24*:33, 1966.
[6] Fisher, R. B.: Proc. Nutr. Soc., *26*:23, 1967
[7] Ingelfinger, F. J.: *op. cit.*
[8] Nassett, E. S.: J.A.M.A., *164*:172, 1957.

Recent studies indicate that the absorption of amino acids through the intestinal mucosa stimulates the release of insulin. Considering that insulin facilitates the movement of amino acids from the capillaries into muscle cells and also stimulates protein synthesis,[9] this new discovery illustrates further the elaborate system of signals and mechanisms by which the human body functions.

Other Nutrients

Simultaneously with the absorption of amino acids, monosaccharides, fatty acids, and monoglycerides, the vitamins, minerals, and fluids are also being absorbed through the intestinal mucosa. About 8 liters of fluid from the body pass back and forth across the membrane of the gut each day to keep the nutrients in solution. This fluid is being continuously reabsorbed. If diarrhea occurs, this fluid is lost to the body, resulting in dehydration and poor absorption.

METABOLISM

When the nutrients in the blood stream pass through the cellular membranes of the body, they enter into the metabolic processes of the cell. Metabolism can be defined as the process by which the cells convert the nutrients from food into useful energy and at the same time create new molecules for tissue synthesis and other vital compounds. The conversion of nutrients into useful energy is called catabolism and the synthesis of new molecules is called anabolism. Since anabolic processes depend on energy from catabolic processes, both proceed simultaneously.

Catabolism

In this metabolic pathway energy is released from the molecules of food—glucose, fatty acids, glycerol and amino acids —through a complex sequence of stepwise chemical enzymatic reactions which take place in the cytoplasmic matrix and the mitochondria of the cell. The energy released in the cell as a result of oxidation is conserved as chemical energy by the compound adenosine triphosphate (ATP). Chemical energy is carried by ATP from the energy-yielding oxidation of food molecules to those processes or reactions of the cell which require it. ATP contains three phosphate radicals, and ADP (adenosine diphosphate) contains two phosphate radicals. It is the change from ADP to ATP that conserves the energy of oxidation. Thus, ATP is the charged form of the energy-transporting system and ADP the discharged form. The oxidation of the food molecules changes the ADP to ATP. Enzymes catalyze the many stepwise chemical reactions that charge and discharge the ATP-ADP system.[10]

The entrance of glucose into the cell is facilitated by insulin. In the cell, glucose is activated by ATP and is broken down in a series of reactions to pyruvate. This process is known as glycolysis. As previously mentioned, cellular enzymes, some of which contain vitamins, are required to catalyze these reactions. One molecule of glucose yields two molecules of pyruvate and a small amount of energy.

In the presence of oxygen pyruvate can be converted to the two-carbon compound acetyl CoA, which is a key substance in the metabolism not only of glucose but also, as will be shown, of fatty acids and certain amino acids. Thiamine is required as part of the coenzyme in this reaction. Also involved in the conversion of pyruvate to acetyl CoA is an enzyme containing the vitamin pantothenic acid (Coenzyme A). Acetyl CoA combines with oxaloacetate to form citrate and enters the oxidative cycle (Citric Acid, or Krebs Cycle) where the greatest amount of the potential energy from the food is released. In this cycle carbon dioxide and water are produced when energy is released (ADP-ATP) and oxaloacetate is regenerated for continuous cycle operation. Figure 9–3 illustrates schematically this pathway of glucose metabolism. The intermediary steps in this cycle require, as in glycolysis, vitamin-containing enzymes—in this case, riboflavin and niacin (Chap. 8).

The potential energy in fat is also released in a similar catabolic pathway. The glycerol of fat is converted to pyruvate and

[9] Nutr. Rev., 25:41, 1967.

[10] Lehninger, A. L.: Bioenergetics. New York, W. A. Benjamin, 1965.

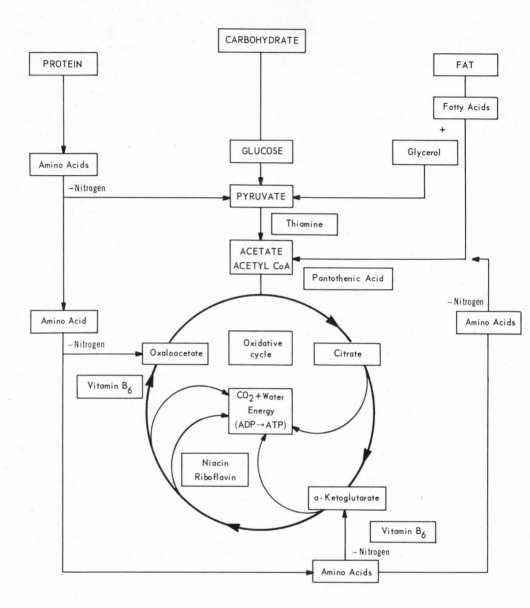

Fig. 9–3. Catabolic pathway of metabolism.

follows the glucose pathway (Fig. 9–3). Through a series of complex stepwise reactions also involving coenzyme A, fatty acids are broken down into acetate or acetyl CoA. In the presence of normal glucose metabolism, the acetate formed from fatty acids enters the oxidative cycle and follows the same pathway as the acetate from glucose. The two-carbon compound acetate is also a key substance in the synthesis of ketone bodies (See Chap. 22) and cholesterol (see Chaps. 3 and 23).

About 50 per cent of the protein of the diet can enter the metabolic pathways which yield energy. After the removal of nitrogen (deamination) certain of the amino acids enter directly into the oxidative cycle while others contribute to the cycle through pyruvate or acetate (Fig. 9–3). Thus, like carbohydrate and fat, the potential energy in amino acids can be released in the oxidative cycle.

Anabolism

In the anabolic pathways of the cell the amino acids are utilized in the synthesis of proteins. This applies not only to the synthesis of new cells but also to the maintenance of already formed cells in tissues and organs. There is a continuous turnover of the amino acids in the cell, with amino acids available from dietary protein to replace similar amino acids being discarded. Not only single amino acids are replaced in anabolic activities; cells also are constantly being renewed. The red blood cell, for instance, is estimated to have a "life" of approximately 120 days. The maintenance of this state of dynamic equilibrium, which is essential for health, is the reason why protein must be included in the diet with each meal. When new tissue is being synthesized, the demand for protein is even greater—for example, the recommendation of protein per Kg. for an infant is 2 to 3 times greater than that for the adult. It is important to recognize that protein synthesis also requires energy, vitamin-containing enzymes, particularly vitamin B_6, and minerals.

Protein Synthesis—DNA-RNA Genetic Control. The ability to produce the many different kinds of proteins needed by the body is determined by the pattern for protein synthesis which is carried in the DNA (deoxyribonucleic acid) of the cell's nucleus. Since this pattern is genetically determined, the various diseases which result from enzyme deficiencies are often referred to as "inborn errors of metabolism" (Chap. 34). For each protein a set of directions is carried on a specific segment, a gene, of the very long DNA molecule. The DNA itself does not leave the nucleus but its "message" is carried by RNA (ribonucleic acid) to the cytoplasm of the cell where the protein is synthesized. Each of these messenger-RNA's contains all the directions for one kind of protein— and there are many different kinds of proteins. Another type of RNA, transfer-RNA, is able to recognize a specific amino acid, pick it up and transfer it to the messenger-RNA which acts as an assembly line in attaching all the amino acids in their proper sequence to form the specific protein needed. Since the cells of the body are constantly manufacturing a wide variety of proteins, each of which must have available all the amino acids it requires for synthesis, the need of the body for a regular supply of the essential amino acids becomes obvious.

Other Anabolic Processes. Glycogen may be synthesized from glucose (glycogenesis) in liver or muscle cells to be available when needed. This is a limited but essential supply of energy when compared with the potential in adipose tissue. Glucose at the pyruvate level with the addition of nitrogen may be utilized to synthesize a nonessential amino acid (Fig. 9–4).

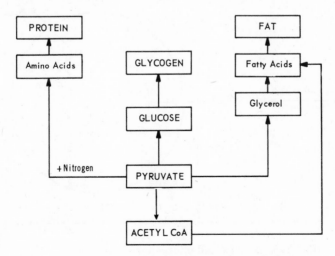

Fig. 9–4. Anabolic pathway of metabolism.

Various lipid compounds are also synthesized by the cells of the body. The fatty acids are synthesized by combining acetate molecules in the numbers which are needed to make up a specific fatty acid. Stearic acid, which contains 18 carbon atoms, uses 9 molecules of acetate. Biotin, a B vitamin, is required for this synthesis. Adipose tissue contains fatty acids synthesized by this method as well as fatty acids obtained directly from food sources. This tissue is the major way in which the body stores reserve energy. Phospholipids also contain fatty acids made available through the same pathways. The glycerol required by both these substances may be synthesized from pyruvate.

The Body's Use of Energy

In the constant round of catabolism and anabolism within the cell, chemical energy is used to perform work. Much chemical energy is converted to mechanical energy for the work performed by the musculature of the body. When a nerve impulse is transmitted, chemical energy is transformed into electrical energy. Chemical energy as such is used for the synthesis of new compounds. All chemical energy produced in the body is eventually converted to heat energy either directly from chemical reactions or indirectly from work energy. The heat energy is used to maintain body temperature, and when more heat than necessary is produced for this purpose, the body rids itself of such by way of the skin, the lungs and the excreta.

DISPOSAL OF END PRODUCTS OF METABOLISM

As the blood transports nutrients to support cellular metabolism, it also participates at the same time in the disposal of the end products of metabolism. The carbon dioxide formed in the oxidative cycle is transported to the lungs where it is lost to the body in the expired air. The nitrogen, from amino acids which have undergone deamination, is synthesized into urea in the liver and is excreted by the kidney in urine together with the water formed in cellular metabolism. Water and some other nutrients may also be lost to the body through the skin and lungs.

SUMMARY OF DIGESTION, ABSORPTION AND METABOLISM

Figure 9–5 summarizes the sequence of processes food undergoes to support the cellular processes we know as growth, maintenance and repair, as well as to supply the chemical energy required for these processes. The ingestion of food followed by the digestive-absorptive processes are basic to the support of the body's metabolic processes.

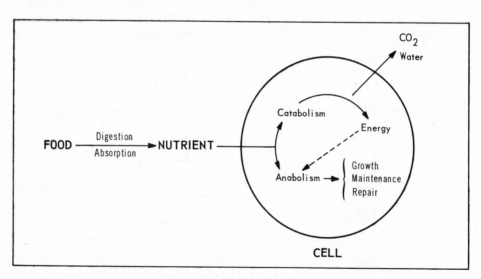

FIG. 9–5. How the cell utilizes nutrients from food.

STUDY QUESTIONS AND ACTIVITIES

1. What is an enzyme? Where are enzymes found in the body?

2. What is a substrate?

3. How does the structure of the mucosal cell in the gastrointestinal tract aid in absorption?

4. Describe the suggested mechanisms for absorption in the gastrointestinal tract.

5. How are short-chain fatty acids absorbed? Long-chain fatty acids?

6. Where in the gastrointestinal tract does most of the absorption take place? Exceptions?

7. What is the meaning of the word catabolism? Of anabolism?

8. What is the relationship between enzymes and vitamins?

9. What happens to ingested carbohydrate, fat, or protein if it is more than the body can use for energy at that time?

10. What are the sources of fat in adipose tissue?

11. Explain the synthesis of protein as controlled by the genetic code. What is meant by an "inborn error of metabolism"?

12. Which vitamins are essential for the catabolic metabolism of carbohydrate? Of fatty acid synthesis? Of protein synthesis?

SUPPLEMENTARY READINGS ON DIGESTION, ABSORPTION AND METABOLISM

Danielsson, H.: Influence of bile acids on digestion and absorption of lipids. Am. J. Clin. Nutr., *12*:214, 1963.

Ingelfinger, F. J.: Gastrointestinal absorption. Nutrition Today, *2*:2. 1967.

Jukes, T. H.: Present status of the amino acid code. J. Am. Dietet. A., *45*:517, 1964.

Kimber, D. C., *et al.*: Anatomy and Physiology. Chaps. 20, 21. New York, Macmillan, 1966.

Mead, J. F.: Present knowledge of fat. Nutr. Rev., *24*:33, 1966.

Review: Carbohydrate digestion and absorption. Nutr. Rev., *21*:279, 1963.

————: Factors affecting amino acid absorption. Nutr. Rev., *24*:332, 1966.

————: Metabolic interrelationships of dietary carbohydrate and fat. Nutr. Rev., *22*:216, 1964.

————: The role of carbohydrates in the diet. Nutr. Rev., *22*:102, 1964.

For further references see Bibliography in Part Four.

CHAPTER 10

Food to Meet Recommended Dietary Allowances

Estimation of Human Dietary Needs • Interpretation and Use of Recommended Dietary Allowances • A Daily Food Guide • Pattern Dietary • Suggested Menus • Foods Fortified or Enriched • Economy Hints • Food Fads

In preceding chapters about the various nutrients needed for health, the Recommended Dietary Allowances have been referred to frequently. The establishment of a yardstick of good nutrition by which to measure progress has long been recognized by scientists as desirable. The foods used to supply the nutrients recommended may vary with preference, availability and cost.

ESTIMATION OF HUMAN DIETARY NEEDS

The idea of setting up standards for planning family meals and food supplies is not new. However, some early estimates were based on what people actually were eating, not on what they needed.

Even after needs were recognized, many years elapsed before methods were developed for quantitative assays. Decades of labor by thousands of research workers have made possible the present-day dietary recommendations.

In 1933 some attempts were made to define human requirements for specific nutrients, first by the British Medical Association and later by Stiebeling and co-workers in the United States Department of Agriculture. The standards formulated by the League of Nations Health Committee in 1935 were the first to represent group opinion and were based on the limited data then available.

When the Food and Nutrition Board was appointed by the National Research Council in 1940, it undertook as one of its most important projects the establishment of a set of figures for human requirements

in terms of specific nutrients. As a result of long and careful consideration, Recommended Dietary Allowances (RDA) were first published in 1943. Since then, they have been revised several times as new research data became available. The objectives are stated as follows in the latest revision[1]:

The allowances are intended to serve as goals toward which to aim in planning food supplies and as guides for the interpretation of food consumption records of groups of people. Actual nutritional status of groups of people or individuals must be judged on the basis of physical, biochemical, and clinical observations combined with observations on food or nutrient intakes. If the recommended allowances are used as reference standards for interpreting records of food consumption, it should not be assumed that food practices are necessarily poor or that malnutrition exists because the recommendations are not completely met. . . .

The allowances recommended are those which, in the opinion of the Food and Nutrition Board, will maintain good nutrition in essentially all healthy persons in the United States under current conditions of living. . . .

The allowances are designed to afford a margin of sufficiency above average physiological requirements to cover variations among essentially all individuals in the general population. They provide a buffer against the increased needs during common stresses and permit full realization of growth and reproductive potential; but they are not to be considered adequate to meet additional requirements of

[1] Recommended Dietary Allowances. National Research Council. Pub. No. 1146. pp. v and vi. Washington, D. C., 1964.

TABLE 10—1. Food and Nutrition Board, National Academy of Sciences-National Research Council
Recommended Daily Dietary Allowances,* Revised 1964
Designed for the Maintenance of Good Nutrition of
Practically All Healthy Persons in the U. S. A.

(Allowances are intended for persons normally active in a temperate climate)

Age† (Yrs.)	Weight Kg.	Weight (Lbs.)	Height Cm.	Height (In.)	Calories‡	Prot. (Gm.)	Calc. (Gm.)	Iron (Mg.)	Vit. A (I.U.)	Thiamine (Mg.)	Riboflavin (Mg.)	Niacin (Mg. Equiv.§)	Ascorbic Acid (Mg.)	Vit. D (I.U.)
Men 18–35	70	(154)	175	(69)	2,900	70	0.8	10	5,000	1.2	1.7	19	70	...
35–55	70	(154)	175	(69)	2,600	70	0.8	10	5,000	1.0	1.6	17	70	...
55–75	70	(154)	175	(69)	2,200	70	0.8	10	5,000	0.9	1.3	15	70	...
Women 18–35	58	(128)	163	(64)	2,100	58	0.8	15	5,000	0.8	1.3	14	70	...
35–55	58	(128)	163	(64)	1,900	58	0.8	15	5,000	0.8	1.2	13	70	...
55–75	58	(128)	163	(64)	1,600	58	0.8	10	5,000	0.8	1.2	13	70	...
Pregnant (2nd and 3rd trimester)					+200	+20	+0.5	+5	+1,000	+0.2	+0.3	+3	+30	400
Lactating					+1,000	+40	+0.5	+5	+3,000	+0.4	+0.6	+7	+30	400
Infants‖ 0–1	8	(18)			Kg. × 115 ±15	Kg. × 2.5 ±0.5	0.7	Kg. × 1.0	1,500	0.4	0.6	6	30	400
Children 1–3	13	(29)	87	(34)	1,300	32	0.8	8	2,000	0.5	0.8	9	40	400
3–6	18	(40)	107	(42)	1,600	40	0.8	10	2,500	0.6	1.0	11	50	400
6–9	24	(53)	124	(49)	2,100	52	0.8	12	3,500	0.8	1.3	14	60	400
Boys 9–12	33	(72)	140	(55)	2,400	60	1.1	15	4,500	1.0	1.4	16	70	400
12–15	45	(98)	156	(61)	3,000	75	1.4	15	5,000	1.2	1.8	20	80	400
15–18	61	(134)	172	(68)	3,400	83	1.4	15	5,000	1.4	2.0	22	80	400
Girls 9–12	33	(72)	140	(55)	2,200	55	1.1	15	4,500	0.9	1.3	15	80	400
12–15	47	(103)	158	(62)	2,500	62	1.3	15	5,000	1.0	1.5	17	80	400
15–18	53	(117)	163	(64)	2,300	58	1.3	15	5,000	0.9	1.3	15	70	400

*The allowance levels are intended to cover individual variations among most normal persons as they live in the United States under usual environmental stresses. The recommended allowances can be attained with a variety of common foods, providing other nutrients for which human requirements have been less well defined. See text for more detailed discussion of allowances and of nutrients not tabulated.

†Entries on lines for age range 18–35 years represent the 25-year age. All other entries represent allowances for the midpoint of the specified age periods, i.e., line for children 1–3 is for age 2 years (24 months); 3–6 is for age 4½ years (54 months), etc.

‡Table 5-4, Chapter 5, shows the calorie adjustment to be made for weight and age of men and women.

§Niacin equivalents include dietary sources of the preformed vitamin and the precursor, tryptophan; 60 mg. of tryptophan represents 1 mg. of niacin.

‖The calorie and protein allowances per Kg. for infants are considered to decrease progressively from birth. Allowances for calcium, thiamine, riboflavin and niacin increase proportionately with calories to the maximum values shown.

(Food & Nutrition Board Pub. 1146, National Research Council.)

persons depleted by disease or traumatic stresses. On the other hand, the allowances are generous with respect to temporary emergency feeding of large groups under conditions of limited food supply and physical disaster.

The margin of sufficiency above normal physiological requirements is different for each nutrient because of differences in the body storage capacity, in the range of individual requirements, in the precision of assessing requirements, and in the possible hazard of excessive intake of certain nutrients.

Patterns of food consumption and food supplies in the United States permit ready adaptation to and compliance with the recommended allowances.

Many writers, teachers of nutrition and especially advertising copy writers, tend to misinterpret the RDA and the purposes expressed in the preceding quotation. One must be cautious in the use of these figures. It is wrong to translate a failure to achieve the goals of the RDA into terms of malnutrition, without knowledge of the nutritional status of the people under investigation. A study of the nutritional status of groups in the United States[2] gives valuable information of this kind and is an example of appropriate use of the RDA.

The British and the Canadian committees working independently arrived at somewhat lower figures for certain nutrients than the United States Food and Nutrition Board and a slightly different philosophy of interpretation. Thus, the British recommendations are believed to be sufficient to maintain good nutrition for the average individual rather than "for essentially all healthy persons" as in the U. S. The Canadian standard represents a minimum for each nutrient or a probable physiologic requirement below which maintenance of health could not be assumed.

Several other countries also have established appropriate nutrition goals in attempts to improve national food habits.

The R.D.A. (See Table 10–1) as adopted by the U. S. Food and Nutrition Board are expressed in nutrients rather than specific foods because these goals can be

---

[2] Morgan, A. F.: Nutritional Status U.S.A. Cal. Agr. Exp. Station Bull. 769. Berkeley, 1959.

attained from a variety of different food patterns. The sample menus, Tables 10–3 and 10–4, show two patterns of eating which approximate the recommended allowances. Many cultural patterns exist in the United States and other countries, and it would be enlightening for students from other cultures to see how well their dietary pattern could serve to provide the nutrients recommended and what minor changes might be needed for improvement. (See Chap. 16.)

INTERPRETATION AND USE OF RECOMMENDED DIETARY ALLOWANCES

Caloric Allowance

The body requires food energy for basal metabolism, synthesis and function of body tissues and for growth and physical activity. Caloric allowances should be sufficient to maintain body weight or rate of growth at levels best for health and well-being. Energy needs vary greatly with the size and activity of the person. Thus it was necessary to adopt the device of using a "reference" man (wt. 70 Kg. or 154 lb.) and a "reference" woman (wt. 58 Kg. or 128 lb.) with three different age groupings. They are presumed to live in an environment with a mean temperature of 20° C. (70° F.). They are considered to be moderately active physically, but caloric allowances are somewhat lower than previous estimates, to fit modern American living patterns.

Adjustment must be made when individuals or population groups differ from the size and activity pattern defined above. A more detailed table of adjustments for age and size is given in Table 5–4. Adjustment of caloric needs to activities is not simple. Dictates of appetite and maintenance of body weight help. For extreme degrees of activity such as heavy physical work, the allowance may be increased as much as 50 per cent; for sedentary people it may be reduced by 25 per cent. For example, a large teen-age boy, active in athletics, may require 3,600 calories, whereas his grandmother, aged 70, cannot use more than 1,200 calories (⅓ as many) without gaining weight. (See Table 5–1.)

Recommended Allowances for Other Nutrients

The specific nutrients included in the 1964 RDA and the quantities of each for the several categories of persons were based upon the best consensus of authorities at the time the table was published. The next edition of the RDA will probably include some additional vitamins but figures are not available at the date of this publication. Other nutrients not listed in the tabulation are apt to be present in adequate amounts in the usual diet, or they are trace elements or vitamins for which there are insufficient data to serve as a basis for recommendations at this time. (See Chaps. 6, 7 and 8.)

The allowances of nutrients are given for the age and sex groups previously mentioned. Attention is called to the calcium and iron figures which are higher proportionally for growing boys and girls than for adults; the B vitamin recommendations are proportional to caloric needs. Of course, some adjustments may need to be made for unusual situations, but, in general, less adjustment is necessary for specific nutrients than for calories; the margins provided take care of ordinary variations.

The allowances for children are listed separately for the sexes after age 9 years, when levels of activity are apt to differ. Allowances are based on needs for the middle years in each age group and for normal activity and weights as given in the table.

The recommended allowance values in the table are for nutrients in foods as consumed and do not take into consideration prior losses in storage, cooking and serving. Provision should be made for these losses in planning practical dietaries. The allowances do provide for incomplete availability or absorption of nutrients such as iron and carotene.

When the table of allowances is used to calculate the needs of population groups, the total estimate should take into account the composition of the population, i.e., the age and sex categories. Emergency conditions may necessitate some modification in the interpretation of recommendations. The liberal margins of safety desirable in normal times may become untenable when whole nations are starving. It then becomes desirable to raise the food allowances of as many people as possible to maintenance levels. Rationing at such times should give special attention to the most vulnerable groups.

Personal Eating Habits Must be Considered

It is possible to obtain the recommended dietary allowance of nutrients in many different diet patterns because of the wide variety of foods yielding similar nutrients. Anyone attempting to evaluate or teach nutrition should be conscious of this fact and avoid any tendency to use stereotyped diet yardsticks for judging individual diets.

If a patient's calcium intake is being estimated and only his milk intake is scrutinized, an entirely erroneous evaluation may be made. It is possible for some people to get enough calcium from the daily use of cheese, fish, legumes and leafy vegetables, even though the more usual pattern would be from the use of simple milk. Thus, although nutrition guides such as the Four Food Groups are valuable, their limitations when applied to an individual must be recognized.

The manner in which foods are stored or prepared may alter nutritive values. Table I in Part Four gives the average values for nutrients in most foods. Averages, however, do not tell, for example, that half of the ascorbic acid in potatoes is lost after several months' storage and that an additional amount is lost in cooking and reheating. Other vitamins are more stable than ascorbic acid, and nutrients such as protein and minerals are stable to cooking. Soluble minerals in vegetables may be lost in cooking water. Another example: a zealous mother who carefully heats the orange juice or dilutes it with boiling water because she has been told to feed her baby only warm food may be giving her infant the recommended daily serving of orange juice but not of ascorbic acid. (See Chap. 13.)

Food values for prepared dishes are based on standard recipes, but people do not always use standard recipes. Obvi-

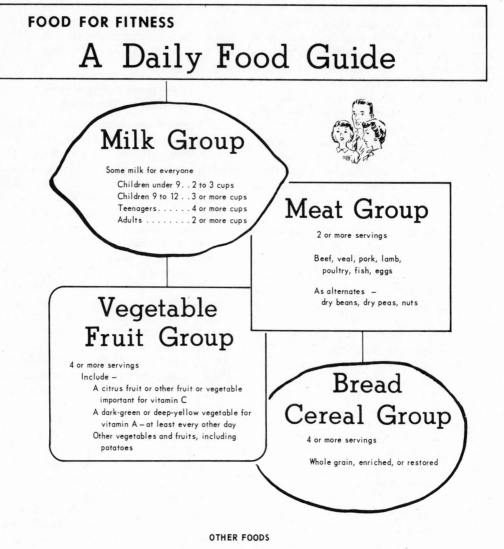

FIG. 10–1. (Modified from Leaflet 424, Institute of Home Economics, U.S.D.A., Washington, D. C.)

TABLE 10–2. Evaluation of a Pattern Dietary for Its Nutritive Content[1]

Food Group	Amt. in Gm.	Household Measure	Calories	Protein Gm.	Fat Gm.	Carbohydrate Gm.	Minerals Calcium Mg.	Iron Mg.	Vitamins A I.U.	Thiamine Mg.	Riboflavin Mg.	Niacin Mg.	Ascorbic Acid Mg.
Milk or equivalent[2]	488	2 c. (1 pint)	320	17	17	24	576	.2	700	.16	.84	.3	5
Egg	50	1 medium	81	7	6	..	27	1.2	590	.05	.15	Tr.	..
Meat, fish or fowl[3]	120	4 ozs., cooked	376	30	31	..	13	3.3	280	.14	.23	6.1	..
Vegetables:													
Potato, cooked	100	1 medium	65	2	..	15	6	.5	..	.09	.03	1.2	16
Deep green or yellow, cooked[4]	75	1/2 c.	27	2	..	6	45	.8	4,700	.05	.10	.5	25
Other, raw or cooked[5]	75	1/2 c.	45	2	..	10	18	.8	300	.08	.06	.6	12
Fruits:													
Citrus[6]	100	1 serving	43	1	..	10	11	.2	140	.06	.02	.3	43
Other[7]	100	1 serving	85	..	..	22	10	.8	365	.03	.04	.5	4
Bread, white, enriched	70	3 slices	189	6	2	35	59	1.7	..	.17	.15	1.7	..
Cereal, whole grain or enriched[8]	130 30	2/3 c. cooked or 1 oz. dry	89	3	1	18	12	.9	..	.08	.03	.7	..
Butter or margarine	14	1 tablespoon	100	..	11	..	3	..	460	..	..	..	..
Totals			1,420	70	68	140	780	10.4	7,535	.91	1.65	11.9[9]	105
Compare with recommended allowances[10]												Niacin Equiv.	
Moderately active man (70 Kg., 18–35 yrs. old)			2,900	70	..	..	800	10.0	5,000	1.20	1.70	19	70
Moderately active woman (58 Kg., 18–35 yrs. old)			2,100	58	..	..	800	15.0	5,000	0.80	1.30	14	70

[1] Calculations from Composition of Foods. Handbook No. 8. U. S. Department of Agriculture, Rev. 1963.
[2] Milk equivalents means evaporated milk and dried milk in amounts equivalent to fluid milk in nutritive content; cheese, if water-soluble minerals and vitamins have not been lost in whey; and food items made with milk.
[3] Evaluation based on the use of 600 Gm. of beef (chuck, cooked), 150 Gm. of pork (medium fat, roasted), 150 Gm. of chicken (roaster, cooked, roasted) and 100 Gm. of fish (halibut, cooked, broiled).
[4] Evaluation based on figures for cooked broccoli, carrots, spinach and squash (all varieties).
[5] Evaluation based on figures for raw tomatoes and lettuce, and cooked peas, beets, lima beans, and fresh corn.
[6] Evaluation based on figures for whole orange and grapefruit, and orange and grapefruit juices.
[7] Evaluation based on figures for banana, apple, unsweetened cooked prunes and sweetened canned peaches.
[8] Evaluation based on figures for shredded wheat biscuit and oatmeal.
[9] The average diet in the United States, which contains a generous amount of protein, provides enough tryptophan to increase the niacin value by about a third.
[10] From the National Research Council Recommended Dietary Allowances, revised 1964.

ously, a fish chowder made with salt pork and heavy cream will have a higher calorie and fat value per serving than a chowder made with diluted evaporated or dried skim milk.

The popularity of between-meal snacks picked from lunch counters or vending machines has created a change in eating patterns. The contribution made by snacks to the total diet should be taken into account. Sometimes the snack adds unneeded calories for the overweight person or it may be merely a refreshing pick-up. Thus, the nurse or the nutritionist must discover not only what and how much a person eats, but when and how it was prepared, if possible. Otherwise, misleading evaluations may be made.

A DAILY FOOD GUIDE

The recommended allowances for nutrients for most people can be obtained from a well chosen variety of ordinary foods including those in our markets which are commonly fortified or enriched with vitamins and minerals. The Daily Food Guide[3] (Fig. 10–1), prepared by nutritionists in the U.S.D.A., presents one way to select food. With this aid almost anyone can get the nutrients needed from everyday foods.

Most foods contain more than one nutrient, but no single food contains all the nutrients in the amount we need. The Daily Food Guide suggests the kinds that together supply nutrients in the amounts needed. In using the Guide one selects the main part of his diet from the four broad food groups. To this one adds other foods as desired to make meals appealing and satisfying. The additional foods should add enough calories to meet energy needs, which will vary widely for different members of the family.

PATTERN DIETARY

The accompanying pattern dietary planned according to the Daily Food Guide provides only about 1,400 calories—less than needed by an active person—but meets or approaches the recommended al-

lowances for all nutrients for an adult. Supplementary foods such as extra milk for children will help meet the calcium level recommended for them. In general, the foods added to meet caloric needs of individuals will provide additional nutrients as well as contribute to taste and satisfaction of meals.

The iron provided in the sample dietary is low for women when compared with the 15 mg. recommended. This amount of iron is difficult to obtain unless a special effort is made to include iron-rich foods. It is suggested that perhaps women might use dried fruits for snacks instead of candy if calories permit, and try to include some type of liver in the diet twice a month. The level of the B vitamins which appears to be slightly low for men and boys will be raised to RDA when calories are increased to meet their needs.

In Part Two it will be noticed that hospital diets are also based upon this pattern dietary, modified as required to meet specific needs.

SUGGESTED MENUS

The first suggested menu for a moderately active woman is of moderate cost and of a type used in a large part of the United States, particularly northern and central areas. The menus for the 3 meals are suggested, and the nutritive value is calculated in Table 10–3. It will be noted that the food values of Menu No. 1 exceed the recommended allowances in most instances.

The second menu for a moderately active woman is low cost and typical of certain groups, especially in the southern part of the United States. This menu also meets the recommended allowances although it is quite different from Menu No. 1 in food items. (See Table 10–4.)

The second list of foods contains less milk, no fruit, no egg and less variety, but it measures up to recommended allowances almost as well as the first. It must be remembered that the calcium from greens may not be as readily available as that from milk, but the liberal supply allows for some of the calcium to be lost. Also the larger proportion of the vitamin A in the form of carotene may not be as effi-

---

[3] Consumer and Food Economics Research Div. Agr. Res. Service. Washington, D. C., (rev.) 1964.

cient as preformed vitamin A but the supply is more than ample.

In addition to these two sample menus, numerous other combinations could be equally adequate and adapted to available food supplies and dietary customs.

Suggested menus for a week for a family are given on pages 134-135.

When enough money is available, the allowances for meat, fresh fruits and vegetables, butter and certain luxuries may be increased. In that case the amounts of potatoes, dried vegetables, bread and cereals will decrease automatically. The homemaker who has the responsibility of planning and preparing meals for a family of varying ages and activities, with perhaps some dietary restrictions in the group, may need some help from a nutritionist or a dietitian. The nutritive requirements of children and elderly people are somewhat different from those of adults in the prime of life. It would be folly to give a small child everything that appears on the family menu. However, the menu should be planned in such a way that few special foods need be prepared for him. The question of food for children, is discussed in detail in Chapters 13 and 14. Of course, any member of the family who is ill must have special consideration. However, all diets should be planned around the family menu, as the essentials are similar for all. Therapeutic diets are discussed in Part Two.

Menu No. 1

Breakfast:

> Orange juice
> Oatmeal
> Whole milk
> Toast and butter or margarine
> Coffee with cream and sugar

Snack: Coffee and cinnamon toast

Lunch:

> Egg salad
> Roll and butter
> Stewed prunes
> Milk

Snack: tea and cookies

Dinner:

> Pot roast of beef
> Potatoes, boiled
> Stewed tomatoes
> Peas, canned or frozen
> Custard pie
> Coffee with cream and sugar
> Peanut brittle

Menu No. 2

Breakfast:

> Grits and pork gravy *or*
> Corn-meal pancakes, fat pork and
>   molasses
> Coffee with evaporated milk

Snack: Coffee and corn bread

Lunch:

> Hot biscuits
> Peanut butter
> Molasses
> Turnip greens

Dinner:

> Pork shoulder
> Sweet potatoes
> Tomatoes
> Cowpeas or black-eyed peas
> Buttermilk
> Corn bread and margarine

TABLE 10–3. Menu No. 1
Moderate-cost menu for moderately active woman, age 25—pattern of Northern U. S. A.

Foods	Amt. Gm.	Approximate Measure	Calories	Protein Gm.	Ca Mg.	Iron Mg.	Vitamin A I.U.	Thiamine Mg.	Riboflavin Mg.	Niacin Mg.	Ascorbic Acid Mg.
Milk	488	2 c.	320	17	576	.2	740	.16	.84	.3	5
Oatmeal, cooked	100	⅔ c.	63	2	9	.7	...	.10	.02	.2	..
Bread, white, enriched	46	2 slices	126	4	36	.8	...	.12	.08	1.0	..
Orange juice	100	½ c.	44	1	19	.2	190	.08	.03	.2	49
Egg	54	1	77	6	26	1.3	550	.05	.14	Tr.	..
Salad dressing	15	1 tbsp.	58	..	1	.1	20	Tr.	Tr.	..	..
Large roll	57	1 large	176	5	31	1.0	...	.14	.09	1.3	..
Prunes, stewed	100	6 prunes, 2 tbsp. juice	165	1	22	1.5	75	.05	.06	.6	1
Cookies, butterscotch	25	2 small	120	1	11	.5	20	.05	.03	.3	..
Beef pot roast	75	med. serving	231	19	9	2.4	...	.03	.15	3.0	..
Potato, boiled	100	1 med.	83	2	11	.7	20	.09	.03	1.0	14
Peas, canned	100	½ c.	68	5	32	2.1	670	.12	.06	1.0	8
Tomatoes, cooked	100	½ c.	19	1	11	.6	1,050	.06	.03	.7	16
Butter or margarine	42	3 tbsp.	300	..	9	..	1,380	..	..	..	..
Pie, custard	135	1/7 of 9" pie	266	7	162	1.0	290	.07	.21	.4	..
Cream	30	2 tbsp.	60	1	30	..	240	..	.04	..	..
Sugar	12	1 tbsp.	48	..	..	..	...	..	..	..	..
Candy—peanut brittle	15	1 piece	66	1	6	.3	...	.01	Tr.	.8	..
Totals			2,290	73	1,001	13.4	5,245	1.13	1.81	10.8	93
Compared with recommended allowances for a woman of 58 kg. (128 lbs.)			2,300	58	800	12	5,000	1.2	1.5	17*	70

* Niacin equivalents include dietary sources of the preformed vitamin and the precursor tryptophan.

TABLE 10—4. Menu No. 2

Low-cost menu for a moderately active woman, age 25—pattern of Southeastern U. S. A.

Foods	Amt. Gm.	Approximate Measure	Calories	Protein Gm.	Ca Mg.	Iron Mg.	Vitamin A I.U.	Thiamine Mg.	Riboflavin Mg.	Niacin Mg.	Ascorbic Acid Mg.
Corn grits, enriched, cooked......	200	1 c.	102	2	2	.6	..	.08	.06	.8	..
Salt pork, cooked................	50	small serving	250	2	..	.3	..	.09	.02	.4	..
Evaporated milk.................	50	¼ c., scant	69	3	121	.1	200	.02	.18	.1	..
Molasses........................	60	3 tbsp.	139	..	174	3.6	..	..	..	..	..
Turnip greens, cooked...........	150	1 c.	45	4	388	3.6	15,900*	.09	.61*	1.0*	87*
Black-eye peas or cowpeas, cooked...................	100	⅔ c.	94	7	37	2.5	390*	.29	.08	.8	20*
Corn bread, enriched............	150	3 pcs., 2½x3"	330	10	209	2.9	195	.25	.35	1.9	..
Biscuits, enriched	100	3 (2" diam.)	342	8	218	1.8	..	.23	.22	2.0	..
Buttermilk......................	244	1 glass	87	9	288	.2	..	.09	.43	.2	2
Pork, fresh.....................	75	1 med. serving	300	18	9	2.4	..	.62	.18	3.7	..
Margarine......................	42	3 tbsp.	300	..	9	..	1,380	..	..	..	..
Peanut butter	32	2 tbsp.	184	8	24	.6	..	.04	.04	5.2	..
Sugar..........................	12	1 tbsp.	48	..	..	..	..	..	..	..	..
Totals........................			2,290	71	1,479	18.6	18,065	1.80	2.17	16.1	109
Compared with recommended allowances for a woman of 58 kg. (128 lbs.)			2,300	58	800	12	5,000	1.2	1.5	17†	70

* If cooked for a long time in a large amount of water, these factors may be reduced considerably; Some is retained if pot liquor is used.

† Niacin equivalents include dietary sources of the preformed vitamin and the precursor tryptophan.

Suggested Menus for a Week for a Family

Sunday

Breakfast:

Orange juice
Scrambled eggs
Toast and butter or margarine
Marmalade or preserves
Milk or coffee

Dinner:

Fried chicken
Boiled rice
Broccoli, cranberry sauce
Celery and apple salad
Ice cream and chocolate sauce
Coffee or milk

Supper:

Grilled cheese and bacon sandwiches
Shredded cabbage and grape salad
Fruit, fresh or canned
Milk or coffee

Monday

Breakfast:

Grapefruit
Hot oatmeal with milk
Milk or coffee

Snack: Coffee, and toast and marmalade

Lunch:

Cream of tomato soup with crackers
Tuna fish and celery salad
Rolls with butter or margarine
Orange sherbet
Coffee or milk

Dinner:

Pot roast with carrots, onions, celery, potatoes
Cole slaw
Deep dish apple pie
Milk or coffee

Tuesday

Breakfast:

Orange or orange juice
Soft cooked eggs
Toast and butter or margarine
Milk or coffee

Lunch:

Baked macaroni and cheese
Carrot and raisin salad
Rolls and butter or margarine
Prune whip with topping
Milk or coffee

Snack: Tea and cookies

Dinner:

Broiled liver and bacon
Mashed potatoes
Corn and lima beans
Tossed green salad
Fruit Jello with custard sauce
Milk or coffee

Wednesday

Breakfast:

Grapefruit juice
Cold cereal with banana
Milk or coffee

Snack: Coffee and toasted English muffin

Lunch:

Vegetable soup
Hamburger on roll, with relishes
Apple sauce and cookies
Milk or coffee

Dinner:

Spaghetti and meat balls
Carrots and peas
Hearts of lettuce with dressing
Chocolate cake
Milk or coffee

Thursday

Breakfast:

Orange juice
Oatmeal and raisins with milk
Milk or coffee

Snack: Tomato juice and crackers

Lunch:

Pizza or grilled cheese sandwich
Cabbage salad
Fresh or canned fruit
Milk or coffee

SUGGESTED MENUS FOR A WEEK FOR A FAMILY (*Continued*)

Dinner:

Roast pork and apple sauce
Baked potatoes
Zucchini (squash)
Perfection salad, jellied
Corn bread and butter or margarine
Peach cobbler
Milk or coffee

FRIDAY

Breakfast:

Grapefruit
Eggs and bacon
Toast and butter or margarine
Milk or coffee

Lunch:

Cream of mushroom soup
Cottage cheese and peach salad
Rolls and butter or margarine
    or toasted English muffin
Milk or coffee

Snack: Tea and molasses ginger cookies

Dinner:

Baked fish (haddock, cod or halibut)
Baked potatoes

Asparagus, fresh or frozen
Cucumber and tomato salad
Bread and butter or margarine
Cheese cake
Milk or coffee

SATURDAY

Breakfast:

Orange juice
Pancakes or waffles with syrup
Preserves or marmalade
Milk or coffee

Lunch:

Tomato juice
Peanut butter and grated carrot sandwiches
Baked custard
Milk or coffee

Dinner:

Corned beef and cabbage or baked beans
    and brown bread with frankfurters
Cole slaw
Green beans
Lemon pie or pudding
Milk or coffee

FOODS FORTIFIED OR ENRICHED TO HELP MEET NUTRITIONAL NEEDS

About 50 years ago nutritionists began to investigate how certain nutritional limitations in our food supplies could be corrected. The first large scale experiment was the addition of iodine to salt to prevent goiter. This program was so successful in the Great Lakes area and in the Pacific Northwest, where goiter was endemic, that iodized salt is available in most markets today (see Chap. 6).

In the 1930's the fortification of homogenized milk with Vitamin D was started in an attempt to prevent rickets in infants. Today most of the homogenized milk on our markets is fortified with 400 I.U. of vitamin D per quart (see Chap. 7).

In the 1940's the increased use of margarines prompted the addition of vitamin A to make the content equivalent to average butter. Today all margarines on our markets are fortified with 15,000 I.U. of vitamin A per pound.

During World War II the enrichment of bread and flour with iron and three of the B-vitamins was initiated when it was realized that repeated attempts to persuade people to use whole grains was unsuccessful. The modification of natural grains by milling had produced a more acceptable product, whiter, with better keeping qualities and more easily digested, but reduced the vitamin and mineral content. Now the practice of enrichment of milled grains and breads has expanded to include not only wheat, but also corn and rice and ready-to-eat foods such as breakfast cereals, macaroni, spaghetti, noodles and infant foods. Standards for enrichment of various products were established by the Food and Drug Administration as given in the accompanying table. Enrichment of white flour and bread is now mandatory in 30

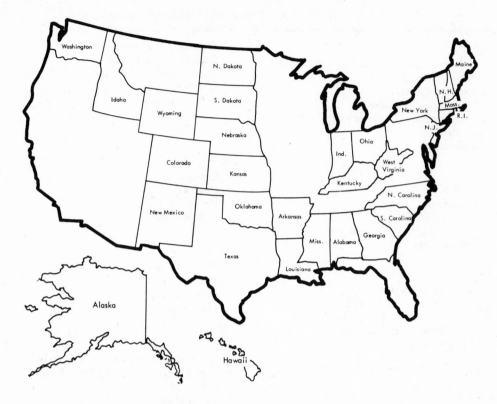

Fig. 10–2. The 30 states designated on this map and Puerto Rico passed enrichment laws prior to 1965. (American Institute of Baking)

states (see map) and in Puerto Rico, and enrichment of cornmeal is common in 12 southern states. Actually, most of the flour and bread sold today in the United States is enriched, although this is not mandatory in all states.

The enrichment of bread and cornmeal is believed to have been an important factor in almost eliminating pellagra as a deficiency disease in the southern states.

The practice of enrichment of bread and other cereal products is now widespread in other countries where public health problems warrant such action and where industry will cooperate.

Some conception of what fortification and enrichment of food has meant in the U. S. may be gained by noting the trend in the per capita consumption of nutrients (Fig. 1–3, Chap. 1). The mandatory enrichment of bread and flour during World War II caused the sudden rise in consumption of iron and the B vitamins and they have never dropped back to the prewar level.

ECONOMY HINTS

Modifications in the family menus may be made when it is necessary to reduce costs. Intelligent adjustments can ensure that meals are still nutritionally adequate and acceptable to the family.

Milk and Dairy Products. Either evaporated or dried skim milk is cheaper than fresh milk and is entirely satisfactory for cooking. Both products have some use as a beverage. When dried skim milk (fat-free milk solids) is used in place of whole milk, some source of vitamin A, such as more generous amounts of green or yellow vegetables or fortified margarine, should be used. Cream is an expensive food. For economy, homogenized milk or sometimes evaporated milk may be used in place of cream. Inexpensive cheese is as good a source of protein as more expensive types.

TABLE 10–5. Standards for Enrichment of Cereal Products in the U. S. A.[1]
To be used whenever claims for enrichment are made.
(Given as milligrams per pound)

Class of Foods	Thiamine Min.	Thiamine Max.	Riboflavin Min.	Riboflavin Max.	Niacin Min.	Niacin Max.	Iron Min.	Iron Max.
Breads and other baked goods...............	1.1	1.8	0.7	1.6	10	15	8.0	12.5
Flour, white..............	2.0	2.5	1.2	1.5	16	20	13.0	16.5
Macaroni and noodle products..............	4.0	5.0	1.7	2.2	27	34	13.0	16.5
Cornmeal, white or yellow, and grits..............	2.0	3.0	1.2	1.8	16	24	13.0	26.0
Rice and related products...	2.0	4.0	1.2	2.4	16	32	13.0	26.0

Calcium and vitamin D may be added as optional enrichment to farina, cornmeal products or rice, and, if so, this must be stated on the label, and the enrichment levels shall be as follows: Calcium—min. 500 mg., max. 750 for cornmeal, max. 1,750 for self-rising cornmeal and for rice max. 1,000; Vitamin D min. 250 U.S.P. units and max. 1,000 U.S.P. units.

Wheat germ and yeast may be added in the enrichment process as partial sources of the B vitamins but with the total amount of each regulated by law for each food product.

[1] From Definition and Standards under the Federal Food, Drug and Cosmetic Act. U. S. Dept. H.E.W., Oct. 1964.

Meats, Fish, Poultry and Eggs. Cheaper cuts of meat may be used when it is necessary to cut food costs. A rough estimate of the cost of the edible portion of some of the apparently cheapest cuts may disclose that the cheapest is not always the cut which has the lowest price tag per pound. Variety meats, such as pork or lamb liver, pork heart and beef tongue, are often good buys, for protein, minerals and vitamins. Fish may be cheaper than meat and is a good source of protein. Poultry today is less expensive per pound than good-quality meats, but the proportion of bone is large. When meats are high, main dishes of beans or peas and peanut butter for sandwiches may be used occasionally. Grade B eggs are as nutritious as Grade A and usually are cheaper. Eggs of graded size show considerable variation in price—sometimes small eggs are the best buy, sometimes large ones. Fat from bacon and other meats can be saved and used for many cooking purposes.

Fruits and vegetables in season and when plentiful are better nutritionally and usually cheaper than canned or frozen. However, home-frozen foods are good economy if home produced, and they can be prepared to suit family tastes. As a rule, carrots and cabbage are inexpensive and can be used raw or cooked. Fresh greens in season and wild greens in some areas may be used in place of more expensive green vegetables. Canned fruits and vegetables can replace fresh products when these are expensive or out of season. Canned tomatoes are cheaper and often higher in vitamin C than raw tomatoes out of season. During some seasons either canned or frozen orange juice is cheaper than fresh and has about the same nutritive value. Sectioned or sliced orange provides more nutritive value than the juice extracted from the same orange. Canned tomatoes, tomato juice, grapefruit juice and low-cost fresh fruits may be used in place of orange juice. The nutritive value of cheaper standard grades of canned fruits and vegetables is essentially the same as that of the more expensive fancy grades, and they are equally sanitary.

Bread, Cakes and Cereals. In general, foods prepared at home are less expensive than foods purchased ready to eat. Sweet rolls, buns, and coffee cakes are expensive types of bread. Breakfast cereals cooked at home are cheaper than the ready-to-eat varieties, but the latter are preferred by many. Large packages are economical for big families but not for small ones, as the contents may become stale and have to be discarded.

RESIST FOOD FADS IN MARKETING AND MEAL PLANNING

In this enlightened age quackery is still flourishing in the field of nutrition as well as in drugs and medical devices. The science of nutrition, although offering sound guidance, has not put the quacks out of business; instead they thrive by misinterpreting scientific facts and by quoting scientific authorities to sell their ideas and their products. In fact, quackery in several phases of medical science has become so serious that the American Medical Association in conjunction with federal and other agencies has sponsored three national congresses on the subject. It is estimated that some 10 million Americans are swindled out of $1 billion a year spent on worthless and sometimes dangerous drugs, treatments, dietary fads and other quackery. Our attention here is focused on the dietary fads, which are the most widespread.

The promotion of vitamin supplements and special diet foods is misleading millions who have little need for such products. And this golden age of quackery seems to have a special appeal to the "golden agers" in our population who often can ill afford it. Such people are attempting self-medication for imaginary or real illnesses with a multitude of irrational products.

So-called natural foods are quite apt to be recommended along with raw foods: raw in place of refined sugar, sea salt in place of table salt, olive oil in place of other fat, lemon juice in place of vinegar. Except for price, there is no objection to these, but neither is there anything poisonous or harmful in the foods for which they are substituted.

One cult recommends that only foods grown according to so-called "organic" farming methods should be eaten. Scientific tests have shown that these foods show no significant difference in the nutritive value from those grown with commercial fertilizers. The chief effect of the fertilizer is an increase in the total amount of the crop and thus an increase in the total nutrients obtained from each acre of land.

It should be noted that solar radiation, climate and genetic factors have an influence on plant composition.

Quacks promoting food supplements usually condemn modern food processing. Yet food technology today has done much to retain food values during processing or to fortify foods where nutrient losses are inevitable.

Certain vegetable juices have been credited with more virtues than they actually possess. An increased consumption of vegetables may be advised for some people, but there is no scientific foundation for such claims as: celery juice for indigestion and rheumatism, carrot juice for the complexion, parsley juice as a building tonic, garlic juice for high blood pressure, white radish and lemon juice for the gallbladder. If and when specific curative properties are found in foods, medical literature will report it with supporting evidence.

Special food combinations are "prescribed" in certain systems of eating. He who dares to indulge in protein and starches or perhaps starches and acid fruits at the same meal faces dire consequences, we are told. There is no physiologic basis for the notion that the normal human digestive apparatus is not equipped to deal with these foods, individually or together. Most natural foods are combinations; even the diet faddists cannot avoid them, but, if they are aware of this, they neglect to tell their disciples.

There is no magic in any specific food item. It makes little difference whether one obtains his nutrients from fluid milk or milk powder, from milk products such as cheese, yoghurt or ice cream, or whether he gets them from meat, fish or fowl, wheat germ, whole grains or blackstrap molasses. The essential point is to get an adequate supply of each nutrient from food that tastes good.

Complicating and encouraging the food fads today are the growing number of false nutrition ideas, or folklore, built up by pseudo-scientific books, pamphlets and periodicals on diets of various sorts. Some tell us that calories don't count or that arthritis can be cured by oils to lubricate your joints; others tempt the unwary with a drinking-man's diet or with martinis and whipped cream. In some unreliable books there is enough of the true mixed with the false regarding food values and human needs to make it difficult for the average person to judge what is valid. As an aid to librarians and others interested, several state health departments and other agencies have published lists of reliable or recommended books for lay readers and in some cases have also listed unreliable or non-recommended books.

Many dietary fads may be relatively harmless but senseless. Too often they detract from the pleasure of eating, an important element in good nutrition. Variety is in itself a safeguard, and, when variety is severely limited, as it is by some fads and self-imposed restrictions, certain nutritive factors are apt to be low or absent. When fads lead to delay in seeking necessary medical advice they can be dangerous indeed. In any event, food fads may increase food costs unduly and result in the omission of foods really needed. The consequences are the same whether one is led to dietary foolishness by the enthusiasms of the uninformed neighbor or of the profit-seekers.

Protection. The Food and Drug Administration maintains strict control over the labeling of foods and drugs so that we may have confidence in the information on a label or a folder enclosed in the package. However, too many consumers fail to read or to understand the label.

The FDA is also clamping down on advertisers of multivitamin and mineral preparations. They will prohibit extravagant promotion of "shotgun" supplements that meet no specific dietary need and tend to deceive or give false hope to the consumer. It is proposed that all preparations bear the following label[4]:

Vitamins and minerals are supplied in abundant amounts by the foods we eat. The Food and Nutrition Board of the National Research Council recommends that dietary needs be satisfied by foods. Except for persons with special medical needs, there is no scientific basis for recommending routine use of dietary supplements.

[4] FDA Release. June 17, 1966.

The FDA is also proposing to establish classes of foods which may be fortified with minerals and vitamins, stipulating that these must state on the label the nutrients and amounts of each used in fortification, and what proportion of the RDA is provided in one serving.

In addition to the Food and Drug Administration, the agencies especially responsible for safeguarding the public are the Federal Trade Commission, The United States postal authorities, Better Business Bureaus, state and national health agencies, and the American Medical Association through its Bureau of Investigation and Council on Foods and Nutrition. New fads will spring up continually and quacks will discover new devices for circumventing the law. The best protection for the consumer is some knowledge of the simple principles of nutrition and some intelligent scepticism and sales resistance when presented with extravagant claims. Money is better spent for good food (protective food), for well-planned and carefully prepared meals, than for pseudo health foods and fads.

STUDY QUESTIONS AND ACTIVITIES

1. The Food and Nutrition Board of the National Research Council has recommended dietary allowances for certain specific nutrients. Which ones are listed in this table?

2. These allowances are listed for different age and sex categories. For which of these are the allowances as great for young children as for a grown man? Why?

3. For which factor do the allowances vary directly with the caloric requirements?

4. The recommended allowances for children are estimated for age groups. How is the average value for each age group computed, and what values would you use for a 13-year-old boy large for his age?

5. Choose any dietary pattern with which you are familiar and plan a day's menu to meet the recommended allowances, using foods well liked by the people for whom it is intended.

6. Which nutrients are most difficult to obtain in sufficient quantities in low-cost meals in your locality at the season of year when you are studying this chapter?

7. Choose any person of your acquaintance whose diet is restricted in certain foods and make the necessary substitutions to provide a diet that meets the recommended allowances.

8. List the food you ate yesterday and check to see whether all four food groups were adequately represented.

9. Visit a local bookstore or your local library and look at the available books on nutrition and diet. Do any of them seem to be unreliable? Can you state why?

10. What food fads have you heard discussed or seen practiced? How would you help a layman to distinguish between fact and fad or between true and false ideas about food?

11. What agencies are attempting to protect the public against misleading advertising?

12. From what sources could you get reliable information about a new food product advertised for a specific diet purpose?

13. Can the average person obtain sufficient vitamins and minerals from food or should supplements be taken regularly?

SUPPLEMENTARY READING ON MEAL PLANNING TO MEET RECOMMENDED DIETARY ALLOWANCES

Food and Nutrition Board: Recommended Dietary Allowances. Pub. 1146. Nat. Research Council. Washington, D. C., 1964.

Jalso, S. B., Burns, M. M., and Rivers, J. M.: Nutrition beliefs and practices. J. Am. Dietet. A., 47:263, 1965.

Johnson, O. C., Nutrition education—what is the goal? Nutr. Rev., 23:353, 1965.

Kaplan, J.: A therapy of chaos. Today's Health, 41:38, 1963.

Mitchell, H. S.: Don't be fooled by fads. Food, The Yearbook of Agriculture, pp. 660-668, U. S. D. A. Washington, D. C., 1959.

Monge, B., and Throssell, D.: Good nutrition on a low income. Am. J. Nursing, 60:2190, 1960.

Sailor, N. M.: Nutrition knowledge applied to everyday living. Nursing Outlook, 9:756, 1961.

Stare, F. J.: Good nutrition from food, not pills. Am. J. Nursing, 65:86, 1965.

CHAPTER 11

Regional, National and Religious Food Patterns

Understanding the Significance of Food Habits • Meeting Nutritional Needs Around the World • Regional Food Patterns in the United States • Cultural and Religious Food Patterns • Dietary Patterns of Some Nationality Groups • Nutritional Problems of Transplanted Peoples • Therapeutic Diet Problems in Other Countries • Understanding Through Sharing of Favorite National and Regional Foods

UNDERSTANDING THE SIGNIFICANCE OF FOOD HABITS

A problem that often confronts the public health nurse or the nutritionist in the U. S. is that of regional or national food habits. Our population has come from all parts of the world and has brought a variety of dietary habits and tastes quite as fixed as our own. Dietary problems among foreign-born or even second generation families are bound to arise because of the fact that foods that have been staples in their diet may now be expensive, while foods that have been considered luxuries are comparatively cheap. Sugar and white bread, for instance, are among the least expensive foods in this country, while milk, vegetables and fruit are often comparatively expensive. The public health nurse often will have an opportunity to guide families of foreign extraction toward an adequate choice of food. Food customs and religious regulations must be considered when the nurse gives advice in regard to food selection. Also, special dishes associated with specific family or holiday events have psychological overtones which

should be appreciated. In an interview with the family or the patient a nurse or a social worker may discover some of these food customs if she shows genuine interest in their traditions and does not antagonize by attempting to judge them critically.

While the majority of the foreign-born or second generation families tend to follow some of their native food patterns they also adopt many American customs of eating. They are, of course, dependent on local markets and though they may find a few familiar items missing, many new ones bid for their attention. The children of such families, associating as they do with Americans and other nationalities, are exposed to many new foods. Not knowing that one food is more valuable than another, or that certain things are essential while others are merely pleasant adjuncts, such families may choose their new diets unwisely.

In the past, many of the immigrants who came to our shores were of the farming class. Some had been accustomed to raising their own produce, to having their own goats or cows for milk and cheese, their own chickens, ducks and geese, and their own fruit trees and vineyards. It is difficult for them to realize that milk, for instance, can possibly be worth from 26 to 35 cents or more a quart, especially since they believe it to be a drink and not a food. Therefore, milk often is one of the first foods on which the family economizes. The children may drink coffee, or possibly tea in its place. On the other hand, second generation families from many countries have adopted the use of milk, even for adults, although this was not the custom in their own country.

Most nationality groups are accustomed to cooking vegetables with meat; but here again the prices of vegetables and meat in this country may seem to be exorbitant and their use may be reduced far below what is necessary for health. In the majority of instances, the great problem of the nutrition worker and the nurse is to recognize the nutritive value of the foods being used and

recommend other foods as supplements when necessary.

Nurses, nutritionists or health workers in other countries are faced with similar but even more perplexing problems, i.e., the availability and cost of foods to meet nutritional needs.

MEETING NUTRITIONAL NEEDS AROUND THE WORLD

In Chapter 1 world food problems have been discussed, especially those in the developing countries. In this chapter some specific suggestions are offered as to how these needs may be met with a wide variety of food patterns. The first eight chapters of the book deal with the fundamental principles of nutrition and are applicable to human needs in any country. The later chapters concerning the application of nutrition in health and disease are naturally oriented toward the people of the U. S. A.;

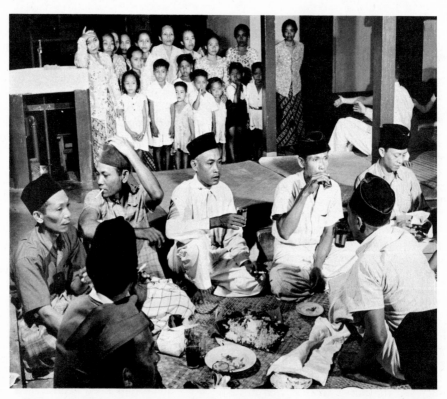

Fig. 11–1. In Sumatra a *salamatan* is a party given to celebrate the beginning of a new venture. Note that the women and the children stand and wait until the men finish eating. (Standard Oil Co., New Jersey)

therefore some adaptation is necessary when this book is used in other parts of the world. These adjustments must always be made in terms of the food patterns of the culture and the country. Whether a large or a small breakfast is customary, whether starches are consumed in the form of bread, rice, spaghetti or casava, whether eggs, fish, and beans are common sources of protein rather than meat—all must be taken into consideration in adapting nutrition principles to meet the nutrition needs of a specific area or condition.

Characteristic food habits of every regional or national group should be respected, because there are good nutritional practices in each of them and nutritional needs may be met by many different patterns of eating. Emphasis should be placed on the desirable features of the established food pattern and on methods of preparation that preserve maximum food values. Although the choice of foods and the methods of preparation may differ from those to which we are accustomed, it often happens that the foods used fall into the Four Food Groups and provide nutrients that meet recommended allowances.

When using any of the chapters about food nutrients in another country, it would be useful to develop charts of local food sources of each nutrient similar to those in Chapters 3 through 8.

Since the supply of protein foods particularly is one of the crucial shortages in various parts of the world, it is worthy of special attention where such shortages exist. The Nutrition Division of the Food and Agriculture Organization, nutrition institutes and university research agencies may be able to supply specific information about the quality and the quantity of protein in locally produced foods and suggest new sources of protein which might be made available. In the chapter on "Energy Metabolism" it needs to be noted that the figures on expenditure of energy for various tasks were derived from research done in western countries. Thus the figures for household tasks and manual labor may have to be modified for application in countries other than the United States.

Unfamiliar foods and methods of preparation need to be studied and possible values recognized before changes are suggested. For example, the use of small whole fish, including bones, as is common in many Asiatic countries, supplies calcium which otherwise might be deficient. A family may be encouraged to continue its own methods of preparation and seasoning when these are not incompatible with health and then gradually be helped to institute necessary changes to correct poor practices, if these exist.

It will be noted that the diets of countries where little or no milk products are available tend to be low in good quality protein, calcium and riboflavin. Most of the localities where fresh fruits and vegetables are used for a long season have more than ample supplies of vitamins A and C. Countries having cooler climates, where grains other than rice are staple and where fruits are less plentiful, will encounter different problems.

Total nutrients provided by any national or regional diet should be compared with the recommendations for that country or locality if such are available. To compare the nutrient value of other national diets with RDA, of the U. S. which provide wide margins above actual need, is unrealistic. Comparative dietary standards for adults in 13 selected countries have been made available by FAO[1] in a table prepared by Dr. L. A. Maynard.

To do an effective job it is necessary to know the nutritive value of foods used in each country or locality. To meet this need the nutritional services in many countries have prepared tables of food composition for use in their country. FAO has published a bibliography of such tables from around the world as well as Food Tables for International Use. These and a few others of the most useful food tables are listed in the Bibliography, Part Four, with the source from which each may be obtained.

Therapeutic diets should be interpreted for the patient or the homemaker in terms

[1] From Nat. Research Council Pub. 1146 Recommended Dietary Allowances. p. 58. Washington, D. C., 1964.

of the regional or the national food pattern. A woman of foreign birth or one from a different part of the country may have little contact outside her home and little opportunity to learn how to use foods that are new to her. The marked improvements in homes where the mother has had the opportunity to learn to adjust to local foods and customs show that instruction as well as understanding is an important phase of nutrition work.

In this chapter special attention is given to regional and national food patterns which are distinctive. A knowledge of these food preferences and attention to them may help to build the bridge of understanding between the health worker, the nurse or the nutritionist and the family that she is trying to assist.

REGIONAL FOOD PATTERNS IN THE UNITED STATES

Anyone who has traveled in different parts of the United States and has eaten meals typical of various regions is aware of differences in menus, food preparation and local terms for foods or special dishes. Part of the joy of travel is in eating the traditional foods of each locality. However, national advertisng in magazines and on TV has tended to popularize certain foods so that diets are not as "regional" as they once were.

People who are ill are much more likely to want familiar foods cooked in a traditional manner with familiar seasoning. Therefore, the dietitian and the nurse should recognize some of these regional differences which exist in our own country so that she can make some adjustments of the diet on the basis of the essential nutrients in terms of familiar foods.

In the South, hot breads are served at nearly every meal, and baker's yeast breads are not popular. There is a preference for vegetables that have been cooked a long time and often with fat pork. Undoubtedly some vitamins are destroyed by this process, but the common use of pot liquor conserves the nutrients which are in solution. The wide variety of greens used compensates in a measure for the low consumption of milk and cheese as sources of calcium and vitamins. The scarcity of fresh milk in some localities has encouraged the use of evaporated and dry milk. Buttermilk is liked and is used when available.

In the Southwest, the Mexican influence is shown in the use of beans and highly seasoned dishes. Again, milk production is limited, and, while the drinking of fresh milk was not part of the original pattern of eating, it is being introduced gradually. Mexican foods such as tortillas, tamales, enchilada and a wide variety of beans are popular in American homes of the Southwest as well as in Mexican families. More details of Mexican foods are given later in this chapter.

In the Far West, the infiltration of oriental cultures has influenced food habits. The use of a wide variety of garden produce and locally grown citrus fruits, the short-time cooking of vegetables typical of oriental cooking, and the serving of generous salads as the first course are features to be commended.

In the north central states, there is a mixed racial background with a strong northern European and Scandinavian heritage in many localities. Even third-generation homes still maintain characteristic native dishes, perhaps modified by regional choice of ingredients. Many of these states produce and use large quantities of dairy products, especially cheeses of several varieties closely resembling European types. The so-called typical American diet is really an adaptation of much of the northern European food pattern. This is only natural since climatic conditions and crops are similar. Locally grown fruits and vegetables are used in season and preserved for winter use. This is a good custom and should be encouraged.

On the east coast and in New England, many traditional dishes have come down from the Pilgrim settlers. The use of corn meal in Indian pudding and johnnycake was acquired from the Indians by their new neighbors. Baked beans, cod-fish cakes, clam or fish chowder and turkey for festive occasions are all old New England traditions, some of which have been adopted nationally. A smaller variety of green, leafy vegetables is used in New England than in many other areas, but yellow vegetables, such as squash, turnips and carrots, are popular.

In isolated communities in any part of the country, unusual food habits may be encountered. Malnutrition may result from a limited variety of foods grown locally, especially if the economic status prohibits extensive use of foods from other producing areas. Sporadic outbreaks of actual deficiency diseases have been reported occasionally. Such instances are less common today, since state health departments are recognizing their responsibilities for these conditions quite as much as for the control of communicable disease.

In metropolitan areas a great variety of food patterns may be found. In large cities, there may be whole sections in which the inhabitants follow as closely as possible the food customs of the country of their origin. This influence is retained to some extent by the second generation. People who come to the city from regions of the United States where definite types of foods are preferred continue to attempt to follow the diet to which they have been accustomed. Usually they can be persuaded to supplement their meals with the foods that are more generally available in the city than they were in the part of the country where their food habits were established.

CULTURAL OR RELIGIOUS FOOD PATTERNS
Jewish Dietary Habits and Laws

In the United States today Jewish family food habits differ according to whether they belong to Orthodox, Conservative or Reform groups. Their food habits may also be influenced by the country from which they or their forefathers came as well as by Biblical and rabbinical regulations, known as the Jewish dietary laws.

According to Kaufman[2]:

Variations in observance are due largely to differences in interpretation and importance placed on dietary laws by the three schools of thought among American Jews today. Ortho-

---

[2] Kaufman, M.: Adapting therapeutic diets to Jewish food customs, Am. J. Clin. Nutr. 5:676, 1957.

dox Jews still place great value on traditional and ceremonial practices of their religion, and observe the dietary laws under all conditions. Reform Jews place much less emphasis on rules which they consider to be purely ceremonial and tend to minimize the significance of the dietary laws. Conservative Jews stand between these two groups and, while nominally adhering to dietary laws, sometimes draw the distinction between the observance of the rules in the home and outside.

The Jewish dietary laws pertain chiefly to selection, slaughter and preparation of meats and the types of fish allowed, and are based on Mosaic law as recorded in several Biblical references. These ordinances are interpreted in the Talmud as specific instructions concerning foods which are fit and proper for people to eat.

Kaufman comments further:

Regulations include selection, preparation and service of the foods involved. The Bible gives no reason for these rules, but observant Jews feel that the rules known as Kashruth and hallowed since the time of Moses, are a positive means of self-purification and of service to their God. Although many hygienic and ethical bases have been alleged for these rules, the spiritual factors of sanctification and self-discipline are the primary motivations for those who adhere to them.

Miss Kaufman also gives some definitions of Jewish terms and special foods.

A brief outline of some of the specific rules to which the Orthodox Jews conform follows:

Foods Allowed or Prohibited. MEATS AND POULTRY. Quadrupeds with the cloven hoof who chew a cud are allowed. These include cows, sheep, goats and deer. Pork in all forms including lard and bacon are prohibited. The poultry allowed includes chicken, turkey, goose, pheasant and duck. All meats and poultry must be freshly slaughtered according to prescribed ritual and soaked in salted water to remove all trace of blood. This process is known as koshering (meaning clean) and many Jewish markets sell koshered meat and poultry. Prescribed methods of preparing meats and other foods are given in most Jewish cook books.

FISH. The fish prescribed in the Bible are those with fins and scales. Thus all shellfish and eels are excluded.

Food Combinations Allowed or Prohibited. The command "Thou shalt not seethe a kid in its mother's milk," repeated several times in Exodus and Deuteronomy, is the basis for never combining meat and milk in the same meal, or even cooking them in the same utensils. Eggs, fruits, vegetables, cereals and all other foods may be used without restrictions.

A striking characteristic of the Jewish diet is the richness of the food, including pastries and cakes, foods rich in fats, and preserves and conserves, as well as stewed and canned fruits. Butter, being a product of milk, must not be served with meat. Most vegetables, therefore, are cooked with the meat. Cooked vegetables are more often served in soup than otherwise. Borscht, a soup made with "sour salt" (tartaric acid) and vegetables to which sour cream is added, is a favorite dish but is not served with the meat meal. Cereals, especially barley and millet, are frequently served as a vegetable with meat or in soup.

Noodles and other egg-and-flour mixtures are used extensively. Rye and whole-wheat breads are well liked, as well as crusty rolls.

Dried fruits, as well as fresh, are used by those who can afford them.

Fish is served frequenty, especially cod, haddock, carp, salmon and white fish, as well as the smoked and the salted fishes—herring, salmon and sturgeon. Gefüllte fish is a delicacy prepared in almost all Jewish homes. Chicken is considered almost an essential for the Sabbath evening meal.

Because milk in any form cannot be served with meat at the same meal, the diet of children in Jewish families that rigidly observe the dietary laws may lack the proper amount of milk. The use of more green vegetables and canned vegetables and fresh and canned fruits for the whole family and more milk for the children should be stressed. The continued use of rye bread, legumes, coarse cereals, dried fruits and a variety of fish which are characteristic of the Jewish diet is advantageous.

Dietary laws for the Jewish Sabbath and religious holidays are often observed by even the less orthodox groups and therefore merit comment.

Sabbath: No food may be cooked on the Sabbath. This means that all cooking for both days is done on Friday. This need has led to the development of foods such as Sabbath Kugel or Sholend, Petshai, and many others.

Passover: During Passover week no leavened bread or its product, or anything which may have touched leavened bread, may be used. A complete new set of dishes is used during the week. Cutlery, silver, or metal pots may be used during this holiday if properly koshered or sterilized. In actual practice this means that in every orthodox Jewish household there are four sets of dishes—the usual set for meat and the set for milk food, in addition to duplicate Passover sets.

Fast days: Yom Kippur (the Day of Atonement); no food or drink may be taken for 24 hours. Fast of Esther; this precedes the Feast of Purim and is now observed only by the very pious. The Feast of Purim is universally observed.

Roman Catholic

The Pope has recently liberalized the dietary restrictions and fast days so that customs vary in different localities. It is well to conform to local custom with regard to foods allowed on fast days and days of abstinence.

Greek Orthodox

The Orthodox laws have not changed in recent years but are interpreted somewhat more liberally. The use of meat, fish, poultry, eggs and dairy products is still restricted on Fridays and certain Wednesdays and during the first and last weeks of the Greek Orthodox Lent.

Seventh Day Adventists

Adventists in general are lacto-vegetarians; thus, they allow the use of eggs, milk and cheese as good sources of animal protein but they use no meat, fish or poultry. They use nuts and legumes as sources of protein.

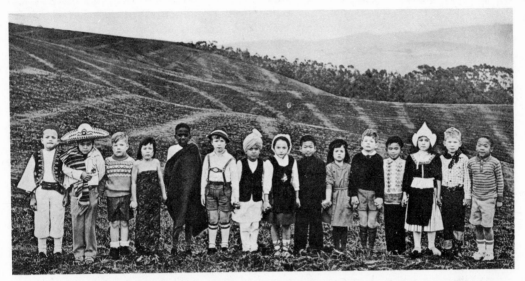

Fig. 11–2. What did you have for breakfast this morning? The children in the picture are (from left to right): Greek, Mexican, Scandinavian, Indonesian, African, Austrian-German, Indian, Basque, Chinese, French, English, Filipino, Dutch, U. S. Caucasian, U. S. Negro. (Courtesy of Olin Mathieson Chemical Co.)

Latter-Day Saints

The Mormons make no food restrictions but prohibit the use of alcohol, tobacco, tea and coffee.

DIETARY PATTERNS OF SOME NATIONALITY GROUPS IN THE U. S. AND IN THEIR OWN COUNTRIES

Space does not permit comment on the food habits of many nationality groups but a few have been chosen to illustrate how nutritional needs may be met with varied food choices. These 15 well-nourished first grade youngsters of different nationalities may have made quite diverse answers when asked "What did you have for breakfast this morning?" (See Fig. 11–2.)

Four sample dietary patterns from Puerto Rico, Lebanon, India and Taiwan, included later in this chapter, are examples of widely diverse ways of meeting nutritional needs.

Dietary Habits of Mexicans and Other Latin Americans

The Mexicans use freely many varieties of beans, as well as rice, potatoes, peas and some vegetables. Chili, a variety of pepper, is also popular. The chili plant is sacred to

the Mexican, who is supposed to be blessed in health if he uses it plentifully. The tomato always is prominent in Mexican cookery. Mexicans use little meat and practically always cook it with vegetables. They have a strong aversion to meat that is not perfectly fresh and slaughtered in the approved Mexican style. Chili con carne is a favorite meat dish. It consists of beef seasoned with garlic and chili peppers and cooked several hours. Tamales also are popular. They are made of corn meal and ground pork, highly seasoned; they are rolled in corn husks and steamed. Tortillas, made with ground whole corn which has been soaked in lime water and baked on a griddle, serve as a bread. Thus some calcium is provided in tortillas and in beans in a diet which includes very little milk or cheese. The use of milk for the children should be encouraged when and if a change to the American type of bread is made.

The influx of Cuban refugees into our southern states creates a need to recognize and adjust nutrition advice and special diets to Cuban preferences when counseling these people. Their food pattern is

TABLE 11–1. Moderate Cost Food for a Day for a Puerto Rican Adult

Food	Amount of Edible Portion	Weight Gm.
Rice...................	3 cups cooked	668
Plantain or root veg.......	1 serving	200
Bean, broad, kidney or other type...........	1 cup	256
Onion..................	1 medium	110
Egg Plant..............	1 small	100
Green Pepper...........	2 small	100
Tomato.................	1 medium	100
Mango.................	1 medium	200
Banana.................	2 medium	300
Salt Codfish.............	1 oz. dry	30
Goat's Milk..............	1 cup	244
Lard...................	½ cup	50
Olive Oil...............	2 Tbsp.	28

The value of this diet is approximately:

Calories	2,506		Vitamin A	33,500	I.U.
Protein	69	Gm.	Thiamine	1.0	mg.
Fat	77	Gm.	Riboflavin	1.0	mg.
Calcium	0.6	Gm.	Niacin	13.3	mg.
Iron	12.5	mg.	Vitamin C	195	mg.

Adapted from information provided by Dr. Lydia Roberts, University of Puerto Rico, and Miss Ethel Robinson, formerly a teacher in rural Puerto Rico.

similar to that of other West Indian groups where the Spanish influence predominates.

It is notable, however, that many of the more prosperous eastern South American peoples have a meat and milk consumption as high or higher than the United States. Spanish and Portuguese influences are evident in the liberal use of peppers and spices.

On the west coast of South America the situation is quite different. A few cities are prosperous, but agriculture is handicapped by desert, mountains and jungles. The native Indian populations of the Andes in Ecuador, Peru and Chile are short of food and especially of some adequate sources of protein.

Puerto Rican Dietary Habits

The dietary pattern in Puerto Rico is similar to that in other Caribbean Islands and to some of the Latin American coun-

tries. From the extensive work of Dr. Lydia Roberts in Puerto Rico information is available on a typical moderate-cost food supply for an adult for one day. The nutrient value comes close to meeting the U. S. recommended allowances.

When Puerto Ricans migrate to the United States, as they do in great numbers, they may modify this pattern considerably according to what is available and what they can afford.

Rice and beans are the staple foods, used almost daily and often cooked together. Salt codfish is used more often than fresh fish. Pork and beef are the favorite meats. Plantain and some root vegetables, along with fresh tomatoes, peppers and onions, are used commonly. Bananas, oranges and pineapple are popular and relatively inexpensive in Puerto Rico, and much to be preferred to canned fruits, which have been widely introduced. Even more important are some of the native fruits which are not familiar in the north, such as the mango and the West Indian cherry or acerola which is now recognized as the richest known natural source of ascorbic acid.

Puerto Ricans living in the north may have to adjust to different fruits in season and to canned fruits. They may well be encouraged to use more milk and cheese, and cheaper cuts of meat to supplement the protein at meals when rice and beans are served. Acceptance of canned tomatoes in place of more expensive fresh ones out of season, margarine in place of butter and cheaper cuts of meat would provide better nutrition for the same cost.

Puerto Ricans in New York City and other urban areas are often among the lower economic groups because many of them are unskilled laborers. Their poor and crowded housing may provide inadequate cooking and refrigeration facilities. Thus they may be unable to provide their families with as good food as they had at home. Malnutrition, rickets and tuberculosis are not uncommon among Puerto Rican children living under such conditions. The nurse or the social worker can offer suggestions as to how they can improve their nutrition within their budgets.

Italian Dietary Habits

Italian-Americans, few of whom today were born in Italy, have adopted many food customs of the United States. Likewise, the popularity of Italian spaghetti and pizza in this country testifies to the influence that Italian food customs have had on Americans. Italians here continue to use pastas in a great variety of shapes and with many different sauces and cheeses. Similarly, bread is still an essential part of an Italian meal, although crusty white bread is now more popular than the dark breads that were a former standby.

Southern Italians may use more fish and highly seasoned foods, while northern Italians use more root vegetables and more meat. The liberal use of eggs, cheese, tomatoes, green vegetables and fruits by all Italians is to be commended. They may well be encouraged to use more milk and meat, both of which they like. In general, the northern Italians have better food habits than those from the south.

Italians have a strong sense of individuality. We may think of spaghetti as a typically Italian food, but not all Italians like spaghetti. They dislike foods that are not prepared to their particular tastes. They are particularly sensitive to the lack of close family ties in a hospital and therefore dread hospitalization more than one may suspect. Most Italians eat a very light breakfast: black coffee for adults and milk for children, with perhaps bread without butter. Some like the main meal at noon, others at night, but bread and cheese with coffee or wine are an acceptable light meal.[3]

Western European and Scandinavian Dietary Habits

Most of the western European peoples, including the Scandinavians, have food patterns not unlike those of northeastern and central North America where immigrants from these areas have settled during the past two centuries. Many American food customs of today have been derived from

---

[3] Italian Food Habits, abstr. J. Am. Dietet. A. 40:342, 1962.

these countries. The lists of meats, vegetables, fruits and grain products used by them would be a mere recital of those in our markets. To be sure, they make more frequent use of dark breads, potatoes, fish and cheese than native Americans do. For western Europeans the differences in culinary methods, seasonings and attitudes toward food are never serious hurdles in adjusting to American food patterns.

Central European Dietary Habits

In many of the central European countries grains and potatoes provide 60 to 70 per cent of the total calories for the rural and the lower income groups. They use rye and buckwheat as well as wheat for their breads. Pork and pork products including highly seasoned sausages are popular. Cabbage may be used raw, cooked or as sauerkraut, and other vegetables—onions, turnips, peppers, carrots, beans, squash and greens—are often cooked with a little meat. Eggs, fresh milk, sour cream and yoghurt (called by a different name in each country), cottage cheese and other cheeses are widely used. Central Europeans bring with them many good food habits which are to be encouraged.

Dietary Habits of the Middle East— Lebanese, Armenian, Turkish, Greek and Syrian

The inhabitants of the Middle East are outdoor people. Most of them are farmers: they raise their own sheep, goats, cattle, chickens, ducks and geese; they produce their own grains and grow fruits and vegetables in abundance, wherever water is plentiful. Grains, rice or wheat, furnish the major source of calories. The whole wheat is parboiled and cracked for use as a staple starchy food at the main meal. Eggs, butter and cheese also are produced on the farm. Lamb is the favorite meat. The food is not highly spiced but is rich in fat. The fat is cooked with the food and this serves in place of butter. Matzoon, leban or yoghurt, a sour-milk preparation, is used almost universally by these people; sweet milk is seldom used. Black coffee, heavily sweetened, in which the pulverized bean is retained—often called Turkish cof-

TABLE 11–2. Calculation of Moderate Cost Food for a Day for an Adult—Lebanon

Food Items	Wt. Gm.	Cal- ories	Pro- tein Gm.	Cal- cium mg.	Iron mg.	Vitamin A I.U.	Thia- mine mg.	Ribo- flavin mg.	Niacin mg.	Ascorbic Acid mg.
Bread, Arabic round loaves.........	400	1,080	36	360	8.8	....	1.1	.32	1.0	...
Burghul, parboiled wheat.........	200	140	5	18	1.4	....	.2	.06	1.8	...
Broad beans......	250	230	15	102	4.9	260	.12	.12	2.0	...
Leban..........	200	106	6	240	.2	660	.18	.42	.8	...
Cheese, variety....	15	34	2	80	.1	240	.02	.06	...	0
Mutton...........	50	130	9	5	1.5	....	.1	.15	4.5	0
Tomato..........	100	20	1	11	.6	900	.08	.03	...	30
Egg plant........	100	20	1	15	.4	280	.06	...	...	...
Onions...........	100	45	1	32	.5	50	.03	.04	.2	9
Mallow (maloukhieh)	50	25	3	...	...	7,000	.25	.16	...	40
Banana..........	100	88	1	8	.6	900	.06	.02	...	...
Orange..........	100	45	1	33	.4	190	.08	.03	.2	49
Olives, ripe......	65	106	1	48	.9	40	...	...	...	...
Olive oil and semnih	55	486	0	0	0	0	0	0	0	0
Total........	...	2,555	83	950	20.3	10,720	2.0	1.4	10.5	128

Adapted from information by Miss Ruth Hembekides, formerly Home Economics Advisor with U. S. Operations Administration to Lebanon, and by Dr. William H. Adolph, late Professor of Nutrition, American University at Beirut, Beirut, Lebanon.

TABLE 11–3. Low-Cost Vegetarian Diet for an Adult Man in Rice-eating Area of India[1]

Food Items	Quan- tity Gm.	Cost ps	Cal- ories	Pro- teins Gm.	Cal- cium mg.	Iron mg.	Vita- min A I.U.	Thia- mine mg.	Ribo- flavin mg.	Ascorbic Acid mg.
Rice............	260	20	1,070	20.4	24.0	7.26	36	0.58	0.28	0
Ragi............	200	15	472	13.1	699	31.3	126	0.75	0.18	0
Black gram dhal..	30	4	104	7.2	46.2	2.73	19	0.12	0.11	0
Bengal gram.....	45	14	166	10.1	2.61	4.27	85	0.09	0.22	0
Roasted ground- nut...........	5	1	28	1.5	2.5	0.08	0	0.01	0.006	0
Red gram dhal...	60	8	200	13.38	44.0	3.48	132	0.26	0.20	0
Amaranth.......	60	6	47	2.4	238.0	15.3	5,520	0.01	0.06	59.4
Mint............	120	12	57	5.7	240.0	18.7	3,240	0.06	0.96	42.4
Onion..........	33	2	17	0.43	59	0.23	0	0.22	0.004	3.63
Brinjal + Ladies finger.........	60	3	40	0.84	23.0	0.36	74	0.02	0.66	7.2
Brinjal.........	120	4	29	1.6	22.0	1.08	148	0.04	0.13	14.4
Banana.........	40	4	43	0.44	4.0	0.20	52	0.02	0.06	2.4
Guava..........	50	4	25	0.45	5.0	0.7	0	0.01	0.01	106
Buttermilk.......	100	3	8	0.40	15.0	0.4	...	...	...	...
Green chillies....	9	2	3	0.24	2.7	0.10	36	0.01	0.03	9.9
Oil.............	60	20	540	...	...	...	...	...	...	...
Total.......	Rs. 1.22		2,849	78.18	1,447.5	86.19	9,468	2.29	2.91	245.33
Recommended Allowances for a Reference Indian adult (moderate work)			2,800	55.0	1,000.0	20 to 30	3,000 to 4,000	1.0 to 2.0	1.5	50

[1] Courtesy of Dr. Rajammal P. Devadas, Sri Avinashlingam Home Science College, Coimbatore, India.

fee—is the preferred beverage in many countries of the Middle East.

Calculation for the nutrients of a diet of moderate cost for one day for an adult in Lebanon is given herewith.

Chinese Dietary Habits

The Chinese diet is varied, consisting of eggs, meat, fish, cereals and a large variety of vegetables. Many plants and weeds, such as radish leaves and shepherd's purse, are used, as well as various sprouts (bean, bamboo, etc.). None of these vegetables is ever overcooked, and no cooking water is discarded; thus, nutrients are well retained. The soybean is abundant, and some 30 or more products are manufactured from it. The protein is high and of good quality for a vegetable protein.

Rice is used freely and takes the place of American bread, particularly in southern China. In northern China, wheat, corn and millet seed are used in abundance. The millet seed (ground or whole) is made into cakes or a thin mush, the latter being the

form in which it is given to children. Noodles are widely used. Grains and, in some areas, sweet potatoes constitute the chief source of calories in the Chinese diet; grain and potato together provide from 70 to 90 per cent of the total calories.

The quantity of meat eaten is small, and usually it is served with vegetables. All ingredients are cut into small pieces in conformity with an ancient law laid down by Confucius, the philosopher, specifying that food should not be eaten unless it had first been chopped or cut into small pieces. Pork is the chief meat of the poorer classes. Lamb and goat meat and other animal foods are used when available, but beef is uncommon.

In certain parts of China, a child rarely tastes cow's milk, but water-buffalo milk is used to some extent. Soybean milk and cheese are more common. When transplanted to this country, the Chinese readily accepts the use of dairy products for children and adults.

The Chinese use practically every part of the animal as food (with the exception of the hair and the bones); even the brain, the spinal cord and the various internal organs, as well as the skin and the blood, are utilized. Coagulated blood is sold on the market in pieces similar to liver and,

TABLE 11–4. Moderate Cost Food for a Day for an Adult of Taiwan

Food	Amount of Edible Portion	Weight Gm.
Rice..................	7 cups cooked	1,176
Pigs Feet..............	1 serving	100
Soy bean curd.........	1 serving	100
Soy Sauce............	2 Tbsp.	25
Bean Sprouts.........	1 cup	100
Cowpeas, green........	1 serving	100
Cabbage, cooked......	1 serving	200
Squash, winter........	1 serving	100
Peanuts, roasted.......	¼ cup	50
Gourd, white..........	1 serving	100
Plantain..............	1 serving	100
Watermelon..........	Large wedge	925
Orange..............	1 medium	215

The value of this diet is approximately:

Calories	2,533		Vitamin A	9,980	I.U.
Protein	83	Gm.	Thiamine	2.1	mg.
Fat	49	Gm.	Riboflavin	1.2	mg.
Calcium	0.6	Gm.	Niacin	23.4	mg.
Iron	17.0	mg.	Vitamin C	196	mg.

Adapted from information provided by Miss Yueh-Hwa Chen, from Taipei, Taiwan.

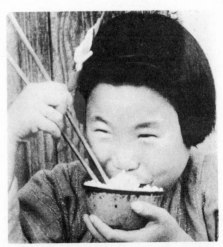

Fig. 11–3. Familiar foods give children of other nationalities a feeling of security. (FAO, from UN film *Battle for Bread*)

since this is one of the inexpensive foods, it is used freely. Fish and shellfish are also in common use. They are sold alive, for the Chinese have a strong aversion to dead fish and consider them unfit for food.

Eggs, including hen, duck and pigeon eggs, are used in abundance, when they can be afforded. The Chinese prepare what are known as fermented eggs, much relished by them, as well as other types of "preserved" eggs, which are eaten much as we in this country eat sweets.

Japanese Dietary Habits

During the past 20 years there have been spectacular changes in Japanese food habits, influenced by Western culture. Typical diets formerly included rice, bean paste soup, raw or cooked fish and pickles. Now the trend is to bread as well as rice, milk, cheese, meat, eggs, vegetables and fruits. Instant foods and frozen items are available. Seafoods are served raw, smoked, fried and, recently, as fish sausage. Japanese make a whole meal of wheat or buckwheat noodles cooked in broth and garnished with a few bits of vegetables and fish sausage and served with salty pickles. Although they are traditional tea drinkers, many of them now prefer coffee, and they like to drink milk when it is available. Many kinds of crisp salty snack foods made from rice or wheat flour, seaweed and other delicacies are popular. A Japanese or Chinese meal is complete without dessert, but at New Years' and other holidays the Japanese relish their "decoration cakes." Even the simplest one-dish meal is attractively served, and an elaborate party meal, served in 10 or 12 separate and colorful dishes of different shapes, is truly a work of art.

The Japanese today are extremely nutrition conscious as prosperity makes it possible for more of their people to have an adequate diet. The result is that Japanese youth today are taller and heavier than a generation ago. This change parallels an increased intake of animal protein, calcium and certain other nutrients without much change in caloric intake. Japan has an almost universal school lunch program ex-

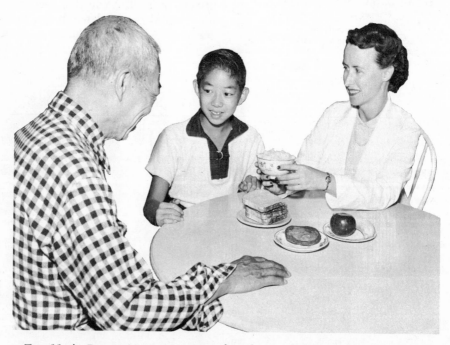

Fig. 11–4. Boy acting as interpreter for Chinese diabetic patient who is being instructed regarding the carbohydrate equivalent of his favorite bowl of rice. (Frances Stern Food Clinic of the Boston Dispensary)

cept in isolated areas, and the lunches are good nutritionally. There is widespread concern for maintaining good health at all ages, with a marked decrease in infant mortality and increased life expectancy.

The Japanese have developed their own table of recommended dietary allowances similar to that in the United States. General interest is such that newspapers carry this table as news whenever it is revised.

NUTRITIONAL PROBLEMS OF TRANSPLANTED PEOPLES IN THE U. S.

The southern Negroes moving to northern cities have special nutritional problems. Vegetables and fruits which were cheap or homegrown in the south may be expensive in the north, and it is thus difficult for people to choose adequate and acceptable foods among those which they can afford. Southern markets may provide a variety of greens which are used abundantly, but cost in northern markets may discourage their use. The limited consumption of milk may not have been as serious for the children eating more of such greens as it is when they move north and fail to make the necessary compensation.

In the case of dark-skinned races, Negroes, Mexicans and others, the children seem to be especially susceptible to rickets in the north, possibly due to lessened exposure to sunlight. Thus more attention to milk and adequate sources of vitamin D is paramount. These same people show increased susceptibility to tuberculosis in the north, and, again, protective foods are important. Thus a marked change in climate may involve adjustments in food to meet modified requirements.

THERAPEUTIC DIET PROBLEMS IN OTHER COUNTRIES

Food may play an important role in the treatment of disease and in the prevention of deficiency diseases. Part Two of this book deals with dietary modifications recommended for specific diseases or metabolic disorders. The principles of diet modification for a disease are valid in any country; however, the specific diets for each condition described in Part Two are based upon the American dietary pattern. It is particularly important that the application of dietary restrictions in other countries be made in terms of their foods in common usage.

An example of this is the adaptation made by one of the authors of the milk and cream regimen often used in the treatment of peptic ulcer. In the Middle East neither sweet milk nor cream is a common food. However, people eat frequently, and are fond of, a very soft cheese made from artificially soured milk and commonly eaten with olive oil. This combination meets the specifications of a bland, nonresidue, high-protein, high-fat diet and was found to be completely satisfactory, both by the patient and in the dietary treatment of peptic ulcer. Other such adaptations of therapeutic diets should be made, based on the principles underlying the dietary care, whenever the foods suggested are not available or not in common usage in the locality where the text is being used.

It is to be remembered that medical opinion and the application of diet therapy may vary by countries and from time to time, as new scientific discoveries alter our present concepts. Therefore, it is urged that instructors consult local medical authorities as to whether the suggested diets in the section on "Diet in Disease" conform to local scientific opinion. This is always a safe procedure even in different parts of the United States.

UNDERSTANDING THROUGH SHARING OF FAVORITE NATIONAL AND REGIONAL FOODS

The traveler in this and other countries may often sample and enjoy the favorite dishes of the locality. Many restaurants offer foods of one nation or region exclusively and give us the opportunity to try dishes from foreign lands. More rewarding is the exchange of ideas and recipes with nationals of different countries. In one city where many nationalities lived but did not mix socially, a project entitled "What's Cooking in Your Neighbor's Pot" served to provide these homemakers with mutual respect and enjoyment.

The thousands of students coming to our colleges and universities from around the world give us unusual opportunities to become familiar with the food habits of other countries. Students usually adjust fairly well to American food customs depending on how drastic a change of diet is involved, although some of the Asiatics lose weight and are quite miserable for a while. One way for Americans to enjoy foreign foods without travel and, at the same time, give pleasure to these foreign students is to invite them into our homes to help prepare a meal including some of their favorite dishes. Even the men students often have the knowledge and the skill to prepare and serve such dishes though they may never have done so at home. Though they most often use the foods available in our markets, they combine and season them differently and add an exotic touch. Actually, it is fun to prepare and eat dishes which are the favorites of other nationalities or regions. The United Nations Cook Book[4] offers an opportunity to try dishes from most of the countries which belong to the UN.

Numerous other regional and foreign cookbooks are available for those who enjoy trying their culinary skills on unfamiliar dishes.

STUDY QUESTIONS AND ACTIVITIES

1. Why is it essential that a public health nurse or a nutritionist be able to adjust her advice on nutrition to various regional and national food patterns?

2. What evidence is there that stature may be influenced by nutrition as well as by racial inheritance?

3. After noting the regional dietary habits in the United States, which ones in the South and the Southwest would you recommend and encourage, and what changes would you recommend?

4. How has the infiltration of various cultures influenced the food habits of those in various regions of the United States?

5. Why is the Jewish diet one of the most difficult problems for the health worker? What are some of the dietary laws which must be respected?

6. How does the use of grains, potatoes and meat vary among the different regions of Europe and Asia?

7. How can you help others to gain respect for the food habits and the favorite dishes of nationality and regional groups other than their own?

8. What source materials are there for food values of foods used in various parts of the world?

9. Plan a suitable menu for a Seventh Day Adventist teen-age boy, making sure to supply adequate protein for his needs.

SUPPLEMENTARY READING ON REGIONAL, NATIONAL AND RELIGIOUS FOOD PATTERNS

Anderson, L. and Browe, J. H.: Nutrition and Family Health Service. Chap. 2. Philadelphia, Saunders, 1960.

Cantoni, M.: Adapting therapeutic diets to the eating patterns of Italian Americans. Am. J. Clin. Nutr., 6:548, 1958.

Fathauer, G. H.: Food habits—an anthropologist's view. J. Am. Dietet. A., 37:335, 1960.

Favorite Recipes from the United Nations, 1960. U. S. Committee for U. N., 816 21st St., N. W., Washington, D. C.

Hacker, D. B., and Miller, E. D.: Food patterns of the Southwest. Am. J. Clin. Nutr., 7:224, 1959.

Kaufman, M.: Adapting therapeutic diets to Jewish food customs. Am. J. Clin. Nutr., 5:676, 1957.

Korff, S. I.: The Jewish Dietary Code. Food Tech., 20:76, 1966.

Macgregor, F. C.: Uncooperative patients: some cultural interpretations. Am. J. Nursing, 67:88, 1967.

Phillips, M. G., and Dunn, M. M.: Toward better understanding of other people: Their folkways and foods. Nursing Outlook, 9:498, 1961.

Torres, R. M.: Dietary patterns of the Puerto Rican people. Am. J. Clin. Nutr., 7:349, 1959.

Valassi, K. V.: Food habits of Greek-Americans. Am. J. Clin. Nutr., 11:240, 1962.

Visiting Nurse Ass. of Chicago: Eating in Different Languages.—A Handbook for Public Health Nurses. Chicago, Ill., Feb., 1960.

---

[4] Favorite Recipes from the United Nations, 1960. U. S. Committee for U. N., 816 21st St. N. W., Washington, D. C.

For Further References see Bibliography in Part Four.

CHAPTER 12

Nutrition in Pregnancy and Lactation

Nutritional Demands of Pregnancy • *Food Selection in Pregnancy*
• *Complications of Pregnancy Involving Diet* • *Diet During Labor*
• *Diet Following Delivery* • *Diet in Lactation*

NUTRITIONAL DEMANDS OF PREGNANCY

Pregnancy makes many demands on the prospective mother, not the least of which are her nutritional needs and those of the unborn infant. Although an undernourished mother may produce a healthy child, studies of nutrition of women during pregnancy have shown a definite relationship between the diet of the mother and the condition of the baby at birth. These studies have also shown that some of the complications of pregnancy, such as anemia, toxemia, and premature delivery, may result from a diet inadequate for the nutritional needs of the mother and the baby.[1] Moreover, if the mother has always eaten a diet adequate in all essentials and is in good health, she has a much better chance of bearing a healthy baby than does the mother who consistently has had a poor food intake.

The Teen-Age Mother. One of the problems today centers on the young girl having her first baby. Young people marry and become parents at an earlier age today than did their parents. In 1962, an estimated 38 per cent of all first-born children in the United States were born to mothers under 20 years old. This group includes the unmarried teen-age girl, who presents special problems.

We do not know if the Recommended Dietary Allowances for pregnancy are adequate for the needs of the adolescent pregnant girl. Certainly, if she has not eaten a proper diet during her own period of rapid growth, which is the case with many girls in this age group, the additional demands of pregnancy may not be met.

Many more complications of pregnancy and early infancy occur when the mother is an early teen-ager than when she is a more mature woman.[2] Marchetti,[3] studying over 600 young mothers 16 years of age or under, found that toxemia was a frequent complication and that there was an increased number of premature deliveries. He comments in this study on the "inability of a considerable number of these young pregnant girls to appreciate the importance of diet and rest" and notes that the diet selected often consisted of cola drinks, potato chips, peanuts and hot dogs. Another study was made by Clough[4] of 175 primiparas 13 to 16 years old. It was found that pre-eclampsia and essential hypertension were increased in the white teen-age patients over patients between 21 and 25 years of age. Weight gain over 25 pounds was commoner in the young Negro girls, and ane-

[1] Stearns, G.: J.A.M.A., *168*:1655, 1958.

[2] Hassan, H. M., and Falls, F. H.: Am. J. Obst. Gynec., *88*:256, 1964.

[3] Marchetti, A. A., and Menaker, J. S.: Am. J. Obstet. Gynec. *59*:1013, 1950.

[4] Clough, W.: Obstet. Gynec., *12*:373, 1958.

mia and essential hypertension were frequent complications in this group.

Many young people do not seek the guidance of a physician or a prenatal clinic early in their pregnancy, so that adequate instruction often comes too late for the prevention of complications. This is due partly to the mobility of young families today, which discourages continuous contact with clinic or physician and in part to ignorance of available services.

Nutrition Studies in Pregnancy. The effect of the food intake on the condition of the newborn baby is best illustrated by the now classic studies of Burke and her coworkers[5] at the Harvard School of Public Health and the Boston Lying-In Hospital. Figure 12–1 shows the relationship of the mother's diet to the health of the baby. In a study of 284 women, it was found that those on good or excellent diets (42 mothers) had babies in good or excellent condition at birth, with only 2 exceptions. The mothers on fair diets (202 patients) had babies rated largely as good or fair. Those mothers on poor to very poor diets (40 patients) had babies rated as fair or

poorest, with only 3 exceptions. The poorest infants were those who were stillborn or born prematurely, who died within 3 days of birth, who had congenital defects or who were functionally immature.

The question sometimes is asked, what is meant by a "poor" diet? Such a diet is usually low in most necessary food nutrients; there may even be one food group, such as milk, entirely missing. An example is that of a young, pregnant mother, living in a housing development, whose husband leaves for work early. Usually she gets up and joins him in a cup of coffee and a piece of Danish pastry for breakfast. In the morning and again in the afternoon, she visits her neighbors, at which time more pastry and coffee are consumed. Often she is not hungry at lunch, nor does she enjoy preparing food only for herself, so that frequently lunch either is skipped or takes the form of a piece of fruit. Fortunately, this patient has a good dinner when her husband returns in the evening, but this is not sufficient to meet her nutritional needs, except perhaps for calories. Another patient drank up to 15 cups of tea daily, each with 2 teaspoonfuls of sugar, and consequently was seldom hungry for other food.

[5] Burke, B. S., *et al.*: J. Nutr., 38:453, 1949.

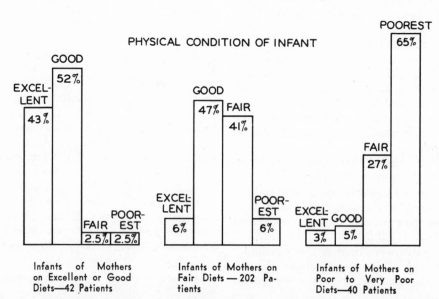

Fig. 12–1. Condition of infants at birth in relation to the prenatal diet of the mother. Note the decrease in excellent and good ratings for infants and the increase in fair and poorest infants as the diet goes from good to poor. (Adapted from Burke, B. S., *et al.*: J. Nutrition, 38:453, 1949)

TABLE 12–1. Recommended Daily Dietary Allowances for a Moderately Active Woman
During Pregnancy and Lactation

(Food and Nutrition Board, National Research Council, Revised 1963)

Essential Nutrients	Nonpregnant Woman 58 Kg.—25 Yrs. Old	Pregnancy Second and Third Trimester	Lactation (850 ml. Daily)
Calories*.............................	2,100	2,300	3,100
Protein, Gm...........................	58	78	98
Calcium, Gm...........................	0.8	1.3	1.3
Iron, mg..............................	15	20	20
Vitamin A, I.U.........................	5,000	6,000	8,000
Thiamine, mg..........................	0.8	1.0	1.2
Riboflavin, mg........................	1.3	1.6	1.9
Niacin Equiv.,† mg....................	14	17	21
Ascorbic acid, mg....................	70	100	100
Vitamin D, I.U........................	..	400	400

* Energy requirements will vary with size, age and activity.
† Niacin equivalents include dietary sources of the preformed vitamin and the precursor tryptophan. (See Chap. 8.)

It will be seen from the foregoing that the importance of nutrition in pregnancy is poorly recognized by a large section of the population, and that nurses, as well as many others in the medical field, must assume more responsibility for teaching this group better nutrition.

Nutritional Requirements. Table 12–1 shows the Recommended Dietary Allowances for pregnancy and lactation compared with those for the young nonpregnant woman. These will vary with the weight, the age and the activity of the mother, and should be used only as a guide. The adolescent pregnant girl, depending on her age and own stage of growth, may require higher allowances than the 25-year-old pregnant woman. See Chap. 10 for the Recommended Dietary Allowances for the various age groups and the additions for pregnancy and lactation.

CALORIES. If the physical activity of the woman remains the same during the second and third trimesters of pregnancy, an additional 200 calories is suggested to meet the energy costs of pregnancy. The building of new tissue in the placenta and fetus, an increased work load associated with the activity of the mother and an increased basal metabolic rate contribute to increased calorie needs. However, decreased physical activity, particularly during the third trimester, may more than compensate, to the point that no additional calories may be needed. The physician, by carefully observing weight changes, is best able to recommend necessary calorie modifications. In any case the calorie increase is small, and foods must be carefully chosen if the other nutrient increases are to be met while keeping the total calories within the recommended allowance. Table 12–2 shows

TABLE 12–2. Suggested Dietary Pattern During Pregnancy

Whole or skimmed milk: 1 qt. (one oz. of Cheddar cheese is equivalent to 8 ozs. milk.)

Lean meat: One liberal or two small servings (4 ozs.) of meat, fish or fowl; liver is desirable at least once each week.

Egg: One each day.

Fruit: Two or more servings (1-1½ cups, 200-300 Gm.) each day. One serving should be citrus fruit or other good source of ascorbic acid.

Vegetables: Two or more servings of cooked or raw vegetables (1-1½ cups, 200-300 Gm.) each day; these should include dark green leafy or deep yellow vegetables; in addition, a medium potato (150 Gm.) should be eaten daily.

Bread and cereal: Whole-grain or enriched bread, at least 4 slices daily (½ cup of cereal is equivalent to 1 slice of bread).

Butter or margarine: 1 to 2 tablespoons.

Additional foods: Consisting of either more of the foods already listed or other foods of one's own choice adjusted to individual energy needs and in relation to desired weight gain.

Vitamin D: Some form of vitamin D to supply 400 I.U.

TABLE 12–3. Sample Menus for the Second Half of Pregnancy

For Pregnant Woman of Normal Weight	For Pregnant Adolescent Girl of Normal Weight
Breakfast Orange slices Shredded wheat Scrambled egg Toast—1 slice Butter or margarine Milk—½ pint Coffee	**Breakfast** Orange juice—8 oz. Shredded wheat Scrambled egg Toast—2 slices Butter or margarine Marmalade Milk—½ pint
Lunch Meat sandwich Carrot and green pepper sticks Oatmeal cookies Milk—½ pint	**Lunch** Meat sandwich on whole wheat bread Carrot and green pepper sticks Cheese cubes Oatmeal cookies Fresh fruit Milk—½ pint
Midafternoon Milk—½ pint	**Midafternoon** Chicken sandwich Milk—½ pint
Dinner Broiled beef or pork liver Steamed broccoli Baked potato Tomato salad with French dressing Baked apple	**Dinner** Broiled beef liver Steamed broccoli Baked potato Vegetable salad with French dressing Baked apple with raisins Milk—½ pint
Bedtime Hot milk or cocoa—½ pint	**Bedtime** Milk or cocoa—½ pint

From Prenatal Care, Children's Bureau Publ. No. 4, 1962, U.S. Dept. of Health, Education and Welfare.

a suggested dietary pattern during pregnancy.

PROTEIN REQUIREMENT. The protein intake must be increased in pregnancy because of its specific contributions to growth and because, as a rule, a diet low in protein is lacking in other nutrients. An additional allowance of 20 Gm. of protein is therefore recommended to provide the protein which is accumulated by the fetus and accessory tissues during pregnancy.

Extra protein in the diet will be supplied by additional milk, meat, poultry, fish and eggs (Table 12–2). Skim milk, liquid or dried, can be used to increase protein without adding considerably to the total calorie intake. Inexpensive dried skim milk can be used in creamed soups and casserole dishes; one or two tablespoons can also be added to regular milk to increase the protein content (some suggestions for adding dried skim milk to food will be found in Chapter 36). Sample menus which meet the recommended dietary allowances for pregnancy are shown in Table 12–3.

CALCIUM AND PHOSPHORUS REQUIREMENTS. The pregnant woman must be supplied with calcium and phosphorus in quantities large enough for her own needs and those of the bony framework of the body of the growing fetus and for the formation of its teeth. An additional allowance of 0.5 Gm. is recommended at this time. Again, a quart of milk a day will supply a large proportion of the needed calcium and phosphorus, as well as a good proportion of the necessary protein.

IRON REQUIREMENT. An adequate iron supply during pregnancy is no less important that that of calcium. The allowance for the second and third trimesters of pregnancy is increased 5 mg. over that for the nonpregnant female. Besides the mother's need for iron, the developing fetus is building its own blood supply. When the baby is born, his blood has a hemoglobin content of from 20 to 22 Gm. per 100 ml. This high level is needed in fetal life for oxygen uptake at the placenta, where oxygen is at lower pressures than it is in the lungs. Soon after birth some of the hemoglobin begins to break down until a normal level of 13 to 14 Gm. per 100 ml. of blood is reached. The iron from the hemoglobin breakdown is stored in the infant's liver to serve as a supply during the first few months of life when his diet of milk provides little iron. If the mother's intake of iron is low, this will reflect itself in the level of her own hemoglobin and in the level of hemoglobin—and, eventually, in the available iron for storage—of the baby.

Foods especially high in iron are the livers of beef, chicken and pork, one of which should be included in the pregnant woman's diet at least once a week. Other good sources are heart, kidney, tongue, all lean meats, chicken, eggs, most green, leafy vegetables, potatoes, whole-grain or enriched bread, dried fruits and dried peas and beans. It is not always easy to include sufficient iron in the daily diet, especially in the low-income group. The physician may prescribe some type of supplementary source of iron.

IODINE REQUIREMENT. Iodine is also an important element in the diet of the pregnant woman. A deficiency of this element during pregnancy may cause goiter in the child or in the mother. The use of iodized salt is suggested for those who live in areas in which the soil and the drinking water are known to be deficient in iodine.

VITAMIN REQUIREMENTS. All vitamins are essential for the metabolism of living tissue, and doubly so in growth. In research studies done on animals, it was possible to produce specific congenital defects by depleting the mother animal of a single vitamin. By creating a severe deficiency of vitamin A in experimental animals, young without eyeballs and with other severe eye

defects were obtained. Warkany,[6] by depleting mother rats of their stores of riboflavin, was able to produce severe skeletal anomalies, such as fused ribs, fingers and toes, and cleft palate. Such conditions are not likely to occur in human mothers, but the findings do emphasize that good nutrition in pregnancy is important from the very moment of conception and, indeed, even before it takes place.

Foods rich in vitamins are those which have been discussed as essential for other nutrients: milk and milk products, eggs, meat, fish and poultry, and especially liver, whole-grain and enriched breads, green and yellow vegetables, citrus fruits, tomatoes, cabbage and potatoes. All these must be supplied liberally in the diet of the pregnant woman if she is to meet her own nutritional needs as well as those of the growing fetus.

The proper utilization of calcium and phosphorus depends on the inclusion of a certain amount of vitamin D in the diet. Most areas today offer both whole and skim fluid milk to which 400 I.U. of vitamin D per quart have been added. Some physicians order vitamin D for their patients as a medication, although not all obstetricians subscribe to this practice. Because of recent evidence indicating a relationship between abnormal calcium deposition in infants and excessive vitamin D intakes during pregnancy, the pregnant woman should be cautioned against overdosage with supplements.

Mineral oil in any form interferes with the absorption of the fat-soluble vitamins and should be avoided, if possible.

In addition to increased amounts of thiamine, riboflavin, niacin, and ascorbic acid (Table 12–1) the pregnant woman may also require larger amounts of other water-soluble vitamins such as pyridoxine and folic acid. Additional pyridoxine corrects the altered tryptophan metabolism which is observed in pregnancy and possibly protects against dental caries. The megaloblastic anemia of pregnancy may be prevented by adequate amounts of folic acid (see Anemias of Pregnancy). The use of vita-

---

[6] Warkany, J.: J.A.M.A. *168*:2020, 1958.

min supplements (except possibly for vitamin D) is not necessary unless, because of illness or other problems, the mother is unable to eat a sufficient diet. The physician is best able to determine whether or not supplements are needed.

FOOD SELECTION IN PREGNANCY

Table 12–2 lists the foods and the quantities of each that, if consumed daily by the pregnant woman, will meet the Recommended Dietary Allowances. Such a food intake represents the so-called excellent diet found by investigators to be most likely to produce a superior infant and to maintain the mother's health at an optimum. Routine salt restriction or too rigid weight control should not be necessary if the pregnancy is proceeding normally.

Two menus based on the foregoing table, one for the adult pregnant woman and one for the pregnant adolescent girl are presented in Table 12–3. It is assumed that both are of normal weight. Note that calories, protein and calcium have been increased in the menu for the pregnant adolescent girl to provide for her own growth needs and those of the fetus.

Adaptations for Cost and Food Habit Patterns. It may be difficult for the mother to follow the suggested diet pattern if she has a strong dislike for a food such as milk or liver, if her food habits are culturally very different, or, most frequent of all, if the cost of the diet is higher than she can afford. However, some adaptations can be made without impairing the nutritive value of the diet too greatly. The use of dried skim milk for part or all of the whole milk will lower the cost substantially. The use of chocolate and coffee flavor, a dash of vanilla extract or of cinnamon or nutmeg may change the taste of milk sufficiently so that the mother will drink it. Milk, either fluid or dried, may be used in desserts, creamed soups and scalloped dishes. As has already been indicated, a 1-oz. slice of Cheddar (hard) cheese has approximately the same protein and calcium content as an 8-oz. glass of milk. This may be an acceptable substitute for Italian patients, who use cheese somewhat more readily than large quantities af milk. Liver, another food sometimes heartily disliked, may be eaten as liverwurst or as a liver spread in a sandwich, or it may be disguised in a variety of ways in cooked dishes. (See Chap. 35.)

In general, meat and eggs are expensive foods. Dried beans and peas, used by many groups in the United States as well as in many other countries, serve as a partial substitute at much lower cost. However, they must not replace the use of animal protein to too great a degree, for the legumes do not supply as good a quality of protein. Fish and eggs are excellent meat substitutes in areas and at times of year when they are cheap. Meats such as heart and tongue are less expensive than other cuts and add variety to the diet.

Fruits and vegetables, bought fresh in season, are usually least expensive. However, the frozen fruit juices, especially orange and grapefruit juice, and canned tomato juice are comparatively inexpensive sources of vitamin C all the year round. In the southeastern section of the United States, the frequent use of greens with their accompanying "pot liquor" provides a considerable source of calcium and vitamin C in the diet. Carrot sticks and celery strips, stored in the refrigerator, will provide the mother with a low-calorie snack to satisfy her craving for nibbling and at the same time help to meet her vegetable requirements.

Desserts made from milk, eggs and fruit, unsweetened or flavored with noncaloric sweetening, give a psychological "lift" to the prenatal diet. See Chapter 37 for recipes.

Pica. An abnormal craving for non-food substances (pica), such as starch and clay, has been reported by certain women during pregnancy. This practice appears to be most prevalent among Negro women, particularly in the south where it is often a traditional practice accepted within the immediate community. A recent study[7] by Edwards and associates in Alabama showed that the caloric intake of pregnant women who consumed starch and clay was reduced when these substances were omitted from

---

[7] Edwards, C. H., *et al.*: J. Am. Dietet. A., *44*: 109, 1964.

the diet, indicating that they were either appetite stimulators or that deprivation of them was so emotionally upsetting as to reduce appetite. In general, the diets of these women tended to be low in protein, iron and calcium. Although the birth weight and length of the infants born to these mothers were similar to those of the control groups' infants, fewer babies born to the starch- and clay-eating mothers were rated in good condition at birth. An irritating effect of starch ingestion on the salivary glands has also been reported.

Nutrition Education. The need of the pregnant girl or woman for nutrition information will vary with each patient. The mother having her second or third baby who feeds her family with good judgment will probably do the same for herself. All she may need is a review of dietary essentials with perhaps some suggestions for the less costly foods if her income is limited. On the other hand, a mother with a large family and a low income may need considerable guidance in wise spending. National and cultural dietary patterns will influence the choice of foods in many families and need to be reckoned with. Chapters 10, 11, and 35 will be of help in this matter.

The most urgent nutritional problem is that of the very young pregnant woman. It has been said that "nutrition for pregnancy begins before conception," and, above all, this is true of the mother under 20. The diet of many teen-age girls is low in calcium and vitamin C. There is also a tendency to an inadequate iron intake.

The nurse, the dietitian and the doctor will have to use patience, imagination and

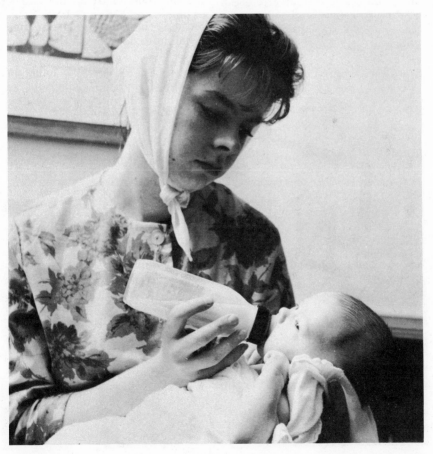

Fig. 12–2. Many of todays' new mothers are teen-agers. (Children's Bureau photograph)

persistence in persuading mothers who are not doing so to follow an adequate diet. The woman who asks for calcium pills because she does not like milk needs to be taught that milk is a rich source of other needed nutrients besides calcium, and be encouraged to use a variety of methods for including it in her diet. The young girl needs help in understanding her body's new needs, and possibly the help of the social worker or community agency in providing a good diet. The use of the attractive health literature available may aid the mother in following an improved diet, both for herself and for her family.[8] It is very possible that the foundation for good nutri-

tion for the whole family may be laid in the obstetrician's office or the prenatal clinic.

COMPLICATIONS OF PREGNANCY INVOLVING DIET

Vomiting. During the first trimester of pregnancy the mother-to-be may be troubled with nausea. Certain foods which previously have been eaten without difficulty now may cause distress. Fats are a common cause of upset. Fluids taken with meals may also precipitate vomiting. Dry toast or a few unsalted crackers eaten before arising may be of help. Fluids should be drunk between meals, not with the meal. Skim milk may be tolerated better than whole milk. Often the nausea disappears by the middle of the day, and the mother can make up her dietary needs by increasing her food intake in the late afternoon, at dinner and before bedtime.

---

[8] Good examples are Prenatal Care, Children's Bureau Publication No. 4, 1962, and When Your Baby is on the Way, Children's Bureau Publication No. 391, 1961, U. S. Dept. of Health, Education and Welfare. Local and state health departments also have good material available.

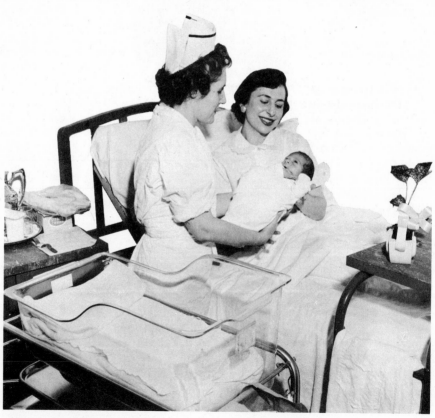

FIG. 12–3. The desirable outcome of pregnancy: a healthy, happy mother and baby. (The New York Hospital)

TABLE 12–4. Diets for Pregnancy Varying in Caloric Content*

	2,300 Calories	1,800 Calories	1,500 Calories
Milk...............	1 qt. whole	1 qt. whole	1 qt. skimmed
Meat, fish and poultry.	4 ozs.	4 ozs. lean	4 ozs. lean
Eggs...............	1	1	1
Fruit...............	2 servings citrus, 1 other	2 servings citrus, 1 other	2 servings citrus, 1 other
Vegetables..........	4 servings, including potato and dark green leafy or yellow vegetable	4 servings, including potato and dark green leafy or yellow vegetable	4 servings, including potato and dark green leafy or yellow vegetable
Bread and cereals....	4 servings whole grain or enriched	4 servings whole grain or enriched	4 servings whole grain or enriched
Butter or margarine...	3 teaspoons	3 teaspoons	3 teaspoons
Other foods.........	Sugar, desserts, fat for cooking; other foods to meet caloric needs	None. Saccharin or Sucaryl may be used for sweetening.	None. Saccharin or Sucaryl may be used for sweetening.

These diets may be restricted in sodium as follows: (See Chap. 24 for details of food restriction.)

1. *Moderate sodium restriction*—1,000 to 1,500 mg. sodium. Prepare all food without salt; do not add salt at table; omit all salted foods such as salt butter and bacon.

2. *Severe sodium restriction*—300 to 400 mg. sodium. Prepare all food without salt; do not add salt at table; omit all salted foods such as salted butter and bacon. Use only low sodium milk. Use only fruit for dessert.

*From the Woman's Clinic of The New York Hospital. The above diets meet the Recommended Dietary Allowances of the National Research Council for pregnancy with the exception of calories for the 1,800 and the 1,500 calorie diets.

Vomiting, if it persists and becomes pernicious, should be treated by a physician.

Overweight in Pregnancy. Pregnancy usually is a time of well-being and often is accompanied by an excellent appetite. Most doctors guard against excessive weight gain as being detrimental to both the mother and the fetus. Overweight may lead to complications during delivery, and, even more serious, there is a marked increase in the incidence of toxemia in overweight women.

If the mother is overweight at the beginning of pregnancy or is gaining weight too rapidly, she should have a diet restricted in calories but otherwise meeting all her nutritional needs. That it is safe and actually beneficial to do so has been shown by Jacobson, Burke and their co-workers.[9] In a study of 92 pregnancies of 89 obese women placed on a 1,500 calorie diet supplemented with iron and thiamine, they

found that those women who followed the diet, as indicated by weight loss, had fewer complications of pregnancy and that the dieting had no demonstrable adverse effect on the condition of the infant at birth.

Care must be taken that a weight-reduction diet in pregnancy is not so low in calories that the protein in the diet is used partly for energy instead of for growth. Oldham[10] has shown that this occurs when the diet is below 1,500 calories, even when the protein of the diet is adequate. Probably no diet in pregnancy should fall below 1,500 calories, and it may be more realistic to allow the mother an 1,800 calorie diet. If she adheres to this, there should be no impairment of her health or of the baby's, and her weight gain should remain at a minimum.

If weight reduction is needed, or if there is a tendency to gain weight too rapidly, such foods as sugar, candy, jelly and other sweets, oil salad dressings, fried foods, fatty

[9] Jacobson, H. N., Burke, B. S., *et al.*: Am. J. Obstet. Gynec., *83*:1609, 1962.

[10] Oldham, H.: Bull. Matern. Welf., *4*:10, 1957.

meats, cake, pie and desserts, and carbonated beverages should be limited or omitted entirely. It may be necessary to limit bread and potatoes; and skim milk may be substituted for whole milk.

A problem arises with the mother who believes that milk is "fattening" and reduces or omits it in her diet. As explained earlier, the substitution of calcium pills for milk markedly lowers the protein and the vitamin content of the diet and should be emphatically discouraged.

Table 12–4 shows a comparison of the recommended diet for pregnancy for a woman of normal weight, containing approximately 2,300 calories, and the restrictions necessary to bring this down to 1,800 and 1,500 calories. All these meet the Recommended Dietary Allowances for specific nutrients, except for calories in the latter two diets. For someone on the 1,500 calorie diet, the physician may wish to prescribe vitamin and iron supplementation as a precaution.

Underweight in Pregnancy. The severely underweight woman and the woman who does not gain normally during her pregnancy are of as great concern as the obese mother. The reason for the underweight may be economic; this may often be discovered by the nurse, who will direct the patient to the social worker or a community agency for help. If the cause is psychological—such as a severe depression—or physical, the doctor will take the appropriate measures. Undernutrition can be as dangerous to the health of both the mother and the baby as overnutrition.

Anemias of Pregnancy. In the latter months of pregnancy there may be a slight lowering of the hemoglobin content of the mother's blood due to physiologic adjustments. By this time her total blood volume has increased considerably to provide for the placental circulation. This may not be accompanied by a corresponding increase in red blood cells; consequently, a degree of hemodilution occurs. However, it is of slight degree and usually is not mistaken for anemia of pregnancy.

True anemia occurring during pregnancy is due most often to an iron deficiency. Frequent pregnancies, depleting the mother's store of iron, may be a factor. Usually, however, anemia occurs in mothers who have an inadequate food intake, particularly of protein and iron. Iron medications will aid greatly in restoring the hemoglobin to normal levels in these patients. It is essential, however, that the mother be urged to include foods rich in iron and protein in her diet, or other deficiencies may appear.

As explained earlier in this chapter, the infant's level of hemoglobin at birth and the supply of iron available for storage for use in the first few months of life are curtailed when the mother's iron intake is inadequate. The result is anemia of infancy, which is not an uncommon finding.

Megaloblastic anemia of pregnancy may be due to a poor food intake, vomiting, the fetal demands for the vitamin, or an unknown metabolic defect in the absorption or synthesis of folic acid coenzymes.[11] It is characterized by an extremely low red blood cell count and an equally low hemoglobin and has some other findings associated with pernicious anemia, with which it may be confused. The administration of folic acid causes an immediate and a dramatic rise in red blood cells and hemoglobin, and in appetite. Recent studies indicate that the folic acid requirement during pregnancy is between 200 and 400 mcg. per day as compared with the minimal adult requirement of 50 mcg. per day.[12] If the mother does not receive treatment before the birth of the baby, the infant also will show some of the symptoms of megaloblastic anemia. It may be treated with folic acid, or, if the mother is being treated while nursing, the infant will receive enough folic acid from its mother's milk to restore its blood components to normal.

Toxemia of Pregnancy. The cause of toxemia of pregnancy is not known. It is characterized by an elevation in blood pressure, albuminuria and rapid weight gain due to edema. In the eclamptic stage

---

[11] Recommended Dietary Allowances, Revised 1963. National Research Council, Washington, D. C., Pub. 1146, p. 41.

[12] Alperin, J. B., *et al.*: Arch. Int. Med., *117*:681, 1966. Willoughby, M. L. N., and Jewell, F. J.: Brit. Med. J., *5529*:1568, 1966.

there may be convulsions and coma. There is considerable controversy over the influence of nutrition on the development of toxemia. Toxemia seems to occur more frequently in pregnant women on poor diets, and particularly on low protein intakes, than in corresponding groups on good diets. Burke's findings[13] show that 44 per cent of the women on poor or very poor diets, 8 per cent on fair diets, and none on good or excellent diets developed symptoms of toxemia. Tompkins and Wiehl[14] have shown that supplementation of the diet with protein and vitamins greatly reduced the incidence of toxemia in their patients. (See Fig. 12–4.) Although McGanity[15] and his group in Nashville, Tenn., were not able to relate nutritional status to the health of the mother during pregnancy as clearly as other investigators, they do report an increased incidence of toxemia in mothers who ate less than 1,500 calories and 50 Gm. of protein per day during the last trimester. Obesity, too, contributes to the development of toxemia. The incidence of toxemia in obese patients is highest when the initial obesity is combined with high levels of weight gain during pregnancy. All these findings reinforce what was said earlier in this chapter; we have not so far made nutrition education in pregnancy as effective a tool as we might in maintaining the health of the mother during this period and ensuring a healthy infant at birth.

Once toxemia has occurred, the dietary treatment of it varies, depending on the severity of the symptoms. In the early stages, a diet high in protein, minerals and vitamins, and low in sodium may best meet the needs of the patient. If the mother is markedly overweight, the calories should be restricted. Suggestions for the restriction of sodium and calories, while maintain-

---

13 Burke, B. S., and Kirkwood, B. B.: Am. J. Pub. Health, *40*:960, 1950.

14 Tompkins, W. T., and Wiehl, D. G.: Am. J. Obstet. Gynec. *62*:898, 1951.

15 McGanity, W. J., *et al.*: Am. J. Obstet. Gynec., *67*:501, 1954.

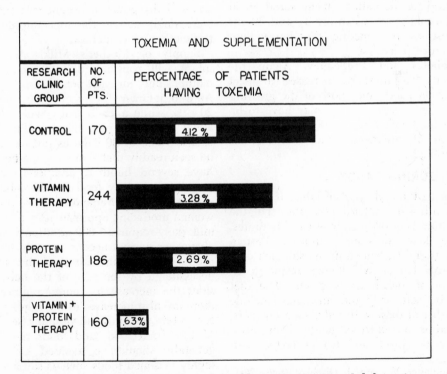

RESEARCH CLINIC GROUP	NO. OF PTS.	PERCENTAGE OF PATIENTS HAVING TOXEMIA
CONTROL	170	4.12 %
VITAMIN THERAPY	244	3.28%
PROTEIN THERAPY	186	2.69%
VITAMIN + PROTEIN THERAPY	160	.63%

TOXEMIA AND SUPPLEMENTATION

Fig. 12–4. (Tompkins, W. T., and Wiehl, D. G.: Nutritional deficiencies as a causal factor in toxemia and premature labor. Am. J. Obst. & Gynec., *62*: 898, 1951)

ing the protein intake, will be found in Table 12–4 on page 163. See Chapters 24 and 39 for suggestions for making the low-sodium diet more palatable.

In the past few years a question has arisen about the relation of salt intake to toxemia. Robinson,[16] studying over 2,000 pregnant women, advised half to increase their salt intake and half to lower it. He found a lower incidence of toxemia in those having the higher salt intake. More recently, Mengert[17] placed 48 patients with proven toxemia either on a high salt intake or on a very low one. No difference in the progress of the disease was noted between the two groups of women in this study.

Cardiac Disease and Pregnancy. It should be remembered that the nutritional requirements of the pregnant woman with cardiac disease are the same as those of the non-cardiac pregnant patient. If it is necessary to limit the mother's salt intake, note the suggestions for moderate sodium restriction in footnote of Table 12–4. The very low sodium diet probably should be reserved for the patients being cared for in the hospital. See Chapters 24 and 39 for suggestions for making the low-sodium diet more palatable.

Diabetes and Pregnancy. Again the mother's diet must be increased to meet her larger needs and those of the growing fetus. The insulin dosage may have to be augmented accordingly. For further discussion of pregnancy and diabetes see Chapter 22.

DIET DURING LABOR

During the early part of labor, if feeding by mouth is permitted by the physician, the diet should consist mainly of carbohydrates, as they leave the stomach quickly. Protein and fat tend to remain in the stomach considerably longer, which may result in aspiration if anesthesia is given. The diet may be soft or liquid and may include white-bread toast with jelly, soda crackers, canned or cooked fruits, gelatin, fruit juices, ginger ale, broth and tea or coffee with

[16] Robinson, M.: Am. J. Obstet. Gynec., 76:1, 1958.

[17] Mengert, W. F.: Am. J. Obstet. Gynec., 81: 601, 1961.

sugar but no milk or cream. By the time the patient is in active labor, most obstetricians prefer that no food be given by mouth so as to prevent the possibility of vomiting, and of aspiration of food into the trachea. Intravenous fluids are given to maintain water balance if labor is prolonged.

DIET FOLLOWING DELIVERY

A liquid diet usually is given for the first meal after delivery. After that, there is a return to the normal diet. If the mother nurses the baby, there must be an even greater allowance of food than there was during pregnancy.

DIET IN LACTATION

Lactation makes even greater demands in some respects on the maternal organism than does pregnancy After birth the child still may be fed from the mother's body, the food now being produced by the mammary glands instead of being supplied through the blood stream, as before birth. As the baby gains in weight and becomes increasingly active, the food supply from the mother must increase.

Supply of Mother's Milk. A normal infant will consume daily 2½ ounces of mother's milk for each pound of his weight. An 8-lb. infant will consume approximately 20 ozs., while a 15-lb. baby will consume about 30 ozs. Since human milk has a caloric value of 20 calories per oz., it will be seen readily that a nursing mother must have several hundred additional calories per day to supply food for the infant.

Dietary Requirements. The nursing woman producing approximately 850 ml. of milk daily requires 1,000 additional calories above her normal needs, not only for milk production, but also for the extra activity necessitated by the care of the baby. Besides the increase in energy requirement, there are also increases in the requirements for protein, minerals and vitamins (see Table 12–1). Fried foods and foods rich in fat generally should be avoided, as should highly seasoned foods such as sausages and pickles. Highly flavored vegetables and dried beans, except in soup form, may also cause disturbances.

TABLE 12–5. Sample Menu for a Day for a Lactating Mother

Breakfast	Noon Meal	Supper or Luncheon
Stewed prunes	Tomato juice	Cream of pea soup
Shredded-wheat cereal with milk (sugar if desired)	Baked ham	Tomato and cottage cheese salad
Scrambled eggs	Scalloped potatoes	Biscuit with butter or margarine
Toast with butter or margarine	Green beans	Apple sauce
Milk. Coffee if desired	Raw carrot sticks	Gingerbread
	Whole-wheat bread and butter or margarine	Milk. Coffee or tea if desired
	Cup custard	
	Milk. Coffee or tea if desired	
Midmorning	*Midafternoon*	*Before Retiring*
Milk	Orange or grapefruit juice	A glass of milk

Between-meal feedings often are advisable during lactation in order to include all the necessary foods. Plenty of water as well as other liquids should be taken. A typical sample menu for a day is shown in Table 12–5.

It should be remembered that the mother must return to a normal food intake when she weans the baby from the breast or she will gain excess weight.

STUDY QUESTIONS AND ACTIVITIES

1. Even the normal healthy woman who has been eating an adequate diet will require more dietary essentials during pregnancy. Review the Recommended Dietary Allowances for women under various conditions. Which allowances increase in ratio to the caloric allowance? What other essentials should be increased during pregnancy?

2 What do nutrition studies show concerning the adequacy of diets in pregnancy of large groups of women in the United States? What is the role of the nurse in the correction of this situation?

3. Give several reasons why the adolescent may have serious nutrition problems in pregnancy. Name some of the ways in which these can be met. How can the nurse be of help?

4. Why is the nutrition of the mother previous to pregnancy so important?

5. Discuss the results of an inadequate intake of protein in pregnancy. In what forms may extra protein be added to the diet?

6. The mineral requirement is naturally larger during pregnancy. How may the calcium and the phosphorus requirements be fulfilled? What are the food sources of iron? How may the iodine requirements be met?

7. What danger to the infant may result from nutritional anemia in the mother? Explain.

8. List the foods and the quantity of each that must be included daily in the diet of the pregnant woman.

9. Plan a menu for a day for a healthy pregnant woman of average weight. Make necessary modifications for a woman who is underweight; for one who is overweight; for a patient with a limited income.

10. Using Chapter 11 as a guide, write a menu for a day for a pregnant patient with a food pattern not typically American. Be sure that it is adequate for the needs of pregnancy.

11. During the first trimester there may be trouble with nausea. How may the menu be modified to relieve this?

12. If for any reason the quota of fluid milk cannot be taken each day, how may milk be used otherwise in the diet? Suggest appetizing, easily digested dishes which may be used in the menu.

13. During the latter part of the second trimester, the pressure of the enlarged uterus may cause constipation. How will you advise the mother? (See Chap. 27.) Why should mineral oil not be used?

14. During the third trimester toxemia may appear. Is there anything to indicate that diet may act as a preventive? If so, state the evidence.

15. How may the diet in pregnancy be restricted in sodium? Should salt be restricted routinely in pregnancy?

16. Lactation makes greater demands upon the mother than does pregnancy. What food increases should be made to provide for the supply of milk? Which foods may cause digestive disturbances? Plan a menu differing in content from the sample menu in Table 12–5, but equivalent to it in other respects.

17. What would you say to the mother who asks about substituting calcium pills for milk?

SUPPLEMENTARY READING ON NUTRITION IN PREGNANCY

Causes and prevention of prenatal mortality. WHO Chronicle, *21*:43, 1967.

Everson, G. J.: Basis for concern about teen-agers diet. J. Am. Dietet. A., *36*:1, 1960.

Macy, I. G., and Kelly, H. J.: Food for expectant and nursing mothers. Food: Yearbook of Agriculture. p. 273. U.S.D.A., Washington 25, D. C., 1959.

McCollum, E. B.: Symposium on prenatal nutrition. J. Am. Dietet. A., *36*:236, 1960.

Maternity Care: The world situation. WHO Chronicle, *21*:140, 1967.

Payton, E., *et al.*: Dietary habits of 571 pregnant southern Negro women. J. Am. Dietet. A., *37*:129, 1960.

Pike, R. L.: Sodium intake during pregnancy. J. Am. Dietet. A., *44*:176, 1964.

Prenatal Care. Children's Bureau Publication No. 4, U. S. Dept. of Health, Education and Welfare, Washington, D. C., 1962.

Rust, H.: Food habits of pregnant women. Am. J. Nursing, *60*:1636, 1960.

Seifrit, E.: Changes in belief and food practice in pregnancy. J. Am. Dietet. A., *39*:455, 1961.

Semmens, J. P.: Implications of teenage pregnancy. Obstet. Gynec., *26*:77, 1965.

For Further References see Bibliography in Part Four.

CHAPTER 13

Nutrition During Infancy

Growth and General Development the First Year • Nutritional Requirements of Infants • Breast Feeding vs. Formula Feeding • Formulas—Types and Sources • Feeding Difficulties in Infants • Feeding Infants of Low Birth Weight • Supplementary Foods • Other Considerations in Infant Feeding

GROWTH AND DEVELOPMENT DURING THE FIRST YEAR

During the early months of life growth is more rapid than at any other time of life. The infant will double his birth weight in about 4 months. After that the weekly gain is slower—4 to 5 ounces—for the rest of the year, but he will be likely to triple his birth weight by the end of the first year.

The infant will grow in length, from 20 to 22 inches at birth to 30 to 32 inches at the end of the year. At birth the head is large in proportion to the rest of the body and will continue to grow. This is the time when the brain and nervous system are developing rapidly and during this period a supply of essential nutrients are crucial for normal mental development.

The gastrointestinal system of a full-term infant can digest protein, emulsified fats and simple sugars, but starches and most other fats are poorly tolerated until the digestive enzymes are more fully developed in later months.

The body of the newborn infant contains a higher proportion of water than that of older children. The muscles are poorly developed and the amount of subcutaneous fat is limited but will increase during the year. The skeleton is not fully calcified and there is still a high percentage of water and cartilage. A full-term infant has a store of iron and a high hemoglobin level—nature's way of providing for the early months on milk which is low in iron. The iron stores are gradually depleted, however, unless either the milk is supplemented with iron in some form or iron-rich foods are added two or three months after birth.

The critera for judging adequate nutrition in an infant are: a steady gain in weight; a moderate increase in subcutaneous fat; the development of firm muscles; good elimination; and a baby that is happy, sleeps well and shows a normal curiosity about his surroundings.

NUTRITIONAL REQUIREMENTS OF INFANTS

The energy requirement of infants is much greater per unit of body weight than it is for older children or adults.

The suggested caloric allowance for the very young infant ranges from 150 to 110 calories per Kg. of body weight and decreases toward the end of the first year to 100 calories per Kg. This is from 3½ to 2½ times the adult requirement.

The reason for this is that the infant has more active tissue and a greater body surface area in proportion to his weight than the adult; consequently, there is a greater heat loss. Additional calories are also needed for growth and activity. The accompanying table shows the approximate distribution of the caloric needs of the infant at the 120 cal./Kg. level.

	Calories/Kg. of Body Weight/24 Hrs.
Basal metabolism.........	60
Activity.................	25
Growth..................	30
Loss in stools.............	5
Total...............	120

The **fluid requirement** for young infants is about 150 ml., or 5 ozs., per Kg. of body weight in 24 hours. At first this usually is calculated into the formula, but later boiled water is given to the baby between feedings.

The **protein requirement** in the first year of life is greater per unit of body weight than at any other time of life. The predominant protein of human milk, lactalbumin, forms a soft flocculent curd, while casein, the predominant protein of cow's milk forms a larger and harder curd when subjected to the action of digestive juices. However, in homogenized, pasteurized cow's milk the fat globules are reduced in size and the curd formed is smaller and softer than in raw cow's milk.

TABLE 13–1.
Recommended Dietary Allowances
for Calories and Nutrients for Infants
During the First Year (Infant 8 Kg. or 18 lb.)

Calories*................	115 ± 15 per Kg.
Protein*................	2.5 ± 0.5 Gm./Kg.
Calcium*................	0.7 Gm.
Iron....................	1.0 mg./Kg.
Vitamin A...............	1,500 I.U.
Thiamine*...............	0.4 mg.
Riboflavin*..............	0.6 mg.
Niacin*.................	6.0 mg.
Ascorbic acid............	30 mg.
Vitamin D...............	400 I.U.

* The calorie and protein allowances per Kg. for infants are considered to decrease progressively from birth. Allowances for calcium, thiamine, riboflavin and niacin increase proportionally with calories to the maximum values shown.

Taken from N.R.C.—Recommended Dietary Allowances 1963.

TABLE 13–2. Estimated Requirements and Advisable Intakes of Protein*

Age (months)	Estimated Requirement		Advisable Intakes†	
	Gm./day	Gm./Kg./day	Gm./day	Gm./Kg./day
1	10	2.2	14	3.0
2	11	2.0	15	2.7
4	12	1.7	16	2.3
6	12	1.6	16	2.2
8	12	1.2	16	1.8
10	12	1.2	16	1.6
12	12	1.2	16	1.6

* From Formon, S. J.: Infant Nutrition, p. 74. Philadelphia, W. B. Saunders, 1967.

† For infants not breast-fed but receiving protein of high nutritional quality.

TABLE 13–3. Comparative Nutritive Value of Human, Cow's and Goat's Milk
(Nutrients per 100 grams of fluid milk)

	Human	Cow's	Goat's
Calories.........	77	65	67
Protein (gm.)......	1.1	3.5	3.2
Fat (gm.).........	4.0	3.5	4.0
Carbohydrate (gm.)	9.5	4.9	4.6
Water (gm.)......	85.2	87.4	87.5
Total ash.........	0.2	0.7	0.7
Calcium (mg.).....	33	118	129
Phosphorus (mg.) ..	14	93	106
Sodium (mg.).....	16	50	34
Potassium (mg.)....	51	144	180
Iron.............	0.1	0.05	0.1
Vitamin A (I.U.)....	240	140	160
Thiamine (mg.)....	0.01	0.03	0.04
Riboflavin (mg.)...	0.04	0.17	0.11
Niacin (mg.)......	0.2	0.1	0.3
Ascorbic acid (mg.)	5	1	1

Figures from Watt, B. K., and Merrill, A. L., Agr. Handbook No. 8. Composition of foods, raw, processed, prepared. U.S.D.A., 1963.

Although cow's milk has a greater quantity of total protein than human milk, both can meet the infant's requirement for protein. The Recommended Dietary Allowances suggest 2.5 ± 0.5 Gm. of protein per Kg. of body weight during the first year of life (see Table 13–1). Human milk provides approximately 2 Gm. of protein per Kg. while cow's milk and some formulas based on it provide approximately 3 to 3.5

Gm. of protein per Kg. Fomon[1] gives estimated requirements and advisable intakes of protein for ages one through twelve months (see Table 13–2). His advisable intake at one month is 3.0 Gm./Kg. and at 12 months, 1.6 Gm./Kg., which illustrates the progessive decrease in requirement from birth to one year of age.

Fat Requirement. No specific requirement for fat can be stated but the caloric value of fat appears to be an asset during the early months of life when energy requirements per unit of body weight are high. The fat must be in easily digestible form, however, preferably emulsified. Fat is also a carrier of fat-soluble vitamins. Human milk provides about 48 per cent of its calories as fat, cow's milk 46 per cent (see Table 13–3). Most commercial formulas provide 35 to 50 per cent of the calories as fat. The essential fatty acid, linoleic, constitutes about 10.6 per cent of the fatty acids of human milk, and 2.1 per cent of the fatty acid of cow's milk.[2] In the preparation of commercial formulas, a combination of corn, coconut and other oils is used.

Carbohydrates in Infant Feeding. Lactose, the natural carbohydrate of mammalian milks, has many advantages. It provides calories in non-irritating and easily available form. Its slow breakdown and absorption probably has a beneficial effect upon calcium absorption in the intestinal tract. Most commercial formulas use lactose as the preferred carbohydrate. However, for economy and convenience of the mother preparing a formula at home, cane sugar (sucrose) or corn syrup is usually recommended by the physician, the amount calculated according to the caloric need. Dextri-Maltose (malt sugar or maltose) formerly used commonly is less often recommended now.

Minerals—Recommended or Advisable Intakes. The differences in mineral and vitamin *requirements* of infants as determined by balance studies and the *recommended* or *advisable* intakes listed by au-

thorities may need some explanation. The recommended Dietary Allowance table lists maximum values for the first year to provide for a wide margin of safety. Fomon[3] gives as advisable intakes, about twice the estimated *minimum* requirements at several age levels, taking into account the per cent of each nutrient absorbed under normal conditions. In general, Fomon's figures are slightly lower than the RDA (see Table 13–1).

CALCIUM. Although breast milk is lower in calcium than the amounts usually recommended for artificial feeding, it must be in an easily available form because breast-fed infants seem to get enough calcium. Cow's milk formulas and all commercial preparations provide at least twice the amount in breast milk (see Table 13–3). According to Fomon[3] an advisable intake for infants under one year is 500 mg. per day. The RDA gives 700 mg. per day as a maximum for artificially fed infants as the level to be approached at the end of the first year of life.

IRON. Iron deficiency appears to be prevalent among infants throughout the world, especially in areas where food is scarce or where the family lacks the money to purchase enough food. The iron requirement of an infant is related to the amount of iron stored during the late prenatal period, to perinatal or subsequent losses of blood, and to the rate of growth in early infancy. Those infants at special risk are the low-birth-weight infant, infants born of anemic mothers, or infants who are twins or the product of other multiple births. Iron-fortified formula, together with infant cereals which are fortified with iron, are desirable for these special risk situations.

Fomon points out that "every normal full-term infant should receive a cumulative intake of iron amounting to 2,000 mg. during the first year of life, of which at least 1,000 mg. should be given between age six to 12 months."[4] To accomplish this, from three months of age a daily intake of 8 mg. of iron should be provided. The fortified infant cereals and the baby meats,

---

[1] Fomon, S. J.: Infant Nutrition. Philadelphia, Saunders, 1967.

[2] Fomon, S. J.: op. cit.

[3] Fomon, S. J.: op. cit., p. 179.

[4] Fomon, S. J.: op. cit.

fruits and vegetables, used in appropriate amounts for age, can provide an adequate iron intake for the normal full-term baby.

For example, some fortified baby cereals provide as much as 3.6 mg. of iron in 3 tablespoons. A 4-month-old baby can be expected to eat at least 6 tablespoons (7.2 mg. of Fe). This, plus the iron in fruits, vegetables and meat, will provide 8 mg. of Fe per day from food. If such foods are used, there is no need for any iron supplement.

TRACE MINERALS. Chromium, cobalt, copper, iodine, manganese, molybdenum, selenium and zinc are discussed briefly by Fomon.[5] Of these *iodine* is unique because it might vary in either human or cow's milk according to amount consumed in food or water. Only in isolated areas where the iodine content of the soil is low and where mostly locally produced food and milk is used would there be much danger of an iodine deficiency. Most commercial formulas and infant foods provide sufficient iodine.

FLUORIDE. In technically advanced countries the magnitude of the dental caries problem exceeds that of all other nutritional diseases. It has been dramatically demonstrated that 6-year-old children born after fluoridation started in one community had significantly fewer cavities than 10- or 11-year-old children using the same water supply but born before fluoridation started.[6] These differences suggest that fluoride prophylaxis during infancy is desirable. The advisable intake tentatively proposed by Fomon,[5] 0.5 mg. per day, is approximately the amount which would be ingested by infants fed formulas diluted with equal parts of water fluoridated at the usual level of 1 p.p.m.

ELECTROLYTE AND FLUID BALANCE. The chief electrolytes that maintain osmotic equilibrium in the body are sodium, potassium and magnesium. The fluid volume of the infant formula or of water consumed as such is usually adequate. Diarrhea is a common cause of water and electrolyte disturbance in infants. The large loss of liquid in the stools can seriously deplete the young child's extracellular fluid volume, especially when it is combined with vomiting.[7] Symptoms of fluid volume deficit due to diarrhea and its treatment will be discussed more fully in Chapter 34. Lytren,[8] a complete electrolyte preparation for oral use, is often prescribed. A pediatric nurse needs to be on the alert to recognize symptoms, which may develop rather rapidly. In one case an experienced nurse noted the ashen gray color, the cold extremities and sunken eyes of a small infant brought to the hospital in a comatose state. Quick referral to the pediatrician and the replacement of fluid and electrolytes saved the child's life.

Vitamins—Advisable Intakes. In technically advanced countries infants seldom suffer from vitamin deficiencies. The requirements are usually met by breast milk or cow's milk formulas consumed at a rate of approximately 800 ml. per day, except for ascorbic acid and vitamin D. Ascorbic acid is a limiting factor for bottle-fed infants whose formula is subjected to high heat during processing. According to Guthrie[9] infants should receive a supplementary source of ascorbic acid by the tenth day of life. A synthetic source of this vitamin rather than orange juice is recommended for small infants because it minimizes any sensitizing reaction.

The 400 I.U. of vitamin D recommended by RDA is generally accepted as a desirable supplement after five days of age unless the child is regularly exposed to sunlight. If the infant is bottle fed with a formula already fortified with vitamin D providing this amount, no further supplement is necessary.

Precautions are necessary in the use of the fat-soluble vitamins, which should be given in the amounts recommended but not more than that, because an excess of

[5] Fomon, S. J.: op. cit.

[6] Dunning, J. M.: Current status of fluoridation. New Eng. J. Med., 272:30, 1965.

[7] Metheny, N. M., and Snively, W. D.: Nurses Handbook of Fluid Balance. Philadelphia, J. B. Lippincott, 1967.

[8] Lytren (Mead Johnson). A complete electrolyte preparation for oral use.

[9] Guthrie, H. A.: Introductory Nutrition. St. Louis, C. V. Mosby, 1967.

TABLE 13–4

	Advisable Intakes of Vitamins for Infants under One Year of Age*			RDA Maximum for Infant at One Year†
Vitamin	**1 Month**	**6 Months**	**12 Months**	**12 Months**
Vitamin A (I.U.).................	600	600	600	1,500
Vitamin D (I.U.).................	400	400	400	400
Vitamin E (mg.).................	1.3	1.8	1.8	0.5 mg./Kg. body wt.
Vitamin K....................	....	....	....	....
Thiamine (mg.).................	0.12	0.16	0.21	0.4
Riboflavin (mg.)................	0.27	0.34	0.44	0.6
Niacin equivalent (mg.)..........	3.7	4.7	6.2	6.0
Vitamin B6 (mcg/gm. protein)....	18	18	18	20
Ascorbic acid (mg.).............	20	20	20	30

* Fomon, S. J.: Infant Nutrition, Phila., Saunders, 1967.
† Recommended Dietary Allowance. National Research Council, Washington, D. C., 1963.

these factors can be toxic (see Chaps. 7 and 10). Fomon[10] gives advisable intakes at three age levels during the first year as shown in Table 13–4. The RDA figures are also given for comparison. As discussed earlier in regard to minerals, the figures suggested by Fomon are estimates of twice the minimum requirements whereas the RDA figures provide for a liberal but safe margin.

BREAST FEEDING VS. FORMULA FEEDING

There is much evidence that the earliest experiences of the newborn baby are of great importance in his later adjustment to the world in which he must live. This is particularly true of the way he obtains his food. Even at this early stage, he will react to the emotions of the mother, and this is of more importance than whether he is breast- or formula-fed. If the mother is relaxed and confident, the baby will respond to her and, through her, to the world about him with trust and confidence. Conversely, if the mother is tense and overanxious, or if the feeding is hurried, the baby becomes aware of discomfort. In response, there may be fretfulness or crying, which may prevent his taking the food he needs.

A mother should be encouraged to breast-feed her baby, but she should not be made to feel guilty if she prefers to bottle-feed him. If he is cuddled and made comfortable when he is being fed, whether by breast or by bottle, his feelings will be those of warmth and comfort.

Actually, breast-feeding is easier than bottle-feeding if the mother has to prepare the formula with special utensils and sterilized bottles and nipples. With commercial formulas ready bottled available today the mother may be relieved of much worry and trouble by formula feeding.

According to Fomon[11] "When a young infant is breast-fed by a healthy well-nourished mother and receives an adequate caloric intake from this source, requirements for most specific nutrients appear to be fulfilled. With the exception of iron, fluoride and vitamin D, there would seem to be no justification for supplementation of the diet of the breast-fed infant."

While breast-feeding is nature's way to feed the baby, relatively few young mothers in the U. S. today nurse their infants for more than a few days and often not at all. In poor areas or where medical aid is not available breast milk may be safer than a poor formula or one unhygienically pre-

---

[10] Fomon, S. J.: op. cit.

[11] Fomon, S. J.: op. cit. p. 42.

pared. Breast milk also has the advantage of freedom from contamination, is economical and requires no preparation. It has the advantage of immunizing the baby against certain infectious diseases through antibodies received in the mother's milk and is less likely to cause allergic reactions.

Certain psychological advantages have been attributed to breast-feeding. Many mothers derive satisfaction from feeling they are the source of their baby's nutriment. Also, breast-feeding permits an early establishment of an intimacy with the child that promises well for the mother-child relationship.

The lactating woman will find that she needs more food than a non-lactating woman of her age and size and it may cost her from $2.50 to $3.00 more per week to feed herself during the time that she is sharing her nutriment with her infant.

The decision to breast-feed or bottle-feed the baby should be made during pregnancy. If the mother desires to breast-feed her infant, instructions for the preparation of her breasts prior to delivery should be given by the nurse. Some young mothers will breast-feed their infants if careful

teaching and psychological as well as physical preparation is instigated early in pregnancy. Moreover, the nursing mother must be sure to have the proper diet (see Chap. 12) and get sufficient sleep and relaxation, otherwise she will not produce enough milk.

The following table shows the approximate quantity of milk consumed by an average baby under normal conditions. This shows why the mother must eat properly if she is going to produce this quantity of milk:

	Gm.	Ozs.
1st day	10	⅓
2d day	90	3
3d day	190	6⅓
4th day	310	10
5th day	350	11½
6th day	390	13
7th day	470	15⅔
3d week	500	16
4th week	600	20
8th week	800	26½
12th week	900	30
24th week	1,000	33

The thick, yellowish fluid which appears the first few days of nursing (colostrum) will nourish the baby until the milk comes a few days later. The baby should be laid beside the mother with his cheek close to her breast. He will turn his head toward the breast trying to find the nipple, and the mother can help him by holding the breast so that he can get the nipple into his mouth. Nursing the baby will in itself increase the milk supply of the mother, and she will be able to satisfy his needs with an ever-increasing supply as he keeps on growing. At first the baby may be satisfied after he has emptied only one breast, but if he does not give signs that he is full, he should be given the other breast. He should be started on this breast at his next feeding so as to be sure to empty it.

If the baby is not getting enough to satisfy his hunger from the breast feeding, the doctor may prescribe an additional formula for him, to be given after he has been at the breast. For one reason or another, the mother may wish to skip a breast feeding occasionally, and in such case a formula feeding may be substituted.

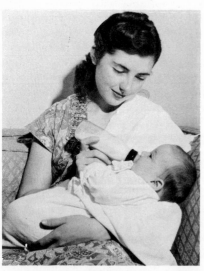

FIG. 13–1. Feeding time should be enjoyed by both mother and baby, whether he is breast- or formula-fed. (Children's Bureau photograph by Philip Bonn)

In some circumstances it may be advisable to substitute bottle-feeding for breast-feeding, even when the mother has an adequate supply of milk. This would be in case of another pregnancy or the development of chronic illness or severe long-lasting infectious disease in the mother.

If the mother is feeding her baby by bottle, she should hold him as though she were breast-feeding him, cradled in her arm (Fig. 13–1), in order to give him the same sense of nearness and companionship. It is important that she feel relaxed and unhurried, and that she enjoys this time with her baby. She should never allow him to eat by himself by propping the bottle up beside him. In this way his nutritional needs will be met but not his need for love and contact.

As he gets older, the baby may want to hold his bottle himself while feeding. There is no reason why he should not eat alone sometimes, but this had better not be when he is going to sleep afterward, or he will come to depend on his bottle in connection with sleeping.

FORMULAS: TYPES AND SOURCES

Milks Used in Infant Feeding. Cow's milk usually is chosen because it can be modified easily to resemble the composition of human milk, and a safe supply is generally available. Fresh pasteurized, canned evaporated or dried whole milk powder may be used in the preparation of a formula.

The choice of the type of milk for infant feeding will be determined by circumstances. Sometimes a safe, dependable fresh milk supply is not available, or home refrigeration is inadequate. Evaporated milk is distributed widely and will keep without refrigeration until the can is opened, after which it must be stored in a cold place, as is the case with fresh milk. Dried milk also will keep without refrigeration until the can is opened, but it must be kept covered and cold afterward. Some physicians prescribe evaporated milk for the formula, even when a supply of fresh milk is available, as they consider it to be more satisfactory. It is possible to obtain each of these milks fortified with vitamin D.

In processing canned and dried whole milk, the fat is blended thoroughly with the other milk solids. When fresh whole milk is used for the formula, it is best to use the homogenized type, in which, during the process of preparation for the market, the cream is thoroughly blended and distributed throughout the milk. Most homogenized milk is fortified with 400 I.U. of vitamin D per quart. Homogenized milk forms a softer curd than cream-line milk, and there is no danger that the mother will use "the top of the bottle" with its high fat content to make the baby's formula. Cow's milk is adapted to the needs of an animal that reaches maturity in a few months, while the human offspring does not reach maturity for some years. Therefore, it is to be expected that cow's milk will be richer in body-building materials than human milk. By analysis, it is found to be richer in protein and in the mineral salts but less rich in milk sugar (see Table 13–3). For this reason it is often modified by dilution with water and the addition of some form of sugar. However, the tendency today is to feed whole cow's milk much earlier than was formerly advocated.

Evaporated milk contains 400 I.U. of vitamin D per reconstituted quart and is less expensive than fresh milk. It is available in two sizes: 5½-ounce and 13-ounce cans. Condensed cow's milk with its high carbohydrate content, and skimmed cow's milk are considered undesirable for infant feeding. Skim milk is deficient in essential fatty acids and in vitamins A and D unless fortified.

The cost of the baby's formula differs widely, depending on the milk and the sugar used. In a study entitled Economy in Nutrition and Feeding of Infants[12] it was shown that a formula using evaporated cow's milk and cane or beet sugar was least expensive, and that the cost of a formula calling for homogenized whole cow's milk with cane or beet sugar cost about half again as much. Directions for the preparation and storage of infant formulas are given in the Appendix of this publication.[12]

---

[12] Food and Nutrition and Maternal and Child Health Sections, American Public Health Association: Am. J. Public Health, 56:1756, 1966.

TABLE 13–5. Nutrients in Selected Premodified Milks*

Product	Sugar	Fat	Amount of Nutrient Per Quart (After Dilution If Indicated)					
			Protein (Gm.)	Calcium (mg.)	Iron (mg.)	Vitamin A (I.U.)	Vitamin D (I.U.)	Ascorbic Acid (mg.)
Baker—Infant Formula (L&P)†	lactose, dextrose, maltose, dextrins	coconut, corn, soy oil	21.4	825	7.5	2,500	400	50
Borden—Bremil (L&P)	lactose	corn, coconut, peanut oil	14.7	630	8.0	2,500	400	50
Carnation—Carnalac (L)	lactose	butterfat	26.6	804	Trace	1,035	400	80
Gerbers—Modilac (L)	lactose, dextrose, maltose, dextrins	corn oil	21.4	800	10.0	1,500	400	45
Mead-Johnson—Enfamil (L&P)	lactose	oleo, corn, coconut oil	14.7	615	1.4	1,500	400	50
Mead-Johnson—Enfamil with iron (L&P)	lactose	oleo, corn, coconut oil	14.4	615	8.0	1,500	400	50
Pet—Formil	lactose	butterfat, coconut oil, corn oil	16.0	590	Trace	2,500	400	50
Pet—Formil with iron	lactose	butterfat, coconut oil, corn oil	16.0	590	8.0	2,500	400	50
Ross—Similac (L&P)	lactose	corn, coconut oil	16.3	630 (L) 730 (P)	Trace	2,500	400	50
Ross—Similac with iron (L&P)	lactose	corn, coconut oil	16.3	630 (L) 730 (P)	12,0	2,500	400	50
Wyeth—SMA S-26 (L&P)	lactose	oleo, soy, corn, coconut oil	14.7‡	400	8.0	2,500	400	50
Recommended Daily Dietary Allowances (5.5-Kg. Infant)			11-16.5	700	5.5	1,500	400	30

* February, 1966, taken from published materials by the indicated company, from Baker Laboratories: Handbook of Infant Formulas. New York, Pfizer, 1964; Meyer, H. F.: Infant Foods and Feeding Practices. Springfield, Ill., Charles C Thomas, 1960.

† L&P—Liquid and powder.

‡ 40 per cent casein.

From Economy in Nutrition and Feeding of Infants. Am. J. Pub. Health, 56:1766, 1966.

In recent years commercially prepared formulas have become widely available. They come in powdered or canned evaporated form, needing only the addition of boiled water. Some have iron and vitamins added. These preparations are convenient for the busy mother, though more expensive than an ordinary formula.

In hospitals where labor costs and space are a consideration commercial formulas are now widely used and the cost is even less than for formulas made in the hospital formula room.

Comparisons of commercial formulas available in 1966 are given in Table 13–5.

PREMODIFIED MILKS. A large variety of premodified milk formulas are now available. They have been modified in one or more of the following ways:

Butterfat is removed and a vegetable oil or oils are added to increase the amount of unsaturated fatty acid, particularly the essential fatty acid, linoleic acid. This makes the cow's milk formula more like breast milk in essential fatty acid content, and fat in this form is better tolerated by the infant.

The protein is treated to produce a softer, more flocculent curd which is more easily digested by the infant.

The milk is diluted to reduce the calcium and, to make up for this dilution in terms of calories, sugar—usually lactose—is added. Both these modifications make the formula more like breast milk.

Dialysis may be used to reduce the sodium content of cow's milk.

Supplements of vitamins A, D and C are usually added and, sometimes, also iron. Another development in a few urban areas is a commercial formula preparation service, which delivers the prepared formula to the home each day. These cost from $0.90 to $1.25 a day, which is prohibitive for most families.

GOAT MILK, seldom used today in the U. S. for infant feeding, is still used in many parts of the world. Experience shows that it is nutritionally adequate in most respects (see Table 13–3). It was formerly used to feed infants who had an allergy to cow's milk. Goat-milk fat differs from cow's milk in that it contains more essential fatty acids and has a greater percentage of medium- and short-chain fatty acids. These differences suggest that the fat of goat milk may be more readily digested than that of cow's milk.[13]

Milk Substitutes. Certain infants are born with a sensitivity to the proteins of all milks. This may be mild enough to cause only irritability, or it may be severe enough to cause violent illness and even death. Several preparations have been devised as foods to approximate human milk in carbohydrate, protein, fat, mineral and vitamin content. These contain no milk at all. Soybean preparations are used most commonly.[14] Usually, the protein in the soybean can be taken by infants allergic to the proteins of milk A milk substitute having meat protein as a base, with added vitamins and minerals, has also proved to be adequate nutritionally for such infants. Milk must also be eliminated from the diet of infants who have galactosemia, a disease in which they cannot metabolize galactose, one of the sugars found in milk. A meat-base formula or a mixture of amino acids[15] must be substituted for milk for these infants (see Chap. 30).

If these milk substitutes are properly supplemented, infants do as well on them as on other bottle feedings. A discussion of the nutritive adequacy of milk substitutes and an excellent table of composition has recently been prepared by the Committee on Nutrition of the American Academy of Pediatrics.[16]

Lactose intolerance in infants and children is discussed in Chapter 34.

Temperature for Feeding. The formula may be given at room temperature or warmed to body temperature if desired. If the formula has been stored in the refrigerator it should be allowed to stand long enough to reach room temperature, or the bottle may be placed in warm water until it reaches the desired temperature.

13 Fomon, S. J.: op. cit.

14 Two such products are ProSobee made by Mead Johnson and Co.; Mull-Soy made by Borden Co.

15 Nutramigen, Mead Johnson & Co. Meat Base Formula, Gerber Prod. Co.

16 Pediatrics, *31*:329, 1963.

The temperature of milk should be tested by shaking a few drops on the inside of the wrist.

How Often to Feed. Much has been said in recent years about so-called "self-demand schedules of feeding." For many years babies were fed by the clock, regardless of whether they were hungry earlier or later than the scheduled time. Today we recognize that when a baby is hungry, that is the time to feed him, whether the interval is 2, 3, 4 or even 5 hours. A newborn baby may wake to be fed 8 to 10 times in 24 hours. By the time he is a month old, there may be 3 hours between feedings. Most babies establish themselves on a schedule of 4-hourly feedings by the time they are between 2 and 3 months old. During this time, too, the baby will begin to sleep through the night after a late evening feeding.

"Burping" the Baby. Once or twice during a feeding, the baby should be given a chance to bring up any swallowed air. Holding him up so that his stomach is against the mother's shoulder and gently patting him on the back will help to eliminate the air. An even better way is to hold the baby in a sitting position on the mother's knee, with his chin held in the palm of her hand. By leaning the baby forward and gently stroking or patting his back swallowed air is released.

FEEDING DIFFICULTIES IN INFANTS

Vomiting and Regurgitation. Vomiting may result from a number of causes and may or may not be a serious symptom. In regurgitation only small amounts of food are lost, while in vomiting the contractions of the stomach are sufficiently strong to empty the stomach. Regurgitation may be avoided by "burping" the infant once or twice during a feeding. Occasional vomiting is usually caused by overdistention of the stomach due to the ingestion of too large or too frequent feedings or to the swallowing of air. It may also be due to an imbalance of the food constituents, especially to an oversupply of fat, causing delayed emptying of the stomach. Persistent vomiting may be a symptom of infection, obstruction or other serious ailment and should be referred promptly to the physician. The cause should be determined and the feedings adjusted accordingly.

Colic. A baby who has hard crying spells shortly after eating is said to be "colicky." The colic, or severe abdominal cramping pain, may be caused by distention due to the swallowing of air; to gas formed by bacterial fermentation of undigested food; to overfeeding or underfeeding; to cold, excitement or only to being tired. The baby may have to be "burped" again. Making sure he is warm may help. Mothers are apt to think that his feeding is wrong, but changing the feeding usually does not help. Spock[17] says that these babies seem to grow and gain weight better than most, and that generally the condition disappears at the age of 3 to 4 months.

Diarrhea. Loose stools may be serious, and the doctor should be consulted at once. See Chapter 34 for diseases in which diarrhea is a symptom.

The lower infant mortality rate and the larger number of well babies are attributed in large part to the great advances made in the last decades in methods of feeding, especially among infants who must be fed artificially. The simplification of the formula and the early supplementation of milk with other foods is partly responsible. However, the reduction of bacterial contamination of the formula has been a major factor in lessening infant morbidity and mortality from gatrointestinal infections during the first year of life.

Constipation. Constipation in infancy is not infrequent, specially in formula-fed babies. Mother's milk, because of a higher lactose content than cow's milk, is more laxative than the latter. Many mothers are concerned when the baby has only one bowel movement per day or on alternate days. The number of movements per day is not of so much importance as the consistency of the stools. If the feces are hard and expelled with difficulty, then the child may be said to be constipated and should be treated accordingly.[18]

---

[17] Spock, B.: Baby and Child Care. New York, Duell, 1957.
[18] Your Baby's First Year. Children's Bureau, U. S. Department of Health, Education and Welfare, Publ. No. 400, Washington, D. C., 1962.

The formula may be made more laxative by changing the type of sugar used. Prune juice or strained prunes, given once or twice a day, may remedy the situation. For the older child, an increase in the diet of whole-grain bread and cereals and of vegetables and fruits may be of help. If the constipation persists, the doctor should be consulted.

FEEDING INFANTS OF LOW BIRTH WEIGHT

The premature infant needs more care in every respect than does a full-term baby. The sucking and the swallowing reflexes may be absent or sluggish, the capacity of the stomach is small, the gastric acidity is low, the absorption of fat is poor, and the digestive enzyme system is incompletely developed. Human milk was long considered to be the ideal food for premature infants. However, it has been found that a high-protein, low-fat cow's milk formula will ensure better weight gain and development in these infants than does human milk, and it is far easier to obtain.

Because of the incomplete antenatal storage and the demands of rapid growth, the premature infant has greater need of iron, calcium, phosphorus and protein than has the full-term infant.

Because the sucking or swallowing reflexes may be sluggish, a very small premature infant may be fed entirely by gavage until he is capable of taking a formula. A somewhat larger baby may be fed with a medicine dropper covered with rubber tubing until he is able to suck. As soon as premature infants are found to suck well, they should be fed by bottle.

Infants of low birth weight are individual problems and the physician will usually prescribe the concentration and the amount of the formula. Davidson,[19] commenting on current practices in feeding premature infants, notes that polyunsaturated fatty acids such as those in corn oil seem to be better absorbed than saturated fats such as milk fat and that such infants can tolerate more fat and thus more calories in this form.

Hassan *et al.*[20] have reported a syndrome in premature infants consisting of edema, skin lesions and hematologic abnormalities resulting from the use of formulas with a relatively high content of polyunsaturated fatty acids (PUFA). These findings were associated with low plasma vitamin E levels. The abnormalities disappeared rapidly after administration of vitamin E and were not observed in infants receiving similar formulas with vitamin E. These results suggest that when the formula is high in PUFA, as recommended by some for premature infants, a vitamin E supplement should be added to the formula.

Fomon[21] recommends that infants of low birth weight be observed during the first 24 hours without feeding. The physician may recommend a 10 per cent glucose solution by gastric tube the second day.

The caloric concentration of the formula will depend upon the physician's judgment and the desired rate of gain in weight. In general, Fomon recommends for infants weighing less than 2,000 Gm. that the initial formula should provide 100 cal./100 ml. (30 cal./oz.) and for the infant weighing 2,000 Gm. or more, the initial feeding should provide 80 cal./100 ml. (24 cal./oz.). After about a week caloric concentration may be increased if the rate of gain is not satisfactory.

For further discussion of rate of gain the reader is referred to Fomon[21] pp. 249 and 250.

The picture (Fig. 13–2) on page 180 is convincing evidence that premature infants can grow into sturdy boys and girls if given proper care.

SUPPLEMENTARY FOODS

The time for the addition of supplementary foods to the diet of the breast or formula fed infant has undergone marked changes in the past 20 years. Whereas earlier no solid foods were introduced until the end of the first year, the pendulum has swung all the way to offering the baby solids during the first month of life. Beal[22]

---

[19] Davidson, M.: J. Pediat., 57:604, 1960.

[20] Hassan, H., *et al.*: Am. J. Clin. Nutr., 49:147, 1966.
[21] Fomon, S. J.: op. cit.
[22] Beal, V. A.: Pediatrics, 20:448, 1957.

has found that the average baby's willing acceptance of cereal is at 2½ to 3 months, of vegetables at 4 to 4½ months, of meat and meat soups at 5½ to 6 months, and of fruit at 2½ to 3 months. Earlier introduction of solid foods tended to meet with resistance by the infant. Beal also has shown that the age of transition from baby foods to the family diet has decreased from approximately 2 years to 13 months.

Guthrie,[23] six years later, reported that some of the young mothers (college personnel) in her survey introduced solid food to their infants at 3 weeks and all had done so by 9 weeks. The contribution of these supplements to total calories was small at first but amounted to 21 per cent of the calories by 13 weeks. The Filer and Marti-

nez study[24] showed that by 6 months of age 30 per cent of the calories fed to their infants came from supplementary feedings.

After discussing the varying patterns and timing of supplementary feeding Guthrie comments: "A rational approach to the question of timing and sequence of additions to the infant's diet should involve a consideration of the nutritional needs of the infant, his physiologic readiness to use foods other than milk, his physical capacity to handle them, and the relative advantages and disadvantages of adding semisolid or solid foods."[25]

In the following paragraphs, the authors have indicated the approximate age at

[23] Guthrie, H. A.: Nutritional intake of infants. J. Am. Dietet. A., 43:120, 1963.

[24] Filer, L. V., and Martinez, G. A.: Clin. Pediat., 3:633, 1964.
[25] Guthrie, H. A.: Introductory Nutrition. p. 343, St. Louis, C. V. Mosby, 1967.

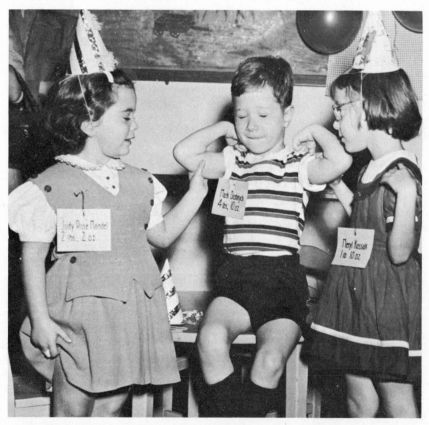

FIG. 13–2. Judy and Meryl, who were prematures weighing 2 lb. 2 oz. and 1 lb. 10 oz. at birth respectively, feel the muscle of another former "preemie," Mark. (The New York Hospital, Cornell Medical Center, New York, N. Y.)

which new foods may be introduced, but in the light of the above paragraphs it can be seen that there may be considerable variation.

Cereals. The baby should be introduced to cereals when he is 2 to 3 months old. If he finds them very distasteful, cooked strained fruits may be given first, and cereal added a week or two later. Dry, precooked cereal preparations and canned cereals especially prepared for infant feeding are available.

The dry, precooked cereals must be mixed with warm formula or whole milk, while the others need only be warmed. The cereals eaten generally by the family may be cooked according to the directions on the package and given to the baby. Some physicians advise longer cooking. The coarse cereals must be strained, and all of them should be thinner than those prepared for the family—thin enough to drop from a spoon. Only a small amount of cereal should be used at first, and this generally is given with the midmorning feeding. The original small amount may be increased gradually, and in a few months it may be of a thicker consistency. By the 7th or the 8th month, the baby will be taking from ¼ to ½ cup twice during the day.

Fruits. Cooked, strained fruits and ripe banana may be added to the baby's diet when he is 3 months old. Like cereals, these may be purchased in cans or jars, all ready for infant use, or they may be prepared at home. Cooked fruits should be put through a purée sieve or strainer. Strained apple sauce, prunes, peaches, pears and apricots are suitable. Ripe mashed banana, thinned out with a little milk, may also be given. Starting with a teaspoonful once or twice a day, the baby will soon take 2 to 3 tablespoonfuls. Most babies like fruit and take it readily. This helps them to accept other solid foods, the taste of which may not appeal to them quite as much.

Vegetables. By the 4th month, or even earlier, strained vegetables are usually introduced. Those added first are peas, string beans, spinach, carrots, beets, tomatoes and squash. Fresh, frozen or canned vegetables are suitable. If prepared at home, they should be cooked in a small amount of water, as would be done for the family meal, and the baby's portion put through a purée sieve or a strainer. Again, these and other varieties of vegetables are available in cans or jars in most grocery stores prepared and ready for serving after they are warmed. Starting with a teaspoonful at one feeding—and, later, as part of lunch—the baby will soon be taking 2 to 3 rounded tablespoonfuls. Potatoes, both sweet and white, may be added a little later, but potatoes in any form are one of the last vegetables to be accepted by most babies.

Egg Yolk. Egg yolk is a good source of iron, but since other infant foods are now fortified with iron, eggs can be deferred until other foods have been given. Eggs are a common cause of an allergic reaction, the white more so than the yolk, which is the reason for the yolk being given first. The egg may be cooked hard by placing it in boiling water, turning off the heat and letting it stand, covered, for 20 minutes. Cooking changes the protein to make it less allergenic.

Egg yolks should be crumbled and given by spoon, or mixed with cereal or vegetables at first. A fourth of a yolk is a good

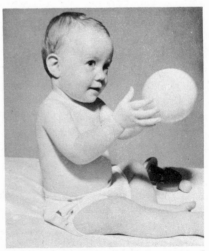

Fig. 13–3. Signs of good nutrition. Note the straight back, well-developed body, alertness and good coordination of this child. (The New York Hospital)

quantity with which to start. If the baby accepts it well and there are no signs of allergy, it may be increased until he is taking a whole yolk, usually at the breakfast feeding. Whole egg may be given by the time he is a year old.

Prepared egg yolk is now available in jars ready to serve as are other infant foods.

Meat. Meats may be added as early as 3 to 4 months or as late as 6 months, depending on the doctor's judgment about the baby's need for them. The most convenient way of serving meat to the baby is by way of the canned, strained beef, beef heart, liver, lamb, chicken, veal and pork preparations available in cans and jars at most grocery stores. To prepare meat for the baby at home, the mother should buy a lamb chop or a slice of beef top round, wipe the surface with a clean damp cloth and scrape off the meat fibers with a tablespoon or a dull knife. The resulting meat pulp may be heated in a custard cup set in a small pan of water over a flame, until it is brown. Liver should be parboiled in water until it is brown, cut in small pieces and put through a sieve. A small amount of salt may be added for flavor to home-prepared meats and water or milk if the mixture is too dry. Salt has been added to the canned meats.

Meats add protein, iron and some of the B complex vitamins to the baby's diet. Again, it is best to begin slowly, with a tea-

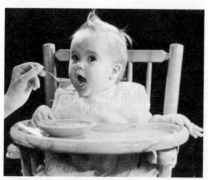

Fig. 13–4. The right start for the baby. Liking comes through learning to like. Teach the flavor of a variety of foods early. (Gesell and Ilg: Behavior of Infants. Philadelphia, J. B. Lippincott)

spoonful or less, at the evening feeding, increasing the quantity as the baby grows older.

Widening Variety in the Infant Diet

By the time they are 6 months old, most babies will be eating all the supplementary foods discussed so far. Besides this, they will be getting either the breast or formula feedings or whole milk, and they will have started to take some fluids, especially orange juice and water, and probably milk, from a cup. A good meal plan for a baby of this age is to give him cereal and egg yolk at breakfast, vegetable and meat for lunch, and cereal and fruit for supper. The quantities will depend on his appetite. If there is a tendency to constipation, giving fruit at breakfast as well as at supper may help. Prunes are particularly good for this.

Additional Foods, 6 to 12 Months. The baby will welcome a piece of dried bread, toast or zwieback to hold in his hands and chew on, particularly if his teeth are beginning to appear. If potato has not already been given, it can be added at this time, mashed fine. It should be thinned out with milk at first until he is used to it. A piece of crisp bacon or a bit of raw, *peeled* apple is also often enjoyed by babies, when they are allowed to hold it in their hands and suck on it. Puddings made mainly with milk, such as junket, cornstarch, tapioca and rice pudding, may also be added occasionally for variety. A small piece of a white, non-oily fish, such as flounder, haddock or halibut, may be substituted for meat now and then. It should be boiled gently in water to cover until it flakes, and *all bones carefully removed.*

By the time he is 9 months old, it is time to try serving some of the junior foods or foods mashed with a fork instead of strained through a sieve. The change should be made gradually and should not be forced. Vegetables and fruits may be tried this way first. Meat had better be served strained until after the first year, because it is so much more difficult to swallow.

As the baby becomes acquainted with a variety of things, including his food, he will want to explore it with such tools as he has at his command. To quote Rabinovitch[26]: "In the second half of the first year, the baby will begin to mess with food, to feel its texture and consistency, to finger-feed himself as he recognizes his growing dexterity. Such experimentation, often difficult for the cleanliness-and-germ-conscious mother, is essential for the child as he learns to relate to food by messing, smelling and pouring. That a high degree of parental fortitude is necessary to allow for these developmental realities goes without saying."

Weaning. The weaning of a baby from milk to other food is not an abrupt transition as infants are fed today. As soon as the baby is introduced to the supplementary foods discussed earlier he is on the way to being weaned. He will have learned to drink from a cup by the time he is 4 or 5 months old. If he still shows a desire to suck he may have a bottle once a day. He will be drinking whole pasteurized milk and eating a variety of foods. The proportion of calories derived from milk will de-

crease gradually as he obtains more of his nutrients from other foods—junior foods for a time and then simple foods from the family table.

OTHER CONSIDERATIONS IN INFANT FEEDING

Satiety, the mechanism by which the infant is made aware that he has had enough, varies widely in babies. In some babies, the reaction is sharp and they actively resist further feeding attempts. In others, satiety is less sharply defined and interest in eating wanes gradually after a period of playfulness. Still others do not seem to know when they have had enough and will vomit what they cannot handle.[27]

Weight Gain

It needs to be pointed out again that a well baby will set his own rate of gain regardless of any so-called "average" tables. When the child is not making a steady gain, something is wrong. He should gain, during the first 6 months, from 4 to 8 ozs. per week, with an average gain of about 6 ozs. Many babies double their birth weight in 4 months.

---

[26] Rabinovitch, R. D., and Fischhoff, J.: J. Am. Dietet. A., 28:614, 1952.

[27] György, P.: Am. J. Clin. Nutr., 8:344, 1960.

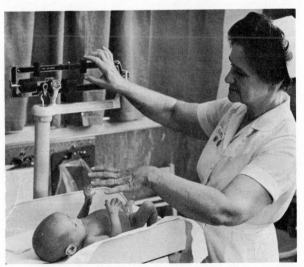

FIG. 13–5. The rate at which a child gains weight is dependent on many factors. As long as he gains weight and length steadily, and exhibits the other signs of good nutrition, there is no cause for worry. (Broadribb, V.: Foundations of Pediatric Nursing. Philadelphia, J. B. Lippincott, 1967)

During the second half of the first year the weight gain will be slower, but most babies will have trebled their birth weight at the end of the first year. The rate of gain will vary with the size of the parents, the sex of the baby—boys are a little heavier than girls—and the type of body build of the child.

Overnutrition

The problem of overnutrition and its hazards in the adult are well known. Lately there has been some question whether our present infant feeding practices may not contribute to the development of overnutrition in later life. It is known that experimental animals whose nutritional needs were met with a minimum of calories during the growth period were healthier, had fewer degenerative diseases and lived longer than similar animals which had been allowed a liberal diet from birth.

We have made great strides in the nutrition of infants in the past 20 to 30 years, but there may be a point at which increasingly rapid growth and development may actually be detrimental in terms of future health.[28] The nurse can help the mother understand that a steady gain in weight, growth and development, within normal limits, is the desirable nutritional pathway for her baby and that this can be achieved by the proper use of ordinary foods.

Radiation and Fallout

Two radioactive elements, strontium-90 and iodine-131, have greatly increased in the atmosphere, and therefore in the soil, as the result of nuclear testing. Cows ingesting a certain amount of Sr^{90} and I^{131} from grass and hay which have absorbed these elements from the soil will secrete them in small quantities in their milk. Careful and constant testing of the quantities of radioactive elements in foods is being done by a number of government agencies. The danger is, of course, that infants and children drinking such milk will ingest enough radioactive material to damage their rapidly growing bodies.

Recently, the Committee on Environmental Hazards of the American Academy of Pediatrics[29] has minimized the danger of fallout at present levels, so far as strontium-90 and iodine-131 are concerned.

Strontium-90. Both cows and man excrete 80 per cent of ingested strontium, so that the actual amount retained in the body is very small. Strontium is normally deposited and therefore localized in bone. If it is radioactive, it emits only beta particles which have little penetrating power. At present levels there is believed to be no danger either to the bone or to the near-lying gonads, the tissues most sensitive to radiation effects. It is possible to remove Sr^{90} from milk, but it is costly and does not seem to be warranted at present.

Iodine-131. This has a carcinogenic effect on the thyroid gland when absorbed in large quantities. The Committee believes that present levels present no danger.

STUDY QUESTIONS AND ACTIVITIES

1. Under what circumstances is breast feeding considered to be an advantage for both mother and baby?

2. What must the mother's attitude be if she bottle-feeds the baby?

3. Under what circumstances should breast feeding be discontinued?

4. What foods in what quantity should be included in the mother's diet if she is nursing her baby? (See Chap. 12.)

5. How much iron should a 4-month-old infant get per day? Can this be supplied by food or is a supplement necessary?

6. Is there evidence that fluoride in an infant's diet has any prophylactic effect during later childhood?

7. Which vitamins are most apt to be the limiting factors in bottle-fed infants?

8. Formerly there were problems in weaning an infant from formula. Why and how has this situation changed with recent methods of infant feeding?

9. Why is the feeding of egg yolk deferred until late in the first year after other supplementary foods are given?

---

[28] Bakwin, H.: Nutrition News, 28:9, 1965.

[29] Pediatrics, 29:845, 1962.

10. Cow's milk is used generally in artificial feeding. How does it compare in composition with human milk? Which forms of cow's milk may be used, and what reasons may influence the choice?

11. In preparing the milk formula, there must be dilution and additions. For what reasons? What are the additions generally used?

12. What is the consensus about the very early supplementation of the infant diet? What did Beal discover in her studies on the acceptability of supplementary foods by infants?

13. Supplementary foods are introduced into the baby's diet gradually. What is the first supplement generally advised and in what amount? In what order are other foods introduced?

14. What do we mean by the term "the baby's own rate of growth and development"? What are some of the factors which will determine his size?

15. There is some concern over the effect of radiation and fallout on the rapidly growing infant and child. How would you reassure a mother about this?

16. Why are we concerned today about overnutrition in infants?

SUPPLEMENTARY READING ON NUTRITION DURING INFANCY

Children's Bureau: U. S. Dept. H.E.W., Washington, D. C. Breast Feeding Your Baby. C. B. Pub. No. 8, 1965; Your Baby's First Year. C. B. No. 400, 1962; Recent Demographic Trends and their Effects on Maternal and Child Health Needs and Services. C. B. 1966.

Committee on Nutrition, American Academy of Pediatrics: Prepared infant formula service. Pediatrics, 36:282, 1965. Vitamin D intake and the hypercalcemia syndrome. Pediatrics, 35:1022, 1965.

Economy in Nutrition and Feeding of Infants. Am. J. Pub. Health 56:1756, 1966.

Filer, L. J.: Current problems in pediatric nutrition. Borden's Review, 27:(Oct.-Dec.) 1966.

Gerber Products Co.; Nutritive Values of Gerber Baby Foods. Fremont, Mich., 1966.

Holt, L. E. Jr. *et al.*: Symposium on infant nutrition. J.A.M.A., 175:100, 1961.

Howley, M. P. F., and Lewis, M. N.: Comparison of hospital-prepared formulas and pre-bottled infant formulas. Hospitals, 39:97, 1965.

Illingsworth, R. S., and Lister, J.: The critical or sensitive period, with special reference to certain feeding problems, in infants and children. J. Pediat., 65:839, 1964.

Lubchenko, L. O.: Formulas and nutrition. Am. J. Nursing, 61:73, 1961 (May).

Meyer, H. F.: Survey of hospital nursery ready-to-eat milk mixtures. Hospitals, 39:60, 1965 (Jan.).

Review: Solid foods in the nutrition of infants. Nutr. Rev., 25:233, 1967.

Richardson, F. H.: Breast or bottle feeding. Today's Health, 40:62, 1962 (May).

For further references see Bibliography in Part Four.

CHAPTER 14

Nutrition of Children and Youth

Growth and Development • Evaluation of Growth and Nutritional Status • Nutritional Needs of Specific Age Groups • School Lunch Program • Nutrition Education

Nutritional requirements change as the infant grows through childhood into adolescence. In this chapter these changes are followed from preschool ages to the late teens. Nutrition influences all phases of growth and development—physical, functional and mental. Poor nutrition may retard any or all of these phases of growth.

Growth and Development. Physical growth is usually measured by changes in height and weight with age. Stature is the more significant criterion because variations in build and the amount of adipose tissue may cause wide variations in weight. Development other than physical growth is more difficult to measure: it deals with muscle strength and coordination, with mental health, with adaptations and attitudes. Different tissues grow at different rates, as shown in Figure 14–1. The nerve and lymphoid tissue grow most rapidly in the early years, the body as a whole more slowly and genital tissues remain almost dormant until puberty.

The rapid rate of growth of the brain which starts before birth persists in the infant and stays well in advance of the growth of the rest of the body. By the time a child is four years old some 90 per cent of the brain has been formed. Along with the increase in size there is a continuous complex evolution of the anatomy, biochemistry and physiology of the brain. The formation and functioning of the brain and nerve fibers and the laying down of the myelin sheaths of the nerves demands that adequate nutrients of the right type be available at this critical period.[1]

During the early formative years, the brain acquires each new specific function and integrates the process into its total pattern of performance and experience. Experimental evidence suggests that the timing of this over-all procedure is of utmost importance. Each new function seems to make its appearance chronologically at a critical period of development. Therefore, any disruption of the normal sequence may result in limitation of the capacity of the brain in some specific ability. This damage may not be evident immediately but may show up at a later age and cannot then be remedied.

A variety of testing procedures is being developed to measure neuromuscular activity and behavioral and intelligence performance. Such tests will allow comparisons among infants and children of different races and geographic origins. Psychological and intelligence tests commonly used in this country have cultural ramifications and are valid only in countries for which standards have been established. They cannot be used in underdeveloped countries.

---

[1] Coursin, D. B.: Undernutrition and brain function. Borden's Rev., *26*:1, 1965.

It has been recognized for some time that certain inborn errors of metabolism may result in brain damage and consequent mental retardation (see Chap. 34). This is understandable if the wrong nutrients reach the brain cells and the essential ones do not. More recently, reports from various parts of the world where malnutrition is common indicate a close relationship between poor central nervous system performance and physical symptoms of undernutrition in height, weight and head circumference[2] (see Chap. 16).

While severe mental retardation is apt to be most evident where protein-calorie malnutrition is most serious, lesser degrees of early malnutrition may result in a child having a lower intellectual capacity than his genetic potential. A few studies of the physical growth of "dull" children found them of shorter stature on the average than normal children of similar racial and environmental background.[3] "Every child born alive is entitled to the normal development of his or her physical and mental potentials."[4] Thus Dr. György prefaces his recommendation that a crash program for better nutrition in early childhood be followed by a long-term educational program toward this same goal.

Growth occurs continuously from conception to full maturity but it is not a uniform process. It consists of two periods of rapid growth separated by a period of more or less uniform but slower increase in size. The first period of rapid growth occurs in fetal life and early infancy, the second during adolescence.

In many countries school children are given physical examinations, are weighed and measured regularly and records are kept which make possible interesting comparisons. Unfortunately, the United States does not have as adequate and complete records as some other countries. In most of the prosperous countries secular increases

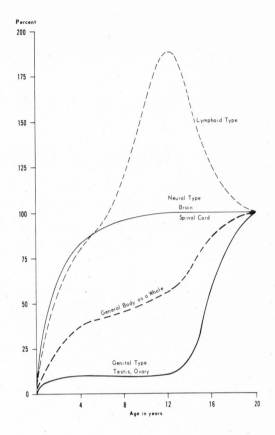

Fig. 14–1. Growth of various body tissues. (Scammon, R. E.: The Measurement of Man. Minneapolis, Univ. Minn. Press, 1930)

in the height and weight of school children of all ages have been reported over several decades. Various explanations are offered for such increases—control of communicable diseases, improved sanitation, and more attention to child nutrition, especially in the early years. When war or economic depressions have interfered with food supplies, the stature of children of a given age has not increased and has even decreased as in Japan during World War II (see Fig. 14–7).

EVALUATION OF THE NUTRITIONAL STATUS OF CHILDREN

Accurate data are lacking on the nutritional status of children in all parts of the U. S. The Children's Bureau is supporting some current work in this area and has

---

[2] Cravioto, J.: Chap. 7, Pre-school Child Malnutrition; Primary Deterrent to Human Progress. Nat. Acad. Science-Nat. Res. Council. Washington, D. C., 1966.

[3] Mosier, H. D., Jr.: Pediatrics, *36*: Suppl. 465, Sept. 1965.

[4] György, P.: Am. J. Clin. Nutr., *14*:65, 1964.

issued guidelines[5] for evaluating the status of preschool children. Similar guidelines might well be set up for school-age children.

In judging the nutritional status of a child there are many factors to look for. Besides a steady gain in height and weight in conformity with his own pattern, there should be good bone and tooth development, good posture, shiny hair, firm muscle turgor, clear skin and eyes, plus alertness and curiosity—all indications of good health and proper nutrition. Nutrient intake calculated from food records is also important but does not tell the whole story.

From 1947 to 1958 a cooperative study was conducted in six states on children under 13 years of age.[6] There was good correlation between the 7-day food intake data and the biochemical and physical examinations. Regional and cultural differences affected the findings slightly. Thus the diets of Spanish-American children in New Mexico were poorer than those of Anglo-American children in the same state, but similar poor diets were found in states and areas with more homogeneous dietary patterns.

The sparsity of our data and the limited number of children in the surveys leave many questions unanswered. Moreover, averages fail to show up the status of children in our poverty groups in cities and isolated rural areas. Current anti-poverty programs have uncovered real malnutrition in this country where food is abundant but not available to disadvantaged families. Also certain age groups, particularly adolescent girls, suffer from self-imposed nutritional inadequacies which will be discussed later.

Longitudinal studies of a limited number of children from birth through adolescence have been carried out—notably at the Harvard School of Public Health in Boston and at the Child Research Council in Denver—which give us information on the variations in food intake and in growth and development of individual children. These studies emphasize the great variability of children, even within the same family. For example, 20 early- and 20 late-maturing boys and girls were chosen from the Harvard study to compare stature changes and caloric intakes during the adolescent growth spurts.[7] The differences between these two groups would be hidden if the two groups were averaged (see Figs. 14–5 and 14–6).

Because of these findings it is now considered better to check all measurements of a child's growth and development against his own previous rate of development, rather than put the major emphasis on comparisons with other children of his age and sex (the custom for many years). Height and weight tables often have served as the only criteria by which growth has been measured. However, this tells us nothing of the child's growth in relation to his hereditary background, or of environmental factors which affect his rate of growth and development.

Growth Charts. Today the preferred method for following a child's rate of growth is by recording it on a chart such as is shown in Figure 14–2. The chart shown is for boys from age 2 to 13. Similar charts have been constructed for girls of this age, for infants, both boys and girls, and for adolescent boys and girls. They are based on careful measurements of a selected group of children followed for the years specified and, as can be seen, show a wide range of variation.

The 50th percentile in both the height and the weight curves represents the median of all children measured. A child of stocky build will be below the median for height and may be slightly above the median for weight. On the other hand, the tall, rangy child will be well above the median for height and may or may not be below the median for weight.

The height and the weight recorded on such a chart at 6 month or yearly intervals will show graphically how a child is progressing within his particular growth pattern. Also, it will show any deviation from

---

[5] Suggested Guidelines for Evaluation of Nutritional Status of Preschool Children. Washington, D. C., Children's Bureau, U. S. H.E.W.

[6] Morgan, A. F.: Nutritional Status, U.S.A. Bull. No. 769, Cal. Agr. Exp. Sta. Oct., 1959.

[7] Mitchell, H. S., *et al.*: Proc. VII Int. Cong. Nutrition. 1967.

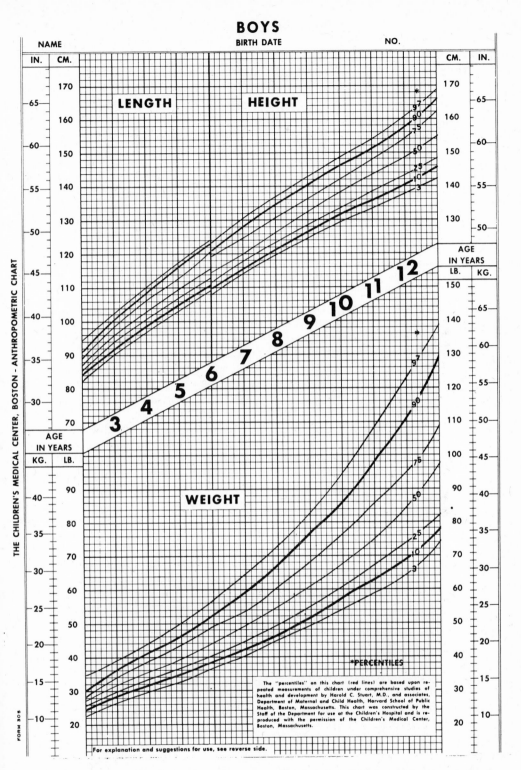

FIG. 14–2. For explanation of use see text. The break in height at the 6 year level occurs because up to that time the length of the child has been measured as he lay recumbent, while after this age the standing height is measured. The 50th percentile is the median range. Most children will fall somewhere between the 10th and the 90th percentiles. From Children's Medical Center, Boston, Mass.

this progress, whether due to illness or other causes, and will alert the examining physician to determine the reason.

NUTRITIONAL NEEDS OF SPECIFIC AGE GROUPS
Preschool Ages 1-6

The one year old, whom we discussed in the last chapter, will already have begun to show a decided change in appetite and interest in food. Beal[8] has shown that, on the average, girls at 6 months and boys at 9 months decrease their milk intake markedly. For girls this persists until 2 to 3 years of age and then slowly begins to rise. In contrast, boys have a somewhat steeper decrease in milk intake than girls but recover more rapidly and by 2½ years have reached a higher level than girls. Other foods, too, are not taken as eagerly as formerly, and some may be refused altogether. This should not be interpreted as a "poor" appetite but rather the decreased appetite of that age.

All this is due in large measure to a decrease in growth rate and, therefore, to the quantitative need for food. At this age, also, the young child is becoming increasingly intrigued by his surroundings—parents, sisters and brothers and the paraphernalia of the home, all of which vie for his attention. He will want to play with his food, to feel its texture, and he will try to feed himself with his hands, refusing the same food when it is offered on a spoon.

This can become an anxious time for the inexperienced mother, accustomed to the voracious appetite of infancy (or to the busy nurse facing a ward full of restive children). Unless the mother is guided correctly, food and eating may become a battleground between herself and the baby and may lay the groundwork for some of the anorexia and the emotional upsets related to food and eating which so often occur in the preschool years. It is important for her to understand that changes in food acceptance and the need for exploration are a part of the normal growth pattern and that all babies go through this process.

[8] Beal, V. A.: J. Nutrition, 53:499, 1954.

Physically, the baby is learning motor mastery of his body—eye, hand and mouth coordination, chewing, swallowing, the use of mouth and throat muscles. He "puts everything into his mouth." From his earliest days his mouth has served him as a sensory organ. He now uses it to explore whatever is within reach. Moreover, from the very beginning his feedings established his primary relationships with other people. If the mother is helped to understand and is able to enjoy her baby's developing skills and interests even when she is frustrated by the spilled milk, the dropped spoons and the gleeful contrariness, she will be less likely to worry over the food which he does or does not eat.

The diet of the 1 year old differs only slightly from that described in the previous chapter. It will include not much more than a pint of milk a day plus the supplementary foods already discussed. His vegetables and fruits will be mashed instead of strained, and he will have started on "finger foods," such as bread crusts, toast and zwieback, and an occasional piece of peeled raw apple. He will have been introduced to the family meal schedule with a midmorning and a midafternoon lunch of fruit juice or milk. The cup will largely have supplanted the bottle, and he may have started to try feeding himself with a spoon.

During the second year more solid foods will be added, such as finely chopped fruits and vegetables in place of mashed ones; ready-to-eat cereals as well as hot cereals; chopped liver, lean meat, fish and poultry instead of the strained variety. Whole egg will have replaced egg yolk, and a child of this age may be ready to eat 1 egg a day. Cottage cheese and mild American cheese, in combination with other foods may be used occasionally. Butter or fortified margarine is used with toast or zwieback. He will also enjoy custard and simple puddings. The 2 year old's food should be prepared simply, and fried foods, rich pastries and most forms of cake should be avoided. Coffee, tea and soft drinks containing caffeine—i.e., colas—should not be given to young children.

Making foods easy to eat for beginners helps them to develop independence in feeding themselves and will prevent accidents. Small plastic cups or tumblers are easier to handle than glass or china. If they are not filled too full, there will be less spilling. Vegetables and meat cut into bite-size pieces can be managed either with fingers or with a spoon. Bread and butter cut into strips are easy to hold and eat.

Over-use of Milk. Earlier in this chapter it was stated that most children decrease their milk intake in favor of other foods sometime during the first year. Because milk has been the center of the diet in infancy, there is a tendency to think that it must continue to be so. Smith[9] has warned that when milk continues to provide the largest part of the 1 to 2 year old's diet, nutritional anemia may result. The need for iron in the diet begins at about 3 months of age, and milk supplies very little of this. The 1 to 2 year old may cut his milk intake down to a pint or even less a day and, instead, eat a variety of other foods, many of which supply his need for iron. He will slowly resume milk drinking, but it will be some years before he is able to consume a full quart and still eat a variety of other foods.

Abnormal Cravings—Pica. Pica is a craving for unnatural foods or for non-food substances such as clay or chalk. It is most apt to occur in children between the ages of 18 and 24 months of age. Lourie *et al.*[10] found no correlation between the occurrence of pica and nutritional deficiencies. Gutelius *et al.*[11] supplemented the diet of some pica children with vitamins and minerals but failed to reduce the incidence of this craving among their subjects. These workers agree that pica is a complicated environmental, cultural and psychological problem most apt to occur among children of mothers who also practice pica themselves. (See Chap. 12.)

For the 3 to 5 year old the basis of the diet should remain the same, but the child should be introduced gradually to most of the foods on the family table. He should be encouraged to drink 1 to 1½ pints of milk a day. Some of this may be used in creamed soups and custards or other desserts included in his meals. Whole fruits and vegetables, both cooked and raw, should begin to appear on his menu. Meat should be cut in small pieces rather than ground. Bacon, if it has not been used earlier, often is a welcome addition. Remember that often at this age a child will gladly eat such foods as raw carrots and lettuce with his fingers but refuse them if he has to use a fork or a spoon, because it is too difficult to manage the food with them.

At this age the child may join the family for two or three meals, but a midmorning, midafternoon and bedtime snack also may be desirable. Some pediatricians feel that there is room for further study and research on the question of the number of meals best suited to the needs of the preschool child. Stitt[10] wonders "whether good nutrients distributed fairly evenly over the waking hours may not be what many children seem to reach toward." Milk, if not consumed at a regular meal, or fruit juice accompanied by bread, crackers or plain cookies, may form a good light meal or snack. Rich cookies, cake and candy should not be given as snacks but, if used at all, should be served in small portions as dessert at the end of a meal.

Vitamin D. The need for 400 I.U. of vitamin D for all age groups may be partially or completely supplied by vitamin D milk which contains 400 I.U. per quart. The child may get some from cereals, candies or other foods fortified with vitamin D. It is recommended that children not be given more than 400 I.U. because of the risk of overdosage. If a vitamin preparation is used as a supplement, it is a good idea to calculate the total amount of vitamin D obtained from all sources.

9 Smith, C. A.: J.A.M.A., *172*:567, 1960.
10 Lourie, R. S., *et al.*: Children, *10*:143, 1963.
11 Gutelius, M. F., *et al.*: Am. J. Clin. Nutr., *12*: 388, 1963.

12 Stitt, P. G.: Nutrition Education Conf. Jan. 29, 1962. Washington, D. C.

TABLE 14–1. Suggested Meal Plan for the 1 to 3 Year Old

Breakfast	Lunch or Supper	Dinner
Fruit or juice	Main dish—mainly meat, eggs,	Meat, poultry or fish
Cereal with milk	fish, poultry, dried beans or	Vegetable
Toast	peas, cheese, peanut butter	Relish or salad
Butter or margarine	Vegetable or salad	Bread
Milk	Bread	Butter or margarine
	Butter or margarine	Fruit or pudding
	Dessert or fruit	Milk
	Milk	

Snacks between meals:

Dry cereal, with milk or out   Fruit sherbet or ice cream
  of the box   Toast, plain or cinnamon
Simple cookie or cracker   Fruit juice
Raw vegetables   Fruit drinks made with milk
Canned, fresh or dried fruit   and juice
Cheese wedge

From *Your Child from 1 to 3*, Children's Bureau, U. S. Dept. of Health, Education and Welfare, 1966.

Although there is no evidence that doses of 3 to 5 times the amount recommended are in any way deleterious after infancy, the long-term effect of large doses is not known.

Establishing Good Food Habits

Children differ greatly in their natural preferences for food, but some patterns emerge clearly. "Finicky" food habits and food jags are characteristic of the 2 to 4 year olds. They may want to eat nothing except peanut butter sandwiches and fruit juice, or two to three hard cooked eggs at a sitting, but these patterns usually do not persist for very long, and soon they will settle down again to normal meals. The overall pattern of food intake from week to week and month to month is more important than the occasional food binge or refusal.

From 5 to 7 years of age there is a dislike of casserole dishes, mixtures of all kinds, fat meats and gravies. This group likes raw vegetables better than cooked ones, and tends to dislike strongly flavored and root vegetables. They prefer plain food such as meat, potatoes, raw vegetables, milk and fruit. By 6 or 7 they are willing to try new foods and to accept foods previously disliked. By 8 there is a ravenous appetite with few refusals but strong preferences. Food may be judged by odor or color, and food served attractively makes an impression. By 9 the child usually has a keen interest in food, likes to help prepare it and is positive in his likes and dislikes. Some will eat everything at this age, but plain foods still are preferred.

One of the best methods for developing good food habits in children is for the whole family to eat wisely. Chapter 10 offers some nutrition yardsticks for different age groups and suggestions for meal planning. If the mother and the father, knowing that they can expect certain variations in food acceptance by their children, can maintain a reasonably firm stand about over-all behavior, mealtimes can and should be one of the pleasant times of day for the whole family.

Children are great imitators. Although they may object, on the one hand, to being asked to conform, on the other they may be heard to say proudly to some friend, "My mother won't let me eat that."

Project Head Start, serving children from 3 to 5, has offered an opportunity of studying the food preferences of children from low-income families. These children usually lack experience with a wide variety of foods. The breakfast and/or lunch at school is a good chance to introduce them to fruit juices, fruits in season, and raw vegetables. They are pretty sure to like the familiar and simple main dishes, bread and butter and milk. Eating in company with other children, perhaps for the first time, often encourages the less venturesome to try something new. A story about a new food and a small sample served attractively may make the difference between rejection and acceptance.

Elementary School Age

In the elementary school years, the child has activities which are often intense, and fatigue becomes a problem. Earlier, at home, he could determine his own activities and rest whenever he was tired. At school, keeping up with the young Joneses is a challenge that may take all his energy. He gets along quite well provided that he has good food, enough rest and does not have severe illnesses.

Inadequate breakfasts or none at all, due to the rush and the excitement of leaving for school and new experiences, may contribute to fatigue. The increasing number of working mothers, who may not have the time or the inclination to prepare breakfast for their school-age children, may mean that some children must shift for themselves before school. On the other hand, if time is allowed and a child is encouraged to help with preparation and the choice of the menu, breakfast may become a relaxed and desirable start for the day. Children of this age can certainly prepare a simple breakfast of cold cereal and milk. Perhaps schools should consider providing mid-morning snacks especially for those children who have not had or are not hungry for breakfast before school but who need something before lunchtime.

There should be time for eating an adequate lunch also, when there are two school sessions and the child comes home for this meal. If he takes lunch to school when there are no provisions for school lunch, the box lunch which he carries should be planned to supplement the home breakfast and dinner. The evening-meal plan for the child must take into consideration the type of midday meal which he has had. He may need an afternoon snack when he returns from school, but it should not be of such a nature as to take away appetite for dinner.

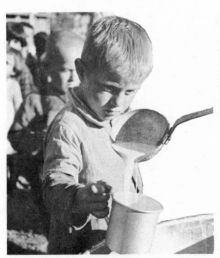 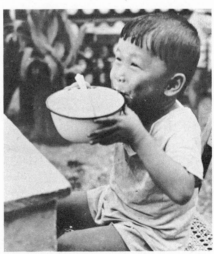

Fig. 14–3. Milk supplied by the United Nations Children's Fund (UNICEF). (*Left*) With tense anticipation, a Greek refugee child watches as his cup is filled with milk. (*Right*) At the feeding center in Barrio Fugoso, Manila, this small boy relishes his daily lunch—a porridge made from rice and milk.

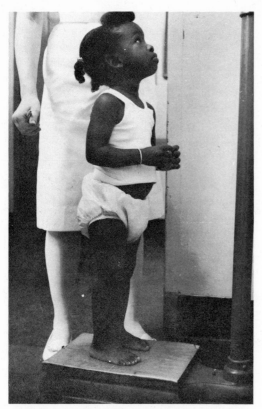

Fig. 14–4. A healthy child at the Pediatric Clinic, The New York Hospital. Note sturdy build, straight back, and alert interest in being weighed. (Children's Bureau photograph)

Figure 14–4 shows a child in this age group with excellent nutritional status.

Nutritional Requirements

Table 14–2 presents a guide to the foods needed by children to meet the RDA which increases with age, until at the 12 to 15 year old level they are equal to and, in some instances, surpass those for the adult (see Table 14–2).

Calories. The basic foods listed in Table 14–2 need to be supplemented by butter or margarine, salad oils, jams, jellies, additional bread and potatoes and desserts, and occasionally by other sweets, to meet the total caloric needs.

Adequate calories must be supplied if growth is to occur. When the caloric intake is below the requirement, protein foods will be used for energy instead of for tissue building. Macy and Hunscher[13] have shown that "a difference in intake of as few as ten calories per kilogram of body weight per day (or approximately four calories per pound) may make the difference between progress and failure in satisfactory growth."

Protein. Protein needs to be increased with growth, and protein intake will rise as calories are increased if a variety of foods is eaten. The milk and meat groups, including fish, eggs, cheese and peanut butter will meet the protein needs adequately. However, if the calories are obtained largely from carbohydrates, including candy and soft drinks in excess, both the quantity and the quality of the protein intake will suffer.

Calcium and Iron. Milk in the amounts recommended will be the main source of calcium and also provides good quality protein and some of the essential vitamins. Iron needs are met by an adequate intake of meat, eggs, green leafy vegetables, whole-grain and enriched breads and cereals and potatoes. Dried peas and beans will contribute a share of iron if these foods form a staple article of the diet.

Vitamins. Vitamin needs are more likely to be met when a variety of foods is included in the diet. Milk, butter, fortified margarine and green and yellow vegetables and fruits will provide vitamin A. Milk fortified with vitamin D will ensure a sufficient intake of this vitamin. The B complex vitamins will be included if good-quality protein foods, as well as enriched bread and cereals, appear frequently in the diet. In our Southern states, where cornmeal rather than wheat flour is frequently used, it is important to obtain enriched cornmeal when this is possible. In at least one Southern state, rice must be enriched by law. Vitamin C needs are not met as easily as other nutritional requirements as shown by the Nutritional Status Study. Citrus fruits and tomatoes are excellent sources but are not available in some communities except during the growing season. Potatoes are a good, cheap

---

[13] Macy, I. G., and Hunscher, H. A.: J. Nutrition, 45:189, 1951.

TABLE 14–2. A Daily Guide to Foods Needed by Children and Their Families*

Type of Food	Each Day
Milk Group	
Milk..Children under 9.......	2 to 3 cups
Children 9–12.........	3 or more cups
Dairy products such as:	
Cheddar cheese, cottage cheese, and ice cream..........................	May be used sometimes in place of milk
Vegetable-Fruit Group...	4 or more servings
Include—	
A fruit or vegetable that contains a high amount of vitamin C: Grapefruit, oranges, and tomatoes (whole or in juice), raw cabbage, green or sweet red pepper, broccoli' and fresh strawberries.	
A dark green or deep yellow vegetable or fruit for vitamin A: You can judge fairly well by color—dark green and deep yellow: broccoli, spinach, greens, cantaloupe, apricots, carrots, pumpkin, sweet potatoes, winter squash.	
Other vegetables and fruits, including potatoes.	
Meat and Meat Substitutes...	2 or more servings
Include—	
Meat, poultry, fish, or eggs..	1 or more servings
Dried beans or peas, peanut butter, and nuts can be used as meat substitutes.	
Breads and Cereals	4 or more servings
Whole grain, enriched, or restored bread and cereals or other grain products such as corn meal, grits, macaroni, spaghetti, and rice.	
Plus Other Foods	
To round out meals and to satisfy the appetite, many children will eat more of these foods, and other foods not specified will be used, such as butter, margarine, other fats, oils, sugars, and unenriched refined grain products. These "other" foods are frequently combined with the suggested foods in mixed dishes, baked goods, desserts, and other recipe dishes. They are a part of daily meals, even though they are not stressed in the food plan.	

* From Your Child from 6 to 12. Children's Bureau, H.E.W., Pub. No. 324. Washington, D. C., 1966.

source of this vitamin, but they are not a staple article of diet in some of our regional and national dietary patterns. Cabbage and other leafy vegetables, particularly raw, will contribute some of this vitamin to the diet whenever these foods are served.

Getting Ready for the Growth Spurt. During the later elementary school period children's bodies begin to get ready for the growth spurt of the early teens. They will begin to eat more and will supplement their meals at the vending machine, the soda fountain or the candy store. A filled cookie jar and fruit juice or milk ready in the refrigerator at home is a better way of meeting the increasing caloric needs of this period.

High School Age—Adolescence

It is during adolescence that the second very rapid growth period occurs. This is usually between the ages of 11 and 14 for girls and 13 and 16 for boys, although it may be sooner for early-maturing children and somewhat later for late-maturing children. The growth spurts at widely different ages and the corresponding caloric intakes are shown in the accompanying chart

TABLE 14–3. Recommended Dietary Allowances,* for Children and Youth,
Ages 1 to 18 years from the Food and Nutrition Board, National Research Council, 1964.
(Designed for maintenance of good nutrition for practically all healthy children in the U.S.A.)

| | Age† (Yrs.) | Weight | | Height | | Calories | Prot. (Gm.) | Calc. (Gm.) | Iron (Mg.) | Vit. A (I.U.) | Thiam. (Mg.) | Ribo. (Mg.) | Niacin (Mg. Equiv.‡) | Asc. Acid (Mg.) | Vit. D (I.U.) |
		Kg.	(Lbs.)	Cm.	(In.)										
Children........	1–3	13	(29)	87	(34)	1,300	32	0.8	8	2,000	0.5	0.8	9	40	400
	3–6	18	(40)	107	(42)	1,600	40	0.8	10	2,500	0.6	1.0	11	50	400
	6–9	24	(53)	124	(49)	2,100	52	0.8	12	3,500	0.8	1.3	14	60	400
Boys..........	9–12	33	(72)	140	(55)	2,400	60	1.1	15	4,500	1.0	1.4	16	70	400
	12–15	45	(98)	156	(61)	3,000	75	1.4	15	5,000	1.2	1.8	20	80	400
	15–18	61	(134)	172	(68)	3,400	85	1.4	15	5,000	1.4	2.0	22	80	400
Girls..........	9–12	33	(72)	140	(55)	2,200	55	1.1	15	4,500	0.9	1.3	15	80	400
	12–15	47	(103)	158	(62)	2,500	62	1.3	15	5,000	1.0	1.5	17	80	400
	15–18	53	(117)	163	(64)	2,300	58	1.3	15	5,000	0.9	1.3	15	70	400

* The allowance levels are intended to cover individual variations among most normal persons as they live in the United States under usual environmental stresses. The recommended allowances can be attained with a variety of common foods, providing other nutrients for which human requirements have been less well defined. See text for more detailed discussion of allowances and of nutrients not tabulated.

† Allowances for the midpoint of the specified age periods, i.e., line for children 1–3 is for age 2 years (24 months); 3–6 is for age 4½ years (54 months), etc.

‡ Niacin equivalents include dietary sources of the preformed vitamin and the precursor, tryptophan; 60 mg. of tryptophan represents 1 mg. of niacin.

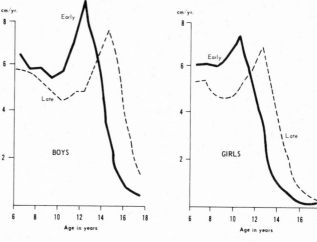

Fig. 14–5. Increments in the height of early and late maturing boys and girls (means of 20 in each group). Mitchell, H. S., *et al.*: The Adolescent Growth Spurt and Nutrient Intake. Presented at the International Congress of Nutrition, Hamburg, Germany, August 8, 1966)

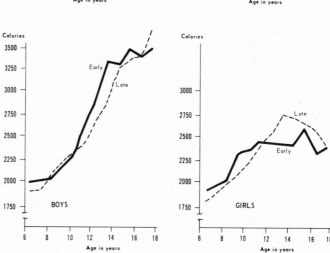

Fig. 14–6. Total caloric intakes of early and late maturing boys and girls (means of 20 in each group). Mitchell, H. S., *et al.*: The Adolescent Growth Spurt and Nutrient Intake, Presented at the International Congress of Nutrition, Hamburg, Germany, August 8, 1966)

from the Harvard Growth Study (Figs. 14–5 and 14–6).

Physical growth occurs in all directions, in length of bones, in muscle mass, in the laying down of body fat in the soft tissues, and in the widening of the shoulders in boys and the broadening of the hips in girls. The total period of rapid growth seldom lasts more than 2 or 3 years, when adult build and stature are reached. However, growth in skeletal muscle mass continues, particularly in the boy. A further "lengthening out" may occur in the late adolescent period in both boys and girls.

Nutritional Needs—Met or Not

As may be expected, the nutritional needs to meet this rapid growth process are tremendous. A look at the Recommended Dietary Allowances in Table 14–3 shows that they markedly exceed those for grown men and women. Anyone who has ever seen a teen-ager eat during this growth spurt will attest to his voracious appetite. If plenty of suitable foods are available, they will be eaten, especially by boys. Unfortunately, enough of even a poor choice of foods will also satisfy the appetite, but will not supply all the necessary materials for optimum growth.

A minority of both boys and girls have the habit of consuming more calories than they can utilize and thus become overweight for their height and age. Sometimes this seems to be due to an inclination to be inactive—to read or play inactive games while their contemporaries are active. At other times, the very fact that a child is overweight makes him the object of ridicule, and he is less acceptable to his peers in sports and other activities. In either situation, the child needs advice and motivation to meet his nutrition needs with fewer calories (see Chap. 21).

During this period of rapid physical growth, there is a concurrent maturing of the whole personality, with its attendant strains and stresses. There is a striving for independence from parental restriction, coupled with an increased need for guidance and reassurance. The adolescent must be given the opportunity to make his own decisions, and parents must be understanding of this urge for independence, yet be willing to help when asked. At this time coffee and tea may begin to appear in the diet as an indication of being "grown up." There is no harm in this if the intake is not excessive, and if it is not substituted for milk. The habits of the parents in this, as in many other matters, are often the deciding factor, as the child patterns himself on the adults whom he knows best.

Because boys and girls differ in their response to this growth period, they will be discussed separately.

The Adolescent Growth Spurt

Boys. The diets of adolescent boys, at all ages, are generally found to be adequate for protein, calcium, iron, vitamin A, riboflavin and niacin. However, some of the groups studied had diets low in calories and ascorbic acid at all age levels, and tended to be somewhat low in thiamine at 15 to 18 years of age.

The adolescent spurt stimulates appetite, as is well recognized. The energy and nutrient requirement for this spurt in any one boy is not known. If the increments of height gained as shown in Figure 14–5 are compared with the caloric intake for the same boys (Fig. 14–6), it is not surprising that the early maturers experienced an earlier increase in food intake than the late maturers.[14]

That serious undernutrition in boys still exists is known from the number of army recruits rejected as being physically unfit, but, on the whole, the nutritional outlook for boys is good.

Girls. With many girls the story is different. Despite the abundance of food in the United States and the inclusion of nutrition education in most elementary and high schools, the Nutritional Status Study[15] found that teen-age girls, at all ages, comprise one of the most poorly fed groups in our population. The most serious deficiencies were in calcium and iron, with smaller deficits in calories, protein, thiamine and ascorbic acid. This finding is particularly critical in view of today's early marriage and childbearing ages (see Chap. 12), with the additional nutritional demands being made on the young mother's body.

The caloric intake of adolescent girls shows quite a different picture from that of the boys. One can almost read into these graphs the psychology of the early-maturing girls who were concerned about their rapid growth and increase in height ahead of the boys their age. Thus they curtailed their total food and often chose unwisely with respect to essential nutrients (Figs. 14–5 and 14–6). The late-maturing girls did not make as drastic a reduction in caloric intake until much later.

The concern of teen-age girls often centers on weight reduction, whether necessary or not. There is probably no great harm in this, if the essential foods to meet nutritional needs are included in the diet. However, as the Nutritional Status Study indicates, it is milk, eggs, vegetables, bread and potatoes that are low in, or omitted from, the diet. Often soft drinks, candy and other sweets are substituted.

Girls have an increased need for iron as soon as their menses begin, yet the study shows that the diet of many girls was inadequate in iron as evidenced by food intake studies and hemoglobin levels.

The diet of teen-age girls needs to be improved in many respects, yet girls seem to have a greater urge than do boys to

---

[14] Mitchell, H. S.: Op. cit.

[15] Morgan, A. F.: Op. cit.

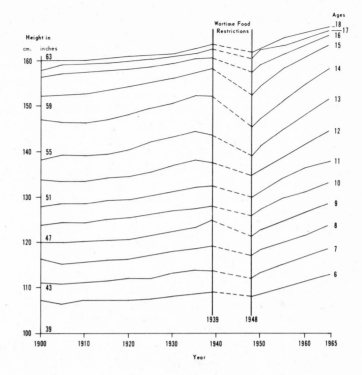

FIG. 14–7. Secular changes in the height of Japanese boys of school age, 1900-1965. (Data from the Japanese Ministry of Education Report for 1965. Tokyo)

assert their independence and break away from family food patterns. How to counteract this is one of the problems in nutrition education confronting parents, teachers, nutritionists and nurses alike.

The adolescent growth spurt is a unique phenomenon, triggered by the endocrine system and timed earlier for girls than for boys. The lengthening of the long bones, particularly the femur and tibia, is largely responsible for the rapid increases in stature. The trunk grows more slowly and over a longer period of time. The time during which this rapid growth occurs and the rate of lengthening of the long bones determine the adult stature. The rate of growth is the crucial factor because the time during which this rapid growth takes place does not seem to be extended sufficiently to compensate when the rate is slowed down by environmental factors.

When the nutrients supplied by the blood stream are inadequate to permit optimum growth of these long bones, merely shorter stature may be found without obvious signs of malnutrition. Protein is essential for the formation of the new cartilage cells in the epiphysis of the long bones which later become calcified to form bone. Evidence that the adolescent growth spurt may be slowed down by nutrient and especially protein limitation has been reported by Mitchell.[16] The changes in stature over 65 years of Japanese youth show a remarkable parallelism with the food limitations during the war years and subsequent increase in consumption of animal protein, which has more than doubled during prosperous years. Fig. 14–7, showing the changes in stature in Japanese boys over a period of 65 years (including World War II and later), seems to show that teenagers were more susceptible than younger children to limitations and more responsive to postwar improvements in food. The response of girls was similar but not quite as striking. The commonly accepted association of calcium with bone growth needs to be supplemented by the concept of the need for good quality protein for the lengthening of bone before calcification occurs.

---

[16] Mitchell, H. S.: J. Am. Dietet. A., *44*:165, 1964.

A study of Japanese children in 22 orphanages of the Island of Hokkaido[17] found that 41 per cent of the boys and 37 per cent of the girls were more than 5 per cent shorter than the average for Hokkaido public school children of the same ages. The limited budgets for food in the orphanages had not allowed the improvement in the diet which the prosperity in general had permitted. The amount of animal protein was less than 30 per cent of the total protein in most of the institutions, and vitamin A, riboflavin and ascorbic acid were below 75 per cent of the recommended allowances in several of the schools.

Various studies in the U. S. and elsewhere indicate that boys and girls seem to be maturing earlier than they did a generation or two ago. This earlier maturing does not necessarily mean taller adults, although there has been a slight increase in stature of men and women in this country during the past 60 years. There is undoubtedly a genetic potential beyond which environmental factors cannot stimulate further growth. Evidence indicates relatively little change in adult stature of the upper socioeconomic classes in recent years. There is less than an inch change in height of boys entering Amherst or Yale, or for girls entering Vassar or Smith colleges in the 25 years, 1932-1957[18]

Foods to Meet Nutritional Needs of Adolescents

All the foods listed under Daily Food Needs of the 6 to 12 Year Old are essential in the diet of the adolescent, but in markedly increased quantities. A rapidly growing boy will need a quart or more of milk or its equivalent a day to meet his calcium requirement, and girls during their period of rapid growth also need a quart of milk daily. Skim milk may be substituted for whole milk if excess weight, real or imaginary, is a factor. The increased milk intake will provide good-quality protein for growth as well. All the other foods listed, eaten in sufficient quantity, will provide for the greatly increased physiologic needs during this period of growth and stabilization.

Besides adequate calcium, protein and calories, girls need an increased iron intake when menses begin. An adequate amount of foods high in iron, such as lean meats, liver, eggs, green, leafy vegetables, enriched breads and cereals and potatoes, should be included in the daily food intake. This is a period when the young girl, beginning to look forward to eventual marriage and motherhood, should be helped to realize that good nutrition is an important factor in the bearing of healthy babies.

THE SCHOOL LUNCH PROGRAM

School lunch programs originated in Europe in the early 1900's, and have since spread throughout the world. In the United States, Federal assistance became available first in 1933. The National School Lunch Act of 1946 put the school lunch program on a permanent basis and made use of surplus farm commodities. The Child Nutrition Act of 1966 has opened up new dimensions in school feeding. The act gives the U. S. Department of Agriculture legal authority to:

1. Provide food service equipment for schools in low-income areas that have been unable to finance even minimal equipment.

2. Begin a pilot program to offer a nutritious breakfast to hungry children whether in low-income areas or because they must travel long distances to school.

3. Extend the Special Milk Program for another three years.

4. Extend the benefits of federal school feeding programs to children in preschool activities operated by part of any regular school system.[19]

The Type A Lunch[20]

Lunches served under the National School Lunch Program, in order to be eli-

[17] Mitchell, H. S., and Santo, S.: J. Faculty of Agriculture, Hokkaido Univ., 52:483, 1962 (Dec.).

[18] Hathaway, M. L., and Ford, E. D.: Heights and Weights of Adults in the United States. U.S.D.A., Washington, D. C., 1960.

[19] Agricultural Marketing. Jan., 1967.

[20] National School Lunch Program. Agricultural Marketing Service, U.S.D.A., Washington, D. C., 1959.

gible for reimbursement, must contain as a minimum:

1. One-half pint of fluid whole milk as a beverage.
2. Two ounces (edible portion as served) of lean meat, poultry, or fish; or two ounces of cheese; or one egg; or one-half cup of cooked dry beans or peas; or four tablespoons of peanut butter; or an equivalent quantity of any combination of the above-listed foods. To be counted in meeting this requirement, these foods must be served in a main dish, or in a main dish and one other menu item.
3. A three-fourths cup serving consisting of two or more vegetables or fruits or both. Full-strength vegetable or fruit juice may be counted to meet not more than one-fourth cup of this requirement.
4. One slice of whole-grain or enriched bread; or a serving of cornbread, biscuits, rolls, muffins, etc., made of whole-grain or enriched meal or flour.
5. Two teaspoons of butter or fortified margarine.

It is estimated that the National School Lunch Program reaches one third of the schoolchildren in the United States. Allowing for children receiving a school lunch not subsidized by the National School Lunch Program, and for those living in small towns and villages, who can go home for lunch, there is still a large number of children in the United States who are without the benefit of a good school lunch.

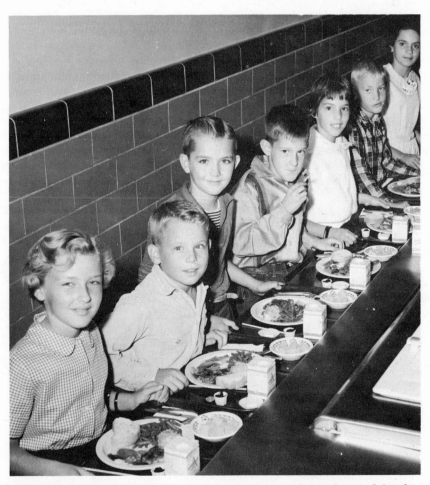

Fig. 14–8. The national School Lunch Program helps make good lunches available to school children. (U. S. Department of Agriculture photograph)

The benefits of this program are both direct and indirect. Children receive food which improves their nutritional status and general health, contributing to better performance in school and later as adults at work or in the home. At the same time the school lunch program provides a unique opportunity for nutrition education.

The Special Milk Program

A second activity of the Department of Agriculture, through the Agricultural Marketing Service, is the Special Milk Program, designed to increase fluid milk consumption among children attending schools of high school grades and under. Since 1956 non-profit child care institutions and summer camps have also been eligible for this program. The Department reimburses the school or agency for part of the cost of the milk so that it may be sold to the children below the regular price, or given to them at less expense to the institution.

Influence of Vending Machines

Food habits are influenced by many factors other than education; by advertising, convenience, cost and changes in cultural patterns or surroundings. One of the developments conspicuous during the last decade—the vending machine—has had a marked impact on food habits. Vending machines have encouraged piecemeal eating of a wide variety of snack foods. Our children grow up with the expectation that the family does not stop for gas—they stop for gas and pop; if Johnny bowls or skis, he snacks on a hot dog and pop; if he is waiting for a bus, he has a candy bar. To be sure, a few schools have recognized the health hazard to the children and have controlled the types of food sold in the self-service machines.

Not all foods sold in vending machines are to be discouraged, some are nutritious such as fruit, milk, ice cream and sandwiches, but the variety is apt to be limited to the few foods that are most popular or on which the most profit can be made —peanuts, candy bars, chewing gum, cookies, crackers and, above all soft drinks; with or without calories. It is not surprising that consumption of soft drinks has increased tremendously while that of fluid milk has decreased slightly since 1955.

The excessive consumption of sweets and other carbohydrates not only spoils the appetite for the more nutritious food of the next meal but provides mostly calories—largely empty calories. Moreover, it is generally agreed that dental caries is aggravated if not initiated by excessive consumption of candy, cookies and sweetened drinks (see Chapter 16).

Since the soft drink, the confectionery and the baking industries dominate in the food vending field, there is little chance of the nutritionist changing the present pattern. Therefore, we must work with children and their families—the ultimate consumers—to help them make wise choices and create a demand for more nutritious items in vending machines.

NUTRITION EDUCATION

Since food, nutrition and health cut across many areas of learning, these subjects lend themselves to integration into the school program without requiring large and special allocations of time in the already crowded school curriculum. Nutrition is required as a part of health education in the secondary schools of about half of the states, but the attention given to this varies with the place and the teacher. In other states no effort is made to introduce any nutrition instruction for all pupils. High school students in home economics get the most systematic courses in nutrition, but these students constitute a small proportion of the total. Every girl and boy in junior and senior high school deserves and needs some knowledge of nutrition.

Approach By Age

Experienced teachers and educational authorities recognize that nutrition education must be approached differently for the various age levels. Programs in both elementary and secondary schools have a good potential for promoting better food habits if geared appropriately to the age groups.

In the elementary grades nutrition subject matter is easily integrated into English composition, mathematics and even art classes where colorful educational posters can be made. Activities such as observation of food choices made by children in the school cafeteria, animal feeding demonstrations and plant growing projects have been used as bases for nutrition teaching. Cooperation of parents is essential if the information gained at school is to be put into action at home. Well-planned meetings can show parents food sources of nutrients, methods of preparation used for the school lunch and favorable cost comparisons.

In one New York City school attended by many newly arrived Puerto Ricans a special project was conducted for Spanish-speaking parents. They were shown how to use foods available on the New York market when familiar items could not be obtained. Recipes were distributed in both English and Spanish. Both parents and students enjoyed tasting the vegetables and other foods prepared.

The approach to the teenagers must be quite different from that used in the elementary grades. At this age youth has begun to assert a certain amount of independence and to throw off parental and other authority. A boy is concerned about his physique and how tall he will be; a girl, about her personality and figure.

Roth [21] offers ten suggestions for parents and other adults who counsel teenagers about good nutrition or other health measures. Abbreviated and slightly modified, they are:

1. Give the teenager credit for knowing something.

2. Give him a chance to talk and ask questions.

3. Allow him to accept or reject an idea while talking about it; then he won't have to reject it by action.

4. Don't fall into the trap of "taking sides" in an argument between generations that probably is not really based on food.

5. Don't force-feed food or ideas to teenagers. Force will make them resist or become more childish and less able to be responsible adults.

6. Don't be afraid to express your honest feelings about what is important.

7. Realize that the best teaching is by example, not by talking.

8. Remember that good nutrition is a

long-term thing, not a meal-by-meal or even a day-by-day emergency.

9. Remember that there is no perfect food and that there may be some value in the snacks we worry about.

10. Help the adolescent aim for acceptance of himself.

For this age group a program should be planned cooperatively by parents, teachers, school lunch personnel and, if available, the school nurse, together with the young people themselves. Again, regularly organized school activities should be used insofar as possible. The home economics teacher or a knowledgeable science instructor should be an advisor. A local or state nutritionist may be available as a consultant.

There are numerous appropriate teaching aids available from local and state health departments and from the federal government. Many commercial agencies publish attractive and reliable literature. In the area of mass media, newspapers sometimes carry useful feature articles on nutrition and some radio and television stations offer good programs. Even when there is misleading material, it can be used to teach students to discriminate between correct information and the questionable pseudo-scientific nutrition propaganda so often reaching the public today. Simple food guides such as the Four Food Groups described in Chapter 10 or the more technical Recommended Dietary Allowances discussed in Chapter 10 can be used with appropriate demonstrations to fit the intellectual level of the student group. Whatever teaching aids are used, one needs to be selective and mindful of their proper use and limitations.

STUDY QUESTIONS AND ACTIVITIES

1. At what ages is good nutrition most important in the development of the central nervous system? When may the result of poor nutrition show up?

2. What is meant by the term "growth"? By "development"? Are they the same? What are some of the criteria by which we judge good growth and development?

---

[21] Roth, A.: J. Am. Dietet. A., *36:*27, 1960.

3. How has the nutritional status of the people of the U. S. been studied? What are some of the findings?

4. What is meant by the term "longitudinal study" of growth and development? What information have we obtained from these studies?

5. Why are individual growth charts preferred to comparison of a child with others of his age group? How is a growth chart used? What does it tell us?

6. What changes take place in the small child's food habits at about 1 year of age? Why does this occur?

7. Why do later emotional problems with food and appetite often have their origin at this period?

8. How can the nurse help to allay the mother's anxiety and sense of frustration about her child's food habits at ages 1-3 years?

9. How much milk is the 1 to 2 year old likely to be willing to drink? What may happen if he is forced to drink a quart of milk daily?

10. What are some food preferences and prejudices of children at various ages?

11. What is the probable effect of a poor breakfast on the total food intake? Why do American families so often eat an inadequate breakfast?

12. What very serious problem was uncovered by the Nutritional Status Study? What nutrients were particularly low?

13. Why do you think adolescent girls eat so much more poorly than boys in the same age group? Have you had experience with this problem yourself?

14. What are the food needs of the teenager? Do girls have additional nutritional needs compared with boys? What are these, why do they occur and how may they be met?

15. How is the school lunch program organized in the United States? What constitutes a Type A lunch? Of what educational value is the school lunch?

16. How have food vending machines influenced food habits? What can be done to minimize the health hazards of snack foods offered in vending machines?

17. To what extent is nutrition education included in the curriculum of the grade schools, and the junior and senior high schools in your community? How can the school nurse be of help in such a program?

SUPPLEMENTARY READING ON NUTRITION OF CHILDREN AND YOUTH

Beal, V. A.: Dietary intake of individuals followed through infancy and childhood. J. Public Health, *51*:1107, 1961.

Breckenridge, M. E.: Food attitudes of five-to-twelve-year-old children. J. Am. Dietet. A., *35*:704, 1959.

Children's Bureau: Your Child from 1-3. 1966. Your Child from 6 to 12. 1966. Moving into Adolescence. 1966. Washington, D. C., U. S. Dept. H.E.W.

Dairy Council Digests: Nutritional status of the teen-ager. D.C.D. *35*: No. 1 (Jan.-Feb.) 1964. Effect of nutrition on growth and development. D.C.D. *36*: No. 2 (March-Apr.) 1965. Nutrition and physical fitness. D.C.D. *36*: No. 5 (Sept.-Oct.) 1965. The formation of bone. D.C.D. *36*: No. 6 (Nov.-Dec.) 1965. The effect of nutrition on body composition. D.C.D. *37*: No. 1 (Jan.-Feb.) 1966.

Daniels, A. M.: Training school nurses to work with groups of adolescents. Children, *13*: 210, 1966 (Nov.-Dec.).

Everson, G. L.: Bases for concern about teenagers diets. J. Am. Dietet. A., *36*:17, 1960.

Hammar, S. L.: The role of the nutritionist in an adolescent clinic. Children, *13*:217, 1966 (Nov.-Dec.).

Hill, M. M.: Food Choices: The Teen-age Girl. Brochure. Nutrition Foundation. New York. 1966.

Lowenberg, M. E.: Between infancy and adolescence. Chap. 26. Food; The Yearbook of Agriculture. Washington, D. C., 1959.

Morgan, A. F.: Nutritional explorations. J. Home Econ., *52*:631, 1960.

Obert, J. C.: When the bell rings. Am. J. Nursing, *61*:89, 1961.

Peckos, P. S., and Heald, F. P.: Nutrition of adolescents. Children, *11*:27, 1964 (Jan.-Feb.).

For further references see Bibliography in Part Four.

CHAPTER 15

Geriatric Nutrition

Gerontology and Geriatrics—Defined • *Nutrition of Older People* • *Planning Meals for Older People*

GERONTOLOGY AND GERIATRICS

Sound nutrition in the mature person and the older adult is not fundamentally different from normal nutrition in earlier years. However, because the aging process gives to each age group unique character- istics, geriatric nutrition is worthy of spe- cial consideration. *Gerontology*—the scien- tific study of problems of aging from birth to death in all its aspects—emphasizes keys to health for the older adult: nutrition, mental health, adequate housing, a safe liv- ing environment, moderate and well-bal- anced personal habits, physical activity, recreation, a useful and productive role in society and a sense of personal security. Good nutrition is allied with all of these— in fact, it is of first importance in realizing some of the satisfactions that come with age.

Geriatrics is that phase of medicine that deals with the prevention and the treat- ment of the diseases of old age. Geriatric nutrition is concerned with conserving health with advancing years and with the delay of some of the degenerative changes that are associated with aging. Thus, the time to start practicing good nutrition for the later years is in young adulthood— better still, in childhood.

Our Aging Population

The aged and aging should be clearly distinguished: the aged are people; aging is a continuous process. It begins at con- ception and terminates at death. Thus birth, growth, maturation and senescence are all part of the normal aging process. Aging proceeds more rapidly during the growing years because change is more rapid at that time. In the adult the aging process slows down and the rate of this change may be further retarded and the active period of life may be extended by good health practices.

Life expectancy has increased at an un- precedented rate in the 20th century. Dur- ing the period of the Roman empire infants had a life expectancy of only 23 years. The slow increase over many centuries brought the figure to 47 years in New England in 1900. Since then, however, scientific prog- ress in all matters pertaining to health has increased life expectancy so that in 1964 it was 66.9 years for men and 73.7 for women in the United States. In Vietnam it is still 25 to 30 years.

The figure of 19 million persons over 65 years of age in the United States in 1965 was about double the number of that age group 25 years earlier in 1940. Of these, over 60 per cent were widowed or un- married, with many living alone. Medical science, which is largely responsible for this increase in the number of senior citi- zens today, is also challenged to learn more about the degenerative and chronic dis- eases common in this group, and the social sciences have a responsibility to help make later years of life more livable.

Inevitable Changes With Age

Behind the obvious changes of aging are invisible changes within the body that may develop as gradually as the hair turns gray. Therefore, authorities emphasize that an adult's nutrition must be considered in terms of the past, the present and the future. The nutritional state of a person at 70 or 80 reflects not only his current food practices but all of his previous dietary history as well. This can be observed by anyone with a close and long association with older persons. As Dr. Swanson[1] comments:

The older a person grows, the longer and more complex is his dietary history. The variations in nutritional status and dietary needs of a group of adults thus are bound to be greater than corresponding variations in a group of young people. Recommendations for the food needs of this age group must be pointed especially to the needs of individuals.

The same nutritional principles that describe adequate diets for earlier periods of life apply to the diets of adults. Even though the adult has grown up—matured—his basic food supply still must provide all the nutrients necessary for maintaining body structure and for operating its machinery.

Good nutrition is only one of the practices which help to maintain strength and vigor, but it can be practiced three times a day—and it is abused more frequently than any other.

Occasionally, persons with exceptional inherited traits may be able to maintain vigorous health throughout life without apparent effort or precautions. It is satisfying to note the number of retired people today who live active, productive lives, who are well adjusted, accept their limitations, and continue to enjoy life. Certainly the surest foundation for a long period of usefulness and activity is that laid in childhood and preserved through youth and adult life. The health and the increased stature of our youth today are undoubtedly due to better nutrition and fewer diseases in childhood. The effects of these same factors will be reflected in the health of the adult population in the future.

[1] Swanson, Pearl: Nutrition Needs After 25. Food. The Yearbook of Agriculture. Chap. 28. U.S.D.A., Washington, D. C., 1959.

H. C. Sherman, a pioneer in scientific nutrition, was a strong advocate of "the nutritional improvement of life." He believed that, just as a farmer may improve his livestock by better feeding, so good nutrition for humans can make for better health. To give this concept a scientific name he called it "the principle of the improvability of the norm."

It has been recognized for centuries that signs of senility might be deferred, but few people were concerned until it was too late. Roger Bacon, the scientific monk of the 13th century, claimed that the three causes of old age were infection, negligence and ignorance. With regard to aging, Bacon wrote:

No one wishes to take thought in regard to methods of prevention, not even physicians, since we see that scarcely one physician in a thousand will give this matter even slight attention. Very rarely does it happen that one pays sufficient heed to the rules of health. No one does so in his youth, but sometimes one in three thousand thinks of these matters when he is old and approaching death, for at that time he fears for himself and thinks of his health. But he cannot then apply a remedy because of his weakened power and senses and his lack of experience.

It is not surprising that this complex human machine of ours gets out of order occasionally; the wonder is that it does not do so more often when it is given so little intelligent care. The delicate organs and tissues of the body continue to do their respective jobs for many decades if given half a chance. No one expects a man-made machine to last as long as that without special care and renewal of parts. Nature has a remarkable ability to repair or compensate for worn-out or injured parts if given the opportunity and the right materials.

It has been demonstrated repeatedly that older people can adjust to circumstances, learn new skills and adopt new food habits. We cite a few examples: the 80-year-old man who learned to eat salads when a thoughtful housekeeper chopped them to make them easier to eat yet kept them colorful and attractive; the two women in Figure 15–1 serving as volunteers in the hospital, feeling useful and adapting themselves to needed tasks; the elderly homemaker who still liked to try new gadgets and ready-prepared foods to make work easier and yet provide interest and variety in meals for two. "Never too old to learn" is a far truer adage than "You can't teach an old dog new tricks."

None of us is too young to begin thinking about improving the health of later years. People buy annuities and life insurance for the future; why not consider other steps which may give even greater security and comfort?

Agencies Concerned with the Care of Older People

The United States government in recent years has assumed more and more responsibility for the comfort and welfare of the elderly. Under the Department of Health, Education and Welfare, the Medicare program provides hospital insurance to help with the cost of hospitalization and related care, and medical insurance to help with the doctor bills and other health expenses. Good nutrition, including special diet if necessary, is an important part of both hospital and nursing home care and has been provided for in the plan.

Also under H.E.W. the Administration on Aging (AOA) was established in 1965 to work closely with other units of H.E.W. and especially with local voluntary organizations to develop programs at the community level for the benefit of our senior citizens. The Home Health Agencies, also under Medicare, provide for skilled nursing services and other therapeutic services at a person's place of residence. Local organizations may also provide nutrition advisory services through the public health nurse or nutritionist.

NUTRITION OF OLDER PEOPLE
Food Habits and the Consequences

Food habits of older people do not always fall in line with their food needs. Several surveys of the food choices of older people have been made in different localities; all report much the same trends. In a Boston survey of 104 geriatric patients, most of them over 70, Davidson[2] found a marked decrease in consumption of meat and milk and an increased use of eggs, but no caloric deficit. In fact, 84 per cent of the men and 71 per cent of the women

---

[2] Davidson, C. S.: Am. J. Clin. Nutr., *10*:181, 1962.

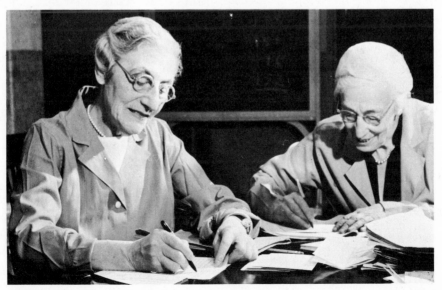

Fig. 15–1. Two long-faithful volunteers happy doing a needed job. (The New York Hospital)

were above desirable weight. He observed factors that seemed to affect the food habits of these elderly retired people: social situation (over half of them lived alone), reduced income, limited cooking and refrigeration facilities, marketing difficulties, condition of the teeth, sense of smell, problems of swallowing, food faddism and long-standing misconceptions concerning what constituted good nutrition.

Another survey was conducted of 283 older households in Rochester, N. Y.[3] All were beneficiaries of Old Age, Survivors, and Disability Insurance (OASDI) and ate most of their meals at home. While many of this aging, low-income group had nutritionally adequate diets, one fourth of them had food that provided less than two thirds of the RDA in one or more of the eight nutrients studied (see Fig. 15–2). Shortages of calcium and ascorbic acid were most frequent. Over one third of the households were using vitamin preparations but only a few were choosing supplements that would have lessened their nutritional faults.

Susceptibility to Fads. Unfortunately, many adults in late middle age, or older, are duped in their search for "eternal youth" or relief from their aches and pains. They hear and believe the glamorous TV and radio promotions of various panaceas —elixirs or multivitamin and mineral mixtures claimed to be remedies for all sorts of ills. They read and believe the faddy

health books, especially those that have been flooding the book market during the past decade. It is well-known that food and nutrition quackery thrives in areas where middle income retired people congregate. So-called health food stores may carry many desirable food items, but they also stock a variety of items ("health foods") promoted by the faddists.

A special study of nutrition beliefs and practices was made in four counties in New York State.[4] The authors found misinformation prevalent in all areas but most often among the older age and lower income groups. Their misconceptions most frequently concerned "health foods," soil depletion, chemical fertilizers and insecticides (see Chap. 10).

Food Requirements Change with Age

The dietary requirements of later life are influenced by a number of factors such as general health, degree of physical activity, changes in ability to chew, digest and absorb food, efficiency in the use of nutrients by the tissues, alteration in the endocrine system, emotional state and mental health. The nutrient and calorie allowances that maintain one person in optimum health may be inadequate or more than adequate to meet the needs of another apparently similar individual. Dr. Swanson's comment is especially pertinent:[5]

---

[3] LeBovit, C.: The food of older persons living at home. J. Am. Dietet. A., *46*:285, 1965.

[4] Jalso, S. B., *et al.*: Nutrition beliefs and practices. J. Am. Dietet. A., *47*:253, 1965.

[5] Swanson, Pearl: Op cit.

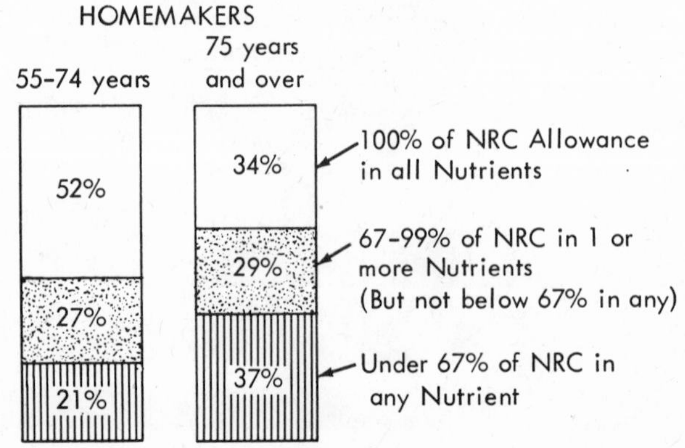

HOMEMAKERS

FIG. 15–2. Diet quality as related to aging (LeBovit, C.: J. Am. Dietet. A., *46*:285, 1965)

CALORIE NEEDS CHANGE WITH AGE

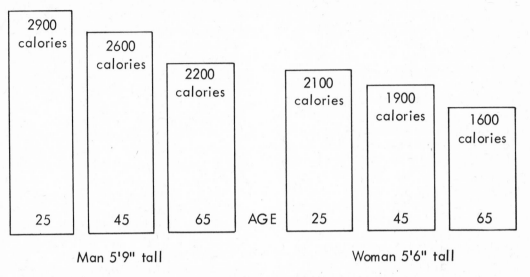

Man 5'9" tall   Woman 5'6" tall

Fig. 15–3. Calorie needs change with age. (Data from Recommended Dietary Allowances, National Research Council, 1964)

A person at 70 is an historical record of all that has happened to him—his injuries, infections, nutritional imbalances, fatigues and emotional upsets. Old people, therefore, differ from each other much more than do younger folk. All this needs to be considered in food planning for any old person. Each one is an individual, quite unlike anyone else.

In a later article Dr. Swanson[6] reported studies on a group of older women in Iowa. She found both deficits and excesses in food energy, low protein intakes and deficient calcium at all ages. The last finding may be significant in the development of osteoporosis.

Calorie Needs

As age advances there is a progressive decrease in metabolism coincident with less physical activity; thus the calorie need is some 22 per cent lower at 65 than at 25 years of age. The Food and Nutrition Board has tabulated some general calorie allowances for men and women of different weights and ages. (See table, Chapter 5, and Fig. 15–3.) For example a woman of 65 weighing 128 pounds may need only

[6] Swanson, P.: Adequacy in old age. Part 1. Role of nutrition, J. Home Econ., 56:651, 1964.

1,600 calories, whereas she needed 2,100 or more at 25, when she weighed the same but was more active. If she does not reduce her caloric intake to conform to her needs, she will store the excess as fat—so common in older people, particularly women.

When Calories Need to be Reduced

The food sources of these reduced calories must be chosen with care to include all essential factors and in higher proportion than in former years because the total food consumed is less. There is an obvious need for foods which carry a full quota of proteins, minerals and vitamins. The day is past when a reduction in the amount of all foods was a satisfactory solution. It is essential to reduce consumption of empty calories—sugar, rich desserts, cakes, candies, fats and alcohol.

Reduction in total calories involves a most difficult task of alteration of food habits. For the majority of persons, habit is perhaps one of the greatest obstacles in the path of an optimal diet. The longer the habits are continued the more fixed they become. The food habits of older people are apt to be so fixed that it is difficult to change them unless the way is made easy and temptation to eat the wrong foods is mastered.

Whoever is planning or preparing the meals for *overweight* persons—the home-maker herself, a health aide or housekeeper —can eliminate some calories behind the scenes—if necessary—while still keeping meals attractive and in the familiar pattern. If people do not see the forbidden foods, one psychological barrier has been over-come. By substituting for rich cakes and pastries such items as puddings and cus-tards made with skim milk, angel food cake and more fruit desserts, gelatins, whips, etc., calories are saved without sacrificing flavor. Also low-calorie salad dressings, less but-ter on vegetables, and gravies made with a minimum of fat are devices for the cook to use before the food reaches the table.

When appropriate, the nurse concerned with the continuing education of the pa-tient may make specific suggestions along this line in keeping with the socioeconomic status of the patient and his cultural pat-tern of eating. (See Chap. 37.)

Surplus calories are not the only reason for curtailing the carbohydrates and the fats in the diets of older people. Some of them seem to have a reduced capacity for metabolizing sugars, and this may result in a fluctuating blood sugar level. When this is true, fewer sweets are advisable. Other foods in moderation such as potatoes, cer-eals and bread are better tolerated to meet the caloric needs.

Fats are the most concentrated source of calories and often the invisible component of common foods. For those who eat out, foods fried in deep fat are apt to be popu-lar since fats give flavor and satiety value to meals, but too much fat may result in indigestion or discomfort for some elderly people. The most serious problem for the middle aged and past middle aged group concerns the type and the amount of fat in the diet and their relation to the blood cholesterol level and to the incidence of atherosclerosis. There are still many uncer-tainties and misconceptions concerning this problem, which is discussed in Chapters 3 and 23.

When Calories Need to be Increased

Quite another problem exists for the really elderly, or the disabled and shut-in who may not get enough food to meet his caloric or other nutritional requirements. If he lives alone or has poor cooking facili-ties, there is little incentive or opportunity to market and cook for himself. In such cases, home care programs such as de-scribed by Piper[7] may come to the rescue. Many of the patients served by these pro-grams are indigent or on low incomes. Another service to shut-ins that is gaining in popularity is the "Meals-on-Wheels" pro-gram which, in 1966, was in use in some 50 to 100 communities and was being con-sidered by several others. This service pro-vides one hot meal a day and a packed lunch for a night meal. The people served must be able to help themselves in the home although unable to get out to market.[8]

Sometimes appetite fails to tempt the very elderly to eat enough food or the right kind of food. The reduced calories in such cases seldom carry enough of the essential nutrients.

The undernutrition which may occur can often be relieved by attention to foods with low bulk and concentrated calories, high in protective values and prepared in a way which the person enjoys. This may not be easy for the person living alone or as a member of a large family where at-tention to the younger members of the family seems more important to the home-maker than tempting the appetite of an elderly grandmother. For others the same problem may stem from the necessity of eating in hotels or restaurants where food does not appeal to the appetite.

Protein Requirements

Apparently, protein needs are not re-duced appreciably with age, and yet many older people eat less protein than when they were younger. This is most likely to

[7] Piper, G. M.: J. Am. Dietet. A., 39:198, 1961.
[8] Keller, M. D., and Smith, C. E.: Geriatrics, 16: 237, 1960. Phillips, E. C.: Nursing Outlook, 8:76, 1960.

happen when marketing is difficult, cooking facilities are poor or the money for food is limited. It can also happen among those of better economic status when denture troubles, lack of appetite or too little energy prevent the preparing or the eating of meats or other protein foods.

Nitrogen balance studies on elderly men and women show that clinical protein deficiencies are not uncommon. Mild deficiencies may be manifested by a sense of habitual fatigue, slow healing of wounds and lowered resistance. Real protein starvation for an extended period is rare, but, if it occurs, it may result in wasting and edema.

Some good-quality protein is essential at each meal regardless of age. The Recommended Dietary Allowances suggest no reduction in protein with age, as they do in calories. Thus, the proportion of protein making up the total calories is increased.

The requirement for certain amino acids may even be increased to meet changes in body function with age. Bigwood[9] found the methionine and lysine requirements of six male subjects 50 to 70 years of age to be substantially greater than for younger males.

Settel[10] found a combination of steroid hormones, enzymes and vitamins to be an effective method of promoting protein formation and weight gain in 25 malnourished elderly patients. It has also been suggested that hormonal disturbances may be responsible for defective synthesis of the organic matrix of bone in osteoporosis.

Special attention may need to be given to meeting the protein requirements of the older person if he is sharing in the family meals planned to meet the higher caloric food habits of the younger members of the family. An extra glass of milk (perhaps reconstituted dry skim milk) at meals or between meals may be the answer. If the person lives alone, milk, cheese and eggs are often used as alternates for meat, fish or poultry because of ease in preparation.

Adequate calories tend to spare protein, so that the total food intake should always be taken into account.

Mineral Requirements

The calcium needs of older people seem to be as great as the needs of younger adults.

Inadequate calcium intake along with some endocrine disturbance may cause the loss of calcium from the bones and lead to osteoporosis and resulting fragility, so frequently responsible for fractures. Lowered gastric acidity and hepatic and pancreatic insufficiency may contribute by impairing calcium absorption.

Dr. Swanson's comments are pertinent[11]:

We cannot consider bony tissue in the adult as static material. It is a dynamic substance, which constantly remodels itself. Formation of new bone and destruction of old bone go on simultaneously. These processes approximately balance each other in the healthy adult. . . . As a person grows older, however, the process of bone destruction may overbalance that of bone building. That this occurs is suggested by observations that the average weight of the skeleton decreases gradually after age 35. The extent to which such decalcification may proceed without injury is not known. We do know that it does not always occur in all individuals.

But we cannot ignore the fact that osteoporosis, or deficient bone substance, certainly is not uncommon in later life. . . . It is commoner among older women than among men. Persons with marked osteoporosis tend to eat food poor in a number of nutrients, including calcium. They also tend to improve in health and to store calcium when the diet is improved.

Nordin[12] reported 29 calcium balance studies on osteoporosis patients in which he found positive balances continuing for at least a year when a liberal allowance of calcium was provided.

Impairment of intestinal absorption of calcium may be responsible, according to Caniggia,[13] for the progessive resorption

[9] Bigwood, E. J.: Senescence and nutrition. Nutritio et Dieta, 8:226, 1966.

[10] Settel, E.: Correction of malnutrition in the aged; comparative efficacy of an anabolic hormone and an enzyme-vitamin complex. Geriatrics, 21:173, 1966.

[11] Swanson, Pearl: Nutrition Needs After 25. Food. The Yearbook of Agriculture, U.S.D.A., Washington, D. C., 1959.

[12] Nordin, B. E. C.: Am. J. Clin. Nutr., 10:384, 1962.

[13] Caniggia, A.: Senile osteoporosis. Geriatrics, 20:300, 1965.

of the skeleton to maintain the homeo-stasis of the plasma calcium level. A diet rich in calcium over a long period seemed to promote some storage of calcium in the osteoporotic skeleton.

Osteoporosis is prevalent among older people around the world and especially so in countries where calcium intakes are rela-tively high. The reasons for poor calcium absorption or utilization in older people is still subject to speculation. There is a pos-sibility that traces of fluorine in drinking water may improve calcium utilization and thus decrease the incidence of osteoporosis. A survey of people living in high- and low-fluoride areas of North Dakota[14] showed osteoporosis more common in the low-fluoride areas than in the higher fluoride areas. This finding served to confirm earlier suggestions of the benefit of fluoride for older people.

More research is needed on why older women seem to fracture bones, especially hips, more often than men. Is it that men tend to drink more milk than women, or is there a sex difference in the aging of bones? For further discussion of osteoporosis see Chapter 32.

At present the best suggestion is to pro-vide liberal amounts of milk and milk prod-ucts. These may be used in cooking, creamed soups, milk desserts, etc. The use of nonfat dry milk is to be encouraged in cooking as an inexpensive source of good protein and calcium. Present evidence favors about 0.8 Gm. of calcium per day.

Another mineral disturbance in older peo-ple is the occurrence of kidney and bladder stones. Stare[15] suggests that diets low in pyridoxine and magnesium may cause or aggravate this condition.

Needs for other minerals are apparently similar to those for all adults, as discussed in Chapter 6.

Vitamin Requirements

Unfortunately, little is known regarding the vitamin requirements of older people

[14] Bernstein, D. S.: Prevalence of osteoporosis in high- and low-fluoride areas in North Dakota. J.A.M.A., *198*:499, 1966.

[15] Stare, F. J.: Good nutrition from food, not pills. Am. J. Nursing, *65*:86, 1965.

and whether there is a change with age or associated with chronic disease. However, there is no evidence that vitamin require-ments are reduced with advancing years, and it is safe to assume that older people need all the vitamins that they did in earlier years.

If there has been merely a marginal sup-ply of any of the vitamins in the diet for many years, then a reduction in total food eaten may be sufficient to precipitate minor nutritional deficiencies. The time factor which is inevitable with advancing age may permit cumulative effects to show up.

The B complex requirement of older peo-ple has been the subject of clinical investi-gation. The apparent lift which extra B vitamins seems to give to some people when no other therapy relieves chronic fatigue and other vague symptoms has not been explained. Perhaps people inadver-tently reduce the B complex intake with reduced calories and fail to make it good from other sources. As a result, slow de-pletion of body reserves is likely, since these factors are not stored to any extent.

The use of vitamin concentrates is dis-cussed in Chapters 7 and 8.

PLANNING MEALS FOR OLDER PEOPLE

The planning of food to meet the needs of the older age group presents many prob-lems, which are as varied as the circum-stances in which such people are living. They may be living alone, or with one or two other older people, and marketing and preparing meals for themselves; they may be the older member in a younger family; they may be cared for by a practical nurse or a housekeeper. Whoever is responsible for planning and preparing food should be aware of likes and dislikes, special needs and limitations. There are numerous fac-tors such as ignorance of nutritional facts, food prejudices, fear of new foods, lack of money, limited cooking facilities and poor appetite which should be considered. The public health nurse may be able to advise or help with the planning where such problems seem to interfere with ob-taining adequate food.

The elderly person, too often a forgotten member of the household, may require some special foods or food preparation, but so far as possible he or she should be a member of the family at mealtime and eat foods prepared for the family. If digestive ability is limited, the family meals should be so planned that the older person may avoid fried foods, rich sauces, pastries and other foods that disagree with him. When lack of mealtime appetite makes an adequate food intake difficult, a midmorning and a midafternoon lunch of something light, such as hot malted milk or orange juice, may be offered. A hot drink at bedtime may be welcomed by an older person and may help to induce sleep.

The older handicapped person, living alone, may encounter real difficulties in preparing meals for himself. *Homemaking for the Handicapped* offers many suggestions to those with physical limitations to assist them in homemaking skills.[16]

16 May, E. E., Waggoner, N. R., and Boettke, E. M.: Homemaking for the Handicapped. New York, Dodd, Mead and Co., 1966.

The nutritional well-being of an increasing number of older people is threatened by one or more of the problems mentioned above. To meet this situation several cities or communities have initiated some type of service for shut-ins or group feeding for aged residents of a neighborhood. Meals-on-Wheels is a program which serves meals to aged or incapacitated persons in their own homes. This idea is spreading but as yet only a small proportion of the older persons who need such a type of service are being reached.

Both normal and modified diets should be planned with the cooperation of a nutritionist and the nurse who knows the patient. Fat or sodium restricted diets or diabetic diets present real problems not easily solved. And, of course, some foods are much more popular with older people than others. For instance, in one city sandwiches, fruits, juices, pies, puddings and cakes were found to be the most popular items and ground meat, casserole dishes and fish were less popular.

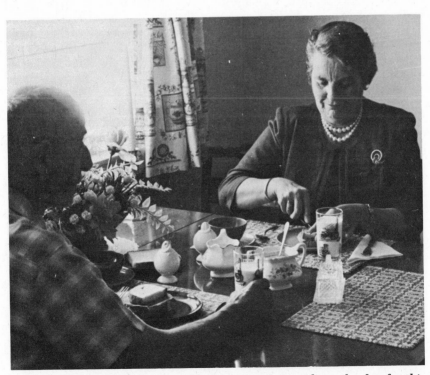

Fig. 15–4. Good food and a pleasant environment enliven the day for this retired couple. (Administration on Aging, U. S. Dept. H.E.W., Washington, D. C.)

When groups of older people are confined in institutions or nursing homes they sometimes become depressed. Volpe and Kastenbaum[17] reported on a ward of 34 confused and deteriorated older men who were agitated and hostile and had poor appetites. They were transferred to a larger ward where a record player was installed and games provided and with large tables for meals. They dressed in white shirts and ties and had an afternoon snack of beer, crackers and cheese. Within a month the atmosphere changed and behavior improved.

Bulletins and pamphlets published by national and state agencies and by insurance companies give simple information about food for older people.

One publication reminds us that making simple food attractive and appropriate to the specific needs of an elderly person is appreciated far out of proportion to the effort involved. An example of good planning occurred at the golden wedding of the parents of one of the authors. One parent was a partial invalid and had a denture problem. The dinner menu of fruit cocktail, turkey croquettes, mashed potatoes, peas, aspic salad, ice cream and a beautiful anniversary cake was a meal that all guests could enjoy, including the guests of honor, who would have been embarrassed by a different menu. Senior members of most families enjoy the young folks at family parties, but they do not want to be conspicuous because of their infirmities. With a little preliminary planning of an appropriate menu, the party can be fun for young and old.

STUDY QUESTIONS AND ACTIVITIES

1. Surveys have shown that older people are apt to omit certain foods from their diets. Which ones are these and which nutrients are deficient as a result?

2. What disease in older people may result from failure to absorb or utilize cal-cium? What suggestions are offered that may help to improve calcium utilization?

3. Why is the caloric requirement of older people reduced? How much reduction in caloric intake is recommended between age 25 and 65?

4. If an elderly person shares the family fare but eats less of everything than younger members, which nutrients may be lower than recommended?

5. In what circumstances may the use of vitamin concentrates be justified?

6. If an older person with whom you are associated is a food faddist or a follower of some of the quack books, how would you attempt to correct his false ideas? What reliable sources of information would you recommend? (See Chap. 10.)

7. What federal, state or local agencies are concerned with care of the aged in your community?

SUPPLEMENTARY READINGS ON GERIATRIC NUTRITION

Beeuwkes, A. M.: Studying the food habits of the elderly. J. Am. Dietet. A., *37*:215, 1960.

Eating is Fun . . . For Older People, Too.: Am. Dietet. A., Chicago, 1961.

Jalso, S., Burns, M., and Rivers, J. M.: Nutrition beliefs and practices. J. Am. Dietet. A., *47*:263, 1965.

King, C. G., and Britt, G.: Food Hints for Mature People. Pub. Affairs Pamphlet No. 336, 1962.

Lane, M. M.: The ideal geriatric diet. Nursing Homes, *16*:27, 1967 (Jan.).

LeBovit, C.: The food of older people living at home. J. Am. Dietet. A., *46*:285, 1965.

Piper, G. M.: Nutrition in coordinated home care. J. Am. Dietet. A., *39*:198, 1961.

Piper, G. M., and Smith, E. M.: Geriatric nutrition. Nursing Outlook, *12*:51, 1964.

Stare, F. J.: Good nutrition from food, not pills. Am. J. Nursing, *65*:86, 1965.

Volpe, A., and Kastenbaum, R.: Beer and TLC. Am. J. Nursing, *67*:100, 1967.

Review: Fluoride, bony structure, and aortic calcification. Nutrition Rev., *25*:100, 1967.

For further references see Bibliography in Part Four.

---

[17] Volpe, A., and Kastenbaum, R.: Beer and TLC. Am. J. Nursing, 67:100, 1967.

CHAPTER 16

Malnutrition—A World Problem

Protein-Calorie Malnutrition • Vitamin Deficiencies—Severe and Marginal • Mineral Deficiencies • Early Diagnosis and Treatment of Nutritional Failure

Lifetime handicaps, starvation and death may result from poor or inadequate food. This we know from the work of hundreds of scientists in many countries. Nutritional deficiencies may be the cause of mental retardation, blindness and physical deformities. Professional help is needed to understand the underlying causes of these and other abnormalities due to improper food, and how they can be relieved. The improvement in the health of children or of whole communities that can take place when practical application of present-day scientific knowledge is put to work is truly dramatic. International, national and private agencies mentioned in Chapter 1 are helping to make this possible.

The concept of nutritional deficiencies as causes of specific diseases evolved from the early work with scurvy and beriberi. It was decades before other diseases related to malnutrition were recognized as the result of specific deficiencies. Only after thorough study of the pathology resulting from controlled lack of specific nutrients in animals or man was it possible to understand the function of each nutrient in metabolism—discussed in earlier chapters.

During the last quarter century the synergistic effect of the combination of malnutrition and infection has been reported in hundreds of scientific articles. One reason that this problem still exists may be, as Scrimshaw has often emphasized,[1] that medical personnel in developing countries fail to recognize malnutrition as an underlying factor in deaths reported as due to infections. Even marginal malnutrition may predispose or make children more susceptible to infections.

It would be a big step forward if it were possible to recognize marginal malnutrition before true clinical signs appeared. There is still much to be done in this field. A deficiency of one nutrient may increase the requirement for or interfere with the metabolism of another and thus precipitate symptoms that are not easily identified. In the U. S. today there is relatively little frank deficiency disease but there are marginal types of malnutrition which are too often ignored. Public health nurses and nutritionists are often in the position to bring suspected cases of malnutrition to the attention of the physician.

Surveys have shown that many people are nutritionally below average by dietary, biochemical and clinical criteria but are not aware of it.[2] One reason for the occurrence of such conditioned malnutrition in this country is the failure of physicians and other professional people as well as the

[1] Scrimshaw, N. S.: J. Am. Med. Women's Assoc., 17:422, 1962.
[2] Sebrell, W. H.: Am. J. Clin. Nutr., 20:653, 1967.

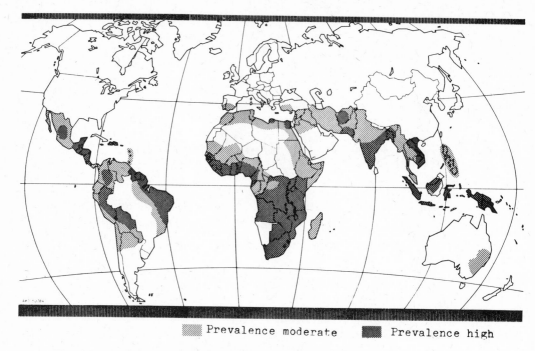

Fig. 16–1. Geographic distribution of protein-calorie deficiencies in young children (general impression). (WHO Chronicle, Nov. 1965)

subjects themselves to recognize the problem and seek assistance.

The medical history and physical examination remain the most important tools of the physician in diagnosing nutritional problems. A good medical history can provide information which will call special attention to the need for examining certain areas of the body and will indicate the need for pertinent laboratory tests. In order to determine whether manifestations of nutritional disease are due to inadequate diets or are secondary to metabolic or physiologic abnormalities, every medical history should record the dietary practices of the person as well as his food dislikes and intolerances.

PROTEIN-CALORIE MALNUTRITION

Protein-calorie malnutrition (P-CM) is the most serious and widespread form of deficiency disease in the world today and occurs most frequently in children during the years of rapid growth. National and international agencies are working to-gether to eradicate this deficiency disease. At the same time they are studying its causes, prevention and treatment; a 1966 publication[3] gives an extensive report on the world picture and progess being made in combating P-CM.

The terms used to describe P-CM are kwashiorkor and marasmus. Kwashiorkor results from a diet inadequate in protein but generally adequate in calories, while marasmus results from a diet inadequate in protein and calories. It is impossible to estimate the number of children throughout the world who are affected by these two forms of malnutrition. One estimate[4] is that 350 million children—70 per cent of the world population under six—are stunted in their early years by these disorders. The accompanying map (Fig. 16–1) shows the geographic distribution of P-CM as estimated by WHO.

[3] Pre-School Child Malnutrition: National Academy of Sciences–National Research Council, Washington, D. C., 1966.

[4] Randal, J.: Current, Jan., 1967.

Kwashiorkor

In 1933 Dr. Cicely Williams, a British pediatrician working in West Africa, first described this protein-deficiency disease in children from 1 to 4 years. She called it by its local name, "Kwashiorkor," and found that it was curable by giving the children milk. The name means "the disease the deposed baby gets when the next one is born."[5] The picture of a mother from Uganda (Fig. 16–2) is a striking example: the healthy infant in arms and the "deposed" one by her side.

While kwashiorkor was first described and named in Africa, it has been recognized in many parts of the world including

[5] Went, L. N.: Doc. Med. Geogr. Trop., 7:139, 1955.

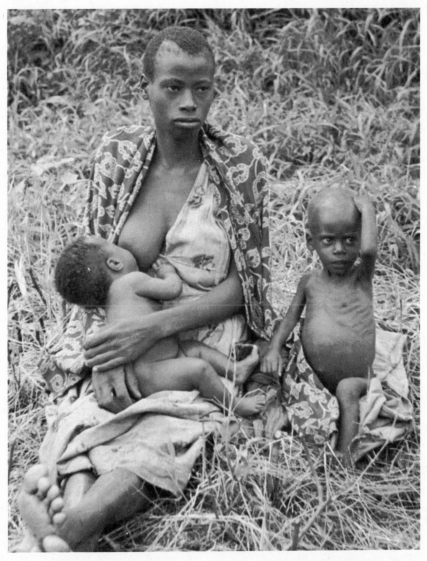

FIG. 16–2. The older child in this picture shows the protein deprivation and the malnutrition that occurred when he was "deposed" or replaced at the mother's breast by the new baby. He is subsisting on starchy foods and a few vegetables. (From Dr. John Bennett, Nutrition Unit, Ministry of Health, Kampala, Uganda)

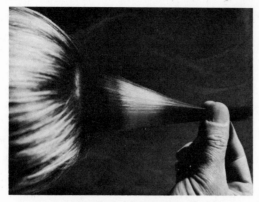

FIG. 16–3. Hair depigmentation typical of ʹkwashiorkor. (Scrimshaw, N. S., and Behar, M.: Malnutrition in underdeveloped countries. New Eng. J. Med. 272:137, 198, 1965)

Central America, parts of South America, some countries in the Middle East, and Southeast Asia and India. It was originally described by various terms such as multiple deficiency or protein deficiency but now it is quite generally known as kwashiorkor. It is always associated with a low-protein high-carbohydrate diet the small child is given at weaning. In Mexico and Latin America this consists of corn and arrowroot; in Asia, and India, rice; in much of Africa, manioc and cassava; in India, also root vegetables. In these countries there is seldom any food suitable for the weaned child who needs approximately 3 grams of protein per kilogram of body weight per day between the ages of 1 and 2 years.

In developed countries milk is so closely associated with the weaning of babies that it is difficult to realize that many of the world's children are weaned directly from human milk to a diet primarily of carbohydrate from grains or roots. Often these foods are unappetizing or are too coarse and bulky for an infant to digest. Either he fails to eat enough or his mother makes a thin gruel from these foods. In either case the infant receives a moderately calorie-deficient and grossly protein-deficient diet.

The signs of kwashiorkor vary from country to country, depending on the nature of the food given at weaning. Invariably growth is retarded and there is some degree of edema, and the child is miserable. In addition there may be disorders of pigmentation of the skin and hair (see Fig. 16–3). The liver may be enlarged.

Marasmus

In addition to the many children who suffer from kwashiorkor there are even more who develop marasmus. The diets of these children are inadequate in calories and protein. Marasmus usually develops in children under 1 year of age when breast-feeding fails or (like kwashiorkor) when the child suffers from some disease, usually diarrhea.

Marasmus differs from kwashiorkor in various ways. According to a WHO account:[6]

The marasmic child is wasted, not swollen. His hair is dull and dry, but not discolored. The skin is thin and wrinkled and has lost its elasticity, but does not break down. The child does not refuse food and does not show the same resentful apathy as in kwashiorkor. The terrible wasting makes the eyes look enormous and staring, and there may be, in some cases, a stiffness of limbs, due to muscle spasm. Why marasmus develops, rather than kwashiorkor, is not understood. . . . The child who has marasmus is much less likely to be depleted of proteins, and dies chiefly because diarrhea and vomiting . . . have brought great losses in body fluids. . . . Only too often marasmic children are brought to the hospital in such a moribund state that nothing can be done to save them.

Synergism Between Malnutrition and Infection

Children who suffer from inadequate protein intake are often exposed to contaminated food and water and unhygienic home conditions. According to Scrimshaw:[7]

Synergism between malnutrition and infection is responsible for much of the excess mortality among infants and preschool children in less developed regions. Two types of relationships can be identified as synergistic. Infections are likely to have more serious consequences among persons with clinical and subclinical

---

[6] Malnutrition and Disease. Geneva, Switzerland, WHO, 1963.

[7] Scrimshaw, N. S.: Recent advances in international nutrition. Presented Oct. 27, 1966. Annual Meeting Am. Dietet. Assoc. Boston.

malnutrition, and infectious diseases have the capacity to turn borderline nutritional deficiencies into severe malnutrition. Thus malnutrition and infection can be mutually aggravating and can produce more serious consequences for the patient than would be expected from the summation of the independent effects of the two.

Malnutrition and Mental Development

Since the earlier surveys which pointed up retarded and abnormal physical development in children who survive one or more episodes of kwashiorkor, more recent studies have emphasized the effect upon *behavior* and *mental development*. Intensive studies are now in progress in several countries in which education and relief measures may have reduced mortality from P-CM but where many of the children may have suffered irreparable damage to the central nervous system. Dr. Cravioto of Mexico City makes several pertinent observations:[8]

The accounts given by several authors from different countries show that apathy probably constitutes the most common finding. The kwashiorkor patients seem to have lost all normal curiosity and desire for exploration that is natural to a child. . . . The possible adverse effects of protein-calorie malnutrition on the development of the human central nervous system can readily be appreciated when one considers that, of the two main processes morphologically associated with growth of the human brain at the time of birth, increase of cell cytoplasm with extension of axons and dendrites and myelination, the former is largely a process of protein synthesis. . . . Perhaps an easy way to grasp the magnitude of these processes may be simply to recall that at the time of birth the human brain is gaining weight at a rate of 1 to 2 milligrams per minute. [1.5 Gm. per day]

A glance at Figure 14–1 (p. 187) will show that nervous tissues continue to grow faster than other tissues during the first four years of life. If essential amino acids are lacking during this period, the brain and nerve cells cannot develop normally.

Even the head circumference of these children indicates retarded brain growth. Research now in progress in several countries is trying to determine at what ages the damage to the nervous system is most severe, to what extent recovery of normal mental function is possible, and how to detect evidence of brain damage at an early age when recovery may be possible.

Coursin says, in summary:

Today's pressing challenge is to solve the intricacies of the roles of nutrients in normal central nervous system metabolism and to clarify the relationships of nutritional deficiencies to the pathogenesis of mental retardation. With better understanding of these problems, it would be possible to develop appropriate measures for prevention and correction that could be instituted for preschool children in developing countries.[9]

P-CM in Older Children and Adults

Older children and adults may also suffer from protein-calorie malnutrition, but fortunately the damage may not be as permanent if food and treatment become available later. In adults emaciation and lethargy are the most common signs of semistarvation and, if protein intake is also inadequate, as is commonly the case, there may be edema and increased susceptibility to infection.

Children deprived of adequate food, especially when the diet is markedly deficient in protein, become emaciated, and growth is definitely retarded. Occasionally they show some edema, but it is less frequent and often less marked than in adults. Even after they have been receiving adequate food long enough to have regained average weight for height, they may still be under height for their age. A relief worker reported surprise on learning that a little fellow who appeared to be about 8 years old was actually 12, and this happened repeatedly. On the other hand, the facial expression of such children is mature for their age.

In teenagers a protein deficiency in either quantity or quality may result in retarded

[8] Cravioto, J.: Pre-school Child Malnutrition. Chap. 7. National Acad. Sci. Nat. Res. Council, Washington, D. C., 1966.

[9] Coursin, D. B.: Undernutrition and brain function. Borden's Rev. Nutrition Res., *26*:1, 1965 (Jan.-Mar.).

growth during the adolescent spurt. This situation seems to have occurred in Japan from 1939 to 1948, resulting in shorter stature, especially among teenagers, at the end of the war than before.[10] Yet there were no reports of obvious deficiency disease (see Chap. 14).

Treatment of P-CM

While the emphasis thus far has been on protein and calories, it must be remembered that the quality and quantity of protein as well as all nutrients must be considered in the treatment and prevention of P-CM (see Chap. 9). For infants the ideal diet would include a liberal supply of fresh milk or, if necessary, dried skim milk fortified with vitamins A and D, and accompanied by adequate non-protein calories and other nutrients. Unfortunately, milk is not available nor can it be readily distributed in the areas where kwashiorkor and marasmus are prevalent. Therefore, attention is focused on improving the quality of the protein in the diets of infants and children in the first year of life as they progress from human milk to other foods.

---

[10] Mitchell, H. S.: J. Am. Dietet. A., *44*:165, 1964.

In several countries where P-CM is recognized as a public health problem and where milk is not easily available, palatable vegetable protein mixtures have been developed using locally grown and familiar products. One of the first of these was prepared at the Institute of Nutrition of Central America and Panama (INCAP) in Guatemala City. This mixture is composed of cornmeal, ground sorghum, cottonseed flour, Torula yeast and leaf meal blended according to a formula that provides the best amino-acid balance and fortified with calcium and vitamins. This is known as *Incaparina* and is now available on the market in several Central American countries where it has proved to be useful and popular. Dr. Behar of INCAP is shown in Figure 16-4 examining a child with kwashiorkor who shows some of the typical lesions—edema, sparse hair and an apathetic expression. The second picture (Fig. 16-5) shows the same child after being fed Incaparina for 6 weeks.

Other mixtures of vegetable proteins with or without the addition of small amounts of dried skim milk, casein or fish meal have been developed in other countries: in India, from Indian pulses, cereals and leafy veg-

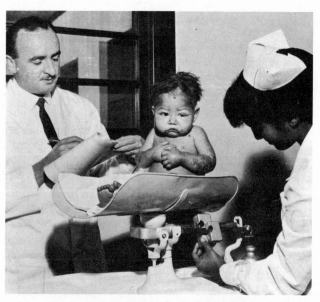

Fig. 16-4. Dr. Moises Behar of INCAP examines a child suffering from kwashiorkor, showing edema, skin lesions, and lethargic expression. (UNICEF photo)

etables; in Indonesia, from soybean and sesame seed; in Nigeria, from peanut flour and some milk casein. Usually, these mixtures have been tested first on animals for adequacy for growth and maintenance. Subsequent experience in feeding these vegetable protein mixtures to children suffering from P-CM has demonstrated that recovery, as well as prevention of P-CM, is quite possible if the blend contains a good balance of essential amino acids. Recovery may not be as rapid as is possible when milk or other animal proteins are fed, but these mixtures of locally grown foods have the advantage of being cheap and available to many more people. Through education and an aroused interest in the problem, real progress is now being made toward the eradication of P-CM.

A major chemical company in the U. S. has developed an instant soybean product, similar to our instant cereals, for export to areas faced with P-CM. As well as supplying nutrients, this product has the distinct advantage of reducing the fuel required to prepare food. Probably as important to the solution to P-CM in the world as food is a fuel supply and pots in which to cook food.

Great credit is due to the technical agencies of the United Nations—FAO, WHO, UNICEF and UNESCO (see Chap. 1)—for their active and practical assistance to the health agencies of the many countries where P-CM is a public health problem. By working cooperatively with local authorities, a better understanding of prevailing food usage and child feeding practices has made it possible to approach a solution without depending on imported foods. The same approach applies to meeting the needs of older children and adults.

Research groups around the world continue to study the problem of P-CM. Dr. Jelliffe expressed the hope of many working to combat P-CM when he said; "What I hope will develop in the next few years, is an increased interest in and emphasis upon scientific investigation of the methodology of prevention, so that important discoveries that have been made in the laboratories can be applied rapidly and effectively, in the field.[11]

The prevention of malnutrition in the world today requires the efforts of various disciplines. Agriculture and food production, processing and distribution are key

[11] Jelliffe, D. B.: WHO Chronicle, *21*:127, 1967.

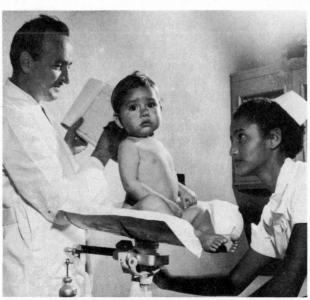

Fig. 16–5. The same child being examined at INCAP in Guatamala, after being fed Incaparina for six weeks. (UNICEF photo)

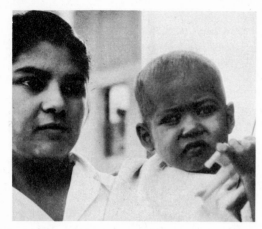

FIG. 16–6. Keratomalacia in a Central American child. (Photo by Marcel Ganzin, FAO)

factors, but economics, education and politics are also involved. Population planning is one of the most critical factors. The International Planned Parenthood Federation and numerous health agencies are focusing on the world-wide population explosion. Educational programs are in progress in many countries to provide birth control information and devices.

VITAMIN DEFICIENCIES— SEVERE AND MARGINAL

Vitamin-A Deficiency

Avitaminosis A and Xerophthalmia

Among the nutritional disorders affecting infants and children, vitamin A deficiency comes second in importance to protein-calorie malnutrition. Very often the two occur together, with serious consequences. Of the effects ascribed to vitamin A deficiency, those involving the eye are specific and can be generally described by the inclusive term "xerophthalmia"; this covers the whole range of ocular changes, from mild local or generalized xerosis of the conjunctiva to the most severe type involving the cornea, i.e., keratomalacia, which may result in partial or complete loss of vision. A mortality of nearly 30 per cent has been reported in young children suffering from keratomalacia. . . . It is estimated that about 25 per cent of the survivors become totally blind, while about 60 per cent are left with reduced vision in one or both eyes.[12]

In 1961, with financial assistance from the U. S. National Institutes of Health, WHO attempted to collect information on the occurrence of the disease in different regions of the world. . . . The data obtained, although incomplete, revealed what had always been suspected: that xerophthalmia occurs in varying degrees of severity, often in association with protein-calorie malnutrition, in a majority of the developing countries. . . . It was the considered view of the WHO experts who undertook this survey that a majority of pediatricians and ophthalmologists in most of the countries visited were in general not very well informed about the problem and that diagnosis and treatment of xerophthalmia were defective.[13]

McLaren,[14] referring to this WHO survey, considers xerophthalmia a neglected problem overshadowed by the attention recently given to P-CM. Yet when xerophthalmia accompanies P-CM, as it does in many areas, the mortality may be as high as 80 per cent, whereas it is only 15 per cent in a group equally malnourished but not deficient in vitamin A. From this survey of nearly 50 countries it was estimated that tens of thousands of children become blind every year from this cause. The worst areas are Central America, northeast Brazil, Haiti, northern and central Africa, Egypt, Sudan, Jordan, Syria, Iraq, Indonesia, East Pakistan, Vietnam, Ceylon and South India. Another report from India[15] estimates that 40 per cent of the blindness there is due to keratomalacia (Fig. 16–6).

Symptoms and Pathology. The first symptoms of xerosis are itching and burning, with a mild light sensitivity, usually accompanied by redness of the lids and some inflammmation. There is probably a secondary infection, but this is not as severe as in xerophthalmia. Xerophthalmia is due to a secondary infection of the cornea which occurs when the protective secretions of the eye are decreased as a result of keratinization of the epithelial cells due to a vitamin A deficiency.

[12] Caddell, J. L., and Goddard, D. R.: New Eng. J. Med., 276:533, 1967.

[13] The WHO Programme in Nutrition, 1948-64. WHO Chronicle, 19:467, 1965.

[14] McLaren, D. S.: Nutr. Rev., 22:289, 1964.

[15] Sinha, B. N.: J. Indian Med. Assoc., 47:67, 1966.

In children affected with these eye conditions, usually there are numerous other evidences of malnutrition, such as stunted growth and anemia. Adults usually develop hemeralopia (glare blindness) before the ophthalmic symptoms appear. The cornea becomes dry and lusterless, and eventually opaque and soft. This infection, once started, may spread rapidly and destroy the eye before the deficiency can be corrected or the infection conquered (Fig. 16–7).

Treatment. Food sources of vitamin A are sufficient as preventives but not as curatives. For treatment of xerophthalmia "large doses of vitamin A (5,000 I.U. per Kg. of body weight daily for five days

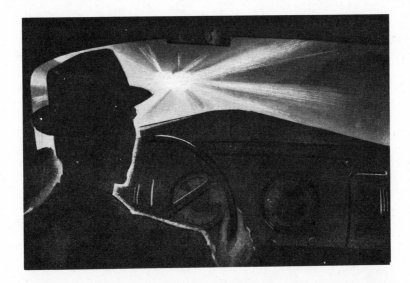

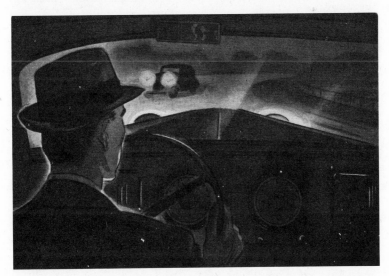

FIG. 16–7. (*Top*) "Glare blindness" often is a symptom of vitamin A deficiency. Headlights dazzle the eyes and cause discomfort. The driver is blinded temporarily by oncoming headlights, and the edge of the road is seen with difficulty. (*Bottom*) An adequate intake of vitamin A protects against "glare blindness" or remedies it. Properly focused headlights no longer dazzle so blindingly, and the road edge can be seen almost immediately after the headlight glare has passed.

orally in a water dispersible form preferably, combined with 25,000 I.U. per Kg. of body weight of palmitate in oil in one intramuscular injection) should be given followed thereafter by 25,000 I.U. daily until cure or discharge."[16]

As a preventive it is now general policy of UN and U. S. agencies to fortify all dry skim milk with vitamin A when it is to be sent as a relief food to such areas.

Night Blindness (Nyctalopia) and Glare Blindness (Hemeralopia)

Incidence. Mild deficiencies of vitamin A with a variety of manifestations still occur in more prosperous areas of the world. One of the early signs long associated with this deficiency is night blindness. In Labrador and Newfoundland, where this condition has been recognized for generations, the popular remedy is fish liver, which the people rarely eat as food but will take as medicine. Varying degrees of night blindness are discovered among children and adults in the U. S. when instruments for detecting and measuring adjustment to dull light are used for routine examinations of large groups. In general, it tends to be more prevalent among low-income groups, but some cases are found in almost any group.

Glare blindness (hemeralopia), closely related and essentially similar to night blindness, was recognized when automobile drivers complained of being unable to drive at night because of the glare of headlights (Fig. 16–7). During World War II pilots were examined especially for this condition, and a liberal intake of vitamin A was recommended as a preventive.

Etiology and Pathology. Both nyctalopia and hemeralopia are functional disorders resulting from the slowed regeneration of visual purple in the retina of the eye. The difficulty is usually due to insufficient vitamin A to combine with the protein of the retina for the regeneration of visual purple, which is bleached to visual yellow under the influence of bright light. Regeneration of visual purple takes place in the dark, but replenishment of vitamin A from the blood stream is essential to continue the reaction, i.e., to permit the adaptation in the shortest possible time (see Chap. 7).

Symptoms and Diagnosis. A person may have a mild degree of either night or glare blindness and not be aware of it unless his attention is drawn to it by some circumstance or special test. One person may be slower than another in adjusting to the dull light of a movie theater, but neither is aware of a difference. This is not a condition which causes sufficient discomfort to prompt one to seek medical advice unless it reaches an advanced stage.

Treatment. A daily intake of 5,000 I.U. of vitamin A is more than enough to prevent night blindness or any related condition, unless for some reason the person is unable to use this vitamin or convert carotene into vitamin A. Usually, a food source of this vitamin is sufficient to clear up a mild pathologic state, but numerous fish-liver-oil concentrates are available as more potent sources if their use is advised.

Other Conditions Due to Vitamin A Deficiency

Cutaneous lesions may appear early in adults and have a characteristic appearance. Papules tend to form around hair follicles on outer surfaces of arms, legs, shoulders and lower abdomen, and are described as having a "gooseflesh" appearance. They usually disappear when an adequate food source of vitamin A is provided.

Epithelial tissue changes may occur as a result of vitamin A deficiency; normal secretory epithelium is replaced by dry, kertinized epithelium which is more susceptible to invasion by infectious organisms.

Genitourinary-tract changes also may occur as a result of vitamin A deficiency. In the female, the epithelial cells in the vagina undergo changes which interfere with the normal estrus cycle, and in the male atrophic changes in the testes may result in permanent damage. More research is needed to explain complications due to epithelial cell changes resulting from this deficiency.

For food sources of vitamin A and further discussion of the subject see Chapter 7 and Table 1, Part Four.

---

[16] McLaren, D. S.: Op. cit.

Thiamine Deficiency

Incidence. Mild or chronic thiamine deficiency is more often part of a depletion of the whole group of B complex vitamins. Such a chronic multiple deficiency may be a contributing factor in malnutrition in children. It also should be recalled that the thiamine allowance is related to total calorie intake (see Chap. 8).

Beriberi

The frank deficiency disease known as beriberi is of special significance among the rice eaters of the Orient, where it still occurs, although less frequently than formerly.

Beriberi is described in Chinese history, and some of the earliest attempts to treat it are reported from Japan and the Philippines. The recognition of its cause and of its possible cure by better diet is one of the landmarks in the history of nutrition. The story is well told by Dr. R. R. Williams in his book entitled *Toward the Conquest of Beriberi.*[17] This account of Dr. Williams's own 26-year search for what proved to be a vitamin, of its identification and eventual synthesis is a classic in nutrition research. Dr. Williams prior to his death in 1965 had been the moving spirit behind the practical use of thiamine and other factors of the B complex for the enrichment of rice in the Philippines and some other oriental countries. This has resulted in a marked reduction in the incidence of beriberi. In fact, beriberi has almost disappeared from Japan where the prophylactic use of thiamine and enrichment of rice are common.

"In Thailand, Malasia, and Vietnam, however, beriberi has increased in recent years as more efficient small mechanical mills replace hand pounding, which left some of the germ and hull. Moreover, most of the increase has been in infantile beriberi, with its recognized high mortality."[18]

According to Scrimshaw:

. . . infantile beriberi is one of the most dramatic deficiencies, for a child may be apparently well and die from this condition in a few hours. It is due to low thiamine levels in breast milk. Recovery is equally dramatic when the mother is given thiamine. [The initial stage is characterized by] vomiting, restlessness, pallor, anorexia and insomnia. . . . In the subacute form further vomiting, puffiness of the face and extremities, oliguria, abdominal pain, dysphasia, aphonia and convulsions may appear. This type may go on to a fatal episode or may become chronic.

There need be no signs of beriberi in the mothers of infants affected. Reports coming to the World Health Organization suggest that infantile beriberi is more of a problem today than clinical beriberi in older children and adults.[19]

Symptoms and Pathology. Beriberi in adults and older children is of three main types: the chronic dry, atrophic type generally found only in older adults, often associated with prolonged consumption of alcohol; the fulminating acute type which is more serious and dramatic but rarely found; and the mild subacute form which is most common. This third type

. . . has characteristic nervous manifestations, including alterations in tendon reflexes. Paresthesia is common. . . . Sensations of fullness and tightening of the muscles and muscle cramps are common at night. Cardiovascular signs and symptoms range from breathlessness on exertion and palpitation to tachycardia, cardiac dilation and some degree of congestive heart failure. Coexisting deficiencies of ascorbic acid, riboflavin, niacin and vitamin A are common.[20]

Treatment. Adequate food sources of thiamine are sufficient to prevent any of the deficiency conditions described, but, when the pathologic symptoms appear, more concentrated sources of thiamine usually are necessary for prompt recovery. Anorexia and nausea are often so severe as to preclude an adequate food intake until symptoms have been relieved by the administration of concentrates.

Since most of the cases diagnosed as beriberi in regions where it is prevalent are suffering from multiple deficiencies, it is customary for the physician to prescribe

[17] Williams, R. R.: Toward the Conquest of Beriberi. Cambridge, Harvard University Press, 1961.
[18] Scrimshaw, N. S.: New Eng. J. Med., 272:137, 1965.

[19] Op. cit.
[20] Scrimshaw: Op. cit.

B-complex concentrates rather than pure thiamine and to seek improvement in the diet. The dosage for therapeutic purposes is often several times the recommended allowance of 0.8 to 1.2 mg. of thiamine with other factors in proportion. (See Chap. 10 for recommended allowances of vitamins for different age and sex categories. See Chap. 8 for rich food sources of thiamine and other fractions of the B complex.)

Beriberi Heart Disease

Beriberi heart disease is described as a distinct clinical entity by Gubbay.[21] The pathology includes right heart failure, edema and peripheral vasodilation. Beriberi heart disease is due to a deficiency and is curable if the deficiency is corrected in time.

Nutritional Disorders of the Central Nervous System

Several acute disorders of the central nervous system have been associated with alcoholism. Similar disturbances may also occur in the absence of alcoholism when there is a prolonged deficiency of food intake, as in gastric carcinoma or when anorexia is a complication of other conditions such as pregnancy.

Experimental work in pigeons in 1938 first demonstrated that a severe thiamine deficiency could produce brain lesions. In 1942 British prisoners-of-war developed nervous disorders which disappeared with small doses of thiamine.

Subsequent clinical research has identified the lesion in man as polioencephalitis, an inflammatory disease of the gray substance of the brain. This is due in most, if not all, cases to a thiamine deficiency.

Polyneuropathy is defined as a disease which involves many nerves and affects the peripheral nerves. The symptoms are remarkably similar to those of classical beriberi and are usually relieved by thiamine or vitamin-B-complex therapy. Under some circumstances a deficiency of pyridoxine or pantothenic acid may give rise to similar symptoms. The chief ones are weakness, numbness, partial paralysis and pain in the legs. The legs are affected earlier than the arms. Motor, reflex and sensory reactions are lost in most cases. Recovery is a slow process involving weeks or months, and a year may pass before a patient is able to walk unaided.

Wernicke's disease is closely associated with Korsakoff's psychosis, and the combination is often referred to as the Wernicke-Korsakoff syndrome. The specific nutritional factor mostly concerned is thiamine. This syndrome may occur apart from alcoholism but is most frequently encountered in chronic alcoholics. The chief symptoms are ophthalmoplegia (paralysis of the eye muscles), nystagmus (involuntary rapid movement of the eyeballs) and ataxia (failure of musclar coordination). The ophthalmoplegia is relieved promptly after a few adequate meals; the other symptoms respond more slowly to thiamine therapy, indicating, perhaps, some structural damage to the nerve tissue. Wernicke's disease is a medical emergency and massive doses of thiamine (as much as 250 mg. per day) may be prescribed. Mental symptoms such as apathy, drowsiness, inattentiveness, inability to concentrate or sustain a conversation seem to clear up upon thiamine administration.

The Korsakoff syndrome is characterized by memory defect and confabulation (a form of mental confusion consisting of giving answers and reciting experiences without regard to truth). These symptoms may not respond to thiamine therapy as do the other mental symptoms mentioned in the preceding paragraph. There is evidence that the damage to the nervous system in the Korsakoff syndrome may be structural rather than biochemical and that thiamine deficiency of long standing may be responsible.

The amblyopia (dim vision) accompanying alcoholism and formerly attributed to the toxic effects of alcohol and tobacco is probably of nutritional origin.[22] Clinical experiments have demonstrated recovery following improved nutrition, with vitamin B complex—and, more specifically, thiamine, the important factor.

---

[21] Gubbay, E. R.: Canad. M. A. J., 95:21, 1966.

[22] Victor, M., and Adams, R. D.: Am. J. Clin. Nutr., 9:379, 1961.

PLATE 1

(*Top, left*) Dermatitis of hands and neck in a case of pellagra. (New York)

(*Top, right*) Beefy red glossitis in a patient with multiple B complex deficiency. This is characteristic of pellagra or sprue. (New York)

(*Center, left*) Late chronic glossitis with complete papillary atrophy, probably resulting from prolonged B complex deficiency. (Newfoundland)

(*Center, right*) Angular stomatitis and dermatitis, probably due to a riboflavin deficiency. (Grace A. Goldsmith, M.D., Tulane University)

(*Bottom, left*) Advanced gingivitis: marked swelling of papillae with loss of tissue and retraction of gums (Newfoundland). Nutritional factors most apt to be associated with such a condition in Newfoundland are ascorbic acid and some of the B vitamins.

(*Bottom, right*) "Granulated" eyelids, or conjunctival follicular hypertrophy, is common in malnourished children. It begins with reddening and thickening of the lower lid. (Florida)

(Plate 1 from Jolliffe, Norman, Tisdall, F. F., and Cannon, Paul R.: Clinical Nutrition, New York, Hoeber.)

PLATE 1

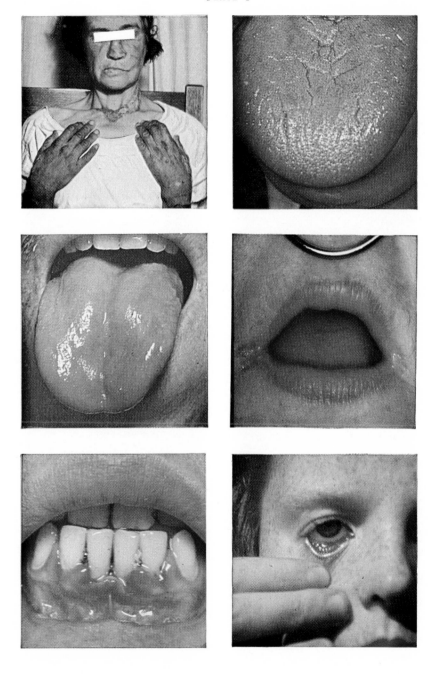

Riboflavin Deficiency

Incidence. No well-defined deficiency syndrome or disease with a long history, such as scurvy or beriberi, is associated with a lack of riboflavin. However, dietary and clinical evidence of riboflavin deficiency or borderline intake have been reported from Taiwan, Korea, the Philippines, East Pakistan and Turkey[23] within the last 15 years. Riboflavin deficiency was the deficiency most commonly reported from these countries, which are predominantly rice-eating. The chief symptoms were nasolabial seborrhea and angular stomatitis (See Plate 1). Ariboflavinosis as it exists today is seldom fatal, but it is a serious handicap. It must be remembered that a person with a riboflavin deficiency is likely to have associated deficiencies of thiamine and niacin.

Symptoms and Pathology. Before any true clinical symptoms appear, a mild riboflavin deficiency may be responsible for a type of light sensitivity and dimness of vision, followed later by itching, burning and eyestrain. Later clinical manifestations are a shiny red mucosa of the lips with cracking at the corners of the mouth, known as cheilosis, a beefy red tongue and roughened skin around the mouth and the nose, often accompanied by sebaceous exudate.

A riboflavin deficiency in certain animals may interfere with normal fetal development. Even though we need to know more about human need for riboflavin during pregnancy, an adequate supply is certainly recommended. The physiologic significance of riboflavin is discussed in detail in Chapter 8.

Treatment and Prevention. Common food sources of riboflavin are listed in Chapter 8, but it is pertinent to emphasize that this factor is perhaps more difficult to obtain in adequate amounts in low-cost diets than are other vitamins. Milk and organ meats are the richest natural sources. Enriched bread made with at least 6 per cent of dry-milk solids is also a good economical source.

Niacin and Tryptophan Deficiency— Pellagra

Incidence. "Pellagra is still found seasonally in Egypt, Yugoslavia and some parts of Africa, where corn supplies more than 60 per cent of the daily calories. Because of the niacin supplied by beans and coffee it is not seen in Mexico and Central America, even among populations deriving up to 80 per cent of the calories from corn."[24]

Isolated cases of pellagra may occur in any area in a person confined to a restricted diet low in protein and niacin. This can happen in older people with self-imposed restrictions or in a person with allergies to a number of protein foods. Alcoholic pellagra is essentially identical with endemic pellagra. It is caused by the substitution of alcohol for food.

Symptoms and Pathology. On exposure to sun, persons whose diets supply inadequate tryptophan and are deficient in niacin acquire a scaly, pigmented dermatitis over the exposed areas. Depending on the type of clothing and exposed skin, the areas most affected are face, neck, back of hands, elbows, knees and ankles. The classic "three D's" *dermatitis, diarrhea* and *dementia* may still describe the symptoms although dementia is rare. Anemias are frequent, probably owing to associated deficiencies. Glossitis (sore tongue) suggests the relationship to the disease blacktongue in dogs (See Plate 1).

Treatment and Prevention. The lethargy characteristic of many of the victims of pellagra, together with ignorance and poverty, has limited the effective introduction of adequate preventive measures in many areas. Severe cases are given multiple-vitamin therapy plus an adequate diet, with the result that they recover in due course.

The dosage of niacin and other B-complex factors is usually well above the recommended allowance of 13 to 19 mg. of niacin equivalent daily and other factors in proportion. Niacinamide is the form in which this factor is administered when large doses are required.

[23] Williams, R. R.: J. Am. Dietet. A., 36:31, 1960.

[24] Scrimshaw, N. S.: New Eng. J. Med., 272:137, 1965.

Milk, eggs, meat, nuts and certain vegetables would supply the factors missing in the typical pellagra-producing diet. A Negro educator in talking to his people recommended:

A garden and a cow, a smoke-house and a sow,
Twenty-four chickens and a rooster and you'll live better than you uster.

Ascorbic Acid Deficiency and Scurvy

History and Incidence. Scurvy is probably the oldest recognized deficiency disease. Although its specific relationship to ascorbic acid was not recognized until the 20th century, its prevention by the use of fresh foods was practiced much earlier. Prevalent in Europe during the 19th century and earlier, for centuries scurvy was attributed to a limited food supply. On the long voyages which followed the discovery of America, sailors were often obliged to subsist for long periods on salt fish and meats, hardtack or other breadstuffs, entirely deprived of any fresh food. The outbreaks of scurvy on such voyages were frequently so severe that there was scarcely enough of the crew left to man the vessel. In 1772, however, Captain Cook took a voyage which lasted 3 years, during which time not one man was lost because of scurvy. This fact he attributed to the use of a "sweet wort" made from barley and sauerkraut. Subsequently, limes or lemons were included in the supplies, since they had been found to be antiscorbutic, i.e., scurvy preventive.

Scurvy probably was responsible for most of the deaths among the pilgrims in the Massachusetts Bay Colony during that first hard winter. There was an outbreak of mild scurvy in northern Maine during the depression years, the early 1930's. Other outbreaks of the disease have been associated with famine or war areas, when the food supply was limited. Its occurrence in earlier years was reported during polar expeditions or other circumstances in which supplies of fresh food were unavailable. Expert dietetic advice was sought in planning the food supplies for the more recent polar expeditions in order to avoid the possibility of a vitamin-C shortage, because scurvy is greatly dreaded by explorers.

Eskimos seldom have scurvy on their native diets but are susceptible to it when they adopt the "white man's diet." On their native diets they may include organ meats and mosses that supply some ascorbic acid. It is also reported that some groups eat meat raw or undercooked, thus retaining the slight amount of ascorbic acid that may be present.

The only cases of scurvy in adults reported in this country are in men living alone and preparing inadequate meals or in psychoneurotic individuals on bizarre diets. With our present knowledge it thus seems incredible that during the 1960's an

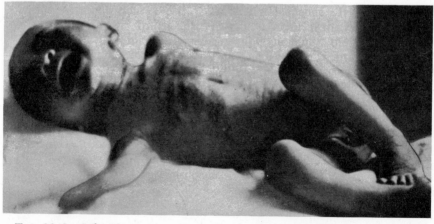

Fig. 16–8. Infantile scurvy. Typical contractions of extremities from pain. (Hoffmann-La Roche, Inc.)

increasing number of cases of infantile scurvy have been reported in the medical literature from such countries as Canada, Newfoundland, and Australia. A survey in Canada during 1961-1963 found 87 cases of infantile scurvy.[25] These cases occurred mostly in small communities where there was ignorance, poverty and poor health supervision. As a result of these findings Canada has enacted a regulation permitting the addition of ascorbic acid to evaporated milk, commonly used in infant feeding.

Scurvy is relatively rare in the underdeveloped areas of the world. Many of these countries are in the tropical and subtropical zones where fruits and vegetables are plentiful and widely consumed.

Frank scurvy is so rare in the U. S. today that medical students seldom have a chance to observe the disease. Yet the history of this disease and its prevention is worthy of note.

Symptoms and Pathology. The principal symptoms of scurvy are restlessness, loss of appetite, general soreness to touch, sore mouth and gums with bleeding and loosening of the teeth, petechial skin hemorrhages, and swelling of the legs with special tenderness about the knee joints (see Fig. 16–8). Anemia may occur as a result of the loss of blood.

Marginal symptoms of this disease are sallow skin, muddy complexion, lack of energy, and fleeting pains in limbs and joints, so often noted in adolescence. Irritability, retarded growth and tooth defects may also accompany this dietary deficiency.

Mild manifestations of ascorbic acid deficiency in adults may easily be overlooked or ignored. Tendency to bruise easily, slow healing of minor wounds and pin-point hemorrhages may be indications of tissue depletion of this factor.

Treatment. An adequate supply of ascorbic acid is the obvious treatment for all these conditions, but what is an adequate supply? There is probably a wide gap between the amount of ascorbic acid necessary to prevent scurvy and the amount essential for optimum health. The recommended allowance of 70 mg. for normal adults with more during adolescence, pregnancy and lactation may be enough to saturate depleted tissues or to meet increased demands associated with fevers and infections. It is more than enough to prevent any symptom of scurvy.

Food sources of this factor are entirely adequate for the prevention of scorbutic symptoms or milder manifestations. For rich food sources of ascorbic acid and for a discussion of its properties and losses in cooking, see Chapter 8. Ascorbic acid in tablet form is stable and relatively inexpensive. It is useful when fresh foods are not available or must be omitted from the diet for any reason. This synthetic form has been used extensively during wars to promote wound healing and to act as a food supplement in emergency rations.

Vitamin D Deficiency—Rickets

"The disappearance of rickets" is the title of a recent article[26] reviewing the history and prevention of vitamin-D–deficient rickets as a triumph of medicine and nutrition. As late as 1940 rickets was still a common disease of early childhood in northern climates.

One cannot be complacent, however, about the over-all decrease in rickets for within the last decade a survey by the Committee on Nutrition of the American Academy of Pediatrics[27] reported 843 cases of rickets in 5 years among hospital pediatric admissions. It would seem that the general use of antirachitic supplements in infant feeding would have precluded the possibility of this deficiency still being a public health problem. Of course, the widespread use of vitamin D supplements in infant feeding has reduced the incidence in northern climates. It is rare in our southern states and in tropical countries in general, where children spend more time out of doors and expose more of their skin to the sun. However, children of dark-skinned races living in northern climates are even more susceptible to rickets than those of the white race.

---

25 Demers, P., *et al.*: Can. M. A. J., 93:573, 1965.

26 Harrison, H. E.: Am. J. Pub. Health, 56:734, 1966.

27 Report: Pediatrics, 29:646, 1962.

Symptoms and Pathology. Rickets is a disease of infancy and early childhood in which the bones do not calcify properly as they grow. They become pliable, malformed and distorted, the result being such evident deformities as pigeon chest, enlarged wrists and ankles, and bowed legs or knock knees which result when the leg bones are not strong enough to support the child learning to walk. All these symptoms are pointed out in the schematic drawing of a child with rickets (Fig. 16–9). The enlargement or beading of the ribs, frequently called "the rachitic rosary," may be less evident in a plump infant than in an emaciated one, but it is characteristic. Profuse sweating and restlessness are early symptoms of rickets in infants. Growth may not be retarded at first, since nature seems to allow the bones to increase in length to keep up with growth in soft tissues if other nutrients are adequate. Prolonged and severe cases usually show stunted growth.

Treatment and Prevention. The major factors involved in the prevention of rickets —calcium, phosphorus and vitamin D— have been discussed in Chapters 6 and 7. Since the geographic incidence of rickets and practical experience indicate that it is more often a deficiency of vitamin D which causes rickets in children, attention is directed to the problem of adequate and reliable sources of this factor in regions where sunshine cannot act as the natural preventive agent. Obviously, when children can be exposed to an adequate source of ultra-violet light (sunshine or ultraviolet lamp), sufficient vitamin D may be synthesized to regulate the utilization of minerals for bone building. Vitamin preparations containing vitamins A and C in addition to vitamin D are readily available for infants in the U. S.

The present popularity of vitamin D milk as a convenient and a reliable antirachitic agent is well founded. Since milk contains the minerals calcium and phosphorus and it is a natural food for children, it seems to be the most suitable carrier for added vitamin D. Fortified evaporated milk is especially convenient for use in vicinities where fresh vitamin D milk is not available. The Food and Drug Administration in the U. S. regulates the types of foods that may be fortified with vitamin D and the amount of fortification.

Precautions. It is wise to caution mothers against the simultaneous use of several supplementary sources of vitamin D because it is possible to give too much. If a vitamin D concentrate is prescribed, advice should also be given the mother on the use of vitamin D milk as an additional source.

Osteomalacia

Incidence and Pathology. Prolonged deficiency of dietary calcium and vitamin D or sunlight may result in osteomalacia, sometimes called adult rickets. This condition is characterized by poor calcification of the bones with increasing softness, so that they become flexible, and leading to deformities of limbs, spine, thorax or pelvis.

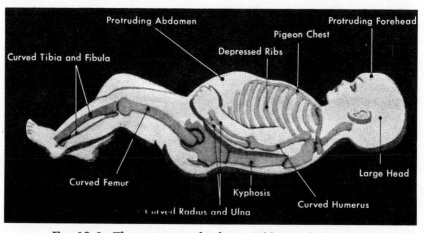

FIG. 16–9. The symptoms of rickets. (Abbott Laboratories)

These bone changes may be accompanied by rheumatic pains and exhaustion.

Osteomalacia is rare in western countries but still occurs in the Middle East and the Orient, especially among women following several pregnancies and when they nurse their infants for extended periods of time. The high incidence of osteomalacia among women in certain parts of India where the rite of purdah is still practiced and among Bedouin Arab women who wear long black garments and live in dark tents testifies indirectly to the protective action of sunshine on exposed skin. In many of these same areas the diet consists largely of cereals and root vegetables low in calcium.

Osteomalacia is often confused with osteoporosis, which may occur in older women in any country, even the most prosperous. The etiology of osteoporosis is not well understood but is more likely due to a metabolic or endocrine disturbance than to a deficiency (see Chap. 32).

Prevention and Treatment. Prevention of osteomalacia, like rickets, is entirely possible by means of a diet adequate in calcium and phosphorus and with a supply of vitamin D or exposure to sunlight. The diet of patients suffering from osteomalacia should be adequate in all respects but especially in calcium and vitamin D. In countries where milk is not readily available other food sources of calcium and the protective vitamin should be supplied.

MINERAL DEFICIENCIES
Nutritional Anemia

There are several types of anemias; their etiology and dietary treatment are discussed in Chapter 31. As a world problem "nutritional anemias due to insufficient intake of hematopoietic factors, their poor absorption or increased demands because of abnormal blood loss are frequent in tropical and subtropical areas. Although these anemias are known to be highly prevalent, little information is available on the magnitude or the nature of the problem."[28] Scrimshaw continues: "The definition of anemia is a major problem since

normal values for red-cell and hemoglobin concentrations of persons living under different environmental conditions, particularly altitude, have not been firmly established. . . . Pregnant women, infants and small children are most seriously affected in the areas where the problem exists."[28]

Iron deficiency anemia is the most common type in tropical and subtropical areas. In some areas hookworm infestation is a cause of anemia even when iron intake seems to be adequate.

Formerly, nutritional anemia was associated chiefly with iron deficiency, but now it is recognized that possibly protein and some of the vitamins are involved. Megaloblastic amenias are less common than the microcytic hypochromic type associated with iron deficiency. They may occur, however, in pregnant women and in severely malnourished children. (See Chap. 31)

"The World Health Organization (WHO) is presently interested in the magnitude and nature of the nutritional anemias as a public-health problem and is coordinating and helping epidemiologic, clinical and experimental studies now in progress in different laboratories around the world."[28]

Simple or Endemic Goiter Caused by Iodine Deficiency

The cause of simple goiter is failure of the thyroid gland to obtain a supply of iodine sufficient to maintain its normal structure and function. The lack of iodine is usually a result of an environmental deficiency of iodine.

Since iodine in surface soil shows a very uneven distribution and plants absorb iodine from the soil, the iodine content of foodstuffs varies with the locality in which they are grown. Thus we find simple goiter most common in those parts of the world where the surface soil is low in iodine and where salt-water fish are not commonly eaten. Due to increased facilities for food distribution in the United States today, city people are less confined to food grown in one locality and the incidence of simple goiter seems to be decreasing.

Iodized salt, which is on the market in most areas of the United States, has proved to be beneficial in reducing the incidence

[28] Scrimshaw, N. S.: New Eng. J. Med., 272:193, 1965.

of goiter, as evidenced by examination of schoolchildren. In one state in which goiter was almost eliminated, it again became prevalent when the emphasis on the use of iodized salt was relaxed. If the spectacular decrease in the incidence of goiter which resulted from the use of iodized salt is to continue, more publicity must be given to it. The use of iodized salt should be emphasized especially in the states where goiter was originally endemic (See Map, Fig. 16–10).

The availability of dietary iodine may be affected by goitrogenic substances which interfere with iodine absorption. These are found in a number of plant species, among them cabbage, Brussels sprouts, soy beans and peanuts. They are of significance only when the intake of iodine is borderline, and their effect can be compensated for by an adequate intake of iodine. The iodine requirement may also be increased by chronic infections, deficiency of vitamin A and, possibly, by other dietary deficiencies or toxic substances.

Dental Caries

Incidence. Dental caries is probably the most common disease affecting the human race. Authorities estimate that only about 2 per cent of the people of the United States have escaped having at least one dental cavity. Contrary to the regional and the endemic incidence of some other deficiencies, dental caries is so common that nearly everyone has experienced it. Few adults in western civilization have absolutely perfect teeth. Figures on incidence of caries among population groups vary according to locality and race. The prevalence among Negroes is lower than among whites of comparable age in the same locality. Primitive peoples as a rule show a lower incidence than do civilized populations. However, as soon as primitive populations are touched by civilization, and native foods are replaced by processed foods, an increase in dental caries follows.

Etiology. Dental caries has been variously attributed to inheritance, metabolic disturbances, specific or multiple food deficiencies, conditions in the mouth, including composition of saliva, and lack of fluorine in the water supply. None of these entirely explains the high incidence or varying degree of susceptibility to caries encountered among children of the same

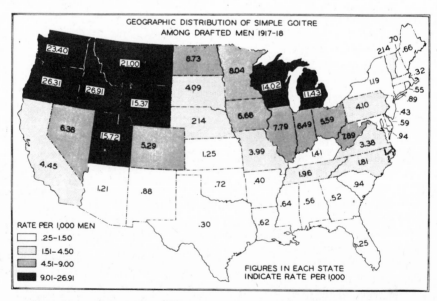

Fig. 16–10. Geographic distribution of simple goiter among men drafted for World War I. These goitrous areas are naturally low in iodine. (U. S. Dept. Public Health)

family with similar dietary and mouth-hygiene habits.

Extensive research has been conducted in an attempt to understand and thus be better able to prevent or inhibit carious changes in teeth.[29] It is now generally agreed that dental caries is unquestionably of bacterial origin with certain other contributing factors. Bacterial metabolism and growth in the mouth lead to destruction of both tooth enamel and dentin. Carbohydrates must be present in the crevices of the teeth for caries-producing organisms to grow. Heredity and nutrition during the period of tooth development will affect the resistance to decay at a later date. Saliva is protective, but much is yet to be learned about hereditary, nutritional, endocrine and other variables that determine the physical consistency, the chemical composition and the rate of flow of saliva. It is now also recognized that teeth are more resistant to caries when the fluoride ion is incorporated in the crystal lattice of the enamel and the dentin.[30]

The inverse relationship between incidence of dental caries and the fluorine content of the drinking water has given impetus to the use of fluorine as a prophylactic agent. A review of caries control in the U. S. by Dunning in 1965[31] indicated that controlled fluoridation had reduced the incidence of caries by 50 to 70 per cent among young people whose teeth were formed during the period of fluoridation.

Prevention. It is generally agreed that fluorine is the only known agent ordinarily included in food and water that is capable of exercising mass control of dental caries. It is effective during the period of calcification of the crown of the tooth and through the period of eruption.

Among the authorities who have studied the problem it is agreed that the simplest, the cheapest and the most far-reaching method of ensuring adequate fluoride is through the fluoridation of the drinking water. This procedure will supplement, but not supplant, other dental health measures.

The level of fluorine which seems to be protective without being harmful is 1.0 part per million (ppm) of drinking water. Mottled enamel (dental fluorosis) is apt to occur when fluorine in the water supply exceeds 2 ppm, as it does naturally in certain communities in several Western states. Indeed, it was the absence of caries in persons with mottled enamel that first called attention to its protective action.

[29] Symposium: Council on Foods and Nutrition. J.A.M.A., *177*:304, 1961.

[30] Dean, H. T.: Fluorine Deficiency in Control of Malnutrition in Man. Am. Pub. Health Assoc., 1960.

[31] Dunning, J. M.: New Eng. J. Med., *272*:30, 84, 1965.

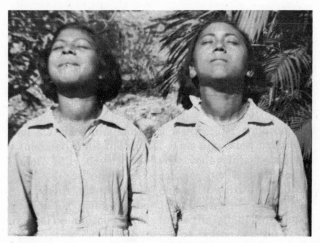

FIG. 16–11. Goiter is so common among youth of mountainous regions of South America that a child without goiter is ridiculed as a "bottle-neck." (Photo FAO, Rome)

TABLE 16–1. Clinical Signs of Nutritional Failure and Suggested Deficiency

Findings	Suggested Deficiencies
General	
Underweight	Calories, protein, Ca, P, vitamins
Underheight (T) for age	Protein limitation
Pallor (T)	Iron, folic acid, B12, ascorbic acid
Lack of appetite (N)	B complex, unknown
Protruding abdomen "pot belly"	Protein-calorie malnutrition
Skin	
Inflammation (perifolliculosis) (N)	Ascorbic acid, vitamin A
Hardening around hair follicles (follicular hyperkeratosis)	Vitamin A
Dermatitis of pellagra (N)	Niacin
Abnormal sebaceous secretion (dyssebacea) in nasolabial folds, behind ears and in body folds (N)	Riboflavin, unknown
Acne vulgaris (T)	Unknown, riboflavin
Hemorrhagic manifestations, petechiae, bruises, etc. (N)	Pyridoxine, vitamin A, ascorbic acid, vitamin K, unknown
Eyes	
Bloodshot (corneal vascularity)	Unknown, riboflavin
Inflammation (conjunctivitis) (T)	Vitamin A, unknown
Night blindness (nyctalopia)	Vitamin A
Light sensitivity (photophobia)	Vitamin A, riboflavin
Lips and mouth	
Cracked lips (cheilosis) (N)	Riboflavin, B complex, pyridoxine
Inflammation of mouth (stomatitis) (N) with cracking at corners	Riboflavin, B complex, iron, niacin
Inflammation of tongue (glossitis) (N)	B complex, protein
Edema of tongue	Niacin, unknown
Teeth	
Caries (N)	Unknown
Malocclusion (T)	Vitamin D, unknown
Scorbutic gums (N)	Ascorbic acid
Gingivitis	Ascorbic acid, unknown
Skeletal	
Rachitic deformities—"squared" head, beaded ribs, bowed legs, knock knees (N)	Vitamin D, Ca and P
Osteomalacia in adults	Vitamin D, Ca and P
Nervous and Mental	
Nutritional polyneuritis	Thiamine, B complex
Combined system disease	B complex, vitamin B12
Degenerative brain disease (encephalopathic states)	Thiamine, niacin, B complex, unknown
Mental retardation	Protein-calories malnutrition
Circulatory	
Beriberi heart disease	Thiamine
Nutritional edema (T)	Protein, thiamine, famine
Endocrine	
Common goiter	Iodine

Teachers (T) and nurses (N) may be instructed to detect the appearance of these signs.
(Adapted from a more detailed table in Jolliffe, N., *et al.*; Clinical Nutrition, ed. 2, New York, Hoeber, 1962.)

Consideration has been given to media other than water as possible means of administering fluorides to children where the community water supply is not fluoridated. Rusoff and co-workers[32] tried milk as a vehicle for fluoride administration in the school lunch program. The amount added was such that ½ pint of milk supplied 1 mg. of fluoride. This was tried on 171 children over a period of 3½ years and resulted in a 70 per cent reduction in caries incidence in teeth erupting after the initiation of the experiment.

Calcium, phosphorus or vitamin D deficiencies during and preceding the eruption of teeth undoubtedly account for some faults in structure. The teeth, once fully developed, are not as apt to be influenced by nutritional intakes later.

Careful observation and accurate data on large numbers of schoolchildren in northern Europe during and after war-imposed restriction of sugar are significant. These findings indicate a lowered incidence of caries during the years of restriction and a marked increase since sweets again became available. However, the younger children, whose teeth developed during the period of low sugar intake, showed a caries reduction in the post-war period, when sugar consumption was again high. Thus, the evidence suggests that the structure of the teeth is involved in determining subsequent caries susceptibility.

Prophylaxis: Successful prophylaxis must be based on a threefold approach: to create an unfavorable medium for bacterial action in the mouth; to increase the resistance of teeth to decay through fluoridation; and to maintain good nutrition in the entire body.

EARLY DIAGNOSIS AND TREATMENT OF NUTRITIONAL FAILURE

Individuals with mild forms of deficiency diseases which usually are not recognized as clinical entities seldom apply to the general practitioner for medical aid unless more serious conditions develop; furthermore, the physician has not had any adequate criteria for recognizing these early signs. The insidious development and the delayed clinical evidence of malnutrition make the problem particularly serious. This subject is of great concern to nutritionists, public-health nurses and others, who frequently are in closer contact than are physicians with children and with families living on low incomes and an inadequate food supply. There is an open field for further study and observation of these marginal deficiencies among all groups of the population, but especially among the lower-income groups, in which the vicious circle of malnutrition, lack of strength and ambition, and continued low income offers little opportunity for real improvement.

Before clinical signs of nutritional deficiencies appear there must be biochemical abnormalities. These are not easily detected but attempts are being made to develop practical and inexpensive laboratory tests to measure such changes. Dr. Goodhart points out: "If ill-health results from intermittent or long-standing deficiencies . . . then the resultant clinical picture is likely to bear little resemblance to any classical acute deficiency."[33] Some conditions not classified as nutritional may be aggravated or even initiated by malnutrition.

Several attempts have been made to tabulate the signs and the symptoms associated with specific deficiencies. Jolliffe, Tisdall and Cannon[34] offer helpful descriptions and pictures of deficiency states. As they say:

Most physicians are familiar with the signs of advanced florid deficiency disease as they occur in classical starvation, protein deficiency, osteomalacia, rickets, scurvy, pellagra and beriberi. Most malnutrition, however, is not this advanced, easily recognized variety but is manifested by signs less fully developed, less severe or less acute than the classic textbook descriptions imply. These lesser signs are frequently overlooked. Consequently much malnutrition remains unrecognized even when it

---

[32] Rusoff, L. L., *et al.*: Am. J. Clin. Nutr., *11*:94, 1962.

[33] Goodhart, R. S., *et al.*: J. New Drugs, *1*:18, 1961.

[34] Jolliffe, N., *et al.*: Clinical Nutrition. Ed. 2. New York, Hoeber, 1962.

is sufficiently advanced to cause anatomic changes detectable without the aid of laboratory or other special technics.

Table 16–1 adapted from Jolliffe *et al.*, suggests that nurses and teachers can help in detecting early signs of malnutrition that should be brought to the attention of the physician.

STUDY QUESTIONS AND ACTIVITIES

1. What is the most widespread nutritional deficiency in the world today? In what countries is it most serious?

2. What age group is most susceptible to this deficiency? Why?

3. What are the most likely symptoms of kwashiorkor? What is the meaning of the word kwashiorkor and where did it come from?

4. What contributions has INCAP made in the control and treatment of P-CM or kwashiorkor? What do the letters INCAP stand for?

5. What effect may P-CM have on mental development? Why is this most serious during ages 1 to 4 years?

6. What other deficiencies may complicate the picture in P-CM?

7. Is there any evidence that marginal hypoproteinemia may exist in the U. S.? Among what groups?

8. Which of the vitamin deficiencies is most widespread and most serious in the world today? What are the consequences?

9. What diseases other than beriberi may result from a thiamine deficiency? What is a common complication?

10. Why is pellagra not as serious a problem in the U. S. today as it was formerly? Is it found elsewhere in the world? What food pattern is most apt to be found associated with pellagra?

11. Is scurvy still a problem in the U. S. or in any part of the world? For what age groups is it most serious?

12. What progress is being made in the control of dental caries? What stands in the way of greater success in this area?

13. What is the world distribution of common goiter? Is there a proved method of control and how successful has it been?

14. What steps might be or are being taken toward earlier diagnosis or detection of mild forms of nutritional failure?

SUPPLEMENTARY READING ON MALNUTRITION—A WORLD PROBLEM

Balcomb, J.: Incaparina—a new protein food. J. Home Econ., *54*:36, 1962.

Coursin, D. B.: Effects of undernutrition on central nervous system function. Nutr. Rev., *23*:65, 1965.

Cravioto, J.: Application of newer knowledge of nutrition on physical growth and development. Am. J. Pub. Health, *53*:1803, 1963.

Horwitt, M. K.: Nutrition in mental health. Nutr. Rev., *23*:289, 1965.

Jelliffe, D. B.: The assessment of nutritional status. WHO Chronicle, *21*:127, 1967.

McLaren, D. S.: Xerophthalmia: A neglected problem. Nutr. Rev., *22*:289, 1964.

McConnell, J. F.: The deposed one. Am. J. Nursing, *61*:78, 1961.

Phipard, E. F., and Kirby, R. H.: Nutritional status of the world. Yearbook of Agriculture 1964, p. 37-43.

Review: Diet, development and intelligence. Nutr. Rev., *22*:244, 1964.

Review: Nutrition and mental development. Dairy Coun. Dig., *37*: No. 5, 1966 (Sept.-Oct.).

Scrimshaw, N. S.: Malnutrition and health of children. J. Am. Dietet. A., *42*:203, 1963.

Scrimshaw, N. S., and Behar, M.: Malnutrition in underdeveloped countries. New Eng. J. Med., *272*:137, 193, 1965.

Sebrell, W. H.: Changing concept of malnutrition. Am. J. Clin. Nutr., *20*:653, 1967.

Sydenstricker, V. P.: History of pellagra: its recognition as a disorder of nutrition and its conquest. Am. J. Clin. Nutr., *6*:409, 1958.

For further references see Bibliography in Part Four.

CHAPTER **17**

Safeguarding Our Food Supply

U. S. Food is Protected by Law • Food Spoilage and Deterioration • Care and Preservation of Foods • Foodborne Disease • Food Additives • Food Laws

U. S. FOOD IS PROTECTED BY LAW

The Yearbook of Agriculture, 1966, entitled *Protecting Our Food*[1] devoted 379 pages to the scientific achievements which assure the people of the United States a safe and plentiful food supply. This chapter can merely summarize how federal agencies established by Congress are attempting to control the quantity, quality and sanitation of the food in our markets.

Agriculture, our biggest industry, depends upon the work of thousands of scientists and experts in other fields to predict needs and regulate food production in the United States. People in general do not have the means or the skills to examine how meats are handled, to check fruits and vegetables for residues of pesticides or processed foods for harmful preservatives or accidental contaminants or packaged goods for insect infestation. Through Congress, however, laws have been passed making certain federal agencies responsible for protecting the safety of our food supplies. Such agencies as the Food and Drug Administration, the Federal Trade Commission and the Department of Agriculture have extensive programs for safeguarding our foods.

A few examples of what has been accomplished may serve to illustrate.

---

[1] Protecting Our Food. The Yearbook of Agriculture. U.S.D.A., Washington, D. C., 1966.

Outbreaks of disease traced to milk and water supplies have gone down steadily since pasteurization of milk, tuberculin testing of dairy cattle, chlorination and filtration of municipal water supplies, and education of the public in the selection of safe rural water supplies have become common practices. One must search with increasing diligence to find a report of sickness traced to milk or water supplies. Milk is now pasteurized for well over 90 per cent of our population. Safe milk flows from the pasteurizer by a closed system of pipes into carefully washed glass bottles or sterile paper cartons, which are promptly sealed and refrigerated for delivery to the consumer.

Foods other than water and milk present a difficult problem of control. They are produced by thousands of processors and handled by millions of people, then may be mishandled by the consumer.

FOOD SPOILAGE AND DETERIORATION

Any change which renders a food undesirable or unfit for human use may be called food spoilage. Although one usually thinks of spoilage as being caused by microorganisms, it can also be caused by chemical or physical changes, by enzymes and by contamination with any foreign matter. A distinction should be made between foods *unfit* for consumption by anyone and foods which may be *distasteful* to

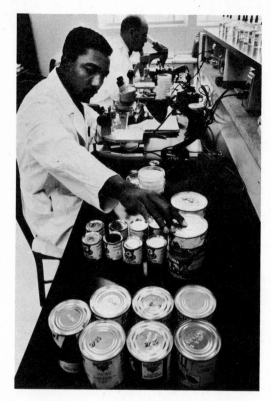

FIG. 17–1. FDA's enforcement effort for foods is mainly concerned with food plant sanitation and the wholesomeness of ingredients and finished products. The Federal Food, Drug, and Cosmetic Act (1938) makes it illegal to ship in interstate commerce a food that comes from unsanitary premises. To enforce this section of the Act, FDA inspects food processors to insure that the factories are sanitary. FDA is responsible for establishing safety standards for additives in foods. (FDA Publ. No. 1. U. S. Dept. HEW, Washington, D. C.)

or *undesirable* by most Americans. For instance: snails, squid, fried grasshoppers and fermented eggs may be delicacies in certain cultures but undesirable in others.

Microbial Food Spoilage

Microbial food spoilage may be caused by three different groups of microorganisms: bacteria, yeasts and molds. The stale odor of spoiled meat, the foul odor of a spoiled egg and the souring of milk are familiar examples of bacterial spoilage. The spoilage of canned foods also is traced usually to bacterial causes.

Yeasts and molds are most familiar as causes of spoilage of fresh foods, dried foods and foods of high sugar content. The fermentation of catsup and cider is due to yeast growth. The fuzzy growths on bread and cheese and on the surface of jams and jellies indicate mold spoilage. The spoilage of citrus fruits and other fruits and vegetables is often due to the growth of molds.

Enzymic Food Spoilage

Spoilage due to enzymic action is much more widespread than most people realize. Enzymic spoilage appears most often in loss of quality rather than as frank spoilage. The haylike flavor of frozen vegetables after long or improper storage is due to enzymic activity. Fruits and vegetables that soften or become overripe during storage may be the result of either enzymic action or mold growth. Difficulty has been encountered with some of the newer methods of food preservation, such as processing at extremely high temperatures for a very short time and preservation by irradiation with ionizing rays, since under the conditions used some enzymes are more resistant to destruction than the most resistant spoilage organisms. These enzymes can cause off odors and flavors, even though the food is perfectly sterile.

Chemical Spoilage

Chemical causes of spoilage include flavor changes due to oxidation; swelling of cans due to production of hydrogen by the action of food acids on the metal of the container; discoloration from the reaction of metal ions from the container with the product to produce discolored crabmeat or corn; and oxidative rancidity of fats.

Most of these situations can be prevented by using a lining in the can to protect the can and the contents; "fruit" enamel prevents the bleaching of highly colored fruits; "corn" enamel prevents corn from discoloring. Antioxidants are added to foods subject to rancidity to prevent oxidation of unsaturated fatty acids.

Physical Causes of Food Spoilage

The spoilage of foods by physical changes usually involves a change of state from a solution to a precipitate, such as is seen in sandy ice cream caused by formation of large lactose crystals during storage at fluctuating temperatures.

Exposure to light can cause spoilage in beer bottled in clear glass, with an off odor described by the industry as "skunky" beer. Sunlight can cause a tallowy off flavor in milk left too long on the doorstep and, at the same time, can destroy a high percentage of its riboflavin content.

Spoilage by Animals and Insects

One means by which the Federal Food and Drug Administration checks the sanitary conditions under which a product has been packed is to examine the product for rat hairs and droppings, insects and insect fragments, and mold hyphae. If any of these is present, they can confiscate an entire shipment of food and prohibit future shipments until the unsanitary conditions are corrected to the satisfaction of the Food and Drug inspector.

Often it would be chemically impossible to show any nutritional difference between a product contaminated with rat hairs and one free of contamination. However, from an esthetic viewpoint, as well as from the public health aspect—as carrier of infections—the product free of rat hairs is naturally preferred.

CARE AND PRESERVATION OF FOODS

The methods of food preservation may be divided into two general classes—bactericidal and bacteriostatic. Bactericidal methods are those which destroy the organisms. These would include cooking, canning, making jams and jellies, smoking, irradiation and the addition of chemical preservatives. Bacteriostatic methods make conditions unsuitable for microbial growth by reducing the temperature (refrigeration and freezing), removing water (dehydration), addition of acid (pickling) or adding substances to inhibit growth (antibiotics, salt or sugar).

Refrigeration

Until the discovery of mechanical refrigeration in the last part of the 19th century, the keeping of fresh foods in northern United States depended on ice cut in winter and stored in insulated ice houses for use in spring, summer and fall to provide refrigeration. Peoples living in warm climates where mechanical refrigeration is not available must depend upon obtaining a fresh supply of perishable foods daily.

A sudden realization of how much we depend on the mechanical refrigerator occurs when a storm disrupts the electrical service to homes and grocery stores. The problem of keeping milk, meat, fish and vegetables becomes acute, for spoilage at room temperature occurs four times more quickly than at 40° F., the temperature of most refrigerators.

Almost all fresh foods sold in the U. S. have been refrigerated during part of their journey from the producer to the consumer.

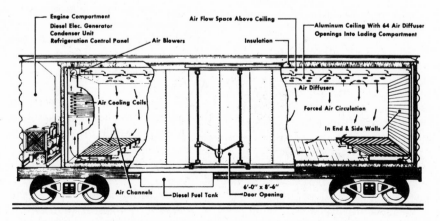

FIG. 17–2. Interior view of a modern mechanical refrigerator car. (From *Railway Age*, February, 1960)

THERMOMETER FOR CONTROL
OF BACTERIA

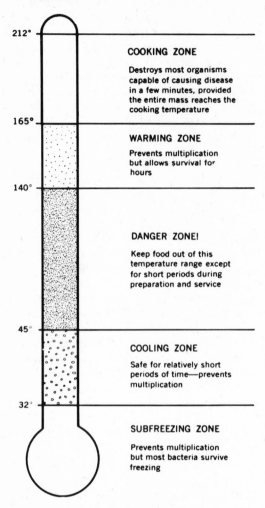

FIG. 17–3. From Protecting Our Food. Yearbook of Agriculture, 1966, p. 189. U.S.D.A., Washington, D. C.

If high-quality foods are to reach the consumer, the enzyme action of the fruits and the vegetables must be reduced (for these products are made up of living cells), growth of microorganisms must be inhibited, and chemical and physical changes must be prevented or slowed down.

Usually, fresh foods are stored at the lowest temperature possible at which no adverse physiologic changes take place. Bananas, for example, are stored at higher temperatures during ripening (62° to 70° F.), then are held at 56° to 60° F. for storage after ripening. If they are chilled below 56° F. before ripening, they develop a smoky, dull color, and if chilled after ripening the skin turns brown rapidly. Apples and some other fruits are usually stored at 30° to 32° F. in a nitrogen atmosphere for best results.

In order to maintain crispness or an attractive appearance, the humidity is usually maintained as high as possible to prevent loss of moisture, but it must also be low enough not to encourage mold growth. Most fruits and vegetables are maintained at 85 per cent to 90 per cent relative humidity.

Freezing

There has been a tremendous rise in popularity of frozen foods, due in part to the increased frozen storage and display capacity of stores and the development of frozen storage space in the modern home refrigerator. The major advantage has been that frozen foods usually retain more of the qualities and the nutrients of fresh foods than those preserved by any other method.

Frozen foods keep because most bacteria will not grow below 32° F., and those enzymes not destroyed by blanching (scalding) are much reduced in activity at 0° F. All bacteria are not destroyed by freezing; they are merely unable to grow at such low temperatures. Trichina, a parasite which may infect pork, however, is destroyed by freezing.

When foods are allowed to thaw and are kept at room temperature, spoilage actually occurs more rapidly than one might expect, since, due to a partial breakdown of cell walls and tissues, the thawed food is an excellent medium for growth of bacteria.

A fairly recent but very active phase of the food industry is the production of frozen prepared foods. It is now possible to have a complete meal from soup to apple pie and ice cream from the freezer and ready to eat in about ½ hour. These prepared meals must be kept solidly frozen until used and then thawed and/or heated just before serving.

The home freezer is convenient for food preservaton. However, most housewives will find that it is not as economical as advertisements indicate.

Cooking and Baking

Nearly all the microorganisms in a food are destroyed by cooking. Since this lengthens the time that a food will keep, cooking may be regarded as a method of preservation. In some cases it is a mixed blessing, as a study of food poisoning will quickly show that most cases of food poisoning are caused by consumption of a cooked food which has not been properly refrigerated. Cooking destroys the organisms that ordinarily would compete with, and hold in check, the growth of food-poisoning organisms. If contamination of the cooked food occurs after cooking, from the hands or the nasal discharge of a food handler, the toxin-producing organisms then can grow without hindrance.

Pasteurization

The time-temperature relationship of pasterization is based on the time at a given temperature in which all the organisms which will produce disease are destroyed. Milk as it comes from the pasteurizer is not sterile. The total bacterial count has been reduced, and all the disease-causing organisms are destroyed.

The reduction in bacterial count plus refrigeration increases the shelf life of many foods other than milk, such as beer, wines, etc. Mild heat treatment of concentrated citrus juices before freezing is practiced by many packers to control the enzymes which may cause clarification and/or gelation of the concentrate if it is mishandled (allowed to remain above freezing) during storage and marketing.

Canning

The original canning method was an art because the causes of food spoilage were not understood. It was not until 1860 that Pasteur determined the relationship between microorganisms and food spoilage. He demonstrated that food that had been sterilized by heat would keep indefinitely if recontamination was prevented.

Canning grew steadily from its beginning as a means of preservation and gained added impetus by the use of pressure-processing equipment introduced in 1874. By using steam pressure, much higher temperatures could be reached (5 lbs. 227°, 10 lbs. 240°, 15 lbs. 250° F.), and processing which had required several hours in boiling water could then be accomplished in less than an hour and result in a product of higher quality.

Canning has probably done more than any other discovery to help mankind maintain an adequate food supply throughout the year.

Canning procedures are continually improving the quality and the retention of nutrients in foods by increasing the rate of heating and cooling. Originally food was preserved by boiling jars of food for hours. Now food can be sterilized in less than a second at temperatures up to 275° F. in a specially designed heat exchanger, cooled immediately and then sealed into sterile containers aseptically. This method, known as aseptic canning, is now used on a small scale to process purées and baby foods, but its use is limited because of the high cost of the equipment required and the short packing periods of most canneries.

Dehydration

In the past dehydration was looked upon as one of the least desirable methods of preservation. Technologic advances during and after World War II have made possible much-improved products with special attributes of low cost, reduced weight, convenience and keeping quality.

The use of dehydrated foods has increased rapidly. Certain dehydrated products are used by some housewives to the exclusion of their counterparts preserved by other methods. An example of this is instant coffee, which now constitutes at least 50 per cent of coffee used.

Of particular interest to the nutritionist is the availability of instant nonfat dried milk, which brings this excellent food to the consumer at a low price in an easily soluble form with good flavor and keeping qualities.

Other items in this multimillion-dollar business are: cake, muffin, cornbread, pancake and roll mixes (which are mixtures of dehydrated ingredients); instant potato, orange juice, tomato juice and dessert mixes; precooked dehydrated cereals, rice and tapioca; soups; and dried active yeast. Dried stabilized eggs (whole eggs, egg yolk or egg white) are used widely in bakery products but have not as yet reached wide distribution on a retail scale.

Cake and cookie mixes often give directions to use fresh eggs because powdered egg included in the mix may not result in as safe and satisfactory a finished product. Spray-drying of egg may not be done at a high enough temperature to ensure that all salmonella organisms are destroyed.

Freeze-Drying

As in the past, the needs of the military continue to stimulate new methods of food preservation and packaging. The freeze-drying of foods is the most recent example. Our modern mobile military forces, often operating in small groups in remote areas, need "quick-serve" meals which can be brought in by airdrop and require no special equipment or skill in final preparation.

Thus freeze-dried foods, developed to serve our armed forces, are beginning to find a place in retail markets. Freeze-dried fruits are now being added to some ready-to-eat cereals. But there are still problems of developing mass production methods to ensure that flavor, texture and color can be retained. At present freeze-drying does not kill the bacteria that may be in the fresh food; they are only inactivated, and therefore reconstituted foods must be used immediately. Since such foods are dehydrated in vacuum they must be packaged in an inert gas such as nitrogen, in puncture-proof containers that can be sealed effectively. In spite of technical difficulties a few foods such as instant coffee and some sea foods are now available as this chapter is being written, and many more may be on the market by the time readers are using this book.

Chemicals As Preservatives

Chemical preservatives are among the oldest forms of food preservation—salt, sugar, vinegar are the most familiar ones. Other types of chemical preservatives are now used in a relatively small proportion of food compared with 60 years ago. Sorbic acid is used to prevent mold growth on cheese, sodium benzoate is used to preserve cider from yeast fermentation and margarine from spoilage by mold. Sodium propionate, calcium propionate or sodium diacetate are used in bread to prevent mold growth. In general, however, chemical preservatives have had a long hard fight to stay in foods, due to adverse public opinion about their use and strict regulation by the Food and Drug Administration. When a food can be preserved satisfactorily without chemicals, chemical preservatives are not allowed. For example, catsup will keep because of the preservative effects of acids, sugars and spices, and for that reason sodium benzoate which for years had been added to catsup may no longer be used. (See section on Food Additives.)

Antibiotics

Various antibiotics have some limited usefulness in food preservation. Growth of spoilage organisms can be inhibited by antibiotics but cannot be completely prevented. These substances are of value in extending the periods for which foods can be kept fresh during processing and storage. For instance, the addition of Terramycin (oxytetracycline) or Aureomycin (chlorotetracycline) to the ice slush in which poultry is cooled after dressing can extend the shelf life of the poultry 7 to 10 days. This is allowed in the United States in the processing of poultry if the residue is no more than 7 parts per million.[2] At this level practically all of the antibiotic is destroyed by cooking.

Because antibiotics are drugs, their use in processing and their presence in foods is carefully regulated by the Food and Drug

---

[2] Stephens, M. R.: Am. J. Pub. Health, 47:341, 1957.

Administration.[3] For use in food processing they must be heat labile and, therefore, destroyed by cooking. It must be demonstrated that residues left in foods will not sensitize individuals and cause allergic reactions. Not only would this create health problems for individuals but would limit the therapeutic value of the antibiotics. Also, tolerance levels for specific antibiotics in specific foods must be established by the Food and Drug Administration before they may be used in processing. Equal care must be taken to ensure that antibiotic residues are not left in animal food products from the treatment of farm animals during their lives.

Radiation

The newest method of food preservation is still in the experimental stage. The Armed Forces Food and Container Institute at Natick, Mass., has been doing extensive research on food irradiation in one of the best equipped laboratories in the world for this purpose. They are testing various types of foods in different designs of containers to determine levels of irradiation which will safeguard the food without changing its flavor. Obviously, food does not become radioactive in the process. F. P. Mehrlich, Technical Director, explains[4]

The radiation preservation process involves exposing food to electrons so the food itself is not cooked in the process. Raw foods remain raw. Different effects are obtained, depending on the level of irradiation provided.

At the lowest levels, in the order of 7,500 rads, sprouting of potatoes and onions is inhibited, extending their postharvest storage life well into the next harvest. At slightly higher levels, human pathogens like trichinosis-causing worms and liver flukes are destroyed, making infested pork and fish safe for human consumption. At still higher levels, insect larvae and eggs are destroyed, eliminating insect damage in packaged cereal and permitting previously infested fruits across quarantine barriers.

At even higher levels, pathogenic bacteria like Salmonella are inactivated. At the same time so are most of the bacteria present, thereby extending the refrigerated shelf life and marketing radius of fresh foods.

Finally, at the highest levels, in the order of 4.5 million rads, all bacteria are killed and prepackaged food can be kept without bacterial spoilage, in the absence of refrigeration. The military and civilian advantages of such a process are readily apparent.

A *rad* is a unit of absorbed ionizing radiation. It corresponds to an energy absorption of 100 ergs per gram of material. A lethal dose for man is between 500 and 600 rads.

Since many foods become unacceptable at radiation levels above 500,000 rads due to off flavor and odor, it is probable that research will develop a combination of heat, radiation and refrigeration to retain the highest quality of certain foods. Heat destroys enzymes which are resistant to destruction by radiation.

FOODBORNE DISEASES AND TOXINS

In addition to contaminants that cause obvious spoilage or deterioration of food as described earlier in this chapter, foods may also be contaminated by helminths and pathogenic microorganisms. These contaminants may be various worms, molds, bacteria, viruses, and other organisms or the toxins produced by them. The appearance, taste and smell of the food so infected may show no change and thus give no warning to the consumer.

These infections may be present in the food at its source, such as animals infected with tuberculosis, brucellosis, salmonellosis, tularemia, tapeworms or trichinae, and may be carried to the consumer if the food is undercooked.

Food may also be infected by food handlers who are convalescent from infectious diseases. They may be in apparent good health but still carry infectious organisms. The organisms may be distributed on food by hands soiled with urine or feces or by spray of oral and nasal secretions by coughing and sneezing over the food being prepared. Contamination may also come from the butcher block or from the handling of an infected animal, before working with the food in question.

Dust falling on uncovered foods and the feces and the bodies of insects may also

[3] What Consumers Should Know About Food Additives. Food and Drug. Adm. Leaflet No. 10, 1961.
[4] Mehrlich, F. P.: Protecting Our Food. Yearbook of Agriculture. P. 204. Washington, D. C., 1966.

TABLE 17–1. Summary of Foodborne and Waterborne Diseases by Types of Infection Reported 1952-1960

Type of Disease	Outbreaks	Per Cent of Outbreaks	Cases	Per Cent of Cases
Typhoid fever......................	65	3.4	603	0.6
Salmonellosis......................	209	11.0	10,699	11.7
Shigellosis........................	99	5.3	10,354	11.0
Botulism..........................	56	2.9	116	0.1
Staphylococcal food poisoning........	633	33.2	28,331	30.0
Gastroenteritis, undetermined........	839	44.2	44,083	46.6
Total......................	1,901	100.0	94,186	100.0

From Moore, A. N.: Meals Away from Home, Protecting Our Food. Yearbook of Agriculture. P. 182. Washington, D. C., U.S.D.A., 1966.

convey pathogenic organisms to a food supply. Covering of cooked foods and refrigeration can do much to cut down on the number of pathogenic organisms in foods. It is wise to put cooked foods promptly into an efficient refrigerator rather than to allow them to cool thoroughly before refrigerating. Often the period required for cooling in a warm kitchen is sufficient for bacteria to grow rapidly.

Transmission of disease by the eating utensils in a restaurant may be eliminated by scalding all dishes and silverware after washing or by rinsing in clean water containing a residual of at least 100 parts per million of chlorine. Drying should be by drainage, since towels frequently are a means of transferring organisms to the utensils rather than of removing them.

Foodborne diseases are not reportable by state law and thus there is no accurate method of determining the incidence. Only major outbreaks in public eating places are apt to come to the attention of newspapers.

Bacterial Contamination of Food and Water

Salmonella infection is a term used to cover a large group of infections caused by several species of the Salmonella organism and common to man and several animals and birds. Salmonellosis is an infection of the intestinal tract and symptoms begin to appear from 12 to 48 hours after contaminated food has been eaten. Symptoms typically are headache, vomiting, diarrhea, fever and cramps. An attack may last a few hours or several days. Infants and debilitated older people may be most seriously affected and death may result. Antibiotics do little to relieve an attack; fluids and a bland diet are the usual treatment.

The National Communicable Disease Center[5] in Atlanta, Georgia, reported in 1967 that salmonellosis has become a major national problem, whereas a generation ago it was a medical curiosity. They reported that some 20,000 cases of salmonella infection were reported in 1966 and in 1967 but that the actual incidence was probably many times that figure. In this decade salmonella have been traced to well water, frozen turkey, fresh chicken, eggs, smoked fish, ground beef and a contaminated batch of powdered milk.

Many varieties of salmonella may be carried by contaminated foods. Since these bacteria grow easily in moist foods of low acidity and may continue to be viable even in some dry foods, strict control of food sanitation and cooking procedures at home and in institutions, especially, is essential. The usual path of infection is from animals or animal products to man. Precautions in regard to utensils, dishwashing and food handling are outlined by Werrin and Kronick.[6] Salmonella are readily destroyed by usual cooking procedures and by pasteurization but not by freezing. Note the incident of turkey-borne multiple infection on the next page.

---

[5] Personal communication, April 1967.

[6] Werrin, M., and Kronick, D.: Am. J. Nursing, 65:528, 1965.

Shigellosis is closely related to salmonellosis. Shigella also are enteric bacteria and are the etiologic agents of bacillary dysentery in man. Young children and newborn animals are most seriously affected.

The typhoid bacillus is another species of Salmonella and may be carried by contaminated water or shellfish. In the United States, however, an outbreak of typhoid fever can usually be traced to a food handler who is a "carrier" of the organism. Fortunately, the disease responds to an antibiotic and the course is not as serious as it once was.

Clostridium perfringens. In addition to the more familiar foodborne disease, salmonellosis, other organisms alone or in combination with salmonella may cause gastrointestinal disturbances. Among the bacteria involved are certain strains of *Clostridium perfringens,* sometimes called the gas-gangrene organism. Although part of the normal flora of the intestines, *Cl. perfringens* may cause gas gangrene in wounds. It is present in soil, water, dust and refuse. It forms spores which are resistant to heat, ordinary cooking, drying, freezing, curing of meats and to irradiation.[7]

The symptoms of *Cl. perfringens* food infection are mild gastroenteritis, abdominal cramps and diarrhea 8 to 16 hours after eating infected food, which may be accompanied by nausea and headache. The illness is usually mild and of short duration, with recovery within 24 hours.

A report of three consecutive outbreaks of foodborne disease in one week was recently investigated and traced to turkey infected with both salmonella and *Cl. perfringens.* The turkey prepared ahead and served at three banquets in one week caused food poisoning in 23 per cent of the persons present at the first, in 35 per cent of those at the second and in 69 per cent of those at the third banquet. The 20 to 22 pound turkeys had been purchased frozen, thawed at room temperature, boiled for 4 hours and allowed to cool in water overnight. They were stored in a refrigerator but were probably at room temperature

for some time during preparation and prior to reheating before service at each banquet. This is an example of poor food handling if not poor sanitation.[8]

Streptococcal Infections. Hemolytic streptococcus is the type most commonly carried by food. Food and utensils may be contaminated by a carrier, from nasal discharge or skin infection. Strep sore throat, strep ear infections and scarlet fever are all caused by strains of hemolytic streptococci.

Tularemia, sometimes called rabbit fever, is caused by infection with *Pasteurella tularensis.* It is transmitted from rodents by flies, fleas and ticks and may be acquired by man from the handling of infected animals. It is characterized by an ulcer at the site of inoculation, followed by inflammation of the lymph glands and by headache, chills and fever. It is recommended that hunters use rubber gloves when dressing wild game.

Parasitic Infections

Parasitic infections are not confined to the tropics as is sometimes thought. They may be transmitted by food or drink, often by infected fish, shellfish or crustacea.

Trichinosis is the parasitic disease most likely to be encountered in the United States and is caused by improperly cooked pork from pigs that were infected with *Trichinella spiralis.* Symptoms of the infection in man include fever, muscle pain, sweating, chills, vomiting and swollen eyelids. Outbreaks have been reported from homemade sausage and other pork products improperly cured. Trichinosis can be avoided if pork is well cooked or properly cured.

Protozoan Infections

Amebic Dysentery, caused by *Entamoeba histolytica,* is another infection that may be carried by food and food handlers. It is common in the tropics. Once it is acquired, the organism remains in the tissues of the intestinal tract and causes intermittent attacks until the individual is treated. Abscesses of the liver may be a complication.

---

[7] Despaul, J. E.: The gangrene organism—a food-poisoning agent. J. Am. Dietet. A., 49:185, 1966.

[8] Three outbreaks of food-borne disease and with dual etiology. Note. Nutr. Rev., 25:94, 1967.

Viral Infections

Infectious hepatitis is the most common of viral infections spread by contaminated food. It may be spread by the consumption of contaminated water, milk or other food or by the blood of persons carrying the hepatitis virus. A food handler who is a carrier may cut his finger and thus contaminate food and this may not be discovered for some time. The incubation period is from 10 to 50 days and the virus may be in the blood 2 to 3 weeks before the onset of the disease.

Toxins Produced by Bacteria and Molds

Bacterial Exotoxins

The bacteria that produce exotoxins in foods are of two types quite different in growth habits and in the clinical symptoms of poisoning. Staphylococci and *Cl. botulinum* both produce toxins that are stable to heat although the organisms themselves are destroyed by cooking.

STAPHYLOCOCCUS FOOD POISONING

Staphylococcus bacteria are responsible for many cases of food poisoning. Most people are sensitive to the exotoxins produced by these bacteria and serious illness can result if enough of the toxin is present in the food. The toxin affects only the gastrointestinal tract and the onset of symptoms occur within 2 to 12 hours after infected food is eaten. The symptoms are severe nausea, vomiting and abdominal cramps. This kind of food poisoning is rarely fatal.[9]

Most outbreaks of this type of food poisoning have been caused by the bacteria in prepared or unheated foods such as custard-filled pastries, cream pies, salads, precooked meats such as ham, sandwiches and creamed dishes. The bacteria get into food from boils, infected cuts, coughing, and sneezing by food handlers followed by improper storage and reheating of foods before service. The flavor and appearance of the food may not change. Control of this type of food poisoning is largely a matter of education of food handlers. An outbreak recently reported aboard a navy ship is of special interest.[10]

BOTULISM

Botulism is a rare form of food poisoning. It occurs when foods have been underprocessed. Botulin (the toxin) may also be found in some meat products such as sausage (the Latin word for sausage is botulus). Since *Cl. botulinum* is a strict anaerobe, it can grow only under conditions in which air is excluded, such as in a can or deep inside a product.

In recent years commercially processed foods have been relatively free of any poisoning caused by *Cl. botulinum*. However, in 1963 two instances of cases were caused by canned tuna fish and one by smoked fish frozen in polyethelene bags.

The few reports of occurrences usually indicate improperly processed, home-canned, low acid foods such as corn, beans, beets, asparagus, meat and fish.

The *toxin* produced is one of the most deadly biologic poisons known. On average, mortality is about 68 per cent and ranges from 50 per cent to 100 per cent in individual outbreaks. Occasionally, entire families are killed by botulism.

Since this is a dramatic disease in which the person may linger on, completely conscious, for a few days before death occurs, much has been made of it for theatrical use, but in reality it is quite rare. A doctor seldom, if ever, sees a case of botulism in his career.

The toxin is absorbed directly from the stomach and the intestinal tract. In about 12 to 24 hours it affects the nervous system, causing double vision, difficulty in swallowing, loss of speech and, when lethal, respiratory failure in from 3 to 6 days.

An antitoxin has been developed for the 5 known strains of *Cl. botulinum*, but it is of little value after advanced symptoms appear.

---

[9] Eshbach, C. E.: Bacterial Food Poisoning. Food Management Leaflet. Coop. Ext. Service, Univ. Mass., 1962.

[10] LaChapelle, N. C., *et al.*: A gastroenteritis outbreak of Staphylococcus aureus type 29. Am. J. Pub. Health, 56:94, 1966.

Toxins from Molds (Mycotoxins)

Aflotoxin, toxin produced by *Aspergillus flavus,* a fungus found in peanuts (groundnuts) which have been improperly dried, has been found to be carcinogenic for rats. No acute illness is caused in man from eating these groundnuts in countries where they are staple food but research is being conducted to investigate the possibility of such mold-producing toxins being carcinogenic in man.[11] Commercial peanut products designed for human consumption are toxin-free, even if produced from contaminated nuts, because any trace of aflotoxin is removed in the refining process.

Naturally Occurring Toxins

It is well known that many varieties of mushrooms are poisonous and have been mistaken for edible types, with disastrous results. There is no simple test which will identify edible types other than botanical characteristics.

A few plants used as foods are safe at one time and not at another. The young white shoots of pokeweed frequently are eaten with safety as greens in the early spring, but the later green shoots may cause severe illness. The green leaves of rhubarb may contain enough oxalic acid to cause illness, but the succulent leaf stems are eaten without any untoward effects. Clams and mussels on the Pacific coast may build up toxins during the summer due to an infection from certain plankton.

FOOD ADDITIVES
Incidental or Accidental Additives or Contaminants

Food additives are prohibited specifically by the Food, Drug and Cosmetic Act where they are used to mask faulty processing and handling technics, to deceive the consumer and to aid processing at the expense of a substantial reduction of the nutritive value of the product, and where good manufacturing practices do not require the use of an additive to produce a food item economically.

The *incidental additives,* usually undesirable, which may appear in food products include:
1. Pesticides (used for plant and animal pest control)
2. Fertilizers (utilized by plants)
3. Feed adjuvants and drugs (antibiotics, hormones, tranquilizers and enzymes)
4. Chemicals used in packaging materials (may migrate into the food)

The legal measures governing the use of intentional and incidental food additives are designed to protect the public from the presence in foods of any substance not demonstrated to be safe under the recommended conditions of use, as judged by competent experts. The major considerations in such judgment are the results of laboratory studies in terms of possible injury to human beings, the amount of additive likely to be present in any reasonable diet, and the extent to which similar or similarly-acting chemicals may be present in the diet. There is no evidence that consumption of food in which approved additives have been used in quantities below tolerance levels in crop production or processing has resulted in epidemics or has endangered health. On the contrary, nutritional quality and sanitary characteristics of foods have been maintained and improved by their use.

There are many chemicals that may contaminate food or water *accidentally* and some of these may be poisonous to man. For this reason, standards have been established for the chemical quality of drinking water by the U. S. Public Health Service.[12] The toxic or other physiologic effects from ingestion of excessive quantities of given substances are outlined and limits for their permissible concentration in drinking water are indicated. The chemicals listed include: alkyl benzene sulfonate (detergent), arsenic, barium, cadmium, carbonchloroform extract, chloride, chromium, copper, cyanide, fluoride, iron, manganese, lead, nitrate, phenols, selenium, silver, sulphate, zinc and total dissolved solids.[13]

[11] English, R. M.: Food and nutr. Notes and Reviews, *21:*3, 1965. Aspergillus flavus toxin. Abs. J. Am. Dietet. A., *47:*48, 1965.

[12] U. S. Public Health Service: J. Am. Water Works A-*53:*935, 1961.
[13] Wright, C. V.: Pub. Health Rep., 77:628, 1962.

Traces of these chemicals and others can get into food in excessive amounts through ignorance or accident in the home: antimony, cadmium, mercury, insecticides, detergents, kerosene, lye, washing soda and silver polish, to name the more obvious. The swallowing of poisons is a common cause of death among children in the United States. It is imperative that poisonous chemicals be plainly marked and kept as far as possible from food supplies. Many manufacturers add coloring to household chemicals to distinguish them from food materials.

The laws and regulations now in effect by our federal government have so effectively controlled the use of pesticides and the sale of foods containing pesticide residues that no harm will result from foods available on the market. Pesticide toxicity results primarily from improper use, from accidental exposure, or from deliberate ingestion with suicidal intent.[14]

Radioactive Fallout

Of special concern with respect to unintentional additives is the possible presence of radioactive materials in foods from fallout resulting from man-made nuclear explosions. Public concern which has centered around the possible presence of strontium-90 in milk does not appear to be

---

[14] Hodges, R. E.: The toxicity of pesticides and their residues in food. Nutr. Rev., 23:225, 1965.

a valid concern under normal peacetime operations of weapons testing. The Federal Radiation Council has established guidelines for safe daily intakes of radioactive substances from natural and manmade sources, based on present knowledge of the biologic effects of exposure to radiation. The average radiation exposure of the bones of the most sensitive segment of our population (the very young children) is estimated to be about one fiftieth of the safe daily intake estimated by the Federal Radiation Council.

For the public protection, a constant "early warning" radiation surveillance program is in operation in the United States. Should radiation levels exceed the guidelines and standards which have been established, steps will be taken to inform and protect the public.

Intentional Food Additives

Intentional food additives include preservatives, anti-oxidants, stabilizers, emulsifiers, coloring and flavoring agents. Well over 1,000 such additives are being used in food processing today and these additives are continually being investigated by the Food and Drug Administration laboratories. The Food Additives Amendment became law in 1958 and is a definite protection for the consumer.

Safety of food additives is a problem of extreme importance that should be consid-

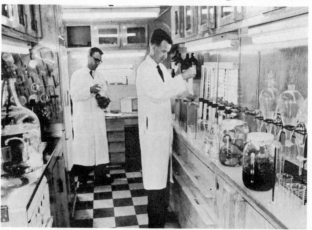

Fig. 17–4. Food and Drug Administration chemists in mobile trailer laboratory analyze raw products for pesticide residues. U.S.D.A., From Protecting Our Food. Yearbook of Agriculture, p. 292. Washington, D. C., 1966.

ered over all other phases of the question. It is practically impossible to demonstrate absolute proof of safety of an additive for all people in a population which may include a few very sensitive individuals and others in poor physiologic condition, as well as those suffering from a disease of one sort or another.

Usually, judgment of safety is based on the result of experiments on three or more types of animals to determine acute toxicity and chronic toxicity at levels far above those intended for use in foods. The maximum level of consumption of an additive in a day's food must be determined or estimated. The minimum level which will produce deviations from normal in animals is studied carefully to determine what effects in humans may be expected, and an adequate margin of safety must be established to reduce to a minimum any hazard to the health of people of varying ages and physiologic states.

The following are examples of the careful checking on additives by the FDA: "chemicals have been found injurious only after they have been in use for a considerable period of time, including a chemical used for flour aging and an ingredient of imitation vanilla extract. Both had to be removed from the market after years of presumed safety."[15]

FOOD LAWS

Food and Drug Administration

Federal Food, Drug and Cosmetic Act

The Federal Food and Drug Administration (FDA) has jurisdiction over the misbranding and adulteration of foods shipped interstate or manufactured in a territory of the United States or the District of Columbia. Federal regulations also control imported and exported foods. Foods manufactured and sold within a state's boundaries are not subject to Federal regulation but are controlled by the food regulations of the state in which they are produced.

A food is considered to be misbranded if the label is false or misleading; if the name and the address of the manufacturer or the distributor are not on the package; if the weight or the volume of food contained is wrong or omitted; if the label does not comply with regulations or the container is misleading in size or shape.

The label must contain the common or usual name of the food and the name of each ingredient other than spices, flavoring and colorings, unless a standard of identity has been established by the FDA.[16] The standard of identity places a lower limit on the amount of the expensive ingredients in the product (e.g., chicken in chicken soup) and an upper limit on the inexpensive items in the product. In addition, the standard of identity lists the optional ingredients which may be used in the product at the discretion of the manufacturer. If a standard of identity has been established for a food, the list of ingredients does not have to be on the label except for a statement of the presence of artificial flavoring and coloring or chemical preservatives, if added.

Special Dietary Food Regulations

Some major changes in requirements for special diet foods and diet supplements were initiated in 1966. Some of these limit content, others limit the claims that may be made on the label. The revised regulations are aimed at providing the consumer with more facts about the food he buys for weight control, for dietary supplementation with minerals and vitamins, and for other special diet needs, such as controlling salt or sugar intake. (Watch for final F.D.A. decisions.)

Changes will include the adoption of the National Research Council's Recommended Dietary Allowances (RDA) in place of the outmoded concept of "minimum daily requirements." The new regulations will probably establish the following classes of foods that may be "fortified with vitamins and minerals: processed cereals, fruit and vegetable juices, infant and junior **fruit products, fluid** or powdered whole

---

[15] Facts for Consumers—Food Additives. Food and Drug Adm. U. S. Dept. H.E.W. Pub. No. 10, 1964.

[16] What Consumers Should Know About Food Standards. Food and Drug Adm. Pub. No. 8, 1961.

milk (or milk product), fluid skimmed and fluid or powdered low-fat milk, table salt.[17]

Not only are infant foods especially protected against unnecessary additives by United States laws but also caution is expressed by a Joint FAO/WHO Expert Committee on Food Additives.[18]

Foods that are specially prepared for babies require separate consideration from all other foods as regards the use of food additives and toxicological risk. . . . The reason for this is that the detoxicating mechanisms that are effective in the more mature individual may be ineffective in the baby. . . . If the use of a food additive is necessary in a baby food, great caution should be exercised both in the choice of additive and in the level of use.

The Committee also urges the governments of the member nations to promote further research on food additives and also recommends that another Joint FAO/WHO Committee draw up specifications for substances that may be used as additives.

Adulteration of Foods

A food is considered to be adulterated if it is filthy, putrid or decomposed, if noncertified colors are used, if the container is made of a substance injurious to health (e.g., lead), if there is dilution or substitution, or if there is omission of a valuable ingredient. Food is also considered to be adulterated if it contains meat from a diseased animal or one that died by means other than slaughter. If a poisonous substance in any amount is added to a food when it is not necessary in good manufacturing practices, the food will be considered adulterated.

False advertising of foods, drugs and cosmetics through media such as television and radio is under the jurisdiction not of the FDA but of the Federal Trade Commission.

An amendment to the Food, Drug and Cosmetic Act of 1938 was passed in 1954 to establish safe limits of pesticide chemical residues on fresh fruits and vegetables.

The chemical pesticide sprays range in toxicity to man from virtually harmless to extremely toxic and dangerous poisons. To control their use the FDA has published a list of more than 2,000 tolerance levels for pesticide chemicals and has established a zero tolerance for certain pesticides such as cyanides, mercury-containing compounds and selenium-containing compounds which are extremely dangerous.

To protect the consumer, foods which are shipped in violation of FDA regulations are subject to seizure. The manufacturers may be fined and/or imprisoned, depending on the circumstances.

U. S. Department of Agriculture
Federal Meat Inspection Act

Through the Bureau of Animal Industry (BAI), the Secretary of Agriculture administers regulations concerning the meat industry. Formerly, laws provided for the inspection of all cattle, sheep, swine and goats slaughtered for transportation or sale as articles of interstate or foreign commerce. A new law, passed in late 1967, provides for similar inspection and regulation of all meats sold for human consumption anywhere in the United States. The carcasses and parts of all such animals found to be sound, healthful, wholesome and fit for human food are stamped "Inspected and Passed." Animals found to be unfit for human food are separated and stamped "Inspected and Condemned." Carcasses which have been condemned for food purposes must be destroyed under the supervision of a Federal inspector.

The Secretary of Agriculture also has charge of regulations concerning imported and exported meat and meat products, as well as the regulation concerning the labeling of horsemeat. Horsemeat may be used for human food, but strict labeling is required to prevent its use as a substitute for beef.

A law passed in 1957 provides for compulsory inspection of poultry and poultry products, and is similar in nature to the Meat Inspection Act.

---

[17] Fortified Foods. FDA Fact Sheet. June 17, 1966.

[18] News Note: J. Am. Dietet. A., *41*:350, 1962.

HOW FOODS GET TO THE CONSUMER—THE PRINCIPAL SUPPLY ROUTES

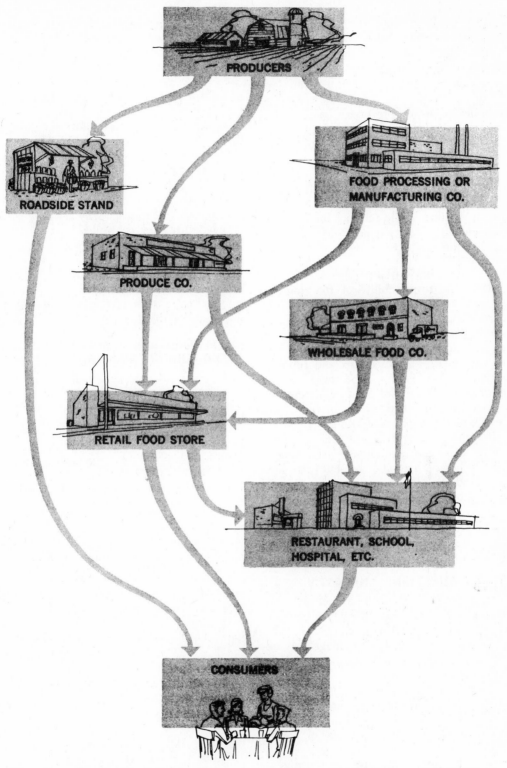

(From Protecting Our Food, Yearbook of Agriculture, 1966. p. 239, Washington, D.C. U.S.D.A.)

FIGURE 17–5

USDA Grade Standards and Inspection Service for Processed Foods

The Fruit and Vegetable Division of the Agricultural Marketing Service, United States Department of Agriculture, develops grade standards for processed foods and supplies an inspection service for processed fruits, vegetables and related foods.

The Federal grading of foods aids in informing processors, sellers, brokers, distributors and buyers concerning the class, the quality and the condition of the product. The grades serve as a basis for arriving at a value of the product for purposes of securing a loan, payment of damages or sale of the product.

State Regulations

It is the responsibility of the states to regulate food production and processing of certain products which do not leave the state. The state also controls such things as pasteurization of milk, inspection of cattle and goats for brucellosis and tuberculosis, and regulations concerning sale of margarine. Many state food regulations are similar to the Federal regulations, but others may prohibit some things which are allowed by Federal law. Food processors must satisfy the regulations of the state in which they operate and the states in which the food is sold, as well as the Federal regulations.

Local municipal sanitary codes may also regulate food production and processing to the extent that they may be more restrictive than state or federal, not less so.

STUDY QUESTIONS AND ACTIVITIES

1. How is food likely to become contaminated? What precautions can be taken to prevent this from happening?

2. What types of food spoilage may occur and under what circumstances? How can each be prevented?

3. Name the various methods of food preservation and the most common ones today. What are the limitations of freeze-drying, irradiation and the use of antibiotics?

4. What foodborne diseases are due to toxins produced by organisms in the alimentary tract?

5. Which foodborne bacteria, carried most often in eggs or poultry, have been responsible for recent outbreaks of gastrointestinal disease?

6. What disease carried by water, milk or food is due to a virus? How long after exposure may it take to develop?

7. Why are certain molds dangerous? What foods are most susceptible?

8. Are pesticide residues in foods available on our markets today likely to be harmful? Why or why not?

9. What types of food additives may be considered "intentional," why are they used and how are they controlled?

10. What regulations in regard to special dietary foods are being revised by the Food and Drug Administration?

11. What new regulations are proposed by the FDA for the fortification and labeling of special diet foods?

SUPPLEMENTARY READING ON SAFEGUARDING OUR FOOD SUPPLY

Anderson, E. C., and Nelson, D. J., Jr.: Surveillance for radiological contamination. Am. J. Pub. Health, 52:1391, 1962.

Council on Foods and Nutrition, A.M.A.: General policy on addition of specific nutrients to foods. J.A.M.A., 178:1024, 1961.

————: Safe use of chemicals in foods. J.A.M.A., 178:749, 1961.

Food and Drug Administration, U. S. Dept. H.E.W.: Facts for Consumers; Food Additives, Washington, D. C., 1964.

————: Fact Sheets (available from FDA consumer representative).

Hodges, R. E.: The toxicity of pesticides and their residues in food. Nutr. Rev., 23:225, 1965.

Milstead, K. L.: Science works through law to protect consumers. J. Am. Dietet. A., 48:187, 1966.

Public Health Service, U. S. Dept. H.E.W.: You Can Prevent Food Borne Illness. Folder, 1967. Hot Tips on Food Protection. Folder, 1966. Government Printing Office, Washington, D. C. 20201.

Werrin, M., and Kronick, D.: Salmonella control in hospitals, Am. J. Nursing 65:528, 1965.

Woodburn, M.: Safe food versus food-borne illness. J. Home Econ., 59:448, 1967.

For further references see Bibliography in Part Four.

PART TWO
Diet in Disease

Introduction

Setting the Climate • Interpretation of the Diet Plan • Patient Education • Knowledge • Patient-Centered Care • Communication Skills

Under the guidance of the physician and the diet order which he devises the nurse and dietitian share with him the responsibility for the dietary component of patient care. Each brings to this responsibility his own professional orientation and functions but for each the focus is the patient.

It is helpful to consider dietary care under three major headings: (1) setting a climate in which it is possible for the patient to eat; (2) interpreting or reinforcing the physician's explanation of the purpose of the dietary plan of care; and (3) assisting the patient through education to accept and to carry out a modification of his food practices. Patient education is not limited to those requiring therapeutic diets; it includes those individuals who are faced for any reason with modifying food practices to ensure an appropriate intake of nutrients.

SETTING THE CLIMATE

For the nurse, setting the climate means the skillful application of those comfort, hygiene, and safety measures she is taught early in her educational experience with patients—for example, positioning the bed patient so that he may feed himself or be fed comfortably, or scheduling treatments and medications so that he is ready to eat when food is served. Whether the nurse herself sets the climate or directs those who assist her, she influences, to a great degree, the acceptance of food by the patient.

For the dietitian, setting the climate includes the establishing of food service schedules for the convenience of the patient, and the planning of the menus and the preparation of foods that are acceptable to him. It is well to recognize that individuals under stress of illness may not be able to accept new and unfamiliar foods or methods of food preparation. The dietitian's creativity is not to be denied but it should be creativity acceptable to the patient by virtue of his past experiences with food.

Setting the climate for patients is a joint responsibility of the administrative personnel in the nursing and dietary departments. Providing a climate for the acceptance of food requires careful planning of nursing and dietary routines and procedures, based on a mutual appreciation of each other's day-to-day responsibilities and pressures. But, with service to the patient as the major goal, coordination of functions often results in both effective nursing and dietary care.

INTERPRETATION OF THE DIET PLAN

In her continuous and close contact with the patient the nurse is often the first to become aware of a patient's anxiety or confusion about his physician's diet order, be it a "normal" or a therapeutic one. Many of the expressions of concern which may come to the nurse's attention are of the moment, and a simple explanation or answer to a question often reassures the patient at that time.

When the dietitian is in the patient area at mealtime and at other times during the day she will also become aware of patients'

255

concerns and will need to help them understand the "whys" of their doctors' diet orders.

To reduce, rather than add to, a patient's anxieties or confusion, close communication among physician, nurse, and dietitian is essential. Also, it is important to recognize that reassurances of the moment to relieve anxiety should not be equated necessarily with education. In a stressful situation what the patient hears today may be forgotten tomorrow.

PATIENT EDUCATION

When a patient needs instruction in normal nutrition, or in a minor modification of his diet, it is expected that physician, nurse or dietitian are all able to do this. When the diet of a patient is, for therapeutic reasons, complex, it is expected that the dietitian will assume the major responsibility for educating the patient. She alone is the member of the health team qualified by education and training to assume this function. For example, a patient with renal disease, who requires a diet modified in protein, sodium and potassium, will need to be instructed by a highly skilled dietitian if he is to manage this complicated diet successfully at home. And, just as important, his diet instruction cannot be done satisfactorily on the day he is discharged from the hospital.

Diet instruction for any patient must be anticipated by physician, nurse, and dietitian and done well in advance of his discharge from the hospital. Education to change behavior takes time and, as Stone points out, the patient needs time to learn how to cope with a diet he may have to use for many years to come.[1] The nurse, in many situations, coordinates the planning for discharge. She may also be the one who knows and shares with the physician and the dietitian how the patient feels about his diet, what his problems will be when he goes home, and what he needs to be taught.

Sharing the responsibility for dietary care and patient education implies that both the

nurse and the dietitian will possess: (1) knowledge of the science and art of foods and nutrition; (2) personal attitudes which will be reflected in patient-centered care; and (3) equal skill in communicating with the patient, and with each other.

KNOWLEDGE

Knowledge of the science and art of foods and nutrition is basic to creating a climate for the acceptance of food, interpreting the physician's diet plan, and educating the patient. The way in which the nurse and the dietitian use their knowledge will vary. The effect of a cerebral vascular accident on the swallowing reflex of a patient will be viewed differently by each: the nurse will consider the effect when positioning the patient for feeding; the dietitian, when selecting food of the right consistency for this same patient.

The degree to which both will apply their knowledge of foods and nutrition will also vary. The nurse applies her knowledge of the diet modification in chronic renal disease to interpret the diet plan to the patient correctly and to reinforce the dietitian's instructions when necessary. The dietitian will apply the same principles in devising the diet plan and in educating the patient. Both nurse and dietitian need to understand the metabolic aberrations in renal disease. At the same time both need to know the nutrient composition of foods at the per serving level—the dietitian, however, in more detail than the nurse.

PATIENT-CENTERED CARE

A true commitment to patient-centered care is required of both nurse and dietitian. Chapter 11, Regional, National and Cultural Food Patterns, explains how the food habits of an individual will reflect his social and cultural heritage, and how one patient's food habits will be different than another's. The nurse and dietitian will demonstrate their acceptance of these individual differences when they take the time to discover what a patient usually eats, and use this information properly in meeting his nutritional needs. Also, if the nurse or dietitian is to gain the confidence of the patient, each must question the patient and

---

[1] Stone, D. B.: The true role of the dietitian: A scholar of nutrition. J. Am. Dietet. A., 49:26, 1966.

listen to his answers in a way that makes it possible for him to tell them what he really eats.

COMMUNICATION SKILLS

Nurses and dietitians use the same communication skills. Both learn about the patient by reading his record, by observing him and listening to him, and by interviewing him. Both are committed to sharing their knowledge of the patient through appropriate notations in his record, through team conferences in the clinical unit, and through a variety of other institutional routines. Without communication with the patient and with each other in behalf of the patient, patient-centered care is not achieved.

CHAPTER 18

Assessment of Patient Needs

Introduction • Cultural Factors • Psychological Influences • Physical Condition • Potential for Learning

Some of the modifications of the normal diet that are commonly made in the treatment of disease will be described in the chapters in this section of the book. To achieve their purpose these modified diets must be followed as accurately and carefully as the physician's orders for medication and other treatment. However, unlike a medication, food is a part of everyday life. It is not primarily associated with illness, and it has many meanings besides that of satisfying hunger. For this reason there may be severe stumbling blocks to the patient's acceptance of a therapeutic diet, whereas he will accept a distasteful medication or a painful treatment without question.

The dietary modification prescribed for the patient must be translated successfully into foods with which he is already familiar, and into a meal pattern similar to that of his family. When this is done there is a far greater probability of the diet being followed and thus being successful in regard to its therapeutic goal. At the same time, both the nurse and the dietitian must recognize that they may encounter a patient whose previous food practices may need to be drastically changed, not modified, to meet the therapeutic goal of his diet. A patient facing this problem requires special support and understanding as he struggles to change his food habits.

As one seeks to help a patient to accept a therapeutic modification of his food practices as part of the treatment of his disease,

it must be kept in mind that his food habits are part of his social and cultural heritage. In addition, certain psychological factors and his physical condition will influence his acceptance of food during his illness. The following sections of this chapter discuss some of the factors which one needs to consider in assessing a patient's needs, and in planning his diet with him.

CULTURAL FACTORS

Cultural heritage, family background and status, religious customs, family patterns of food preparation and service, emotional experiences with food, as well as exposure to nutrition education, food fads, and superstitions all contribute to the individual's food habits. A variety of ethnic patterns may be encountered in the hospital (see Chapter 11). The Orthodox Jewish, the Puerto Rican, the Mexican, the Polish and the Italian patient may have food habits different from each other's and from those of other Americans. Even in the United States food patterns may vary widely by region. A patient from the South who finds himself in a Northern hospital may feel that, because of the way vegetables are cooked, they are insipid and uninteresting and he may flatly refuse to eat them. These differences may well be the first problem confronting the nurse and the dietitian when they are helping the patient to adjust to needed diet modifications in the hospital.

Most people's lives are set in families, and to eat in bed and by one's self may accentuate the patient's illness in his mind. Some hospitals try to meet this problem by having as many patients eat together as possible, and here the hospital ward, with several patients in a room, may actually be a better setting than a single room with its lone private patient. Even a low-sodium diet may be accepted when its restrictions are shared with a fellow patient.

PSYCHOLOGICAL INFLUENCES

Illness may change a person's psychological orientation to everyday occurrences and personal relationships; the need for the familiar and the customary is immeasurably increased. Because what, how and with whom we eat is an everyday occurrence, illness, which interrupts this pattern, may have serious psychological repercussions. The fear, the worry, the insecurity and the frustration that possess the patient as he changes from an independent, healthy individual to one dependent on others in illness is often expressed through regressive behavior. Fussiness, anorexia or demands for extra attention are traits that may be exhibited by the worried patient. Babcock says that "it is easier to show discouragement through anorexia than it is to explain that one is feeling inadequate and depressed in the presence of a frightening disease or a disheartening experience."[1]

The apparent apathy or uncooperativeness of a patient may mean not that he does not want to eat, but that the food offered to him is unacceptable because of its emotional connotations. His food habits have developed slowly through the years and have become a personal and guarded part of himself, so that many foods may be associated with specific feelings and emotions separate from their nutritional significance. Such foods as milk, cocoa, custards, junket, creamed and strained foods, first met with in infancy, become associated with the dependency and the security of that period. Some adults will refuse such foods despite their apparent nutritional value simply because they resent the dependency of illness. Because of the sense of security they convey, others may cling

to using these same foods, even though they may not be desirable nutritionally or psychologically.

Desserts, sweets and delicacies have become reward foods to many people because they first were received as a reward for cleaning one's plate or being a good child. It is not surprising that adolescents, and older people too, indulge in excessive intake of such foods when they are under stress and in need of psychological reward.

In the United States some foods have gained special status. Steaks, chops, green salads and butter are four examples of these foods. Patients may resent suggestions to reduce the cost of food by substituting ground meat for steaks and chops, or margarine for butter. On the other hand the young homemaker who is well aware of the cost of food uses ground meat and margarine.

Tea, coffee and alcoholic beverages may be thought of as adult foods by some patients because they were forbidden to them as children. Excessive use of these beverages, to the exclusion of milk, may be an expression of a desire to seem mature. On the other hand, some cultural groups use tea, coffee and alcoholic beverages regularly as part of the daily diet for the whole family, including the children.

It must not be forgotten that the appearance of the food and the tray also will produce a psychological effect which may determine acceptance or rejection of the meal. Hot food must be served *hot* and cold food *cold*. A pot of *hot* coffee or tea may make the remainder of a restricted diet acceptable. It tells the patient, as no words can, that those about him really care about him and are making every effort to make his food as palatable as possible.

The therapeutic diet itself may have meaning for the patient that is not evident to the professional staff. Everyone rejoices with the patient who progresses from a liquid diet to one containing solid food as concrete evidence that he is getting better. But, should that patient ask if he must follow a sodium-restricted diet for the rest of his life, are we aware that he may be inquiring in reality if he is going to have cardiac disease permanently, with all that

[1] Babcock, C. G.: J. Am. Dietet. A., 28:222, 1952.

this implies? The therapeutic diet which must be of long duration may give to the patient a real sense of deprivation, with depressing overtones that are difficult to resolve.

All those concerned with the nutrition of people need to be cognizant of what food means to people under various circumstances. Attempts to change long-established and deeply ingrained patterns may be met with resistance. The overzealous nurse, dietitian or physician who is trying to teach a patient "what is good for him, nutritionally," may interpret the patient's response as "ignorance" or "lack of cooperation." Pumpian-Mindlin writes[2]: "To accomplish the prime purpose of regulating and guiding what goes into a patient's mouth, one must learn to listen carefully to what first comes out of the same mouth. . . . Otherwise one may find himself in the

position of having more than mere words thrown back in one's face." We must be able to interpret what the patient says or does not say about food, what he does with food, and how he reacts to food service in the light of his emotional as well as his metabolic needs. Whatever dietary changes may be necessary for his therapy must be made within this framework if they are to be successful.

PHYSICAL CONDITION

Through observation the physical characteristics of the patient which may influence his acceptance of food or ability to feed himself may be identified. Because of her constant contact the nurse, more readily than the dietitian or even the doctor, will often be the one to make these observations.

Older patients may have lost some of their teeth, making chewing difficult if they are placed on a general house diet. Some individuals will use poor fitting dentures

---

[2] Pumpian-Mindlin, E. J.: Meanings of food. J. Am. Dietet. A., 30:576, 1954.

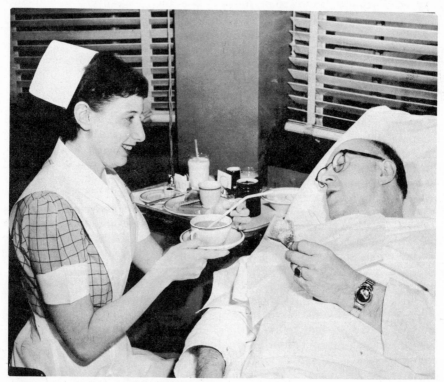

FIG. 18–1. The patient who must be fed is more likely to eat and enjoy his meal if the person assisting him is cheerful and unhurried. (The New York Hospital)

for cosmetic reasons and remove them at meal time. The adolescent boy with a fractured jaw may complain bitterly of hunger because his liquid house diet has not been modified sufficiently in calorie content or frequency of feeding to satisfy his needs. Patients recovering from oral surgery will not be appreciative of the effects of citrus juices on a sore mouth. Assessment of the ability to swallow is critical for certain patients if aspiration and its adverse effects are to be avoided.

Patients with emphysema and other respiratory difficulties may be forced to eat and drink slowly and, therefore, may need their trays for a longer period of time than other patients. Providing adequate nutrients and fluids for these individuals may require four or five meals per day.

Many individuals with sight problems, including the blind, can and prefer to feed themselves. They will need to be oriented to the placement of dishes and other articles on their trays. They may need help in pouring beverages, in opening milk cartons, and in removing protective coverings from foods. Individuals with poor manipulative skills such as the arthritic or the multiple sclerosis patient may need the same kind of assistance. Assessing the ability of any handicapped individual and providing the proper assistance not only will reduce his frustrations and promote his independence but also may help him to achieve a reasonable nutrient intake.

Every patient does not require the same size serving of food. A nursing note which states "appetite poor" may really mean that the patient was served too much food not, as this note is usually interpreted, that the patient did not eat enough food. A high-calorie diet for an 82-year-old, 5-foot 1-inch chronically ill woman may be 2,000 calories and for a 27-year old, 6-foot 2-inch man after an hemorrhoidectomy, 3,500 calories.

The long-term or chronically ill patient presents a special challenge to both the nurse and the dietitian. The scheduling of treatments and nursing care are often critical factors in obtaining a proper food intake. The best meal of the day for some of these patients is breakfast because they are rested or, for some of the older patients, because breakfast has always been an important meal. As the day progresses they may become increasingly tired and tend to eat less. Therefore, treatments should be planned so that the patient may rest before the noon and evening meals. Some of these patients may require only minimal assistance at breakfast and considerably more at the evening meal.

Interval nourishments for the chronically ill patient need to be carefully planned. A 400-calorie milkshake at 10:30 A.M. may result in the patient's refusal of an 800-calorie meal at 12:00 noon. Four meals, with the last one served at 8:00 or 9:00 P.M., may be a more effective plan for providing for his nutrient needs, especially if he is accustomed to an evening snack at home.

The patient restricted to prolonged bed rest benefits from nursing care procedures which promote the maximum movement by, or of, himself. Research has shown us that immobilization, even with adequate food intake, promotes negative nitrogen and calcium balance which may result in progressive muscular weakness. Turning and positioning the patient as ordered by the physician and providing passive exercise during personal care will help to prevent the adverse metabolic effects of immobility.

Cycle menus which repeat the same menus every four to six weeks are used in many hospitals. The long-term or chronically ill patient presents real problems to the dietitian, especially if he experiences two or three periods of a cycle menu plan, even though the menu items are familiar and acceptable to him. For some patients this will not be a problem; for others, it will. Family members or friends can often be helpful when a patient becomes bored with the hospital's food by occasionally providing a favorite dish from home, although they will need direction from the dietitian so that their contribution will fit his diet plan.

The wife of a patient who will require a sodium-restricted diet for the years ahead may demonstrate her understanding of the dietitian's instructions and her skill in adjusting her methods of food preparation by bringing her husband the "fruits" of her labors. At the same time she may feel a certain satisfaction from participating in her husband's care.

POTENTIAL FOR LEARNING

The nurse and the dietitian in their roles as educators will begin by discovering, through observation, listening, and interview, what the patient knows about nutrition and diet; his attitudes toward his illness and diet; and his readiness for learning, when necessary, how to manage a complex therapeutic diet.

Studies tell us that, as our nutrition education programs in elementary and secondary schools have been improved, we have a better educated young adult population today than in the past. If we are to avoid boring patients by giving them nutrition information they already have, we need to find out what they know and how they use it. In this way we can discover the problem, if any, and focus our teaching on the patient's real need.

As we listen to the patient his vocabulary will give us numerous clues as to the words and kinds of explanations we will need to use in teaching him. For example, if the patient is a newly diagnosed diabetic who is an organic chemist he may expect the nurse or dietitian to use the word "carbohydrate"; whereas, the mother of six children who reads and understands at the 6th grade level will need to be approached quite differently. In helping her to understand diabetes and her diet we would more likely use the word "sugar."

With the increasing use of programmed instruction both the nurse and the dietitian will want to watch for clues as to whether or not a patient is literate, in English or any other language. We have not always been aware of this in the past as we used printed instructions, since children, friends, or other patients may have interpreted such instructions for the patient.

The dietitian, who begins diet instruction as early as possible during the patient's hospitalization, can use the trays served each day to demonstrate to him the kinds and amounts of food he will be eating at home. At the same time, she can involve him or a member of his family in the planning of his daily menu. This approach to patient education not only prepares the individual and his family for his discharge but also, in many instances, stimulates the patient's interest in learning about his diet.

STUDY QUESTIONS AND ACTIVITIES

1. Select a patient who has been identified as a "feeding" problem. With the assistance of your instructor determine what the patient's problem really is. Either through your nursing care plan or communication with the appropriate individual(s) how can you work toward a solution to the problem?

2. With a classmate and with the help of your nursing instructor choose two patients with whom neither of you has had previous contact. The patients should be the same sex, about the same age, and, if possible, from the same socioeconomic class. Each student should select and study one patient's chart. Using the information gained from your study of Part I of this book and from courses in the social sciences, list the food practices you expect of your patient. Through observation and interview discover what his practices actually are. In clinical conference you and your classmate will report how each of these patients met your individual expectations and how each one differed from these expectations.

3. Obtain a 24-hour intake of all food and nutrient beverages from a patient. Estimate the calorie and nutrient intake using Table 2, Short Method of Dietary Analysis, in Part IV. Was this a reasonable intake for this patient?

4. For class discussion list the foods which have emotional significance for you; the menu your mother would plan for dinner when she expects guests; and the food you would serve to your gang on Friday night.

5. What are some of the physiologic effects of immobilization? How may these be minimized? Name some of the foods which should be included in liberal amounts to meet this specific need.

6. How may the nurse help the patient who has a poor appetite?

7. How may one be sure that the patient understands directions that have been given him?

8. At what time of day does the chronically ill patient have the best appetite?

SUPPLEMENATRY READING ON ASSESSMENT OF PATIENT NEEDS

Babcock, C. G.: Attitudes and the use of food. J. Am. Dietet. A., 38:546, 1961.

Bermosk, L. S.: Interviewing: A key to therapeutic communication in nursing practice. Nurs. Clin. of N. Am., 1:205-214, 1966 (June).

Cantoni, M.: Adapting therapeutic diets to the eating patterns of Italian-Americans. Am. J. Clin. Nutr., 6:548, 1958.

Fathauer, G. H.: Food habits—an anthropologist's view, J. Am. Dietet. A., 37:335, 1960.

Guidelines for the therapeutic dietitian in making notations on the medical record. J. Am. Dietet. A., 49:215-216, 1966 (Sept.).

Hacker, D. B., and Miller, E. D.: Food patterns of the Southwest. Am. J. Clin. Nutr., 7:224, 1959.

Johnson, D.: Effective diet counseling begins early in hospitalization. Hospitals, 41:94, 1967 (Jan. 16).

Kaufman, N.: Adapting therapeutic diets to Jewish food customs. Am. J. Clin. Nutr., 5:676, 1957.

MacGregor, F. C.: Uncooperative patients: some cultural interpretations. Am. J. Nursing, 67:88-91, 1967 (Jan.).

Morris, E.: How does a nurse teach nutrition to a patient? Am. J. Nursing, 60:67, 1960 (Jan.).

Paynich, M. L.: Cultural barriers to communication. Am. J. Nursing, 64:87, 1964 (Feb.).

Simon, J.: Psychologic factors in dietary restriction. J. Am. Dietet. A., 37:109, 1960.

Stitt, P. G.: Helping medical students find the strength in people. Children, 13:104, 1966 (May-June).

Torres, R. M.: Dietary patterns of the Puerto Rican people. Am. J. Clin. Nutr., 7:349, 1959.

Valassi, K. V.: Food habits of Greek-Americans. Am. J. Clin. Nutr., 11:240, 1962.

Wilson, N. L., et al.: Nutrition in pulmonary emphysema. J. Am. Dietet. A., 45:530, 1964 (Dec.).

For further references see Bibliography in Part Four.

CHAPTER 19

Progressive Hospital Diets

The Diet Order • The Diet Manual • Progressive Hospital Diets
• Therapeutic Diets • Nutritional Adequacy of Hospital Diets

INTRODUCTION

The Diet Order. A patient's diet prescription is ordered by the physician, and will be found in the orders written by him at the time the patient is admitted to the hospital. The order will depend on the patient's condition and may vary from nothing-by-mouth to a normal or regular diet. The diet order is changed as the patient's condition changes. If he is known to have a disease which requires the modification of the normal diet as part of his treatment, or if diagnostic procedures during hospitalization discover this, a therapeutic diet will be ordered.

The Diet Manual. The diet manual is a compilation of routine and therapeutic diet plans and is used for ease of communication among the physician, the nurse, and the dietitian. The manual serves as a guide to the kinds and amounts of food the dietary department will serve to a patient to fulfill his physician's diet order. Under Medicare in the Conditions of Participation for Hospitals,[1] the dietary department is required to have an up-to-date manual which has been approved jointly by the medical and dietary staffs. A copy of the manual used by a hospital is usually available in the Ward Office or at the head nurse's desk for the convenience of physicians and nurses.

---

[1] Health Insurance for the Aged: Conditions of Participation for Hospitals. Soc. Sec. Adm. HEW HIM—1, 1966, p. 20.

In teaching hospitals and in many large hospitals, physicians and dietitians, working together in committee, frequently compile a diet manual for use in their institutions. Some of these manuals are used only by the hospital in which they were written, while others have been published and are used by a variety of institutions. Diet manuals have also been compiled by the combined efforts of a State Department of Health and the State Dietetic Association, for use by small hospitals and nursing homes in a particular state. (See Part Four, Bibliography, for a partial list of diet manuals.)

As a general rule the first section of a manual will describe routine or standard diets for infants, children and adults, including soft and liquid diets; the following sections will describe a variety of therapeutic diets used in the treatment of disease. Diet manuals often differ in the terms used to describe diets, and in the recommendations for the foods to be used in a diet plan. The nurse should become thoroughly familiar with the diet manual used by the hospital in which she is located.

This chapter will discuss the general principles used in setting up the routine diet plans—sometimes referred to as house diets or progressive house diets—and the general principles used in setting up therapeutic diet plans.

TABLE 19–1. Evaluation of a Pattern Dietary for Its Nutritive Content[1]

Food Group	Amt. in Gm.	Household Measure	Calories	Protein Gm.	Fat Gm.	Carbohydrate Gm.	Minerals Calcium Mg.	Iron Mg.	Vitamins A I.U.	Thiamine Mg.	Riboflavin Mg.	Niacin Mg.	Ascorbic Acid Mg.
Milk or equivalent[2]	488	2 c. (1 pint)	320	17	17	24	576	.2	700	.16	.84	0.3	5
Egg	50	1 medium	81	7	6	..	27	1.2	590	.05	.15	..	..
Meat, fish or fowl[3]	120	4 ozs., cooked	376	30	31	..	13	3.3	280	.14	.23	6.1	..
Vegetables:													
Potato, cooked	100	1 medium	65	2	..	15	6	.5	..	.09	.03	1.2	16
Deep green or yellow, cooked[4]	75	½ c.	27	2	..	6	45	.8	4,700	.05	.10	0.5	25
Other, raw or cooked[5]	75	½ c.	45	2	..	10	18	.8	300	.08	.06	0.6	12
Fruits:													
Citrus[6]	100	1 serving	43	1	..	10	11	.2	140	.06	.02	0.3	43
Other[7]	100	1 serving	85	..	..	22	10	.8	365	.03	.04	0.5	4
Bread, white, enriched	70	3 slices	189	6	2	35	59	1.7	..	.17	.15	1.7	..
Cereal, whole grain or enriched[8]	130	⅔ c. cooked or	89	3	1	18	12	.9	..	.08	.03	0.7	..
	30	1 oz. dry		3			3						
Butter or margarine	14	1 tablespoon	100	..	11	..	3	..	460	..	..	..	..
Totals			1,420	70	68	140	780	10.4	7,535	.91	1.65	11.9[9]	105
Compare with recommended allowances[10]												Niacin Equiv.	
Moderately active man (70 Kg., 18–35 yrs. old)			2,900	70	..	..	800	10.0	5,000	1.20	1.70	19	70
Moderately active woman (58 Kg., 18–35 yrs. old)			2,100	58	..	..	800	15.0	5,000	0.80	1.30	14	70

[1] Calculations from Composition of Foods. Handbook No. 8. U. S. Department of Agriculture, rev. 1963.
[2] Milk equivalents mean: evaporated milk and dried milk in amounts equivalent to fluid milk in nutritive content; cheese, if water-soluble minerals and vitamins have not been lost in whey; and food items made with milk.
[3] Evaluation based on the use of 600 Gm. of beef (chuck, cooked), 150 Gm. of pork (medium fat, roasted), 150 Gm. of chicken (roaster, cooked, roasted) and 100 Gm. of fish (halibut, cooked, broiled).
[4] Evaluation based on figures for cooked broccoli, carrots, spinach and squash (all varieties).
[5] Evaluation based on figures for raw tomatoes and lettuce, and cooked peas, beets, Lima beans and fresh corn.
[6] Evaluation based on figures for whole orange and grapefruit, and orange and grapefruit juices.
[7] Evaluation based on figures for banana, apple, unsweetened cooked prunes and sweetened canned peaches.
[8] Evaluation based on figures for shredded wheat biscuit and oatmeal.
[9] The average diet in the United States, which contains a generous amount of protein, provides enough tryptophan to increase the niacin value by about a third.
[10] From the National Research Council Recommended Dietary Allowances, revised 1963.

PROGRESSIVE HOSPITAL DIETS

Regular, Standard, General. A variety of terms are in current use to describe the normal hospital diet which will provide a patient with the calories and nutrients he needs. It is intended for ambulatory patients and for those whose condition does not require a therapeutic diet.

The foods chosen for the regular diet menu will reflect the preferences characteristic of the cultural background and the economic status of the majority of those served by the institution. The choice of food will be further determined by its suitability for quality and quantity preparation, seasonal availability and local market costs and conditions. It is not surprising, therefore, that patients and staff members coming from backgrounds different from that of the local area may find some unfamiliar items on the menu.

The pattern dietary, Table 19–1, reproduced on the preceding page for the convenience of the reader (see Chapter 10), constitutes the basic pattern on which the regular hospital diet is planned. This pattern furnishes the nutrients recommended by the National Research Council for an adult, with the exception of calories. It is assumed that when the menu for the regular diet is planned, "other foods" as desired and as required by a patient will be added. For example, cream or milk and sugar will be served with the breakfast cereal and coffee; or other beverages may be served with the 3 meals, either with or without sugar and cream. Jelly with the toast may add pleasure to the meal as well as additional calories. Soup and crackers are desirable additions. Two more vegetables may be added, one of them raw, if the patient's condition permits. If not, additional citrus fruit, such as orange or grapefruit juice, is desirable. Desserts also furnish not only calories but other important nutrients as well. It is well to remember that some patients may require fewer calories than usual, since even ambulatory patients are less active during hospitalization than they are at home or at work.

The nutritional adequacy of a regular diet depends not only on the selection of foods and the amounts served but also on the protection of the nutrients in food during preparation and cooking, including the time and temperature of these processes.

The regular diet may be modified in food selection and methods of food preparation and in consistency for patients who cannot tolerate it but do not require a therapeutic diet. These modifications of the regular diet are the light or convalescent diet; the soft diet, including the surgical soft, medical soft, and dental soft diets; and the full liquid and clear liquid diets. Foods Used in Progressive Hospital Diets (Table 19–2) illustrates the types of food used in planning regular, light, soft and full liquid diets; and Table 19–3, Typical Menus for Progressive Hospital Diets, illustrates how these foods are used in menu plans.

Light or Convalescent Diet. A light, or convalescent, diet is intended for convalescent patients not yet able to tolerate the regular diet and for those with minor illnesses. It must be appetizing and readily digested. The chief difference between this diet and the regular diet is the method of preparation. The foods are cooked simply, and fried foods and rich pastries are omitted. Other fat-rich foods, such as pork (except bacon) and salad dressing, are avoided. Bran and strong or gas-forming vegetables are avoided, as well as most raw vegetables and fruits. All foods included in the soft and the liquid diets may be served on the light diet. In some hospitals this classification is omitted.

Soft Diet. The soft diet is soft in texture and consists of liquids and semisolid foods. It is an intermediate step between the liquid and the light diets. It is indicated in certain postoperative cases, in acute infections and in some gastrointestinal conditions; also, it may be ordered for the debilitated patient for ease of eating.

It is low in residue and is readily digested. Little or no spices or condiments are used in the preparation. It is somewhat more restricted than the light diet in fruit, meat and vegetables.

TABLE 19–2. Foods Used in Progressive Hospital Diets

Type of Food	Regular Diet	Light Diet	Soft Diet	Full Liquid Diet
Fruits	All	All cooked and canned fruits, citrus fruits, bananas	Fruit juices, cooked and canned fruits (without seeds, coarse skins or fiber), bananas	Fruit juices, strained
Cereals and cereal products	All	Cereals: dry or well cooked, spaghetti and macaroni, not highly seasoned	Same as light diet	Gruels, strained or blended
Breads	All	Enriched and whole-wheat bread, crackers	Same as light diet	
Soups and broths	All	All	Broth, strained cream soups	Same as soft diet, or blended
Meat, fish and poultry	All	Tender steaks and chops, lamb, veal, ground or tender beef, bacon, chicken, sweetbreads, liver, fish	Tender chicken, fish and sweetbreads; ground beef and lamb	
Eggs	Eggs cooked all ways	Soft-cooked eggs	Same as light diet	Eggnogs*
Dairy products	Milk or buttermilk; cream; butter; cheese, all kinds	Milk or buttermilk; cream, butter; cottage and cream cheese, Cheddar cheese used in cooking	Same as light diet	Milk or buttermilk, cream
Vegetables	All, including salads	Cooked vegetables: asparagus, peas, string beans, spinach, carrots, beets, squash Salads: tomato and lettuce Potatoes: boiled, mashed, creamed, scalloped, baked	Cooked vegetables: same as light diet Salads: none Potatoes: same as light diet	
Desserts	All	Ices, ice cream, junket, cereal puddings, custard, gelatin, simple cakes, plain cookies	Same as light diet	Ices, ice cream, gelatin, junket and custard
Beverages	All	Tea, coffee, cocoa; coffee substitutes; milk and milk beverages; carbonated beverages	Same as light diet	Same as light diet

* Because of the danger of salmonella infection when raw egg is used, a pasteurized commercial eggnog preparation is recommended.

TABLE 19–3. Typical Menus for Progressive Hospital Diets

Regular Diet	Light Diet	Soft Diet	Full Liquid Diet
Breakfast			
Fresh pear	Orange	Orange juice	Orange juice, strained
Oatmeal with milk or cream	Oatmeal with milk or cream	Oatmeal with milk or cream	Strained oatmeal gruel with milk or cream
Scrambled eggs	Soft scrambled eggs	Soft scrambled eggs	Coffee with cream and sugar
Buttered whole-wheat toast	Buttered whole-wheat toast	Buttered whole-wheat or white toast	
Coffee with cream and sugar	Coffee with cream and sugar	Coffee with cream and sugar	*10 A.M.*
			Eggnog*
Dinner			
Vegetable soup	Vegetable soup	Strained vegetable soup	Broth with rice
Roast veal	Roast veal	Ground beef	Ginger ale with ice cream
Mashed potato	Mashed potato	Mashed potato	Coffee with cream and sugar
Buttered broccoli	Buttered carrots	Buttered carrots	
Tomato salad with French dressing	Tomato salad with French dressing	Bread: whole-wheat or white	
Bread: whole-wheat, rye or white	Bread: whole-wheat, rye or white	Butter	
Butter	Butter	Vanilla ice cream with chocolate sauce	
Peppermint stick ice cream	Peppermint stick ice cream		
Milk	Milk	Milk	
			3 P.M.
			Malted milk or buttermilk
Supper			
Cream of pea soup with crackers	Cream of pea soup with crackers	Cream of pea soup with crackers	Strained cream of pea soup
Macaroni au gratin	Macaroni au gratin	Macaroni au gratin	Plain gelatin with whipped topping
Head lettuce salad with Russian dressing	Head lettuce salad with French dressing	Buttered beets	Tea with cream and sugar
Bread	Bread	Bread	
Butter	Butter	Butter	*9 P.M.*
Fruit gelatin	Fruit gelatin	Plain gelatin with whipped topping	Hot cocoa
Tea with cream and sugar	Tea with cream and sugar	Tea with cream and sugar	

* See note, Table 19–2.

The foods used in the medical soft diet are generally the same as those used in the soft diet in Table 19–2. In the surgical soft diet less tender meats and certain vegetables and fruits may be puréed or blenderized.

Dental or Mechnical Soft Diet. The regular diet may need modification for patients with poor teeth or none, or with dentures which they are unable or unwilling to wear. The nurse can be of help by seeing that the term "dental soft" is included in the diet order. Additional cooked vegetables or juices should be substituted for salads, and no whole meats should be served, unless the physician approves of the patient eating whole tender meats. Otherwise the diet should follow the foods used in the Light Diet.

The Full Liquid Diet. Liquid diets are usually prescribed for the postoperative patient, or the patient acutely ill with an infection, gastrointestinal tract disturbances, or a myocardial infarction. See Table 19–2 for the kinds of fluids used and Table 19–3 for a suggested menu.

Clear Liquid Diet. If the patient's condition requires it, only clear fluids may be offered him. In addition to water, clear broth, ginger ale, thin gruels made with water, plain gelatin, and tea and coffee are generally used. Carbonated beverages may or may not be used, depending on the policy set by the physicians and dietitians.

Both the clear and the full liquid diet are low in nutritive value. The clear liquid diet is used for only limited periods of time, usually no longer than 24 to 36 hours. When the full liquid diet must be used for a period of time special attention must be given to improving its nutritive value. Skim milk powder, protein supplements, cream, and sugars may be used to increase its protein and calorie content. Some suggestions for doing this are included in Chapter 36.

Patients receiving liquid diets will require a feeding every 2 to 3 hours during the day and evening. When it is not possible for the dietary department personnel to serve these patients other than at regularly scheduled meal times, nurses have found it helpful to remind themselves of a patient's need for an interval feeding by noting this at the proper time interval in the nursing care plan. Also, when the nurse observes that a patient is ready for more than a liquid diet, she can often tactfully suggest this to the physician so that he will revise the patient's diet order.

THERAPEUTIC DIETS

Therapeutic diets are planned as part of the treatment, in the following situations:

1. **Abnormalities of digestion and absorption:** Foods offered are modified in texture and consistency in the treatment of diseases of the gastrointestinal tract such as peptic ulcers and diarrhea. Also, food may be modified because of the lack of a digestive enzyme(s); the lack of bile to emulsify fat: or because an end product of digestion cannot be absorbed.

2. **Energy needs:** The calorie content of the diet is modified for overweight and underweight patients.

3. **Utilization of nutrient(s) by the body:** The treatment of a variety of diseases requires a specific modification of one or more nutrients—for example, carbohydrate in diabetes mellitus; sodium in cardiac disease; protein and sodium in kidney disease and cirrhosis of the liver; and a specific amino acid, phenylalanine, in phenylketonuria.

4. **Correction of malnutrition:** The nutritionally debilitated patient needs special attention to help him re-establish good food habits.

The pattern dietary is used, insofar as possible, as the foundation for therapeutic diets, except those used in emergencies or for short periods of time such as test diets. This not only helps to ensure the nutritional adequacy of the therapeutic diet but also serves to teach the patient how his particular diet order is met from his family's foods. When the therapeutic diet plan cannot for any reason provide an adequate intake of vitamins and minerals the physician should be informed so that he can supplement the diet with vitamins and other medicinal concentrates.

NUTRITIONAL ADEQUACY OF HOSPITAL DIETS

In the previous chapter some of the problems which may be encountered in feeding the hospitalized patient were discussed. There is further need for observation of the patient's appetite, particularly in the long-term, chronically ill patient. In a study by Goodman and Dowdell[1] it was found that of 431 chronically ill patients, 138 suffered from undernutrition. Duncan[2] has reported that a survey of the medical wards of the hospital with which he is connected showed that 37 per cent of the patients consumed grossly inadequate diets, including 13 per cent who ate less than 1,000 calories a day. These findings show the need of constant watchfulness of both chronically and acutely ill patients.

The diet as the dietitian writes and serves it may meet all the doctor's specifications and be adequate for the nutritional needs of the patient, but, unless the patient eats and retains it, little has been accom-

[1] Goodman, J. I., and Dowdell, W.: Ann. Int. Med., 43:1241, 1955.
[2] Duncan, G. G.: Am. J. Gastroent. 36:309, 1961.

plished. Here again the nurse and the dietitian must work hand in hand. Not only must the diet be made as acceptable as possible by catering to the patient's likes and dislikes, but, if he still finds it difficult to eat, every effort must be made to meet his nutritional needs in other ways.

The nurse's observations are of great practical value in helping the dietitian and the physician become aware of the patient's lack of appetite, and in helping to determine its cause. The very ill patient, or the patient who lacks appetite, will take fluids more easily than solid food. Small servings on his tray supplemented with a high-protein or a high-caloric beverage may help to meet the problem. Occasionally a patient will accept a high-protein, high-caloric beverage 6 times a day for a few days and then return to a tray with a renewed appetite. Even tube feeding may need to be used to maintain the patient's nutritional status, although this should never be done in a punitive fashion. Directions for such feedings will be found in Chapter 29.

STUDY QUESTIONS AND ACTIVITIES

1. Compare the menu selections of a patient on a regular diet with the pattern dietary. Will his selections provide adequately for his nutrient needs?

2. Record the 24-hour intake of a patient on a clear liquid diet. Using the food tables in Part IV estimate his calorie and nutrient intake. How adequate was this diet for him?

3. Compare the soft diet in the diet manual your hospital uses with the soft diet in Table 19–2. Are there any differences in the foods used in the two plans? With the help of your instructor determine the reasons for these differences.

4. In which ways may diets be modified to meet therapeutic needs? Illustrate with the diet of a patient observed by you.

5. Have you observed any patients with poor appetites? What are some of the causes? What attempts are being made to improve the patient's food intake? Have these been successful?

SUPPLEMENATRY READINGS ON PROGRESSIVE HOSPITAL DIETS

Coston, H. M.: Dining room service for hospital patients. Nursing Outlook, 7:425, 1959.

Newton, M. E., and Folta, J.: Hospital food can help or hinder care. Am. J. Nursing, 67:112-113, 1967 (Jan.).

For further references see Bibliography in Part Four.

CHAPTER 20

Fevers and Infections

Fevers of Short Duration • Chronic Fevers and Infections • Acute Infection

Fever is a condition that is characterized by an elevation of body temperature above normal. It always is accompanied by an increase in metabolism. In most febrile conditions the metabolic rate is increased 7 per cent for each degree Fahrenheit rise in temperature. (12 per cent for each degree Centigrade). As a result, the carbohydrate stores are quickly exhausted, and body protein and stored fat are used for energy if insufficient food is eaten. There is also a loss of body fluids and electrolytes, especially sodium chloride. In planning the diet for such patients, these factors must be kept in mind.

The advent of the antibiotics has shortened the course of many fevers from weeks to days. Typhoid fever is such an infection, and so is pneumococcic pneumonia. These now can be classed with fevers of short duration such as colds, grippe and influenza. Subacute bacterial endocarditis may run a somewhat longer course, even with antibiotics. Recently, the course of rheumatic fever has been much curtailed by the use of the hormone ACTH (adrenocorticotropic hormone) and the steroid hormones. The fever that accompanies poliomyelitis may be of short duration, but it is extremely destructive of body tissues. Pneumonia due to one of the viruses may be accompanied by a low-grade fever for several weeks. However, we still have fevers that may last for months—even years—and, therefore, may be classed as chronic. Tuberculosis is a fever of this type. Another is malaria. Although this disease is not common in North America and northern Europe, it is found in many other parts of the world despite efforts to eradicate it. Because it is accompanied by intermittent high fever, it makes great demands on the nutritional stores of the body.

If an infection accompanied by fever is superimposed on malnutrition, the nutritional consequences may be critical. In countries like the United States this may occur among elderly people living on limited incomes; among any of the low income groups, particularly in the children; among teenagers with erratic food habits; and among patients suffering from a chronic disease. In underdeveloped countries, particularly where protein intake is low and calories limited, the onset of infection presents a much more serious problem than in well-nourished individuals.

Effect of Infection on Appetite. Loss of appetite and intolerance to food usually accompany serious infection. Fluids of low caloric value are best tolerated but hardly meet the nutritional requirements. This can be of serious consequence in an already malnourished patient, especially if he is a child.

Special Nursing Problems. The food service to patients with suspected or confirmed contagious disease presents special problems in the hospital, since other patients and staff must be protected from cross-infection. Each hospital will have its own procedure for this which must be rigidly followed. The patient "on isola-

271

tion" often has many fears and anxieties. It is important that his food continue to be palatable and that it be attractively and promptly served, for psychological as well as nutritional reasons.

FEVERS OF SHORT DURATION

Metabolic Changes. In acute febrile conditions both the energy metabolism and the protein metabolism are increased. The longer the fever lasts and the greater the elevation of the temperature, the greater will be the loss of protein from the body tissues. This will be excreted chiefly in the urine in the form of nitrogen compounds. Body fluids also are lost, as well as the electrolytes of the blood and the tissues. There will be an increased need for those vitamins involved in metabolism.

Dietary Treatment

Because of the increased metabolism and the destruction of body protein, it will be necessary, sooner or later, to increase both the caloric and the protein intake. But since the digestion is also disturbed, and because the fever is of short duration, it is often advisable to disregard these needs for a few days in order to lessen the work of the gastrointestinal tract. A liquid diet consisting of 800 to 1,200 calories, adjusted somewhat to the appetite of the patient, will suffice through the early, acute stages of the fever. It is important that the calories be increased as quickly as possible.

The liquid diet (see Chap. 19) is usually prescribed because it is easy to eat and the fluids will contribute to the needed fluid intake of 3 to 4 quarts of liquid a day to prevent dehydration. Feedings should be given every two hours.

Fruit juices, including lemon, orange, pineapple, tomato and grapefruit, are given frequently. Tea and coffee (not too strong) with cream and sugar may be given 2 or 3 times a day. Carbonated beverages may be used to lend variety and to increase fluid consumption.

Broths and strained soups are important for their stimulating effect, and as conveyors of salt (sodium chloride), which will be used to replace body losses of this substance as well as fluids.

Milk and milk drinks should be added to the diet as soon as they are tolerated. The addition of lactose or flavored syrups and one or two tablespoons of dry skim milk or eggnog mixture will contribute protein and calories. Gruels and thin cereals served with milk or cream are warm and bland and often well tolerated by the very sick patient.

Vitamin supplements may be prescribed by the physician, especially if the patient is debilitated or malnourished.

During convalescence solid foods, such as crisp toast with butter, toasted breakfast cereals (without bran), soft-cooked eggs, baked or mashed potatoes and, later, soft-cooked vegetables may be added. In other words, the liquid diet is followed by a soft diet, later by a light diet, and still later by a normal diet. If there has been loss of weight, it is advisable to increase the protein in the diet, with calories adequate for the patient's need.

If the weight and the protein losses have been considerable, the protein intake should be at least 1½ times the normal requirement.

In countries where milk and eggs are not easily obtainable, the use of a vegetable protein mixture devised for infants, such as Incaparina in Central America and L'Aubina in the Middle East, may be of value in meeting the nutritional needs of the patient with a fever.

The diet in typhoid fever may differ somewhat from that in other acute fevers in that it should be high in calories and low in residue (see Chap. 27). Milk and cream, malted beverages and gruel or ginger ale with cream are indicated in frequent feedings if the patient tolerates them. Lactose may be added for extra calories. Fruit juices had best be omitted, as they tend to distend the typhoid patient. Fortunately, the use of antibiotics has greatly shortened the course of the disease, and it is no longer necessary to keep the patient on this diet for several weeks.

The diet in virus pneumonia should follow that described under Fevers of Short Duration. It should be remembered that it may be several weeks before the patient has recovered from the infection and that there may be considerable loss of weight and strength unless care is taken that the diet is as nutritious as possible.

The diet in rheumatic fever should be the same as that in other fevers. In the acute stage, it should be liquid and as high in calories and protein as feasible. If ACTH or one of the steriod hormones is used, the diet may have to be restricted in sodium. (See Chap. 24.) These hormones tend to increase sodium re-absorption in the kidneys, which in turn causes fluid retention and edema. (See Part Four, Table 5, for sodium content of food.) In the chronic stage, the diet may be general or soft and, if carditis is present, low in sodium. (See Chap. 24 for low sodium diets.)

Poliomyelitis. With the introduction of the Salk and the Sabin vaccines, the incidence of this dread infection has diminished markedly in countries where practically all children have been immunized. Even so, cases still occur, and in lands where complete immunization has not yet been achieved, outbreaks of poliomyelitis constitute a serious problem. The need for maintaining good nutritional status in both the acute and chronic phases of the disease is of first importance.

The diet in the acute stage is the same as that in fevers of short duration. Since there may be extremely rapid tissue destruction,[1] protein intake should be at as high a level as it is possible to obtain. In the acute stage, protein supplements may be tolerated better than milk and milk beverages, particularly if there is involvement of the trunk and the neck. Milk may increase the production of mucus in the throat, which is dangerous, because such patients cannot cough. Thin gruels and thinned mashed potatoes sometimes are taken more easily than clear fluids such as tea and broth. Because with cell destruction there are also large losses of potassium from the body, orange juice, which is high in potassium, should be included frequently. (See the suggested diet on this page.)

NURSING PROBLEMS. If in the acute phase of the disease the muscles concerned with

TABLE 20–1. Liquid Diet for the Acute Stage of Poliomyelitis

Breakfast	Strained orange juice with lactose
	Hot gruel with sugar and salt
	Tea with sugar and lemon
10 A.M.	Strained fruit juice with added protein supplement and lactose
Lunch	Hot broth with added gelatin
	Strained vegetable juice with added protein supplement
	Lemon ice
2 P.M.	As at 10 A.M.
4 P.M.	As at 10 A.M.
Supper	Strained clear vegetable soup with added gelatin
	Tomato juice with added protein supplement
	Grapefruit juice gelatin
8 P.M.	Any of the above
10 P.M.	Any of the above

the swallowing mechanism are involved, it may be necessary to give all nutrients by vein in the form of glucose, fat emulsion, protein hydrolysates and electrolyte solutions. As soon as it is possible to pass a plastic tube through the nose into the stomach, tube feedings should be begun. A discussion of tube feedings will be found in Chapter 29. At first the quantities will be small, but they should be increased as rapidly as the patient can tolerate them. When the ability to swallow returns, liquid feedings by mouth may be started.[2]

As soon as the disease subsides, and particularly if there is much tissue damage, an attempt should be made to restore good nutritional status. A high caloric, high protein diet is indicated, and every attempt should be made to get these patients to eat as soon and as much as possible. A general or soft house diet (see Chap. 19) plus high caloric, high protein beverages between meals, if eaten, will go far toward this goal (see Chap. 36 for recipes).

Fortunately, many poliomyelitis patients recover from the disease with little or no permanent nerve damage. These patients

[1] Bower, A. G., *et al.*: Am. J. M. Sc., 223:532, 1952.

[2] Seifert, M. H.: J. Am. Dietet. A., 30:671, 1954.

will do well on the diet described in the foregoing paragraph and present no further nutritional problems. It is the patients with extensive loss of muscle function who need special care. They are often depressed and may be resistant to eating, either because it is too much trouble or because they have lost interest in life. They present a challenge to the dietitian and the nurse which must be met constantly and with unflagging imagination. To talk to these patients about the need for eating meets with little success. The trays must be inviting—the food, if possible of the patient's own choosing and of such consistency and arrangement that it can be managed without spilling. For instance, fingers may be of more importance than forks in the matter of salads. Dishes with hot-water reservoirs beneath them will keep food hot longer than the ordinary dinner plate. All food should be so arranged on the tray that it is easily reached by the patient. If he needs help, it should be given unobtrusively, so as to minimize his need of it. If he must be fed, as with patients in respirators or on rocking beds, the nurse should assume a comfortable position, either sitting or standing, so that the patient will not feel hurried.

If the family lives within visiting distance, they should be encouraged to cook and bring some of the patient's favorite dishes and feed the patient themselves if this can be arranged. These patients present nutritional problems of long duration. It is the patience and the persistence of those caring for them in this as in other matters that may restore them eventually to a useful place in society.

COMPLICATIONS. Patients who are permanently immobilized have a tendency, despite more than adequate diets, to lose nitrogen and calcium from their tissues. This may happen even when they spend much of their time on rocking beds. The loss of calcium from the bones may lead to increased urinary excretion of calcium and the formation of calcium phosphate stones in the kidney. For the moderately low calcium, low phosphorus diet used in the treatment and the prevention of such stones, see Chapter 25.

CHRONIC FEVERS AND INFECTIONS
Tuberculosis

Etiology and Symptoms. Of the chronic infections, tuberculosis is the most prevalent throughout the world. Despite the discovery of antibiotic therapy, and the immunization programs of UNICEF and WHO, the disease affects great numbers of people, particularly in areas of poverty, poor sanitation, ignorance and malnutrition.

The infection is due to the tubercle bacillus, which may involve any or all tissues of the body, but the lungs are most commonly affected. Pulmonary tuberculosis is characterized by the elevation of temperature, by coughing and expectoration, and by loss of weight and strength. Because of the fever, the caloric needs are increased while for the same reason the appetite decreases. The food intake does not keep pace with the need, and weight loss and fatigue result.

Dietary Treatment. Although antibiotics and other medications, where these are available, are doing much to control tuberculosis, they do not effect an immediate cure. Therefore, the diet continues to be highly important in treatment. It should be moderately high in protein to promote healing and high enough in calories to regain lost weight. For example, a man weighing 70 Kg. but confined to bed should receive from 2,500 to 2,800 calories; if he is an ambulatory patient, this should be raised to from 2,800 to 3,000 calories, reduced or modified according to age (see Chap. 10). When the patient has reached his ideal weight, or slightly above, the high protein diet should be continued, but the calories should be sufficient only to maintain the weight.

It is known that the basal metabolism of the tuberculous patient is increased only moderately, and that destruction of body tissues (protein) is not as marked as in some other fevers. Nevertheless, the protein intake should be liberal, averaging from 75 to 100 Gm. per day for adults.

The diet should include all the foods rich in minerals and vitamins. Calcium is important for the calcification of the tuberculous nodes. Brewer and her co-

TABLE 20–2. A Sample Menu for a Tuberculous Patient

Breakfast	Dinner	Supper
Citrus fruit	Soup, vegetable or cream	Tomato or fruit juice
Cereal, enriched, with half milk and half cream, sugar	Meat or poultry	Soup, consomme or cream
Egg and bacon	Potato or substitute	Fish, shellfish or cheese dish
Toast, 2 slices, or muffins	Vegetable, green or yellow, cooked	Vegetable or fruit salad
Butter or margarine	Vegetable, raw, salad	Bread or roll
Jam, jelly or marmalade	Roll or bread	Butter or margarine
Coffee with sugar and cream	Butter or margarine	Sponge cake with ice cream
	Glass of milk	Tea or coffee with cream and sugar
	Dessert, baked apple or other fruit	
10 A.M.	**3 P.M.**	**9 P.M.**
Malted milk made with milk	Eggnog Crackers or cookies	Hot cocoa with sweet roll or crackers

workers[3] have shown the need for a greatly increased intake of calcium in a study of tuberculous women if they are to maintain calcium balance. Iron is necessary if there has been hemoptysis (hemorrhage from the lungs). Getz[4] found low blood levels of ascorbic acid and vitamin A in patients with tuberculosis. Vitamin D is known to be essential for the absorption and the metabolism of calcium. The B vitamins, having a role in the oxidation of food, should be increased if fever is persistent; they may also stimulate the appetite. When marked malnutrition accompanies the disease, the use of vitamin supplements and perhaps iron medication is indicated.

Of the foods especially indicated in tuberculosis, milk stands at the head of the list because of its high content of excellent protein, calcium and vitamins. At least a quart a day should be consumed. This may be taken in any form desired—plain, in cream soups and in desserts. Cultured milks such as yoghurt or buttermilk are digested more easily than sweet milk and have the advantage of introducing variety into the diet.

Eggs, meat, fish, poultry and cheese should be used freely. Fruits and the non-gaseous vegetables should be included because of their richness in vitamins and in minerals. Fats and carbohydrates in abundance will help to meet the caloric needs.

The food should be simply prepared and easy to digest. Table 20–2 shows a day's diet for a patient in the United States requiring 3,000 calories and approximately 100 Gm. of protein.

The use of legumes should be encouraged for patients for whom this is a staple food, and who may not be able to obtain sufficient protein from the more costly animal foods. The vegetable protein concentrates, mentioned earlier in this chapter, have been developed in many areas in the world, and will also be found of value in meeting the nutritional needs of the tuberculosis patient.

It is essential that the economic circumstances of the tuberculous patient be investigated before he is discharged, so that the benefits of his hospitalization are not lost. Especially if the patient is the breadwinner, the family may be living on a much reduced income, and the cost of a high-caloric, high-protein diet at home may be prohibitive. Again, the nurse is often the first person to become aware of this problem, which should be referred promptly to such community services as are available.

DRUG COMPLICATIONS. It has been found that large doses of isoniazid, one of the antibiotics used commonly in the treatment of tuberculosis, causes rapid excretion of pyridoxine or vitamin B_6. The deficiency results in peripheral neuritis and, possibly, anemia. For this reason, pyridoxine may be given along with isoniazid as a preventive measure.[5]

[3] Brewer, W. D., *et al.*: J. Am. Dietet. A., *30*:21, 1954.
[4] Getz, H. R.: J. Am. Dietet. A., *30*:17, 1954.
[5] Ross, R. R.: J.A.M.A., *168*:273, 1958.

Malaria

Malaria is another infection which is endemic in many parts of the world. In most developed countries it has been eradicated, but military personnel returning from affected areas such as Viet Nam show a high incidence of malaria despite preventive drugs. They are carefully screened and treated, if necessary, before they are declared free of the disease. Extensive efforts are being made to erase malaria by national and international health agencies, aided by WHO, but the disease still affects great numbers of people—again, particularly those living in poverty.

Malaria is accompanied by intermittent high fever, which drains the patient of all nutritional reserve. Everything that has been said in the earlier parts of this chapter on the dietary needs in fevers applies here also. During the bouts of fever fluids, calories, mainly in the form of sugars, and salt are of first importance. In convalescence the principles laid down for the diet in tuberculosis apply here also.

ACUTE INFECTION

Cholera

Asiatic cholera is a bacterial infection of the intestine which produces a sudden, massive diarrhea. Loss of sodium and other electrolytes and of water leads within a few hours to profound shock and death. It has recently been reported[6] that this sequence of events can be reversed, after initial rehydration intravenously, by the oral administration of a solution of electrolytes and glucose, and the addition of an antibiotic. The glucose aids in the reabsorption of sodium and water from the intestinal tract and markedly reduces the loss of these substances in the stool, while the antibiotic combats the bacterial infection. This procedure gives rise to the hope that it may become widely available so that recovery from this dread infection may be possible for many more patients than is presently the case.

---

[6] Medical News—World Wide Report. May 15, 1967.

STUDY QUESTIONS AND ACTIVITIES

1. A patient who has a basal caloric requirement of 1,500 calories is running a temperature of 104°. How many more calories will he need because of this increase in temperature?

2. Write a day's liquid diet menu for a patient with an acute fever of short duration. How frequently should he be fed?

3. Has the procedure for the prevention of cross-infection for patients "on isolation" affected the food intake of any patient under your observation? How? What could be done about it?

4. What are the characteristics of the diet used for typhoid fever? Explain the reason for each one.

5. Plan a high-caloric soft diet for a patient with typhoid fever.

6. What problems may be encountered in feeding the poliomyelitis patient?

7. Plan a high-protein semisoft diet for a patient recovering from poliomyelitis who has difficulty feeding himself.

8. How can the moderately low calcium, low phosphorus diet be increased in protein? In calories? (See Chap. 25.)

9. What factors should be considered in the feeding of patients with tuberculosis?

10. Suggest 5 different high-caloric between-meal feedings that a patient may use to increase his caloric intake.

11. What additions can be made to the regular diet to increase the calories?

12. What foods may be used to increase the protein content of the diet when sufficient animal protein is not available?

13. Why are malarial patients in underdeveloped countries often very malnourished? What are the principles of dietary treatment?

14. What is the mechanism by which glucose aids in the absorption of sodium in the intestinal tract? (See Chap. 9.)

SUPPLEMENTARY READING ON FEVERS AND INFECTIONS

Andrews, J. M.: Perspective on malaria today. J.A.M.A., *184*:873, 1963.

Everson, G. J.: Bases for concern about teenagers diets. J. Am. Dietet. A., *36*:17, 1960.

Getz, H. R.: Problems in feeding the tuberculous patient. J. Am. Dietet. A., *30*:17, 1954.

Plum, F.: Prevention of urinary calculi after paralytic poliomyelitis. J.A.M.A., *168*:1302, 1958.

Ross, R. R.: Use of pyridoxine hydrochloride to prevent isoniazid toxicity. J.A.M.A., *168*: 273, 1958.

Scrimshaw, N. S.: Malnutrition and infection. Borden's Rev., *26*: No. 2, 1965.

Seifert, M. H.: Poliomyelitis and the relation of diet to its treatment. J. Am. Dietet. A., *30*:671, 1954.

For further references see Bibliography in Part Four.

CHAPTER 21

Weight Control

Health Implications of Weight Status • Obesity • Causes • Prevention • Dietary Treatment • The Calorie-Restricted Pattern Dietary • Treatment Other Than Diet • Patient Education • Underweight

INTRODUCTION

The concept of what constitutes correct weight has undergone marked revision in recent years. Even today the definition of the terms *normal* or *desirable* weight is sharply debated. To assess the weight status of individuals we have traditionally used height-weight tables derived from experience with life insurance policy holders. The first tables for adults were based on the heights and weights of men and women at various ages. The figures in these tables were averages and reflected the actual weights of the individuals. Since the data showed an increase in weight with age the recommended weight for height in the tables increased with each age group. For example: it was recommended that a woman 5 feet 4 inches tall weigh 131 pounds at age 30, and 144 pounds at age 55.[1]

In recent years the height-weight tables have been re-evaluated and revised. It is recognized that, when growth in height has been achieved, there is no biological need to gain weight in excess of that which is satisfactory for the individual. Also the best health prognosis is found in individuals of average or less than average weight in their early 20's who maintain this weight throughout their adult years. Studies indicate that certain diseases in adults are associated with excessive weight, and that

fat people are more likely to die at a younger age than people of normal weight (see Fig. 21–1).

It must be remembered that body weight is made up of a number of components: fat, muscle, organs, bone and fluid. At the same time as height and weight data have been re-evaluated, body build and body fatness have been studied. As yet there is no method for estimating body build easily. Given two men of the same height, the one with a large frame will normally weigh more than the one with a small frame.

As sophisticated methods for studying body composition have been developed over the past twenty years, we are learning that, in the assessment of an individual's weight status, we must be as concerned with the estimation of total body fatness as with the measurement of height and weight. It is possible for an individual, for example an athlete, to weigh more than recommended due to a greater than expected amount of muscle, not to excessive body fatness. On the other hand, an individual of "desirable" weight for height and age may have an excess of body fatness. The measurement of skinfold thickness with calipers determines body fatness. Research workers are presently establishing norms for this measurement, and it can be expected that physicians, nurses, and dietitians will be trained to use calipers just as

---

[1] Cooper, Barber and Mitchell, 7th ed., 1940.

they are now trained to weigh and measure patients accurately (see Fig. 21–2).

The revised weight tables in current use reflect the concern for maintaining over the life span the weight appropriate for an individual at age 25 and, at the same time, take into consideration body build. The Metropolitan Life Insurance Company's Desirable Weight Tables, published in 1960, give desirable weight ranges for heights for men and women 25 years of age and over, and allow for differences in body frame, which is designated as small, medium, and large. The range for a 5'4" woman with a small frame is 108 to 116 pounds; with a medium frame, 113 to 126 pounds; and with a large frame, 121 to 138 pounds.

OVERWEIGHT SHORTENS LIFE

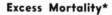

Excess Mortality*

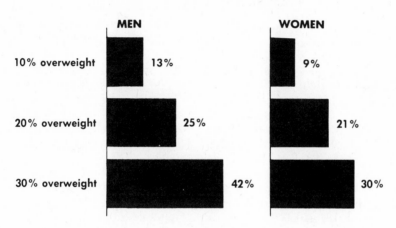

	MEN	WOMEN
10% overweight	13%	9%
20% overweight	25%	21%
30% overweight	42%	30%

EXCESS MORTALITY DUE CHIEFLY TO HEART AND CIRCULATORY DISEASES

Excess* for Principal Diseases Among Persons About 20% or More Overweight

	Men	Women
Heart disease	43%	51%
Cerebral hemorrhage	53%	29%
Malignant neoplasms	16%	13%
Diabetes	133%	83%
Digestive system diseases (gall stones, cirrhosis, etc.)	68%	39%

*Compared with mortality of Standard risks
(Mortality ratio of Standard risks = 100%)

FIG. 21–1. (From Overweight—Its Significance and Prevention. Metropolitan Life Insurance Company. Derived from The Build and Blood Pressure Study, Society of Actuaries, 1959)

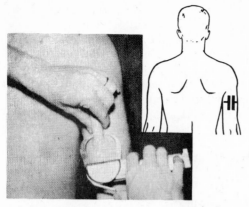

FIG. 21–2. Skinfold measurement at back of upper arm (triceps). Hertzberg, H. T. E., Churchill, E., Dupertius, C. W., White, R. M., and Damon, A. (Aerospace Medical Research Laboratories, U.S.A.F.): Anthropometric Survey of Turkey, Greece and Italy, 1963. p. 120. Pergamon Press.

In 1960 Hathaway and Foard published a table of suggested weights for heights for men and women.[2] (See Part Four, Table 12.) The weights in this table are based on those of men 25 to 29 years old and women 20 to 24 years old measured in a study carried out in 1948-1950. The weights for heights are given in ranges of low, median and high, and body build determines where within the ranges a given normal weight will fall. For example, for a woman 5′4″ tall, and of small frame, the recommended weight is 113 pounds; with a large frame, it is 132 pounds. It is advised that weight should not vary with age by more than 5 pounds for shorter adults and 10 pounds for taller individuals.

Overweight—Obesity. Although there is not as yet general agreement, the following description of overweight and obesity are being used. *Overweight* is "over-heaviness" and the term does not carry any direct implications with regard to fatness. *Obesity* is described as a bodily condition marked by excessive generalized deposition and storage of fat or adipose tissue. Until we are able to estimate with some degree of accuracy an individual's fatness it will con-

tinue to be difficult to identify the obese individual, except for those individuals who are obviously obese.

Underweight. In the United States in recent years the problem of *underweight* in the population has received little attention. We continue to regard 20 per cent or more below desirable weight to be dangerous. Underweight is a major problem for many of the world's populations and is being studied extensively in infants and children in various parts of the world (see Chap. 16).

Health Implications of Weight Status

The adverse effects on health of excessive body fatness have been mentioned in the preceding paragraphs. The evidence from mortality and morbidity data presently available to us indicates that certain hazards to health are associated with obesity. These hazards can be classified as follows: (1) changes in normal body functions; (2) increased risk of developing certain diseases; (3) detrimental effects on established diseases; and (4) adverse psychological reactions.

The changes in normal body function most frequently observed in the obese are respiratory difficulties; cardiovascular dysfunction including cardiac enlargement, congestive failure, and elevated blood pressure; menstrual abnormalities; and impaired carbohydrate tolerance that may be severe enough to classify as diabetes mellitus (see Chap. 22).

In the obese, both men and women, an increase in mortality over the expected has been associated with diabetes, heart and circulatory diseases, digestive diseases, and nephritis. The markedly obese experience a higher mortality than individuals who are slightly obese. Obese pregnant women are more prone than non-obese women to toxemia and to complications during delivery, including still-births.

Loss of excessive fat benefits the individual who has had a myocardial infarction, or who has circulatory problems, diabetes mellitus, or problems of the skeletal system, including osteoarthritis, ruptured intervertebral discs and many other varieties of bone and joint disease.

---

[2] Hathaway, M. L., and Foard, E. D.: Home Ec. Report No. 10, U.S.D.A. August, 1960.

Some, though not all, obese patients have psychological disturbances. It is difficult to determine whether the obesity is the result of the disturbance. For some, the problem may result from a conflict with the standards of society—for example, the acceptance of the standards for weight set by models, entertainers and other public figures.

The health hazards of underweight are less well understood. Underweight people often suffer from non-specific symptoms such as fatigue and mild infections. Statistics indicate that tuberculosis is found more frequently in underweight persons than those of normal weight.

It will be remembered from the information presented in Chapter 5, Energy Metabolism, that the energy needs of an adult are determined primarily by his basal metabolism and degree of physical activity; while infants and children, adolescents and pregnant women require calories for growth as well.

OBESITY

Prevalence and Incidence. Obesity is considered a major public health problem today although there are no statistics for the general prevalence and incidence in the total population. However, the available data indicate a substantial prevalence of obesity at every age in both sexes. Excessive weight gain occurs more frequently at certain ages or periods in the life cycle. In women it occurs after the completion of growth, during pregnancies, and after the menopause. In men there is no one period when they are apt to be obese. They tend to gain weight between 25 to 40 years of age with some acceleration after age 40.[3] Individuals who become obese as children are apt to be obese adults and have more difficulty losing fat and maintaining the loss than those who become obese as adults.

Causes

Food Intake

Obesity is the result of a positive energy balance and can be due to a calorie intake

which exceeds the energy need. While excessive food intake does account for most obesity, not every obese person necessarily eats large quantities of food. Based on the fact that a pound of body fat contains approximately 3,500 calories, an intake in excess of even 100 calories a day will add up to 3,000 calories a month, or almost a pound of body weight. Over a year this will amount to a weight gain of 10 pounds.

Physical Activity

Energy expenditure is as important in the development of obesity as food intake. In the past 25 to 50 years life in the highly developed areas of the world has undergone great changes. Work hours have been shortened, labor-saving machinery has been installed in homes and factories, transportation is easier, homes are well heated, and even our leisure-time occupations are sedentary rather than active. This has reduced the energy needs of the body markedly, but, by and large, food habits have not changed sufficiently to offset the decreased need. Although the American breakfast is considerably smaller today than that which our forefathers were accustomed to eating, the coffee break, morning and afternoon, the increased use of sugar, the ubiquitous candy bar and the TV "snack" have more than compensated for the change in breakfast patterns. (See Table 21-1, Calorie Values of Common "Snack" Foods.)

A number of investigators have observed that the obese person, and particularly the obese child and adolescent, is less active than his counterpart of the same age. Whether this is due to his inability to keep pace with other children or to apathy born of emotional conflict, the inactivity lowers the energy need of the body and in this way contributes to the overweight. The above is also true of obese women as compared to women of normal weight. In obese men the difference in activity is less striking but still of significance.

Family Patterns

Studies show that overweight and obesity tend to exist as a family pattern. Mayer[4]

[3] Obesity and Health. P.H.S. Pub. No. 1485, 1966.

[4] Mayer, J.: Am. J. Clin. Nutr., 9:530, 1961.

TABLE 21–1. Caloric Values for Common "Snack" Foods

	Amount or Average Serving	Calorie Count
"Just a Little Sandwich"		
Hamburger on bun..................................	3-in. patty	330
Peanut butter......................................	1 tbsp. P.B.	330
Cheese...	1-oz. cheese	280
Ham..	1-oz. ham	320
Beverages		
Carbonated drinks, soda, root beer, etc..............	6-oz. glass	80
Cola beverages....................................	12-oz. glass (Pepsi)	150
Club soda..	8-oz. glass	5
Chocolate malted milk..............................	10-oz. glass (1¾ c.)	500
Ginger ale...	6-oz. glass	60
Tea or coffee, straight.............................	1 c.	0
Tea or coffee, with 2 tablespoons cream and 2 teaspoons sugar........................	1 c.	90
Alcoholic Drinks		
1 Ale..	8-oz. glass	155
1 Beer...	8-oz. glass	110
1 Highball (with ginger ale—ladies' style).............	8-oz. glass	185
1 Manhattan.......................................	Average	165
1 Martini..	Average	140
Wine, Muscatel or Port..............................	2-oz. glass	95
1 Sherry...	2-oz. glass	75
Scotch, bourbon, rye...............................	1½-oz. jigger	130
Fruits		
Apple..	1 3-in.	75
Banana..	1 6-in.	130
Grapes..	30 medium	75
Orange..	1 2¾-in.	70
Pear...	1	65
Salted Nuts		
Almonds, filberts, hazelnuts.........................	12-15	95
Cashews...	6-8	90
Peanuts..	15-17	85
Pecans, walnuts....................................	10-15 halves	100
Candies		
Chocolate bars,		
Plain, sweet milk...............................	1 bar (1 oz.)	155
With almonds................................	1 bar (1 oz.)	140
Chocolate-covered bar..............................	1 bar	270
Chocolate cream, bon bon, fudge....................	1 piece 1-in. square	90-120
Caramels, plain....................................	2 medium	85
Hard candies, Lifesaver type........................	1 roll	95
Peanut brittle......................................	1 piece 2½ x 2½ x ⅜ in.	110

(Adapted from Smith, Kline and French Laboratories)

TABLE 21–1. Caloric Values for Common "Snack" Foods (Continued)

	Amount or Average Serving	Calorie Count
Desserts		
Pie:		
Fruit—apple, etc..................................	1/6 pie 1 average serving	375
Custard..	1/6 pie 1 average serving	265
Mince..	1/6 pie 1 average serving	400
Pumpkin pie with whipped cream..................	1/6 pie 1 average serving	460
Cake:		
Chocolate layer...............................	3-in. section	350
Doughnut, sugared.............................	1 average	150
Sweets		
Ice Cream:		
Plain vanilla.................................	1/6 qt. serving	200
Chocolate and other flavors......................	1/6 qt., ⅔ c.	260
Orange sherbet...................................	½ c.	120
Sundaes, small chocolate nut with whipped cream..........	Average	400
Ice-cream sodas, chocolate..........................	10-oz. glass	270
Midnight Snacks for Icebox Raiders		
Cold potato	½ medium	65
Chicken leg.......................................	1 average	88
Glass milk..	7-oz. glass	140
Mouthful of roast.................................	½ in. x 2 in. x 3 in.	130
Piece of cheese....................................	¼ in. x 2 in. x 3 in.	120
Leftover beans....................................	½ c.	105
Brownie..	¾ in. x 1 ¾ in x 2 ¼ in.	140
Cream puff.......................................	4 in. diam.	450

found that 8 to 9 per cent of children of normal weight parents became obese. When one parent is obese, the likelihood of the child becoming obese is 40 per cent, and this proportion rises to 80 per cent when both parents are obese. There may be a genetic component, since this distribution is not true for adopted children. However, in most such families the pattern of food intake tends to be excessive and the body image of a "well fed person" is the preferred one. Such families may eat because plenty of food denotes prosperity or success in life, or because increased food intake has become an established pattern for relieving tension, boredom or emotional stress.

Emotional Problems

Many people who are overweight eat because they have nothing else to do. They may eat when they are under strain or when they feel unappreciated or lonely. Food now becomes a symbol of love, of satisfaction, or security. Stunkard and his co-workers[5] have described a so-called *night-eating syndrome* in some gravely obese patients. Such a patient eats little during the day, but in the evening and in the early night hours he consumes large quantities of food. Some of these patients exhibited symptoms of severe emotional stress when an attempt was made to reduce their weight. The investigators concluded that it might be wiser to allow such patients to remain obese than to precipitate an emotional illness with a weight reduction program.

Endocrine Glands

In a small percentage of patients obesity is caused by a disturbance of function of one or more of the endocrine glands, such

[5] Stunkard, A. J., *et al.*: Am. J. Med., 19:78, 1955.

as the thyroid (hypothyroidism) or the pituitary. In hypothyroidism part of the excess weight is due to fluid retention. Obesity should not be attributed to glandular abnormalities unless this is determined by specific diagnostic tests, e.g., the protein-bound iodine in plasma for thyroid function.

Balance Between Hunger and Satiety

In recent years there has been renewed interest in the physiologic control of hunger and satiety. Many individuals maintain a balance between food intake and energy expenditure which keeps their weight comparatively stable over a period of many years. Research indicates that the hypothalamus regulates food intake. Destruction of the ventromedial nuclei of the hypothalamus in the rat results in marked hyperphagia and extreme obesity, while the destruction of the outer part of the lateral hypothalamus in the rat results in a complete absence of food intake. There are many other factors which suggest that the hypothalamus may be involved in the balance of hunger and satiety and, therefore, in the maintenance of normal weight and, possibly, in the development of obesity.

Prevention of Obesity

Successful weight reduction and the maintenance of weight loss are not easily achieved. It is hoped that, as we learn more about the causes of obesity, health workers will focus their attention on the prevention of obesity at all stages in the life cycle.

Infants and Children

Studies indicate that many obese adults were obese children. Prevention of obesity begins with the careful supervision of the feeding of infants and children. The nurse in the pediatrician's office, the public health nurse in the clinic and home, and the school nurse can all play a role in prevention. Accurate weighing and measuring of infants and young children combined with a diet interview of the mother will give the physician clues to the development of a weight problem. Effective nutrition counseling of the mother may correct the problem in its earliest stages. At the same time it must be remembered that the weight status of a child may reflect a problem of mother-child relationships, not solely a nutrition problem.

For the school-age child the physical education programs in elementary and secondary schools should be directed to helping both boys and girls develop a lifetime pattern of physical activity. The present emphasis on team sports, which provide activity for only a few students, does not always help the individual to be active in his adult years.

Adults

As adults settle into a routine of daily living in their late twenties and early thirties, and if physical activity is limited because of the demands of their employment, a conscious effort should be made to limit calorie intake. For many of these adults this means decreasing their intake of such foods as sugar, high-calorie desserts and snacks, cream and other fats. The Pattern Dietary (Chap. 19, p. 265) with reasonable additions of food to maintain weight provides a guide for these individuals. For example: a man who maintained his normal weight at age 20 with a calorie intake of 3,000 calories may find at age 30 he will maintain his weight on 2,500 calories. Both the activity and the time devoted to it must be taken into consideration when exercise is combined with food intake to control body weight. It is the daily increase in physical activity rather than the occasional vigorous activity which is effective in controlling weight. Table 21–2

TABLE 21–2. Calorie Expenditure for Some Types of Activity*

	70 Kg. Man Cals./hour	58 Kg. Woman Cals./hour
Painting furniture.....	200	160
Walking (3 mi./hr.)...	240	190
Skating.............	340	285
Swimming (2 mi./hr.)..	685	570

* Calculated from the table *Energy Expenditures for Everyday Activities* in Chapter 5.

shows the calories expended by the 70-Kg. man (154 pounds) or the 58-Kg. woman (128 pounds) in various activities. It must be noted that these figures are for a full hour of continuous activity. For many adults in our society it is difficult to devote 1 hour every day to walking or swimming. A conscious effort to increase activity throughout the day may be possible—for example, walking to the second bus stop instead of the first, walking to the nearby grocery store or newsstand in place of driving the car, or walking up one flight of stairs instead of taking the elevator. In our society today finding a place to walk is often the real problem: many of our suburban areas have no sidewalks.

Controlling weight by diet and exercise is a family affair. The home-maker is often the one who bears the major responsibility for food. If her family has a tendency to gain weight easily she will have to pass up the recipes on the women's page of the newspaper which require 1 pint of whipping cream, 1 pint of sour cream, six ounces of cream cheese or ½ to ¾ pound of butter.

Dietary Treatment

Since an abnormal amount of adipose tissue is a storage of energy in excess of need, the calorie intake must be less than the actual daily energy need if the body is to draw upon and reduce its surplus of fat.

Determination of Present Practices. The first step in helping the obese patient is to determine, through individual interview, how he usually has lived his day and, specifically, his food and beverage intake and physical activity. An appraisal of his habitual food intake will give an indication of his daily calorie intake and the kinds of food he eats; an appraisal of his activity pattern will give an indication of his energy expenditure. From this information one can estimate a reduced calorie intake for him which should promote weight loss.

Calories. Considerable difficulty may be encountered in determining the level of reduced calorie intake for an individual. His previous intake may have been underestimated, or his energy expenditure overestimated. In theory, without increasing activity a deficit in intake of 500 calories per day, compared with previous intake, should

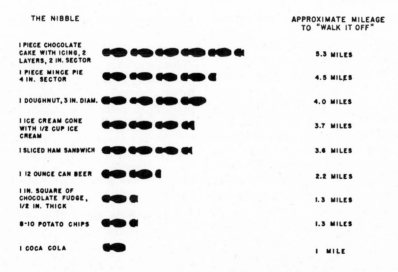

MILEAGE TO WALK OFF THAT NIBBLE

THE NIBBLE		APPROXIMATE MILEAGE TO "WALK IT OFF"
I PIECE CHOCOLATE CAKE WITH ICING, 2 LAYERS, 2 IN. SECTOR		5.3 MILES
I PIECE MINCE PIE 4 IN. SECTOR		4.5 MILES
I DOUGHNUT, 3 IN. DIAM.		4.0 MILES
I ICE CREAM CONE WITH 1/2 CUP ICE CREAM		3.7 MILES
I SLICED HAM SANDWICH		3.6 MILES
I 12 OUNCE CAN BEER		2.2 MILES
I IN. SQUARE OF CHOCOLATE FUDGE, 1/2 IN. THICK		1.3 MILES
8-10 POTATO CHIPS		1.3 MILES
I COCA COLA		I MILE

Fig. 21–3. Mileage to walk off that nibble (from Peyton, A. B.: Practical Nutrition. 2nd ed., p. 178. Philadelphia, J. B. Lippincott, 1962; adapted from Hauck, H. M.: How to control your weight. Ithaca, N. Y., New York State College of Home Economics).

promote a weight loss of approximately one pound per week. (500 Calories × 7 = 3,500 calories = 1 pound of fat.) A relatively sedentary obese woman 55 years old and 5 feet, 4 inches tall, who has been consuming approximately 1,700 calories per day, should lose weight on a 1,200-calorie diet, while a moderately active obese business executive 35 years old and 6 feet tall, who has been consuming 2,500 to 3,000 calories, should lose weight on a 2,000-calorie diet.

A deficit of 1,000 calories per day should promote a loss of 2 pounds per week. It is considered unwise for an individual to lose more than 2 pounds per week unless he is under the close supervision of his physician. It is generally considered unwise for a patient to be given a diet of less than 1,000 calories unless he is hospitalized.

Regardless of the level of calorie restriction prescribed by the physician, it must be recognized that, through variations in daily food selection and serving size, the actual calorie intake at home will not be exactly the number of calories ordered. For example a 1,200-calorie diet may vary by chance from 1,000 to 1,400 calories. Also, physical activity may vary from day to day. To be successful in carrying out a calorie restriction the patient needs careful diet instruction. Patient education is discussed later in this chapter.

Protein. At least one gram of protein per kilogram of desirable body weight for adults is used to supply the body's needs for this nutrient. Some doctors will prescribe a higher intake, 1½ grams of protein per kilogram. This allows for a more liberal use of meat, fish, eggs, and cottage cheese in the diet plan. At a very restricted level of calories (1,000 calories) this requires the careful selection of lean meat and fish.

Fat and Carbohydrate. Since these two nutrients constitute the greatest source of calories in the diet, they must be reduced. However, there is considerable difference of opinion as to whether carbohydrate or fat should be cut to a minimum. The usual calorie restricted diet will derive approximately half its calories from carbohydrate, as in the normal diet, and the calories from fat will be considerably reduced. One ad-

vantage of this division is that it permits the use of commonly accepted foods such as bread.

On the other hand, both Young and Cederquist and her co-workers advocate a diet with less carbohydrate and more fat than is usually included in the diet plan. They claim that patients find that such a diet has greater satiety value and, therefore, it is easier for the patient to follow. Recently, a limit of sixty grams of carbohydrate for calorie restricted diets has been recommended.[6] Counting grams of carbohydrate has become almost as popular with lay persons as counting calories.

Minerals and Vitamins. Care should be taken to see that the calorie restricted diet plan provides all the other essentials of a normal diet, such as minerals and vitamins, in quantities at least equivalent to the Recommended Dietary Allowances. If the calorie intake is very restricted (less than 1,000 Cal.) vitamin and mineral supplements may be needed.

Alcohol. One gram of alcohol provides 7 calories. Also, in some alcoholic beverages carbohydrate contributes calories. If these beverages are to be used, their calorie value must be calculated in the Calorie Restricted Pattern Dietary. For some patients the calories from the alcoholic beverages they consume may be the difference between losing and not losing weight. (See Table 7, Part Four.)

Water. Water and other non-nutritive fluids are not restricted unless there is some heart or kidney complication. Sometimes there is fluid retention in women prior to menstruation, which may temporarily mask the real loss of body fat. Early weight loss in some patients may be fluid loss rather than loss of adipose tissue.

Planning the Calorie-Restricted Pattern Dietary

1,200-Calorie Diet. Table 21–3, Composition of a 1,200 Calorie Diet demonstrates one way in which the Pattern Dietary in Chapter 19, p. 265, may be modified for calorie restriction. The daily amounts of

---

[6] Gordon, E. S., *et al.*: J.A.M.A., *186*:50-60, 1963.

TABLE 21–3. Composition of a 1,200-Calorie Diet[1]

Food Group	Amt. In Gm.	Amt. Household Measure	Calories	Protein Gm.	Fat Gm.	Carbohydrate Gm.	Minerals Calcium Mg.	Minerals Iron Mg.	Vitamins A I.U.	Vitamins Thiamine Mg.	Vitamins Riboflavin Mg.	Vitamins Niacin Mg.	Vitamins Ascorbic Acid Mg.
Milk, skim...........	492	2 c. (1 pt.)	176	17.6	..	26	594	0.4	..	0.20	0.88	0.4	4
Egg.............	50	1 medium	81	7	6	..	27	1.2	590	0.05	0.15	..	..
Meat, fish, fowl, lean ..	120	4 ozs., cooked	376	30	31	..	13	3.3	280	0.14	0.23	6.1	..
Vegetables:													
Deep green or yellow, cooked[2]....	150	2 servings	54	4	..	12	90	1.6	9,400	0.10	0.20	1.0	50
Other, cooked[2]	150	2 servings	90	4	..	20	36	1.6	600	0.16	0.12	1.2	24
Fruits:													
Citrus...........	100	1 serving	43	1	..	10	11	0.2	140	0.06	0.02	0.3	43
Other[3]..........	200	2 servings	146	1.4	1	38	22	1.6	740	0.06	0.08	1.0	8
Bread, white, enriched.	46	2 slices	124	4	2	24	38	1.2	..	0.12	0.10	1.2	..
Butter or margarine...	14	1 tablespoon	100	..	11	..	3	..	460	..	..	..	..
Totals............			1,190	69	51	130	834	11.1	12,210	0.89	1.78	11.2[4]	129
Compare with recommended allowances[5]												Niacin Equiv.	
Moderately active man (70 Kg., 18–15 yrs. old)			2,900	70	..	..	800	10.0	5,000	1.20	1.70	19	70
Moderately active woman (58 Kg., 18–35 yrs. old)			2,100	58	..	..	800	15.0	5,000	0.80	1.30	14	70

[1] Calculations from Composition of Foods. Handbook No. 8, U. S. D. A., Rev. 1963.

[2] See Pattern Dietary, Page 265, for basis of evaluations.

[3] Evaluation based on figures for apples, bananas, unsweetened prunes, water-pack peaches.

[4] The average diet in the U. S., which contains a generous amount of protein, provides enough tryptophan to increase the niacin value by about one-third.

[5] From the National Research Council Recommended Dietary Allowances, Rev. 1963.

TABLE 21–4. Food for a 1,200-Calorie Pattern Dietary

Food	Amounts
Milk, skim............	2 cups (1 pint)
Egg[1]................	1 medium
Meat, fish, or fowl, lean .	4 ounces (cooked)
Vegetables...........	4 servings (½ cup each)
Fruit[2]	
Citrus.............	1 serving
Other.............	2 servings
Bread, white, enriched[3]..	2 slices
Butter or margarine.....	1 tablespoon (3 tsps.)

[1] One ounce of meat may be substituted for one egg.
[2] See Exchange Lists, pp. 306-307, for size servings of various fruits.
[3] See Exchange Lists, pp. 306-307, for substitutes for one slice of bread.

food used in this 1,200-Calorie Restricted Pattern Dietary are summarized in Table 21–4. The food in this diet plan may be distributed among three meals, three meals with an evening snack, or 5 or 6 small meals a day. The suggested menu in Table 21–5 shows how the amounts of food might be used in three meals.

It must be stressed that no food other than non-caloric beverages and seasonings may be added to the 1,200-Calorie Restricted Pattern Dietary. For example, if fat is added to a serving of cooked vegetables, it will be part of the fat calculated in the pattern (1 tbsp. butter or margarine). When canned fruits are used, they

TABLE 21–5. Suggested Menu— 1,200-Calorie Diet

Breakfast	Noon Meal	Evening Meal
4 ounces orange juice	¼ cup cottage cheese	3 ounces lean roast beef
1 egg	tomato and lettuce	½ cup beets with 1 tsp. butter
1 slice toast	1 slice of bread	
1 tsp. butter	1 tsp. butter	cucumber and lettuce
coffee without cream or sugar	8 ounces skim milk	salad with vinegar
	1 small apple	8 ounces skim milk
		2 medium apricots, canned, without sugar

must be those which have been canned without sugar. Also, care must be taken to use the size serving defined in the Household Measure column, Table 21–3.

Of the calories in this diet, approximately 20 per cent are derived from protein, 35 per cent from fat; and 45 per cent from carbohydrate. If eggs are to be omitted from a calorie restricted diet one ounce of meat may be substituted for one egg.

If one compares the kinds and amounts of food in the 1,200-Calorie Pattern Dietary with those in the Pattern Dietary in Chapter 19, it will be observed that this calorie restricted diet plan varies from the normal in the following food groups:

Milk—skim milk is used in place of whole milk (176 Calories vs. 320 Calories).

Meat—meat is lean.

Vegetables—potatoes are *not* used and the servings of deep green and yellow and of other vegetables are each *increased* from one to two.

Fruits—the serving of other fruit is *increased* from one to two.

Bread and cereals—the total of four servings is *reduced* to two.

Table 21–7 shows the kinds of foods used in calorie-restricted diets; recipes and guides to food preparation are given in Chapter 37.

1,800-Calorie Diet. Table 21–6, Composition of an 1,800-Calorie Diet demonstrates one way in which The Pattern Dietary (p. 265), may be modified for a more liberal restriction than a 1,200 Calorie Diet. It will be noted that in this 1,800-Calorie Diet whole milk is used in place of the skim milk in the 1,200-Calorie Diet. Also, one tablespoon of sugar and two, rather than one tablespoon of butter are included in this plan. These two items may be used to flavor other foods or provide for calories in a simple dessert. The daily amounts of food for this 1,800-Calorie Diet are listed in Table 21–8. Of the calories in this diet plan approximately 15 per cent are derived from protein, 40 per cent from fat, and 45 per cent from carbohydrate.

TABLE 21–6. Composition of an 1,800-Calorie Diet[1]

Food Group	Amt. in Gm.	Household Measure	Calories	Protein Gm.	Fat Gm.	Carbohydrate Gm.	Minerals		Vitamins					Ascorbic Acid Mg.
							Calcium Mg.	Iron Mg.	A I.U.	Thiamine Mg.	Riboflavin Mg.	Niacin Mg.		
Milk, whole	488	2 c. (1 pt.)	320	17	17	24	576	0.2	700	0.16	0.84	0.3		5
Egg	50	1 medium	81	7	6	..	27	1.2	590	0.05	0.15	..		..
Meat, fish, fowl, lean	120	4 ounces	376	30	31	..	13	3.3	280	0.14	0.23	6.1		..
Vegetables[2]:														
Potato, cooked	100	1 medium	65	2	..	15	6	0.5	..	0.09	0.03	1.2		16
Deep green and yellow, cooked	150	2 servings	54	4	..	12	90	1.6	9,400	0.10	0.20	1.0		50
Other, cooked	150	2 servings	90	4	..	20	36	1.6	600	0.16	0.12	1.2		24
Fruit[2]:														
Citrus	100	1 serving	43	1	..	10	11	0.2	140	0.06	0.02	0.3		43
Other	200	2 servings	170	..	..	44	20	1.6	730	0.06	0.08	1.0		8
Bread, white enriched[2]	100	4 slices	270	9	3	50	84	2.5	..	0.25	0.21	2.4		..
Cereal, whole grain[2]	30 / 130	1 oz. dry or ⅔ c., cooked	89	3	1	18	12	0.9	..	0.08	0.03	0.7		..
Butter or margarine	28	2 tablespoons	200	..	22	..	6	..	920	..	..	..		..
Sugar	12	1 tablespoon	46	..	..	12	..	..	..	..	..	..		..
Totals			1,804	77	80	205	881	13.6	13,360	1.15	1.91	14.2[3]		146
												Niacin Equiv.		
Compare with recommended allowances[4]														
Moderately active man (70 Kg., 18–35 yrs.old)			2,900	70	..	..	800	10.0	5,000	1.20	1.70	19		70
Moderately active woman (58 Kg., 18–35 yrs.old)			2,100	58	..	..	800	15.0	5,000	0.80	1.30	14		70

[1] Calculations from Composition of Foods. Handbook No. 8. U. S. D. A., Rev. 1963.

[2] See Pattern Dietary, page 265, for basis of evaluation.

[3] The average diet in the United States, which contains a generous amount of protein, provides enough tryptophan to increase the niacin value by about one-third.

[4] From the National Research Council Recommended Dietary Allowances, Rev. 1963.

TABLE 21—7. Kinds of Foods Used in Calorie-Restricted Diets

Principle: To meet all the nutrient needs of the individual except calories

Foods Used:

Milk..........................	Milk, buttermilk, skim milk, as calculated
Cheese........................	Made of skim milk (cottage cheese). Other as calculated
Butter or margarine..............	As calculated
Eggs..........................	Cooked in all ways except fried or otherwise prepared with butter, cream or fat
Meats, fish, poultry, lean...........	Lean roast or boiled beef, lamb, veal, pork, chicken, turkey; broiled beefsteak or lamb chops (lean meat only); fish, boiled or broiled
Soups.........................	Clear broths and strained soups
Bread, cereals, potato, macaroni products	Whole grain or enriched as calculated. One slice of bread is approximately equivalent to ½ cup potato or ½ cup of rice, macaroni, spaghetti or breakfast cereal, and may be substituted for one of these
Vegetables.....................	See Exchange Lists, pp. 306-307
Fruits.........................	All fresh fruits and fruits canned without sugar
Beverages......................	Milk, buttermilk, skim milk as calculated. Coffee, tea or cereal beverage, all without sugar and cream
Desserts.......................	Fruit as above; gelatin desserts made without sugar
Condiments....................	As desired. Saccharin or Sucaryl may be used as sweetening in place of sugar

(See some suggested recipes for low caloric diets in Chapter 37)

Foods To Be Avoided:

Fats..........................	Meat fats, salad dressings, nuts, cream, fried foods, pastries. Butter or margarine as calculated
Sugars........................	Sugar, candy, jellies, jams, honey, all sweetened fruits and desserts. Saccharin or Sucaryl may be used in place of sugar if desired
Miscellaneous..................	Alcoholic and sweetened carbonated beverages, "snack" foods

TABLE 21—8. Food for an 1,800-Calorie Pattern Dietary

Food	Amounts
Milk, whole................	2 cups (1 pint)
Egg[1]......................	1 medium
Meat, fish, or fowl, lean	4 ounces (cooked)
Vegetables:	
Potato.................	1 medium
Deep green or yellow.....	2 servings
Other..................	2 servings
Fruit[2]:	
Citrus.................	1 serving
Other..................	2 servings
Bread, white, enriched[3]......	4 slices
Cereal, whole grain.........	1 serving
Butter or margarine.........	2 tablespoons
Sugar...................	1 tablespoon

[1] One ounce of meat may be substituted for one egg.
[2] See Exchange Lists, pp. 306-307, for size servings of various fruits.
[3] See Exchange Lists, pp. 306-307, for substitutes of one slice of bread.

Carbohydrate- and Calorie-Restricted Diets. If the diet prescription for a patient restricts carbohydrate to 60-80 Gm. per day, the 1,200-calorie pattern dietary can be adjusted in the following way:

Milk—skim milk, no change
Egg—no change
Meat, fish, fowl—*increase* from 4 ounces to 7 ounces, lean
Vegetables—*decrease* to one serving of deep green or yellow only
Fruit—citrus fruit, no change
  other fruit, *decrease* to one serving
Bread—*omit* all bread
Butter or margarine—no change

The carbohydrate content of this diet is approximately 60 grams. The increase in meat, fish, and fowl from four to seven ounces will compensate, to some degree, for the decrease in the contributions of fruits and vegetables to the daily intake of iron and the B vitamins. The ascorbic acid in the pattern will average 70 mg. per day and the calcium and vitamin A content are within reasonable levels in terms of the Recommended Dietary Allowances for these nutrients. Vitamin and mineral supplements may be needed to ensure an adequate intake of iron and the B vitamins, particularly thiamine.

Meal Planning With Exchange Lists. This method was set up to facilitate the calculation of pattern dietaries for diabetic patients and is very useful for planning calorie-restricted patterns. It is explained in detail on pages 305-310 in Chapter 22, Diabetes Mellitus.

Starvation Regimens. Recently, workers in metabolic research have used this method to study obesity.[7] Water and other non-caloric fluids together with vitamin and mineral supplements have been allowed. Hospitalized patients appear to tolerate this approach for periods of 30 days or more. During fasting weight loss is rapid, averaging 1 to 3 pounds per day. There are no long-term follow-up reports of this regimen to show whether or not this drastic approach is effective in the treatment of obesity. Because of the potential hazards of this method of weight reduction—e.g., anemia and gout—it is used only with closely supervised hospitalized patients. It should never be self administered.

Formula Diets. Liquid formula diets fortified with vitamins and minerals are now available in most supermarkets. They contain approximately 225 calories per 8-ounce serving; and four 8-ounce servings per day yield 900 calories. Their advantage lies in the fact that they provide a specific number of calories per serving: their disadvantage is the monotony of a bland liquid diet. Some people have found it helpful to use the formula diet for one meal a day and eat a calorie-restricted diet at other mealtimes. These formulas generally made from non-fat dry skim milk, are relatively expensive. The same type of formula can be made at home for less cost by adding non-fat dry skim milk to fluid skim milk.

---

[7] Drenick, E. J., *et al.*: J.A.M.A. *187*:100, 1964.

Maintenance of Weight Loss

Once the patient has achieved his weight loss, he should be warned not to return to his previous dietary practices. He will need assistance in establishing a pattern dietary that suits his situation. Unless he has increased his physical activity significantly, most adults will discover that the calorie-restricted diet, especially if it was a moderate and not a drastic restriction, is his basic normal diet with only minor modifications for weight maintenance.

Treatment Other Than Diet

Drugs

Drugs or proprietary preparations to decrease weight should be taken only under the supervision of the physician. Anorexigenic agents—the amphetamines and other drugs—have been used to promote weight loss. They depress appetite but it has been observed that their effectiveness decreases after about six weeks. In increasing doses they have unpleasant side effects. For the obese person who also has cardiac disease these drugs are dangerous.

Thyroid hormone has been used as an adjunct to diet therapy on the grounds that obese patients are in a hypometabolic state and need this metabolic stimulant if weight loss is to be accomplished. When an individual has hypothyroidism, hormone preparations are required to achieve a weight loss. For obese individuals with normal thyroid function—the majority of patients—thyroid hormone is dangerous.

Diuretics and Laxatives. The indiscriminate use of diuretics and laxatives, which promote a fluid loss, may give the patient a false sense of accomplishment when he weighs himself. His weight loss will reflect a water loss, not a decrease in adipose tissue. Only when the physician observes an abnormal fluid retention in a patient will a diuretic be part of the patient's therapy.

Physical Activity

Physical activity is as important an adjunct to dietary therapy in weight reduction and maintenance as it is in prevention. The more obese the individual doing the exercise, and the more strenuous the exercise, the greater will be the energy expended. Strenuous exercise may be dangerous for the obese, especially if they are past middle age and the exertion is spasmodic. The type and the amount of exercise should depend on the age and the specific condition other than obesity. Cardiovascular disease may limit the patient's activity.

Patient Education

Diet Instruction. Before participating in the diet instruction of the obese patient both the nurse and the dietitian must have an extensive knowledge of the calorie content of average servings of commonly used foods. One problem confronting the nurse and the dietitian is the average lay person's lack of this knowledge. On the other hand, individuals who have tried a variety of reducing diets may be highly expert at counting calories.

The lay person who lacks any specific information about the calorie value of foods at the per serving level often incorrectly classifies a food or food group as "fattening." For example, many people classify bread as "fattening." One regular-sized slice of bread weighing about 23 Gm. contains 60 to 70 calories. "Diet" bread, weighing about 18 Gm. per slice, contains 45 to 50 calories. For an individual bread will be "fattening" when his excessive daily calorie intake can be attributed to an excessive intake of calories from bread.

The definition of "average size" servings will also vary with the individual. For one man a serving of meat may be three ounces (approximately 250 calories if cooked without the addition of fat); for another man, six ounces (450 calories). A serving of pie, for one man, may be one sixth of a 9-inch pie; for another, one quarter of a 9 inch pie (apple pie: 380 calories vs. 590 calories).

Obese patients may also need considerable assistance with food selection and methods of food preparation. Chapter 36 in Part Three offers information on food selection and recipes for certain low-calorie items. Since the monotony of the diet is often a problem these suggestions and recipes may help a patient enjoy his meals.

Each meal served to the hospitalized patient should be planned to show him the variety possible in his diet.

Helping the obese patient to acquire knowledge of the calorie and, also, the nutrient values of food at the per serving level is the first step in patient education. This approach alone, however, will not ensure success: the nurse and the dietitian must be prepared to give unstinted support and understanding to the obese patient—even the well educated patient—who fails to adhere to the diet. Successful weight reduction is a long-term process and the monotony of the diet, due to the limitations in food choice, becomes intolerable to some patients.

Predicting Success. Since it can be said by many obese patients that "it is easy to lose weight, I have done it ten times," attempts have been made to identify the characteristics of those persons who can lose and maintain a weight loss. From the evidence available today the person who is most likely to lose weight successfully:[8]

1. Is slightly or moderately above a desirable weight for him, due to excess adipose tissue.

2. Gained weight as an adult.

3. Never attempted to lose weight as an adult.

4. Is well adjusted emotionally.

5. Accepts weight reduction as a realistic goal.

Bruch[9] indicates from her experiences that there are those patients who prefer to be obese and who meet the stresses of daily living more successfully when they are obese. Young[10] has shown in a series of studies that the reasonably stable individual is the most likely to achieve weight reduction, the anxious, tense or insecure person is less successful, and those who had little or no success presented deep emotional problems.

---

[8] Health and Obesity. P.H.S. Pub. No. 1485, 1966.

[9] Bruch, H.: The emotional significance of the preferred weight. Am. J. Clin. Nutr., 5:192, 1957.

[10] Young, C. M., *et al.*: J. Am. Dietet. A., *31*: 1111, 1955.

Fads and Fashions in Reducing Diets. Wyden,[11] in his book, The Overweight Society, presents an excellent review of the fads and fashions in diets over the past years. All those involved in patient education should read this book so that they will be able to recognize the return of old fads and fashions in reducing diets.

Extremely restricted diets, such as often become fashionable for a time, may promote weight loss, but they are seldom successful over a period of time. The monotony of the diet cannot be tolerated and the individual returns to his previous food practices. The formula diet is one recent example of this ineffective approach to weight reduction.

The search for familiar and acceptable foods without calories has been with us for many generations. Numerous attempts have been made by manufacturers to produce non-foods. The speed with which many of the products disappear from the grocer's shelves attest to their non-acceptance. The artificially sweetened carbonated beverage is one exception.

[11] Wyden, P.: The Overweight Society. New York, Wm. Morrow & Co., 1965.

UNDERWEIGHT

Leanness or underweight may be due to an inadequate caloric intake. A contributing factor may be excessive bodily activity, which increases the energy requirements beyond the caloric value of the food eaten. Thin people are usually of a so-called nervous temperment. Others are weak (asthenic leanness), with muscles poorly developed and lacking in stamina.

Leanness may be due to some other contributing factor within the body, such as malignancy, gastrointestinal disorders, chronic infectious diseases and endocrine disturbances. An increase in metabolic rate due to hyperthyroidism is frequently a cause of progressive weight loss. In such cases, rest and medical treatment or surgery may be necessary, as well as a high caloric diet.

Underweight Owing to Malnutrition or an inadequate caloric intake may be a serious condition, especially in the young. Growth is retarded, efficiency is impaired, and resistance to disease is reduced. It has been found that despite the general decrease in tuberculosis in the last few years, the disease has increased among

---

TABLE 21–9. Kinds of Foods Used for Increased Calories

Principles:
1. High in caloric value: 25-50 per cent above normal
2. High in protein: 90-100 Gm. for adults
3. High in vitamins, especially in the vitamin B complex
4. Nourishment may be served between meals and before retiring

Foods Used:

Milk	Milk and cream
Cheese	All kinds
Fats	Butter and margarine; all other fats
Eggs	Cooked in all ways
Meats, fish and fowl	All varieties; bacon and fat meats are indicated if the patient tolerates them
Soups	Preferably creamed or thick soups
Bread, cereals, macaroni products	All kinds; preferably whole grain or enriched
Vegetables	All vegetables, including potatoes
Salads	All kinds; oil dressings especially desirable
Fruits	All fresh and cooked fruits and juices, jellies, jams and marmalades
Desserts	Ice cream, custards, tapioca and rice puddings, cake, fruit desserts, other desserts
Beverages	Tea, coffee, cocoa, served with cream and sugar; fruit juices; malted preparations
Vitamin concentrates	If ordered by the physician

(See Chapter 36 for high caloric foods and beverage recipes)

young women between 15 and 24 years of age.

Underweight, like overweight, is a relative term, being based on the ideal weight for a given height, build and sex. More than 10 per cent below the ideal usually is considered to be abnormal, especially in persons under 25, and is worthy of medical investigation.

Diet for Underweight

The usual cause of underweight is an inadequate diet, the inadequacy being due to either the quantity or the quality of the food supply. A deficiency in calories, protein or its component amino acids, minerals or vitamins may produce faulty nutrition, with loss of weight. A careful survey of the dietary habits of the patient should reveal such inadequacies. The most common dietary cause is insufficient intake of calories to meet the energy requirements. Therefore, calories must be increased. Not only must the normal requirement be met, but an increase of from 400 to 800 calories must be made to allow for storage. Fifty per cent above the normal is sometimes prescribed, but this may be more than the patient can or will eat.

Vitamin supplements are sometimes prescribed, especially thiamine hydrochloride, for stimulating the appetite and improving digestion.

Table 21–9 shows the kinds of foods used to increase calorie intake. The objectives of this diet are:

1. An adequate diet, as described in Chapter 19.

2. Additional calories, which may be obtained by: (a) increasing the quantity of the foods listed in the normal pattern, (b) increasing the carbohydrates and, to some extent, the fats, and (c) frequent feedings to include nourishment between meals and before retiring at night.

3. An increase in protein to approximately 90 to 100 Gm. for adults in order to combat the deficiency due to previous malnutrition, with loss of body tissue.

4. An abundance of vitamins and minerals, especially thiamine.

5. A reduction in bulk, if not needed as a laxative, in favor of foods with higher calorie value.

6. Easily digested foods. Carbohydrate-rich foods are especially indicated, since carbohydrate is both easily digested and quickly converted into body fat. Foods rich in fat may be used to increase the fuel value without unduly increasing the bulk, but they must be used with discretion. Fat-rich foods will lessen the appetite of many patients, and too much fat in any form is frequently distasteful unless cleverly disguised. The uncooked fats, such as cream, butter and salad oils, are more easily digested than the fat in fried foods.

It will be noted that the diet described here is a house, or regular, diet supplemented with cream, extra butter, high caloric desserts and nourishment between meals.

Nursing Problems

The diet must be built up gradually, otherwise the patient may not be able to tolerate the sudden increase. Care must be taken to ascertain the likes and the dislikes of the patient and to prepare the food as appetizingly as possible, both as to methods of cooking and appearance when served. Above all, the patient must be encouraged to accept the necessity for his cooperating by consuming all food served to him. Low caloric soups, salads and beverages should not be eaten at the beginning of a meal, as they tend to give temporary satiety and to diminish appetite for the more substantial part of the meal.

Anorexia Nervosa

A very severe form of underweight is occasionally found in young people, most frequently young women, which is due to mental illness. Although these patients may seem to be physically well, and may protest that they eat sufficient amounts of food, they are often 30 per cent or more underweight, and their actual food intake is negligible. Since rejection of food is part of their illness, it is best not to press the need for calories on such patients but to serve pleasing meals without comment, in the hope that, as they recover, their food intake will increase. (See section on Mental Illness in Chapter 32.)

STUDY QUESTIONS AND ACTIVITIES

1. In conversation with the adult patients to whom you give nursing care this week ask each patient to recall what he or she weighed at age 12, 18, 25, 35, 45, and 55. For some patients it will be easier for them to relate weight to some event in their lives—e.g., graduation from high school, the time of marriage, induction into the armed forces, or, for women, their weight at the time of the birth of their first baby. Do any of these patients illustrate: (1) normal weight over their life span thus far; (2) obesity throughout their life span; (3) obesity which developed during their adult years?

2. In conversation with adult patients discover what foods they consider "fattening." In clinical conference with your classmates and instructor discuss these ideas.

3. Calculate a 1,500-calorie pattern dietary for yourself. For 3 days, use this pattern to select your food in the hospital dining room, at your favorite snack bar, and any meal you might eat at home or in a restaurant. Record all food and beverages you consume each day. Appraise the calorie value of each day's intake. In clinical conference with your instructor discuss the problems you met and your feelings about "counting" calories each day.

4. With the assistance of your instructor make appointments to accompany the dietitian when she does the diet interview and when she gives diet instruction to an obese patient. Observe and talk with this patient at one meal time for at least three days and report your observations to the dietitian. Summarize this experience and with the dietitian report to your classmates in clinical conference.

5. Write a day's menu for the 1,800-Calorie Pattern Dietary in Table 21–8.

6. Why is obesity considered a public health problem?

7. What is the direct cause of overweight? What are some of the factors which may play a role in overeating?

8. How can the nurse help in the prevention of obesity?

9. Why might an obese physician, nurse or dietitian be ineffective in helping a patient lose weight?

10. What role does exercise play in weight control?

11. What are the criteria for successful weight reduction as given by Young?

12. What approaches should the nurse use in working with a patient with a diagnosis of anorexia nervosa?

SUPPLEMENTARY READINGS ON WEIGHT CONTROL

Cederquist, D. C.: Comments on fad dieting. J. Am. Dietet. A., *40*:535, 1962.

Hathaway, M. L., and Sargent, D. W.: Overweight in children. J. Am. Dietet. A., *40*: 511, 1962.

Mayer, J.: Obesity: Causes and treatment. Am. J. Nursing, *59*:1732, 1959.

Monello, L. F., and Mayer, J.: Obese adolescent girls, an unrecognized "minority" group. Am. J. Clin. Nutr., *13*:35-39, 1963.

Moore, M. E., Stunkard, A., and Srole, L.: Obesity, social class, and mental illness. J.A.M.A., *181*:962, 1962.

Obesity and Health: U. S. Dept. H.E.W.-U.S.P.H.S. Pub. No. 1485, 1966.

Seltzer, C. C., and Mayer, J.: Body build and obesity: who are the obese? J.A.M.A., *189*: 677, 1964.

Young, C. M.: Some comments on the obesities. J. Am. Dietet. A., *45*:134, 1963.

The end of the rainbow may be tragic—scandal of the diet pills. Life, p. 23, Jan. 26, 1968.

For further references see Bibliography in Part Four.

CHAPTER 22

Diabetes

*Classification · Metabolic Aberrations · Symptoms · Therapy:
Goal and Approaches · Insulin · Oral Hypoglycemic Agents · The
Diet Prescription · Planning the Diabetic Pattern Dietary · Teaching the Diabetic Patient · Special Concerns*

INTRODUCTION

Diabetes mellitus is a chronic disease, the history of which goes back many centuries. The word *diabetes* was derived from a Greek word meaning "to siphon; to pass through," and *mellitus* came from the Latin word "honey." Thus the copious urination (polyuria) and sugar in the urine (glycosuria), two characteristic symptoms, gave the name to the disease. Until recently, diabetes mellitus, or "sugar diabetes," as the layman often refers to it, has been described as a chronic disorder of carbohydrate metabolism due to a lack of insulin.

It is generally agreed that insulin, secreted by the beta cells (Islets of Langerhans) of the pancreas, exerts some control of carbohydrate metabolism by effecting the transfer of glucose from the spaces around the cell (extracellular) into the cell interior. Present research indicates that while, in some persons, diabetes may be due to a lack of beta cells or to the inability of the beta cells to secrete enough insulin, it may also be due to the inability of the pancreas to synthesize and excrete effective insulin; or, after the secretion of effective insulin, some factor(s) may interfere with its function.[1] It has also long been

observed that physical activity appears to reduce the body's requirement for insulin.

Carbohydrate metabolism is the prime concern in the diagnosis and treatment of diabetes mellitus. As we have come to appreciate the complex relationships of protein, fat, and carbohydrate in intermediary metabolism in the cell (see Chap. 9), and as the effect of insulin and other hormones on these processes is becoming known, diabetes mellitus is better described as a complex metabolic disorder characterized by a lack of adequate, effective insulin. Moreover, persons with diabetes experience more vascular disease than normal individuals and for this reason the description of diabetes may also include "associated with accelerated vascular disease."

Predisposing Factors. It is generally accepted that diabetes mellitus is inherited; and it is suspected that many genes rather than a single gene may be involved. It is characteristic of a patient with diabetes to know of other members of his family who have the disease or who had it during their lives. It has also been observed that the disease occurs at a progressively earlier age with each passing generation of affected individuals.[2] For these reasons rel-

---

[1] Levine, R., and Mahler, R.: Production, secretion and availability of insulin. Ann. Med., *15:* 413, 1964.

[2] Sunder, J. H.: *in* Diabetes Mellitus, Diagnosis and Treatment, N. Y., Am. Diab. A., 1964.

atives of known diabetics are advised to be tested by their physicians each year.

Statistics show that diabetes in the adult is frequently associated with obesity. It is possible that the susceptibility to diabetes mellitus is enhanced by obesity combined with inactivity. Weight reduction alone results in the improvement of the disease in some obese adult diabetics. Members of families with a history of diabetes should be advised to maintain their weight at desirable or slightly below desirable levels throughout the life cycle (see Chap. 21).

Prevalence and Incidence. The Public Health Service estimates that by 1970 in the United States there may be 4.7 million or more persons with diabetes mellitus, and WHO reports that there are signs of increasing prevalence of the disease in most parts of the world.[3] In the United States it is thought that about one half of the persons with diabetes have never been diagnosed and are unaware of their condition. Case-finding programs conducted by health departments and other agencies seek to discover these individuals and to guide them to treatment in the hope of retarding the complications associated with this disease.

Diabetes occurs in all age groups from young infants to the elderly. The greatest incidence occurs in middle or older aged adults. In these groups more women than men, and more married than single women over 45, have diabetes.[4] The higher incidence in married women may reflect factors related to pregnancy (see p. 312). With today's longer life expectancy and the greater salvage of babies of diabetic mothers, and, therefore, the "seeding" of the diabetic potential, the number of people who will develop diabetes is expected to increase.

Associated Vascular Disease. It has been observed that disease of the heart and of the large and small blood vessels appears to occur more frequently in diabetics than in non-diabetics.[5] In the diabetic there is a tendency to recurrent myocardial infarction and an increase in the incidence of congestive heart failure. Peripheral vascular disease, retinopathy, nephropathy and neuropathy also occur more frequently than in the non-diabetic. The reason for this associated pathology is at present poorly understood.

Classification of Diabetes Mellitus. Primary diabetes mellitus may be classified as (1) growth-onset (juvenile) type, and (2) maturity-onset (adult) type.[6] These two types of diabetes vary not only by age, but particularly in the characteristics of the disease process.

Juvenile-type diabetes occurs in children from 0 to 14 years of age. The onset is sudden; the child has usually lost some weight and may be at or less than his normal weight, and the course of the disease is characterized by instability in the response to insulin and diet, especially in relation to activity. Insulin production by the pancreas is minimal or lacking and the administration of insulin is required by all juvenile diabetics. This type of diabetes may also be observed in adolescents and in adults to approximately age 40.

Maturity-onset diabetes is less sudden and dramatic than the growth-onset type. It occurs usually in individuals over age 40 and most frequently in the older age groups, age 55 and up. Approximately 85 per cent of patients are overweight. The course of the disease is usually stable. Although adequate insulin may be produced by the pancreas, it may be ineffective.

Secondary diabetes mellitus may occur due to damage or removal of the pancreas, or to disorders of other endocrine glands, e.g., the pituitary, the adrenals and the thyroid.

Metabolic Aberrations. The disorders in intermediary metabolism which occur in untreated diabetes mellitus, due either to a lack of insulin or to ineffective insulin, are

---

[3] Diabetes Mellitus. WHO Tech. Rep. 310, 1965.
[4] Newill, V. A.: *in* Diabetes Mellitus; Diagnosis and Treatment. N. Y., Am. Diab. A., 1964.

[5] Goldenberg, S., and Blumenthal, H. T.: *in* Diabetes Mellitus; Diagnosis and Treatment. N. Y., Am. Diab. A., 1964.
[6] Marble, A.: *in* Diabetes Mellitus; Diagnosis and Treatment. N. Y. Am. Diab. A., 1964.

presented in Figure 22–1. With the decrease in the entry of glucose into the cell, the amount of glucose circulating in the blood increases. The normal level of fasting blood glucose (FBS, fasting blood sugar) ranges from 60 to 100 mg. per cent. The untreated diabetic will have a fasting blood glucose greater than 100 mg. per cent (hyperglycemia). When the blood glucose exceeds approximately 160 mg. per cent the excess is excreted in the urine (glycosuria). Thus the potential energy of the glucose, which is not available to the cell, is lost to the body. At the same time water is lost from the body because it is required for the excretion of the glucose.

This sequence of events—hyperglycemia followed by glycosuria—accounts for the excessive thirst (polydypsia), copious urination (polyuria), and hunger (polyphagia) accompanied by weight loss which many untreated diabetics experience. As Figure 22–1 indicates, sodium is also lost with the water. If the water and sodium loss is great enough, dehydration results.

The oxidative cycle, as explained in Chapter 9, requires acetate derived from glucose. In untreated diabetes mellitus the cells in the body compensate for this lack up to a point by deriving the compounds required by the oxidative cycle from amino acids and fatty acids. As indicated in Figure 22–1 there is an increased excretion of

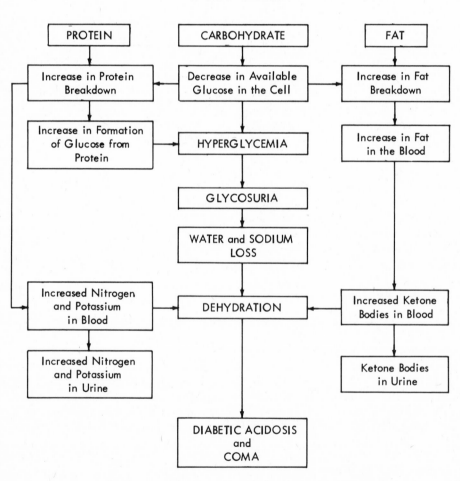

Fig. 22–1. Metabolic aberrations in untreated diabetes.

potassium and of nitrogen, as urea, from the increase in breakdown of protein. These products of catabolism require water for excretion and, therefore, this aberration also contributes to the dehydration which can occur in untreated diabetes.

The increase in fatty acid breakdown in untreated diabetes results in the production of an abnormal amount of ketone bodies which appear in the blood (ketonemia). The synthesis of ketone bodies is a normal intermediary metabolic reaction in the breakdown of fatty acids (see Chap. 9) and occurs to a large extent in the cells of the liver. However, the cells of the liver do not contain the necessary enzyme to metabolize ketone bodies. Instead the liver releases these compounds into the blood stream. The blood, in turn, transports them to other cells which can metabolize them. In untreated diabetes ketonemia occurs because the liver releases more ketone bodies than the cells can metabolize.

Two of the three compounds classified as ketone bodies—acetoacetic acid and beta-hydroxybutyric acid—are organic acids. The accumulation of these acids in the blood leads to diabetic acidosis or ketosis. At the same time, the kidney excretes these acids in the urine (ketonuria) which, like the excretion of glucose in the urine, increases the loss of water from the body. The third ketone body, acetone, is volatile and is excreted by the lungs, giving a "fruity" odor to the breath of the individual in diabetic acidosis. If severe enough the acidosis leads to diabetic coma and, if untreated, ultimately to death.

One pathway of the metabolism of acetoacetate is the synthesis of cholesterol. Some investigators attribute the associated vascular disease of diabetes mellitus to an increased synthesis of cholesterol from the excess of acetoacetic acid which occurs in ketonemia.

Symptoms. In the adult diabetic the onset of symptoms is usually slow. Acidosis will not develop unless the individual is under stress from an overwhelming infection or an acute vascular episode such as a myocardial infarct. There will be mild hyperglycemia and some glycosuria. Without an annual physical examination the disease may go undetected for a number of years. Anderson[7] estimates that maturity-onset diabetes may go undiagnosed for as long as ten years. When medical care is finally sought, the presenting symptoms are usually fatigue, thirst, increased urination, and weight loss despite hunger. Sometimes skin infections, such as furuncles, or impaired vision may be the reason for seeking medical care.

With growth-onset diabetes in children and younger adults the individual will usually experience all the classical symptoms of diabetes: polydipsia, polyphagia, polyuria and weight loss. Soon after the onset of these symptoms diabetic acidosis may occur. Mothers of children young enough to need help in getting a drink of water can often recall when the polydipsia first began.

Diagnostic Tests. When diabetes is suspected two laboratory tests will be done routinely: (1) urine will be tested for sugar, and (2) blood will be tested for glucose. Glycosuria is considered indicative but not diagnostic for diabetes. In addition to diabetes, sugar may occur in the urine in the following conditions: when the renal threshold for glucose is low; when too much sugar has been ingested at one time for the liver to convert to glycogen; in pentosuria, when the body is unable to metabolize 5-carbon sugars; in fructosuria, when fructose cannot be metabolized; in galactosuria, in infants with galoctosemia; and in lactosuria in nursing mothers, when lactose is produced in excess. Older individuals may have a high renal threshold and may not spill sugar into the urine even when blood sugar levels are above normal.

The blood sugar is tested either after a fast of eight to fourteen hours or after an intake of a known amount of carbohydrate or glucose. An elevated fasting blood glucose is usually but not always diagnostic of diabetes. Duncan[8] states that a fasting blood sugar level of 110 mg. per cent determined by the Symogyi-Nelson method,

---

[7] Anderson, T. W.: Diabetes, *15*:160, 1966.
[8] Duncan, G. G. (ed.): Diseases of Metabolism. 5th ed. p. 956. Philadelphia, W. B. Saunders, 1964.

which measures true glucose, indicates diabetes. A blood sugar level of 140 mg. per cent, or greater, two hours after a meal (post prandial) indicates diabetes. The test meal contains at least 100 Gm. of carbohydrate. Duncan[8] reports that the fasting blood sugar in the average untreated diabetic without acute complications will range from 180 to 300 mg. per cent. In the individual in or approaching acidosis, the fasting blood sugar will be greatly in excess of 300 mg. per cent. Recently it has been observed that there may be an increase in normal blood sugar levels with age, so that a slight increase in blood sugar levels in the older age group does not necessarily denote diabetes.[9]

When the fasting blood sugar determinations are inconclusive a glucose tolerance test (GTT) is done. For three days prior to the test the patient is required to eat 250 to 300 Gm. of carbohydrate daily. This is done to ensure adequate carbohydrate stores prior to the test. On the morning of the test after a 12-hour fast the patient is given 100 Gm. of glucose (1.75 Gm. per Kg. in children) in 300 ml. of water.[10] This solution is usually flavored with the juice of one lemon. Some individuals experience nausea and even vomiting after drinking the glucose solution. If vomiting occurs the test should be discontinued. Blood and urine samples are collected before giving the glucose solution and ½ hour, 1, 1½, 2, and 3 hours after ingestion. Figure 22–2 illustrates the results of a glucose tolerance test in a normal person and in a diabetic.

When it is suspected that a patient is in diabetic acidosis, or when he is being treated for acidosis, the urine and the blood will be tested for sugar and for ketone bodies.

9 Streeten, D., *et al.*: Diabetes, *14*:579, 1965.

10 Duncan, G. G.: Op. cit., p. 960.

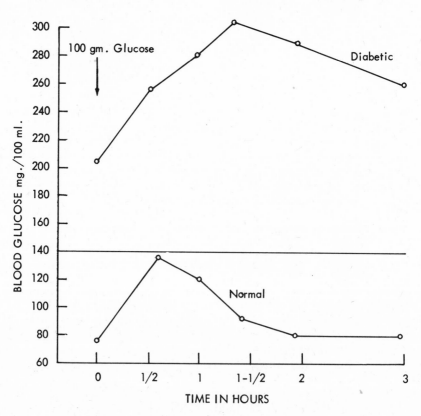

FIG. 22–2. Results of glucose tolerance tests in 2 normal persons and a diabetic.

THERAPY

Goal of Therapy. The basic goal of therapy in the treatment of diabetes mellitus is to help the patient achieve and maintain a normal blood sugar level with the hope of delaying the onset of associated vascular disease. The basic elements of this therapy are: (1) diet, which is presented in the next sections of this chapter; (2) insulin or oral hypoglycemic agents if needed; (3) physical activity appropriate to the individual; (4) personal hygiene, and (5) constant medical supervision. Personal hygiene will not be discussed in this book.

Approaches to Therapy. There is a sharp controversy among physicians in the United States as to the best method of treating the patient with diabetes mellitus. The disagreement centers on the control of blood sugar levels. A group of conservative physicians believe that blood sugar levels higher than normal, resulting in the presence of sugar in the urine, contribute to the onset and the severity of vascular disease in diabetes. Hence diet and insulin therapy are regulated carefully so that the blood sugar levels will be kept within normal limits and no sugar will be found in the urine. This careful treatment of diabetes is known as chemical regulation; it is achieved by the use of a weighed diet for at least a year and intermittently thereafter.

A group of liberal physicians believe, from the evidence available to them, that

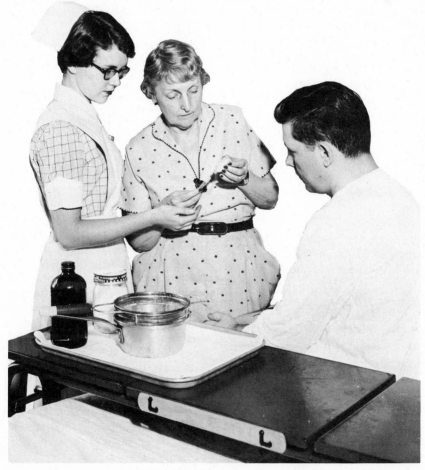

Fig. 22–3. Both the patient and his wife are learning about the administration of insulin. (The New York Hospital)

careful regulation does not delay the onset of vascular disease. They treat their patients with insulin, if needed, and a liberal diet as long as no symptoms of diabetes other than glycosuria, without ketonuria and weight loss, are present. The physicians who advocate this approach to treatment claim that the patient lives a more nearly normal and satisfying life. This regimen is called the clinical method of regulation, and the patient is placed on an unmeasured or "free" diet, restricting only sugar and foods high in sugar.

A third group, the majority of physicians who treat diabetic patients, have adopted a middle-of-the-road approach. Their treatment plan is neither as limiting as the chemical method nor as liberal as the clinical method. They use the Exchange Lists for diet planning, a somewhat liberal yet moderately accurate method, which is based on standard household measures.

Regardless of the method used, the nurse and the dietitian must be aware that diet is an integral part of the treatment of any patient with diabetes mellitus. Mild diabetes, especially if the patient is obese and his diagnosis and treatment are not delayed, may be controlled by diet alone, whereas the severe diabetic will require diet plus insulin or an oral hypoglycemic agent to control his disease. In either case the diet, in addition to helping to control the disease, must meet the individual's nutritional needs.

Insulin. Since the discovery of insulin by Banting and Best in 1922 many advances have been made in the preparation of insulin from the pancreas of animals. The development of standards for its commercial production and its effectiveness in the control of diabetes are some of the greatest contributions to medical science in this century. Insulin is a protein and therefore cannot be taken orally, since it would be digested by the enzymes in the gastrointestinal tract and rendered ineffective. It is administered hypodermically and most patients need careful instruction in learning how to prepare and give the injection (Fig. 22–3).

TABLE 22–1. Insulin Action*

Type	Onset of Action Hours	Maximum Action Hours	Duration of Action Hours
Regular (Crystalline)..	1 hour or less	2-4	6-8
Semi-lente.....	1-2	5-7	8-12
Globin........	2-3	6-10	10-16
NPH..........	2-4	8-12	18-24
Lente..........	2-4	8-12	18-24
Protamine zinc..	4-6	16-24	24-36
Ultra-lente.....	4-6	16-24	24-36

* The hours given are average. Other authors may give slightly different figures. The duration of action of all insulins can vary somewhat according to the size of the dose, the severity of the diabetes, the amount of exercise the person takes, and whether the individual is in a fed or fasting state.

ONSET, PEAK, AND DURATION of insulin activity depend on whether an insulin is of the regular or unmodified type and, therefore, fast-acting, or whether it has been modified to prolong its activity over a long time. Most insulin reactions occur during the period of maximum insulin activity. Assuming that insulin injections are given in the morning before breakfast, reactions following regular (crystalline) or semilente insulins are most likely to occur during the late forenoon. Reactions from insulins of intermediate activity such as globin, NPH, or lente are most apt to occur in mid- or late afternoon. And reactions which are caused by the slow-acting protamine zinc or ultra-lente insulins occur most frequently during the evening, night, or early morning hours.
From Martin, M. M.: Insulin reactions. Am. J. Nursing, 67:328, 1967 (Feb.).

The first insulin developed is now known as regular or crystalline insulin. As can be seen in Table 22–1, it acts quickly but over only a short period of time. When it was the only insulin available, it had to be injected three and sometimes four times a day in order to be effective. The next insulin to be developed was protamine zinc insulin. This is an insulin with a prolonged action (see Table 22–1) and could be given in one dose in place of the three to four doses per day of regular insulin.

Today, there are a variety of moderate-acting insulins available for the treatment of diabetes. Those most commonly used are Lente, Globin and NPH (Neutral Protamine Hagedorn). Most patients require only one injection of these insulins per day, although the occasional patient may require two.

The insulin requirement varies with each individual and is influenced primarily by the severity of the disease. A number of other factors affect the requirement, of which physical activity is foremost. Activity increases the body's ability to metabolize glucose, although the mechanism is not well understood. Duncan[11] considers that the total insulin dose needed by an individual is related to total calorie intake, whereas other investigators consider that it is related to total carbohydrate intake.

Infections, including the common cold, may increase the insulin requirement, especially in growth-onset diabetes. Emotional stress can also affect the insulin requirement. Either metabolic or emotional stress may be more important factors for some patients in controlling their diabetes than dietary indiscretions. As Hinkle[12] points out, anxiety is often accompanied by fluctuations in blood glucose levels. Physicians, nurses and dietitians must guard against accusing patients of "cheating on their diets" when the real problem may be an emotional conflict.

Insulin Reactions. Insulin reactions result from depressed blood glucose levels (below 60 mg. per 100 ml.) and they occur when too much insulin is given, when the patient does not eat all of the prescribed diet, or when he engages in excessive exercise before a meal.

With the moderate-acting insulins the onset is gradual and is characterized by weakness, fatigue and headache, sometimes nausea, dizziness and double vision, and, eventually, stupor. The treatment when the condition is discovered is the immediate administration of sugar in some form, either as one of the fruit juices or as sugar and water. This should be followed by a more slowly absorbed food mixture such as crackers or toast and milk, which will continue to feed carbohydrate into the system. It may be necessary to repeat both the rapidly and the slowly absorbed feedings for some time until all danger of insulin reaction is past. If the individual has lost consciousness, intravenous glucose will be used.

With regular insulin, the onset of an insulin reaction is rapid and more dramatic. The patient may complain of nervousness and hunger, perspire profusely and become inarticulate. If untreated, stupor will result here also. Immediate administration of rapidly absorbed carbohydrate such as fruit juices or sugar in other forms is effective.

The danger of an insulin reaction is that permanent brain damage may result, especially if the reactions are frequent, or if it is severe and extended so that the patient becomes unresponsive. Patients taking insulin are advised to carry 2 lumps of sugar or hard candies for such emergencies.

Oral Hypoglycemic Agents. In the past ten years research workers have discovered a number of synthetic compounds which lower blood sugar in both normal and diabetic individuals. The first two of these compounds are tolbutamide (Orinase) and chlorpropamide (Diabinese) which are related in structure to the sulfa drugs and belong to a group called sulfonylureas. A third member of this group, acetohexamide (Dymelor) is also in current use. The advantage of these drugs is that they can be taken by mouth and, therefore, for some diabetic patients hypodermic injections are no longer necessary. Since these agents act to depress the blood sugar level and hypoglycemic reactions can occur, it is essential that the patient maintain his diet as carefully as if he were taking insulin.

It is generally accepted that the sulfonylureas stimulate increased production or release of insulin by the beta cells of the pancreas. Hence, these compounds are effective only in those diabetics who have beta cells which can respond to the stimulus, generally the patient with maturity-onset type diabetes (see p. 297).

In a 5-year study of almost 2,000 patients on the effectiveness of tolbutamide in the control of diabetes,[13] it was found that about one quarter were "secondary failures." After an initially good response, for

[11] Op. cit.
[12] Hinkle, L. E., Jr.: *in* Diabetes Mellitus: Diagnosis and Treatment. N. Y., Am. Diab. A., 1964.

[13] Camarini-Davalos, R. A., and Marble, A.: J.A.M.A., *181*:1, 1962.

a number of reasons their diabetes was no longer well controlled by the drug. With a few exceptions, these patients were able to return to their original dosage of insulin with good results.

More recently another oral compound, the phenethyldiguanide, phenformin (DBI), has been shown to have hypoglycemic activity. Although the function of this compound is not well understood, it is generally accepted that it enhances the action of insulin. It was originally considered that this compound used in combination with insulin in growth-onset diabetes reduced the requirement of insulin. This has not proved effective in long-term treatment.[14] In the treatment of some maturity-onset diabetics a sulfonylurea is used in combination with phenformin. They complement each other, since the sulfonylurea stimulates the production of insulin and the phenformin enhances the action of insulin.

DIET THERAPY

The Diet Prescription. CALORIES. The calorie requirement for the non-obese adult diabetic is the same as for normal individuals of the same sex, age, height, and activity. However, the diabetic is cautioned to maintain his weight at a level slightly below his desirable weight. Therefore, his calorie prescription may be somewhat less than for a normal individual. It is usually based on 30 to 35 calories per Kg. (2.2 pounds) of ideal body weight (1,750 to 2,000 calories for a woman whose ideal weight is 58 Kg.). The calorie requirement for a child or adolescent diabetic, neither of whom is usually obese, will be the same as others of his age group.

The calorie prescription for an obese adult diabetic will be designed to promote a weight loss. It will be based on 20 to 25 calories per Kg. of ideal body weight, depending on his activity (1,150 to 1,450 calories for an obese woman whose ideal weight is 58 Kg.).

CARBOHYDRATE. Forty to fifty per cent of the calorie prescription is usually derived from carbohydrate. For example: at 40 per cent a 1,200-calorie diet will contain 120 Gm. of carbohydrate, and a 2,000-calorie diet will contain 200 Gm. of carbohydrate.

The distribution of the carbohydrate in the day's diet is equally as important as the total quantity. For patients who do not require insulin, the day's carbohydrate is divided equally between his three meals, or four if he is accustomed to a bedtime snack. This distribution is used to promote, in so far as possible, a constant level of blood sugar throughout the day. Such division also applies to patients using oral hypoglycemic agents.

For patients using moderate-acting insulins (Lente and NPH), the distribution of carbohydrate in the day's diet is usually ordered by the physician. As a general rule about one half of the total carbohydrate is given prior to the time of peak action, about 8 hours after injection, and one half of the carbohydrate is given after this time. One example of dividing the day's carbohydrate by this method is 1/6 for breakfast, 2/6 for the noon meal, 2/6 for the evening meal, and 1/6 at bedtime. The bedtime snack is used to protect the patient against insulin reactions during the night.

Another method commonly used to distribute the day's carbohydrate is to subtract 10 to 30 Gm. from the total. This amount of carbohydrate is used for a bedtime snack. The remaining grams of carbohydrate in the diet prescription may be distributed equally among three meals (see Calculation of Diabetic Pattern Dietary, p. 308); or by some other division required to regulate the patient's blood sugar level. It is expected that there will be a reasonable distribution of protein and fat and, therefore, total calories, throughout the day's meal plan. Some physicians require that protein and fat as well as carbohydrate be distributed in the day's diet according to the figures for distribution in the diet orders. For example: an order for 1/6 at breakfast means 1/6 of the day's carbohydrate, protein and fat for breakfast.

PROTEIN. The protein requirement for the adult diabetic is the same as for the normal person, 1 Gm. per Kg. of body weight. For the child or adolescent the

[14] Krall, L. P.: *in* Diabetes Mellitus; Diagnosis and Treatment. N. Y., Am. Diab. A., 1964.

TABLE 22–2. Nutrient Composition of Food Exchanges*

Group†	Amount	Weight Gm.	Protein Gm.	Fat Gm.	Carbo-hydrate Gm.	Calories
Milk, whole	½ pt. (8 oz.)	240	8	10	12	170
Vegetables, Group A	as desired	..	..	..	..	..
Vegetables, Group B	½ cup	100	2	..	7	35
Fruit Exchanges	varies	..	..	..	10	40
Bread Exchanges	varies	..	2	..	15	70
Meat Exchanges	1 oz.	30	7	5	..	75
Fat Exchanges	1 tsp.	5	..	5	..	45

* Table 22–2 and Food Exchange Lists modified from Caso, E. K.: Calculation of diabetic diets. J. Am. Dietet. A., 26:575, 1950 (August).

† For lists of foods in each exchange, see Table 22–3.

requirement is the same as for his age group. In practice the amount of protein in a diabetic diet prescription is usually greater than the amount in a normal one because the amount of carbohydrate and, therefore, of calories from carbohydrate, is restricted. The amount of protein in a diabetic diet for an adult will usually not exceed 1½ Gm. per Kg. of body weight. Larger amounts of protein are not needed and, as they are expensive, they add to the cost of the diet plan. If severe renal or liver disease is present the protein will be restricted.

FAT. After establishing the protein and carbohydrate of the diet, fat is used to supply the remainder of the calories. This will vary from 35 to 45 per cent of calories from fat. Since it seems that the kind of fat in the diet, i.e., the quantity of saturated vs. polyunsaturated fatty acids, may have a relationship to the development of atherosclerosis, some physicians are modifying the type of fat included in the diet of the diabetic (see Chap. 23).

To summarize: Given a non-obese 58-Kg. woman, aged 55, who requires 1,800 calories, her diet order may be as follows: 1,800 calories; 180 Gm. of carbohydrate; 80 Gm. of protein; 80 Gm. of fat. Thirty grams of the carbohydrate are used for a bedtime snack. (See Calculation of Diabetic Pattern Dietary, Table 22–4.)

Planning the Pattern Dietary
With the Diabetic Patient

The first step in translating a physician's diet prescription into a pattern dietary for a newly diagnosed diabetic patient is to discover where he lives and works and with whom and what he eats each day. The foods he likes, accepts, and can afford should be used whenever possible in setting up his diet, because this or a similar diet will be the way he will eat for the rest of his life. In the following pages the three methods of diet planning—the exchange method, chemical control and clinical control—will be presented, with the major emphasis on the most commonly used one: meal planning with exchange lists. Both the nurse and the nutritionist should be aware that, regardless of the method used, the diet must meet all of the patient's nutritional needs.

Meal Planning With Exchange Lists. This method for planning diabetic pattern dietaries, sometimes referred to as the Exchange System, was prepared in 1950 by a committee of the American Dietetic Association, and received the approval of the American Diabetes Association and the United States Public Health Service.

In the Exchange Lists, foods of similar nutritive composition per serving are grouped together: milk, vegetables, fruit, bread, meat and fat. (See Table 22–2, Nutrient Composition of Food Exchanges.) The size serving of each food given in the lists is defined in household measures—8-ounce measuring cup and standard measuring spoons—except meat, which is given in ounces, and bread, which is listed in units, e.g., bread in slices, rolls in numbers, etc. With the exception of meat, the size servings of the items within each list are aver-

TABLE 22–3. Exchange Lists for the Diabetic Diet

(Adapted from Meal Planning with Exchange Lists, The American Dietetic Association,
620 N. Michigan Ave., Chicago, Ill. 60611)

Foods That Need Not Be Measured

(Insignificant carbohydrate or calories)

Coffee

Tea

Clear broth

Bouillon (fat free)

Lemon

Gelatin (unsweetened)

Rennet tablets

Cranberries (unsweetened)

Mustard (dry)

Pickle (unsweetened)

Saccharin and other noncaloric sweeteners

Pepper and other spices

Vinegar

Seasonings

To season your food, you may use chopped parsley, mint, garlic, onion, celery salt, nutmeg, mustard, cinnamon, pepper and other spices, lemon, saccharin and Sucaryl and vinegar. All of these may be used freely.

List 1. Milk Exchanges

One exchange of milk contains 8 Gm. of protein, 10 Gm. of fat, 12 Gm. of carbohydrate and 170 calories.

This list shows the different types of milk to use for one exchange:

Type of Milk	Amount to Use
Whole milk (plain or homogenized)...	1 c.
*Skim milk......................	1 c.
Evaporated milk..................	½ c.
Powdered whole milk..............	¼ c.
*Powdered skim milk (nonfat dried milk).........................	¼ c.
Buttermilk (made from whole milk)....	1 c.
*Buttermilk (made from skim milk)......	1 c.

You can use one type of milk instead of another. For example, you may use ½ cup of evaporated milk in place of 1 cup of whole milk.

* Skim milk and buttermilk have the same food values as whole milk, except that they contain less fat. Add 2 fat exchanges to your meal when you use 1 cup of skim milk or buttermilk made from skim milk in place of whole milk.

List 2. Vegetable Exchanges: Group A

Group A contains little protein, carbohydrate or calories. You may use as much as 1 cup at a time without counting it.

Asparagus	Greens (*Continued*)
*Broccoli	Kale
Brussels sprouts	Mustard
Cabbage	Spinach
Cauliflower	Turnip greens
Celery	Lettuce
*Chicory	Mushrooms
Cucumbers	Okra
*Escarole	*Pepper
Eggplant	Radishes
*Greens	Sauerkraut
Beet greens	String beans, young
Chard	Summer squash
Collard	*Tomatoes
Dandelion	*Watercress

* These vegetables contain a lot of vitamin A.

List 2. Vegetable Exchanges: Group B

Each exchange contains 2 Gm. of protein, 7 Gm. of carbohydrate and 35 calories.

½ cup of vegetable equals 1 exchange:

Beets	Pumpkin
*Carrots	Rutabagas
Onions	*Squash, winter
Peas, green	Turnip

* These vegetables contain a lot of vitamin A.

List 3. Fruit Exchanges

One exchange of fruit contains 10 Gm. of carbohydrate and 40 calories.

This list shows the different amounts of fruits to use for one fruit exchange:

Fruit	Amount to Use
Apple (2″ diam.)................	1 small
Applesauce......................	½ c.
Apricots, fresh.................	2 medium
Apricots, dried.................	4 halves
Banana.........................	½ small
Blackberries....................	1 c.
Raspberries.....................	1 c.
*Strawberries...................	1 c.
Blueberries.....................	⅔ c.
*Cantaloupe (6″ diam.)...........	¼
Cherries.......................	10 large
Dates..........................	2
Figs, fresh.....................	2 large
Figs, dried....................	1 small

TABLE 22-3 (Continued)

Fruit	Amount to Use
List 3 (Continued)	
*Grapefruit....................	½ small
*Grapefruit juice................	½ c.
Grapes........................	12
Grape juice....................	¼ c.
Honeydew melon...............	⅛ medium
Mango........................	½ small
*Orange.......................	1 small
*Orange juice..................	½ c.
Papaya.......................	⅓ medium
Peach........................	1 medium
Pear.........................	1 small
Pineapple.....................	½ c.
Pineapple juice................	⅓ c.
Plums........................	2 medium
Prunes, dried.................	2 medium
Raisins.......................	2 tbsp.
*Tangerine....................	1 large
Watermelon...................	1 c.

* These fruits are rich sources of vitamin C. Try to use one of them each day.

List 4. Bread Exchanges

One exchange contains 2 Gm. of protein, 15 Gm. of carbohydrate and 70 calories.

This list shows the different amounts of foods to use for one bread exchange:

Bread, Cereal, etc:	Amount to Use
Bread.........................	1 slice
Biscuit, roll (2″ diam.)...........	1
Muffin (2″ diam.)..............	1
Cornbread (1½″ cube).........	1
Cereals, cooked.................	½ c.
Dry, flake and puff types........	¾ c.
Rice, grits, cooked...............	½ c.
Spaghetti, noodles, cooked........	½ c.
Macaroni, etc., cooked...........	½ c.
Crackers, graham (2½″ sq.).......	2
Oyster (½ c.).................	20
Saltines (2″ sq.)................	5
Soda (2½″ sq.)................	3
Round, thin (1½″).............	6
Flour.........................	2½ tbsp.
Vegetables:	
Beans and peas, dried, cooked...	½ c.
(Lima, navy, split pea,	
cowpeas, etc.)	
Baked beans, no pork...........	¼ c.
Corn.........................	⅓ c.
Popcorn......................	1 c.
Parsnips......................	⅔ c.
Potatoes, white................	1 small
Potatoes, white, mashed...........	½ c.

Bread, Cereal, etc:	Amount to Use
List 4 (Continued)	
Potatoes, sweet, or yams..........	¼ c.
Sponge cake, plain (1½″ cube).....	1
Ice cream (omit 2 fat exchanges)....	½ c.

Use these foods carefully because they have a lot of carbohydrate.

List 5. Meat Exchanges

One meat exchange contains 7 Gm. of protein, 5 Gm. of fat and 75 calories.

This list shows the different amounts of foods to use for one meat exchange:

Meat	Amount to Use
Meat and poultry (medium fat).....	1 oz.
beef, lamb, pork, liver, chicken, etc.	
Cold cuts (4½″ x ⅛″)...........	1 slice
salami, minced ham, bologna, liver-	
wurst, luncheon loaf	
Frankfurter (8-9 per lb.)..........	1
Egg...........................	1
Fish: haddock, etc................	1 oz.
Salmon, tuna, crab, lobster......	¼ c.
Shrimp, clams, oysters, etc.......	5 small
Sardines.......................	3 medium
Cheese: Cheddar type...........	1 oz.
Cottage.....................	¼ c.
*Peanut butter..................	2 tbsp.

* Limit peanut butter to 1 exchange a day unless the carbohydrate in it is allowed for you in your meal plan.

List 6. Fat Exchanges

One fat exchange contains 5 Gm. of fat and 45 calories.

This list shows the different foods to use for one fat exchange:

Fat	Amount to Use
Butter or margarine................	1 tsp.
Bacon, crisp.....................	1 slice
Cream, light.....................	2 tbsp.
Cream, heavy....................	1 tbsp.
Cream cheese....................	1 tbsp.
Avocado (4″ diam.)................	⅛
French dressing...................	1 tbsp.
Mayonnaise.....................	1 tsp.
Oil or cooking fat.................	1 tsp.
Nuts..........................	6 small
Olives.........................	5 small

Note: See Chapter 37 for recipes based on Exchange Allowances.

TABLE 22–4. Calculation of Diabetic Pattern Dietary

Diet Prescription: Protein, 80 Gm.; Fat, 80 Gm.; Carbohydrate, 180 Gm.; Calories, 1800

Meal		Protein Gm.	Fat Gm.	Carbo-hydrate Gm.	Calories
Breakfast...............	1 Fruit Exchange	..	..	10	40
	2 Bread Exchanges	4	..	30	136
	1 Meat Exchange	7	5	..	73
	1 Milk Exchange	8	10	12	170
	2 Fat Exchanges	..	10	..	90
	Total for Meal	19	25	52	509
Noon meal.............	2 Meat Exchanges	14	10	..	146
	2 Bread Exchanges	4	..	30	136
	Any A Vegetable	..	..	..	..
	2 Fruit Exchanges	..	..	20	80
	2 Fat Exchanges	..	10	..	90
	Total for Meal	18	20	50	452
Evening meal............	3 Meat Exchanges	21	15	..	219
	3 Bread Exchanges	6	..	45	204
	Any A Vegetable	..	..	..	..
	1 B Vegetable	2	..	7	36
	2 Fat Exchanges	..	10	..	90
	Total for Meal	29	25	52	549
Bedtime snack	1 Bread Exchange	8	10	12	68
	1 Milk Exchange	2	..	15	170
	Total for Meal	10	10	27	238
	Total for Day	76	80	181	1,748

age servings. The basic unit for the meat list is one ounce. For an adult, this unit is multiplied by the number of ounces which are required to make an average serving. Depending on the diet prescription for an individual this may be two, three or four or more ounces. This method facilitates the calculation of diabetic pattern dietaries. It it also used widely today to calculate calorie-restricted pattern dietaries (see Chap. 21).

The values for calories and nutrients in Table 22–2, are not exactly the same as those in the Pattern Dietary (Chap. 19, p. 265), because the values for the food exchanges are averages which have been rounded to the nearest whole figure. From the evidence available to them the committee that set up the exchange system felt justified in recommending these values for the nutritive composition of the food ex-changes.[15] With repeated use, the nurse and the dietitian will discover that they have memorized the figures in Table 22–2 and can easily calculate a pattern dietary for a diabetic patient. They will also discover that they will use them in answering patient's questions about food, as well as in making an on-the-spot estimate of any patient's calorie, protein, fat, or carbohydrate intake. These figures are not applicable, however, when greater accuracy is required.

The various Exchange Lists in Table 22–3 on pages 306-307 show the foods included in each group. Any special directions should be carefully checked, such as the notation that when skim milk is used 2 fat exchanges should be added. This applies only when whole milk is calculated

---

[15] Caso, E. K.: J. Am. Dietet. A., *26*:575, 1950.

in the pattern dietary and skim milk is substituted for whole milk. When skim milk
is calculated in the pattern dietary this notation does not apply.

Vegetables are divided into two lists.
Vegetable Exchanges—Group A are those
having 3 to 5 Gm. of carbohydrate per one
half cup serving, cooked (100 Gm.), and
are not calculated in the diet. Vegetable
Exchanges—Group B are those which provide 7 Gm. of carbohydrate per one half
cup serving, cooked (100 Gm.) and are
calculated in the diet. It will be noted that
certain vegetables are listed with the Bread
Exchanges. These contain 15 Gm. of carbohydrate per serving as listed, such as ⅓ cup
of corn. The items in the Fruit Exchanges
are listed by serving size that yields 10
Gm. of carbohydrate. Bacon and nuts are
listed in the Fat, not in the Meat Exchanges
as might be expected. Their primary contribution is fat rather than protein. (See
Table 1 in Part Four.)

When a patient customarily uses a food
that does not appear in one of the Exchange Lists, for instance pinto beans which
are not listed in the Bread Exchanges, the
size serving that gives the same nutritive
value as the exchange can be calculated
from a food table. (See Table 1 in Part
Four, or Handbook 8, U.S.D.A.) Exchange
Lists modified for various cultural food patterns are available from state and city health
agencies, social welfare agencies, and the
visiting nurse services in large cities; or the
dietitian can set up Exchange Lists to meet
a patient's cultural food practices.

When a patient's preferences or limited
income is a factor, the number of fruit and
vegetable exchanges included in the diabetic pattern dietary need not exceed the
quantity required for an adequate daily intake of ascorbic acid and other vitamins.
The remainder of the carbohydrate may
then be distributed among bread, spaghetti, potatoes, etc., which are lower in
cost, and which may be preferred to large
quantities of vegetables and fruits.

Table 22–4 (Calculation of a Diabetic
Pattern Dietary) illustrates a way in which
a diet prescription for an 1,800-calorie diet
with 180 Gm. of carbohydrate, 80 Gm. of

TABLE 22–5. Suggested Menu for Diabetic Pattern Dietary

Breakfast	Noon Meal	Evening Meal
½ small grape-fruit	2 ounce ham-burg pattie	3 ounces sliced turkey
1 poached egg on 1 slice of toast	1 hamburger roll (large)	1 cup mashed potato
1 slice of toast with 1 tsp. butter	1 tsp. mayon-naise	½ cup peas
8 ounces of milk	1 thin slice bermuda onion	tossed salad with vinegar and 1 tsp. oil
2 cups of coffee with 2 tbsp. coffee cream	lettuce and mustard	1 dinner roll and 1 tsp. butter
	1 medium apple	coffee without cream
	1 cup coffee with 1 tbsp. coffee cream	**Bedtime Snack**
		8 ounces milk
		1 piece of sponge cake

protein, and 80 Gm. of fat might be translated into a diabetic pattern dietary for a
patient. It will be noted that part of the
prescription is used for a bedtime snack
and the rest distributed in three approximately equal meals. Daily menu choices
are selected by the patient from the Exchange Lists. (See Table 22–5, Suggested
Menu.)

For those learning how to calculate a diabetic diet the first step is to distribute
those exchanges—milk, vegetables, fruit,
and bread—that will fulfill the carbohydrate prescription in the physician's diet
order. As previously explained (p. 304),
the amount of carbohydrate for each meal,
and snack if included, will be indicated by
the diet order. The second step is to distribute the protein, primarily the meat exchanges; the last step is to distribute the
fat exchanges.

The totals of the grams of protein, fat
and carbohydrate in the pattern dietary
calculations may vary by approximately 5
grams from the figures in the diet prescription. Some protein and fat should be included in each meal and in the evening
snack. Parts of exchanges should not be
used in calculating the diet unless they
reflect the patient's preference. For example, a patient may want only one half
of a milk exchange (4 ounces) at break-

fast for his cereal. This is practical only if he usually eats his breakfast at home. In a restaurant he would use only part of a 6 to 8 ounce serving of milk yet would pay for the whole serving.

Exchanges may be used in the preparation of "mixed" dishes. These can be prepared for the whole family, with the patient receiving his correct portion. See Chapter 37 for recipes. The patient or his family may also find *A Cookbook for Diabetics*[16] useful in adding variety to the diabetic diet.

Weighed Diets. The physician who uses the chemical method to treat the diabetic will require his patients to purchase a scale which weighs in grams. The patient will weigh each serving of food at each meal. The instruction materials for the patient will give the gram weight of each serving of food. The equivalent household measure may also be included. Many physicians have adapted the exchange system or constructed a similar system for this method of diet instruction. The nutrient values of foods used by some physicians may vary to some degree from those used in the exchange system, therefore the nurse or dietitian will need to use the nutrient values used by the physician when calculating the pattern dietary for a patient. As the patient acquires experience in weighing his food he becomes expert in judging serving size and may be advised by his physician to weigh his food only one day a week to check his practices. Even some physicians who use the exchange system have their newly diagnosed patients weigh foods for a short time in order to learn to judge serving size.

The Unmeasured or "Free" Diet. The physician who uses this method usually guides his patients to establish daily food practices very similar to the Pattern Dietary (Chap. 19, p. 265) at the calorie level required by the individual. The patient actually sets up his own diet pattern and the physician adjusts the insulin to the intake. Concentrated sweets such as sugar, jelly, honey, candy, sweetened fruits, frosted cakes, pies, and sweetened fruit juices and sweetened carbonated beverages are omitted. Concentrated sweets are excluded because they are quickly absorbed, raise the blood sugar level above the kidney threshold and are then excreted in the urine. The patient derives no benefit from the calories so lost.

Special Diet Foods. At present the regulations of the Federal Food and Drug Administration covering Foods for Special Dietary Purposes are under revision. Diabetic patients should be warned that, other than the non-caloric carbonated beverages, those foods advertised as low or reduced in sugar may still contain too much carbohydrate from sources other than sucrose to be used in their diets.

Diet Planning and Associated Diseases. The diabetic diet may need to be modified if other disease is also present. In the case of an elderly, debilitated patient, the diet may have to be Soft as outlined in Chapter 19. If there is disease of the intestinal tract a low residue (see Chap. 27) or a bland diet (see Chap. 26) may be indicated. In cardiac disease sodium may need to be restricted (see Chap. 24). The American Dietetic Association has available supplements to the exchange lists which are modified in texture for bland, low fiber diets, and low in sodium for those patients who require a sodium-restricted diet.[17]

The amount and kind of fat in the American diet as it relates to cardiovascular disease, particularly coronary heart disease, is under careful study (see Chap. 23). Diabetic diets containing 1,800 calories or more tend to have the same per cent of calories from fat as the ordinary American diet (40 to 45%). In the diabetic diet this amount of fat is used to compensate for the restriction of carbohydrate to 40 per cent of total calories. Since it has been observed that coronary artery and other vascular disease is associated with diabetes, the kind and amount of fat included in the diabetic diet is also being studied. Some physicians are modifying the kind of fat in the diabetic diet from primarily satu-

---

[16] Behrman, D. M.: Am. Diabetes A., 1959. 18 E. 45th Street, N. Y., 10017. Price $1.00.

[17] Caso, E. K.: J. Am. Dietet. A., 32:929, 1956.

rated fats to a greater use of polyunsaturated fat. A modified fat exchange list which reflects this trend is available from the American Dietetic Association. If research shows that the amount of fat in the diabetic diet should be reduced, it can be expected that the amount of carbohydrate in the diet will be increased. With the insulin now in use this is possible.

TEACHING THE PATIENT

The diabetic patient must be helped to face the fact that his disease cannot be cured but that, with proper dietary care, and the use of insulin or one of the oral drugs if necessary, he can live a comfortable and productive life. Teaching the patient in simple terms what his disease is and why his dietary restrictions are necessary is often a responsibility shared by the physician and the nurse. As soon as the patient's diabetes is stabilized, actual dietary instruction should begin, with the doctor, the nurse and the dietitian working closely together. Stone has demonstrated that given adequate instruction and time to learn, the majority of diabetic patients can manage their diets successfully.[18]

The patient's trays are an important first step in teaching. From them he will learn the size of food portions and the foods which have approximately the same composition and, therefore, may be exchanged for each other. The foods that do not appear on the tray, such as sugar, jelly, canned or cooked sweetened fruits and desserts with sugar added, are also points to be emphasized in teaching. The approximate quantity of food served at each meal, particularly if the patient is receiving insulin or one of the oral drugs, needs to be pointed out.

When a specific plan for the patient's diet is constructed, care must be taken that it fits into his life situation. The diet for a small child will differ from that of an active adolescent; both will differ from the diet of the man who works. Again, adjustments must be made for the older man or woman, often with other serious disease as well, who lives alone, perhaps on a very small income. The dietary pattern should be fitted to the person for whom it is designed, not the person fitted to the pattern. Economic necessity, cultural preferences and personal likes and dislikes must all be incorporated insofar as possible. There is no reason why an Italian patient may not have "pasta" and the Chinese or Arabic patient rice in place of bread and potatoes. Fortunately, "Meal Planning and Exchange Lists" (see Table 22–3) allow for a considerable amount of choice.

Also available to help the diabetic adjust to the new demands being made on him is the bimonthly magazine published for patients by the American Diabetes Association.[19] It contains information about the disease, stories of patients and recipes based on the Exchange Lists. It has a fine section for children with diabetes.

The family, too, may need encouragement and support in the adjustment to the diagnosis of diabetes in one of its members. This is particularly true for parents when one of their children develops the disease.

In all this the nurse, the dietitian and the physician, as well, must work as a team. The nurse will often elicit questions and information from the patient which will help to fit his diet restrictions to his need. And, most of all, those who teach the diabetic patient must realize that it is not only difficult to change one's dietary pattern, but also difficult to adhere to the new pattern. Patience, support and encouragement are needed until the diabetic has accepted the restrictions of his disease and has learned to live comfortably with them.

SPECIAL CONCERNS

Diabetic Acidosis and Coma. Diabetic acidosis and coma require emergency treatment by the physician and the nurse to re-establish fluid and electrolyte balance and normal metabolism. If the patient is in coma, or if he is nauseated and vomiting, insulin and intravenous fluids will be used to treat him. As his hyperglycemia and

---

[18] Stone, D. B.: Am. J. Med. Sci., *241*:436, 1961.

[19] ADA Forecast, Amer. Diab. A., 1 E. 45th Street, N. Y. 17, N. Y.

ketonemia decrease, and when he can tolerate it, he will be offered a variety of fluids by mouth. When his condition is stabilized he will be given a diabetic diet and insulin.

Replacements. It is expected that diabetic patients receiving insulin or an oral hypoglycemic agent will consume all the food served at each meal to prevent the possibility of insulin shock. When a patient refuses a food, especially one which is primarily carbohydrate, he should be provided with a substitute equal in carbohydrate to the food refused.

If a patient refuses the major portion of a meal for any reason, the physician may require that the total available glucose of the meal be replaced. To calculate the total available glucose in a meal, the number of grams of carbohydrate calculated in the patient's pattern dietary are added to the number of grams of carbohydrate equal to 58 per cent of the grams of protein and 10 per cent of the grams of fat. It is estimated that 58 per cent of the protein and 10 per cent of the fat in a diet give rise to glucose. For example: a meal calculated to provide 30 Gm. of protein, 30 Gm. of fat and 60 Gm. of carbohydrate has 80 Gm. of available glucose (30 Gm. of protein $\times$ 0.58 = 17.4 Gm. of glucose; 30 Gm. of fat $\times$ 0.1 = 3 Gm. of glucose; and 60 Gm. of carbohydrate = 60 Gm. of glucose). This amount of carbohydrate may have to be given in several small feedings within the next two or three hours to prevent insulin shock.

Surgery. Today diabetic individuals undergo surgery with comparative safety. In emergencies, such as an acute appendix, there is usually no reason to delay surgery because of diabetes. In these situations the patient is given insulin and intravenous fluids and glucose.

When there is time to prepare for surgery the status of the patient's diabetes is carefully evaluated and, if his disease is not well controlled, the proper diet and insulin treatment is instituted before he undergoes surgery. On the day of surgery breakfast and insulin are withheld. If required a small dose of regular insulin may be given before surgery. After the operation glucose and fluids with sufficient insulin are given intravenously. Oral feedings of liquids such as fruit juices, broth, tea and ginger ale are started as early as possible. Later the patient's usual diet is resumed.

Diabetes in Pregnancy. Diabetes in the mother has always been a special hazard in pregnancy. There is increased fetal loss in the course of the pregnancy as well as an increased loss of infants carried to term as compared with the non-diabetic patient. In the past few years, however, by keeping close watch on the mother, obstetricians have been able to secure a far greater number of successful pregnancies than formerly.

Early prenatal care is an important factor in the salvage of these babies as well as in the maintenance of the health of the mother. Again there is a difference of opinion about the type of dietary control, but all physicians agree that the nutritional needs of pregnancy must be adequately met (see Chap. 12), with sufficient insulin to cover the increased food intake.

Diabetes in Children. Although it is estimated that children under 14 years of age make up approximately only 5 per cent of the known diabetics, they present the most serious problems in the management of the disease. Their disease is more severe and less stable than the maturity-onset type.

The outlook for children who develop diabetes has changed markedly from the pre-insulin days when the disease invariably was fatal. White[20] reported on 1,072 patients whose onset of diabetes occurred before the age of 15 and who had had the disease 20 years or more. Of these, 879 were living at the time of the study. Of the 879 patients, 71 per cent had had diabetes from 20 to 29 years, 24 per cent had had diabetes from 30 to 34 years and 5 per cent had had the disease for more than 35 years.

However, in a large percentage of such patients, complications develop after 15 to 20 years or more of diabetes. These include diminished vision and heart and kidney disease, all attributable to blood-vessel

---

[20] White, P.: Diabetes, 5:445, 1956.

changes. In a later paper[21] White states that 90 per cent of patients who developed diabetes before the age of 15 and had had the disease for 30 years or more could be shown to have such blood-vessel changes. Thus, although much has been gained in lifespan for the young diabetic, much remains to be done.

The controversy over the best approach to treatment applies particularly to this age group of patients (see p. 301). Those physicians who advocate chemical control direct the parents and children to weigh food; and those advocating clinical control have the children share the family meals. Some physicians use Meal Planning with Exchange Lists.

Whatever the school of thought is in regard to control of the diet, all physicians agree that the nutritional needs of the diabetic child are the same as those of the non-diabetic (see Chaps. 13 and 14). If there has been any marked weight loss before the disease is discovered, which is usually the case, the diet prescribed should be such as to allow the child to recover this loss. As he grows and develops, there must be periodic readjustment of the diet and the dosage of insulin. Strenuous physical activity may be compensated for by small amounts of food before the exercise.

Particularly in the adolescent years, when girls and boys grow very rapidly, it is essential that the diet keep pace with the nutritional needs, and that insulin be increased accordingly.

Both the diabetic child and his parents will require long-term and constant instruction and support if the disease is to be kept under control. Tact, sympathy and understanding will do much to help them in the acceptance and the adjustments which will be necessary over the years.

STUDY QUESTIONS AND ACTIVITIES

1. Find out the total number of adult diabetic patients in your hospital today. The therapeutic dietitian's records of diet orders will give you this information most readily. How many of these diets are also calorie restricted? (1,500 calories or less)

How many are also restricted in sodium? Do any diet orders for these diabetics also require modification of fatty acid composition?

2. Using the patient's chart and the physician's daily orders, summarize and present to your classmates in clinical conference the insulin and diet changes in a post-partum woman who is a diabetic. Include the pediatrician's progress notes and orders for her infant, especially feeding changes.

3. Through observation and interview discover how a patient with well-controlled diabetes, who has been admitted for elective surgery, has managed his activities of daily living including his diet prior to admission to the hospital. What resources has he used in the past for guidance and counseling? If indicated, what further help does he need, and who should help him, during his convalescence from surgery?

4. Record the 24-hour food and nutrient beverage intake of a patient with diabetes. Using the appropriate food value system appraise his calorie and nutrient intake. Compare his actual intake of calories, protein, fat, and carbohydrate with the diet order prescribed by his physician. Compare his mineral and vitamin intake with guidelines appropriate for him. If there is any significant discrepancy between intake and order, seek the assistance of your instructors in identifying the reason and in solving the problem.

5. What symptoms does a patient with diabetes have? Why does he show each one of these symptoms?

6. A patient has a fasting blood sugar of 300 mg. per cent and shows sugar and acetone in his urine. What has happened to his metabolism to bring about these two conditions?

7. What percentage of carbohydrate is metabolized as glucose in the body? Of protein? Of fat? How much glucose will the body obtain from the Pattern Dietary which contains 90 Gm. of protein, 100 Gm. of fat and 200 Gm. of carbohydrate?

8. The carbohydrate allowance for a diabetic patient is 150 Gm. He is receiving insulin. How will the carbohydrate of his diet probably be divided for the day?

[21] White, P.: Diabetes, 9:345, 1960.

9. Plan a diabetic diet with the following diet order: protein 75, fat 110, carbohydrate 200, carbohydrate divided for insulin, using the Exchange Lists in this chapter. The patient is a man with a large appetite.

10. Give 5 substitutions that a diabetic can make for a slice of bread.

11. What is meant by the chemical regulation of diabetes? The clinical regulation? Why is there controversy over these two methods of regulation?

12. What is meant by a "free" diabetic diet? What advantages are claimed for it?

SUPPLEMENTARY READING ON DIABETES

Caso, E. K., and Youland, D. M.: An apple for an orange. Am. J. Nursing, 55:942, 1955.

————: Supplements to diabetic diet material. J. Am. Dietet. A., 32:929, 1956.

————: Diabetic meal planning—a good guide is not enough. Am. J. Nursing, 62:76, 1962 (Nov.).

Diabetes Mellitus: A Guide for Nurses. U. S. P. H. S., Pub. No. 861, 1962.

Etzwiler, D. D.: Who's teaching the diabetic? Diabetes, 16:111, 1967 (Feb.).

Hinkle, L. E.: Customs, emotions and behavior in the dietary treatment of diabetes. J. Am. Dietet. A., 41:341, 1962.

Hodges, R. E.: Present knowledge of nutrition in relation to diabetes mellitus. Nutr. Rev., 24:257, 1966 (Sept.).

Kaufman, M.: A food preference questionnaire for counseling patients with diabetes. J. Am. Dietet. A., 49:31, 1966 (July).

————: Programmed instruction materials on diabetes. J. Am. Dietet. A., 46:36, 1965 (Jan.).

Krysan, G. S.: How do we teach four million diabetics? Am. J. Nursing, 65:105, 1965 (Nov.).

Martin, M. M.: Diabetes mellitus: current concepts. Am. J. Nursing, 66:511, 1966 (Mar.).

————: The unconscious diabetic patient. Am. J. Nursing, 61:92, 1961 (Nov.).

————: Insulin reactions. Am. J. Nursing, 67:328, 1967 (Feb.).

Moore, M. L.: Diabetes in children. Am. J. Nursing, 67:104, 1967 (Jan.).

Stone, D. B.: A rational approach to diet and diabetes. J. Am. Dietet. A., 46:30, 1965 (Jan.).

Watkins, J. D., et al.: A study of diabetic patients at home. Am. J. Pub. Health, 57:452, 1967 (Mar.).

Weller, C.: Oral hypoglycemic agents. Am. J. Nursing, 64:901, 1964 (Mar.).

For further references see Bibliography in Part Four.

CHAPTER 23

Atherosclerosis

Definition • Coronary Risk Factors • Role of Diet • Diet Prescription • Planning the Fat-Controlled Diet • Patient Education • Planning the Cholesterol-Restricted Diet

INTRODUCTION

The term atherosclerosis is derived from two Greek words: athere meaning "porridge" or "mush," and skleros meaning "hard." The atheromatous lesion, which develops in the arterial blood vessels, begins as a soft deposit and hardens as it ages. With time these lesions, known as plaques, gradually grow and thicken the arterial walls, thus narrowing the lumen of the blood vessel (see Fig. 23–1). The atherosclerotic plaque is composed of a variety of substances which include cholesterol, fatty acids, lipoproteins (a complex molecule of protein and fat), calcium deposits, complex carbohydrates, fibrous scar tissue, and blood.[1] How and why these plaques develop is not well understood and numerous theories have been under intensive study for the past fifteen years.

Coronary occlusion, or heart attack, occurs when a blood clot forms suddenly and occludes the lumen of a coronary artery already narrowed by an atheromatous plaque. This event deprives the surrounding tissue of its blood supply. Depending on the extent of damage to the tissue of the heart in the area of the occlusion, the patient may survive or die suddenly. If the occlusion of a blood vessel occurs in the brain the result is a cerebral hemorrhage or "stroke." Other arterial blood vessels in the body may also be occluded and cause serious disease or death.

Atherosclerosis is a major public health problem because the sequelae to the formation of atheromata—coronary occlusion and cerebral hemorrhage—are the leading causes of disability and death in the United States and in many of the countries of the western world. In the U. S. in 1965 about 600,000 persons died from heart attacks. About one third of these individuals were under 65 years of age and victims of a first attack. It is estimated that these 600,000 deaths reflect 30 to 40 per cent of the total number of individuals who had heart attacks[2] in 1965 and, therefore, approximately 1,400,000 individuals survived heart attacks during that year.

We do not know with certainty, as yet, the cause or causes of atherosclerosis, particularly the involvement of the coronary arteries in coronary heart disease. However, many medical and public health workers consider that the evidence from the studies and research of the past fifteen years is sufficient to help us identify the coronary-prone individual, and to undertake programs to prevent heart attacks. At the same time many physicians are using this research in the treatment of individuals who have an attack.

---

[1] Spain, D. M.: Scientific American, 215:48, 1966 (Aug.).

[2] Stamler, J., et al.: Am. J. Nursing, 66:1788, 1966 (Aug.).

CORONARY RISK FACTORS

Epidemiologic studies such as the Gas Company Study in Chicago,[3] the Framingham Study,[4] and the Tecumseh Michigan Study,[5] have identified certain coronary risk factors. Although the data do not permit absolute prediction that an individual will have a heart attack, those factors which appear to be most strongly associated with coronary heart disease are elevated blood serum cholesterol levels (hypercholesterolemia), hypertension and excessive cigarette smoking.[6] There is also evidence that diabetes mellitus, obesity, diet, physical inactivity, diminished glucose tolerance without frank diabetes, elevated serum triglyceride levels as well as elevated serum cholesterol levels, genetics, and social and psychological stresses are associated with the disease. Men 45 years of age and older are, in general, more susceptible to coronary heart disease than women.

---

[3] Stamler, J., *et al.*: Med. Clin. N. Am., *50*:229, 1966.
[4] Kannel, W. B., *et al.*: Ann. Int. Med., *55*:33, 1961.
[5] Epstein, F. H., *et al.*: Ann. Int. Med., *62*:1170, 1965.
[6] Epstein, F. H.: J. Chron. Dis., *18*:735, 1965.

At this point it does not appear that any one of the factors listed above is the cause of coronary heart disease in an individual. Rather, the epidemiologic studies indicate that it is the presence of two or more risk factors in an individual which determine his coronary proneness. For example: there is strong evidence that for men the multiple risk factors are hypercholesterolemia, hypertension and excessive cigarette smoking. A man with a serum cholesterol of 250 mg. per 100 ml. or greater, a blood pressure of 160 systolic or greater and who smokes twenty or more cigarettes per day is at greater risk than when only one or two of these risk factors are present.[7]

ROLE OF DIET

The precise role of diet in the development of coronary heart disease is not known at this time. There is considerable evidence, however, from both clinical and epidemiologic studies which relates diet to blood lipid levels. The amount of cholesterol and the amount and type of fat in the diet appear to be related to serum cholesterol and other lipid levels.

---

[7] Epstein, F. H.: Op. cit.

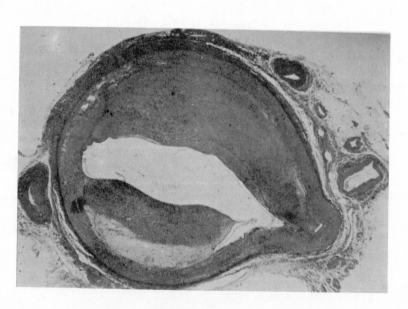

FIG. 23–1. Atherosclerotic obliteration of the lumen of the iliac artery. (Bailey, C. P., *et al.*: Rheumatic and Coronary Heart Disease. p. 41. Philadelphia, Lippincott, 1967)

Cholesterol. It must be kept in mind that the cholesterol in the diet is not the only source of serum cholesterol: it is synthesized principally in the liver from acetyl coenzyme A (see Chap. 9). Early studies in humans indicated that dietary cholesterol did not influence the amount of serum cholesterol. More recent work, however, indicates that the level of dietary cholesterol may have an effect on serum levels. It now appears that, as the intake of cholesterol from food increases from 0 to 800 mg. per day, the serum cholesterol level increases progressively.[8] The American diet

[8] Hegsted, D. M., *et al.*: Am. J. Clin. Nutr., *17*: 281, 1965.

contains on the average 800 to 1,000 milligrams of cholesterol per day from meat, eggs, milk and other dairy products.

Fats and Fatty Acids. The information gathered after World War II from the study of food intake and the incidence of coronary heart disease in a number of countries showed that the incidence of disease in the populations studied seemed to be related to the amount of fat in the national diet. For example, the Japanese, who at that time consumed about 10 per cent of their total calories as fat (see Fig. 23–2), had a low incidence of coronary heart disease compared with Americans who were consuming about 40 per cent of their total

DEGENERATIVE HEART DISEASE IN MEN

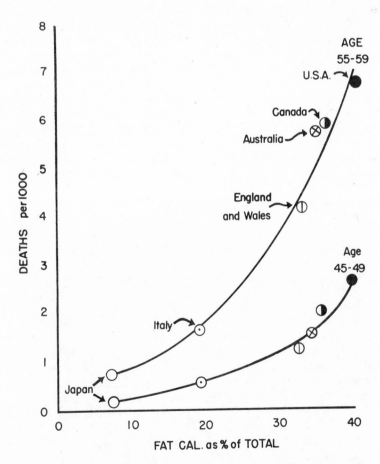

Fig. 23–2. Mortality from degenerative heart disease in two age groups, as related to percentage of fat calories in total calories of the national diet. (From Keys, A.: Atherosclerosis: a problem in newer public health. J. Mt. Sinai Hosp., *20*:118)

TABLE 23–1. Critical Limits of Dietary Fat Composition for Serum Cholesterol Reduction*

Component	Diet With 36-40 Per Cent Fat Calories	Diet With 25-30 Per Cent Fat Calories
Saturated fatty acids	less than 14% calories	less than 11% calories
Polyunsaturated fatty acids (linoleic)	more than 14% calories	more than 13% calories
Cholesterol	less than 350 mg.	less than 300 mg.

* Brown, H. B., and Farrand, M. E.: J. Am. Dietet. A., 49:303, 1966.

calories as fat. At the same time it was observed that in populations with low fat intakes the serum cholesterol levels were appreciably lower than in Americans with high fat intakes. It was also observed that the polyunsaturated fatty acids provided a significant amount of the fat in the low-fat diets.

These observations of the relationship of the amount and type of fat in the diet to coronary heart disease did not apply equally to all the groups studied. For example, certain pastoral tribes in Africa who have a high milk intake and, therefore, a high saturated fat intake have a relatively low serum cholesterol level and incidence of coronary heart disease. It is suspected that physical activity may explain this difference, since the members of these tribes are more active than the other populations which were observed.

Following these population studies, extensive research was done to determine the effect of polyunsaturated fat on serum cholesterol levels in man and animals. The results of these investigations indicate that saturated fats tend to increase serum cholesterol, while fats containing primarily polyunsaturated fatty acids tend to decrease serum cholesterol.[9] Monounsaturated fats appear to have no effect on serum cholesterol levels. (See Chapter 3 for explanation and food sources of saturated and unsaturated fatty acids.) There is, as yet, no agreement on the mechanism(s) by which the degree of saturation of fats affects serum cholesterol levels.

Diet Studies. As a result of the population studies and the research on fatty acids, other research workers have studied

the effect of modified diets on serum cholesterol levels. A number of investigators have studied individuals, primarily men, under metabolic research conditions, while other investigators have studied groups of men living and eating at home with their families.

The work of Page and Brown and their co-workers in Cleveland is one example of the first type of research. These investigators have determined critical limits for the fat and cholesterol composition of a diet effective in reducing serum cholesterol. Their research involved 134 normal, free-living, active subjects who were served test diets prepared in a research kitchen. All but fifteen of the subjects were men between the ages of twenty and fifty-five years.[10] Table 23–1, based on their work, shows that there are critical limits in the fatty acid and cholesterol composition of diets which had a significant effect on lowering the serum cholesterol levels of their subjects. A diet with 36 to 40 per cent of calories from fat was effective in lowering serum cholesterol when less than 14 per cent of total calories were provided by saturated fatty acids, more than 14 per cent of total calories were from polyunsaturated fatty acids (linoleic), and the diet contained less than 350 mg. of cholesterol. A diet containing 25 to 30 per cent of calories from fat was effective when less than 11 per cent of total calories were provided by saturated fatty acids, more than 13 per cent by polyunsaturated fatty acids, and the diet contained less than 300 mg. of cholesterol. The section in this chapter Planning Fat-Controlled Diets is based on this research.

[9] Ahrens, E. H., Jr., et al.: J.A.M.A., *164*:1905, 1957.

[10] Brown, H. B., and Farrand, M. E.: J. Am. Dietet. A., *49*:303, 1966 (Oct.).

Christakis[11] and his group in New York have studied 814 men ages 40 to 59 years who were placed on a diet relatively rich in polyunsaturated fatty acids. This diet resulted in a significant decrease in serum cholesterol levels, and maintained the decrease for as long as five years. A control group of 463 men was also studied. Compared with the control group the diet group had less morbidity from new coronary disease.

At present the National Heart Institute is supporting the National Diet-Heart Study.[12] The first step in this study has been a feasibility trial with 1,500 healthy male volunteers to determine whether or not a large-scale study to test the fat-controlled diet would be possible. The volunteers, ages 45 to 58, and their families have followed diets lower in saturated and higher in polyunsaturated fat than the usual American diet. The results of this trial and the plans for a larger trial are not known to date.

Present Recommendations. From the evidence presently available from epidemiologic, experimental and clinical studies, it is generally accepted that, compared with usual present practices, a decrease in the intake of saturated fatty acids, an increase in the intake of polyunsaturated fatty acids and a reduction in the intake of cholesterol is most likely to benefit the coronary-prone individual. There appears to be a trend toward recommending this modification of diet for those individuals who are identified as at risk for coronary heart disease. This diet recommendation is combined, when appropriate, with the recommendations to decrease cigarette smoking and to increase physical activity.

DIET PRESCRIPTION

No one diet order for hospitalized patients with a heart attack (myocardial infarction) can be anticipated. The order for a patient will be determined by his condition, and by the physician's decision as

to the therapy he requires. In this section those orders which can be anticipated will be discussed.

Calorie Restriction. For many years the restriction of calorie intake has been a part of the medical plan of care for the patient with an acute myocardial infarct. Calorie restriction combined with bed rest is used to reduce the work of the heart.

Many patients, during and immediately after a heart attack, are nauseated. When they can tolerate food by mouth the diet may be liquid as well as calorie-restricted. Some physicians prefer that neither very hot nor very cold liquids nor carbonated beverages be offered to these patients. If a patient's condition requires it, the liquids may also be restricted in sodium. As the patient's condition improves he will progress to a calorie-restricted soft or regular diet (see Chap. 21). Some physicians will require that six small meals, rather than the traditional three, be served to the patient convalescing from a recent heart attack. Foods which are gas-forming or any food the patient knows he cannot tolerate should be avoided. If the patient is obese it can be expected that calorie restriction will be a part of any diet prescription.

Sodium Restriction. Sodium restriction will be prescribed for the patient who has a myocardial infarct complicated by congestive failure. (See Chapter 24). This complication occurs most frequently in patients experiencing a second or third myocardial infarct. Some physicians also prescribe sodium restriction to guard against congestive failure at the time of the acute event, and then liberalize this restriction as the patient recovers.

The Fat-Controlled Diet. A variety of written orders for this diet are presently in use. The order may read "low animal fat–high vegetable fat diet." This order came into use as the result of the early research which indicated that vegetable oils were effective in reducing serum cholesterol. Another order, which can be found in many diet manuals, states a specific P/S ratio. A 2:1 ratio is a common order. Early work related the effectiveness of modifying the fatty acid composition to the ratio of polyunsaturated to saturated fat. The re-

[11] Christakis, G., *et al.*: J.A.M.A., *198*:129, 1966.
[12] Dietary Fat and Human Health. National Academy of Science–National Research Council, Pub. 1147, 1966.

TABLE 23–2. Nutrient Composition of Exchanges for Fat-Controlled Diet*

Food Group	Amount	Gm.	Protein Gm.	FAT Total Fat Gm.	FAT Saturated Fat Gm.	FAT Linoleic Fatty Acid Gm.	Cholesterol mg.	Carbohydrate Gm.	Calories
Milk, skim...........	½ pt. (8 ozs.)	240	8	tr.	..	..	7	12	80
Vegetables Group A..	as desired	..	..	..	..	..	..	..	..
Group B...	½ cup	100	2	..	..	..	..	7	35
Fruit...............	varies	..	..	..	..	..	..	10	40
Bread and Cereal....	varies	..	2	0.5	..	..	..	15	70
Meat, lean only......	1 oz.	30	8	2	0.6	0.1	21	..	50
Egg (3/week)........	3/7	21	3	3	0.9	0.2	118	..	35
Fat (Veg. oil)[1]........	1 tablespoon	14	..	14	2.0	8.0	..	..	125
Fat ("Special Margarine" Corn oil etc.)...	1 tablespoon	14	..	11	2.5	3.7	..	..	100
Fat ("Special Margarine" Safflower oil) ..	1 tablespoon	14	..	11	1.9	6.3	..	..	100

* Compiled with the assistance of M. C. Zukel.
[1]Corn, cottonseed, safflower, soybean oil.

cent work of Brown shows that the amount of fat as well as the P/S ratio and the amount of cholesterol are all critical factors. Planning the Fat-Controlled Diet is presented in the next section of this chapter.

Cholesterol Restriction. A diet restricted in cholesterol may be prescribed for some patients, either alone or in combination with other restrictions. The cholesterol in the diet is usually restricted to 150 to 250 mg. per day.

Fat-Reduced Diet. The total fat in this diet plan may be severely restricted to 10 per cent of total calories. An 1,800-calorie diet which derives 10 per cent of its calories from fat contains 20 Gm. of fat. No visible fat or fat for cooking or flavoring foods can be used at this level of restriction, and only skim milk is allowed.

More commonly, the diet order will allow a more liberal intake of fat, e.g., 25 per cent of total calories from fat (50 Gm. of fat in an 1,800-calorie diet). See Chapter 38 for planning the fat-reduced diet.

PLANNING THE FAT-CONTROLLED PATTERN DIETARY

Foods for the Fat-Controlled Diet. It is well to recognize that this is a therapeutic diet which requires significant changes in an individual's food practices. The most critical changes in food selection required by this diet occur in the following groups: (1) milk and other dairy products; (2) meat, fish and poultry; (3) eggs; and (4) fats. Table 23–2, Nutrient Composition of Food Exchanges for Fat-Controlled Diets, is a modification of Table 22–2, Nutrient Composition of Food Exchanges (Chap. 22) used in the calculation of diabetic diets.

It will be observed that there are major differences between the two tables in the nutrient values of the milk, meat and fat exchanges, and that values are given for saturated fat and linoleic fatty acid in addition to values for total fat. Adding the figure for saturated fat to the figure for linoleic fatty acid in an Exchange will not give the same figure as the one in the fat column because the figure for monounsaturated fat is not given. (See Part Four, Table 3.) Linoleic fatty acid is used to calculate the polyunsaturated fat in a diet because it is the one which occurs in food in significant amounts. The cholesterol values are given for those foods which contain this nutrient.

The nutritive composition of the Vegetable and Fruit Exchanges and the foods in these two Exchanges are the same for both the diabetic and the fat-controlled diets. These Exchange lists will not be reproduced in this chapter (see Chap. 22, Table 22–3).

TABLE 23–3. Food Exchange List for Fat-Controlled Diets*

MILK EXCHANGES

(One serving contains 8 Gm. of protein, 12 Gm. of carbohydrate, 7 mg. of cholesterol, and 80 calories)

Skim milk. . . . .   1 c.
Non-fat dried milk. . . . .   ¼ c.
Buttermilk (made from skim milk)   1 c.

VEGETABLE EXCHANGES

See Exchange Lists, Chapter 22, Table 22-3.

FRUIT EXCHANGES

See Exchange Lists, Chapter 22, Table 22-3.

BREAD EXCHANGES

(One serving contains 2 Gm. of protein, 0.5 Gm. of fat, 15 Gm. of carbohydrate and 70 calories)

Bread (white, whole wheat, raisin,
   rye, pumpernickel, French,
   Italian or Boston brown bread)   1 slice
Roll (2 to 3 inches across).   1
†Biscuit, muffin (2″ diam.).   1
†Cornbread (1½″ cube).   1
Melba toast (3½″ x 1½″ x ⅛″)   4
Matzo (5″ x 5″).   1
Bread sticks, rye wafers. . . . . . .   ¾ oz.
Cereal, cooked. . . . .   ⅓ c.
   dry, flake or puffed. . . . .   ¾ c.
Rice, grits, cooked. . . . .   ½ c.
Spaghetti, noodles, cooked. . . . .   ½ c.
Macaroni, cooked. . . . .   ½ c.
Dry bread crumbs. . . . .   ¼ c.
Flour. . . . .   3 tablespoons
Cornmeal. . . . .   2½ tablespoons
Bean, peas, dried, cooked. . . . . .   ½ c.
Corn, kernels or creamstyle. . . . .   ⅓ c.
Corn on the cob, medium ear. . .   ½ c.
Potatoes, white (2″ diam.).   1
Potatoes, sweet. . . . .   ¼ c.

MEAT, FISH AND POULTRY EXCHANGES

(One ounce contains 8 Gm. of protein, 2 Gm. of fat, 0.6 Gm. of saturated fat, 0.1 Gm. of linoleic fatty acid, 21 mg. of cholesterol, and 50 calories)

Meat selections from the following list are limited to 3 meals a week and to 3 ounces per serving

Beef—lean. . . . .   1 oz.
   Hamburger—ground round or
   chuck

Roasts, pot roasts, stew meats—
   sirloin tip, round, rump, chuck,
   arm
Steaks—flank, sirloin, T-bone,
   porterhouse, tenderloin,
   round, cube
Soup meat—shank or shin
Other—dried chipped beef

Lamb. . . . .   1 oz.
   Roast or steak—leg
   Chops—loin, rib, shoulder

Pork. . . . .   1 oz.
   Roast—loin, center cut ham
   Chops—loin
   Tenderloin

Ham. . . . .   1 oz.
   Baked, center cut steaks, pic-
   nic, butt, Canadian bacon

Meat selections for 11 of the 14 main meals each week are made from the following list:

Poultry (without skin). . . . .   1 oz.
   Chicken, turkey, cornish hen,
   squab

Fish—any kind (not shellfish). . . .   1 oz.

Veal—any lean cut. . . . .   1 oz.

Cottage cheese, preferably
   uncreamed. . . . .   ¼ c.

Peanut butter. . . . .   2 tablespoons

  *Eggs—limit to 3 per week (3/7 of an egg contains 3 Gm. of protein, 3 Gm. of fat, 0.9 Gm. of saturated fat, 0.2 Gm. of linoleic fatty acid, 118 mg. of cholesterol, and 35 calories.)

FAT EXCHANGES

(One tablespoon of vegetable oil contains 14 Gm. of fat, 2.0 Gm. of saturated fat, 8.0 Gm. of linoleic fatty acid, and 125 calories)

Corn oil.   1 tablespoon
Cottonseed oil. . . . .   1 tablespoon
Safflower oil. . . . .   1 tablespoon
Soybean oil . . . .   1 tablespoon
French dressing (made with any
   of the oils listed above). . . . . .   1½ tablespoons
Mayonnaise (made with any of
   the oils listed above). . . . .   1 tablespoon
Special margarine. . . . .   1 tablespoon

(One tablespoon of special margarine, corn oil, contains 11 Gm. of fat, 2.5 Gm. of saturated fat, 3.7 Gm. of linoleic fatty acid, and 100 calories.)

(One tablespoon of special margarine, safflower, contains 11 Gm. of fat, 1.9 Gm. of saturated fat, 6.3 Gm. of linoleic fatty acid, and 100 calories.)

---

  * Adapted from Zukel, M. C.: Fat-controlled diets. Am. J. Clin. Nutr., *16*:270, 1965 (Feb.).

  † See recipes, Chapter 38.

---

  *If the cholesterol in the diet is limited to 200 mg. per day eggs cannot be used.

TABLE 23–3. Food Exchange List for Fat-Controlled Diets* (Continued)

SUGAR AND DESSERT EXCHANGES	
(One serving contains about 50 calories)	

Sugars

White, brown or maple......	1 tablespoon
Corn syrup or maple syrup...	1 tablespoon
Honey....................	1 tablespoon
Molasses.................	1 tablespoon
Jelly, jam or marmalade.....	1 tablespoon

Desserts

Tapioca or cornstarch pudding ¼ c.
(Made with fruit and fruit juice
or with skim milk from milk calculated in diet plan)

Fruit whip................. ¼ c.
(Made with egg whites, no
cream)

Gelatin dessert.............	⅓ c.
Water ice.................	¼ c.
Sweetened canned or frozen fruit.....................	⅓ c.
(Equals 1 fruit exchange and 1 tablespoon sugar)	
Angel cake, plain...........	1 small piece
Sweetened carbonated beverages................	6 ounces

Candies

Gumdrops.................	3 medium or 14 small
Marshmallows..............	3 large
Hard fruit drops...........	4

Milk Exchanges. The only item in this list in the Fat-Controlled Diet is skim milk. This may be fluid skim milk, non-fat dried milk or buttermilk made from skim milk. Milk fat contains a significant amount of saturated fat (see Part Four, Table 3). Therefore, milk fat in any form—whole milk, cream, butter, cheese made from whole milk, or ice cream—is not used in this diet plan. There is no vitamin A in skim milk, since it is in the milk fat. Vitamin A has been added to some skim milks and it is wise to use these products to ensure an adequate vitamin A intake. Also the cholesterol in skim milk is much less than the amount in whole milk. Eight ounces of skim milk contains approximately seven mg. of cholesterol while 8 ounces of whole milk contains approximately 26 mg.

Bread Exchanges. The major modification in the items in this list compared with the Bread Exchanges for diabetic diets is in the type of fat used in making hot breads, e.g., biscuits, muffins and cornbread. Only the fats and oils in the Fat Exchange list in Table 23–3 are used in the recipes for these breads. (See recipes in Chap. 38.) The amount of fat in a serving of these products is counted as part of the fat planned in a diet pattern. For example, if a diet plan contains 3 tablespoons of oil, the one teaspoon of oil in one biscuit made

from the recipe in Chapter 38 will count as one teaspoon of this amount of oil. The 0.5 gm. of fat for Bread Exchanges is included to account for the fat in cereals.

Plain cake and ice cream which are included in the Bread Exchanges for diabetic diets are omitted from the Bread Exchanges for fat-controlled diets. Because of the egg and milk fat in cake and the milk fat in ice cream these foods are not included in this exchange list. It will be noted that only crackers made without fat such as rye wafers and bread sticks are included in these lists. Bread crumbs, flour and cornmeal have been added for use in food preparation, especially for cooking meat and fish.

Meat Exchanges. There is considerable difference between the nutrient values and the items in this Exchange list compared with the Meat Exchange for diabetic diets. If a Fat-Controlled pattern dietary is to provide the amount of the polyunsaturated fatty acid, linoleic, required by the physician's diet prescription, careful selection of the kinds and amounts of meat must be made. Only lean cuts of those items listed in the Meat Exchange in Table 23–3 can be used in order to avoid an intake of saturated fats in excess of the prescribed amount.

The calorie and nutrient values for one Meat Exchange in Table 23–2 were derived from weighted averages of the values for the meat, fish and poultry items in the Meat Exchange list. All the items in this list contain less than 13 Gm. of total fat per 100-Gm. portion.* Lean beef, lamb, pork and ham contain more saturated fat than poultry, fish and veal. Therefore, beef, lamb, pork and ham are limited to three meals and poultry, fish and veal are used for the other eleven main meals in a week. If beef, lamb, pork and ham are used more frequently, the weighted values for one meat exchange will not apply and the intake of saturated fat will be in excess of that calculated in the diet plan.

Liver is not included in the Meat Exchanges due to its cholesterol content. Poultry without skin is used since the major amount of the fat in poultry is in the skin. Eggs are limited to three per week not only because of the saturated fat content but also because of the cholesterol content. When cholesterol is limited to 200 mg. or less per day eggs will be omitted from the diet plan entirely, with adequate protein provided by the Milk and Meat Exchanges.

Fat Exchanges. Together with the Meat Exchanges these are critical factors in achieving a fat-controlled intake. The items in the Fat Exchange list (Table 23–3) are certain vegetable oils; French dressing and mayonnaise made with these oils; and special margarines. The oils are limited to cottonseed, soy, corn, and safflower. These are the vegetable oils with the most significant amount of linoleic fatty acid (see Table 23–4).

Commercial French dressings can be used because they are made with cottonseed, soy or corn oils. Commercial mayonnaise can be used because it is also made with these oils. The amount of cholesterol from eggs in commercial mayonnaise is not significant (8 mg. per 1 tablespoon) but if used in excessive amounts could add to the total cholesterol in a diet,

---

* U.S.D.A. Handbook No. 8, 1963 revision.

TABLE 23–4.
Approximate Fatty Acid Composition of Vegetable Oils*

Vegetable Oil	Saturated Fatty Acids†	Mono unsaturated Fatty Acids†	Polyunsaturated Fatty Acids†
Coconut......	86	7	—
Cocoa butter..	56	37	2
Olive........	11	76	7
Peanut.......	22	43	29
Cottonseed....	25	21	50
Soy..........	15	20	59
Corn.........	10	28	54
Safflower.....	8	15	72

* From USDA Home Economics Report No. 7.
† Grams per 100 Gm. ether extract or crude fat.
Brown, H. B. and Farrand, M. G.: J. Am. Dietet. A., 49:303, 1966.

especially if cholesterol is limited to 200 mg. per day.

The "special" margarines are those made either from corn or safflower oil. It will be observed that Table 23–2 gives separate values for corn oil and safflower oil margarines, and shows that the safflower oil margarine contains more linoleic fatty acid than the kind made with corn oil. These margarines are usually soft and are packaged in a tub. The first ingredient named on the label of the package will state either liquid corn or safflower oil. Unfortunately, this does not necessarily, under present labeling regulations, ensure that the margarine will contain the amount of linoleic fatty acid given in Table 23–2. As a general rule, the best guide to purchasing margarine with a significant amount of linoleic fatty acid is to look for the soft type in a tub, with safflower oil as the first ingredient listed on the label.

Sugar and Dessert Exchanges. This exchange provides calories from sugars and simple desserts, and is useful in planning diets containing 1,800 calories or more. It must also be remembered that milk fat in any form cannot be used in the desserts listed.

TABLE 23–5. Nutrient Composition of a 1,500-Calorie Fat-Controlled Diet

| | | | | | Fat | | | |
Food	Amount	Weight Gm.	Protein Gm.	Total Fat Gm.	Sat- urated Fat Gm.	Linoleic Fatty Acid Gm.	Chole- sterol Gm.	Carbo- hydrate Gm.	Calories
Milk, skim .... 1 pt. (2 c.)		480	16	tr.	..	..	14	24	160
Vegetables, Group A.. as desired		varies	..	..	..	..	..	..	..
Group B.. 1 cup		200	4	..	..	..	..	14	70
Fruit................ 3 servings		varies	..	..	..	..	..	30	120
Bread and cereal..... 6 servings		varies	12	3.0	0.6	..	..	90	420
Meat, lean .... 6 ounces		180	48	12	3.6	0.6	126	..	300
Egg................ 3/wk. (3/7)		21	3	3	0.9	0.2	118	..	35
Fat (veg. oil)[1] .... 2 tablespoons		28	..	28	4.0	16.0	..	..	250
Fat (Special margar- ine safflower) ...... ½ tablespoon		7	..	5.5	1.0	3.1	..	..	50
Sugar (dessert)....... 1 tablespoon		12	..	..	..	..	..	12	50
Totals			83	51.5	10.1	19.9	258	170	1,455

[1]Corn, cottonseed, safflower, soybean oil.

CALCULATION OF FAT-CONTROLLED DIET

Table 23–5, Nutrient Composition of a 1,500-Calorie Diet, illustrates the calculation of a fat-controlled pattern dietary. Approximately 22 per cent of the total calories are provided by protein, 46 per cent by carbohydrate, and 30 per cent by fat. About 13 per cent of the total calories are provided by linoleic fatty acid, and less than 11 per cent by saturated fats. It will be observed that this diet contains approximately

TABLE 23–6. Suggested Menu for 1,500- Calorie Fat-Controlled Diet

Breakfast	Noon Meal	Evening Meal
8 ounces orange juice	Chicken sand- wich	4 ounces roast veal
1 cup cooked oatmeal	2 slices bread	½ cup peas ½ cup winter squash
8 ounces skim milk	2 ounces chicken	Sliced tomato with 1 tsp. French dress- ing
	1 tbsp. may- onnaise	
	Lettuce	2 biscuits*
	Fresh peach	½ tbsp. saf- flower mar- garine
	8 ounces skim milk	¼ cup fruit whip

* See recipe, Chapter 38.

260 mg. of cholesterol and, if eggs are not used three times per week, the cholesterol in the diet would be less than 200 mg. per day. Table 23–6 offers a suggested menu for a 1,500-Calorie Fat-Controlled Diet.

For the hospitalized patient careful precautions must be taken to ensure that the patient is not served vegetables which have been seasoned with butter, meat which is well marbled with fat or meat from which the visible fat has not been removed, or hot breads made with other than vegetable oil shortening. At the same time, relatives and friends should be instructed to avoid offering the patient chocolate candies and ice cream or beverages made with whole milk and ice cream.

PATIENT EDUCATION

The patient who requires a fat-controlled diet will need careful, detailed diet instruction. The first step is a complete diet history to determine his previous food practices. Since this diet requires extensive changes in the average American diet, a comprehensive diet history will help to identify more readily those food practices of a patient which can be continued as well as identify those which will of necessity be changed.

It is also important to discover where and with whom the patient eats his meals. These patients will not be able to adhere to their diets if they eat all or most of their meals in restaurants. With careful selection an occasional meal in a restaurant is possible. For example: a possible restaurant meal might be roasted or broiled lean meat, green salad with vinegar and oil dressing, fruit and skim milk.

Since the majority of patients who experience heart attacks are men, it is essential that the wife be present for the diet history and all diet instruction. It is possible that many of her food-buying practices and methods of food preparation will need to be changed. For example, if she has always made fruit whip with whipped cream, she will need to be instructed to make it with egg whites. Or if she has found it convenient to use frozen dinners frequently, she may need help in planning the preparation of meals which require more of her time in the kitchen.

Many of these patients and their wives will be well motivated to learn how to cope with the fat-controlled diet. The press, popular magazines and television, have all helped to make the middle-aged American conscious of the need for "polyunsaturates" in their diets. Unfortunately, some of these media have oversimplified the problem by emphasizing only one food—for example, changing from butter to "special" margarines without considering the need also to change to skim milk and lean meat.

A very useful teaching aid is the booklet, Planning Fat-Controlled Meals for 1200 and 1800 Calories (revised 1966). This booklet, prepared in cooperation with the American Dietetic Association and the Heart Disease Control Program, U. S. Public Health Service, is published by the American Heart Association.* Copies are available to the patient on a physician's prescription only. They are available to physicians, dietitians, and other professional persons on request.

_____
* A.H.A., 44 East 23rd Street, N.Y., N.Y. 10010.

TABLE 23–7. Cholesterol Content of Food*
(per Exchange-size serving)

Food	Household Measure	Weight in Gm.	Cholesterol mg.
Whole milk.......	8 ozs.	240	24
Egg.............	1	50	275
Meat, fish........	1 oz.	30	21
Chicken (with skin).	1 oz.	30	18
Cheese, Cheddar..	1 oz.	30	30
Liver............	1 oz.	30	90
Butter...........	1 tbsp.	14	35
Margarine....... (All veg. fat)	1 tbsp.	14	0

* Calculated from Table 4, Handbook No. 8, U.S.D.A., 1963.

PLANNING THE CHOLESTEROL-RESTRICTED PATTERN DIETARY

Cholesterol in Food. Meat, organ meat, shellfish, eggs, and dairy products are the major contributors of cholesterol to the American dietary. Plant foods generally do not contain cholesterol.

Table 23–7, Cholesterol Content of Food (per Exchange-size serving), lists the average number of milligrams of cholesterol in the meat, milk and fat exchanges. It can be seen that egg, liver and butter are the most significant contributors of cholesterol at the per serving level. The substitution of two eggs (550 mg. of cholesterol) for two ounces of meat (42 mg. of cholesterol) in a day's menu plan significantly increases the total cholesterol intake.

The Pattern Dietary. The Pattern Dietary (p. 265, Chap. 19) contains approximately 500 mg. of cholesterol per day provided that liver is not selected as a serving of meat, and the selection of other foods to meet an adult's allowance for calories does not contain additional eggs, butter, or whole milk. This means that cakes, cream pies, milk puddings, ice cream and whipped cream cannot be used for dessert in the daily menu plan.

A significant reduction in cholesterol in the Pattern Dietary can be achieved by omitting the egg each day (minus 275 mg. of cholesterol) and adding one ounce of meat (plus 21 mg. of cholesterol). Egg white, which does not contain cholesterol, can be used. All organ meats and shellfish contain a greater amount of cholesterol than muscle meat and fish and, therefore, cannot be used. (See Table 3, Part Four.) The use of margarine in place of butter will also reduce the amount of cholesterol in the pattern dietary.

STUDY QUESTIONS AND ACTIVITIES

1. Why is atherosclerosis a public health problem of major importance?

2. List the foods which contain the greatest per cent of linoleic fatty acid.

3. Is it correct to say that all plant oils contain only linoleic fatty acid and that all animal fats contain only saturated fat? (See Chap. 3 and Table 3, Part Four.)

4. List some of the foods commonly used in the American diet which are omitted on the fat-controlled diet.

5. What epidemiologic study is being carried out to test the fat-controlled diet for the prevention of coronary heart disease?

6. Accompany the dietitian when she takes the diet history and instructs a patient who requires a fat-controlled diet. While giving nursing care to this patient, discover how well he understands his diet instructions. Share your observations with the dietitian before her next appointment with this patient. Report this experience to your classmates in clinical conference with them, your nursing instructor and the dietitian.

7. Which food, if any, did the patient on the fat-controlled diet miss most?

8. Calculate a 2,000-Calorie Fat-Controlled Diet containing 38 per cent of fat, more than 14 per cent of linoleic fatty acid and less than 14 per cent of saturated fat.

9. Estimate the cholesterol in the food you consumed in one day. (See Table 3, Part Four.)

SUPPLEMENTARY READING ON ATHEROSCLEROSIS

Brown, H. B., et al.: Design of practical fat-controlled diets. J.A.M.A., 196:205, 1966.

Brown, H. B., and Farrand, M. E.: Pitfalls in constructing a fat-controlled diet. J. Am. Dietet. A., 49:303, 1966 (Oct.).

Christakis, G., et al.: Effect of the Anti-coronary Club program on coronary heart disease risk-factor status. J.A.M.A., 198:129, 1966 (Nov. 7).

Council on Foods and Nutrition: Diet and the possible prevention of coronary atheroma. J.A.M.A., 194:1149, 1965.

Dietary Fat and Human Health. National Academy of Sciences—National Research Council Pub. 1147, 1966.

Editorial: Changing Dietary Habits. J.A.M.A., 196:281, 1966 (Apr. 18).

Planning Fat-Controlled Meals at 1200 and 1800 Calories, Revised 1966. Am. Heart A., New York, N. Y.

Stamler, J., et al.: Coronary proneness and approaches to preventing heart attacks. Am. J. Nursing, 66:1788, 1966 (Aug.).

Zukel, M. C.: Fat-Controlled Diets. Am. J. Clin. Nutr., 16:270, 1965.

For further references see Bibliography in Part Four.

CHAPTER 24

Cardiac Disease; Hypertension

Cardiac Disease • Principles of Dietary Treatment • Sodium in Foods and Beverages • Sodium in Medications • The Diet Prescription • Planning the Sodium-Restricted Pattern Dietary • Teaching the Patient • Hypertension • Dietary Treatment

CARDIAC DISEASE

Disease of the heart is found among all age groups, although it is most common in older individuals. The causes are many. It may be due to a congenital defect, in which case the patient will be in the younger age group. Rheumatic fever, a frequent cause of cardiac damage in the past, has responded to antibiotics, and cardiac disease from this origin now occurs mostly in the middle age group. Arteriosclerotic heart disease, due to hardening of the arteries and usually accompanied by high blood pressure, occurs in older patients. Atherosclerosis is one of the major causes of heart disease and is most frequently found from middle age onwards (see Chap. 23). Because heart disease is the first cause of death in the United States, it is considered a primary public health problem.

Severity of Cardiac Involvement. Cardiac disease may be acute, as in coronary occlusion, with a sudden onset and no previous history of cardiac insufficiency; or it may be chronic, of long standing, with increasing loss of cardiac reserve. The severity of cardiac disease depends on the degree to which the heart is damaged and the extent to which this interferes with its function. If damage is slight, and the heart is able to maintain adequate circulation to all parts of the body, the disease is said to be mild or "compensated." The patient may have to avoid strenuous activity but otherwise will be able to perform his daily tasks without discomfort.

Decompensation, or severe heart disease, is said to occur when the heart is unable to sustain adequate circulation of blood to the tissues. The blood flow to the lungs is slowed, and oxygen uptake and carbon dioxide excretion are inadequate. The patient suffers from shortness of breath and chest pain when he performs any sort of activity. As decompensation progresses, both the liver and kidneys may become involved and edema may appear in the dependent parts of the body and, sometimes, in the pleural and the peritoneal cavities. Severe cardiac disease of this magnitude is called congestive heart failure.

When patients are chronically ill with severe heart disease, their activities must be severely restricted, and they may even have to spend much of their time in bed so that the limited oxygen supply will be sufficient for whatever activity is allowed. Drugs to strengthen the heart muscle are commonly prescribed. If edema is present, diuretic drugs to increase sodium and water excretion are usually given, and a diet restricted in salt must be followed.

Salt and Water. The sodium of salt (sodium chloride) is the water-holding mineral of the body fluids and is found

327

abundantly in the blood and in the fluid spaces between the cells (interstitial space). Normally we ingest a good deal of sodium each day, some of it found in the food itself and most of it added as salt in cooking processes and at the table. It is estimated that the average person consumes from 2 to 3 level teaspoons of salt per day, or about 8 to 15 Gm. This is equivalent to 3,000 to 6,000 mg. of sodium. Except for a small amount needed to replace normal sodium losses, this intake is excreted in the urine and lost in perspiration. If all salty foods such as bacon, ham, salted crackers and salted butter are omitted and no salt is used at the table, the diet will contain approximately 2,000 to 3,000 mg. of sodium.

The patient with severe impairment of cardiac function may retain sodium and, therefore, fluid in his tissues, causing edema. As the circulation becomes less efficient, there is venous stasis and increased venous pressure. This prevents the return of sodium and water from the interstitial spaces to the blood stream to be carried to the kidneys for excretion. With poor circulation, the rate of flow of blood to the kidney is diminished and kidney function is impaired. Aldosterone, the adrenal cortex hormone which causes sodium retention and potassium excretion by the kidney, and the pituitary antidiuretic hormone, which aids the kidney in the reabsorption of water, are out of balance and contribute to the production of edema.

By lowering the sodium in the diet, there will be a decrease in the quantity of sodium circulating in the blood. This will help to draw the sodium, and therefore water, from the interstitial spaces back into the blood stream to be excreted eventually by the kidneys, relieving the edema. The use of diuretic drugs by the physician aids in this process.

Even the patients with mild cardiac disease are usually placed on some degree of sodium restriction in order to prevent the development of edema.

WATER. As has been said, when sodium is excreted from the body, there will be a corresponding loss of water. For this reason fluids are usually not restricted. See the discussion of the sodium content of water supplies later in the chapter.

Principles of Dietary Treatment

Nutritional Adequacy. As in all therapeutic dietary regimens which must be used for a long period of time, the diet for the cardiac patient should meet all of his nutritional needs. Certain foods which are high in sodium may need to be omitted or replaced with others, but the foods that are chosen should provide all the nutrients in sufficient quantity to maintain health. (See Pattern Dietary, Chap. 19.)

Weight. If the cardiac patient is overweight, it is essential that the caloric intake be diminished and that the patient lose weight. This measure tends to reduce basal metabolism and, thus, the work of the heart. Even for the cardiac of normal weight it may be beneficial to reduce the weight slightly below this level, in order to lessen the work of the heart. (See Chap. 21 for low caloric diets.)

Some cardiacs, especially those suffering from rheumatic heart disease, may be underweight and undernourished. Although it may not be possible or desirable to have them gain weight, every effort should be made to make the diet nutritionally adequate in calories, protein, minerals and vitamins.

General Suggestions. The diet for the patient with heart disease may be ordered as fluid, soft or general, depending on the severity of his illness, on his physical condition, on whether he has teeth and whether he is confused or alert. If the patient tires easily, it may be best to serve the diet in five meals. The cereal and milk from breakfast and the dessert and part of the fluid from lunch and dinner may be served as between-meal nourishment. The evening nourishment may have to be omitted if the patient is too tired to eat. It will be remembered that the appetite of most chronically ill patients is best at breakfast, when they are rested, and gradually decreases throughout the day.

Foods which cause a patient to have discomfort or distention should not be served. These foods may be members of the cabbage family, dried peas and beans, or any other food the patient feels he cannot tolerate. Distention of the abdomen presses the diaphragm upward and "crowds the heart" lying just above it. Constipation must be avoided to prevent straining at stool. Simple remedies such as prune juice, hot water or hot water and lemon juice are often effective. Laxative drugs should never be used except by order of the physician, since many of them contain sodium.

Coffee and tea are usually allowed. However, very hot or very cold fluids may affect heart action as they flow down the esophagus, and are sometimes omitted. Alcoholic beverages may be used by the patient at the discretion of the physician.

Sodium in Foods and Beverages

Salt. Salt or sodium chloride, commonly used in cooking and preserving food, is approximately 40 per cent sodium. Thus, 1 Gm. of salt (1,000 mg.) contains 0.4 Gm. or 400 mg. of sodium. It can readily be seen why salt, added to foods during cooking or at the table, must be omitted or used only in very limited amounts on sodium-restricted diets. Also foods which have had sodium added during processing or preservation are avoided. (See Food Processing, pp. 331–332 and Figs. 24–1 and 24–2.)

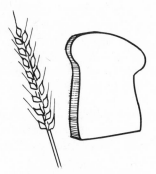

A slice of regular bread contains about 150 milligrams of sodium.

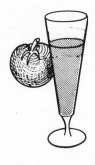

A half cup of canned tomato juice contains about 275 milligrams of sodium.

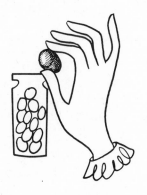

Just one large olive will add 130 milligrams of sodium to the diet.

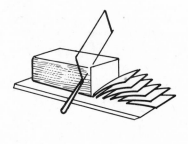

One ounce of processed cheddar cheese contains about 420 milligrams of sodium.

Fig. 24–1. A few examples of foods high in sodium content.

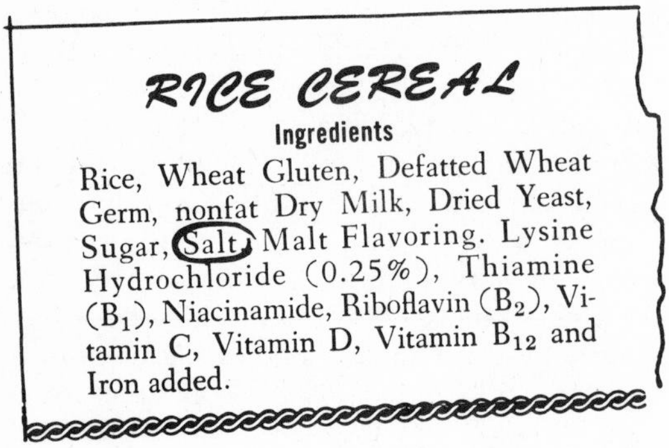

RICE CEREAL

Ingredients

Rice, Wheat Gluten, Defatted Wheat Germ, nonfat Dry Milk, Dried Yeast, Sugar, Salt, Malt Flavoring. Lysine Hydrochloride (0.25%), Thiamine (B₁), Niacinamide, Riboflavin (B₂), Vitamin C, Vitamin D, Vitamin B₁₂ and Iron added.

Some cereals have salt added.

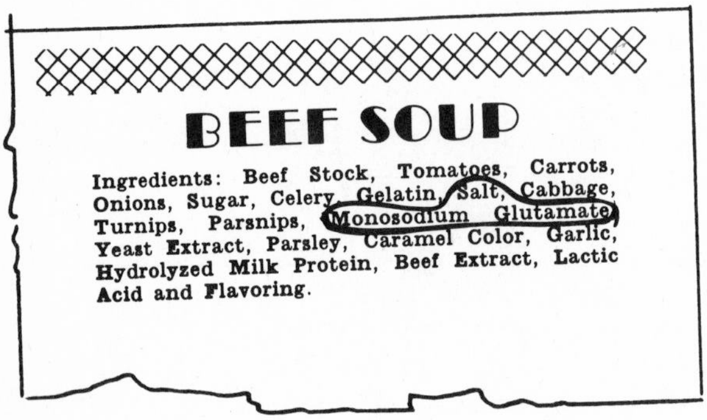

BEEF SOUP

Ingredients: Beef Stock, Tomatoes, Carrots, Onions, Sugar, Celery, Gelatin, Salt, Cabbage, Turnips, Parsnips, Monosodium Glutamate, Yeast Extract, Parsley, Caramel Color, Garlic, Hydrolyzed Milk Protein, Beef Extract, Lactic Acid and Flavoring.

Even if this can of soup did not contain salt it should not be used because of the monosodium glutamate.

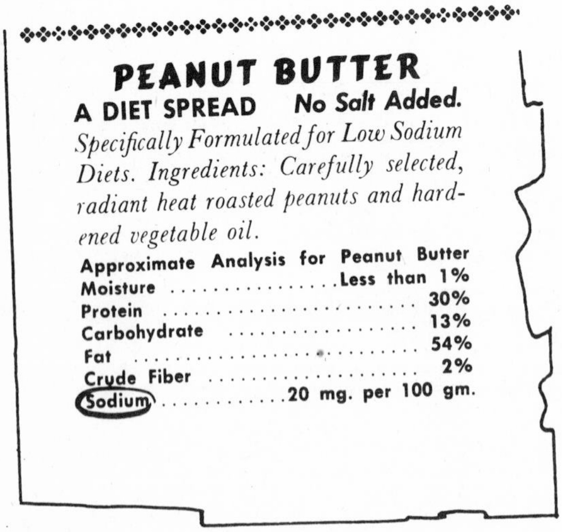

PEANUT BUTTER

A DIET SPREAD   No Salt Added.

Specifically Formulated for Low Sodium Diets. Ingredients: Carefully selected, radiant heat roasted peanuts and hardened vegetable oil.

Approximate Analysis for Peanut Butter

Moisture	Less than 1%
Protein	30%
Carbohydrate	13%
Fat	54%
Crude Fiber	2%
Sodium	20 mg. per 100 gm.

Dietetic foods must be labeled carefully.

FIG. 24–2. Examples of labeling.

Food. With few exceptions all of our food, by nature, contains sodium but the amounts vary by food groups. Animal foods are our most important sources of sodium; plant foods usually contain the least sodium. Milk, meat, fish, fowl, and eggs, processed or cooked without the addition of salt or any other sodium compound, contribute the greatest amount of sodium in the restricted diet. (See Table 24-2, p. 334, Sodium Content of Food Exchanges.)

Animal fats and vegetable oils naturally contain only very little or no sodium. Therefore, at certain levels of sodium restriction salt-free butter and unsalted margarine are used. Vegetable oils and cooking fats made from vegetable oils do not have salt added in processing and may be used in the sodium-restricted diet.

Cereals, breads, fruits, and vegetables, processed and cooked without the addition of salt or other sodium compounds, contribute the least amount of sodium to the restricted diet. There are exceptions in the vegetable group: artichokes; beets, carrots, white turnips; celery; spinach, kale, beet greens, chard, dandelion greens and mustard greens—these contain more sodium per serving than other commonly used vegetables. For example, one half cup of carrots (100 Gm.) cooked without salt contains about 50 mg. of sodium, whereas one half cup of broccoli (100 Gm.) cooked without salt contains about 10 mg. of sodium.

Food Processing. The greatest source of the sodium in our food is the sodium added in food processing and preservation. Easily recognized examples of this are bacon and ham; salted crackers, potato chips, popcorn and other snack foods; and olives, pickles and sauerkraut.

The cereals and bread and other bakery products in our markets have salt and other sodium compounds added in processing or preparation. Bread made without salt or other sodium compounds is now available in many areas because of the great demand by individuals needing sodium-restricted diets. One slice of bread made with salt contains about 150 mg. of sodium (see Fig. 24-1); 1 slice made without salt contains about 5 mg. Unsalted melba toast is also generally available. A recipe for making bread without salt will be found in Chapter 39.

Canned foods, packaged mixes and other convenience foods such as frozen dinners, frozen vegetables with sauces and seasonings added, and frozen waffles and pizza all have sodium added. The same applies to canned soups, gravies and soup mixes; mayonnaise and salad dressings; and condiments such as chili sauce, ketchup, and meat sauces. Sodium is not added to canned fruits; also vegetables naturally low in sodium, and canned without the addition of salt, are generally available in our markets.

Sodium may also be added in food processing where we do not expect it. Fresh peas and lima beans have very little sodium and are used in the sodium-restricted diet. But frozen peas and lima beans are omitted because they are sorted in salt solution in the processing plant and pick up significant amounts of sodium. One half cup of fresh peas cooked without salt has about 1 mg. of sodium; one half cup of frozen peas cooked without salt has about 115 mg. of sodium. This is only one example of an unexpected addition of salt in food processing and illustrates why patients who require a sodium-restricted diet need careful instruction.

Sodium compounds other than salt which may be used in food processing are: disodium phosphate in quick-cooking cereals; monosodium glutamate in a variety of foods, to enhance the flavor; sodium alginate in chocolate milk and ice creams for smooth textures; sodium benzoate as a preservative in jams, jellies, relishes, sauces and salad dressings; sodium hydroxide to soften skins of certain fruits, olives and hominy; sodium proprionate to inhibit mold growth in cheese and bread; and sodium sulfite to bleach certain fruits before coloring such as maraschino cherries.

Baking powder and baking soda (sodium bicarbonate) are also important sources of sodium. A sodium-free baking powder for home use is available in some of our markets. A recipe for sodium-free baking powder, which the pharmacist in the hospital or in a local drug store can make up, will be found in Chapter 39.

Labels and Label Reading. Although the booklets and other materials which may be used in patient education will warn him to "read labels," this may not be as helpful as it sounds. The Food and Drug Administration (see Chap. 17) allows many processed foods such as mayonnaise and ketchup to be sold without listing the ingredients on the label. These and other foods are prepared under a standard of identity which specifies the kind and the minimum content of each ingredient and, therefore, in such cases the listing of sodium on the label is not required.

On many packages and containers, even when properly labeled, the salt content of the food is listed by a variety of terms such as salt, sodium chloride, sodium, Na, or soda. The patient must be cautioned that these terms are synonymous and that foods containing them must be avoided (see Fig. 24–2).

Low-Sodium Dietetic Foods. Products offered as low-sodium dietetic foods come under the regulations of Food for Special Dietary Uses of the Food and Drug Administration. These regulations are presently under revision (1967) but it appears that those which apply to sodium content of food will not be changed. Under the regulations the label must clearly show the content of sodium, in mg. per 100 Gm. of food, and the number of milligrams of sodium in a specified serving of such food. It is helpful to remember that 100 grams is approximately three ounces.

Some of the foods labeled "low sodium" may not be usable on a sodium-restricted diet because, although reduced in sodium as compared with the regular food, they still contain too much sodium per serving. Low-sodium soups, for instance, may still contain too much sodium to be included in the diet. Vegetables, such as those previously listed as having a high natural sodium content, even when canned without salt, should not be used if they are not listed on the sodium-restricted diet.

Seasonings. A variety of spices and herbs which can be used to make the diet more palatable will be found in Chapter 39. For-

tunately, most of these are low in sodium. It must be remembered that some commonly used seasonings and condiments contain salt. These are celery, garlic and onion salt; dried parsley and onion flakes; prepared mustard, worcestershire and soy sauce; and sodium glutamate and meat tenderizers. Patients who have not previously used a variety of spices and herbs should be cautioned to use them sparingly until they are sure they enjoy the new flavors.

SALT SUBSTITUTES. Salt substitutes are available at drugstores and some food markets. They usually contain potassium or ammonium in place of sodium. The potassium substitute may be contraindicated if there is kidney damage and the ammonium ones if there is extensive liver damage. In the hospital they may be offered to patients on sodium-restricted diets routinely or only by order of the physician. Those patients who use a salt substitute need to be advised to use it sparingly because in excessive amounts some individuals find the taste unpleasant. One of the substitutes, labeled "seasoned," has a variety of spices added and is very palatable.

"Koshering" of Food. Jewish patients who follow the orthodox dietary laws salt their freshly slaughtered meat and fowl to extract the blood, allowing it to stand for an hour or so, then washing it thoroughly before cooking. Although this will remove some of the added salt, a good deal will have penetrated the inner portion of the meat. Kaufman[1] states that meat so treated has from 334 to 375 mg. of sodium per 100 Gm., depending on the manner of cooking. She suggests that Jewish patients be taught to salt their meat lightly and allow it to stand for the minimal amount of time; after it has been rinsed and soaked in water, it should be boiled in a generous amount of water and the broth should be discarded. Meat so treated was found to contain 63 mg. of sodium per 100 Gm. As an alternative, she suggests the use of ammonium chloride salt in place of sodium chloride for drawing out the blood.

---

[1] Kaufman, M.: Am. J. Clin. Nutr., 5:676, 1957.

The Drinking Water. In some areas of the country drinking water may present a special hazard because of its high sodium content. This may be due either to the sodium content of the soil from which the water is drawn or to the use of water softeners.

In a recent study of over 2,000 local water supplies,[2] widely distributed throughout the United States and covering approximately 50 per cent of the population, great variation in sodium content was found, as shown in Table 24–1.

TABLE 24–1. Range of Sodium Ion in Drinking Water for a Sampling Period*

Range of Sodium Ion Concentration	Number of Samples	Per Cent of Total Samples
mg./L.		
0- 19.9.........	1,194	58.2
20- 49.9.........	391	19.0
50- 99.9.........	190	9.3
100-249.9.........	178	8.7
250-399.9.........	74	3.6
400-499.9.........	10	0.5
500-999.9.........	14	0.7
Over 1000..........	2	0.1

* From White, J. M., *et al.*: Sodium ion in drinking water. J. Am. Dietet. A., 50:32, 1967.

It will be noted that only 58 per cent or a little over a half the water supply was within the range of none to 20 mg. of sodium per liter (approximately a quart). Water used for coffee and tea, for drinking and for food preparation is estimated at 2½ to 3 quarts per person a day. When water contains more than 20 mg. of sodium per quart, it quickly begins to affect the sodium content of the diet. The patient should obtain information about his community's water by contacting the department of health.

[2] White, J. M., *et al.*: J. Am. Dietet. A., 50:32, 1967.

"Soft Drinks." Bottled "soft drinks" may be high in sodium due to the sodium content of the water in the area where they are manufactured. Low caloric beverages may have their sodium content increased still further by the substitution of sodium cyclamate, an artificial sweetener, for sugar. They are therefore omitted when careful sodium restriction must be maintained.

Sodium in Medications

The physician will avoid prescribing medications which contain sodium. The patient should be cautioned to take no medication, "patent" medicine or home remedy without consulting his physician. Baking soda (sodium bicarbonate) is a popular home remedy for indigestion or "heart-burn"; and many alkalizers, antacids, headache remedies, sedatives and cathartics are high in sodium and should not be used.

The Diet Prescription

Depending on the condition of the patient, the physician's diet order will state in milligrams the specific amount of sodium he wants the patient to have each day. The order for sodium restriction may also be combined with one for calorie restriction (Chap. 21) or for diabetes (Chap. 22). In the past there was considerable confusion because the diet order restricting sodium intake tended to be general, rather than specific. Such terms as salt-poor, low-salt, or salt-free diet gave little indication of the amount of sodium permitted. This confusion has disappeared as we have learned how the body uses sodium, and how to analyze foods for their sodium content. The most commonly used levels of sodium restriction are 500 mg. and 1,000 mg. The term, mild sodium restriction, is used when a level of 2,000 mg. or more of sodium is allowed.

500-Milligram Sodium Diet. A diet order for 500 mg. of sodium or less is considered a severe restriction and will be used with the acutely ill patient. He may be in congestive failure with edema, or have hypertension. Planning the 500-mg. sodium Pat-

TABLE 24–2. Sodium Content
of Food Exchanges*

Food	Household Measure	Gm.	Milligrams of Sodium
Milk Exchanges...	8 ounces (½ pint)	240	120
Meat Exchanges...	1 ounce	30	25
Vegetable Exchanges.......	½ cup	100	9
Fruit Exchanges...	1 serving	varies	2
Bread Exchanges..	varies	varies	5
Fat Exchanges....	1 tsp.	5	negligible

* Foods produced, processed or prepared without the addition of any sodium compound.

tern Dietary is discussed in the next section of this chapter. The water used for drinking or in cooking must contain no more than 20 mg. of sodium per quart, or distilled water must be used.

When less than 500 mg. of sodium (200 to 300 mg.) is required, special low-sodium milk—either Lonalac or dialyzed whole milk, fresh or canned—will be used to ensure an adequate intake of protein, calcium and the other nutrients usually supplied by milk. Dialyzed milk, which contains more potassium than regular milk, may be contraindicated if there is kidney damage, or other reason for restricting potassium. On the other hand if the diuretic being used promotes potassium loss, the dialyzed milk can help replace potassium.

Sometimes 600-, 700-, or 800-mg. sodium diets will be ordered.[3,4] The 500-milligram Pattern Dietary can be modified in various ways to fulfill these orders.

1,000-Milligram Sodium Diet. Diet orders for 1,000 mg. of sodium are used for patients who require only a moderate restriction of sodium intake. Some of these patients may tolerate 1,200- to 1,500-milligram sodium diets, and diets in this range

[3] Mayo Clinic Diet Manual. ed. 3. p. 36.
[4] Johns Hopkins Hospital, Manual of Applied Nutrition. ed. 5. p. 126.

may be ordered. Planning the Pattern Dietary for the 1,000-milligram sodium-restricted diet is discussed in the following section of this chapter.

Mild Sodium-Restricted Diet. The sodium content of these diets may range from 2,000 to 4,500 mg. of sodium and is usually prescribed for the patient who has only moderate cardiac damage. No salt is added to food at the table and foods obviously high in salt are omitted.

Planning the Sodium-Restricted Pattern Dietary

Sodium-Restricted Food Exchange Method

A widely used method for planning the sodium-restricted pattern dietary is based on the Exchange Method such as the one used for planning diabetic pattern dietaries. Table 24–2, Sodium Content of Food Exchanges, gives the average sodium values of the Exchanges. These are values for foods produced, processed and prepared without the addition of salt or any other sodium compound.

The Exchange Lists for the sodium-restricted diet are on pages 335 to 337. If they are compared with the Diabetic Exchange Lists in Chapter 22, it will be seen that there is only one Vegetable Exchange List in the sodium restricted Exchange Lists. The sodium value, 9 mg. per one half cup serving cooked without salt, applies to both Vegetable Exchanges—Groups A and B—in the diabetic exchanges. It will be remembered that certain vegetables in both Groups, A and B, may not be used on sodium-restricted diets because of their high natural sodium content (for example, spinach, kale, carrots, etc.). Although one ounce of meat and one egg are interchangeable for protein and calories, this is not true for sodium. One egg contains 70 mg. of sodium while one ounce of meat, cooked without salt, contains only 25 mg. of sodium. Therefore, one egg cannot be substituted for one ounce of meat in a sodium-restricted diet. Careful study of the Sodium Exchange Lists on the following pages point out these and other variations between the Sodium Restricted and the Diabetic Exchange Lists.

Sodium-Restricted Diet Exchange Lists

Milk Exchanges. One cup (8 ounces) contains 120 mg. of sodium

Use:

Regular (whole) milk

Skim milk (liquid or reconstituted according to directions on the package)

Unsalted buttermilk (ask the dairy)

Evaporated milk (½ cup = 1 cup whole milk)

If skim milk, either fresh or powdered, or buttermilk is used, add 2 teaspoons of fat for each glass unless calories are restricted.

Milk used in cooking must be counted in the day's allowance.

Substitutes for not more than 1 glass of milk a day: 2 ounces of meat, poultry or fish or 6 ounces (¾ container) of plain yogurt.

Do Not Use:

Ice cream	Chocolate milk
Sherbet	Condensed milk
Malted milk	Fountain drinks
Milk shakes	Junket tablets
Instant cocoa mixes	

Meat Exchanges. Each ounce, cooked, contains 25 mg. of sodium

Use:

Meat or poultry, fresh frozen or dietetic canned

Beef	Tongue, fresh	Turkey
Lamb	Liver	Rabbit
Pork	Chicken	
Veal	Duck	

Fish, fresh* or dietetic canned, all except those listed under Do Not Use.

An average serving of cooked meat, poultry or fish is 3 ounces. Allow an extra ounce or two for shrinkage, bone and fat when shopping.

One egg contains 70 mg. of sodium. Egg should not be substituted for meat.

Substitutes for 1 ounce of meat, poultry or fish: ¼ cup unsalted cottage cheese, 1 ounce low-sodium dietetic cheese, or 2 tablespoons low-sodium dietetic peanut butter.

Do Not Use:

Brains, kidneys

Canned, salted or smoked meat:

Bacon	Meats, koshered by
Bologna	salting
Chipped beef	Luncheon meats
Corned beef	Sausage
Frankfurters	Smoked tongue
Ham	

Frozen fish fillets

Canned, salted or smoked fish:

Anchovies	Herring
Caviar	Sardines
Salted cod	

Canned tuna or salmon unless low-sodium

Shellfish:

Clams	Oysters
Crabs	Scallops
Lobster	Shrimp

---

* Fresh fish must be rinsed thoroughly in clear water because it is sometimes kept in salt water or temporarily frozen with salt before it reaches the market.

Vegetable Exchanges. One serving—½ cup—contains about 9 mg. of sodium

Use:

Any fresh, frozen* or low-sodium dietetic canned vegetables or vegetable juices except those listed under Do Not Use.

Some patients may not tolerate strong-flavored vegetables.

Restaurants usually add salt and monosodium glutamate to vegetables.

Do Not Use:

Canned vegetables and vegetable juices unless low-sodium dietetic.

Frozen vegetables if processed with salt.

These vegetables in any form:

Artichokes	Whole hominy
Beet greens	Kale
Beets	Mustard greens
Carrots	Sauerkraut
Celery	Spinach
Chard	White turnips
Collards	
Dandelion greens	

---

* A few frozen vegetables, such as peas and lima beans, have had salt or other sodium compound added during processing. Read labels.

Sodium-Restricted Diet Exchange Lists *(Continued)*

Fruit Exchanges. Each serving contains about 2 mg. of sodium

Use:

Any kind of fruit or fruit juice—fresh, frozen, canned or dried.

The size of a serving of fruit varies, depending on the fruit. Examples of 1 serving: a small apple, ½ cup fruit cup, 2 medium plums.

Substitute for fruit juice: low-sodium dietetic tomato juice.

Do Not Use:

Fruit flavored beverage mixes and powders.
Commercial gelatin dessert

Low-Sodium Bread Exchanges. Each serving contains about 5 mg. of sodium

Use:

Low-sodium bread and rolls, unsalted Melba toast, plain unsalted Matzo

Unsalted cooked cereals:

Farina	Rolled wheat
Hominy grits	Wheat meal
Oatmeal	

Dry cereals:

Puffed rice	Shredded wheat
Puffed wheat	

Macaroni products and cereals:

Macaroni	Barley
Noodles	Unsalted popcorn
Spaghetti	Flour
Rice	

Count as 1 serving 1 slice of bread, 1 roll or muffin, 4 pieces of Melba toast; ½ cup cooked cereal, ¾ cup dry cereal; ½ cup cooked noodles, rice, etc.; 1½ cup popcorn; 2½ tablespoons flour.

Low-sodium bread, rolls, etc., are made without salt and with yeast or sodium-free baking powder or potassium bicarbonate.

Substitute for a serving of bread or cereal one of the following:

Dried beans or peas—½ cup cooked
Corn ⅓ cup or ½ small ear
Potato, white—1 small
Potato, mashed—½ cup
Sweet potato—¼ cup or ½ small

Do Not Use:

Regular breads, crackers, rolls, muffins
Commercial mixes
Cooked cereals containing a sodium compound (read label)
Dry cereals other than those listed or those that have no more than 6 mg. of sodium in 100 Gm. of cereal (read label)
Self-rising cornmeal
Self-rising flour
Potato chips
Pretzels
Salted popcorn

Fat Exchanges. Contain practically no sodium

Use:

Butter, unsalted
Margarine, unsalted
Fat or oil for cooking, unsalted
French dressing, unsalted
Mayonnaise, unsalted
Cream, light or heavy, sweet or sour (see limitation below)
Nuts, unsalted

One serving equals 1 level teaspoon of butter, margarine, fat, oil or mayonnaise; 1 tablespoon French dressing; 1 tablespoon heavy cream*; 2 tablespoons light cream*; 6 small nuts.

Do Not Use:

Regular butter
Regular margarine
Commercial salad dressings or mayonnaise unless low-sodium dietetic
Bacon, bacon fat
Salt pork
Olives
Salted nuts
Party spreads and dips

---

* Cream contains more sodium than other fats and is limited to 2 tablespoons a day.

Sodium-Restricted Diet Exchange Lists (Continued)

Miscellaneous Foods. The following foods contain no sodium

Use:		Do Not Use:
Coffee	Lemons	Beverage mixes, including instant cocoa and fruit
Coffee substitutes	Limes	flavored powders
Tea	Plain, unflavored	Fountain beverages, including malted milk
Cocoa powder	gelatin	Soft drinks, both regular and low caloric
Sugar, brown and white	Vinegar	Bouillon cubes, powders or liquids
Honey	Cream of tartar	Sodium cyclamate, sodium saccharin
Sugar substitutes:	Potassium bicarbonate	Commercial candies
Calcium cyclamate	Sodium-free baking	Commercial gelatin desserts
Calcium saccharin	powder	Regular baking powder
	Yeast	Baking soda (sodium bicarbonate)
		Rennet tablets
		Molasses
		Pudding mixes

500-Milligram Sodium-Restricted Diet Pattern. Table 24–3 shows how the sodium-restricted Exchanges can be combined to provide a 500-mg. sodium pattern dietary and, at the same time, provide the nutrients needed by an adult. It will be seen that milk, meat, fish, fowl and eggs account for four fifths of the sodium intake each day. The remainder of the sodium comes from the foods naturally low in sodium, and from the water used in drinking and cooking. To reduce this pattern dietary to about 250 mg. of sodium one pint of Lonalac or dialyzed whole milk (about 12 mg. of sodium) is substituted for one pint of regular milk (240 mg. of sodium).

When compared with the Pattern Dietary in Chapter 19, it will be seen that the foods in the quantities listed in the 500-Milligram Sodium-Restricted Diet will provide the Recommended Dietary Allowances, with the exception of iron for women. The calories will be approximately 1,650, however, due to an increased quantity of vegetables, fruit and bread. Some patients, those who need to lose weight, will have to omit some of the bread and potato and possibly use skim in place of whole milk. Other patients will need additional food to meet their caloric requirement. This will vary, of course, with size, age and activity. A big-boned man, 6'2" tall, will need more calories than a man who is 5'6" tall, even if both are doing the same type of work. A woman with several small children, doing her own housework,

TABLE 24–3. A 500-Milligram Sodium-Restricted Pattern Dietary

Food	Amount	Sodium Approximate mg.	Calories* Approximate
Milk	one pint	240	320
Meat, poultry, fish	4 ounces, cooked	100	376
Egg	one	70	81
Vegetables	4 ½-cup servings	36	{ 54 { 90
Potato	2 ½-cup servings	10	65
Fruit	4 servings	8	{129 { 85
Bread, unsalted	4 servings	20	252
Cereal, unsalted	1 serving	5	89
Fat	1 tablespoon	..	100
Totals		489	1,641

*Calorie values are based on the Pattern Dietary in Chapter 19.

TABLE 24—4. The 1,000-Milligram Sodium-Restricted Diet Pattern

This diet follows the foods allowed and restricted on the 500-Milligram Sodium-Restricted Diet. In addition the patient may "spend" the other 500 mg. of sodium on one of the following choices:

Equivalents for 500 mg. sodium

¼ *scant* teaspoon salt	Water containing approximately 200 mg. of sodium per quart
¾ teaspoon monosodium glutamate	
2 slices regular bakery bread plus 1 tablespoon salted butter or margarine	Water containing approximately 100 mg. of sodium per quart plus 1 slice of regular bread and 1 teaspoon salted butter or margarine
½ cup serving of cooked cereal, rice, spaghetti, macaroni or noodles, cooked *with* salt plus 1 tablespoon salted butter or margarine	Water containing approximately 50 mg. of sodium per quart plus 2 slices regular bread

has greater energy needs than an older woman of the same size, who lives alone. Foods which will supply calories without adding to the sodium content of the diet are sugar, honey, jams, jellies and marmalades (if made without sodium benzoate), cream for coffee, an increased use of unsalted fats, and desserts made with the allowed ingredients.

Adjustment of the diet will also have to be made for individual preferences and needs. Two additional ounces of meat may be more acceptable to a patient in place of one of the 8-ounce glasses of milk, particularly if he dislikes milk. The remainder of the milk may be used with coffee and on cereal. It may become necessary for a secretary to carry her lunch rather than buy a sandwich at a nearby drugstore if she is to maintain her sodium restriction.

The 500-mg. sodium pattern dietary can serve as the foundation for diets of 600, 700, or 800 mg. of sodium. The patient's preferences, the amount of money he can spend for food, and the ease with which he can buy low-sodium diet foods should be taken into consideration. For example, if a patient who requires a 600 mg. sodium diet is using only two teaspoons of margarine per day, he could substitute two

teaspoons of salted margarine. Two teaspoons of unsalted margarine have little or no sodium, and two teaspoons "with salt added" contain 100 mg. of sodium. The salted margarine is cheaper and generally more readily available.

The 1,000-Milligram Sodium-Restricted Diet Pattern. This diet which is used for many patients, permits a choice of additions and substitutions as shown in Table 24–4.

One fourth *scant* teaspoon of salt contains 500 mg. of sodium. This carefully measured amount of salt can be added to the 500-mg. sodium diet to provide a 1,000-mg. sodium intake. Some physicians are strongly opposed to this method for increasing sodium. They feel that it makes it difficult for the patient, should his condition require it at some time in the future, to reduce his sodium intake again to less than 1,000 milligrams. Also, patients who have accepted foods without added salt and have become used to omitting salt report that they have "lost their taste" for salt and do not enjoy it. For the patient who cannot tolerate food without salt, and if his physician agrees, the one fourth *scant* teaspoon of salt may make it possible for him to have an adequate diet, which he would not have without the salt.

Often additions or substitutions more acceptable to the patient are the use of regular bread and salted butter or margarine, since these are easily available and cheaper than the low-sodium varieties. One slice of salted bread of the usual size, about 3½ inches by 4 inches, and no more than ½ inch thick, contains approximately 150 mg. of sodium. One level teaspoon of salted butter or margarine contains about 50 mg. of sodium. It will be seen that changes or additions to the 500-mg. sodium-restricted diet must be carefully measured in order not to exceed the allowed sodium intake. Notice also the limitations if the water supply contains more than 20 mg. of sodium per quart.

Mild Sodium-Restricted Diet Pattern. This diet permits the use of foods processed and cooked with moderate amounts of salt and other sodium compounds. Highly salted foods are not used. Table 24–5, The

TABLE 24–5. The Mild Sodium-Restricted Diet Pattern

This diet should follow the 500-Milligram Sodium-Restricted Diet, with the following additions:

Salt.............A moderate amount of salt may be used for cooking, but none may be added at the table. Garlic, onion and celery salt may be used if they replace salt in cooking

Meat, poultry, fish,
eggs...........Brains, kidneys, frozen fish fillets, regular canned tuna and salmon and all shellfish are permitted

Vegetables........All vegetables, fresh, frozen or canned, except sauerkraut, are allowed

Bread and cereals..Regular bread and rolls, but none with salt topping, are permitted. All cereals are allowed

Fats.............Salted butter and margarine and commercial salad dressings are allowed

All other restrictions as listed on the 500-Milligram Sodium-Restricted Diet must be observed.

Mild Sodium-Restricted Diet, illustrates the additions which can be made to a 500-mg. sodium diet to provide a reasonably mild sodium-restricted diet.

Teaching the Patient

Teaching Materials. Three excellent booklets are available for helping the patient to understand his sodium-restricted diet. These were prepared by the American Heart Association in conjuction with the American Dietetic Association, the Council on Foods and Nutrition of the American Medical Association, the Nutrition Foundation and the Public Health Service of the Department of Health, Education, and Welfare. The diets are constructed on the Exchange system presented in this chapter. The three booklets are entitled "Your 500 Milligram Sodium Restricted Diet"; "Your 1000 Milligram Sodium Restricted Diet"; and "Your Mild Sodium-Restricted Diet." The first two booklets have also been issued as a simplified leaflet. They are available to the patient through his physician, who may obtain them from his local heart association, or, where there is no local association, from the American Heart Association.[5]

The Patient's Problems. Learning to omit salt from his diet is not an easy process for most patients. Not only do foods taste flat, but they serve as a continual reminder that something is wrong with him. When a patient newly placed on sodium restriction asks the nurse "How long will I be on this diet?" he may be asking in reality if he will have heart disease the rest of his life. Unless he is carefully instructed throughout his stay in the hospital, the cardiac patient may think that, although his diet was instrumental in his improvement, now that he is better he does not need to follow it at home.

Depending on the degree of sodium restriction ordered by the physician, one of the three booklets from the American Heart Association, or one of the two leaflets described above, may be of help to the pàtient in learning how to adapt his food to the prescribed restrictions, but it must be implemented with specific suggestions to meet his own needs. The nurse and the dietitian must be ready to answer questions, to direct the patient's thinking, to give concrete suggestions, and to be ever ready with encouragement and support. Again, the teaching should be begun early in the patient's hospital stay, so that he has a chance to think through the needed adjustments for sodium restriction before he has to adapt to them at home.

In teaching the patient on a sodium-restricted diet it is especially important to find out something about his home circumstances and his cultural background. Both the wife and the husband should be taught what is required if the husband is the patient. Since an older patient may live with a son or a daughter, whoever is the homemaker should receive instruction along with the patient. Chapter 39 will be found helpful for giving specific instructions to the patient and his family about the preparation of food.

---

[5] American Heart Association, 44 East 23rd Street, New York, N. Y. 10010.

Patients who do not have adequate cooking facilities and are accustomed to eating their meals in restaurants will need help in adjusting to the demands made by sodium restriction. Southern patients in the habit of cooking with bacon or salt pork must be warned about this. Jewish patients, following their dietary laws of heavily salting their meats before cooking (koshering) will need help in readjusting their deeply ingrained convictions. (See p. 332 in this chapter.) Italian patients should be warned not to use purchased tomato paste, olives, Italian cheese and Italian bread. Tomato paste can be made at home, omitting salt and spices containing sodium. Occasionally an Italian bakery will make low-sodium bread if there is sufficient demand for it. Japanese and Chinese patients must be cautioned particularly to omit sodium glutamate and soy sauce, both of which are used commonly in the seasoning of their food. Greek patients and those coming from the Near East frequently use heavily salted olives as an accompaniment to meals. When counseling a patient it is essential not only to obtain information on his food habits from him, but also to look up the foods common to his culture which may interfere with his ability to maintain a sodium-restricted regimen. (See Chapter 11 for descriptions of varying food patterns, and also the Supplementary Readings following Chapter 11.)

HYPERTENSION

In a study of blood pressure in a very large number of individuals,[6] it was found that, although there is a small but steady rise in blood pressure with increasing age for both men and women, the average blood pressure remained below 135 mm. Hg systolic and 82 mm. Hg diastolic, even at 60 to 64 years of age. Although there is no commonly accepted definition for hypertension, insurance studies show that systolic pressures of 140 mm. Hg and over and diastolic pressures of 90 mm. Hg and over are associated with an appreciably higher

degree of mortality. In most patients the hypertension remains benign for many years, although eventually cardiac failure, cerebral hemorrhage or chronic kidney disease may follow.

Etiology. Several hormones, produced in the kidney and in the adrenal cortex, are involved in the maintenance of normal blood pressure levels. One of these, aldosterone, regulates sodium excretion by the kidney.

The work of Dahl[7] indicates that the salt intake of the individual may play a role in the development of hypertension. In a study of over 1,300 subjects, he found that less than 1 per cent of those who habitually had a low salt intake demonstrated hypertension, while among those ingesting an average amount of salt the incidence was 6.8 per cent, and among those with a high salt intake the number of individuals with hypertension rose to 10.5 per cent.

There is presently no known organic cause for hypertension although Conn[8] postulates that very small adrenal adenomas, producing an increase in the hormone aldosterone, may be responsible for an increased blood pressure in a considerable number of patients.

Use of Drugs. Drugs with an anti-hypertensive effect and others which aid sodium excretion are now available. They are prescribed by the physician in the hope that the more serious systemic involvement may be averted or delayed.

Dietary Treatment

Overweight. Weight above desirable levels places an extra burden on the heart. For this reason the hypertensive patient who is also overweight should lower his caloric intake until his weight is at normal levels for his height and build. (See Chap. 21 for low caloric regimens.)

The Role of Sodium. Experimental and clinical evidence indicates that rigid restriction of sodium in the diet results in a decided reduction in the blood pressure of hypertensive patients. Kempner,[9] using a

---

[6] Build and Blood Pressure Study, 1961, Society of Actuaries; from Blood Pressure: Insurance Experience, Metropolitan Life Insurance Co., 1961.

[7] Dahl, L. K.: J. Am. Dietet. A., *34*:585, 1958.

[8] Conn, J. W.: New Eng. J. Med., 273:1135, 1965.

[9] Kempner, W.: North Carolina M. J., 5:125, 273; 6:62, 117, 1944-45.

diet of unsalted rice and fruit supplemented with minerals and vitamins and containing less than 200 mg. of sodium, reported beneficial results in 138 of 213 patients. However, this diet is so difficult to maintain that it has largely been abandoned. Other investigators, using a more liberal diet equally low in sodium, were able to obtain decreases in blood pressure in hypertensive patients, showing that sodium restriction was responsible for the results.

Sodium-Restricted Diet. For the patient who has developed cardiovascular-renal disease as a result of his hypertension, a diet restricted in sodium may be prescribed. This will usually be the 500-Milligram Sodium-Restricted Diet, described above. Further sodium restriction, to 250 mg. daily, can be achieved by substituting low-sodium milk, which contains approximately 2 to 5 mg. of sodium in 100 ml. or 5 to 12 mg. in one cup (8 ounces), for regular milk (see Table 24–3). All other restrictions of the 500-Milligram Sodium-Restricted Diet must be observed. If the cardiovascular-renal disease is severe, however, with impending kidney failure, the use of low-sodium milk may be contraindicated because of its increased potassium content (see Chap. 25).

The low-sodium diet is lacking in flavor as are all salt restricted diets. Moreover, the patient is likely to be quite ill and to have a poor appetite. The use of seasonings suggested in Chapter 39 will help to make the diet more palatable. Care taken with preparation, appearance and contrast in color and flavor, and the use of permissible garnishes, may help to tempt the patient's appetite.

SALT SUBSTITUTES may be used, but these should be approved by the physician. Salt substitutes containing potassium are contraindicated if there is kidney disease.

STUDY QUESTIONS AND ACTIVITIES

1. Why may the patient with cardiac disease develop edema?
2. Why will a diet restricted in sodium aid in preventing or eliminating edema in the cardiac patient?

3. Compare the food restrictions between the 500-Milligram, the 1000-Milligram and the Mild Sodium-Restricted Diets. How do they differ, and in what ways are they alike?
4. Give the approximate sodium content of the foods and the quantities allowed on the 500-Milligram Sodium-Restricted Diet. Which food contributes most to the sodium content of the diet? Which foods are next?
5. What advice would you give a patient who dislikes milk?
6. Is low-sodium bread available in your community? How does its price compare with regular bread? How may it be kept fresh?
7. Look at the recipe for low-sodium bread in Chapter 39. Will this be easy or difficult to make?
8. Which foods must be omitted on all varieties of sodium-restricted diets?
9. What is the sodium content of one slice of regular bread? Of one teaspoon of salted butter or margarine? Of one tablespoon?
10. Make out a menu for a day for a soft diet, and 500-Milligram Sodium restriction, for a patient with congestive heart failure, dividing it into 5 meals and observing the precautions you would follow in planning a menu for any very ill patient.
11. Will the foregoing menu meet all of the patient's nutritive needs including calories?
12. List the points you would stress to a patient going home on a mild sodium-restricted diet.
13. Which cooking ingredients and seasonings must a patient on a sodium-restricted diet be warned not to use?
14. Which seasonings, spices and condiments may be used to make a sodium-restricted diet more palatable? (See Chap. 39.)
15. Name the foods that commonly cause distention. Why should these not be served to the cardiac patient?
16. What simple remedies for constipation may the cardiac use? What must he be warned not to use?
17. What should the cardiac patient be told about labeling?

18. What warning must be given a patient about the use of salt substitutes?

19. How may a patient obtain information about the sodium content of the drinking water in his community?

20. What aids are available for teaching patients on sodium-restricted diets? How should these be used?

21. What are some of the regional and cultural food patterns which may make it difficult for a patient to adhere to a sodium-restricted diet?

22. Make out a menu for a secretary on a 1,500-Calorie, 1,000-Milligram Sodium-Restricted Diet who must carry her lunch. For the same secretary who wishes to buy her lunch at a local restaurant.

23. Why may a 250-Milligram Sodium-Restricted Diet be prescribed for a patient with severe hypertension? Is fresh low-sodium milk available in your community? If not, how may the patient obtain low-sodium milk? (See Chap. 39.)

SUPPLEMENTARY READING ON CARDIAC DISEASE; HYPERTENSION

Heap, B.: Sodium restricted diets. Am. J. Nursing, *60*:206, 1960.

Heap, B., *et al.*: Simplifying the sodium-restricted diets. J. Am. Dietet. A., *49*:327, 1966.

Keller, M., and Segner, E. F.: When heart and hands are overburdened. Am. J. Nursing, *62*:92, 1962 (Jan.).

Rimer, D. G., and Frankland, M.: Sodium content of antacids. J.A.M.A., *173*:995, 1960.

Vavra, C. E., *et al.*: Meeting the challenge of educational care in heart disease. Am. J. Publ. Health, *56*:1507, 1966.

Your 500 Milligram Sodium-Restricted Diet (booklet and leaflet); Your 1000 Milligram Sodium-Restricted Diet (booklet and leaflet); Your Mild Sodium-Restricted Diet (booklet); American Heart Association, New York, N. Y.

For further references see Bibliography in Part Four.

PLATE 2

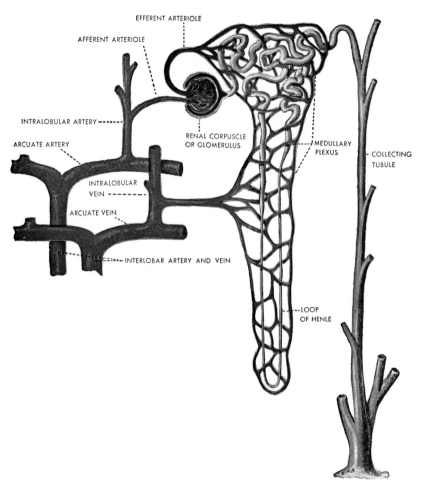

A schematic drawing of the nephron, showing arterial and venous circulation. Water and water-soluble substances are filtered from the glomerular blood capillaries into the tubule. In the tubule, all of the glucose and much of the water, sodium and other components of the glomerular filtrate are reabsorbed into the surrounding capillary bed. The remainder passes from the collecting tubule into the pelvis of the kidney and, finally, by way of the ureters, into the bladder. (Sharp & Dohme's *Seminar,* vol. 9, No. 3, August, 1947.)

CHAPTER 25

Diseases of the Kidney; Kidney Stones

Function of the Kidneys • Diseases of the Kidney • Kidney Failure • Principles of Dietary Treatment • Pattern Dietary for Protein, Sodium and Potassium Restrictions • Teaching the Patient • Kidney Stones: Dietary Treatment

Function of the Kidneys. The kidneys, with the lungs, are the chief excretory organs of metabolic end products from the body. Practically all the waste materials resulting from catabolism, except carbon dioxide which is eliminated by the lungs, are carried by the blood to the kidneys where they are filtered and the waste products excreted.

It is estimated that each kidney contains about 1 million filtering units, called nephrons. The nephron consists of a tuft of capillaries—the glomerulus—surrounded by a covering capsule which merges into a long, winding tubule (see Plate 2). The fluid which filters through the glomeruli is a protein-free filtrate of the blood plasma. It consists of water and all the water-soluble substances in the blood, among which are glucose, amino acids, electrolytes such as sodium, potassium, chlorides, phosphates and many others, as well as the nitrogenous end products of protein metabolism—uric acid, creatinine and urea. The filtrate then passes through the tubules, where over 99 per cent of the water, most of the glucose and the amino acids, a good portion of the electrolytes and even some of the apparent waste products such as urea are reabsorbed into the blood capillaries surrounding the tubules. The remainder passes on through the collecting tubule into the pelvis of the kidney. This fluid is the urine which is passed by the ureters into the bladder, where it accumulates and in due time is eliminated from the body.

Water is the chief constituent of the urine, the quantity varying mainly with the amount taken into the body and the amount excreted by means of the skin and lungs. Normal urine contains about 5 per cent of solids, consisting of a variety of electrolytes, both basic and acid, and the end products of protein metabolism, of which the largest constitutent is urea nitrogen.

The kidneys are subject to disease, as are other organs of the body. There may be congenital malformation and a decreased number of nephrons; or cysts may be present, occluding some of the functioning nephrons. Infection may occur, as in pyelonephritis; there may be inflammation of kidney tissue as in nephritis and nephrosis; kidney damage may result from long continued hypertension, or from decreased blood flow in severe cardiac disease; or the kidney pathways may be blocked by the formation of kidney stones.

Fortunately the kidneys have a large reserve of functioning units. It is estimated that only about one sixth of the total number of nephrons are active at any one time, and that this number is sufficient to clear the blood of waste materials.

In kidney disease the filtering mechanism is usually affected, and substances not normally found in the urine, such as albumin, one of the proteins in the blood, may now be present. Conversely, substances cleared from the blood by the healthy kidney may not be fully eliminated. Two of these are urea, and, in very severe disease, potassium. They will be found in increased quantites in the blood. For these reasons urine analysis, blood chemistry determinations and kidney function tests are common procedures in the diagnosis of kidney disease.

Kidney disease may be acute, followed by healing; or it may be recurrent and eventually become chronic, with an ever decreasing number of functioning nephrons. When the kidney no longer is able to maintain the normal composition of the blood by excreting all of the waste products, the patient is said to have uremia (referring to the retention of urea nitrogen in the blood) and to be in kidney failure. Eventually there will be oliguria (diminished secretion of urine), or even anuria (complete suppression of urine). Death will intervene unless hemodialysis, either by the artificial kidney or via the peritoneum, is available.

GLOMERULONEPHRITIS

The most frequently occurring kidney disease is probably nephritis, or Bright's disease, characterized by inflammation of kidney tissue. Since it is the glomeruli which are first affected, this type of kidney damage is called glomerulonephritis. It usually follows a hemolytic streptococcal infection in another part of the body, or it may be precipitated by a generalized infection. It occurs more often in childhood or early adult life than in later years.

Acute Glomerulonephritis

Acute glomerulonephritis is characterized by hematuria (red blood cells in the urine), oliguria, puffy eyes and swelling of the ankles due to retention of sodium and water, and hypertension. There may be anorexia or nausea and vomiting. The disease is self-limiting, and complete recovery results in 4 to 6 months in the large majority of patients. In a few cases, however, the disease may go on to chronic glomerulonephritis.

Dietary Treatment. Merrill[1] states that the aim of the dietary treatment of acute glomerulonephritis is rest for the kidney by minimizing its excretory work. Protein should be limited to 0.5 Gm. or less per Kg. of body weight. If edema or increased blood pressure is present, sodium must be restricted. In order to prevent tissue breakdown for energy needs, the caloric content of the diet should be adequate. This will depend on the age and size of the patient.

Foods Allowed. In the early stages of the illness, the patient, especially if he is a child, may want little more than fluids. Water, ginger ale, plain or with added corn syrup, sweetened fruit juices and fruit ices are well tolerated. They are low in sodium, unless the local water supply or the water used in ginger ale are high in sodium. Usually the potassium intake need not be restricted. If oliguria is present, fluids are limited to the urine output plus the water loss from the skin, depending on the degree of oliguria and the age of the patient. As urine output increases, so does the fluid allowance.

In a few days other foods may be added such as cereal with a small amount of milk, toast with butter, jelly or jam, baked potato and fresh or cooked fruit. If sodium restriction is necessary, only low-sodium cereals and unsalted bread and butter should be used. No salt should be added in cooking or at the table (see Chap. 24).

As the patient improves, other foods will be added until he is back on his normal diet. On the other hand, he may continue to be somewhat restricted in protein, and possibly, sodium, until the kidney function tests show complete recovery. This may take up to six months despite subjective improvement, and the patient should be warned to maintain whatever dietary restrictions have been ordered by the physician. See the Pattern Dietary for protein, sodium and potassium restriction later in the chapter (Table 25-2).

---

[1] Merrill, A. J.: J.A.M.A., *173*:905, 1960.

Chronic Glomerulonephritis

Chronic glomerulonephritis may follow an attack of acute nephritis, particularly if repeated infections have occurred; or it may be insidious in its onset, the symptoms being so mild at first that the subject is not aware of his condition until his attention is drawn to it, perhaps when undergoing a physical examination for life insurance. The urine is usually abundant in quantity and of low specific gravity, and it may show much or comparatively little albumin and some casts. There may be morning headache, and the patient may be annoyed by the necessity of frequent urination during the night, due to the inability of the kidneys to concentrate the urine.

As time goes on these symptoms become more severe. Increased loss of albumin in the urine lowers the level of serum albumin, and therefore the osmotic pressure of the blood, resulting in generalized edema. This is sometimes called the nephrotic phase of glomerulonephritis.

Dietary Treatment. The physician will usually order a diet increased in protein content to compensate for the loss of albumin. Sodium may be restricted if edema or hypertension is present. See the discussion on dietary prescription later in the chapter.

NEPHROSIS

True nephrosis is characterized by severe loss of serum albumin from the kidney, resulting in marked edema. It occurs only in young children and will be discussed in Chapter 34, Diseases of Children.

NEPHROSCLEROSIS

Nephrosclerosis occurs among older patients and is usually the result of arteriosclerosis and essential hypertension of long standing. The blood supply to the kidney has decreased gradually because of the thickening of the wall and the narrowing of the lumen of the blood vessels. Usually this is accompanied by increased blood pressure and is characterized by urea nitrogen retention in the blood. In the more severe cases, mild or moderate albuminuria also may be present.

Dietary Treatment. Many patients with arteriosclerosis and resulting kidney disease are overweight. If this is the case, the calories in the diet must be limited so that the patient will lose weight. (See Chapter 21 for low caloric diets.) If the patient is of normal weight, the diet should provide the proper amount of calories, depending on the age, size and activity of the patient.

If the urea nitrogen level of the blood is increased only slightly, the patient with nephrosclerosis may be allowed the normal amount of protein in the diet, so that his strength and vigor will be maintained. When the blood urea is elevated markedly, indicating inability of the kidney to excrete sufficient amounts of this waste product of protein metabolism, it becomes necessary to restrict the patient's protein intake.

Sodium intake may be limited by the physician in patients with hypertension (see Chap. 24). Fluids are usually allowed liberally to aid in the excretion of waste products, unless there is a degree of kidney failure with oliguria. In such case the amount of fluid allowed is closely correlated not only with the fluid loss from the kidneys but also with estimated losses from the skin and lungs.

KIDNEY FAILURE

When the kidney cannot maintain its excretory function, either because of a sudden emergency or as the result of permanent damage, of whatever origin, the patient is said to be in kidney failure. It is manifested by scanty urine, or even anuria, with subsequent retention in the blood of all normally excreted substances. These include the end products of protein metabolism—urea, uric acid and creatinine—giving rise to uremia; electrolytes, especially sodium and potassium; and water. In the terminal stages the patient is critically ill, manifested by a number of symptoms including nausea, vomiting and anorexia.

Dialysis. With the advent of hemodialysis techniques, either by the artificial kidney or by peritoneal dialysis, it is possible to rid the blood of accumulated waste products. When this is done regularly, usually twice a week, the patient may be able to return to a reasonable amount of normal

Butter and Sugar Mixtures for Kidney Failure

Frozen Butter and Sugar Balls

200 Gm. cane sugar
200 Gm. unsalted butter
   1 ½ tsp. vanilla extract and 6 drops peppermint
extract or enough lemon juice to flavor the product

Cream sugar and butter together, add flavoring, roll into small balls, place in refrigerator until solid. 2,250 calories

Butter and Sugar Soup

200 Gm. cane sugar
 20 Gm. flour
200 Gm. unsalted butter
600 ml. water
Coffee or rum extract

Mix sugar and flour together. Add enough water to make a paste. Add the melted butter. Cook 20 minutes in double boiler. Add remainder of water and flavor with coffee or rum extract. 2,300 calories

living and activity. There are at present a number of centers in the United States which have the equipment and the skilled staff to perform these procedures in patients suffering from either acute or chronic renal failure, and more centers are being established with the aid of government grants. Unfortunately the number of patients in kidney failure far outstrips the available and even the proposed facilities. Hemodialysis, therefore, may be reserved for those patients for whom recovery of kidney function is possible and for patients who are candidates for kidney transplants.

Acute Kidney Failure

Acute kidney failure may occur in response to severe hemorrhage, in burns, or in poisoning, especially with heavy metals such as mercury, which are deposited in the tubules as the kidney tries to excrete them.

Dietary Treatment. If facilities for hemodialysis are available, the patient's blood will be cleared periodically of waste products until there is healing and kidney function is restored. The dietary regimen will follow that of other hemodialysis patients described later in the chapter.

If hemodialysis is not available, a carefully regulated diet is essential. Protein may have to be entirely eliminated or restricted to 10 to 20 Gm. a day. Calories are provided by infusions of glucose, and as much other carbohydrate and fat are given by mouth as can be included without appreciably increasing the sodium or potassium intake, both of which must be severely restricted during the acute phase. Total

fluids for the day must not exceed the urine output plus the estimated loss from the skin and lungs. It will include not only all fluid given by mouth, but also that given parenterally.

As can be seen in Tables 1 and 5, Part Four, there are few foods which do not contain protein, sodium or potassium. These are limited to white sugar, unsalted butter and margarine and the vegetable oils. The use of a nasogastric feeding of a mixture of glucose and one of the vegetable oils in emulsified form[2] has been reported. Earlier, Kolff[3] suggested butter and sugar mixtures to be taken by mouth. Directions for these will be found on this page. They may be substituted for nasogastric feedings, but most patients find them distasteful, and it is difficult for them to consume the equivalent of 1,800 to 2,000 calories a day. Hard candies may help to raise the intake of calories. Such severe dietary restrictions as have been described here are difficult for the very ill patient, and the nurse and the dietitian must constantly assure him of their necessity.

As the kidney begins to recover its function, other foods very low in protein, sodium and potassium may be added, such as unsalted cooked rice, unsalted bread, crackers and butter, sugar, a few vegetables, ginger ale, root beer and some other carbonated beverages (unless these are bottled in an area with a high-sodium content of the water supply), until the patient

---

[2] Lipomul, Upjohn Co., Kalamazoo, Mich.
[3] Kolff, W. J.: Am. J. Med., *12*:667, 1952; Nutr. Rev., *11*:193, 1953.

can tolerate a more liberal diet. As healing progresses, the patient may be maintained for a considerable length of time on a restricted protein, sodium, potassium and fluid regimen described later in the chapter.

Chronic Kidney Failure With Hemodialysis

As was stated earlier, if facilities either for direct hemodialysis or for peritoneal dialysis are available, patients in chronic kidney failure may be kept comfortable and active for several years. In order to curtail the accumulation of waste products between dialyses as much as possible, while at the same time maintaining the nutrition of the patient, diets limited in protein, sodium, potassium and fluids, but adequate in calories, will be ordered by the physician.

There is some diversity of opinion among the investigators working with patients receiving hemodialysis on the amounts of these nutrients that can be tolerated. One group,[4] working entirely with adult patients, advocates a basic menu pattern of 75 Gm. of protein, 1 Gm. of sodium, and 1 Gm. of potassium, with fluids restricted as necessary. It is claimed that patients are more content with this diet than one lower in protein, and can be more easily persuaded to follow it. Other investigators[5] believe that protein should be restricted to approximately 0.75 to 1 Gm. protein per Kg. of body weight for children and pre-adolescents, and to 0.5 to 0.75 Gm. per Kg. of body weight for adults. The degree of sodium restriction will depend on whether hypertension accompanies renal failure, and on the amout of sodium excreted in the urine. For these reasons, sodium allowance may range from 250 to 2,000 mg. a day. Potassium is limited, depending on kidney excretion, and may vary from 1.5 to 3 Gm. a day. Fluids are limited for the reasons described earlier in the chapter, under Acute Kidney Failure.

Chronic Kidney Failure Without Hemodialysis

When treatment by dialysis is not available for the patient in chronic kidney failure—and, unfortunately, this applies to the greater number of patients—the diet alone must serve to keep him functioning for as long as possible. In 1963 Giordano[6] showed that uremic subjects were able to utilize their accumulated urea nitrogen for protein synthesis, provided that the diet included minimal amounts of essential amino acids and sufficient calories. This regimen resulted in marked clinical improvement, with urea formation and accumulation kept at a minimum.

Subsequently Giovannetti and Maggiore,[7] after performing hemodialysis on their severely uremic patients, placed them on a diet containing 22 Gm. of protein, 600 to 900 mg. of sodium, 1,400 to 2,000 mg. of potassium and 2,000 to 3,000 calories. Part of the nitrogen was supplied by essential amino acids, given in the daily amounts recommended by Rose. The remainder of the protein came from cereals, fruit and vegetables of low protein content. Additional calories were supplied by sugars and fats. These investigators reported considerable success on this diet, with patients in chronic, severe uremia. After the initial dialysis, blood urea nitrogen did not return to previous high levels, patients lost their symptoms of nausea and anorexia, and some were able to return to work.

Similar results have been reported in the United States with a modification of the Giordano-Giovannetti diet.[8] Complete protein, 12 to 13 Gm., was provided by the use of one egg and 6½ ounces of milk daily. The remainder of the protein was obtained from low-protein cereals, especially corn and rice, and from the fruits and low-protein vegetables allowed on the diet. A special bread recipe was devised from a

[4] Jordan, W. L., *et al.*: J. Am. Dietet. A., 50:137, 1967.

[5] Bakke, J., *et al.*: Hospitals, 40:76, 1966; Mitchell, M. C., and Smith, E. J.: Am. J. Clin. Nutr., 19:163, 1966; Silverberg, D. S., and Hunt, J. C.: J. Am. Dietet. A., 49:425, 1966; personal communication.

[6] Giordano, C.: J. Lab. Clin. Med., 62:231, 1963.

[7] Giovannetti, S., and Maggiore, O.: *Lancet,* 1: 1,000, 1964.

[8] Bailey, G. L., and Sullivan, N. R.: J. Am. Dietet. A., 52:125, 1968.

self-rising wheat starch preparation* (see p. 355). Sugars and unsalted fats provided the remainder of the calories to a total of 350 Gm. of carbohydrate and 80 to 90 Gm. of fat. Multivitamins were prescribed as well as folic acid. Basalgel† to absorb the phosphate in the diet was given, and until recently a methionine supplement was prescribed twice a week. The last was later discontinued. Patients lost their gastrointestinal symptoms, were able to return home, to school or to work, and remained for months relatively asymptomatic. Eventually, however, they developed severe cardiac enlargement and decompensation, and had to be placed on dialysis.[9]

These investigators presently propose a diet containing 0.3 Gm. of complete protein per Kg. of body weight, or approximately 20 Gm. for a 70-Kg. man, plus the incomplete protein found in the cereals, fruit and vegetables of the earlier diet. Their rationale is based on the findings of McCracken *et al.*[10] who found it was possible to limit urea production on a diet supplying 30 Gm. of protein, of which 20 Gm. was complete. Directions for this regimen are given later in the chapter.

Terminal Nephritis

When neither hemodialysis nor the dietary measures described are any longer effective, the dietary regimen must be directed entirely to keeping the patient comfortable. The suggestions given under Acute Kidney Failure may be found helpful.

PRINCIPLES OF DIETARY TREATMENT

In the foregoing pages the underlying principles of the dietary treatment of a variety of kidney disease have been described. These may be summarized as follows.

Protein. The protein content of the diet should be normal—that is, 1 Gm. per Kg. of body weight—as long as kidney function is intact. When there is considerable loss of albumin in the urine, the physician may order an increased protein intake to meet the nutritional needs of the patient and to compensate for the albuminuria. On the other hand, when the kidney begins to fail in its function, and protein metabolic end products are retained in the blood in lesser or greater degree, restriction of protein in the diet becomes essential.

To increase the protein content of the diet, increased amounts of milk, eggs, and meat, fish and poultry should be included. When the protein intake must be limited, it is important that as much complete protein—milk, eggs, meat, fish and poultry—be included as possible. These foods are the source of the essential amino acids which the body cannot make. It is equally important that these foods be distributed throughout the three meals in order that they may be used to best advantage (see Chap. 4).

Sodium. The amount of sodium in the physician's diet order will depend on several factors. If hypertension is present and sodium reabsorption from the kidney is normal, sodium in the diet may be considerably restricted, to 500 mg. or less. Because protein foods are naturally high in sodium, a low-protein diet automatically becomes somewhat restricted in sodium. At the 500-mg. level of sodium, however, foods must be cooked and served without salt, and no foods prepared or preserved with salt may be included unless specifically directed. Chapters 24 and 39 list the foods which are permitted and which must be excluded on sodium-restricted diets. Chapter 39 also provides a number of low-sodium recipes. Both lists and recipes should be checked against other restrictions of the protein-, sodium- and potassium-restricted diet, however, before they are used. Low-sodium milks which are processed by dialysis should not be used, because they have a high potassium content. The patient must be warned not to use any salt substitutes containing potassium, since this is generally contraindicated in kidney disease. The sodium content of the drinking water in the locality where the patient resides should also be investigated. If it is high, the use of distilled water for drinking and cooking purposes may be necessary.

In patients with considerable kidney damage, there is danger that the sodium-

---

* McDowell Bros., Ogdensburg, N. Y.
† Wyeth Labs., Phila., Pa.
[9] Personal communication
[10] McCracken, B. H., *et al.*: New Eng. J. Med., 272:1050, 1965.

TABLE 25–1. Protein, Sodium and Potassium Content of Food Exchanges*

Food	Household Measure	Grams	Protein Gm.	Sodium mg.	Potassium mg.
Milk Exchanges	½ cup	120	4	60	90
Meat Exchanges					
Group A	1 ounce	30	7	60	70
Group B	1 ounce	30	7	25	120
Vegetable Exchanges					
Group A	½ cup	100	1	9	120
Group B	½ cup	100	2	9	230
Fruit Exchanges					
Group A	as listed	100	1	2	100
Group B	as listed	100	1	2	145
Bread Exchanges	1 slice	25	2	5	50
Fat Exchanges, salted	1 teaspoon	5	0	50	0
Beverages	1 cup	240	0	varies	varies
Desserts	1 serving	varies (see recipes)			
Low-protein bread	1 slice	25	0.1	84	1

* Adapted from the Department of Dietetics, Peter Bent Brigham Hospital.

depletion syndrome may occur, because the kidney cannot reabsorb sufficient sodium to maintain the normal level in the blood. This in turn causes movement of potassium from the cells into the blood stream, raising the serum levels of potassium and endangering the physiology of heart action. Therefore a more liberal sodium intake is essential. The physician may want to accomplish this by limiting the dietary sodium to a specified amount, and by giving a known quantity of sodium in addition, either as a medication such as sodium bicarbonate, or as salt to be used on food; or he may allow a small amount of salt in cooking, though not at table, omitting such salted foods as ham, bacon, sauerkraut, etc.

Potassium. In the early stages of chronic kidney disease, potassium is excreted normally, and there is no need to limit the dietary intake of potassium. If, however, renal failure causes retention of potassium in the blood, the physician's diet order will include a degree of potassium restriction. As has already been said, an increase in serum potassium affects the action of heart muscle and is therefore dangerous. Both plant and animal foods contain potassium, and it is usually not possible to restrict dietary potassium below 1.5 Gram per day.

Fluids. Fluid restriction may become necessary due to kidney failure. The beverages included in the diet plus the drinking water must not exceed the amount ordered by the physician. This order may change from day to day, depending on the amount of urine output plus the estimated loss from the skin and lungs. Mitchell and Smith[11] suggest that a simple way for a patient to keep track of his allowed fluid intake during a 24-hour period is to measure an equivalent amount of water into a single container; then discard a volume equal to the fluid ingested with and between meals throughout the day. This limits the intake of fluid to the specified amount and is easy for the patient to comprehend and use.

Calories. An adequate caloric intake is essential for the patient on protein restriction to prevent the use of body protein to meet his energy needs. When this occurs, it leads to an increase in urea formation and a rise in serum potassium from cellular breakdown.

PLANNING DIETS OF VARYING PROTEIN, SODIUM AND POTASSIUM CONTENT

The method of using Exchange Lists, as described in earlier chapters, is also helpful in planning diets of varying levels of protein, sodium and potassium content.

Protein, Sodium and Potassium Content of Food Exchanges (Table 25–1) gives the composition for each of the food groups,

11 Op. cit.

averaged from the composition of each item in the group. Since there are three nutrients to be averaged, the figures vary somewhat more widely than in exchanges where only one nutrient needs to be considered. When greater accuracy is desirable than can be supplied by exchange groupings, Table 1, Composition of Foods, and Table 5, Sodium and Potassium Content of Foods, in Part Four, should be consulted.

The figures given for sodium in Table 25–1 apply to foods produced, processed and prepared without the addition of salt or other sodium compounds, except where noted specifically in the Exchange Lists. It can readily be seen that milk, eggs, meat, fish and poultry provide the major part of the protein and the sodium in the diet, and that, with the exception of fats and sugars, almost all foods contain considerable amounts of potassium. It will also be noted that the meat, vegetable and fruit exchanges have been subdivided on the basis of their sodium and/or potassium content.

Exchange Lists. The Exchange Lists for the protein, sodium and potassium restricted diet will be found on pages 350–351. If they are compared with the Restricted-Sodium Diet Exchange Lists in Chapter 24, it will be seen that some foods, not allowed on the diet restricted only in sodium, have been included in the Protein, Sodium and Potassium Exchange Lists because the potassium content of each food group also had to be considered. Salted butter and margarine as well as unsalted fats are included in the Fat Exchanges and make it easier to raise or lower the sodium content of the diet.

Protein, Sodium and Potassium Restricted Diet Exchange Lists*

Milk Exchanges: 1 serving contains 4 Gm. of protein, 60 mg. of sodium, 90 mg. of potassium

Milk	½ cup
Light cream	½ cup
Heavy cream	¾ cup
Sour cream	½ cup
Half and half	½ cup
Ice cream, regular	½ cup (⅛ qt.)
Sherbet, regular	1 cup (¼ qt.)
Creamed cheese, regular	1 tablespoon

Meat Exchanges: Group A. 1 serving contains 7 Gm. of protein, 60 mg. of sodium, 70 mg. of potassium

Egg, prepared any way	1
Cheese, low sodium	1 ounce
cottage, regular	¼ cup
Tuna and salmon, canned in water	¼ cup
Lobster and shrimp, fresh or canned in water	1 ounce
Oysters, fresh	4 in number
Clams, fresh	3 in number

Meat Exchanges: Group B. 1 serving contains 7 Gm. of protein, 25 mg. of sodium, 120 mg. of potassium

Beef, lamb, liver, rabbit, veal	1 ounce
Chicken, turkey	1 ounce
Fish, fresh water	1 ounce
haddock	1 ounce
halibut	1 ounce
swordfish	1 ounce

Vegetable Exchanges: Group A. 1 serving contains 1 Gm. of protein, 9 mg. of sodium, 120 mg. of potassium

Asparagus	6 spears
Beans, green or wax	½ cup
Beets	¼ cup
Carrots	⅓ cup
Lettuce	2 large leaves
Onions	1 medium
Peas	½ cup
Squash, summer, yellow, white	½ cup

Vegetable Exchanges: Group B. 1 serving contains 2 Gm. of protein, 9 mg. of sodium, 230 mg. of potassium

Broccoli	1 stalk, ½ cup
Brussels sprouts	½ cup
Cabbage	½ cup
Corn	½ cup
Cucumber	8 slices ⅛ in. thick
Eggplant	½ cup
Okra	½ cup
Potato	¼ cup
Pumpkin	½ cup
Rutabagas	½ cup
Squash, acorn, Hubbard	½ cup
Tomato	1 small
Tomato juice, low-sodium dietetic	½ cup
Turnips	⅓ cup

Vegetables may be fresh, low-sodium dietetic canned, or home-canned if no salt has been added.

Use only frozen vegetables to which no salt or other sodium compound has been added. **READ LABELS.**

---

* Adapted from the Department of Dietetics, Peter Bent Brigham Hospital. Protein, sodium and potassium figures are averages for each group, from Handbook No. 8, Composition of Foods. U. S. Department of Agriculture, 1963.

Protein, Sodium and Potassium Restricted Diet Exchange Lists* (Continued)

Fruit Exchanges: Group A. 1 serving contains 1 Gm. of protein, 2 mg. of sodium, 100 mg. of potassium

Apple, raw	1
Apple juice	½ cup
Applesauce	½ cup
Blueberries	½ cup
Cherries, Bing and Royal Anne	½ cup
Cranberries	½ cup
Cranberry juice	½ cup
Peaches, canned	½ cup
Peach Nectar	½ cup
Pears, canned	½ cup
Pear Nectar	½ cup

Fruit Exchanges: Group B. 1 serving contains 1 Gm. of protein, 2 mg. of sodium, 145 mg. of potassium

Blackberries, fresh or frozen	½ cup
Fruit cocktail	½ cup
Grapes	½ cup
Grape juice	½ cup
Grapefruit, raw	½ medium fruit
Grapefruit juice	½ cup
Grapefruit sections	½ cup
Orange, raw	½ small fruit
Orange juice	⅓ cup
Peach, raw	1 small fruit
Pear, raw	1 small fruit
Pineapple, canned	½ cup
Pineapple juice	½ cup
Plums, canned or raw	2 in number
Raspberries, fresh or frozen	½ cup
Strawberries, fresh or frozen	½ cup
Tangerine	1 medium
Watermelon	½ cup

Bread Exchanges: 1 serving contains 2 Gm. of protein, 5 mg. of sodium, 50 mg. of potassium

Low-sodium bread	1 slice
Unsalted cooked cereal	½ cup

Cornmeal	Farina
Cream of Rice	Hominy grits
Cream of Wheat	Ralston

May use Instant or Regular. Do not use quick-cooking varieties.

Dry cereal	¾ cup
Puffed rice	Shredded wheat
Puffed wheat	Unsalted cornflakes
Unsalted cooked	½ cup
Rice	Noodles
Macaroni	Spaghetti
Popcorn, unsalted	1 cup

Fat Exchanges: 1 serving contains 0 protein, 50 mg. of sodium, 0 potassium

Butter, salted	1 teaspoon
Margarine, salted	1 teaspoon
Mayonnaise, salted	1 teaspoon

Unsalted butter and margarine and vegetable oil may be used as desired.

Beverages: May be taken as allowed, according to fluid intake.

Ginger ale   Pepsi Cola
Coca Cola   Kool Aide (not orange)
Sodium and potassium content may vary according to local water supply.
Juices, milk, ice cream and sherbet must be counted as fluid in the diet.

Desserts: Content varies depending on recipe. See pages 352 – 353.

Fruit tapioca
   Group A fruit. 1 serving contains 1 Gm. of protein, 2 mg. of sodium, 100 mg. of potassium

Apple pie
   Group A fruit. 1 serving contains 2 Gm. of protein, 5 mg. of sodium, 150 mg. of potassium

Butter Cookies
   3 cookies = 1 serving. Contains 1 Gm. of protein, 2 mg. of sodium, 30 mg. of potassium

Miscellaneous: These items may be used as desired to add flavor.

Allspice	Mustard, dry
Caraway	Nutmeg
Cinnamon	Paprika
Curry powder	Pepper
Garlic	Peppermint extract
Garlic powder (not garlic salt)	Sage
Ginger	Syrup, corn
Hard candy	Sugar, white
Honey	Thyme
Jams	Turmeric
Jellies	Vanilla extract
Lollipops	Vinegar
Mace	

Small amounts of the following may be used to season foods:

Celery	Horseradish, fresh
Green pepper	Mushrooms
	Onion

*Adapted from the Department of Dietetics, Peter Bent Brigham Hospital. Protein, sodium and potassium figures are averages for each group, from Handbook No. 8, Composition of Foods. U. S. Department of Agriculture, 1963.

The Dietary Prescription

As we noted earlier in the chapter, diets of varying protein, sodium and potassium content may be ordered by the physician, depending on the condition of the patient and the treatment he is receiving. A diet containing 40 Gm. of protein, 500 mg. of sodium and 1,500 mg. (1.5 Gm.) of potassium is frequently ordered for the patient with considerable kidney damage, either to promote healing, following an acute attack of kidney disease, or to maintain the pa-

TABLE 25–2. A 40-Gram Protein, 500-Milligram Sodium, 1,500-Milligram Potassium Restricted Pattern Dietary*

Food†	Household Measure	Grams	Protein Gm.	Sodium mg.	Potassium mg.	Calories
Milk	1 cup	240	8	120	180	161
Meat						
Group A	1 ounce	30	7	60	70	⎰188
Group B	1 ounce	30	7	25	120	⎱
Vegetables						
Group A	1 cup	200	2	18	240	⎰108
Group B	½ cup	100	2	9	230	⎱
Fruit						
Group A	½ cup	100	1	2	100	⎰107
Group B	½ cup	100	1	2	145	⎱
Bread, low sodium	4 servings	varies	8	20	200	252
Fat, salted	1⅓ tablespoon	20	..	200	..	135
Totals			36	456	1,285	951

* The addition of beverages and special desserts will increase the calories, and bring the totals for protein, sodium and potassium to the desired amounts. See menu on page 353.
† See Protein, Sodium and Potassium Restricted Diet Exchange Lists.

tient who still has some kidney reserve. The Pattern Dietary given above may also serve as a basis for other diet prescriptions.

The 40-Gram Protein, 500-Milligram Sodium and 1,500-Milligram Potassium Restricted Pattern Dietary. Table 25–2 gives a combination of foods containing 36 Gm. of protein, and approximately 450 mg. of sodium, 1,300 mg. of potassium and 950 calories. The addition of beverages and desserts, and the use of light cream in place of milk, as shown in the menu on page 353, will bring the protein, sodium and potassium to the desired levels, and the calories to 2,100. Recipes for the three desserts used in this menu will be found on pages 352–353.

Recipes*

Fruit Tapioca

Ingredients:

    2 cups peach nectar
    ½ cup water
    ½ cup sugar
    ¼ cup tapioca
    1 cup peach slices, canned

Procedure: Mix peach nectar, water, sugar and tapioca in top of double boiler. Cook over water, stirring constantly until mixture thickens

* Mitchell, M. C., and Smith, E. J.: Am. J. Clin. Nutr., *19*:163, 1966.

slightly, 5 to 8 minutes. Remove from heat and cool. Stir in 1 cup of sliced, canned peaches. A dash of cinnamon or ginger will add flavor. A tablespoon of lemon juice will make the dessert less sweet. Other allowed fruits may be substituted. Yield: 6 servings. One serving contains 1 Gm. of protein, 2 mg. of sodium and 100 mg. of potassium.

Butter Cookies

Ingredients:

    1 cup unsalted butter or margarine
    1 cup sifted confectioners' sugar
    1 teaspoon vanilla extract
    2½ cups all-purpose flour

Procedure: Cream butter and confectioners' sugar together. Add vanilla and mix. Sift flour and stir in. Mix thoroughly with hands. Mold into long smooth roll about 2 inches in diameter. Wrap in wax paper and chill in refrigerator until stiff. With thin, sharp knife, cut into thin, ⅛- to 1/16-inch slices. Place slices a little apart on ungreased baking sheet. Bake at 400° F. until lightly browned. Yield: 6 dozen 2-inch cookies. One serving = 3 cookies and contains 1 Gm. of protein, 2 mg. of sodium, 30 mg. of potassium.

Pie Crust

Ingredients:

    2 cups sifted all-purpose flour
    ½ teaspoon sugar
    ⅔ cup unsalted shortening
    5 to 6 tablespoons ice water

Procedure: Mix flour and sugar. Cut in shortening with two knives or pastry blender. Stir in just enough water to make ingredients adhere together. Pat lightly in hands until dough forms a smooth mixture. Divide in half and roll lightly on floured board, handling as little as possible. If dough is chilled before rolling, it is easier to handle. Yield: makes 9-inch, 2-crust pie.

Apple Pie

Ingredients:

    6 medium apples

¾ cup sugar
2 tablespoons flour
¼ teaspoon nutmeg
1 tablespoon unsalted butter
    or margarine
Add up to 1 tablespoon lemon juice or
    vinegar if apples are very sweet

Procedure: Mix sugar, flour and nutmeg. Alternate with layers of peeled, sliced apples in 9-inch pastry-lined pie plate. Dot with butter or margarine and add lemon juice or vinegar if needed. Add top crust, and seal two crusts together. Bake on bottom shelf of oven

Menu for 40-Gram Protein, 500-Milligram Sodium, 1,500-Milligram Potassium Diet

Food	Household Measure	Grams	Protein Gm.	Fat Gm.	Carbo-hydrate Gm.	Sodium mg.	Potassium mg.	Fluids ml.
Breakfast								
Blueberries	½ cup	100	1	..	10	2	100	..
Shredded wheat	1 biscuit	30	2	..	15	5	50	..
Cream, light	½ cup	120	4	27	5	60	90	120
Coffee, weak	½ cup	120	..	..	..	1	30	120
Sugar, white	1 tablespoon	15	..	..	15	..	..	..
Lunch								
Egg, poached	1	50	7	6	..	60	70	..
Bread, unsalted	1 slice	25	2	..	15	5	50	..
Butter or margarine, salted	1 teaspoon	5	..	5	..	50	..	..
Salad								
Lettuce	1 large leaf	50⎱	1	..	2	9	120	..
Asparagus	3 spears	50⎰						
French dressing, unsalted	1 tablespoon	15	..	5	..	..	..	..
Apple pie	⅛ 9-in. pie	—	2	10	40	5	150	..
Ginger ale	8 ounces	240	..	..	20	20	1	240
Dinner								
Beef, ground, cooked in	1 ounce	30	7	7	..	25	120	..
Butter, salted	1 teaspoon	5	..	5	..	50	..	..
Spaghetti, cooked	½ cup	100	2	..	15	5	50	..
Tomato juice, unsalted	½ cup scant	100	2	..	3	9	230	120
Green beans	½ cup	100	1	..	7	9	120	..
Bread, unsalted	1 slice	25	2	..	15	5	50	..
Butter, salted	2 teaspoons	10	..	10	..	100	..	..
Fruit tapioca peach nectar ⎱ sliced peaches ⎰	1 serving	..	1	..	31	2	100	..
Lemonade	8 ounces	240	..	..	24	..	8	240
Evening								
Cream, light, diluted with water	½ cup	120	4	27	5	60	90	120
Cookies	3	..	1	7	16	2	30	..
	Totals		39	109	238	484	1,459	960

Calories 2,089

at 425° F. for 15 minutes. Change to middle shelf and continue baking until apples are tender, about 20 to 30 minutes. Yield: 8 servings. One serving (⅛ pie) contains 2 Gm. of protein, 5 mg. of sodium, 150 mg. of potassium. Other allowed fruits may be substituted.

On the 40-Gm. protein-restricted diet, servings of milk and meat exchanges are of necessity small, and make the diet difficult to accept by many patients. Combining the meat with some of the other allowed foods, for example an eggplant, tomato and ground meat casserole, served on rice, will stretch the meat allowance as well as provide a method for adding calories by frying the eggplant in oil before combining. It is possible to adapt other "regular" recipes by combining foods for main dishes, as well as for desserts, so long as the limitations of foods, seasonings and quantities of the restricted diet are observed.

Since the milk and meat exchanges are limited, the sodium content of the diet is low, and permits the use of some salted butter or margarine for bread and vegetables, helping to make the diet more palatable.

Variations for Protein Content

Increased Protein Diet. When the main symptom of kidney disease is albuminuria, the physician may order a diet increased in protein, up to 90 to 100 Gm. daily. The use of 1 quart of milk and 6 ounces of meat will increase the protein in the Pattern Dietary to approximately 90 Gm. If all food is processed and prepared without salt or other sodium compounds, and if unsalted fats are substituted for salted, the sodium content of the diet will be approximately 800 mg. and the potassium content 2500 mg. If a lower sodium and potassium content is necessary, the use of Protinal,* a protein concentrate containing 61 gm. of protein, 30 Gm. of carbohydrate, 30 mg. of sodium and 35 mg. of potassium per 100 Gm. may be substituted for some of the milk and meat and the protein content of the diet thus maintained. Protinal may be used in beverages or sprinkled over cereals and vegetables.

_____
* National Drug Co., Phila., Pa.

The 50- to 60-Gram Protein Diet. For patients receiving hemodialysis, the physician may prescribe a diet containing 50 to 60 Gm. of protein. An increase in meat from the B group of the Meat Exchanges to 3 to 4 ounces will raise the protein in the Pattern Dietary to the desired amount. By substituting unsalted butter or margarine for some of the salted variety, the sodium may be kept at 500 mg. The potassium will be increased to approximately 1,800 mg. However, the physician's diet order may allow up to 2,000 to 3,000 mg. (2 to 3 Gm.) of potassium with the amount of protein included in this diet.

The 30-Gram Protein Diet. This diet may be ordered for the patient in kidney failure for whom hemodialysis is not available. The rationale for this degree of protein restriction was discussed earlier in the chapter. Since it is important to include 20 Gm. of complete protein in the diet, the decrease in protein from that in the Pattern Dietary must be made in the vegetables or the bread. The substitution of 4 slices of a bread very low in protein, made from a self-rising wheat-starch flour, for the low-sodium bread exchanges in the Pattern Dietary will lower the protein closely to the desired amount. A recipe for the low-protein bread is given on page 355. It will be noted that this bread is high in sodium content. By using only unsalted butter and margarine, the sodium content of the diet may be kept at approximately 500 mg. The potassium content will be somewhat below that of the Pattern Dietary, approximately 1,300 mg.

The 20-Gram Protein Diet. This diet, which resembles the modified Giordano-Giovannetti regimen described earlier, limits the milk to ¾ cup (6 ounces) and the meat exchanges to 1 ounce in the Pattern Dietary, Table 25-2. Low-protein bread must be substituted for the bread exchanges. Since the low-protein bread is high in sodium, only unsalted fats may be used. The remainder of the protein is contributed by the fruits and vegetables.

Other Considerations

Fluids. Water and beverages are restricted, often quite severely, for patients with oliguria. This may limit the use of beverages included in the menu of the Pattern Dietary, and will also lower the calories they contribute. All beverages, milk, ice cream and sherbet must be counted as fluid in the diet.

Calories. Diets restricted in protein, sodium and potassium seldom meet the caloric needs of the patient, especially if he is reasonably active. A generous use of fats and oils, unsalted if necessary, for frying, in mixed dishes, on vegetables and as dressing for salads will aid in raising calories. For the limited amounts of milk allowed on the diet, half milk, half cream or light cream may be substituted. Jellies, jams and honey for use on bread and fruit increases the calories without adding appreciably to the sodium or potassium content of the diet. Corn syrup added to ginger ale and lemonade, within the fluid allowances, will be of help. The use of desserts made from the foods permitted in the quantities allowed, plus the sugar and fat included in the recipe, will provide calories as well as add variety and interest to the diet.

Nutritional Adequacy. Most diets restricted in protein will be low in minerals and vitamins. Patients who are on hemo-

dialysis may also lose calcium, iron and some of the water-soluble vitamins in the dialysis fluid. Anemia frequently accompanies severe kidney disease. On the other hand, the level of serum calcium may be high. The physician may prescribe an iron medication, and vitamin supplements are usually indicated, whether the patient is being treated by diet alone, or by diet and hemodialysis.

TEACHING THE PATIENT

The Exchange Lists included in this chapter, or those in use in other institutions, are designed to help the patient keep the dietary restrictions ordered for him by his physician. Because of the multiplicity of restrictions, it is a more limited diet than either the diabetic or sodium-restricted diet, and is therefore more difficult to follow. Moreover, most patients suffering from severe kidney disease are anxious and easily discouraged. While they are in the hospital, every opportunity should be sought for teaching, by the physician, the dietitian and the nurse. If the patient is a man, it is essential that his wife be included in the plan for instruction. Both must be given frequent opportunities for questions. The hospital tray becomes the visual aid for teaching not only what foods

Recipe: Low Protein Bread*

Composition:	Calories	Protein Gm.	Fat Gm.	Carbohydrate Gm.	Sodium mg.	Potassium mg.
100 Gm.	293	0.4	7	57	336	5
25 Gm. (1 slice)	73	0.1	2	14	84	1

Ingredients:

    1½ teaspoons baker's dry yeast
    2 teaspoons granulated sugar
    1½ cups warm water
    2¾ cups *self-rising wheat starch flour†*
    ¼ teaspoon salt
    3 tablespoons unsalted shortening
       (Crisco or Spry)

Procedure: Mix yeast and sugar. Add the warm water. Let stand 15 minutes, stirring occasionally. Sift flour and salt together. Cut shortening into flour mixture with two knives

or a pastry blender. Gradually add yeast, sugar and water mixture, beating well, until well blended. Pour dough into well greased loaf pan, approx. 5 in. × 9½ in. × 3 in. Cover with clean towel and place in a warm place. Let dough rise until it doubles in size, approximately 20 minutes. *Caution:* If dough does not rise enough or is allowed to over-rise, loaf will collapse when baked. Bake at 400° F. for 35 to 40 minutes. Remove bread from pan and brush top with unsalted butter or margarine to keep surface soft. The finished product will not be fine-textured but quite coarse. Cut into slices, wrap in wax paper and freeze. Use as needed. Yield: One loaf or 26 slices.

---

* Department of Dietetics, Peter Bent Brigham Hospital.

† McDowell Bros., Ogdensburg, N. Y.

TABLE 25–3. Moderately Reduced Calcium and Phosphorus Diet

(This diet will contain from 500 to 700 mg. of calcium
and from 1,000 to 1,200 mg. of phosphorus*)

Foods Allowed:

Milk......................Limited to 1 cup (½ pint) a day. Cream may be substituted for part of the milk.

Cheese....................Pot or cottage cheese only. Limited to 2 ozs.

Fats......................As desired

Eggs......................Limited to 1 a day; egg whites as desired

Meat, fish, fowl............Limited to 4 ozs. daily of beef, lamb, pork, veal, chicken, turkey, fish. See those To Be Avoided.

Soups and broths............All. Cream soups made with milk allowance only

Vegetables................At least 3 servings besides potato. One or 2 servings of deep green or deep yellow vegetables to be included daily. See list of those To Be Avoided.

Fruits......................All except rhubarb. Include citrus fruit daily.

Breads, cereals, Italian pastes..White, enriched bread, rolls and crackers except those made from self-rising white flour. Farina (not enriched), cornflakes, corn meal, hominy grits, rice, Rice Krispies, Puffed Rice. Macaroni, spaghetti, noodles

Desserts....................Fruit pies, fruit cobblers, fruit ices, gelatin. Puddings made with allowed milk and egg. Angel food cake. (Do not use packaged mixes.)

Beverages..................Coffee, Postum, Sanka, tea, ginger ale

Condiments.................Sugar, jellies, honey, salt, pepper, spices

Foods To Be Avoided:

Cheese....................All except pot or cottage cheese

Meat, fish, fowl............Brains, heart, liver, kidney, sweetbreads. Game (pheasant, rabbit, deer, grouse). Sardines, fish roe

Vegetables................Beet greens, chard, collards, mustard greens, spinach, turnip greens. Dried beans, peas, lentils, soybeans

Fruits......................Rhubarb

Breads, cereals, Italian pastes..Whole-grain breads, cereals and crackers. Rye bread. All breads made with self-rising flour. Oatmeal, brown and wild rice. Bran, Bran Flakes wheat germ. All dry cereals except those allowed

Desserts....................All except those allowed

Beverages..................Carbonated "soft" drinks; cocoa

Miscellaneous..............Nuts, peanut butter, chocolate, cocoa. Condiments having a calcium or a phosphate base. (Read labels.)

* Adapted from Shorr, E.: Aluminum hydroxide gels in the management of renal stone. J. Urol., 53:507, 1945.

may be used, but also the portion sizes. Imagination, patience, understanding and sympathy are demanded of those who are teaching these patients to live within their dietary limitations, and to help them extend their lives for months or even years.

KIDNEY STONES

Kidney stones or urinary calculi are formed because the concentration of a par-ticular substance in the urine exceeds its solubility. A low urine volume and the pH of the urine are also factors. However, in many instances the cause for the formation of kidney stones is not known.[12]

About 95 per cent of all kidney stones contain calcium. They may also contain

12 Krane, S. M.: New Eng. J. Med., *267*:875, 1962; *267*:977, 1962.

magnesium and ammonia combined with phosphates, carbonates and oxalates. Four per cent of renal calculi consist of uric acid, and 1 per cent are cystine stones.[13] They vary in size from fine gritty particles to those which fill the pelvis of the kidney, and they may form either in the kidney or the bladder. The type of stone from which a patient suffers is determined by careful urinalysis and by the chemical identification of crystals in the urinary sediment.

Calcium Phosphate Stones. These may occur in hyperparathyroidism, in which oversecretion of the parathyroid hormone causes loss of calcium from the bones, resulting in a high blood level of calcium with increased excretion of calcium in the urine. Immobilization for long periods of time, osteoporosis, or an abnormally high intake of milk, alkalis or vitamin D may also give rise to the formation of calcium phosphate stones.

DIETARY TREATMENT. A moderately low calcium and phosphorus diet and the use of an aluminum hydroxide gel has been successful in controlling the formation of calcium phosphate stones. The aluminum hydroxide, given by mouth, unites with the phosphates present in food to form insoluble aluminum phosphate which is excreted in the feces. Such calcium as is excreted in the urine is now in the form of soluble salts such as calcium chloride and calcium citrate, which are less likely to precipitate. The diet restricts the intake of calcium and phosphates to minimal levels consistent with maintaining nutritional adequacy. See Table 25–3, Foods Allowed and Foods to be Avoided. Fluid intake should be high to keep the urine dilute.

Sodium phytate, in conjunction with a low-calcium, low vitamin-D diet, has also been used in the treatment of calcium phosphate stones.[14] In this instance it is the calcium which is precipitated in the intestinal tract and excreted in the feces. There is some danger of calcium deficiency if this regimen is continued over an extended period of time. Milk and cheese must be carefully limited in the diet. (See Table 1, Part Four, for other food sources of calcium.) No milk fortified with vitamin D should be used. A number of cereals, margarines, beverage syrups and even candies have been fortified with vitamin D (check labels) and should therefore be omitted.

Calcium Oxalate Stones. Until recently this type of kidney stone has been the most resistant to treatment. Calcium oxalate stones tend to recur and may obstruct the urinary tract, necessitating surgery for their removal. A diet limited in oxalic acid, omitting such foods as rhubarb, spinach, cocoa and chocolate, wheat germ and several varieties of nuts, has been prescribed, but has proved relatively ineffective.

A few years ago, Gershoff and his coworkers[15] noted that in the vitamin-B_6-deficient rats with which they were working, there was a marked increase in urinary oxalate accompanied by calcium oxalate stone formation similar to that found in humans. The feeding of high levels of magnesium to the experimental animals reduced the formation of calcium oxalate stones but did not affect the oxaluria.

Applying their findings to the treatment of patients with demonstrated calcium oxalate stones, they report on the results with 36 patients, treated for a period of 5 years. Besides a diet restricted in milk and cheese, which are high in calcium, and the drinking of 2 quarts of water a day, all patients received a daily medication of magnesium oxide and vitamin B_6, both given by mouth. All but five patients in the group have had no further stone formation, or have shown marked improvement.

These investigators postulate that the magnesium aids in keeping the oxalate in solution, and thereby prevents its precipitation and stone formation. Vitamin B_6 increases citric-acid excretion, which may also serve to keep oxalate in solution. It should be recognized that this disease is not considered a vitamin B_6 deficiency, since the etiology of oxalate stone formation is unknown.

[13] Boyce, W. H.: Borden's Review. Vol. 21, No. 4, 1960.

[14] Boyce, W. H., *et al.*: J.A.M.A., *166*:1577, 1958.

[15] Gershoff, S. N., and Prien, E. L.: Am. J. Clin. Nutr., 20:393, 1967.

Uric acid stones occur in patients who have an increased level of uric acid in the blood (hyperuricemia), and increased urinary excretion of uric acid. It may or may not be accompanied by symptoms of gout. Since uric acid is an end product of purine metabolism, foods with a high purine content are avoided. This is discussed in Chapter 33, under Gout.

The precipitation of uric acid crystals in the urinary tract occurs most readily at a low urinary pH. Krane[16] recommends alkali medications to keep the pH of the urine as high as possible, and a fluid intake which will produce at least 3 liters of dilute urine daily.

Cystinuria; Cystine Stones. Cystinuria is an inborn error of metabolism, characterized by faulty absorption of the amino acids cystine, ornithine, arginine and lysine in the intestinal tract, slightly retarded growth, and the appearance of the four amino acids in the urine, due to defective tubular reabsorption. Of these, cystine is the least soluble. It will precipitate when there is increased concentration in the urine, and form stones. Hydration, alkalies and a low-protein diet has been prescribed, but with little success.

In 1965 McDonald and Henneman reported[17] that the administration of d-penicillamine dramatically reduced the amount of cystine in the urine of three patients with cystinuria and kidney stones, preventing further stone formation and, in one of the patients, resulting in complete dissolution of stones already formed. It is postulated that the d-penicillamine keeps the cystine in solution.

Acid and Alkaline Ash Diets. The mineral elements in food are sometimes referred to as "ash" because they do not "burn" in metabolism. They form a residue which is eventually excreted either in the intestinal tract (most of the calcium and the iron) or in the urine. By changing the composition of the diet, the urine may be made either acid or alkaline. An acid urine may act to limit enlargement of already present alkaline stones, or prevent their further formation. Likewise, an alkaline urine may affect the less common acid stones in the same manner.

Most vegetables and fruits will yield an alkaline ash and, therefore, aid in the formation of an alkaline urine. Meats, fish, fowl, eggs and cereals will give an acid ash when metabolized and cause the urine to be acid. Since much of the calcium of milk is re-excreted in the intestinal tract while the remainder of its mineral content is excreted in the urine, its effect on the acidity or the alkalinity of urine is problematical.

Although most physicians will alter the pH of the urine by prescribing the appropriate medication, occasionally he may order a diet to achieve a change in pH. On an alkaline ash diet, sometimes used for oxalate stones, vegetables and fruits should predominate, while meat, eggs and cereals are somewhat restricted. Conversely, on an acid ash diet, which may be prescribed for calcium phosphate and calcium carbonate stones, meat, eggs and cereals are liberally included and vegetables and fruits are restricted. On either diet milk is restricted to one pint. All foods should be in sufficient quantity for nutritional adequacy. For further details on acid and alkaline ash content of food, see Table 8 in Part Four.

STUDY QUESTIONS AND ACTIVITIES

1. What is the function of the kidneys? Using Plate 3, explain how this is accomplished.

2. What substances are filtered from the blood? Which are largely reabsorbed? Which excreted?

3. Plan a diet menu, fluid to soft, for a day for a 10-year-old boy who has glomerulonephritis. Food must be unsalted, he is allowed 30 Gm. of protein, and fluid is restricted to 800 ml.

4. In which circumstances is protein usually restricted in the diet of a patient with nephritis? What is the purpose of this restriction? When may the protein in the diet be increased over normal needs? Why?

5. Why may sodium be restricted in kidney disease?

---

16 Op. cit.

17 McDonald, J. E., and Henneman, P. H.: New Eng. J. Med., 273:578, 1965.

6. What is the danger of an increased potassium level in the blood?

7. What is meant by the sodium depletion syndrome? How may the physician treat it?

8. Why are fluids restricted in kidney failure? On what basis is the amount of fluid allowed calculated?

9. Using the Protein, Sodium and Potassium Restricted Diet Exchange Lists, make out a Pattern Dietary for a 16-year-old boy who is receiving hemodialysis. His physician has ordered a diet containing 60 Gm. of protein, 750 mg. of sodium, 2,000 mg. of potassium, and fluids restricted to 1000 ml. The boy is in school, continually hungry, and rather anxious.

10. Name some of the seasonings the boy's mother may use on the above diet to make it more palatable. What food combinations can you suggest to use extra fat in the diet?

11. Make out a menu for a day for a patient critically ill with nephrosclerosis and uremia. His physician has ordered: 30 Gm. of protein, 500 mg. of sodium, 1,500 mg. of potassium, fluids restricted to 800 ml. The patient is anorexic and has some nausea. The diet should be bland and semi-soft.

12. Look at Table 5 in Part Four, Sodium and Potassium Content of Foods. What foods are high in sodium? In potassium? Take average servings of foods into account.

13. Make out a menu for a day for a patient who has a calcium phosphate kidney stone, and who has been placed on a moderately low calcium and phosphorus diet. He is young and somewhat of a gourmet.

14. Should the patient with calcium oxalate stones be considered to have a vitamin-B_6 deficiency? If not, why not? Look up vitamin B_6 in Table 6, Part Four. Is it widely distributed in food? What is the function of this vitamin? See Chapter 8.

15. What food groups will tend to produce an aciduria? Which an alkaline urine? How is this effected?

SUPPLEMENTARY READING IN DISEASES OF THE KIDNEY; KIDNEY STONES

Bailey, G. L., and Sullivan, N. R.: Selected-protein diet in terminal uremia. J. Am. Dietet., A., *52*:125, 1968.

Bakke, J., *et al.*: Sodium restricted diets for dialysis patients. Hospitals, *40*:76, 1966.

Editorial: Borrowed Time. New Eng. J. Med., *276*:1206, 1967.

Gershoff, S. N., and Prien, E. L.: Effect of daily MgO and vitamin B_6 administration to patients with recurring calcium oxalate kidney stones. Am. J. Clin. Nutr., *20*:393, 1967.

Jordan, W. L., *et al.*: Basic pattern for controlled protein, sodium and potassium diet. J. Am. Dietet. A., *50*:137, 1967.

Krane, S. M.: Renal lithiasis. New Eng. J. Med., *267*:875, 1962; *267*:977, 1962.

Mitchell, M. C., and Smith, E. J.: Dietary care of the patient with chronic oliguria. Am. J. Clin. Nutr., *19*:163, 1966.

For further references see Bibliography in Part Four.

CHAPTER **26**

Diseases of the Esophagus and the Stomach

Pathway of Digestion • Dietary Terminology • Diagnostic Procedures • Peptic Ulcer • Cancer • Hiatus Hernia • Cardiospasm • Gastritis • Indigestion

The relationship of food to the gastrointestinal tract is an intimate one, since this organ serves as the channel of food into the body. It is not surprising, therefore, that diet therapy constitutes much of the treatment in the diseases which affect the gastrointestinal tract.

Since food carries many emotional overtones, it is to be expected that the emotional state of the individual will affect his digestion. Hurried meals, meals eaten under unpleasant circumstances, and other stressful situations all take their toll of the digestive processes. This may result in temporary discomfort, such as so-called "indigestion" or "heartburn," but if continued for a considerable time it may develop into serious organic disease.

Symptoms ascribed to gastric disorders may be due to pathologic conditions in other organs. It has been well said that the stomach is a mirror reflecting the ailments of the whole abdominal region, and of other parts of the body as well. Chronic appendicitis, gallbladder disease, pulmonary tuberculosis and heart disease are known to be causes of gastric distress. Likewise, many of the neuroses, and even the psychoses, may give rise to gastrointestinal symptoms.

THE PATHWAY OF DIGESTION

Food passes from the mouth via the esophagus into the stomach. Here it is mixed with the constituents of the gastric juice, the hydrochloric acid acidifying the contents and the digestive enzymes beginning the chemical breakdown of food. However, the stomach serves mainly as a storage organ. The rate at which food leaves the stomach depends on its composition. Water and fluids containing only small amounts of nutrients such as broth and fruit juices leave the stomach very quickly. Of solid foods, carbohydrate remains the shortest period in the stomach, protein somewhat longer. Fat delays emptying of the stomach, which is why a meal high in fat gives a feeling of satiety, of being "filled up." It takes as long as 3 hours or more after a mixed meal before the stomach is empty again. During this time small amounts of food are carried into the duodenum each time the pyloric sphincter opens. This is a circular muscle at the junction of the lower end of the stomach and the beginning of the intestinal tract.

In the duodenum the food mass is further mixed with bile and the pancreatic enzymes, and digestion proceeds more rapidly. The digested food materials are absorbed largely in the duodenum and the upper part, the jejunum, of the small intestine, although absorption takes place throughout the whole of the small intestine.

The residue, when it enters the colon, is largely water and waste matter. The main function of the colon is to absorb water, forming the feces into a solid mass. It used to be thought that patients could be fed with nutrient enemas, such as glucose solutions, but actually very little absorption other than water takes place in the colon. For a review of the digestive enzymes and their actions, and a discussion of absorption, see Chapter 9.

DIETARY TERMINOLOGY IN GASTROINTESTINAL DISEASE

There is much popular conviction but not very much basic knowledge associated with the effect of specific foods on the physiology of the gastrointestinal tract. Foods are said to be "hard to digest" or, conversely, "easy to digest." They are classed as "irritating" or "gas-forming." Or they possess a quality described as "blandness." Most of these terms may be traced to reports of individual experience of patients, to incorrectly interpreted results of

early studies of gastrointestinal function, and perhaps most frequently to long usage. Thus the "digestibility" of a food has been equated with the rate at which it leaves the stomach. Because fat remains longest in the stomach, it is thought to be more "difficult to digest" than protein and carbohydrate foods. Fried foods are said to be "irritating" to the gastrointestinal tract although there is little evidence to support this statement. Supposed differences in the "digestibility" of light versus dark meat, for which there is no basis for judgment, is another commonly accepted classification.[1]

On the other hand, we have insisted for years that milk is "easy to digest," despite the protest of the occasional patient that it gives him diarrhea. It is now known that such patients may have a deficiency of the intestinal enzyme lactase, needed for the

[1] Kramer, P., and Caso, E. K.: J. Am. Dietet. A., *42*:505, 1963.

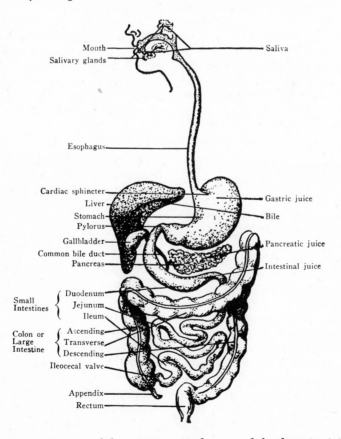

Mouth — Saliva
Salivary glands

Esophagus

Cardiac sphincter — Gastric juice
Liver
Stomach — Bile
Pylorus
Gallbladder
Common bile duct — Pancreatic juice
Pancreas — Intestinal juice

Small Intestines { Duodenum
Jejunum
Ileum
Colon or Large Intestine { Ascending
Transverse
Descending
Ileocecal valve

Appendix
Rectum

Fig. 26–1. Diagram of the gastrointestinal tract and the digestive juices.

breakdown of the milk sugar lactose. When the enzyme is lacking, the undigested and unabsorbed lactose gives rise to the diarrhea.

There is no question but that certain foods may cause gastrointestinal discomfort in the occasional individual. The reason may be due to the specific food, such as the lactose in milk in a lactase-deficient patient, or it may be an unexplained sensitivity to a food. Thus melons and cucumbers, members of the same family, may be gas-forming for an individual who is able to eat baked beans, which are traditionally gas-forming, without any discomfort. The role of emotional stress, anxiety, frustration or boredom, as discussed earlier in the chapter, may also determine whether a food is tolerated or not, but this does not determine its "digestibility" in general terms.

In the discussion of dietary regimens associated with gastrointestinal diseases in Chapters 26 and 27, certain diets, such as those for non-tropical sprue or celiac disease and for disaccharidase deficiencies, have a true physiological basis. They must be carefully followed by the patient if he is to remain free of symptoms. Other diet prescriptions, such as those for peptic ulcer and the composition of a bland diet, have no such rationale. They are included in this chapter because their long usage has been beneficial in practice.

DIAGNOSTIC PROCEDURES IN GASTROINTESTINAL DISEASE

Two common procedures used in the diagnosis of gastrointestinal diseases are (1) the visualization of the gastrointestinal tract by means of a fluoroscope and x-ray photographs after a barium meal has been ingested, and (2) analysis of the gastric juice for the quantity of hydrochloric acid that is being produced.

Roentgenography. Roentgenography of the gastrointestinal tract is an important diagnostic procedure. It may be done by x-ray photography or by direct examination with a fluoroscope, or, usually, by both. By this means the progress of an opaque "meal" of barium sulfate may be followed through the entire digestive tract, and motility (including peristalsis), emptying time,

general tonus (including cardiospasm or pylorospasm), defects of outline indicative of ulcer or carcinoma, and other signs of abnormalities can be studied in detail. The barium meal is given in the morning, or at least 12 hours after the taking of food or drink.

Gastric Analysis. This test is carried out in the morning, before the patient has received any food. A tube is passed from the mouth into the stomach, and any gastric juice present is withdrawn. The patient may then be given an injection of histamine, a drug that stimulates the production of gastric juice, or he may be given a "test meal," consisting of one or two slices of bread and a glass of water. The gastric contents are withdrawn at intervals, for an hour or longer. All samples of gastric juice, including the fasting one, are examined for the presence of undigested food, bile and blood, and tested for the quantity of free and total hydrochloric acid each contains.

In the normal individual no remnants of a previous meal (other than the "test meal," if this is used) or of blood should be present. A small amount of bile is sometimes regurgitated from the duodenum. The amount of acid present in the fasting specimen and after histamine or a test meal ranges from 20 to 70 ml. of N/10 hydrochloric acid per 100 ml. of gastric juice.

If a higher range of acid is found, the condition is called *hyperchlorhydria* and may indicate the presence of an ulcer in the stomach or the duodenum. If the range is much below normal, the term *hypochlorhydria* is used. It may indicate gastric disease in the presence of other findings. *Achlorhydria* denotes that no hydrochloric acid is present. It may occur in gastric disease, and is often found in patients with pernicious anemia.

Gastroscopy. A third diagnostic procedure is the visualization of the gastric mucosa by a gastroscope. This is a rigid tube with a light at the end, which is inserted through the mouth and esophagus into the stomach, and an eyepiece through which the physician can examine the stomach directly.

Other Procedures. Other procedures used in the diagnosis of gastrointestinal disease are the jejunal biopsy, tests for the presence or lack of digestive enzymes, particularly the disaccharidases, and the barium enema. These will be discussed in Chapter 27.

PEPTIC ULCER

The term *gastric ulcer* denotes an eroded lesion in the stomach, usually occurring along the lesser curvature or near the pylorus. A *duodenal ulcer* is the same type of lesion, but is found in the duodenum. It is much more common than a gastric ulcer. Whether an ulcer occurs in the stomach or in the duodenum, the treatment is similar. They will be considered together here under the term *peptic ulcer*. An ulcer is always troublesome and may endanger the life of the patient, as hemorrhage and perforation of the gastric or the duodenal wall are not uncommon occurrences. Cancer, too, may result, more frequently from gastric ulcer than from duodenal ulcer.

Causes of Peptic Ulcer

Many theories have been advanced about the cause of these lesions. Most patients are found to have a marked increase in acid secretion and an engorged and friable gastric or duodenal mucosa.

It is thought that the high acid secretion is responsible for the breakdown of some pinpoint in the mucosal wall with a resulting eating away of the surrounding tissue and the formation of a crater. It is notable that ulcers occur only in areas which come in contact with hydrochloric acid—the stomach and the duodenum, and sometimes the lowest section of the esophagus.

What causes the increase in the secretion of hydrochloric acid is not known. However, it has been observed that the development of an ulcer seems to be related to emotional and other types of stress. Peptic ulcer has sometimes been called the "executives' disease" because it occurs frequently in men whose position in our competitive society subjects them to greatly increased pressures for achievement.

Wolf and Wolff[2] reported their observations on the gastric mucosa in a patient with a gastric fistula. They found that "emotional conflict involving anxiety, hostility and resentment was accompanied by accelerated acid secretion, hypermotility, hypermia and engorgement of the gastric mucosa, resembling 'hypertrophic gastritis.'" Therefore, they concluded that "the chain of events which begins with anxiety and conflict and their associated overactivity of the stomach and ends with hemorrhage or perforation is that which is involved in the natural history of peptic ulcer in human beings."

Symptoms

Pain in the epigastrium, occurring more or less regularly from 2 to 3 hours after meals, is characteristic of peptic ulcer. It is usually of a burning or gnawing type and is relieved by food or alkalis such as sodium bicarbonate.

The diagnosis of ulcer is commonly made by a gastric analysis and by fluoroscopy and x-ray findings. Hyperacidity and hypersecretion of gastric juice are usually found in examination of the stomach contents, and the ulcer crater is often plainly visible on the roentgenogram. The pain complained of by the peptic ulcer patient when the stomach is empty is due to the action of the highly acidic gastric juice on the open lesion when no food is present to dilute and neutralize the gastric juice.

Hemorrhage and Perforation. Sometimes hemorrhage is the first indication of the presence of an ulcer; or this may occur if the ulcer goes untreated. Sudden weakness and tarry tools, the latter due to the presence of blood, are the outstanding symptoms, and the patient is usually hospitalized at once. If perforation of the gastric or the duodenal wall accompanies the hemorrhage, the situation is extremely serious and the patient is subjected to surgery as soon as possible.

Dietary Treatment

The medical treatment of peptic ulcer consists basically of the neutralization of

---

[2] Wolf, S., and Wolff, H. G.: J.A.M.A., *120*:670, 1942.

TABLE 26–1. Progressive Peptic Ulcer Regimen

In the Acute Stage:

Milk and cream, half and half, or
  milk, or skim milk...........3 Oz. every hour alternating with alkaline powders on the half hour
Supplements (given in 3 small meals, adding 2 or 3 foods each day as tolerated, in addition to hourly milk feedings)

Eggs.......................Soft cooked or poached
Cereal.....................Refined, cooked cereals only
Toast and crackers..........White, refined bread and crackers
Cottage and cream cheese....May be substituted for an egg
Strained cream soup.........Made of bland, low residue vegetables such as asparagus, corn (cream), peas, spinach, and strained
Baked or soft custard,
  Jello, junket
Purée fruits and vegetables....Those available as infant foods are suitable

Convalescent Ulcer Diet (Served in 3 meals with 3 between meal feedings)

Milk.......................Milk, cream, buttermilk
Cheese.....................Cottage, cream; other mild, soft cheeses. Cheddar cheese may be added later.
Fats.......................Butter or margarine
Eggs.......................Soft or hard cooked, poached, scrambled
Meats......................Tender beef, lamb, veal; sliced chicken; liver; fish, poached, broiled or baked; crisp bacon; smooth peanut butter
Soups......................Cream soups, using only vegetables listed blow
Vegetables.................Well cooked or canned: asparagus, beets, carrots, peas, green or wax beans, spinach; mashed squash or pumpkin; mashed or baked white and sweet potato (no skins)
Fruits.....................Applesauce, baked apples without skin, ripe or baked bananas, diluted fruit juices, stewed or canned pears, peaches and peeled apricots, purée of all dried fruits except figs
  It is advisable to take citrus fruit juices after eating some of the other foods of the meal, or to dilute them half and half with water.
Breads, cereals, macaroni
  products ....Enriched white bread, fine whole wheat or light rye bread; refined cereals; all ready-to-eat cereals except those containing bran; oatmeal; macaroni, spaghetti, noodles
Desserts...................Ice cream, plain; custard; simple puddings of rice, cornstarch, tapioca or bread without fruit or nuts; gelatin desserts (with fruit as permitted above); sponge and other plain cakes, sugar cookies
Beverages..................Milk, cream, buttermilk. Postum, and decaffeinated coffee if allowed by physician
Condiments.................Moderate amounts of sugar, jelly and salt; others if permitted by physician

Foods To Be Avoided:

Fats.......................All fried foods
Meats and fish.............Smoked and preserved meats and fish; pork; meat gravies
Soups......................All meat soups; all canned soups
Vegetables.................All raw vegetables; all gas-forming vegetables, including cabbage, cauliflower, Brussels sprouts, broccoli, cucumbers, onions, turnips, radishes
Fruits.....................All raw fruits except orange juice and ripe banana
Breads and cereal..........Coarse breads and cereals; hot breads
Desserts...................Pastries, nuts, raisins, currants and candies
Beverages..................Coffee, tea, alcoholic and carbonated beverages
Condiments.................All condiments except salt, unless permitted by physician

Menu for 6-Feeding Convalescent Peptic Ulcer Diet

Breakfast	Dinner	Supper
Orange juice	Chicken, sliced	Cream of spinach soup
Eggs, scrambled	Baked potato (no skin)	Cottage cheese
White toast	String beans purée	White-bread toast
Butter or margarine	White bread	Butter or margarine
Jelly	Butter or margarine	Milk
Milk	Milk	
10 A.M.	**3 P.M.**	**9 P.M.**
Cornflakes with milk	Canned peaches	Baked custard
Milk	Plain cookies	Milk
	Milk	

hydrochloric acid to free the ulcerated area from irritation and to promote healing. For many years this has been achieved by the use of a severely restricted diet, supplemented with antacid drugs, to buffer the highly acid gastric juice. Rest and removal from stressful situations may also be necessary at the beginning of treatment, either at home or in the hospital.

The Progressive Peptic Ulcer Regimen (Sippy Regimen)

The traditional diet of hourly feedings of milk and cream, and more recently of homogenized and even skim milk, alternating with antacids, first proposed by Sippy,[3] has a long history of success. The milk protein buffers the hydrochloric acid and the fat helps to keep food in the stomach to maintain the buffering action. Supplements of cereal, soft-cooked eggs, custard and junket are added within a few days, followed by strained cream soups, white bread toast, cream and cottage cheese and puréed fruits and vegetables. As healing progresses, the patient is placed on six meals a day of carefully selected foods. During the convalescent period, he gradually returns to his regular diet but continues the between-meal feedings of milk, and omits or limits foods high in cellulose and those which stimulate the flow of gastric juice such as broth, coffee, tea and alcoholic beverages. Smoking is also usually prohibited. Table 26–1 lists the foods allowed and the progression of the Sippy regimen.

Nutritional Adequacy. It is obvious that in the early phases of the Sippy regimen the diet is inadequate for nutrients such as iron and ascorbic acid, and will be low in calories, protein and the B vitamins. Especially if the patient is undernourished, the use of vitamin and mineral supplements may be indicated, and it is important that he progress to a convalescent ulcer diet as quickly as possible.

Calories. Not all patients with peptic ulcer are underweight or malnourished. Some will be within normal weight limits, and some may actually be overweight. (See Table 12 in Part Four.) For the latter patients milk should be substituted for milk and cream. Cornwell and Killenberg[4] found that a low-fat, low caloric beverage, frequently used for weight reduction, is equally effective in the healing of peptic ulcer as milk or milk and cream, and may be useful for the markedly overweight patient with a peptic ulcer.

Atherosclerosis. With our increasing knowledge of the relationship of the type of dietary fat to the level of serum cholesterol and the development of atherosclerosis (see Chap. 23), the possible effect of a diet high in milk fat has been questioned. Sandweiss[5] in a study of 180 ulcer patients found the mortality from heart disease 14 per cent higher than in the general population. Hartroft[6] also warns about

---

[3] Sippy, B. W.: J.A.M.A., *64*:1625, 1915.

[4] Cornwell, G. G., III, and Killenberg, P. G.: Am. J. Digest. Dis., *10*:22, 1965.

[5] Sandweiss, D. J.: Am. J. Digest. Dis., *6*:929, 1961.

[6] Hartroft, W. S.: Am. J. Clin. Nutr., *15*:205, 1964.

TABLE 26–2. Bland Diet

Principles:

1. Low in residue and connective tissue
2. Little or no condiments or spices, except salt in small amounts
3. No highly acid foods
4. Foods simply prepared

Foods Allowed:

Milk
　Milk, cream, buttermilk, yoghurt

Cheese
　Cream, cottage and other soft, mild cheeses

Fats
　Butter and margarine

Eggs
　Boiled, poached, scrambled in double boiler

Meat, fish, fowl
　Roast beef and lamb; broiled steak, lamb or veal chops; stewed, broiled or roast chicken; fresh tongue; liver; sweetbreads; baked, poached or broiled fish

Soups
　With milk or cream-sauce foundation

Vegetables
　Potatoes, peas, squash, asparagus tips, carrots, tender string beans, beets, spinach. (In severe cases these vegetables are puréed.)

Fruits
　Orange juice, ripe bananas, avocados, baked apple (without skin), applesauce, canned peaches, pears, apricots, white cherries, stewed prunes

Bread, cereals, macaroni products
　White bread and rolls, crackers, all refined cereals; macaroni, spaghetti, noodles

Desserts
　Custard, junket, ice cream, tapioca, rice, bread or cornstarch pudding, gelatin desserts, junket, sponge cake, plain cookies, prune, apricot or peach whip

Beverages
　Milk, buttermilk, cocoa, malted milk, fruit juices (if tolerated), coffee or tea (if allowed)

Foods To Be Avoided:

Fats
　Fried or fatty foods

Meat, fish
　Smoked and preserved meat and fish; pork

Vegetables
　All raw; all cooked except those listed above

Fruits
　All except those listed above

Desserts, sweets
　Pastries, preserves, candies

Beverages
　Alcoholic beverages; carbonated drinks unless prescribed by the doctor

Condiments
　Pepper, other spices, vinegar, ketchup, horseradish, relishes, gravies, mustard, pickles

Typical Menu for Bland Diet

Breakfast	Dinner	Supper
Banana, ripe	Roast lamb	Cream of potato soup
Farina with milk	Mashed potatoes	Scrambled eggs
1 egg, poached	Peas	Fresh spinach
White-bread toast	White bread	White bread
Butter or margarine	Butter or margarine	Butter or margarine
Coffee or substitute	Canned pears	Applesauce with sugar cookies
Cream	Tea or milk	Milk
	Cream	Small glass orange juice
	Small glass tomato juice	

this incidence, but states that this may not necessarily be cause and effect.

The use of the low-fat, low caloric beverage, described earlier, may be indicated for the potential atherosclerotic subject with a peptic ulcer. A more recent product, consisting of skim milk, soybean oil, minerals and vitamins, was found to have a buffering capacity equal to milk and cream, and produced both relief of ulcer symptoms and a fall in serum cholesterol and triglycerides in over half the patients studied.[7]

The Liberal Diet for Peptic Ulcer

For some years investigators have advocated a more liberal diet in the treatment of peptic ulcer, based on the premise that although all food stimulates the flow of gastric juice to some extent, it is the presence of food itself in the stomach that, aided by antacids, buffers the hydrochloric acid and thereby promotes healing of the ulcer.

As early as 1956, Schneider and his coworkers[8] showed that the addition of considerable amounts of cinnamon, allspice, thyme, sage, paprika, cloves and other spices produced no increase in gastric juice in patients with gastric ulcer. Some difficulty was encountered with chili, black pepper, mustard seed and nutmeg, but only in 5 out of 50 patients. This suggests that we may be more rigid than we need be in the preparation of food for the peptic ulcer patient.

About the same time Kramer[9] in the United States and Doll *et al.*[10] in England found that relief of symptoms and healing of the ulcer were the same for patients on a liberal diet as for those on a restricted, bland diet. Texter[11] states that peptic ulcer tends to run its course regardless of the type of diet used. Not even a bland diet has merit over a more liberal, almost normal diet for patients with peptic ulcer.

Liberal Dietary Regimen. Either the bland diet outlined in Table 26–2, which will be found on page 366, or the patient's own regular regimen provided that this meets the criteria of sensible food choices and regular mealtimes, may form the basis for a liberal ulcer diet. Coffee, tea and broth, and alcoholic beverages, should probably be limited. Highly spiced foods such as Italian pizza or chili con carne had better be omitted. The patient should also be instructed to omit any food which has regularly disagreed with him.

Feedings mid-morning, mid-afternoon and before retiring should be included in order to maintain the buffering action of food in the stomach. These may consist of milk or one of the beverages described above, or if the patient is at home, of part of the regular meal, such as cereal and milk in mid-morning and dessert in mid-afternoon and evening.

In the patient of normal weight, and even more in the patient who is overweight, the total calories of the diet should be such as to maintain weight or to induce weight loss, as needed. Limited use of butter and margarine and other fats, and of sugar and foods containing sugar will help in keeping calories down. See Chapter 21 for further detail of low caloric diets.

Individualization

Most clinicians who have found that a more liberal diet is equally as effective as a rigidly restricted diet in the treatment of peptic ulcer, nevertheless emphasize that the diet should be adjusted to the patient and not the patient to the diet. Careful assessment of the patient's nutritional status and of his cultural and socio-economic background should always precede the dietary prescription.[12]

The personality of the patient may also be a factor in the diet the physician chooses for him. A patient with an ulcer often expects to be placed on dietary restrictions. If he is a worrisome, overanxious individual, he may find a carefully controlled regimen such as the Sippy diet or a bland diet more to his liking than to be told he may eat as

[7] McHardy, G., *et al.*: Am. J. Clin. Nutr., *15*:229, 1964.

[8] Schneider, M. A., *et al.*: Am. J. Gastroenterology, *26*:722, 1956.

[9] Kramer, P.: Med. Clin. N. Amer., *39*:1381, 1955.

[10] Doll, R., *et al.*: Lancet, *1*:5, 1956.

[11] Texter, E. C.: Am. J. Digest. Dis., *2*:130, 1957.

[12] Krehl, W. A.: Am. J. Clin. Nutr., *15*:191, 1964.

he wishes. On the other hand, the patient who is able to take the diagnosis in his stride, or one who is judged to be the type of patient who finds dietary restrictions irksome and is not likely to follow them, may do very well on his regular diet if it meets good dietary practices.

Antacids

The role of antacids in the neutralization of gastric acidity has been indicated as part of the treatment of peptic ulcer. These consist usually of calcium carbonate or aluminum hydroxide. Fortran[13] has recently reported that calcium carbonate is the more effective in lowering gastric acidity, and that when it is given one hour after a meal, its effect will last at least 3 hours.

Surgical Treatment

Peptic ulcer tends to be recurrent, precipitated possibly by nonadherence to sensible dietary habits or by a renewal of emotional tension, or both. If the ulcer proves to be resistant to medical treatment, or if it recurs fairly frequently, surgery is usually resorted to.

For the diet regimen following surgery for peptic ulcer and for the dietary treatment of the "dumping syndrome" see Chapter 29.

OTHER DISORDERS OF THE UPPER GASTROINTESTINAL TRACT
Cancer of the Stomach

Delayed Diagnosis. Because the onset usually is very gradual and there are no distressing symptoms in the early stages of cancer of the stomach, it is frequently overlooked until too late to effect a cure. For this reason, any continued abdominal discomfort should be investigated, even though seemingly inconsequential.

Symptoms and Diagnosis. Lack of appetite over a considerable period of time with loss of weight and strength are symptoms suggestive of carcinoma. Vomiting, particularly of food eaten many hours before, may occur and sometimes newly acquired con-

---

[13] Fortran, J. S., and Collyns, J. A. H.: New Eng. J. Med., 274:921, 1966.

stipation is a symptom. The absence of free hydrochloric acid in the gastric contents is suggestive, although in the earlier stages it may be increased. Occult blood is frequently present in the stools. The most important method in diagnosing cancer is by roentgenogram. The early discovery of this condition, when surgical intervention is more likely to be successful, is of utmost importance.

Dietary Adaptations. When either a subtotal or total resection of the stomach has been performed, the diet should follow that outlined in the chapter on preoperative and postoperative diets (see Chap. 29).

Often in inoperable carcinoma of the stomach, patients feel that if only they could eat they would get well; therefore, the diet is difficult to prescribe. A bland or a convalescent ulcer diet is indicated, or even a liquid diet, particularly if there is obstruction or bleeding. However, the patient's morale may be benefited most by serving a regular house diet as long as possible and letting him choose from his tray what appeals to him.

Hiatus Hernia

The term *hiatus* or *diaphragmatic hernia* refers to herniation of the upper part of the stomach into the thoracic cavity. Since this occurs in the area of the diaphragm through which the esophagus normally passes into the stomach, there may be constriction of the stomach at this point. The resulting discomfort may express itself as substernal pain, heartburn and poor appetite. Sometimes an ulcer will be found at the area of constriction.

The best treatment at present is thought to be conservative and medical, using antacids, and either a bland or a convalescent ulcer diet, described earlier in this chapter. Should the patient be overweight, reduction of weight is important, so that no superfluous tissue presses against the diaphragm. No constricting abdominal garments should be worn. In severe cases, or in those which do not respond to medical therapy, surgery may be advised.

Cardiospasm

Cardiospasm occurs at the junction of the esophagus with the stomach, where the sphincter muscle separates the two organs. Sleisenger *et al.*[14] have shown that this is a disorder of the nervous control of the opening and the closing of the sphincter muscle. Other investigators[15,16] believe that the symptoms of cardiospasm are associated with emotional difficulties. Food does not pass from the esophagus into the stomach, and vomiting and loss of weight are common symptoms. Dilatation and inflammation of the lower end of the esophagus may also result.

The patient may be treated by a series of dilatations of the stricture if the cardiospasm is severe. The diet should be bland and nonstimulating so as not to irritate the esophagus, and may have to be high in calories and protein if much weight has been lost. Frequent small feedings may be better tolerated than 3 regular meals.

Acute and Chronic Gastritis

Acute Gastritis. There is some difference of opinion as to whether acute gastritis is a functional or an organic disease. Gastritis is essentially an inflammation of the gastric mucosa. Acute gastritis may follow the ingestion of toxic substances, such as alkalis, strong acids, alcohol and certain drugs.

THE TREATMENT should include elimination of the offending substance as soon as possible. This is accomplished by induced vomiting or by lavage, and is followed by fasting for an appropriate interval. During this time, fluids usually are given intravenously rather than by mouth, although bits of ice may be held in the mouth to quench severe thirst.

A *liquid diet* should be given the first and possibly the second day following the fast. A start should be made by giving 3 oz. of a bland liquid such as homogenized milk, or buttermilk, or a strained gruel, and repeating in half an hour if no ill effects

result from the first feeding. Both the amount and the interval should be increased until from 6 to 8 oz. are given at 2-hour intervals. Solid foods should be added to the diet slowly, crisp dry toast or crackers being the first addition to the liquid food. Toasted cereal flakes, well-cooked cereals, such as rice or Cream of Wheat, and a soft-cooked egg may be given on the third and the fourth days of feeding.

A convalescent ulcer diet or a bland diet, both described in this chapter, may be given when the acute emergency is over and should be continued until healing is complete.

Chronic Gastritis. Chronic gastritis may accompany organic disease lesions such as ulcer and cancer, or it may be a disease entity of its own. Although no specific lesion may be present, the gastric mucosa is engorged and friable, and the patient complains of continued gastric discomfort. Causative factors other than organic lesions may be long-continued emotional stress, chronic alcoholism, hyperchlorhydria or hypochlorhydria.

THE TREATMENT consists of discovering the cause of the gastritis and treating the patient accordingly. If no specific dietary regimen is indicated, a convalescent ulcer diet or a bland diet will meet the need of these patients. It should be continued until the gastric mucosa has returned to its normal condition.

Indigestion

Discomfort of the gastrointestinal tract may be due to a variety of causes and, if it is persistent, should be thoroughly investigated to determine if organic disease is present.

When no organic disease is found, the indigestion is said to be functional. A common complaint of such patients is "heartburn"; that is, pain high under the sternum. Others have eructation of gastric juice or complain of frequent belching and a sense of fullness. On gastric analysis such patients may be found to have increased gastric secretion, or they may have decreased secretion, but no indication of organic gas-

---

[14] Sleisenger, M. H., *et al.*: Gastroenterology, 25: 333, 1953.

[15] Weiss, E.: Am. J. Digest. Dis., 3:275, 1958.

[16] Wolf, S., and Almy, T. P.: Gastroenterology, 13:401, 1949.

tric disease. Physicians differ as to the importance to be attached to an increase or a decrease of hydrochloric acid in the gastric juice when not accompanied by other findings. Some believe that this condition is not incompatible with good health, while others feel that it may be the precursor of more serious disease.

Functional indigestion may be due to poor food habits and hurried and irregular meals; to food idiosyncrasies and possible allergies; or its cause may be tension and anxiety.

Individuals who live for much of the day on doughnuts and pastries accompanied by frequent cups of coffee or carbonated beverage, with a proper meal only in the evening, are good candidates for indigestion. Overeating, especially of very sweet and fatty foods, may be the cause of indigestion. Rapid eating, particularly when under pressure, resulting in "bolting" of food cannot help but cause gastric discomfort. For all these, the treatment consists of finding time for rest and relaxation and the adoption of more moderate food habits. The nurse may have to persuade patients of the necessity for such changes and to reassure them that it is their food habits and not organic disease which has caused their discomfort.

As discussed earlier in this chapter, certain foods have been labeled as difficult to digest, although the reason is not always clear. Such foods as lobster, crab, sardines, peanuts and other nuts, raw apples, garlic and pickles are in this group. The gas-forming vegetables and fruits may cause discomfort, either because of coarse cellulose or their volatile oils. Common gas-forming foods are cabbage and its relatives —Brussels sprouts, broccoli and cauliflower; dried peas and beans; onions; turnips; green peppers; radishes; cucumbers and melons. If any of these foods are known to be troublesome, they should be omitted from the diet. True food allergies are discussed in Chapter 30.

Disturbed or anxious patients, whose gastric distress is an outcome of their emotional problems, are in need of medical guidance and help. However, the nurse and the dietitian should give the patient sympathetic support and reassurance. A bland diet may be found to be of help in treatment.

STUDY QUESTIONS AND ACTIVITIES

1. Which food groups leave the stomach most quickly? What foods give a sense of satiety? Why?

2. Why are such terms as "hard to digest," "irritating" and "gas-forming" when applied to a specific food open to question? Is there any validity for such classifications?

3. Which component of gastric juice is thought to be responsible for the development of a peptic ulcer? What are some possible causes for its increase in gastric juice?

4. Of what symptoms does the patient with peptic ulcer usually complain?

5. Explain the principles underlying the dietary treatment of peptic ulcer. What is the purpose of the antacid medication?

6. Why are hourly feedings of milk and cream effective in counteracting the hyperchlorhydria of peptic ulcer?

7. What are some of the first foods added to the milk and cream regimen when symptoms subside?

8. Name some of the foods included in a convalescent ulcer diet. What foods are usually omitted?

9. A patient on a convalescent ulcer diet works from 8:00 A.M. to 5:30 P.M. and must buy his lunch. What suggestions can you make to enable him to follow his diet while at work? How can you be sure that the diet will be nutritionally adequate?

10. Using Chapter 11 and the appropriate Supplementary Reading in Chapter 18 as guides, write a convalescent ulcer diet for a Jewish patient who carries his lunch to work; for a Puerto Rican elevator operator who works from 4 P.M. to midnight.

11. Is the Sippy diet in the early stages adequate for normal nutritional needs? What nutrients are likely to be low?

12. How can calories be restricted in an overweight patient with a peptic ulcer who is on a Sippy regimen?

13. Why may the Sippy regimen contribute to the development of atherosclerosis?

14. What is the rationale for the use of a bland or regular diet in the treatment of gastric ulcer?

15. Make out a menu for a day for an overweight patient with a hiatus hernia who has been placed on a bland diet. Keep the number of calories at approximately 1,500.

16. Write out the dietary instructions for a secretary with cardiospasm who has been placed on a bland diet.

17. Name some of the causes of gastritis. Plan a menu for a day for a patient with chronic gastritis. Is it adequate for normal nutritional needs?

18. What are some of the causes of "indigestion" that are not due to an organic lesion? Write a diet for a housewife who complains of heartburn and gastric discomfort. What are some of the questions you would ask her before giving her instruction?

SUPPLEMENTARY READING ON DISEASES OF THE STOMACH AND ESOPHAGUS

Jay, A. N.: Is it indigestion? Am. J. Nursing, 58:1552, 1958.

Kirsner, J. B.: Fact and fallacies of current medical therapy for uncomplicated duodenal ulcer. J.A.M.A., 187:423, 1964.

Kramer, P., and Caso, E. K.: Is the rationale for gastrointestinal diet therapy sound? J. Am. Dietet. A., 42:505, 1963.

McHardy, G., et al.: Effect of polyunsaturated fat diet on serum lipids of hypercholesteremic patients with peptic ulcer, Am. J. Clin. Nutr., 15:229, 1964.

Moeller, H. C.: Conventional dietary treatment of peptic ulcer. Am. J. Clin. Nutr., 15:194, 1964.

Ochsner, S. F.: Gastric ulcer in hiatus hernia. J.A.M.A., 177:892, 1961.

For further references see Bibliography in Part Four.

CHAPTER 27

Diseases of the Intestines

Diarrhea • Malabsorption Syndromes • Disaccharidase Deficiency • Celiac Disease • Tropical Sprue • Cystic Fibrosis • Medium Chain Triglycerides • Regional Ileitis • Ulcerative Colitis • Cancer of the Bowel • Diverticulitis • Hemorrhoids

The small intestine is primarily the organ for the digestion and absorption of food. A discussion of the enzymes and digestive fluids needed for the chemical breakdown of food, and of the mechanics of absorption should be reviewed in Chapter 9. Due in part to our greatly increased knowledge of the microanatomy and the physiologic processes of the small intestine, our understanding of specific diseases of the intestinal tract has steadily increased in the past 20 years.

DIARRHEA

One of the commonest symptoms of malfunctioning of the intestinal tract, of whatever cause, is diarrhea. This is characterized by an abnormally rapid passage of food along the digestive tract, effectively preventing complete digestion and absorption. The total quantity and the water content of the feces are increased, there is a loss of electrolytes, especially sodium, and frequently undigested food is found in the stool. The stools are semifluid and increased in number. When diarrhea persists for more than a few days, dehydration and weight loss result. In infants and children the fluid and electrolyte losses may be critical.

Diarrhea may occur as an acute episode lasting 1 to 3 days, followed by complete recovery; or it may be the symptom of serious disease. In the former case it is usually due to a gastrointestinal infection. When outbreaks of diarrhea occur in groups of people an investigation into the cause usually shows that they had consumed a food which was contaminated with salmonella or staphylococcus. Although individuals may be very ill for a day or so, recovery is complete. Unfortunately, in salmonella infection, an occasional person may become a carrier (see Chap. 17).

When diarrhea lasts more than a few days, or recurs after seeming recovery, the cause should be investigated thoroughly. Infections of the intestinal tract such as typhoid fever, bacillary or amebic dysentery may be the underlying cause of the diarrhea; the first symptom of viral hepatitis is often diarrhea; there may be organic disease such as ileitis or colitis; or one of the malabsorption syndromes may be present.

Diet in an Acute Attack of Diarrhea. Food and fluids by mouth should be withheld for the first 24 hours until the diarrhea subsides. If the fluid and electrolyte loss is critical, intravenous fluids may be ordered. Tea, toast and salted broth are usually well tolerated at the end of this time, and the patient is soon ready for a soft and then a regular diet (see Chap. 19).

In diarrhea of longer duration, such as is found in dysenteries, individuals may require a low-residue diet. Diets varying in residue are presented later in this chapter. (See Table 27–2.) Calories can be increased, if necessary, by the use of high caloric beverages (see Chap. 36).

MALABSORPTION SYNDROMES

Several disease entities of the small intestine, characterized by an inability to digest food or to absorb the end products of digestion, are grouped together under the term "malabsorption syndrome." They are the disaccharidase deficiencies and defective monosaccharide absorption, celiac disease, tropical sprue and cystic fibrosis. Each of these is either known to be or suspected to be due to the lack of a specific enzyme or group of enzymes. In the following pages these diseases will be discussed, together with their dietary treatment.

Disaccharidase Deficiencies and Defective Monosaccharide Absorption

Although the recognition of this malabsorption syndrome is the most recent, it will be discussed first, for it may accompany other disease of the intestinal tract.

However, it usually occurs as a single enzyme deficiency.

The three disaccharides commonly found in food, lactose, sucrose and maltose, the last an intermediate product of the digestion of starch, are normally broken down to their constituent monosaccharides by their respective enzymes in the brush border of the epithelial cells of the villi (see Chap. 9). These enzymes are lactase for the breakdown of lactose to glucose and galactose; invertase for sucrose, yielding glucose and fructose; and maltase and isomaltase, and possibly other forms of maltase, yielding glucose from the breakdown of maltose. The absorption of glucose and galactose into the blood stream occurs by an active transport system in the epithelial cell, but fructose seems to be absorbed by some kind of facilitated transfer.[1] (See Fig. 27–1, Digestion and Absorption of Carbohydrate.)

Symptoms. If one or a group of these enzymes is low or absent, the sugar on which it acts will not be digested and absorbed. It will be acted on by the bacteria in the lumen of the intestinal tract to

---

[1] Lindquist, B., and Meeuwisse, G.: J. Am. Dietet. A., 48:307, 1966.

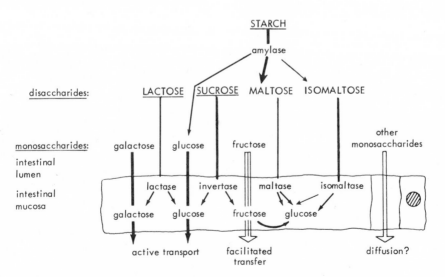

Fig. 27–1. Digestion and absorption of carbohydrates. (Lindquist, B., and Meeuwisse, G.: Diets in disaccharidase deficiency and defective monosaccharide absorption. J. Am. Dietet. A., 48:307, 1966)

form lactic and acetic acids, with subsequent withdrawal of water and cramping pain and diarrhea. Stools are watery and have a low pH.

Diagnosis. An enzyme deficiency may be demonstrated by a sugar tolerance test such as is described in Chapter 22 for diabetes. The patient should be free of diarrhea, and a pre-test diet, omitting the suspected sugar, should be eaten for several days before the test is performed. In the morning, when the patient is fasting, he is given either 50 or 100 Gm. of the suspected sugar suspended in water. Blood samples are withdrawn at 30-minute intervals for 2 hours and tested for glucose. A patient who is intolerant of the sugar being tested will have no increase in his fasting blood sugar following the ingestion of the sugar. He may experience abdominal pain and discomfort, and his stool will contain the disaccharide as well as lactic acid, and have a low pH. A normal rise in blood sugar when the monosaccharide constituents of the suspected disaccharide are given confirms the diagnosis.[2]

Other diagnostic procedures are test diets, omitting the suspected sugar, testing of the stool for the presence of the sugar, and the measurement of disaccharidase activity in a jejunal biopsy specimen.

Lactose intolerance is due to a deficiency of the enzyme lactase. It is the most prevalent of the disaccharidase deficiencies. In infants it seems to occur as a congenital deficiency. In adults it is thought to be an acquired intolerance. It has been suggested that the latter is due to a natural process of aging, as part of a post-suckling syndrome.[3]

Severe milk intolerance may also occur following subtotal gastrectomy in patients who were able to drink milk without symptoms prior to operation. Kern[4] suggests that this may be due to the prompt emptying of the stomach, permitting a comparatively large amount of lactose to enter the

small intestine at once. Lactose intolerance has also been reported in celiac disease, tropical sprue, cystic fibrosis, ileitis, colitis, and kwashiorkor.

The symptoms in infants are immediate and severe on the ingestion of milk, whether the baby is breast or formula-fed, and may become life-threatening. The substitution of a non-lactose-containing mixture of amino acids or of a formula such as one of the soybean "milks" relieves the symptoms dramatically. As the infant grows the restrictions listed under dietary treatment should be observed.

In the adult lactose intolerance may be mild and intermittent, or severe whenever milk is ingested. The symptoms may be of recent origin, or have persisted for years. Often the patient has recognized his intolerance to milk and has excluded it from his diet.

DIETARY TREATMENT. The omission of all forms of milk and cheese, and of foods containing milk such as ice cream, milk chocolate, cream soups and other creamed dishes gives striking relief of symptoms. For infants care must be taken to use only those baby foods to which milk or milk solids have not been added. Medications containing lactose should be omitted. Some adult patients tolerate small amounts of milk, and this should be encouraged for the calcium it contributes to the diet. To date no studies of lactose intolerance report the supplementation of calcium as a medication to the diet of these individuals.

Sucrose intolerance is due to a deficiency of the enzyme invertase, and is comparatively rare. It is manifested most frequently in infancy, although one case of adult deficiency, in a 29-year-old man with a history of symptoms for only two years, has been reported.[5] Burgess et al.[6] describe the finding of the deficiency in 7 infants and young children. There was a history of explosive diarrhea, abdominal distention, dehydration and, in the older children, poor weight gain. Sucrase (invertase) activity

---

[2] Dahlqvist, A.: J.A.M.A., *195*:225, 1966.

[3] Weser, E., *et al.*: New Eng. J. Med., 273:1070, 1965.

[4] Kern, F., Jr., and Struthers, J. E., Jr.: J.A.M.A., *195*:927, 1966.

[5] Neale, G., *et al.*: Brit. Med. J., *5472*:1223, 1965.

[6] Burges, E. A., *et al.*: Arch. Dis. Child., 39:431, 1964; Nutr. Rev., 23:101, 1965.

was virtually absent in all cases. Glucose absorption was normal. Withdrawal of sucrose from the diet promptly relieved all symptoms. These investigators report that in three of their seven patients the diagnosis was not made until the children were 4 to 5 years old.

DIETARY TREATMENT. The omission from the diet of granulated sugar, and of foods such as cakes, cookies, puddings and candy, all of which have sucrose as an ingredient, is relatively simple. Brown sugar, molasses, syrups and jellies should also be omitted. Some fruits and vegetables have a high sucrose content as shown by Hardinge and co-workers.[7] Lindquist[8] suggests the omission of apricots, bananas, dates, melons, oranges, pineapple and peas. Medications such as antibiotic syrups may also contain sucrose.

Invertase-Isomaltase Deficiency. This is a rare disorder in which the patient lacks both invertase and isomaltase. The latter breaks down one of the intermediate products of starch digestion, isomaltose, derived from amylopectin, to glucose. Lindquist[9] suggests the sparing use or avoidance of wheat and potato, both of which contain considerable amounts of amylopectin. The omission of sucrose and foods containing sucrose, as described in the previous paragraph, should also be observed.

Glucose-Galactose Malabsorption. In this rare disorder the mechanism for the active transport of glucose and galactose in the intestinal mucosa is not functioning. The digestion of sucrose and starch each yield glucose, and the end products of lactose digestion are glucose and galactose. Infants with this disorder cannot be kept free from symptoms unless all sources of carbohydrate are omitted with the exception of fructose. Lindquist[10] gives details of a for-

mula and the subsequent diet for children with this disorder.

Celiac Disease (Non-tropical Sprue)

Although the term celiac disease was originally applied only to children who exhibited this malabsorption syndrome, it is generally accepted today that what formerly was called non-tropical sprue is in reality adult celiac disease and may be referred to as celiac-sprue. It has been observed that a number of patients who developed celiac disease in adult life have a history of the disease in childhood.

Symptoms. The celiac syndrome is characterized by diarrhea, with the passing of at least 2 to 3 stools a day. These are described as bulky, foamy, light colored and foul smelling. They contain a high percentage of fat, fatty acids and calcium soaps, resulting from incomplete digestion and absorption in the intestinal tract. The term *steatorrhea* (fatty diarrhea) is applied to this finding.

Due to the loss of fat and other nutrients in the stool a whole complex of symptoms results. There is often marked weight loss, muscle wasting, anorexia and debilitation; in infants and sometimes in adults there is a typical "pot belly"; there is anemia due to poor absorption of iron and folic acid; there may be tetany, bone pain and fractures resulting from the poor absorption of calcium and vitamin D; and hypoprothrombinemia and roughening of the skin may be present because fat-soluble vitamins K and A are not absorbed. Occasionally patients have glossitis and peripheral neuritis, possibly due to an inadequate intake of the B vitamins. More recent findings suggest that there may also be a deficiency of vitamin E due to faulty fat absorption, and of vitamin B_6.

Diagnosis. The finding of unabsorbed fat and fatty acids in the feces and the history and appearance of the patient give the first clue to the diagnosis. A jejunal biopsy, viewed under the electron microscope, reveals marked changes in the jejunal mucosa. Instead of the fingerlike projections of the villi with their brush border, the mucosa is flat and thickened and appears to have

[7] Hardinge, M. G., *et al.*: J. Am. Dietet. A., *46*: 197, 1965.

[8] Lindquist, B., and Meeuwisse, G.: J. Am. Dietet. A., *48*:307, 1966.

[9] Op. cit.

[10] Op. cit. Also note correspondence and correction in regard to this formula in J. Am. Dietet. A., *49*:457, 1966.

varying degrees of epithelial cell atrophy, now recognized as characteristic of celiac disease. (See Figs. 27–2 and 27–3.)

It is suspected that a cellular enzyme, probably a peptidase, may be lacking in the mucosa of individuals with celiac-sprue. In 1953 three Dutch investigators Dicke, Weijers and van de Kamer[11] reported that wheat, rye and oat cereals were responsible for the steatorrhea and other symptoms of celiac disease in children. When they excluded these cereals from the diets of their patients there was prompt and marked improvement. In a subsequent report these same authors[12] showed that the two major components of wheat protein, gluten and gliadin, which are also present in rye protein and, to a lesser extent, in oat protein, were the offending substances. They indicated that the specific substance in the

cereal gluten is the amino acid glutamine when it is bound in a peptide (a partial breakdown product of protein digestion). When they tested their treated patients with bound glutamine the symptoms reoccured. This did not happen when they tested these same patients with glutamine alone.

Glutamine, the amide of glutamic acid, occurs widely in all food proteins but the greatest concentration is found in the gluten of wheat, rye, barley and oats. Although rice and corn also contain glutamine—but in smaller amounts than the other cereals—they are well tolerated in patients with celiac-sprue.

Dietary Treatment

From the work of the Dutch investigators with children, and of others with adults with non-tropical sprue, a "gluten-free" diet which excluded the use of wheat, rye, barley and oats was begun and soon proved

[11] Dicke, W. K., *et al.*: Acta paediat., *42*:34, 1953.

[12] van de Kamer, J. H., *et al.*: Acta paediat., *42*: 223, 1953.

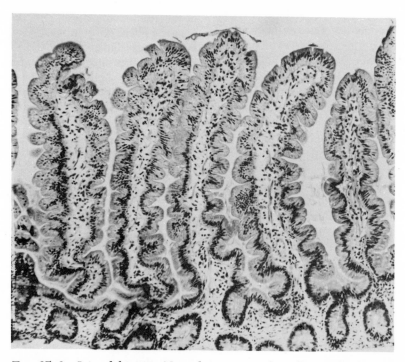

Fig. 27–2. Jejunal biopsy. Normal jejunum. The villi are slender and of uniform size. The epithelial cells are intact in all areas. (Benson, G. D., Kowlessar, O. D., and Sleisenger, M. H.: Adult celiac disease with emphasis upon response to the gluten-free diet. Medicine, *43*:1, 1964)

to be successful in controlling the disease. Foods used in the Gluten-Free diet are presented in Table 27–1. In the patient with severe diarrhea, the diet may be restricted in residue until the diarrhea is controlled.

The exclusion of all cereal grains except corn and rice from the diet may seem to be an easier matter than it actually is. Wheat-flour and wheat-bread products are used in such a variety of ways in food preparation that their elimination poses many problems. Not only must all wheat bread and rolls be omitted, both white and whole wheat, but all breaded products, bread stuffing, gravies and cream sauces thickened with wheat flour, macaroni, spaghetti, noodles, biscuits, crackers, cakes and cookies made from wheat flour must be eliminated from the diet. Rye grain, with the exception of rye breads, pretzels and Ry-Krisp, is less commonly used and, therefore, is omitted more easily. Oatmeal is excluded, as it caused a recurrence of symptoms when reintroduced into the diet. Barley and buckwheat are also excluded, as their effect in the intestinal tract in this disease is not known. For adults, beer and ale must be omitted, since they may contain cereal grain residues.[13]

In place of the cereals which must be excluded, bread, biscuits and cookies made from rice, corn and soy flour and wheat starch are used. (See Chap. 40 for recipes.) Cornflakes, corn meal, hominy, rice, Rice Krispies, Puffed Rice and precooked rice cereals may be used. Cornstarch and potato flour can be used to thicken gravies and cream sauces. Because wheat flour is in such common usage, it is well to check the labels on commercially prepared foods for content before using them on this diet to be sure that no wheat flour has been used in their preparation. Postum, malted milk and Ovaltine are examples of commercial products made from or containing cereal grains. Where such content is not in-

[13] Sleisenger, M. H., Rynbergen, H. J., *et al.*: J. Am. Dietet. A., 33:1137, 1957.

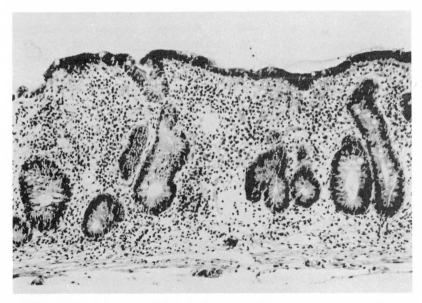

Fig. 27–3. Jejunal biopsy. Adult celiac disease. Pretreatment biopsy showing severe changes. There is complete absence of villi, thinning of the mucosal surface, and disorganization of the epithelial cells. (Benson, G. D., Kowlessar, O. D., and Sleisenger, M. H.: Adult celiac disease with emphasis upon response to the gluten-free diet. Medicine, 43:1, 1964)

TABLE 27–1. Gluten-Free Diet

Characteristics:

   1. All forms of wheat, rye, oatmeal, buckwheat and barley are omitted, except gluten-free wheat starch.

   2. All other foods are permitted freely, including fats and starches.

   3. The diet should be high in protein and calories, and probably in minerals and vitamins if malnutrition is present. After that, the diet should be sufficient to maintain normal growth and development in children, and normal weight in adults.

Foods Allowed:

Milk.....................2 glasses or more. Flavored if desired. More for children

Cheese...................As desired. Cottage and pot cheese only for very young children

Fats......................Butter and other fats as desired. (Note restrictions under "Foods To Be Avoided.")

Eggs.....................1 to 2 a day

Meat, fish, fowl.............1 or 2 servings daily (not breaded, creamed or served with thickened gravy; no bread dressings). Otherwise prepared as desired

Soups....................All clear and vegetable soups; cream soups thickened with cream, corn-starch or potato flour only

Vegetables................As desired, except creamed. Include 2 servings of green or yellow vege-tables and at least 1 raw vegetable daily. (The last may be omitted for very young children.) Rice may be substituted occasionally for potato.

Fruits....................As desired; 2 or 3 servings daily. Include citrus fruit once a day.

Bread and cereals..........Bread made from rice, corn or soybean flour and gluten-free wheat starch only

                                    Cornflakes, corn meal, hominy, rice, Rice Krispies, Puffed Rice, precooked rice cereals

Desserts...................Any of the following: jello, fruit jello, ice or sherbet, homemade ice cream, custard, junket, rice pudding, cornstarch pudding (homemade) or blanc mange if thickened with cornstarch

Beverages.................Milk, fruit juices, ginger ale, cocoa. (Read label to see that no wheat flour has been added to cocoa or cocoa syrup.) Coffee (made from ground coffee), tea, carbonated beverages

Condiments and sweets.......Salt; sugar, white or brown; molasses; jellies and jams; honey; corn syrup

Foods To Be Avoided:

Fats......................Cream sauces made with wheat flour; commercial salad dressings except pure mayonnaise. (Read labels.)

Meat, fish, fowl.............Meat patties or meat, fish or chicken loaf and pies made with bread or bread crumbs; croquettes; breaded meat, fish or chicken. Chili con carne and other canned meat dishes. Cold cuts unless guaranteed pure meat. Bread stuffings

                                      All gravies or cream sauces thickened with wheat flour

Soups....................All canned soups except clear broth. All cream soups unless thickened with cream, cornstarch or potato flour

TABLE 27–1. Gluten-Free Diet (Continued)

Foods To Be Avoided: (Continued)

Vegetables.................	Any prepared with cream sauce or breaded
Bread, cereals, macaroni products.................	All bread, rolls, crackers, cake and cookies made from wheat or rye; Ry-Krisp; muffins, biscuits, waffles, pancake flour and other prepared mixes; rusks, Zwieback, pretzels; any product containing oatmeal, barley or buckwheat Breaded foods, bread crumbs All wheat and rye cereals; wheat germ, barley, oatmeal, buckwheat, kasha Macaroni, spaghetti, noodles, dumplings
Desserts..................	Cakes, cookies, pastry; commercial ice cream and ice-cream cones; prepared mixes, puddings. All homemade puddings thickened with wheat flour
Beverages.................	Postum, malted milk, Ovaltine. For adults: beer, ale
Sweets...................	Commercial candies containing cereal products. (Read labels.)

Warning; Read labels on all packaged and prepared foods.

---

cluded in the label, the food had better be omitted if there is a question.

When the individual has a concurrent lactase deficiency, milk in all forms will also be excluded from the diet.

The physician may augment the diet with mineral and vitamin supplements to correct deficiencies and hasten recovery. Although fat excretion persists to some extent, fat is well tolerated and there is no need to limit it in the diet.

Results and Prognosis. The response of the patient with celiac disease to the elimination of the offending cereal grains is often dramatic, and may occur within 24 hours to a week. The appetite returns, the patient begins to regain lost weight, the stools become less fatty and less frequent, and a sense of well-being is quickly apparent.

The long-term effects of adherence to the gluten-free diet are equally striking. Benson *et al.*,[14] reporting on 32 patients with adult celiac disease followed for a number of years, found that there was improvement in every diagnostic finding, including in most cases a return to normal mucosal structure. The degree of improvement was in direct proportion to the careful adherence to the diet. That the diet does not cure the disease is shown by the fact that symptoms recur if the patient consumes food containing gluten.

Other Findings. Weser and Sleisenger[15] and others have reported that lactase deficiency and the absorption of undigested lactose occurred in some patients in whom celiac disease was untreated or who did not follow their diets carefully. Symptoms were abdominal cramps, distention and diarrhea, and were relieved when lactose as well as gluten were omitted from the diet. That this is not a permanent defect is shown by the fact that patients who had maintained a strict gluten-free diet for two years or more had no symptoms of lactase deficiency.

Celiac disease in infants and children will be discussed in Chapter 34.

Tropical Sprue

Tropical sprue, another malabsorption syndrome, is endemic in the native populations of some tropical and subtropical areas in the world, notably Puerto Rico and

---

[14] Benson, G. D., *et al.*: Medicine, 43:1, 1964.

[15] Weser, E., and Sleisenger, M. H.: Gastroenterology, 48:571, 1965.

Southeast Asia. Military personnel as well as other residents from temperate countries, who are stationed in these areas, also may develop tropical sprue, either during their stay in the host country or on their return home. Sheehy[16] warns that with increased involvement of our military personnel in the tropical areas of the world, we may expect to see this disease in the United States more frequently than in the past.

The symptoms are diarrhea, with loss of nutrients, especially fat, weight loss and macrocytic anemia. If the disease is of long standing, there will be severe malnutrition, megaloblastic bone marrow changes, and villous atrophy of the jejunal mucosa, eventually leading to the typical flat mucosa of celiac disease.

The syndrome responds dramatically to the administration of folic acid and antibiotics. In some patients, despite continuance of therapy, the megaloblastic anemia recurs due to deficient absorption of vitamin B_{12}. There is prompt response to vitamin B_{12} therapy. The response to a gluten-free diet is minimal, and an ordinary, nutritionally adequate diet, increased in calories and protein to counteract malnutrition and weight loss, is sufficient. With treatment, patients become asymptomatic and eventually the intestinal mucosa returns to normal.

The etiology of tropical sprue is still in doubt. It has been thought to be due to a diet deficient in folic acid or to an interference with its absorption, but there is no basis for this other than the response to treatment with folic acid. There is some evidence of the presence of an infective agent, because of the response to antibiotic therapy, but no pathogens have been demonstrated.

Cystic Fibrosis

Cystic fibrosis is an inherited disease affecting the mucous glands and the sweat glands of the body. It is sometimes called mucoviscidosis because of the abnormally thick mucus excreted by the exocrine glands (those excreting to the outside of

the body). The sweat glands produce unusually salty sweat, high in soc chloride.

The disease may first manifest itse the lungs where the thick mucus obst the air passages; or there may be diar with fatty stools and growth failure, to mucus plugs in the fine pancreatic d blocking the release of pancreatic dige enzymes. The diagnostic test for c fibrosis is the determination of the soc chloride content of the sweat. Testing enzyme content of the pancreatic juice also be done.

Until recently cystic fibrosis was tho of primarily as a disease of young chil usually fatal. With the use of techni to clear the lungs of mucus, of antibi to control infections, of pancreatic enz and a nutritionally adequate diet, mc ately restricted in fat, patients are growing into young adulthood.

Dietary Treatment

Protein foods are the foods most rea digested by the patient with cystic fi sis, and fat is digested least well. If disease is discovered in infancy, Matthe recommends a formula of half skim, whole milk to which casein hydroly and sugar are added to bring the for up to 20 calories per ounce. Solid f including meat, is started at 2 months the older child, the diet is increase protein, normal in carbohydrate and stricted in excessively fatty foods sucl butter and margarine, peanut butter, cr fatty meats, vegetable oils, fried food pastry rich in shortening. (See later in chapter on the use of fat made with dium-chain triglycerides.) Pancreatin, taining pancreatic enzymes, is given each feeding. Both water-soluble and soluble vitamins, including vitamin E, prescribed. During the summer mor when there is danger of heat prostra from excessive loss of sodium chlorid the sweat, extra salt must be added to diet. Fortunately under treatment t

---

[16] Sheehy, T. W., *et al.*: J.A.M.A., *194*:1069, 1965.

[17] Matthews, L. W., *et al.*: J. Pediatrics, *65* 1964.

patients eat well and are able to maintain good nutrition.

Care of the patient with cystic fibrosis can be a great financial, physical and emotional drain on the family resources. Fortunately professional help is available from government agencies. A private health agency, the National Cystic Fibrosis Research Foundation,[18] with chapters throughout the United States, also provides services to the family and the patient, as well as financing information and research for the control of this disease.

Medium-Chain Triglycerides

Fat in the ordinary diet contains mainly the long-chain fatty acids, oleic, palmitic and stearic, which are digested and absorbed into the lacteals of the villi, and carried by the great thoracic duct to the general circulation. Digestion and absorption are dependent on the bile salts and the enzyme lipase, and is a complicated process (see Chap. 9). In several of the malabsorption syndromes, it is the long chain fatty acids which are frequently not absorbed, and are lost in the stool.

About 5 per cent of naturally occurring fat contains short- and medium-chain fatty acids, C6:0 to C12:0. Hashim *et al.*[19] showed that these are split to glycerol and fatty acids by the mucosal enzymes and are absorbed directly from the villi into the capillary bed without re-esterification, and are carried via the portal vein to the liver.

The synthesis of a fat containing only medium-chain fatty acids was accomplished by the hydrolysis of coconut oil or butter and the distillation of the fatty acids. The short- and medium-chain fatty acids, C6:0 to C12:0, being the lightest, come off first. They were reconstituted with glycerol to form a fat (an oil) which can replace regular fat in the diet. This product, containing almost entirely caprylic (C8:0) and capric (C10:0) fatty acids, is called medium-chain triglyceride or MCT.

Holt and co-workers[20] report the use of MCT in cystic fibrosis, pancreatitis, biliary atresia and subtotal gastrectomy. In each instance fat excretion decreased or became normal. They also found evidence that the excretion of albumin from the intestinal tract was curtailed. MCT has also been shown to be of value in the treatment of tropical sprue, in massive resection of the small intestine, and in chyluria and chylothorax.

Use of MCT in the Diet. MCT is a liquid fat which yields 8.2 to 8.4 calories per gram. It can be incorporated into recipes in the same fashion as corn oil. Since patients for whom MCT is prescribed are those who do not readily digest and/or absorb long-chain fatty acids, fats containing these must be omitted. Schizas and her co-workers in a recent article[21] list the foods restricted and those allowed on the diet, give recipes using MCT, and include suggestions for menus.

REGIONAL ILEITIS

Regional ileitis is a chronic, progressive disease of the ileum of unknown etiology. It may first involve the terminal loop of the ileum proximal to the ileocecal valve, but, eventually, it will spread along the ileum and may involve the jejunum. For this reason the disease is sometimes called regional enteritis. The term regional refers to the fact that healthy areas of the bowel may alternate with diseased ones. Despite occasional remissions, the disease is progressive.

The condition is characterized by hyperplasia (enlargement due to cell increase) of the lymphatics, which eventually interferes with the blood supply of the mucosa of that section of the intestinal tract which is affected. This in turn gives rise to edema and ulceration, scarring of the mucosa, thickening of the intestinal wall with narrowing of the lumen of the bowel and obstruction. The most common symptoms are persistent diarrhea and pain.[22]

[18] National Cystic Fibrosis Research Foundation, 521 Fifth Avenue, New York, N. Y. 10017.

[19] Hashim, S. A., *et al.*: J. Clin. Invest., *43*:1238, 1964.

[20] Holt, P. R., *et al.*: Am. J. Gastroenterology, *43*: 549, 1965.

[21] Schizas, A. A., *et al.*: J. Am. Dietet. A., *51*:228, 1967.

[22] Crohn, B. B.: J.A.M.A., *166*:1479, 1958.

Because of the persistent diarrhea there may be marked malnutrition. If the disease is extensive, there will be poor absorption of food nutrients, further accentuating the poor nutrition. A chronically ill patient may be markedly underweight and show signs of protein depletion. Anemia may be present due to blood loss and to poor absorption of iron and vitamin B_{12}. There may be insufficient absorption of fat-soluble vitamins as evidenced by hypoprothrombinemia and roughened skin. If medical treatment fails to restore the patient's nutritional status, or if there is obstruction, surgery may be indicated. See Chapter 29 for dietary care in the latter case.

Dietary Treatment

The diet in regional ileitis should be high in protein and calories, and low in residue, as described under Ulcerative Colitis. It is possible that the substitution of medium-chain triglycerides (MCT) for ordinary dietary fat may be of value in this disease. The patient may eat better when the diet is divided into 6 meals during the day and evening, and if he is given some choice. Seasonings and cold fluids are not well tolerated and should be omitted. Vitamin supplements should be given as additions to the diet. Vitamins K and B_{12} and, possibly, iron should be given as parenteral medications, since they are not sufficiently absorbed from the intestinal tract.

Lactose Intolerance. Chalfin and Holt[23] report lactose intolerance in three out of five patients with ileitis. Two of these had a history of milk intolerance previous to the disease. The restrictions for lactase deficiency discussed earlier in the chapter should be observed in cases where the diagnosis has been established.

ULCERATIVE COLITIS

Ulcerative colitis is an inflammatory disease of the colon, encountered in all age groups from very young children to the elderly. It is characterized by friability and hyperemia of the mucosa, leading to many small areas of bleeding ulceration. This may involve only a part of the rectum or the colon, but in advanced stages of the disease it usually involves the entire area of the large bowel. The stools, which may be as frequent as 15 to 20 a day, are semi-liquid and contain blood and mucus. The patient suffers from the discomfort of the frequent stools and the accompanying cramps, and he is usually malnourished, often to an extreme degree. Anemia may be present due to blood loss, and the patient may be severely underweight. The disease is usually treated conservatively by medical means, but in advanced cases surgery may be resorted to and a colostomy performed. See Chapter 29 for dietary care in the latter case.

The etiology of colitis is unknown. No organism has been isolated as a cause of the disease. It has been ascribed to allergy, especially to milk, wheat and eggs. In addition, there are indications that colitis may occur on an emotional basis, since these patients are often very painstaking and meticulous and seem to have more than an ordinary dependence on others.[24]

Dietary Treatment

The dietary treatment in colitis is supportive rather than curative. A patient, previously well controlled by diet and medication, may have diarrhea when emotionally upset, even though he is adhering to his prescribed diet.

The frequency of the stools, the degree of bleeding and ulceration of the colon and the general malnutrition present in all patients with severe colitis demand the use of a diet low in residue and as high in protein and calories as the patient can tolerate. The omission of roughage will prevent irritation of the inflamed colon, and the high protein, high caloric diet will help to restore the patient to a better nutritional status. Vitamin and iron supplements should be given.

Low Residue. Either the moderately low residue diet or the very low residue diet

---

[23] Chalfin, D., and Holt, P. R.: Am. J. Digest. Dis., *12*:81, 1967.

[24] Kirsner, J. B.: J.A.M.A., *169*:433, 1959; Rider, J. A., and Moeller, H. C.: Am. J. Gastroenterology, 37:487, 1962; Fullerton, D. T., *et al.*: J.A.M.A., *181*: 463, 1962.

TABLE 27–2. Diets Varying in Residue

Foods	Soft Diet	Moderately Low Residue Diet	Very Low Residue Diet
Milk	Milk, buttermilk, yoghurt, cream	Same	Same if allowed. Boiled or evaporated milk may be tolerated better than pasteurized milk.
Cheese	Cottage, cream, Cheddar	Same	Cottage, cream only, if tolerated
Fat	Butter, margarine	Same	Same
Eggs	Cooked, poached, scrambled in double boiler	Same	Same
Meat, fish, fowl	Tender chicken, fish, sweetbreads; ground beef and lamb	Same	Ground, tender meat; minced chicken and fish
Soups and broths	Broth, strained cream soups	Same	Broth only
Vegetables	Cooked vegetables: asparagus, peas, string beans, spinach, carrots, beets, squash; potatoes, boiled, mashed, creamed, scalloped, baked	Vegetable juice; vegetable purée; cooked asparagus tips, carrots; potatoes as for soft diet	Unseasoned vegetable juices in limited amounts
Fruits	Fruit juices, cooked and canned fruits (without skins, seeds or fiber); bananas	Fruit juice; fruit purée, ripe bananas; cooked, peeled apples, apricots, peaches, pears, plums	Fruit juices, preferably citrus in limited amounts if allowed
Bread, cereals, macaroni products	Whole-grain or enriched bread and cereals; macaroni, spaghetti, noodles, crackers	Refined, enriched bread and cereals only; macaroni, spaghetti, noodles, white crackers	As in moderately low residue
Desserts	Ices, ice cream, junket, cereal puddings, custard, gelatin, plain cake and cookies; all without fruit and nuts	Same	Same
Beverages	Tea, coffee, cocoa; milk and milk beverages; carbonated beverages	Same	Tea, Postum; coffee as permitted; milk and milk beverages if tolerated
Condiments	Salt, moderate amounts of pepper; other mild spices; sugar	Salt and sugar only	Salt in small amounts; sugar

Menu for a Very Low Residue Diet

Breakfast	Lunch	Supper
Cream of Wheat	Hot vegetable juice	Broth
Light cream	Minced creamed chicken	Cream cheese and jelly
Sugar	on toast	sandwich
Postum	Milk	Fruit juice gelatin
10 A.M.	**3 P.M.**	**8 P.M.**
Warm milk or	Custard, served at	Warm milk or
malted milk	room temperature	malted milk
Cookie		Cookie

listed on page 383 is suitable for the very ill colitis patient. It should be served in six small meals at first. Unfortunately the diet is not very palatable or colorful, and the nurse and the dietitian must do all they can to serve the food as attractively as possible. A suggested menu is given on page 383. Although it contains a good deal of milk, the patient may not tolerate it well at this stage. Buttermilk or yoghurt may be tried, but if they cause discomfort, tea and broth should be substituted even though they contribute few nutrients. A commercially available booklet of recipes, using infant foods, may be found helpful in adding variety and interest to low residue diets.[25]

Increased Protein. As soon as the patient begins to respond to treatment the diet should include two servings daily of tender meats, fish or chicken, with little connective tissue. Two or three eggs may be served, either plain or in desserts. High-protein beverages (see Chap. 36) will aid in raising the protein content of the diet, but the patient may find that concentrated fluids cause discomfort. An inexpensive source of additional protein is dried skim milk powder, which may be added to fluid milk beverages or to other foods such as creamed dishes, mashed potatoes or desserts, provided the patient does not have an intolerance to milk.

Increased Calories. Due to the loss of food substances in the stools and the patient's often capricious appetite, weight loss is a frequent symptom of colitis. Calories may be increased in the diet by more bread and cereals, simple desserts and jellies and also more butter and cream if the patient tolerates them. The high-protein beverages mentioned in the previous paragraph may be made high caloric by the addition of chocolate or other fountain syrup. As the patient improves, his choice of food may approximate that of a soft or even a general diet. However, gas-forming food such as members of the cabbage family, turnips,

onions, cucumbers and dried beans and peas should be omitted.

Self-Selected Diet. Since colitis seems to have strong emotional components, the diet may be used to help the patient to achieve some degree of independence. The doctor may allow him to choose his own diet and to encourage him to try whatever food appeals to him, even those which would seem to be contraindicated, such as foods high in residue. The nurse and the dietitian must be supportive as well as permissive, giving the patient confidence and encouraging him to make his own decisions. As the patient's feeling of security increases, he will eat larger and more nutritious meals, with the subsequent healing of the colon and a gain in weight and strength.

Lactose intolerance may further complicate the dietary treatment of the patient with ulcerative colitis. Chalfin and Holt[26] report improvement of symptoms when lactose was withdrawn in 4 patients with colitis who had flat lactose tolerance curves. One of these had had milk intolerance for many years prior to the onset of colitis.

If lactose intolerance is shown to be present, the restriction of foods, especially milk and medications containing lactose, as described earlier in the chapter, should be followed.

Nursing Problems. Recovery is often slow and there are likely to be setbacks. Patients with colitis are fussy about their food and often extremely hard to please. They wish others to make choices for them, yet refuse to eat the food when it appears on the tray. They have the irritability of the badly nourished patient and need much understanding and encouragement. Fortunately, most patients recover, at least for a time, and can return to a more or less normal diet.

CONSTIPATION

A common disturbance of the digestive tract is constipation. However, there is considerable confusion as to what is meant by this term. Although a daily bowel movement has been stressed as desirable, there

---

[25] McIntosh, E. M.: Making Meals More Appealing for Special Diets, Gerber Products Co., Fremont, Michigan.

[26] Chalfin, D., and Holt, P. R.: Am. J. Digest. Dis., *12*:81, 1967.

are many people for whom an evacuation every other day or even every third day is normal. Moreover, evacuation may occur regularly until an emotional upset occurs, in which case there may either be an increased number of bowel movements, almost a diarrhea, or retention of the feces for a day or two, resembling constipation. The matter usually straightens itself out when the strain is relieved. However, if the person becomes anxious when no daily bowel movement occurs and begins to resort to cathartics or enemas, a vicious pattern is set up, and it may be difficult to effect a return to normal habits.

Chronic constipation may be due to the individual's dietary and living habits. Insufficient rest, hurried, irregular meals, a food intake which does not meet the nutritional needs of the body, and too sedentary a life all may contribute to poor bowel function. The problem here is to help the patient to accept a more regular mode of living, including a diet that meets all his nutritive requirements and a reasonable amount of exercise.

Elderly patients may suffer from constipation because muscle tone is relaxed, the dietary intake is inadequate for nutritional needs, and activity is diminished.

Dietary Treatment

In most cases of so-called constipation, a normal diet (see Chap. 10) containing roughage in the form of fresh and cooked fruit and vegetables and including whole-grain bread and cereals will provide sufficient bulk to maintain regular bowel evacuation. Where such regularity needs to be re-established—for instance, following an illness in which the mobility of the patient has been greatly limited—the addition of stewed fruit and of fruit juices to the ordinary diet will be found helpful. Prune juice, particularly, taken at bedtime or the first thing in the morning, is usually effective.

Elderly patients should not use foods with a high bran content for fear of impaction. Cooked fruits and vegetables are often better tolerated by the older patient than raw ones, except for bananas.

Nursing Problems. Patients in the hospital, particularly those who are confined to bed, may suffer from constipation because of strange surroundings or as a result of inactivity. Older patients on bed rest may develop fecal impaction unless they are carefully checked for regularity of evacuation. Patients with heart disease should be prevented from straining at stool. Immobilized patients, either in a cast or for other reasons, may need help in maintaining regular bowel habits. For such patients the generous inclusion of stewed fruit and stewed fruit juices, especially prune juice, in a well-balanced diet may be all that is necessary to prevent constipation and straining. Other simple remedies are lemon juice in hot water or a cup of hot coffee before breakfast. Whatever procedure has helped a patient in the past should be permitted him in the hospital so long as it is not contraindicated. Only if these methods fail should cathartics be prescribed.

CANCER OF THE BOWEL

In all cases of constipation, or of constipation alternating with diarrhea, particularly if these symptoms are of short duration and in the face of otherwise normal living habits, there is the possibility of neoplastic growth of some section of the colon or the rectum. If this diagnosis is established by the use of proctoscopic and roentgenographic examinations, the patient is subjected to surgery. See Chapter 29 for postoperative diets.

DIVERTICULITIS

Diverticula, or small pouches, sometimes appear along the walls of the intestines. They may occur in the small intestine but are seen much more frequently in the colon. There may be few or many. The condition is known as diverticulosis and may or may not be a source of trouble. However, when one or more of the pouches becomes infected or irritated, the condition is known as diverticulitis. The infection may be due to an accumulation of feces in the pouches and may result in ulceration and perforation. In the latter case surgery is indicated.

In diverticulitis without perforation, but with pain, tenderness and sometimes fever, the treatment is much the same as for appendicitis, i.e., complete abstinence from food for from 24 to 48 hours, with only sips of water or cracked ice. Gradually, liquid foods are added, then a low-residue diet should be followed until all symptoms have subsided (see Table 27–2). When diverticulosis has been diagnosed, even though without acute symptoms, the patient should restrict the amount of residue in his diet.

HEMORRHOIDS

Hemorrhoids are varicose veins around the anal sphincter. They may be internal or external. Some of the causes of the condition are childbearing, constipation, hepatic cirrhosis and the long-continued use of cathartics and enemas. The symptoms are bleeding, itching and pain. The purpose of the treatment is to restore normal function of the intestinal tract. A bland diet, high in nonirritating forms of bulk or fiber, such as puréed fruits and vegetables, is given in addition to local treatment. Surgery is used in severe cases.

STUDY QUESTIONS AND ACTIVITIES

1. What are the functions of the small intestine? Why does disease of the small intestine often result in malnutrition?

2. What are the differences between a soft diet, a moderately low-residue and a very low-residue diet?

3. Plan a high caloric, low-residue diet for a patient suffering from amebic dysentery.

4. What does the term "malabsorption syndrome" mean?

5. Which two tests are most frequently done to determine disaccharidase deficiency?

6. Name six foods or food groups which must be omitted in lactose intolerance.

7. What is the older term for adult celiac disease?

8. What are the symptoms of celiac disease? What does the term "steatorrhea" mean? What pathologic changes are found in the jejunal mucosa?

9. Why is the so-called gluten-free diet used in celiac disease? Which cereals must be omitted?

10. Plan a diet for an adult patient with celiac disease living at home; for a secretary with this disease who eats her lunch at a drugstore counter.

11. What is the difference between celiac disease and tropical sprue? How is the latter treated?

12. How does cystic fibrosis differ from other malabsorption syndromes?

13. Make out a diet plan for a 4-year-old child with cystic fibrosis. She has a good appetite. Her protein should be somewhat increased and the fat restricted.

14. What is medium-chain triglyceride? Why may it be used effectively in some diseases of the small intestine?

15. Why should a patient with ileitis have a low-residue diet? Can such a diet meet all the patient's nutritional requirements? How may additional calories and proteins be included?

16. What problems may the nurse encounter in regard to the food habits of the colitis patient? What should be her attitude toward these?

17. What additions to the diet will help many patients who have a tendency to constipation?

18. Why may hospitalized patients develop constipation? Which groups are especially vulnerable? Name some simple remedies by which the problem may be corrected without the aid of cathartics.

19. Plan a diet for a working man with diverticulosis, using a moderately low-residue diet.

SUPPLEMENTARY READING ON DISEASES OF THE INTESTINES

Crohn, B. B.: Regional ileitis. Postgrad. Med., 38:276, 1965.

Hashim, S. A.: Medium-chain triglycerides—clinical and metabolic aspects. J. Am. Dietet. A., 51:221, 1967.

How to Eat Well on a Gluten-Free Diet. Today's Health, 43:38, 1965 (Oct.).

Lindquist, B., and Meeuwisse, G.: Diets in disaccharidase deficiency and defective monosaccharide absorption. J. Am. Dietet. A., 48:307, 1966.

McKittrick, J. B., and Shotkin, J. M.: Ulcerative colitis. Am. J. Nursing, *62*:60, 1962.

Nutrition Review: Medium chain triglycerides in tropical sprue. Nutr. Rev., *23*:71, 1965.

————: Primary intestinal lactase deficiency. Nutr. Rev., *25*:265, 1967.

Ratcliff, J. D.: America's laxative addicts. Today's Health, *40*:52, 1962 (Nov.).

Schizas, A. A., *et al.*: Medium-chain triglycerides—use in food preparation. J. Am. Dietet. A., *51*:228, 1967.

Sheehy, T. W., *et al.*: Tropical sprue in North Americans. J.A.M.A., *194*:1069, 1965.

Sleisenger, M. H., *et al.*: A wheat, rye and oat-free diet in the treatment of non-tropical sprue. J. Am. Dietet. A., *33*:1137, 1957.

————: Clinical and metabolic studies in non-tropical sprue. New Eng. J. Med., *265*:49, 1961.

Your Child with Cystic Fibrosis. National Cystic Fibrosis Foundation, 521 Fifth Avenue, New York, N. Y. 10017.

For further references see Bibliography in Part Four.

CHAPTER 28

Diseases of the Liver, the Biliary Tract and the Pancreas

Functions of the Liver • Diseases of the Liver • Infectious Hepatitis • Cirrhosis • Complications • Disease of the Gallbladder • Pancreatitis

FUNCTIONS OF THE LIVER

The liver is not only the largest glandular organ in the body but also one of the most important, because of the diversity of its functions. It serves as the entrance into the body, via the portal circulation, of most of the products of digestion. It stores, distributes or metabolizes these to their end products, manufactures needed substances, detoxifies harmful ones and performs numerous other functions.

Metabolism and Storage

Protein. The liver regulates the distribution of amino acids to the tissues, where they are used for growth and tissue maintenance. It synthesizes some of the amino acids absorbed from the digestive tract into the plasma proteins, albumin, fibrinogen, prothrombin and possibly globulin. Excess amino acids are split into the nitrogenous portion to form urea, while the remainder of the molecule is converted to carbohydrate or fat.

Carbohydrate. The liver converts glucose, galactose and fructose to glycogen and stores it. As needed, the glycogen is broken down to glucose and sent as blood sugar to the tissues, particularly the muscles, eventually to be metabolized for energy.

Fat. The liver oxidizes fatty acids to ketones, converts excess glucose to fat for storage in the tissues, and synthesizes lipoproteins and phospholipids, the latter with the aid of choline derived from the amino acid methionine. In the absence of sufficient protein in the diet, fat stasis in the liver results and may become a serious condition.

Minerals and Vitamins. An important function of the liver is the storage of iron and copper for distribution as needed in the synthesis of hemoglobin for the red blood cells. The liver also stores vitamin B_{12}, needed for the development of red blood cells in the bone marrow (see Chaps. 8 and 31). Other minerals such as zinc and magnesium are also probably stored in the liver.

Most of the vitamin A stored in the body is found in the liver. The conversion of carotene to vitamin A takes place here. Vitamin D is also stored in the liver, as is vitamin K, essential for the production of prothrombin, which occurs in the liver. Other vitamins, particularly the B complex and ascorbic acid, are found in considerable amounts in the liver.

Production and Role of Bile

Another of the functions of the liver is the production of bile, which plays an important part in the digestion and the absorption of fat. Bile, after its manufacture in the liver cells, is collected by many small bile ducts and emptied into the hepatic duct, which leads to the cystic duct and to the gallbladder, where the bile is concentrated by the absorption of water and stored. (See Fig. 28–1.)

Bile is composed of bile salts, bile pigments, cholesterol, inorganic salts and water. Approximately 800 to 1,200 ml. of bile are produced daily. Fat in the duodenum stimulates the flow of bile from the gallbladder into the duodenum.

With the aid of peristalsis and segmentation, bile emulsifies the fat in the intestinal tract by breaking up the larger globules into many smaller ones. This creates a greater surface area for the digestive enzymes to act on.

The bile salts aid in "ferrying" the fatty acids across the intestinal wall during absorption. In diseases in which the amount of bile in the intestinal tract is diminished, there is interference with the absorption of fats and also with some of the fat-soluble vitamins (see Chap. 9).

The bile pigments are breakdown products of hemoglobin and have no known role. They give the feces the characteristic green-brown color. When bile is absent from the intestinal tract, so-called clay-colored stools result.

The function of the other constituents of bile is not known. They may be waste products.

Jaundice is a symptom of a number of diseases of the liver and the biliary tract. It is manifested by a yellow pigmentation of the body tissues due to the presence in the blood of more than the normal amount of bile pigments caused by obstruction of the bile ducts.

Detoxification

The liver detoxifies harmful substances into non-toxic compounds. These may be ingested with food or taken as drugs. Bacterial action in the intestinal tract may produce irritating or toxic substances, including ammonia, of which we shall hear more later. When any of these are absorbed via the portal circulation, the liver alters them chemically into non-toxic materials.

Some of the hormones are changed in the liver to inactive compounds to terminate their action. The liver also is involved in the detoxification of metabolic fragments. Among these is ammonia, an intermediate product of the breakdown of amino acids to form urea.

DISEASES OF THE LIVER

It is not surprising that an organ which performs as many functions as the liver should manifest many and far-reaching symptoms when it is diseased. Fortunately, the liver, with adequate treatment, has remarkable capacity for regeneration and repair.

FIG. 28–1. The hepatic duct from the liver unites with the cystic duct from the gallbladder, forming a common bile duct opening into the small intestine. Note also that the pancreatic duct joins the common duct before entering the duodenum. (Greisheimer: Physiology and Anatomy, ed. 8, Philadelphia, Lippincott)

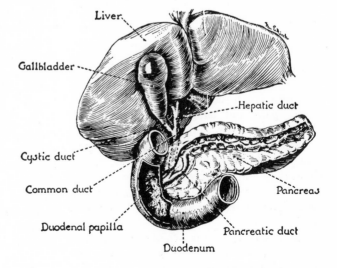

Liver

Gallbladder

Hepatic duct

Cystic duct

Common duct

Pancreas

Duodenal papilla

Pancreatic duct

Duodenum

Two of the principal diseases of the liver in which dietary treatment plays an important role are infectious hepatitis and cirrhosis.

Infectious Hepatitis

Etiology and Symptoms. Hepatitis is a general term which may be used to include injury to the liver cells as a result of bacterial or viral infections, toxins and drugs. The most important example of hepatitis is infectious or viral hepatitis. This disease was a major cause of illness among our armed forces in World Wars I and II. It is also prevalent all over the world among civilians. It may be acquired by direct transmission of the virus or by transfusion of blood from a donor who has had infectious hepatitis. In the latter case the disease is called serum hepatitis.

Acute infectious hepatitis is characterized by elevation of temperature, headache, abdominal discomfort and loss of appetite. After a short period, lasting from a few days to 2 or 3 weeks, jaundice may appear. Usually from 6 to 8 weeks are required for recovery.

Whether the disease is due to a direct infection with the virus or to a blood transfusion, two essentials of treatment are rest and an increased protein, increased carbohydrate, moderate fat diet. If sufficient time for rest and treatment is not provided, a chronic condition such as cirrhosis may be the final outcome. However, most patients recover completely.

Dietary Treatment

In the acute stage of infectious hepatitis it may not be possible for the patient to consume much food because of severe anorexia, pain and nausea, and intravenous fluids, electrolytes and glucose have to be substituted. As soon as possible the patient should be placed on a diet increased in protein and carbohydrate, and of moderate fat content. The diet is maintained until liver function tests return to normal levels.

Increased protein is essential for the regeneration of liver tissues. Double the normal allowance, or 2 Gm. of protein per Kg. of body weight, is considered sufficient for this purpose. For a 50-Kg. woman this would be 100 Gm. of protein per day, whereas a 70-Kg. man would require approximately 140 Gm. of protein daily.

Increased Carbohydrate. The diet is increased in carbohydrate to provide calories and spare the protein for liver regeneration.

Moderate Fat. It used to be thought that the diet had to be low in fat in order to prevent deposition in the liver, but so long as enough protein is ingested there seems to be no necessity to limit the fat. Its presence in the diet enhances palatability and increases the total food intake. See the discussion of foods and a menu for the above regimen under Cirrhosis later in the chapter.

Cirrhosis

Etiology. Cirrhosis is the final stage of liver injury. It may be due to chronic alcoholism, to diseases of the circulatory system, such as Banti's disease, or to chronic infectious hepatitis discussed in the paragraphs above.

The Role of Nutrition. It is thought that in chronic alcoholism, cirrhosis is due to deficiencies in food intake occurring over a long period of time. The individual may get as many as 1,500 to 2,500 calories daily from the alcohol he consumes, since 1 Gm. of alcohol yields 7 calories. (See Table 7, Part Four.) There is little desire for other food, and gross inadequacies in all food constituents result. Vitamin deficiency, particularly of thiamine, may be manifested by polyneuritis. An acute form of thiamine deficiency, known as the Wernicke-Korsakoff syndrome, may occur in sereve alcoholism.[1] It is described in Chapter 16.

The lack of protein, necessary for the metabolism of fat in the liver, leads to fat stasis and eventual necrosis (death) of liver tissue and, finally, to replacement of liver cells by scar tissue. If the diet is changed to supply the needed nutrients, regeneration of the less-damaged liver tissue may take place, or, at least, further degeneration will be prevented.

---

[1] Victor, M., and Adams, R. D.: Am. J. Clin. Nutr., 9:379, 1961 (Part I).

The Role of Alcohol. Whether alcohol itself is damaging to liver tissue is still under debate. Hartroft and Porta[2] report that in untreated alcoholics there was deposition of fat droplets of various sizes in all hepatic cells except those in regenerating areas. There was also marked enlargement of the mitochondria of liver cells. They found that in rats, fed a low fat, normal protein diet with added alcohol calories, they could not induce fatty change in the liver. They conclude that the causative factors in cirrhosis are probably a number of nutritional deficiencies, since these are almost certain to develop when the "empty calories" of alcohol constitute a large part of the daily caloric intake. Conversely, Lieber *et al.*,[3] studying 5 alcoholics under metabolic unit conditions, found that the patients developed fatty livers when an isocaloric amount of alcohol was substituted for carbohydrate in an otherwise adequate diet, and also when alcohol was added to an adequte diet. These investigators conclude that alcohol itself is an etiologic factor in the pathogenesis of fatty liver, independent of nutritional factors. Isselbacher and Greenberger,[4] in a lengthy review of fat metabolism in the liver, state that the pathway to cirrhosis is still unclear. They postulate that, under the influence of alcohol, the metabolic action of fat in the liver, and particularly the increased mobilization of fatty acids from depot fat and their conversion in the liver to triglycerides, favors their accumulation in this organ. They believe this is a factor, in addition to impaired nutrition, in the pathogenesis of cirrhosis.

Symptoms. Many patients with alcoholic cirrhosis suffer from as severe a degree of malnutrition as the nurse is likely to see. Cheilosis, a beefy red tongue and hypoprothrombinemia may all be present. Weight loss may not be marked due to the calories derived from alcohol, although it occurs.

Besides jaundice and marked enlargement of the liver, there may be a low level of serum albumin due to protein starvation and leading to nutritional edema. In advanced cases, portal hypertension (increased blood pressure in the portal system) occurs, because the liver is so filled with scar tissue that circulation is impaired. This, in turn, causes diffusion of fluids and electrolytes from the intestinal capillary bed into the peritoneal cavity, and there may be a large accumulation of fluid in the abdomen. This is called *ascites*. It is thought also that the hormone aldosterone, which affects sodium retention in the body, is more slowly destroyed by the diseased liver, and therefore contributes to the stasis of sodium and water.[5]

The swelling of the abdomen is sometimes the symptom that is noticed first by the patient and that leads him to seek medical advice. Another complication of portal hypertension is the formation of varices (varicose veins) in the lower esophagus, since its veins empty into the portal vein. These varices may hemorrhage and complicate the ravages of this disease.

Dietary Treatment

Since chronic alcoholism is the most frequent cause of hepatic cirrhosis, the discussion of the dietary treatment will focus primarily on this condition. However, cirrhosis from other pathology will usually be treated in the same manner, depending in each instance on the degree of functioning liver tissue that remains.

The physician's diet order for the alcoholic cirrhotic patient will be based on the condition of the patient and of his liver. If there is no immediate danger of liver failure, the diet for these severely malnourished individuals will be increased in protein, up to 2 Gm. per Kg. of body weight. Carbohydrate will be increased to provide calories, and enough fat is included to make the diet palatable. If liver failure threatens or if there are complications from esophageal varices, it is essential that the protein content of the diet be reduced immediately. This is discussed later in the chapter.

[2] Hartroft, W. S., and Porta, E. A.: Nutr. Rev., 24:97, 1966.

[3] Lieber, C. S., *et al.*: J. Clin. Invest., 44:1009, 1965.

[4] Isselbacher, K. J., and Greenberger, N. J.: New Eng. J. Med., 270:351, 402, 1964.

[5] LaLonde, J. B., *et al.*: J.A.M.A., 187:117, 1964.

TABLE 28–1. A Suggested Menu Containing 100 Grams of Protein, 120 Grams of Fat, 300 Grams of Carbohydrate and 2,550 Calories[1]

Food	Household Measure	Calories	Protein Gm.	Fat Gm.	Carbohydrate Gm.
Breakfast					
Citrus fruit	1 serving	43	1	..	10
Cereal	1 serving	89	3	1	18
Milk	8 ounces	160	8.5	9	12
Toast	1 slice	63	2	1	12
Butter or margarine	1 teaspoon	34	..	4	..
Jelly	2 teaspoons	34	..	..	10
Coffee	....	..	..	..	..
Sugar	1 tablespoon	46	..	..	12
		469	14.5	15	74
Midmorning					
Milk	8 ounces	160	8.5	9	12
Chocolate syrup	2 tablespoons	98	..	..	26
		258	8.5	9	38
Lunch					
Meat	1 ounce	94	7.5	8	..
Bread	2 slices	126	4	1	24
Butter or margarine	1 teaspoon	34	..	4	..
Egg	one	81	7	6	..
Salad, lettuce, tomatoes	1 serving	45	2	..	10
Mayonnaise	2 teaspoons	62	..	7	..
Milk	8 ounces	160	8.5	9	12
Fruit	1 serving	85	..	..	22
		687	29	35	68
Midafternoon					
As midmorning		258	8.5	9	38
Supper					
Meat	3 ounces	282	22.5	23	..
Potato	1 serving	65	2	..	15
Vegetable	1 serving	27	2	..	6
Butter or margarine	1 teaspoon	34	..	4	..
Ice cream	⅛ quart	173	4	10	19
Tea	....	..	..	..	..
Sugar	2 teaspoons	32	..	..	8
		613	30.5	37	48
Evening					
Milk	8 ounces	160	8.5	9	12
Cooky	1 3-inch	109	2	3	19
		269	10.5	12	31
Total for day		2,554	101.5	117	297

[1] Calculations based on food groups in Pattern Dietary in Chapter 19, and on Table 1, in Part Four.

TABLE 28–2. Increased Protein and Carbohydrate, Moderate Fat Menu
Semi-Liquid Form

Breakfast	Lunch	Supper
Orange juice	Cream of celery soup	Apricot nectar
Farina, cooked	Poached egg on toast	Farina, cooked
Milk, 1 glass	Creamed spinach	Milk, 1 glass
Cream, light, 2 ounces	Milk, 1 glass	Cream, light, 2 ounces
Coffee	Canned pears	Sugar
Sugar		Baked custard
10 A.M.	**3 P.M.**	**8 P.M.**
High-protein beverage*	High-protein beverage*	High-protein beverage*

* See Chapter 36 for suggestions and recipes.
To lower the protein in this menu, substitute plain milk or buttermilk, or fruit juice for the high-protein beverages.

Increased Protein. The increased protein in the diet will aid in the regeneration of such liver tissue as has not entirely necrosed and become scar tissue. Adequate dietary protein will also lessen the fat stasis in the liver cells by converting the fat to phospholipid to be carried by the blood to the tissues. It is also given in an attempt to increase the low serum albumin of the blood and relieve nutritional edema if it is present.

Increased Carbohydrate. An increase in dietary carbohydrate is well tolerated in liver disease, provides needed calories, and seems to aid in recovery, probably due to its protein-sparing action.

Moderate Fat. Patek[6] first showed that fat, despite fat stasis in the liver, may be consumed in reasonable amounts, from 100 to 150 Gm., without deleterious effects. The fat makes the diet more palatable, encouraging the patient to eat the food so essential for some degree of recovery.

Vitamins and Iron. The use of vitamin supplements and possibly iron is nearly always indicated because of most patients' poor physical condition and previously limited food intake. Deficiencies in the B-complex vitamins as shown by tongue lesions and the presence of polyneuritis, and of vitamin K, indicated by hypoprothrombinemia, are not uncommon. Iron-deficient anemia may also be present.

Alcohol is strictly prohibited.

⁶ Patek, A. J., and Post, J.: J. Clin. Invest., 20:481, 1941.

A SUGGESTED MENU

For 100 Grams of Protein. A Suggested Menu providing 100 Gm. of protein, 300 Gm. of carbohydrate, 120 Gm. of fat and 2,550 calories (see Table 28–1) is based on the Pattern Dietary in Chapter 19 which contains 70 Gm. of protein. The increase in protein is achieved by the addition of 1½ pints of milk and one egg to the Pattern Dietary. The use of sugar, fountain syrup and a dessert accounts for the increase in carbohydrate. The added foods also contribute to the content of fat and total calories. On the basis of 2 Gm. of protein per Kg. of body weight, the Suggested Menu is suitable for a 50-Kg. woman with cirrhosis, who has sufficient liver function to metabolize this amount of protein.

For 140 Grams of Protein. A 70-Kg. man under the same conditions would need 140 Gm. of protein. The addition of two more ounces of meat (15 Gm. of protein), a tablespoon of powdered skim milk to each of the milk beverages (5 tablespoons = 15 Gm. of protein), and the inclusion of some cottage or cheddar cheese to the Suggested Menu on page 392 will accomplish this.

Other variations on the Suggested Menu may be made by consulting the Pattern Dietary in Chapter 19, Tables 36–1 and 36–2 in Chapter 36, and Table 1, Part Four, Food Composition.

FEEDING PROBLEMS

One of the grave problems confronting the nurse is to persuade the patient with cirrhosis of the liver to eat, for his recovery rests almost entirely on his dietary intake. Often he is toxic and may be extremely discouraged and depressed. A soft to semi-liquid diet, consisting of high-protein, high-carbohydrate beverages (see Chap. 36), supplemented with small trays at regular meal hours may best meet his needs at first. Such a menu is suggested in Table 28–2.

As his nutrition improves, it is gratifying to see that the patient will relish a general diet, increased in protein, carbohydrate and calories as outlined on page, 392.

Complications

Ascites; Sodium Restriction. Patients with hepatic cirrhosis often have some degree of ascites. When it is severe, it may be necessary to limit the dietary sodium intake, usually to 500 mg. per day. All food must be cooked without salt, and all foods containing added salt or other sodium compounds must be omitted, as outlined in Chapter 24. The substitution of low-sodium milk for regular milk in the 500-Milligram Sodium-Restricted Pattern Dietary in Chapter 24 will reduce the sodium content to 250 mg. or less. The remaining sodium may then be "spent" on increased quantities of low-sodium milk, and on meat and eggs to maintain the increased protein intake needed by the patient with cirrhosis. The use of Protinal,* a low-sodium protein supplement, will aid in keeping the protein content of the diet high when the patient's appetite is poor. See Chapters 36 and 39 for use of Protinal and for low-sodium recipes.

Salt substitutes containing ammonia should never be used because of the danger of precipitating liver failure or hepatic coma. See later in this chapter.

Esophageal Varices; Tube Feeding. Esophageal varices may occur in the patient with advanced cirrhosis, as explained earlier in the chapter. It may be necessary to avoid roughage in the diet to prevent injury and bleeding. Foods to be omitted are raw vegetables and fruits, except bananas, and whole-grain breads and cereals.

If the varices hemorrhage due to increased portal pressure, a tube, surrounded by a balloon, may be inserted into the esophagus, and the balloon inflated to apply pressure to the bleeding area. The remainder of the tube is passed into the stomach, and the patient must now be tube-fed. It has been found that a tube feeding consisting of a mixture of ordinary foods as eaten daily is not as likely to cause diarrhea or other discomfort. Therefore the foods meeting the physician's diet order may be mixed in a blender, substituting infant meat, vegetables and fruits for those regularly eaten. A sufficient amount of water should be added to make the tube feeding fluid, and it should be strained so that no particles remain to obstruct the tube. It may be fed at 2-hour intervals or 6 times a day. Each feeding should be warmed over hot water before serving. See Chapter 29 for further discussion of Tube Feedings.

Liver Failure; Protein Restriction. The increased protein diet may be contraindicated for the patient with only a limited amount of functioning liver tissue. Moreover, in liver disease of long standing accompanied by portal hypertension, collateral blood vessels from the intestinal tract will develop directly to the general circulation, bypassing the liver. If there has been severe hemorrhage from esophageal varices, the surgeon may connect the portal vein to the vena cava to relieve the pressure on the veins in the stomach and the esophagus. In either case, materials absorbed from the intestinal tract now enter the general circulation before reaching the liver.

Intestinal bacterial action on blood from hemorrhage and on protein of the diet results in the formation of ammonia. Normally, this is quickly converted to urea by the liver. However, if a portacaval shunt or collateral circulation is present, the ammonia first enters the general circulation. Since ammonia is extremely toxic to the nervous system, it will produce serious neurologic symptoms beginning with drowsiness and lethargy and ending in coma. Other symptoms are "liver breath," a flapping tremor of the hands when the arms are extended and, sometimes, disorientation.

---

* National Drug Co.

In order to prevent the development of liver failure and of hepatic coma, the physician may drastically reduce the protein content of the diet, to 60 or even 40 Gm. per day.

If hepatic coma occurs, protein should be omitted completely from the diet. In the recovery period, dietary protein is restored gradually, beginning with 20 to 30 Gm. per day.[7] The diet should be as high in calories as possible to spare the protein for tissue repair and maintenance. As recovery proceeds, the protein of the diet is raised by 20 Gm. amounts to as high a protein diet as the patient can tolerate without again showing signs of hepatic failure. Most patients who have this degree of liver damage will not be able to take more than 60 to 70 Gm. of protein per day.

The 40-Gram Protein-Restricted Diet in Chapter 25 may be found of help in constructing diets limited in protein content. The diet should be as high as possible in calories to spare the protein for tissue repair and maintenance.

DISEASE OF THE GALLBLADDER

Disease of the gallbladder may be due either to infection or to the presence of gallstones. In either case, there is a great deal of pain when fat is ingested.

When fat arrives in the duodenum in the course of digestion it stimulates the production of a hormone—cholecystokinin —in certain cells lining the duodenum. The hormone is carried by the blood stream to the gallbladder and its ducts, causing them to contract and force the bile into the cystic duct and the common duct into the intestine. (See Fig. 28–1 and Chapter 9.)

Dietary Treatment

It can be seen readily that a meal containing much fatty food may bring on an acute attack of gallbladder pain and distress in individuals suffering from inflammation of this organ, from the presence of gallstones, or both. Therefore, the diet should be low in fat. Since homogenized fats are better tolerated than visible fats, it is better to omit the latter.

---

[7] Harper, H. A.: J. Am. Dietet. A., 38:350, 1961.

TABLE 28–3. Restrictions and Omissions on a Low Fat Diet

Foods Limited:

Milk to 1 pint daily
Eggs to 1 daily
Butter or margarine to ½ tablespoon daily
Lean meat, fish or fowl to 1 serving daily
  (If skim milk is used, meat may be increased to 2 servings without altering the fat limitation.)

Foods Omitted:

Cream; cheese other than pot or cottage cheese
All fried foods
Salad oils
All meat high in fat, such as pork, bacon, ham, goose, duck, fatty fish
Pastry
Nuts, olives, avocados

Foods such as milk, eggs and butter should be allowed in limited quantities in order to meet the requirements of the adequate diet. (See Table 28–3.)

The milk and the egg may be used as such in the diet, or they may be incorporated in cooked foods such as plain cake or custard.

Other Considerations. Patients with gallbladder disease often show a tendency to constipation. The use of a diet plentiful in fruit and nondistending vegetables (see Chap. 26) and with added stewed fruit and stewed fruit juices should correct this condition. In many cases these patients are obese. If there is overweight, the low-fat diet should limit the caloric intake somewhat, but sugar, desserts, candy and other foods high in carbohydrate may also have to be limited if weight loss is to be achieved (see Chap. 21). The diet following surgery of the gallbladder is discussed in Chapter 29.

PANCREATITIS

The etiology of pancreatitis, or inflammation of the pancreas, is little understood. Most investigators agree that there is obstruction of the pancreatic duct, possibly due to calculi, to spasm of the sphincter of Oddi, the opening of the common duct into the duodenum, or to inflammation accompanying infection.[8] The reflux of bile

---

[8] Knight, W. A.: Am. J. Digest. Dis., 9:832, 1964; Nardi, G. L.: New Eng. J. Med., 268:1065, 1963.

TABLE 28–4. Very Low Fat, Bland Diet in 6 Meals*

Breakfast	Lunch	Dinner
Stewed prunes	Cottage cheese	Sliced chicken
Cream of Wheat	Toast, slightly buttered, 2 slices	Baked potato
Milk, whole, ½ cup	Jelly or honey	Soft-cooked string beans
Postum	Applesauce	Canned apricots
Sugar	Tea, sugar	Tea, sugar
10 A.M.	**3 P.M.**	**8 P.M.**
Toast, slightly buttered, 2 slices	Junket made with skim milk	Crackers
Jelly or honey	Crackers	Jelly or honey
Skim milk, 1 glass	Jelly or honey	Skim milk, 1 glass

* This diet will contain approximately 70 Gm. of protein, 25 Gm. of fat, 325 Gm. of carbohydrate and 1,750 calories.

into the pancreatic duct causes irritation, and the action of the proteolytic enzymes on pancreatic tissue may be responsible for the necrosis and hemorrhage that may exist. Chronic alcoholism may be a contributing factor in the development of pancreatitis.

The symptoms are pain, severe and constant; nausea and vomiting; and weight loss. There may be diarrhea and steatorrhea. As the disease progresses, diabetes mellitus may develop.

Dietary Treatment

The pancreas is stimulated to produce pancreatic juice by the presence of food and hydrochloric acid in the duodenum. Likewise, fat in the duodenum stimulates the flow of bile. Therefore, the dietary treatment of pancreatitis consists of foods which will not call either of these mechanisms into action.

In severe, acute pancreatitis, the patient is fed nothing by mouth, and intravenous feedings of fluids, electrolytes and glucose must be given. During recovery, and in milder attacks, frequent small meals consisting of easily digested carbohydrate and protein should be given. The use of skim milk may help to neutralize hydrochloric acid and prevent stimulation of the pancreas. Fat should be limited to 25 Gm. or less per day. See Table 28–4 for sample menu.

During remissions of the disease the patient should be maintained on a bland low-fat diet. The Bland Diet in Chapter 26 may be made low in fat by substituting skim milk for whole milk; limiting butter

or margarine to 1 tablespoonful per day and eggs to 1 a day; using only lean meats, fish and fowl; and omitting cream, creamed soups and sauces, and all cheese except cottage cheese.

The substitution of medium-chain triglycerides (MCT, see Chap. 27) for regular fat in the diet has been reported as well tolerated by the patient with pancreatitis.[9]

Alcohol is absolutely prohibited, as it irritates the duodenum and may precipitate an attack.

The problem of keeping the patient with pancreatitis in a good nutritional state is a difficult one. The diet tends to be low in calories due to the fat restriction, and the patient's food intake is poor because of constant pain. Every effort should be made to give the patient the foods that he can tolerate, and in such quantity that his nutritional needs continue to be met.

STUDY QUESTIONS AND ACTIVITIES

1. How does the liver function in the metabolism of foods? As an organ for storage? In detoxification?

2. How does bile function in digestion and absorption? Under what circumstances may a patient have clay-colored stools accompanied by jaundice?

3. Why is a diet increased in protein usually ordered for a patient with infectious hepatitis? What feeding problems may be encountered in the early stages of the disease?

---

[9] Holt, P. R., *et al.*: Am. J. Gastroent., *43*:549, 1965.

4. Why may alcoholic cirrhosis be considered a nutritional deficiency disease? Name some deficiency symptoms that may be manifested.

5. A patient is diagnosed as having cirrhosis of the liver with ascites. The doctor orders a diet increased in protein and carbohydrate and moderate in fat content. Explain why such a diet has been ordered.

6. The patient weighs 65 Kg. and has moderately good liver function. How much protein should the diet contain? Using the Pattern Dietary in Chapter 19, how would you add sufficient protein to bring the diet up to the required amount?

7. Will patients with cirrhosis readily eat this much food? If not, how can the diet be adjusted to encourage him to eat as much as possible?

8. The patient has a moderate degree of ascites, and the doctor has ordered sodium restriction to 500 mg. How can you change his diet to meet this order? Use Chapter 24 to arrive at your answer.

9. Why may the diet of the patient with esophageal varices be low in residue? What foods should be omitted from his diet? Under what circumstances must he be tube-fed? How may such a tube feeding be prepared?

10. Why may a diet increased in protein be a source of danger to the patient with severe liver disease?

11. How may hepatic coma develop? Why is a diet severely restricted in protein essential?

12. Make a diet plan for a day containing 30 Gm. of protein and 2,000 calories. Use Chapter 25 and Table 1, Part Four.

13. Why does a patient with gallbladder disease have pain on the ingestion of fat?

14. Which foods should be avoided, which limited on a low-fat diet?

15. Write a low-fat general diet for a patient with gallbladder disease who is 20 pounds overweight. Use Chapter 21.

16. Why may a low-fat, bland diet be ordered for a patient with pancreatitis? Which foods must be omitted? Which severely restricted?

SUPPLEMENTARY READING IN LIVER DISEASES; PANCREATITIS

Crews, R. H., and Faloon, W. W.: The fallacy of a low fat diet in liver disease, J.A.M.A., *181*:754, 1962.

Davidson, C. S.: Is life worth living: It depends upon the liver. New Eng. J. Med., *274*:894, 1966.

Harper, H. A.: Protein intake in liver disease. J. Am. Dietet. A., *38*:350, 1961.

Jones, D. P., and Davidson, C. S.: Current concepts in therapy: The treatment of hepatic coma. New Eng. J. Med., *267*:196, 1962.

Leevy, C. M., *et al.*: Protein tolerance in liver disease. Am. J. Clin. Nutr., *10*:46, 1962.

Nardi, G. L.: Current concepts in therapy: Pancreatitis. New Eng. J. Med., *268*:1065, 1963.

For further references see Bibliography in Part Four.

CHAPTER 29

Surgical Nutrition; Burns

Preoperative Nutrition • Postoperative Nutrition • Surgery of the Stomach and Duodenum • The Dumping Syndrome • Gastrostomy and Jejunostomy • Surgery of the Lower Intestinal Tract • Cholecystectomy • Tonsillectomy • Radical Surgery of the Mouth and Throat • Tube Feeding • Nutrition Following Burns

PREOPERATIVE NUTRITION

A state of good nutrition is an important asset for the patient who is to undergo surgery. The trauma of the surgery and the effect of a decreased food intake before and following operation will be less acute and convalescence will proceed more quickly than in the undernourished individual.

Many patients come to surgery, however, in a depleted nutritional state. This may be caused by the disease that brings the patient to surgery, by pain and anorexia, by nausea and vomiting and by occult or overt bleeding. The elderly patient particularly, who may have put off surgery for a long time, whose income is insufficient for an adequate diet or whose food habits are poor, may be especially in need of good nutritional care preoperatively.

The needs of each patient will be determined by physical examination, laboratory findings and a dietary history. If he is found to be in poor nutritional state, surgery may be postponed, and measures to improve his nutrition instituted. A diet increased in protein and other protective foods, vitamin supplements if they are indicated, and sometimes blood transfusions are given to improve the patient's ability to withstand and recover from the trauma of

surgery. Adequate stores of protein, glycogen, vitamin K and ascorbic acid are particularly important. For patients unable to take food by mouth, intravenous feedings of electrolytes, glucose, amino acids and vitamins may be given.

The overnourished or obese individual is also a surgical risk. If time permits, he should have a diet restricted in calories but adequate in all other nutrients for several weeks before surgery. (See Chap. 21.)

All food is withheld immediately before an operation as undigested food in the gastrointestinal tract may cause vomiting with the possibility of aspiration of food into the bronchi during recovery from anesthesia; or it may give rise to distention postoperatively. The length of time for the withholding of food depends on the type of operation. Usually, no food or fluid is allowed after midnight of the day before operation.

In preparation for minor surgery no food is allowed on the day of the operation unless the operation is delayed until the afternoon, in which case a light breakfast of cereal, toast, coffee or tea, and fruit juice may be given.

For operations on the gastrointestinal tract, a clear or full fluid diet may be ordered for 2 or 3 days preceding the operation in order to have the tract as clear of partially digested food as possible.

POSTOPERATIVE NUTRITION

During surgery blood, fluids and electrolytes are lost from the body, especially if the operation is a major one. Anesthesia decreases peristaltic action. Therefore food and fluids are not given by mouth postoperatively until peristalsis returns. Vomiting and drainage, and loss of gastrointestinal fluids, if suction by nasogastric tube is used, further deplete the body of some of its essential components. Nausea, pain and the after-effects of anesthesia make it difficult at first for the patient to replenish these losses by mouth. Meanwhile the caloric needs of the body must be met, and this will be done by the breakdown of body stores and tissues.

Intravenous Feeding. After surgery the restoration and maintenance of fluid and electrolyte balance is of first importance. To prevent dehydration and shock, and to provide a minimum of calories, intravenous fluids consisting of physiologic saline combined with 5 per cent glucose are usually started immediately following operation. Water-soluble vitamins, particularly ascorbic acid and thiamine, may be added to aid in wound healing and in metabolism. Other minerals besides sodium chloride may be given if the serum electrolyte determinations show imbalance in these.

Of equal importance may be the need for protein, since it is essential for the healing of wounds. Blood transfusions to supply serum proteins as well as to counteract blood loss are a routine procedure immediately after major operations. Protein hydrolysates may be given intravenously, especially in situations in which the patient was in a poor nutritional state preceding operation or the amount of food taken by mouth following operation is limited.

In patients in whom recovery from surgery is slowed for some reason, the problem of maintaining nutrition may become acute. Holden[1] has shown that both weight and tissue nitrogen losses occur very rapidly when postsurgical patients do not have a sufficient caloric intake.

A glucose-fat emulsion which can be given by vein, Lipomul,[*] which contains 1,600 calories per liter, is effective in providing calories for patients with extensive gastrointestinal or other surgery, or those who are seriously ill or emaciated. However, it must be used with caution, as it may be responsible for latent and undesirable effects in the occasional patient. This is true particularly if a fat emulsion is administered for a considerable time.[2]

Surgeons are increasingly aware of the nitrogen losses from the breakdown of body protein in the immediate postoperative period. In uncomplicated surgery adequate nutritional maintenance by intravenous fluids can minimize or even eliminate this nitrogen deficit. One liter of protein hydrolysate in 10 per cent glucose yields 550 calories. Two liters will provide 75 gm. of protein and 1,100 calories, which may be close to the patient's needs the first day or two postoperatively. More than this cannot be tolerated because of the danger of fluid overloading.

There is a much more severe nitrogen deficit in extensive surgical procedures which are followed by some days of limited nutritional intake. Levey reports on a study of a series of patients undergoing subtotal gastric resection as follows[3]: For the day of operation and 4 days postoperatively, patients receiving only intravenous electrolytes and glucose, totaling 900 calories per 70-Kg. man, had an average daily nitrogen deficit of 11.6 Gm. (equivalent to 72 Gm. of protein) and averaged a weight loss of 7 to 9 pounds in the 5-day period. When protein hydrolysate was added in a second series of patients, the daily nitrogen deficit dropped to 7.6 Gm. (47 Gm. of protein) per day. With the further addition of an intravenous fat emulsion, in a third series, raising the caloric intake to 2,450 calories per 70-Kg. man, the nitrogen deficit averaged 1.5 Gm. (9 Gm. of protein) daily, and the average weight loss was 1 pound during the 5-day period.

[1] Holden, W. D., *et al.*: Ann. Surg., *146*:563, 1957.

[*] The Upjohn Co.
[2] Jones, R. J.: Nutr. Rev., *24*:225, 1966.
[3] Levey, S.: Nutr. Rev., *24*:193, 1966.

TABLE 29–1. Suggested Dietary Regimen Following Operation on the
Stomach or the Duodenum

Day After Operation	Food Allowed
1 and 2	Nothing by mouth
3	30 ml. water every hour while awake
4	60 ml. water alternating with 60 ml. milk every hour while awake
5	90 ml. milk every hour while awake plus Cream of Wheat at breakfast Soft-cooked or poached egg at supper
6	120 ml. milk every hour while awake plus Cream of Wheat at breakfast Cream soup made of puréed bland vegetables such as peas, carrots, spinach or asparagus at lunch Custard with the 3 P.M. feeding Milk toast, made of white bread and warm milk, at supper
7	120 ml. milk every hour while awake, all feedings as under Day 6, plus junket with the 10 A.M. feeding and cottage or cream cheese added at 9 P.M.
8	Six-feeding convalescent ulcer diet, increasing the size of servings and the variety of the foods in the diet as tolerated. See pages 364-365 for Foods Allowed and Foods To Be Avoided. The physican may limit the quantity of food to 200 to 250 Gm. at each meal until the 9th or 10th day.

Sample Diet: Day 8 to 10

Breakfast	Lunch	Supper
Diluted orange juice	Cream of spinach soup	Poached egg on toast
Soft-cooked egg	Sliced chicken	Milk, ½ glass
White-bread toast	White-bread toast	Canned peaches
Butter	Butter	
Sanka, cream	Milk, ½ glass	
10 A.M.	**3 P.M.**	**10 P.M.**
Cream of Wheat	Baked custard	Milk, 1 glass
Sugar	Milk, 1 glass	Lemon gelatin
Milk, 1 glass		Sponge cake

Food by Mouth. Except in operations on the gastrointestinal tract, the first thing given by mouth is water in sips as soon as the nausea stops. If preferred, bits of ice may be held in the mouth; this supplies small amounts of water. If sips of water do not cause vomiting, other clear liquids, such as tea with sugar, ginger ale or broth, are added next.

From this stage the patient will progress to a full-liquid, a soft and, finally, a general house diet. (See Chap. 19.) With intravenous feeding and early ambulation there is usually quick recovery from the postoperative state and, therefore, a rapid increase in the diet. It is not uncommon for a patient to be on a general diet by the second postoperative day. The great advantage of this rapid progression in dietary intake is that there is little loss in the nutritional state of the patient and, therefore, speedy recovery.

DIETS FOLLOWING SPECIFIC SURGICAL PROCEDURES

Surgeons often have their own preferred dietary routines which they wish to have followed. It will be found that these usually incorporate the principles included in the dietary regimens described in the following pages, differing only in detail.

Surgery of the Stomach and the Duodenum

There are a number of surgical procedures which may involve the stomach and the duodenum. The most extensive of these is resection of a part or of all of the stomach as well as a section of the duodenum, either for cancer or for peptic ulcer.

Dietary Regimen

Whatever the operation, the usual procedure is to give nothing by mouth for from 24 to 48 hours afterwards and to provide for the body's nutritional needs by intravenous fluids. After this, water in small amounts is given by mouth from 2 to 4 oz. an hour, as tolerated. The patient may then go on such a regimen as outlined in Table 29–1, incorporating the principles of bland, small frequent feedings and omitting stimulating or mechanically irritating foods.

This routine, while necessary because of the site of the operation, calls for a period of 1 or 2 weeks when food intake is most inadequate. Intravenous feeding will aid in meeting nutritional needs to some extent, but it is important that the patient's food intake be increased as rapidly as possible, so that health and strength may be regained. If the patient's condition warrants it, the regimen outlined in Table 29–1 should be speeded up so that he returns more quickly to an adequate diet.

Precautions. A patient who has had extensive surgery of the stomach may be afraid to eat a sufficient quantity or variety of food. Preoperatively he may have been on a very restricted diet, and the tendency is to continue with this. He may develop mild symptoms of the dumping syndrome (see later in this chapter), which further discourages him from eating enough to meet his nutritional needs. Consequently, many patients fail to gain weight and strength following partial or total gastrectomy unless they are carefully watched and instructed.

Lieber[4] suggests that the gastrectomy patient be limited to the foods outlined in Table 29–1, but that he progress somewhat more rapidly so that by the 6th postoperative day he is on a convalescent ulcer diet. He advises, however, that sugar and all foods containing sugar be omitted for at least 2 months to prevent development of the dumping syndrome.

If the gastrectomy patient fails to gain weight following operation, he should be placed on the same diet as that described under the dumping syndrome, whether the symptoms are present or not.

The Dumping Syndrome

Most patients undergoing gastric surgery develop a new pouch by stretching the remaining stomach tissue. This now acts as a storage reservoir for ingested foods exactly as the original stomach once did. However, a complication is seen to a greater or a lesser degree in a number of patients which has been termed the dumping syndrome.

If the syndrome is severe, the ingested food is not held in the remaining stomach pouch but is "dumped" in its entirety into the jejunum 15 to 30 minutes after eating. Because it is concentrated in comparison with body fluids, water is withdrawn from the circulatory system into the intestines, giving rise to a sense of fullness and distention. The withdrawal of fluid from the blood may lower total blood volume sufficiently to cause lowered blood pressure and symptoms of cardiac insufficiency, characterized by sweating, faintness and nausea.

About 2 hours after a meal, a further effect may appear. Because the quantity of food which has been "dumped" into the jejunum is large, digestion and absorption, especially of carbohydrate, is very rapid. This leads to an overproduction of insulin and to an eventual drop of the blood sugar level below normal fasting levels. The symptoms of mild insulin shock result. Giv-

---

[4] Lieber, H.: J.A.M.A., *176*:208, 1961.

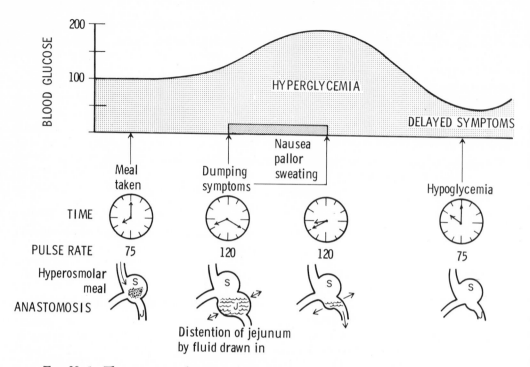

Fig. 29–1. The sequence of events in the dumping syndrome. S—stomach; J—jejunum. (Your Patient, Vol. 3, No. 1, Wyeth Laboratories)

ing carbohydrate in this instance only aggravates the symptoms. See Figure 29–1 for a graphic representation of the sequence of events.

Patients suffering from this syndrome tend to eat less and less, since their discomfort is associated with the ingestion of food. Moreover, the unusual activity of the digestive tract may cause diarrhea and loss of food, further increasing the tendency toward malnutrition and weight loss.

Dietary Treatment

The control of these manifestations by dietary measures is not an easy matter. Some patients may require hospitalization until the exact dietary regimen suited to their needs can be determined; others may recover by strict adherence to a dietary routine at home. An occasional patient may not find relief from the dumping syndrome or achieve favorable weight gain, regardless of the diet prescribed, until his emotional environment becomes more stable.

All investigators agree that the diet should be high in protein (115 to 150 Gm.), high in fat (170 to 225 Gm.) and low in carbo-

hydrate (100 to 125 Gm.). The protein is needed to prevent further wasting and to promote rebuilding of tissue. The fat content is high to provide adequate calories, since the carbohydrate must be consistently low in order to prevent the hypoglycemia (low blood sugar) referred to earlier. No sugar, jellies, jams, or desserts, fruits and beverages sweetened with sugar should be included, since these digest rapidly, are rapidly absorbed and will raise the blood sugar above normal levels.

Such a diet should be given in at least six or possibly eight small, regular, dry meals. No liquids should be taken until 30 to 40 minutes after meals; or they may be taken an hour before meals. Relaxation and rest before and after meals and unhurried eating are most essential to the success of the diet.

Eggs, meat, liver, fish, poultry and cheese are well tolerated, but whole milk sometimes causes difficulty. This may be due to the lactose content of milk, either as a rapidly absorbed carbohydrate or to a deficiency of the mucosal enzyme lactase (see Chap. 27). If there is intolerance to

TABLE 29–2. High Protein, High Fat, Low Carbohydrate "Antidumping" Diet*

General Directions:

1. This diet should be divided into 6 to 8 meals a day.
2. Omit fluids with meals, especially at breakfast. They may be taken half an hour following meals.
3. No food, especially fluids, should be eaten chilled or very cold.

Foods To Be Included and To Be Avoided:

Milk.....................1½ pints whole milk, buttermilk or yoghurt if tolerated.† Should not be taken too cold.

Cream....................¼ pint heavy cream or ½ pint light or sour cream

Cheese...................1 oz. or more. All cheeses are allowed, but cream cheese is preferred.

Fats.....................5 tablespoons butter, margarine, oils, fats, mayonnaise, French dressing

Eggs.....................3 eggs, in any form desired

Meat, fish, fowl.............8 ozs. or 2 large servings. (Do not include bread crumbs or stuffing, or thickened gravies.)

Soups....................None with meals. Broth, bouillon or unthickened soups may be taken between meals.

Vegetables...............2 servings, including 1 green or deep yellow. If tolerated, 1 vegetable may be served raw as a salad, with mayonnaise added. Omit sweet potatoes, corn and lima beans. White potatoes are allowed only as a substitute for bread.

Fruits...................2 servings, including 4 ozs. citrus juice or fruit. Use fresh, cooked or canned unsweetened fruits or fruit juices. Prune juice and banana only if substituted for bread.

Bread, cereals, macaroni
    products...............4 slices of bread or equivalent.
        Equivalents for 1 slice of bread
        Crackers, graham.................2 medium
        Crackers, saltine..................3 2½-inch square
        Matzoth........................⅔ 9-inch square
        Ry-Krisp.......................3 oblong
        Cereal, prepared.................½ c.
        Cereal, cooked...................2 rounded tablespoons
        Rice, macaroni, noodles, spaghetti....⅓ c. cooked
        Banana........................½ medium
        Prune juice.....................4-oz. glass
        Potato, white...................½ medium

Desserts.................Junket, custard and gelatin made without sugar. (Substitute saccharin or Sucaryl. See Chap. 37 for recipes.) Unsweetened fruit as allowed

Beverages................Milk,† tea and coffee

Miscellaneous.............Unsalted nuts, if tolerated. Moderate amounts of salt, spices, ketchup, Saccharin and Sucaryl for sweetening

Foods To Be Omitted:

Sugar, jellies, jams, honey, syrups, molasses, candies; alcoholic and carbonated beverages; cakes, cookies, hot breads, pastries, puddings; frozen fruits; figs, dates; thickened gravies and cream sauces; cornstarch, tapioca, potato flour and barley

    This diet will contain approximately 120 Gm. protein, 200 Gm. fat, 125 Gm. carbohydrate and 2,800 calories.

---

* Adapted from the Antidumping Diet of the Surgical Research Clinic at The New York Hospital.

† If milk is not well tolerated, Liprotein (Upjohn) may be substituted with the permission of the physician.

whole milk, dry skim milk, buttermilk or yoghurt may be ingested without difficulty. If milk and/or milk products give rise to symptoms associated with dumping, the physician may substitute Liprotein,* a commercial food concentrate high in protein and fat and low in carbohydrate.

Butter, cream and salad dressings provide fat along with that found in protein foods. Unsalted nuts are sometimes well tolerated. Vegetables (except gaseous ones), fresh and unsweetened canned fruit, a limited amount of potato, bread and crackers, and occasional cereal make up the carbohydrate allowance. Sugar should not be used in any form. Sucaryl and saccharin may be used for sweetening. (See Foods To Be Included and To Be Avoided, Table 29–2.) Since individual variation in food tolerance is marked in the patient with the dumping syndrome, he should be frequently consulted and the diet adjusted to his progress and preferences. Recovery is often slow, and the nurse and dietitian must exercise skill and patience in helping these patients return to a good nutritional state.

Other Complications

Vitamin B$_{12}$ Deficiency. If a large part or all of the stomach has been resected, pernicious anemia may make its appearance 3 to 5 years following the surgery, when liver stores of vitamin B$_{12}$ are exhausted. The intrinsic factor produced by the normal stomach and essential for the absorption of vitamin B$_{12}$ may be entirely absent. Fortunately, adequate parenteral therapy with vitamin B$_{12}$ is a simple matter if the physician is aware of this possible complication.

Obstruction of the Small Bowel. In gastrectomized patients, obstruction of the small bowel by potato skins, orange pulp, sauerkraut and other plant foods with high cellulose content has been reported.[5] This is thought to be due to the poor condition or complete absence of teeth, with resultant inadequate chewing and maceration, as well as to rapid progress of food into the small bowel. Patients with gastrectomies should be sure to have proper dentures, to chew their food well and to be cautious about including foods that are high in residue.

Gastrostomy or Jejunostomy

When the surgeon finds inoperable cancer in the esophagus, stomach or duodenum, he may perform a gastrostomy or jejunostomy, depending on the site of the cancer. In this procedure an opening is made in the stomach or jejunum which is then sutured to an opening in the abdominal wall. It is this opening through which the patient now will receive most and, eventually, all of his food, and which makes it possible to maintain his nutrition for much of the remainder of his life.

As soon as possible postoperatively 60 to 90 ml. of water alternating with the same quantity of milk are given every hour via the new opening. This is increased gradually over a period of 3 to 4 days until a blenderized tube feeding is tolerated. (See later in this chapter for tube feedings.) This should be given in 300 to 400 ml. quantities in each of 6 feedings.[6] Although such a tube feeding is well tolerated by the patient with a gastrostomy, Machella[7] warns that, for a jejunostomy, the feeding must be diluted so as to be iso-osmolic to the blood and it must be given slowly, or there may be symptoms of the dumping syndrome. It should not contain sugar for the same reason. (See earlier in this chapter.)

The tube feeding should be warmed to room temperature and served in a teapot or other usual eating utensil placed on a tray covered with a tray cloth, so that the feeding may seem as normal as possible. Both the patient and a member of his family should be taught how to give the tube feeding, in order that there be someone trained to take over the responsibility when the patient becomes too ill to care for himself.

---

* The Upjohn Co.

[5] Wilde, W. L.: Am. J. Surg., *109*:649, 1965; Schlang, H. A., and McHenry, L. E.: Ann. Surg., *159*:611, 1964.

[6] Kurihara, M.: Am. J. Nursing, *60*:852, 1960.

[7] Machella, T. E., and Ravdin, R. G.: Am. J. Clin. Nutr., 3:481, 1955.

The patient may enjoy chewing and savoring foods, even if he cannot swallow them. He should be encouraged to take fluids such as water, milk, melted ice cream and eggnogs by mouth for as long as possible, although eventually obstruction will be complete.

Ileostomy

An ileostomy may be performed in the patient with ileitis when there is danger of obstruction (see Chap. 27) or in severe colitis which has not responded to medical treatment. Part or all of the colon and the diseased part of the ileum are resected, and the proximal end of the ileum is brought out on the abdominal wall to form a new pathway through which the feces are discharged.

The immediate postoperative diet consists largely of fluids until the ileostomy bud is healed and is well established. After this, a low-residue diet (see Chap. 27) is usually given. Protein and calories should be as high as the patient can tolerate to compensate for the malnutrition and the weight loss common to these patients. Raw fruits except bananas, all vegetables except those of low fiber content, and whole grain breads and cereals, as well as highly seasoned foods, should be omitted at first. However, the patient should be encouraged to try new foods, one at a time and in small quantity, to see if they are tolerated. Vitamin supplements and iron medication may be needed to ensure adequate nutrition.

If a large section of the ileum has been removed, there will be a correspondingly smaller area for absorption. Moreover, certain nutrients such as vitamin B_{12} and, possibly, a considerable amount of fat are absorbed only in the ileum.[8] Fat may have to be somewhat restricted and vitamin B_{12} may have to be given parenterally if only a short section of ileum remains.

The ileostomy patient faces a number of problems after operation. Since water is normally absorbed in the colon, the ileostomy discharge is fluid and continuous, so that an ileostomy bag must be worn day and night. Moreover, there is constant danger of skin irritation and breakdown due to the digestive enzymes contained in the discharge. Patients with ileostomies are usually young, with most of life ahead of them. They need a great deal of emotional support from those who are involved in helping them to return to a normal existence. Initial care and teaching will be done by the medical team, but the patient may find continued help from ileostomy clubs, composed of people with either ileostomies or colostomies, with chapters in many areas of the country.[9]

Colostomy

When cancer of the large bowel or intractable colitis necessitates the removal of a section of the colon or the rectum, the proximal part of the colon is brought out on the abdominal wall. This colostomy bud now becomes the permanent opening through which the feces are discharged. For a day or two postoperatively the patient is given nothing by mouth, after which a clear fluid diet is given until healing of the colostomy bud is well established. The patient then progresses to a full liquid diet (see Chap. 19) and then to a moderately low residue diet. (See Chap. 27.)

Most patients with colostomies are able before long to return to their regular food habits, provided that these are adequate for their nutritional needs. They should omit foods which caused discomfort before they were ill, among which may be some of the gas-forming vegetables, but no food is contraindicated once the patient has recovered from the operation.

Because a section of the colon remains for water absorption, most colostomy patients are able to establish bowel regularity early in their hospitalization. Dericks[10] notes that there seemed to be a direct relationship between the taking of a normal

---

[8] Cornell, G. N., *et al.*: Bull. N.Y. Acad. Med. 37:675, 1961.

[9] To ascertain where such groups exist, write to the United Ostomy Association, Inc., 1111 Wilshire Blvd., Los Angeles, Calif. 90017.

[10] Dericks, V. C., and Robeson, K. A.: Pub. Health Nursing, 41:16, 1949.

diet and such regularity. An exception is the patient who has had half or two thirds of the colon removed, leaving only a small area for water absorption. Such a patient may have to follow the dietary regimen outlined under Ileostomy.

Most patients with permanent colostomies are in the later decades of life, with firmly established habits of living and eating. These can be continued with relatively little difficulty when the nurse and the dietitian give adequate counsel about the care of the stoma, regulation of bowel evacuation and adequate diet.

Malabsorption Due to Massive Resection of the Small Intestine

When it is necessary for the surgeon to remove a large section of the small intestine because of necrosis or other life-threatening pathology, absorption of nutrients may be seriously impaired, depending on the amount of absorptive surface left. Steatorrhea, weight loss and vitamin-B_{12} deficiency will occur if most of the ileum has been removed. In patients who have less than 10 to 12 inches of remaining jejunum and ileum combined, there will be loss of all nutrients in the stool, malnutrition and severe weight loss.

Recently Zurier *et al.*[11] and Winawer *et al.*[12] have described the use of medium-chain triglycerides (see Chap. 27) in these patients with good results. This fat is absorbed in the duodenum, and is not dependent on the usual mechanisms for fat absorption. Included as part of a high-carbohydrate, high caloric diet, these investigators report good weight gain and relief of diarrhea.

Rectal Surgery

Following operation for hemorrhoids or other rectal surgery, an opiate may be given to prevent defecation, and a clear fluid diet is ordered for 2 or 3 days for the same reason. A low resdiue diet is given for the next 3 or 4 days (see Chap. 27 for diets

[11] Zurier, R. B., *et al.*: New Eng. J. Med., 274:490, 1966.

[12] Winawer, S. J., *et al.*: New Eng. J. Med., 274: 72, 1966.

varying in residue) after which the patient is ready to go back to a regular diet. However, some physicians place the patient on a regular diet immediately after surgery, particularly if a local anesthetic has been used.

Before discharge, the patient should be instructed in a diet which will enable him to avoid constipation. (See Chap. 27.)

Cholecystectomy

After removal of the gallbladder, it is customary to continue moderate fat restriction for from 3 to 6 months. Cholecystokinin, the hormone produced in the duodenum by the presence of fat, stimulates the contraction not only of the gallbladder but also of the smooth muscle in the common duct and of the ampulla of Vater, the opening of the common duct into the intestinal tract. Since these tissues are irritated and inflamed, there is the possibility of pain from contraction on the ingestion of considerable amounts of fat. The low-fat diet found in Chapter 28 may be modified by an increase in butter or margarine and the inclusion of medium-fat meats and all varieties of cheese. The remainder of the restrictions should be followed until healing is complete.

Tonsillectomy

After a tonsillectomy or other minor mouth or throat operation, cold fluids only are allowed for the first 24 hours to prevent bleeding from the operative area. Sharp fruit juices must not be given, as they will cause pain. Toast or other food which may irritate the operative site must be avoided, as it may cause coughing. Water, milk, vanilla ice cream and bland fruit juices such as pear or white cherry juice are permitted. The adult patient may find iced tea or iced coffee refreshing. On the 2nd day, warm but not hot liquids are added. Soft bland foods such as milk toast, custard, soft-cooked egg, soft-cooked cereals and vegetable purées may be permitted on the 3rd and the 4th days. The patient usually discovers what foods will slip down easily; it may be from several days to a week before a regular diet can be resumed.

Radical Surgery of the Mouth and the Throat

Following radical surgery of the mouth or the throat the patient may have to follow a liquid diet for a long period of time or perhaps permanently. At first this may have to consist of a tube feeding such as those described later in the chapter, administered by nasogastric tube. As the patient recovers, he may again be able to take his food by mouth. Even if the diet must be a liquid one permanently, it is important that a varied and nearly normal menu be offered. This can be done by means of a food blender. With such an appliance meat as well as other foods can be liquefied, so that a diet approaching the usual pattern can be served. Instead of a succession of soups, eggnogs and other liquids, dinner may consist of meat, potatoes, vegetables, fruit and pudding, all liquefied and served in separate dishes. A sectioned plate over a hot water container may be found useful, as will a thermos beverage cup or glass.

Soft and liquid diets may also be prepared by putting the food through a food mill or sieve and adding liquids. If these devices are not available, commercially prepared baby foods can be used, since they contain only a small amount of seasoning. The tray should be served in the usual fashion, so that the patient will have the pleasure of sight and odor of food to stimulate his appetite. The food may have to be taken by a syringe placed in the back of the mouth if swallowing is impaired. Whatever the method, the most important aspects in the care of these patients are that a nutritionally adequate diet be eaten and that every effort be made to make the food appetizing and inviting.

If the patient is unable to take sufficient nourishment in the manner described above, because of fatigue or discouragement, the diet should be supplemented with high-protein, high caloric beverages (see Chap. 36) and, if necessary, minerals and vitamins.

Adrenalectomy and Hypophysectomy

See Chapter 33 under Adrenal Cortex Insufficiency.

TUBE FEEDINGS

Feeding by nasogastric tube or by gastrostomy or jejunostomy is instituted when it is not possible for the patient to take food otherwise. This may occur when there is obstruction of the upper part of the gastrointestinal tract; following operation on the head and neck; or in cerebral hemorrhage or other pathology if the patient is unconscious. The tube feeding must be liquid, yet contain all the nutrients essential for adequate nutrition, especially if it must be used permanently or over a considerable period of time.

If the patient is conscious, and as soon as his condition will allow, a variety of liquid food prepared by blender, as described under Diet after Radical Surgery of the Mouth and Throat, is to be preferred in place of a prepared tube feeding.

In the unconscious patient, it is particularly important for the nurse to realize that good nutrition is essential in the prevention of pressure sores and decubitus ulcers. Immobilization causes an increased breakdown of protein tissue and loss of calcium from the bones. These must be replaced by a more than adequate amount of protein and calcium in the diet (see Chap. 18). Unconscious patients sometimes resist feeding, but that should not deter the nurse from seeing that an adequate intake of food is achieved each day. Since in many cases the unconscious patient is unable to cough or otherwise handle secretions, the nurse must observe him closely for signs of regurgitation during and after each feeding to avoid aspiration into the lungs.

Types of Tube Feedings. There are three general types of tube feedings: those prepared from a variety of common foods, mixed in a blender and strained; those with a milk base to which a few other foods are added; and commercial preparations.

BLENDER FEEDING. The tube feeding outlined in Table 29–3 is made up to contain approximately 1,800 calories or ⅔ calories per ml. It is high in protein (120 Gm.), and is well above the Recommended Dietary Allowances with the exception of thiamine, which is adequate for women but not for men.

TABLE 29–3. Blender Tube Feeding*

| Food | Measure | Weight Gm. | Calories | Protein Gm. | Fat Gm. | Carbohydrate Gm. | Minerals | | Vitamins | | | | |
							Calcium Mg.	Iron Mg.	A I.U.	Thiamine Mg.	Riboflavin Mg.	Niacin Mg.	Ascorbic Acid Mg.
Milk	1½ pints	732	480	26	26	36	864	.3	1,050	.24	1.26	.5	8
Pasteurized powdered eggs†	2 tablespoons	30	163	13	12	1	54	2.3	1,180	.11	.30	.1	..
Cream, light, 20%	½ c.	100	211	3	21	4	102	..	840	.03	.15	.1	1
Farina, enriched, cooked	1 c.	200	86	2	..	18	120	10.0	..	.10	.06	.8	..
Bread, white, enriched	3 slices, no crusts	50	135	4	2	25	42	1.3	..	.13	.11	1.2	..
Meat,‡ strained baby food													
Beef	3½ ozs.	100	99	15	4	..	8	2.0	..	.01	.16	3.5	..
Veal	3½ ozs.	100	91	16	3	..	10	1.7	..	.03	.20	4.3	..
Vegetables‡ strained baby food													
Carrots	3½ ozs.	100	29	1	..	7	23	.5	13,000	.02	.03	.4	3
Peas	3½ ozs.	100	54	4	..	9	11	1.2	500	.08	.09	1.2	10
Protinal§	¼ c.	60	216	37	..	18	..	..	..	..	..	..	..
Apple juice	1¼ c.	300	141	1	..	36	18	1.8	..	.03	.06	.3	3
Orange juice	½ c.	100	45	..	..	11	9	.1	200	.09	.01	.3	45
Water added to 2,500 ml.													
Totals			1,750	122	68	165	1,261	21.2	16,770	.87	2.43	12.7‖	70

* Adapted from the Department of Nutrition, The New York Hospital.
† Pasteurized powdered egg is used to avert the danger of salmonella infection. Fifteen grams is the equivalent of one egg.
‡ It is suggested that meats and vegetables be changed daily. This will alter the food composition somewhat. See Table 1, Part Four.
§ A low-sodium, high-protein product derived from casein (National Drug Company).
‖ The protein in the feeding will supply enough tryptophan to increase the niacin value by about a third.

Directions: Place all ingredients in a mechanical blender and mix for 10 minutes. Strain through a fine sieve, place in bottles with covers, label and refrigerate immediately. Shake before pouring. Tube feeding should be warmed to body temperature over hot water before being served to the patient.

Variations. See text for variations of this tube feeding.

Calories may be added by increasing the cream and the farina, or by the addition of small quantities of sugar and/or salad oil. Either may cause diarrhea if added in too great an amount. If there is considerable increase in calories, the tube feeding should be supplemented with thiamine.

Calories may be decreased by omitting the cream, or using skim instead of whole milk, or both.

The protein content of the feeding may be lowered to approximately 85 Gm. by omitting the Protinal. This will decrease the calories to 1,600, and it may be necessary to add sugar or salad oil to bring the calories to the desired level.

The sodium content of this feeding may be lowered to approximately 300 to 400 mg. by the use of low-sodium milk and unsalted farina, bread, meat and vegetables. Canned strained baby foods cannot be used as they have salt added. Sodium restriction may be ordered by the physician for the patient with cerebral hemorrhage to lower blood volume and control further bleeding.

The advantage of using a mixture of foods as they commonly appear in the diet in a blender-type feeding is that it is usually well tolerated, and does not cause the diarrhea which so often complicates the care of the tube-fed patient. The apple juice is included for this reason, even though it contributes less of the essential nutrients than most fruit juices. Moreover, the use of common foods, even though in a tube feeding, may give the patient a feeling of familiarity, which may be of considerable psychological benefit.

MILK BASE FEEDING. This consists of milk to which eggs, skim milk powder, sugar and sometimes liver are added in amounts sufficient to meet the caloric and other nutritional needs of the patient. It is easier to concentrate than a blender feeding, up to 1 calorie per ml., but it may not be as well tolerated.

COMMERCIAL PREPARATIONS. A variety of commercially prepared tube feedings are available. Most of these more than meet the Recommended Dietary Allowances when used in sufficient quantity. They are easier to prepare, but tend to be somewhat more expensive than the tube feedings given here.

Diarrhea is sometimes a complication of tube feeding. It may be caused by feeding a formula that is too concentrated or one which contains too much sugar or oil; or it may be administered too rapidly, or be too cold. Because tube feedings are usually made up in a full day's quantity, it is important that they be kept refrigerated except when a feeding is measured out. Souring and bacterial contamination may follow if this precaution is not observed. Either may be disastrous for the ill or apprehensive patient.

It is not known whether the use of raw eggs in tube feedings, with the possibility of salmonella infection, is responsible for the frequent occurrence of diarrhea in tube-fed patients (see Chap. 17). It is strongly recommended that pasteurized powdered egg be substituted for raw eggs, one tablespoon (15 Gm.) being equivalent to one egg.

All tube feedings should be given slowly to prevent diarrhea. If diarrhea does occur, the addition of 2 tablespoonfuls of strained apple sauce or ½ oz. of fluid pectin (such as Certo) to 1 quart of feeding may be beneficial.

Nursing Responsibilities. It is usually the responsibility of the nursing service to ensure that the patient receives the total quantity of his tube feeding each day. The blenderized tube feeding described above, which contains 2,500 ml. of fluid, might be given in six 400-ml. feedings throughout the day and evening. The feeding should be warmed and served on a tray, as described earlier in the chapter under Gastrostomy and Jejunostomy.

Most patients find it difficult to accept tube feeding. Again the nurse plays a decisive role in the adjustment that the patient makes to this procedure. In an excellent article on the subject of tube feeding, Smith[13] says: "The nursing care of the patient with a nasogastric tube in place may be relatively easy and pleasant for both the nurse and the patient, or it may be difficult, untidy and distressing. Whichever it is

---

[13] Smith, A. V.: Am. J. Nursing, 57:1451, 1957.

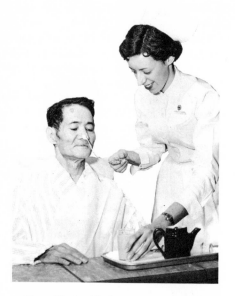

Fig. 29–2. If the patient must be fed by tube, the feeding should be served in an attractive and appetizing manner, so that it reflects that this is food and not a medication. (Paul Parker)

depends in large measure on the nurse's attitudes and her appreciation of the patient's feelings."

NUTRITION FOLLOWING BURNS

Patients with extensive burns present nutritional problems much more far-reaching even than those who have undergone major surgery or sustained severe hemorrhage. There is massive loss of fluids, electrolytes and serum proteins by exudation from the burned areas. There is extensive tissue breakdown, lasting for periods of weeks as evidenced by tremendous losses of nitrogen and potassium in the urine. Soroff[14] reports that in a 25 per cent full thickness burn the nitrogen loss in the first 8 days is equivalent to 190 Gm. of protein a day. Extensive nitrogen losses continue for the first 30 days, then gradually diminish as wound cover is achieved. There is also severe heat loss from the burn area, as shown by the rate of oxygen consumption.

The energy losses may be as crucial to the ultimate survival of the patient as the loss of protein.

The first need is for fluid and electrolyte replacement, followed as quickly as possible by a diet markedly increased in protein and calories, with supplemental vitamins, particularly ascorbic acid to aid in wound healing and the B complex vitamins to meet the tremendously increased metabolic demands.

If flames or fumes have been inhaled, injuring the respiratory and the gastrointestinal tracts, or if there are burns about the mouth and the face, the oral route of feeding may at first be impossible. Tube feeding may be further contraindicated, as badly burned patients frequently have gastrointestinal atony the first few days after injury.

The early part of treatment consists of the intravenous administration of plasma and whole blood, glucose and electrolyte solutions and solutions of protein hydrolysates. Artz[15] warns, however, that fluid replacement must not be excessive, but only sufficient to assure excretion of urine, as burn patients may have temporary oliguria the first 48 hours, and there is danger of tubular kidney damage if there has been hemoglobinuria from red cell breakdown.

No food or fluid is given by mouth except occasional ice chips for the first 24 to 48 hours. Then a hypotonic solution of sodium chloride and sodium bicarbonate may be tried, and if tolerated, the patient will quickly progress from a clear to a full liquid diet.[16] By the 7th postburn day a high-calorie, high-protein diet, supplemented with high-protein, high-calorie beverages, is usually tolerated by the patient. Ascorbic acid, from 1 to 2 Gm., greatly increased amounts of B-complex vitamins and 2 times the requirement of fat-soluble vitamins should be given by medication.[17]

From 2 to 4 Gm. of protein and 50 to 70 calories per Kg. of body weight[18] will

[14] Soroff, H. S., *et al.*: Surg., Gynec. Obstet., *112*: 159, 1961.

[15] Artz, C. P.: Am. J. Surg., *108*:649, 1964.
[16] Larson, D., and Gaston, R.: Am. J. Nursing, 67:319, 1967.
[17] Ibid.
[18] Ibid.

meet the needs of the severely burned patient, but it may not be possible for him to ingest such a large quantity of food, and tube feedings may be necessary for a time. If these are spread evenly over the 24-hour period, the overstimulation of the gastric mucosa and the danger of gastric hemorrhage, both of which may occur in burn patients, will be avoided. See Chapter 28 for high-protein, high-calorie diets, Chapter 36 for high-protein, high-calorie beverages, and earlier in this chapter for tube feeding.

There is a tremendous need for supportive care of the severely burned patient by nurses, doctors, dietitians and all others with whom he comes in contact. The importance of the greatly increased need for food must be carefully explained to the patient. The diet particularly must be individualized to meet his needs and desires, and close cooperation by all who care for him is essential to meet the nutritional and emotional needs of the burned patient.

STUDY QUESTIONS AND ACTIVITIES

1. What are the dangers of a poor nutritional state to the patient who must undergo surgery? What nutritional deficiencies may be found? How may these be corrected?

2. What are some of the possible causes of such a poor nutritional state?

3. Why is it important that food be withheld immediately prior to operation?

4. What nutritional problems occur directly before and after operation? Why may these be serious following major surgery?

5. What nutrient solutions may be given by vein postoperatively? What does each contribute? Which one has to be used with caution?

6. List the foods permitted on a clear fluid diet. Why are fruit juices omitted? What foods are included on a full fluid diet?

7. List the postoperative dietary regimen usually prescribed for a patient who has had gastric surgery. When does it become adequate for the patient's nutritional needs?

8. What is the sequence of events in the dumping syndrome? Why do these occur?

9. What type of diet has been devised to prevent the symptoms of dumping? Which foods must be omitted? Which limited? How should fluids be spaced?

10. What food is sometimes poorly tolerated in the dumping syndrome? Why may this be? What should be substituted?

11. What danger does the patient with poor or no teeth and a gastrectomy face? How should this be corrected and how should the patient be cautioned?

12. Using the antidumping diet in this chapter, make out a menu for a day for a man who is working.

13. What prophylactic measure has been suggested for the dumping syndrome?

14. How should a tube feeding be served to a patient with a gastrostomy or jejunostomy, or with a nasogastric tube?

15. Why may a partient with a jejunostomy suffer from the dumping syndrome? How may this be avoided?

16. How do the effects of a colostomy differ from those of an ileostomy in the type and quantity of food tolerated? In absorptive defects?

17. What are medium-chain triglycerides? Why may they be of value to the patient with massive resection of the small intestine?

18. Why is a low-fat diet prescribed postoperatively for a patient who has had a cholecystectomy? What foods should be omitted? Which limited?

19. Plan a tonsillectomy diet for an adult for the first 2 postoperative days.

20. Plan a menu for a patient with a radical mouth operation who is on a fluid diet, making it as nearly normal as possible.

21. Compare your menu with the Pattern Dietary in Chapter 19. Are all the nutritional needs met? Are there enough calories? If not, what can be added?

22. How may the calories in the tube feeding (Table 29–3) be increased? The sodium content be decreased?

23. What are some possible causes of diarrhea in the tube-fed patient? How may they be prevented?

24. What is the nurse's responsibility to the tube-fed patient? How is this accomplished in your hospital?

25. What are the grave nutritional problems in severe burns? How must they be met?

26. Find 5 different high-protein, high caloric beverages in Chapter 36 that may appeal to a patient with burns.

SUPPLEMENTARY READING IN SURGICAL NUTRITION; BURNS

Dericks, V. C.: Rehabilitation of patients with ileostomy. Am. J. Nursing, *61*:48, 1961.

Fason, M. F.: Controlling bacterial growth in tube feeding. Am. J. Nursing, *67*:1246, 1967.

Fisk, J. E.: Nursing care of the patient with surgery of the biliary tract. Am. J. Nursing, *60*:53, 1960.

Hayden, M. L.: After surgery—rehabilitation for a full life. Nursing Outlook, *7*:21, 1959.

Henderson, L. M.: Nursing care of the patient with facial injuries. Am. J. Nursing, *57*:453, 1957.

Jones, R. J.: Present knowledge of intravenous fat emulsions. Nutr. Rev., *24*:225, 1966.

Katona, E.: Learning colostomy control. Am. J. Nursing, *67*:534, 1967.

Klug, T. J., *et al.:* Gastric resection. Medical and surgical care. Am. J. Nursing, *61*:73, 1961 (Dec.).

Kurihara, M.: The patient with an intestinal prosthesis. Am. J. Nursing, *60*:852, 1960.

Larson, D., and Gaston, R.: Current trends in the care of burned patients. Am. J. Nursing, *67*:319, 1967.

Levey, S.: Reduction of nitrogen deficits in surgical patients maintained by intravenous alimentation. Nutr. Rev., *24*:193, 1966.

Machella, T. E.: Post-surgical problems of the gastrointestinal tract. J.A.M.A., *174*:2111, 1960.

Magruder, L., *et al.:* Gastric resection. Nursing care. Am. J. Nursing, *61*:76, 1961.

Pittman, A. C., and Robinson, F. W.: Dietary management of the dumping syndrome. J. Am. Dietet. A., *40*:108, 1962.

White, D. R.: I have an ileostomy. Am. J. Nursing, *61*:51, 1961.

Zurier, R. B., *et al.:* Use of medium chain triglyceride in management of patients with massive resection of the small intestine. New Eng. J. Med., *274*:490, 1966.

For further references see Bibliography in Part Four.

CHAPTER 30

Allergy; Diseases of the Skin

Allergy • Foods and Allergy • Diagnosis • Treatment • Diseases of the Skin • Vitamin Deficiencies • Fatty Acid Deficiency • Psoriasis • Acne Vulgaris

ALLERGY

Allergy is a condition of hypersensitivity to a substance or substances which do not evoke symptoms in the ordinary individual. There is a significant familial incidence which may aid in diagnosis; and there may be a strong emotional component related to the severity of allergic manifestations.

Causes. Allergic reactions are caused by a wide variety of substances and conditions. These include pollens, dust, cosmetics and animal hair; poisonous plants; serums, vaccines and drugs; physical agents such as heat, cold and sunlight; a variety of foods; and many others. Sensitivity to a given substance may cause a reaction in one individual, and in another person a similar reaction may be caused by an entirely different substance. Or the same substance may cause two widely differing reactions in each of two individuals.

Symptoms of allergy are as varied as the substances causing the reaction. Eczema is most common in infants and young children; rhinitis and asthma occur in both children and adults, and are sometimes preceded by allergic eczema in infancy; urticaria or hives, physical allergies and angioneurotic edema are common in adults. Serum sickness and drug reactions are directly related to the administration of vaccines and drugs, and may occur at any age. The diagnosis of gastrointestinal allergy is both accepted and disputed as a manifestation of allergy.[1] The fact that so many of the allergic attacks are related to the skin and the mucous membranes is explained by the extensive surface exposed to contact with irritating substances or allergens either directly or through the circulating blood.

Foods and Allergy

This chapter is chiefly concerned with food allergies, but it should be borne in mind that any allergy from whatever cause, if severe, may interfere with the nutrition of the individual due to the effect on appetite and thus the general health. This is often the case with a child, whose growth and development may be retarded seriously unless his diet is evaluated carefully and made as attractive and nutritionally adequate as possible.

The protein component of a food is considered to be the causative factor in food allergy, even though foods which cause an allergic reaction may vary widely in protein content. Sensitivity to a food such as honey is explained as due to the associated protein in the pollen grains mixed in the honey, for it has been shown that very minute amounts of a given protein may cause an allergic reaction.

---

[1] Waldmann, R. D., *et al.*: New Eng. J. Med., 276:761, 1967; Editorial: New Eng. J. Med., 276:809, 1967.

TABLE 30–1. Rowe Elimination Diets

(Rowe, A. H.: Elimination Diets and the Patient's Allergies, ed. 2, Philadelphia, Lea & Febiger, 1944)

Diet 1	Diet 2	Diet 3	Diet 4
Rice	Corn	Tapioca	Milk†
Tapioca	Rye	White potato	Tapioca
Rice biscuit	Corn pone	Breads made of any com-	Cane sugar
Rice bread	Corn-rye muffins	bination of soy, lima,	
	Rye bread	potato starch and tapioca	
	Ry-Krisp	flours	
Lettuce	Beets	Tomato	
Chard	Squash	Carrot	
Spinach	Asparagus	Lima beans	
Carrot	Artichoke	String beans	
Sweet potato or yam		Peas	
Lamb	Chicken (no hens)	Beef	
	Bacon	Bacon	
Lemon	Pineapple	Lemon	
Grapefruit	Peach	Grapefruit	
Pears	Apricot	Peach	
	Prune	Apricot	
Cane sugar	Cane or beet sugar	Cane sugar	
Sesame oil	Mazola	Sesame oil	
Olive oil*	Sesame oil	Soybean oil	
Salt	Salt	Gelatin, plain or flavored	
Gelatin, plain or flavored	Gelatin, plain or flavored	with lime or lemon	
with lime or lemon	with pineapple	Salt	
Maple syrup or syrup	Karo corn syrup	Maple syrup or syrup	
made with cane sugar	White vinegar	made with cane sugar	
flavored with maple	Royal baking powder	flavored with maple	
Royal baking powder	Baking soda	Royal baking powder	
Baking soda	Cream of tartar	Baking soda	
Cream of tartar	Vanilla extract	Cream of tartar	
Vanilla extract		Vanilla extract	
Lemon extract		Lemon extract	

* Allergy to it may occur with or without allergy to olive pollen. Mazola may be used if corn allergy is not present.

† Milk should be taken up to 2 or 3 quarts a day. Plain cottage cheese and cream may be used. Tapioca cooked with milk and sugar may be taken.

Among the common allergy-producing foods, particularly in children, are oranges, milk, eggs and sometimes wheat. Other common food allergens are fish and shellfish, chocolate, tomatoes and strawberries. It has been found that members of the same botanic family may have a similar allergic effect. Lemons and grapefruit are likely to cause a reaction if oranges are allergenic. Likewise, if cabbage gives rise to an allergic reaction, so may broccoli, Brussels sprouts and cauliflower.

Other Factors Affecting Allergic Reactions

Whether or not an allergic disturbance follows the eating of a specific food depends in great part upon the individual's physical and often emotional state. This may make the search for the offending food or foods a difficult process. Moreover, there are no specific criteria by which a diagnosis of allergy can be made, and symptoms are sometimes ascribed to allergy when their cause is obscure.

Diagnosis

History. All investigators stress the need for a careful history. This is especially true for the older child and the adult, who eat a variety of foods. In the very young infant ingesting only a limited number of foods, the diagnosis may be more easily

TABLE 30–2. Rowe Elimination Diets
Typical Menus Based on Diets 1 to 3

Diet No. 1

Breakfast	Dinner	Supper
Half grapefruit	Lamb patties	Lamb stew with carrots
Steamed or Puffed Rice with maple syrup or pear juice	Spinach with lemon	Steamed rice
Lamb chop	Sweet potato, baked	Lettuce and grapefruit salad. Dressing of olive oil, lemon juice, salt
Lemonade	Rice bread or biscuit with grapefruit and lemon marmalade	Gelatin made with lemon juice, sugar and pear
	Stewed fresh pear	Grapefruit juice or lemonade
	Pear and grapefruit juice	

Diet No. 2

Breakfast	Dinner	Supper
Stewed prunes or fresh peaches	Roast chicken	Sliced cold chicken
Fried cornmeal mush	Baked squash with bacon	Pickled beets
Bacon	Asparagus vinaigrette, dressed with sesame oil, white vinegar, salt	Ry-Krisp with pineapple jam
Corn and rye muffins	Corn pone with apricot jam	Stewed apricots with sugar
Apricot and pineapple jam	Pineapple, fresh or canned	Pineapple juice
Pineapple juice	Prune juice	

Diet No. 3

Breakfast	Dinner	Supper
Half grapefruit	Roast beef	Bacon
Fried potatoes	Boiled potato with pan gravy	Lima bean casserole with tomatoes, seasoned with bacon fat
Bacon	Glazed carrots, using sugar and sesame oil	Potato flour muffins with apricot jam
Soybean muffins, made without eggs	Lima bean bread with grapefruit marmalade	Peach tapioca
Apricot jam	Sliced peaches	Grapefruit juice
Tomato juice	Lemonade	

established. In all instances a careful history of recent food intake, appearance of symptoms and of other events and conditions relating to the illness is of utmost importance.

Skin Tests. If a careful history does not reveal the cause of the allergic symptoms, the physician may resort to skin tests. Solutions, each containing a small quantity of a common allergen, are applied to a scratched portion of the skin, and then covered with cellophane for 2 to 4 days. Interdermal injections of the suspected allergen may also be used.

In the event that welts, wheals and redness develop from any of these tests, an allergic reaction is indicated. However, it has been observed that many foods may give a positive skin test without causing allergic symptoms.

Elimination Test Diets

Because food allergy is somewhat more difficult to demonstrate by means of skin tests than other forms of allergy, Rowe[2] finds the trial of elimination test diets to be more reliable. As can be seen in Table 30–1, they consist of a series of 3 diets, each containing a cereal or a starch, 1 or 2 meats, a small group of vegetables and

[2] Rowe, A. H.: Elimination Diets and the Patient's Allergies. Ed. 2. Philadelphia, Lea and Febiger, 1944.

fruits, and seasonings and condiments. All the foods included in these diets are known to be unlikely to produce allergic reactions. The fourth diet, consisting only of milk, tapioca and sugar, is used as a last resort.

The patient is placed on one of the test diets for a period of a week. If the symptoms do not abate, he is tried on another one of the diets for the same length of time. If, at the end of the last test diet, relief has not been obtained, it is evident that causes other than food should be sought as allergic agents.

If, on the other hand, the patient is relieved of his symptoms on any one of the elimination test diets, he is kept on this for another week. Other foods, first chosen from the related test diets and then from foods in general, are added one by one, with wheat, eggs and milk last, because these three foods have been found to be the most likely to produce allergy. If the patient shows allergic symptoms after the addition of any one food, that food may be suspected as the cause of the allergic disturbance and must be omitted from the diet.

Table 30–2 shows a typical day's menu based on each of the first 3 diets.

In infants or young children suspected of food allergy, the problem of eliminating the offending foods may be done by placing the patient, if he is an infant, on nothing by mouth except Nutramigen* (protein hydrolysate) and glucose, or on a simple elimination diet consisting of lamb, rice, carrots, pears and soybean milk if he is older. If symptoms clear, additions will be made as described later in the chapter. If there is no improvement, the allergic symptoms may be due to causes other than food.

Treatment

Food Allergy in Infants and Children

Food allergy is much more common in infants and young children than in adults, and is often much more severe. It may express itself as a skin rash developing into severe eczema if untreated, in gastrointestinal symptoms, and in the young child

as asthma. Fortunately, many children outgrow their allergies, although they may retain mild sensitivity to certain foods or substances.

Orange Juice. Allergy to orange juice may appear very early in infancy as a skin rash. The substitution of ascorbic acid usually clears the rash. Orange juice in small doses may be started again when the child is a bit older and may then be well tolerated, or he may continue to be allergic to it.

Milk allergy in the small infant may pose a more serious problem. Sometimes boiled or evaporated cow's milk may be tolerated by such infants because the offending protein has been denatured by heat. If this fails, several milk substitutes are available. The most common of these are the numerous soybean preparations. These are reported to maintain satisfactory weight gain and growth. Commercially available soybean formulas vary considerably in mineral and particularly in vitamin content, and deficiencies of both vitamin A and thiamine have been reported in infants on such formulas. The physician should note the mineral and vitamin content of the specific soybean preparation prescribed, and provide for adequate supplementation. Iodine deficiency has also been reported in infants on soybean formulas, which consequently are now fortified with iodine or iodized salt. An extensive survey of the nutritional adequacy of soybean formulas has been prepared by the Committee on Nutrition of the American Academy of Pediatrics.[3]

A meat base formula* prepared from beef heart, sesame oil, sucrose, tapioca flour and calcium salts may also be prescribed for the infant who is allergic to cow's milk. This seems to be well tolerated and to promote satisfactory growth and gain in weight.

Nutramigen, prepared from casein by hydrolysis, contains only amino acids and polypeptides. It has lost its allergenic properties, and may be substituted for milk in the very young infant with milk allergy. However, weight gain of infants on this

---

* Mead Johnson and Co., Evansville, Ind.

[3] Pediatrics, *31*:329, 1963.
* Gerber Products, Fremont, Mich.

preparation is somewhat below normal, and in some instances there was diarrhea and vomiting.

Goat's milk has also been used as a substitute in infants with an allergy to cow's milk. For these infants evaporated goat's milk is recommended, as fresh goat's milk has been shown to have the same allergenic properties as cow's milk. An occasional infant on goat's milk has developed a macrocytic type of anemia. This responds well to folic acid, although the deficiency in goat's milk is of vitamin B_{12} rather than of folic acid.

A discussion of meat base formulas, Nutramigen and goat's milk is included in the report of the American Academy of Pediatrics referred to earlier in this section.

Additional Foods. For the infant or young child with demonstrated allergic eczema due to food sensitivity, Collins-Williams[4] suggests the progression of commonly non-allergenic foods, through Stage 2, and then the addition of frequently allergenic foods, one at a time, as shown in Table 30-3.

TABLE 30–3

Basic Diet:	Soybean milk, rice cereal, multivitamins
Stage 1:	Barley cereal, carrot, squash, applesauce, banana, lamb, Jell-O
Stage 2:	Oatmeal, cooked vegetables, stewed fruits, bacon
Stage 3:	Wheat cereals and other wheat products
Stage 4:	Beef, evaporated milk, raw and semi-raw vegetables and fruits, hard-boiled egg yolk
Stage 5:	Soft-cooked egg yolk, well cooked egg white, bottled milk
Stage 6:	Other foods

He warns that the basic principle to be followed is to proceed slowly, adding simple (not mixed) foods, one at a time, but not to keep the infant or child indefinitely on a restricted diet. Any food implicated as causing an allergic response such as a rash should be omitted, but may be tried again a few months later.

[4] Collins-Williams, C., *in* Gellis, S. S., and Kagan, B. M.: Current Pediatric Therapy. Philadelphia, Saunders, 1964.

The problem of maintaining good nutrition in the allergic child, whose needs are the same as those of other growing children, is stressed by all investigators. Moreover, there may be loss of fluid, electrolytes and protein from the skin of the child with severe eczema. In both eczema and asthma, irritability and restlessness may be accompanied by anorexia. The constant emphasis on food and the fear of precipitating symptoms may create emotional problems in both the child and his parents. The nurse needs to be aware of these, so that her guidance will help to alleviate overprotection and rigidity in the parents and the sense of frustration in the child.

Food Allergy in Older Children and Adults

Although allergic symptoms may be severe in older children and adults, they are less often due to food allergens than in infants. Sometimes the food allergy is for a single food such as strawberries or chocolate, easily eliminated from the diet.

When patients are sensitive to a food such as wheat, eggs or milk, all of which appear in the diet in many guises, or to several foods, as some allergic patients are, great care must be exercised in planning the diet. Careful food lists need to be prepared so that no food containing the allergen is overlooked.

The patient should be taught where the food allergen or allergens to which he is sensitive may be found, for even minute quantities may produce attacks. He must beware of commercial products of whose composition he is not absolutely certain. This applies not only to the foods and the drinks purchased in the market, but to those served in restaurants and other eating places, for prepared foods are usually mixtures of various products.

The commercial availability of many prepared foods which formerly were made in the home has made us less aware of what such foods contain. An example is mayonnaise, now seldom prepared by the housewife. That it contains a small quantity of egg may well be overlooked, and that it may contain wheat or wheat gluten as a binder would not generally be known.

Many packaged, canned, bottled and frozen foods have their contents listed, which will be of help in determining whether or not the offending substance is present. Other foods are packaged, canned or bottled under a standard of identity approved by the Food and Drug Administration, whereby specified amounts of certain ingredients must be present, but the food processor may add other, optional ingredients. These products do not have to have their contents labeled and had better be omitted from the diet.

The wheat-sensitive patient must learn that baker's rye bread contains some wheat flour; that practically all hot breads, griddle cakes, pastries and crackers are made chiefly or partly from wheat products; that bran and gluten are wheat derivatives. Thickened gravies, cream soups and sauces are to be avoided unless the thickening agent is known. Even meat dishes, such as meat loaf, hamburger, bologna and sausage may contain wheat flour or bread. All malted and cereal beverages must be avoided by the wheat-sensitive individual.

For a complete description of the omissions necessary in wheat sensitivity, see Chapter 27 under Gluten-Free Diet. For the patient allergic to wheat only, the restrictions on rye flour and oatmeal do not apply, but the remaining material will prove helpful in ensuring that all wheat products are eliminated from the diet.

The egg-sensitive patient likewise must investigate carefully all commercial products before partaking of them. He must remember that even the baking powder used in baked goods may contain dried egg white; that egg white may be used in the clearing of coffee and in the preparation of foaming beverages; and that most desserts, especially cakes, cookies, pastries, puddings and ice cream, contain eggs. These patients may also be allergic to chicken, which must then be omitted from the diet.

The milk-sensitive patient may find that he is able to use milk that has been boiled, evaporated or dried; but if sensitive to all milk, he must avoid cheese, butter and margarine (to which dry milk solids usually are added for flavor), as well as all other foods containing even infinitesimal

amounts of milk. Bread as purchased usually contains milk; therefore, bread made at home, with water in place of milk, is preferable.

It is well to note here that so-called soybean milk is an excellent milk substitute. It is made from soybeans, a vegetable protein of good biologic value, and fortified with minerals. Its nutritive value is almost equal to milk with the exception of the vitamin content.

Role of the Nurse

For the nurse in the doctor's office, where most allergy patients are treated, a knowledge of the preparation and the composition of foods may be of the greatest assistance to the physician and the patient.

The nurse and the patient together should explore every possibility in food preparation or composition so that the offending food or foods are sure to be omitted from the diet.

An excellent booklet, "Allergy Recipes," is available from the American Dietetic Association.[5] It contains a number of recipes for diets free of wheat, milk or eggs.

Also see Chapter 41 for recipes for bread, muffins, cake and cookies for wheat, milk and egg free diets. For the patient allergic to wheat only, the recipes in Chapter 40 may also be suitable.

Nutritional Adequacy. When the diet is very restricted, it is essential that it be evaluated for its calorie, protein, mineral and vitamin content. Using the Four Food Groups as a guide (see Chap. 10), it is possible to make a rough estimate of the adequacy of all nutrients in the diet except calories. For instance, if all citrus fruits must be omitted, there is little likelihood that the diet will be adequate in ascorbic acid. Similarly, if milk and cheese must be omitted, the calcium content of the diet is sure to be too low for the patient's needs. In such instances, it is important to stress those foods in the diet which are fair sources of the inadequate nutrient and, if necessary, to supplement the diet with mineral or vitamin concentrates.

---

[5] American Dietetic Association, 620 N. Michigan Avenue, Chicago, Ill. 60611.

Similarly, it is important that the caloric content of the restricted diet be carefully evaluated, so that weight loss does not result unless this is desirable.

Desensitizing the Patient

The difficulties inherent in strict avoidance of allergy-causing foods, especially in a child, may cause the physician to try to desensitize him to such food. This treatment should follow a period of complete abstinence from the offending food. Fortunately, it may be possible to desensitize by mouth; and, beginning with doses so minute that they cause no reactions in the person being treated, gradually the amount is increased until ordinary food portions can be tolerated.

To illustrate, one child sensitive to egg white was desensitized in this way over a period of 7 months by a dosage beginning with 1 mg. of dry or powdered egg white. Another child could tolerate at first only such small amount of egg white as that present in a teaspoonful of a dilution made by adding 1 drop of egg white to a pint of water. In 3 months, however, he was able to include eggs in his diet.

Often adults may desensitize themselves successfully. A man acutely but periodically sensitive to milk desensitizes himself every 3 or 4 years, in the following way. After eliminating milk, he takes daily an increasing number of drops of cream until he can resume the use of both cream and milk in his diet.

DISEASES OF THE SKIN

The relationship of nutrition to the health of the skin is well established. Good skin color and turgor and glossy, fine-textured hair are accepted indications of good nutritional status. Conversely, diseases of the skin, many of them of unknown etiology, are not necessarily a sign of poor nutrition, nor will they, with few exceptions, respond to dietary treatment. A careful nutritional history is important, and correction of poor food habits is as beneficial to patients with skin disease as to any one else, but specific diet therapy is indicated in only a few instances.

Vitamin Deficiencies

Several vitamin deficiencies are accompanied by skin manifestations such as thickening, cracking, eruption and bleeding. These have been described in detail in Chapter 16. The cure depends on the correction of the deficiency.

Fatty Acid Deficiency

Infants with Eczema. Hansen[6] has shown that infants with nonallergic, chronic eczema tended to have serum fatty acids with iodine numbers in a lower range than those of normal infants. Feeding these infants with unsaturated fatty acids, and especially with linoleic acid, was of benefit to a number of them, showing that a deficiency of unsaturated fatty acids may have been an etiologic factor in the eczema. (See Chap. 3.)

Psoriasis

Psoriasis is a chronic skin disease, characterized by red spots or plaques covered with a silvery scale. The lesions may become confluent or, rarely, generalized. The finger and toe nails are frequently affected, with pitting and thickening of the nail plate. A family history can be elicited in about 25 per cent of cases. The sexes are equally affected and the age of onset is variable. Spontaneous remission is common, but exacerbation or reactivation may occur in response to a number of stress factors.

It has been frequently noted that increased animal protein intake may provoke spread of the lesions. This observation was studied by Roe[7] in a series of experiments, designed to determine whether a specific amino acid load could induce the appearance of lesions. Itching, scaling and spread of lesions followed the ingestion of taurine, an intermediary product of the metabolism of cysteine, a sulfur-containing amino acid. Taurine is a normal component of animal protein foods. The mechanism of this reaction has not been elucidated.

---

[6] Hansen, A. E.: Am. J. Publ. Health, 47:1367, 1957.

[7] Roe, D. A.: N. Y. State J. Med., 65:1319, 1965.

TABLE 30—4. Low Taurine Diet*

Food	Allowed	Omitted
Milk	Evaporated milk, limited to ½ to 1 13-ounce can a day; or an equivalent amount of reconstituted powdered dry milk	Whole fluid, skim or buttermilk; cream
Cheese	½ cup cottage cheese or ½-ounce slice American or Swiss cheese or 1 tablespoon (½ ounce) cream cheese	All other cheese
Eggs	None	Any food containing eggs except for the small amounts present in cookies or a 1-egg cake
Meat, fish, poultry	Beef, veal, chicken, turkey: limited to 3 ounces a day†	Pork, lamb, cold cuts of all varieties, liver, heart, kidneys, meat gravies; fish, including canned tuna and salmon; shellfish
Soups	Cream soup made with milk allowance	Meat broth and soup; bouillon cubes and powders; meat extractives
Desserts	Puddings made with milk allowance; fruit ices; Jell-O; cookies, cake	Ice cream

As desired: Vegetables, potatoes, fruits, bread, cereals, macaroni products, butter, margarine, salad oils, beverages, sugars and jellies, salt, pepper, spices and herbs. A generous use of legumes and nuts to increase the protein content is recommended. Meat substitutes derived from vegetable protein are permitted.

* Adapted from Roe, D. A.: N. Y. State J. Med., 65:1319, 1965.

† Meats and poultry should be boiled for 10 minutes and the water discarded before further cooking such as roasting, broiling or frying.

On the basis of these investigations, a low-taurine diet was formulated, and Roe[8] subsequently showed that partial or complete remission of the disease could be accomplished by rigid adherence to this diet. The over-all reduction in protein intake, necessitated by the diet, may contribute to its success.

Low-Taurine Diet. Reduction in taurine intake may be achieved both by restriction of animal protein foods and by leaching out the taurine by boiling the food portion.

MEAT, FISH AND POULTRY. Beef, veal, chicken and turkey are limited to 3 ounces a day. The taurine content of these foods can be lowered by boiling for 10 minutes and discarding the water, before roasting, broiling or frying. Longer periods of boiling does not result in increased taurine loss.

8 Roe, D. A.: J. Invest. Dermat. 46:420, 1966.

All meats except those listed above, gravies, broth, bouillon cubes and powders, cold cuts, to which meat extractives are commonly added, organ meats, fish, including canned tunafish and salmon, and shellfish are omitted.

EGGS. Eggs and all foods containing eggs are omitted from the diet, except for the small amounts present in cookies or one-egg cake.

MILK. One half to one can (13 oz., liquid) of evaporated milk or an equivalent amount of reconstituted powdered dry milk are allowed each day. It may be used as a beverage with or without fountain syrup, in coffee and in food preparation. Cream and ice cream are omitted.

CHEESE. One half cup cottage cheese *or* a ½-ounce slice of American or Swiss cheese, *or* 1 tablespoon (½ ounce) of cream cheese is allowed.

OTHER FOODS. All other foods are allowed as desired. The liberal use of legumes and nuts to raise the protein content of the diet is recommended.

MEAT SUBSTITUTES. There are presently on the market several meat substitutes made from soybean protein, and simulating white chicken meat, beef and ham.[9] These are directed to non-meat eaters such as vegetarians and Seventh Day Adventists. They are low in taurine content and are suitable for inclusion in the diet restricted in taurine. See Table 30–4 for Foods Allowed and to be Omitted.

Nutritional Adequacy. Roe[10] states that the diet meets the Recommended Dietary Allowances for protein, vitamin and mineral content, with the exception of calcium if the full amount of milk is not included. In such case calcium lactate is prescribed.

The diet is not recommended except under medical supervision. It should not be prescribed for pregnant or lactating women, or persons with acute or chronic disease other than psoriasis. In children the diet must be modified to meet requirements for normal growth. Similar modification may be necessary for persons undertaking strenuous physical activity.

Acne Vulgaris

Acne vulgaris is defined as "an inflammation of the sebaceous glands from retained secretions." It is common to oily skins and occurs most frequently on the face, the chest and the back. The condition occurs most commonly in adolescents and young adults, and seems to be associated with abnormal response to hormonal activity in maturing individuals. Because it is so disfiguring, it is a source of real distress to this age group.

The condition has been attributed to a high carbohydrate diet. However, in a study testing two groups with acne (26 in each group), permitting sugar as desired in one group but limiting it sharply in the other, no difference was observed in clinical results.[11] A diet high in fat has also been suggested as a causative factor.

Cormia[12] found that chocolate and nuts aggravated the condition in some individuals. He suggests that, along with good hygiene, probably the most important aspect of treatment is to ensure that these adolescents have a highly nutritious diet adequate to meet their needs during this period of rapid physical development (see Chap. 14).

STUDY QUESTIONS AND ACTIVITIES

1. What are some common allergenic foods? Which of these are the most difficult to eliminate from the diet should they prove allergenic?

2. Why are allergies difficult to diagnose? What factors besides an allergen may affect the reaction?

3. How can the nurse aid the physician and the patient in interpreting the allergic patient's food history?

4. What is the procedure for using the Rowe Elimination Test Diets?

5. What is the danger when patients are kept on test diets such as elimination diets for long periods of time?

6. Plan a week's menu for a patient who must follow Rowe's Elimination Diet No. 3.

7. List an elimination diet suitable for a young child suspected of having a food allergy. Is it adequate for his nutritional needs?

8. What milk substitutes are available for an infant with milk allergy? Are these nutritionally equal to milk? Proof?

9. How may an infant or a young child with food allergy progress to a full diet?

10. What are some of the emotional complications inherent in allergy? How may the nurse be of help to the child and his parents?

11. Name 10 foods in which wheat may be used as an ingredient and of which a patient on a wheat-free diet must be warned; 10 foods in which milk may be the hidden ingredient; 10 foods in which eggs are the hidden ingredient.

12. Look at the label of a package of margarine. Why must a patient on a milk-free diet omit this food?

[9] Hartman, W. E.: Food Technology, 20:39, 1966; Worthington Foods.

[10] Roe, D. A.: Cutis, 2:1013, 1966.

[11] Cornbleet, T., and Gigli, I.: Arch. Dermat., 83:968, 1961.

[12] Cormia, F. E.: Am. J. Nursing, 57:198, 1957.

13. Are all packaged foods labeled, stating their contents? Which are not? Have you found any such foods at home or in a supermarket?

14. What would you advise a patient with a food allergy about the use of unlabeled prepared or mixed foods?

15. How may an allergy diet be evaluated for nutritive content? If milk has to be eliminated, which food nutrient is likely to be inadequate? Which is likely to be low? How can these be provided for?

16. Which foods may be substituted for wheat to retain the caloric value of the diet? Which nutrients are lost to the diet when enriched wheat bread and cereal cannot be used?

17. Which foods equal eggs for nutritive value and may be substituted for them?

18. How may a patient be desensitized to a food allergy?

19. If the physician orders a low-taurine diet for a patient with psoriasis, which foods should be restricted and to what quantity? Are any foods to be omitted entirely?

20. How may the protein content of the low-taurine diet be maintained at adequate levels?

21. What dietary advice should be given to a young boy or girl with acne?

SUPPLEMENTARY READING IN ALLERGY AND DISEASES OF THE SKIN

Allergy

Allergy Foundation of America, 801 Second Avenue, New York, N. Y. 10017.

Gryboski, J. D.: Gastrointestinal milk allergy in infants. Pediatrics, *40*:354, 1967 (Pt. 1, Sept.).

Heiner, D. C., et al.: Sensitivity to cow's milk. Council on Foods and Nutrition, J.A.M.A., *189*:563, 1964.

Kleinman, A. I.: Present status of foods in allergic diseases. N. Y. State J. Med., *63*: 538, 1963.

Krehl, W. A.: Skin disease and nutritional therapy. J. Am. Dietet. A., *35*:923, 1959.

Rapaport, H. G.: Psychosomatic aspects of allergy in childhood. J.A.M.A., *165*:812, 1957.

Diseases of the Skin

Cormia, F. E.: Acne vulgaris. Am. J. Nursing, *57*:198, 1957.

Hansen, A. E.: Role of unsaturated dietary fat in infant nutrition. Am. J. Publ. Health, *47*:1367, 1957.

Roe, D. A.: Nutrient requirement in psoriasis. N. Y. State J. Med., *65*:1319, 1965.

For Further References see Bibliography in Part Four.

CHAPTER **31**

Diseases of the Blood

Anemia Due to Loss of Blood • Iron Deficiency Anemia • Folic Acid Deficiency Anemia • Pernicious Anemia • Anemia—A World Health Problem • Favism • Diseases Affecting the White Blood Cells

The components of the blood are many and varied. (See Table 9, Part Four.) They may be divided into two large groups, the cellular elements and the remaining fluid or plasma, containing the dissolved substances. The blood plasma may have a deficiency, alteration or excess of its normal components, but this is usually a reflection of pathology of other organs, and, where nutrition is involved, has been discussed elsewhere. The cellular elements, comprised of the red and the white blood cells and the platelets, are the factors usually affected in diseases of the blood-forming organs, and are termed blood dyscrasias.

The erythrocytes or red cells in the blood, which normally number about 5,000,000 per cubic millimeter in the male and about 4,500,000 per cubic millimeter in the female, have a life span of only 120 days and must be continually renewed to maintain the normal concentration. As in other tissue repair of the body, food plays an important part in supplying the necessary materials for blood building.

However, many blood dyscrasias are not of nutritional origin, and are not responsive to dietary treatment, although maintenance of good nutrition may be a challenging problem. The diseases of the blood with which we are concerned are the anemias due to blood loss or to an inadequate intake or absorption of some essential nutrients; and leukemia, a disease of the white blood cells.

ANEMIAS

Anemia may be defined as a condition in which there is a decrease in the quantity of hemoglobin, of the number of red cells, of the volume of packed cells (hematocrit) or a combination of these. From the strictly nutritional aspects, anemias may be classified as follows:

1. Hypochromic microcytic anemias (too little hemoglobin)

Due to hemorrhage, acute or chronic

Due to inadequate intake of iron

2. Hyperchromic macrocytic anemias, due to deficiency of substances essential to red cell formation, and the release of these cells from the bone marrow.

Anemia Due to Loss of Blood

Severe Hemorrhage. In severe hemorrhage the immediate treatment is restoration of blood volume by transfusion. The blood must be further restored by an increase in the production of red blood cells and hemoglobin. In an otherwise normal individual recovery is spontaneous, but the red cells are replenished more rapidly than is the hemoglobin. The latter will be restored gradually, but the speed of its restoration seems to depend largely on the diet of the individual. The necessary food materials must be supplied in the diet in order that each of these red cells may contain the normal amount of hemoglobin. (See under Iron Deficiency Anemia.)

Chronic Hemorrhage. Chronic blood loss may accompany such conditions as gastric ulcer, colitis or long untreated hemorrhoids. The important aspect of treatment is to determine the cause of the blood loss and to control it. The dietary care is the same as that described under Iron Deficiency Anemia.

Iron Deficiency Anemia

Iron deficiency anemia is characterized by a low hemoglobin, giving less color than normal to the red blood cell (hypochromia). Red cells are in sufficient number, but are smaller than normal (microcytic) due to inadequate hemoglobin to fill the cell. It is most often due to a diet inadequate in iron, although poor absorption of iron from the intestinal tract may be a factor.

An inadequate iron intake may result owing to insufficient money to buy food; to consumption of food low in iron such as often occurs in children 6 months to 2 years of age, teen-age girls at the time of the menarche and pregnant women; to severe reducing fads, especially if undertaken without the supervision of a physician; and to poor food intake and anorexia accompanying illness.

Food iron is absorbed at any level of the intestinal tract from the stomach on, but is greatest in the duodenum. In malabsorption syndromes, such as are described in Chapter 27, there may be poor absorption of iron as of other nutrients. In disease accompanied by low gastric acidity there may also be insufficient iron absorption, since an acid medium is essential to keep iron in solution. Medications of hydrochloric acid as well as iron may be necessary to maintain a normal level of hemoglobin, although the dietary intake of iron should also be investigated.

Iron deficiency anemia in infants is discussed in Chapters 13 and 34; in pregnancy in Chapter 12; and as a world problem in Chapter 16.

Dietary Treatment of Iron Deficiency Anemias

An increased supply of iron and protein is the important factor to stress in a diet which must be adequate also in all other dietary essentials. Whipple[1] and his co-workers found liver, high in both iron and protein, to be at the top of the list of foods that promote blood regeneration. Other investigators have shown experimentally that diets high in iron but inadequate in protein will not promote hemoglobin regeneration.

Besides liver, which should be included at least once a week, lean meat, eggs, whole-grain and enriched bread and cereals, and potatoes are common and good food sources of iron and, in the case of meat and eggs, of protein. Other foods valuable for iron content which should appear frequently in the diet are kidney, heart, green, leafy vegetables, dried fruits such as apricots, prunes and figs, the legumes and, where it is in common use, molasses. See the bar chart in Chapter 6 for iron content of common foods.

Ascorbic acid (vitamin C) may be instrumental in the absorption of iron from the intestinal tract. Moore[2] found that the absorption of the iron contained in eggs was markedly increased when ascorbic acid, or orange or grapefruit juice were added to the diet.

Medications. When it is necessary to restore the hemoglobin level promptly, iron medication as well as a diet high in protein and iron are indicated. Fortunately, most patients respond well to such a regimen. Simple ferrous sulfate is as effective as more elaborate preparations. Since iron tablets sometimes cause irritation when taken on an empty stomach, they should be taken after meals.

Folic Acid Deficiency Anemia

Whereas iron is essential for the formation of hemoglobin, two vitamins, folic acid and vitamin B_{12}, are necessary for the formation of red blood cells. They are both involved in the building of the nucleoproteins needed for red blood cell structure and maturation. In a deficiency of either of these vitamins, the number of red cells is markedly reduced. The red cells present in the blood are large and filled with hemoglobin, since there is no deficiency of iron.

---

[1] Whipple, G. H., and Robscheit-Robbins, F. S.: Am. J. Physiol., 72:408, 1925.

[2] Moore, C. V.: Am. J. Clin. Nutr., 3:3, 1955.

These anemias are therefore called hyperchromic macrocytic (large cell) anemias.

Free folic acid does not occur naturally, but can be made synthetically and used as a medication. In food, folic acid is part of a much larger molecule. We have little knowledge at present of the manner in which it is absorbed, and some investigators believe that folic acid deficiency may be the result of a defect in absorption rather than an inadequate dietary intake. For this reason the folic acid content of a food as determined in the laboratory may give only a rough approximation of the amount absorbed when a food is eaten.

In the tissues folic acid is part of a folate co-enzyme which is involved in a number of metabolic reactions. Its major role is the transfer of one-carbon units to appropriate metabolites in the synthesis of DNA, RNA, and the amino acids methionine and serine.[3] Vitamin B_{12} is also involved in these reactions.[4] Both folic acid and vitamin B_{12} are stored in the liver. Although folic acid deficiency is closely related to pernicious anemia, it differs from it in a number of respects as described later in the chapter.

The anemia due to folic acid deficiency occurs in tropical sprue (see Chap. 27), and, more frequently than was previously thought, in pregnancy and in infants born of mothers suffering from folic acid deficiency.[5] It is also known to occur in alcoholic cirrhosis.[6] The cause may be either a poor dietary intake or a defect in absorption, as discussed above.

Patients with folic acid deficiency suffer from anorexia, weakness and lassitude. There may be a sore tongue (glossitis), and they have the characteristic yellowish skin color associated with a severe reduction of red blood cells.

The anemia responds dramatically to therapy with folic acid. If the deficiency is due to a poor food intake, it is essential that the diet be improved in all respects.

The Four Food Groups plus an increased intake of green leafy vegetables, liver, meat, fish, legumes and whole grains, all of which are food sources of folic acid, are essential to maintain recovery.

When antimetabolites which interfere with nucleoprotein synthesis are used in drug therapy for cancer, folic acid may be given by medication to protect healthy tissues from the effects of the drug.

Pernicious Anemia

Pernicious anemia is characterized by a marked decrease in the number of red blood cells, but an increase in the size of the cells. Therefore it also is a macrocytic anemia. It is due to the lack of the "intrinsic factor" produced in the mucosa of the stomach and present in gastric juice. The intrinsic factor is essential for the intestinal absorption of vitamin B_{12} obtained in food. Once absorbed, B_{12} is stored in the liver until needed, which is the reason liver administration proved to be the first successful treatment for pernicious anemia.

Vitamin B_{12}, in conjunction with folic acid, is necessary for the maturation and the release of red blood cells from the bone marrow, where they are formed. In pernicious anemia, the cells do not mature normally and they are not released in sufficient numbers. Therefore, the bone marrow becomes overcrowded with immature cells, while the blood is deficient in mature red blood cells. Besides the anemia there is usually a very low gastric acidity, or the hydrochloric acid may be absent altogether from the gastric juice. The patient has the characteristic yellowish skin color, and there is weakness and fatigue. In cases which have gone long untreated there are likely to be neurologic lesions, first evidenced by the tingling of hands and feet.

Liver and liver extract, long recognized as effective therapeutic agents in pernicious anemia, are potent sources of the antianemic factor. When vitamin B_{12} was isolated as the effective agent, it superseded the use of liver preparations. Both the anemia and the neurologic symptoms, if present, respond promptly to its administration.

[3] Vitale, J. J.: Nutr. Rev., *24*:289, 1966.

[4] Herbert, V.: Am. J. Clin. Nutr., *20*:562, 1967.

[5] Streiff, R. R., and Little, A. B.: New Eng. J. Med., *276*:776, 1967.

[6] Leevy, C. M.: Am. J. Clin. Nutr., *20*:570, 1967.

During the first few days of treatment there is a marked increase in the number of immature red cells in the blood. These cells are called reticulocytes, because when they are stained the disintegrating nucleus appears as a mesh or network. After a few days this disappears, and the cells appear as normal erythrocytes. The cell count and hemoglobin continue to increase until the normal levels are reached, and these are maintained as long as therapy is continued. Appetite and digestion also improve.

A good dietary supply of protein and iron is as essential for this type of anemia as it is in other anemias to provide building substances for the rapid increase in red cells and hemoglobin which occurs following the administration of vitamin B_{12}. Moreover, many patients with macrocytic anemias have a long history of a poor food intake. Therefore, the diet should be increased in vitamins and minerals in addition to iron and protein, and be adequate in calories.

Caution. Because the macrocytic anemia of pernicious anemia will respond to folic acid, it has sometimes been used in place of vitamin B_{12}. However, folic acid will not improve the neurologic symptoms, and these may become irreversible if they go long untreated. It has also been found that the indiscriminate use of multivitamin capsules, most of which contain folic acid, may mask a developing pernicious anemia. For this reason vitamin preparations which contain more than 0.1 mg. of folic acid may not be sold without prescription.

Anemia—A World Health Problem

The prevalence of nutritional anemias in underdeveloped and tropical areas of the world is discussed in Chapter 16. The relative roles of dietary deficiencies and parasitism has been under study by WHO since 1949. A recent progress report[7] deals with absorption of iron from tropical dietaries; dermal losses of iron in tropical regions; the role of hookworm infection in anemia; tissue iron stores; the role of protein, as well as iron, vitamin B_{12} and folate defi-

ciency in anemia; anemias in pregnancy; and the incidence of iron deficiency anemia in infants and children in the tropics. It can readily be seen that the impairment of health and working capacity caused by the anemias delays the much-needed economic progress of many of the underdeveloped countries of the world.

FAVISM

Favism is an inborn error of metabolism which has been known from very ancient times. It is found primarily in people who live, or have lived, in the Eastern Mediterranean basin. The eating—or even inhaling the pollen—of the fava or broad bean, a legume widely used as food in this part of the world, causes an acute hemolytic anemia in the affected individual.

These individuals have a decrease in the amount of glutathione and a lack of the enzyme glucose-6-phosphate dehydrogenase (G-6-PD) in their red blood cells. Both are necessary for the metabolism of glucose (see Chap. 9). When fava beans are eaten, the steps necessary for the conversion of glucose to carbon dioxide and water, and the release of energy, are halted partway. Hydrogen peroxide, ordinarily quickly converted to the next metabolic step by glutathione and G-6-PD, now accumulates in the red blood cell and destroys it. The symptoms are dizziness, nausea and vomiting, and sometimes a high fever and collapse, followed by severe anemia.

More recently it has been discovered that a drug used to treat malaria, primaquine, has the same effect as the ingestion of the fava bean on sensitive individuals. Black water fever, so called because of the production of very dark urine, which sometimes complicates the treatment of malaria, is now thought to occur only in individuals who lack G-6-PD. The dark or almost black urine is due to the presence of the breakdown products of hemoglobin from the destroyed red blood cells. A fascinating account of the disease and the discovery of the metabolic processes involved has recently appeared in a non-medical journal.[8]

---

[7] Patwardhan, V. N.: Am. J. Clin. Nutr., *19*:63, 1966.

[8] Marcus, J. R., and Cohen, G.: Harper's Magazine, June, 1967.

DISEASES AFFECTING THE WHITE BLOOD CELLS

Of the diseases affecting the white blood cells, leukemia is the most common. As in all chronic diseases, it is important to maintain good nutrition. Often this is difficult because of the patient's lack of appetite. In far-advanced disease there may be lesions in the mouth which make eating difficult and painful. Therefore, food should be soft so as not to require much chewing. It should not be heavily salted or spiced; sharp fruit juices should be omitted; and such beverages as coffee and tea should not be given to the patient too hot. Milk and milk beverages, eggs, very tender meat, fish and poultry, mashed potatoes and strained vegetables and fruits such as are used for infants are good and usually are well tolerated.

See earlier in the chapter on the use of folic acid when antimetabolic drugs are used in treatment.

STUDY QUESTIONS AND ACTIVITIES

1. Name two causes of iron-deficient anemias. What foods should be stressed in treatment? What other nutrients are essential?

2. Using the Pattern Dietary in Chapter 19 as a base, write a menu for a day for a 20-year-old nursing student of normal weight, containing 15 mg. of iron. Do not include liver or organ meats. Is it easy to obtain this much iron in the diet each day?

3. What may cause folic acid deficiency anemia? In which disease entity and in which groups is it known to occur? How is it treated? What foods are good sources of folic acid?

4. What are the metabolic processes in which both folic acid and vitamin B_{12} are involved?

5. What is the function of vitamin B_{12} in pernicious anemia? How does this disease differ from folic acid deficiency? In what respect are they similar?

6. Why has the amount of folic acid in multiple vitamin preparations been limited to 0.1 mg. unless ordered by the physician?

7. Why are the nutritional anemias a world-wide health problem?

8. What inborn error of metabolism may cause a severe anemia? Which food is involved? What medication?

9. Plan a menu for a day for a patient with leukemia who has developed sore and bleeding gums, making it as adequate nutritionally and as attractive as possible.

10. Why may folic acid be given when antimetabolic drugs are used in the treatment of cancer or leukemia?

SUPPLEMENTARY READING ON DISEASES OF THE BLOOD

Brown, E. B.: The absorption of iron. Am. J. Clin. Ntr., *12*:205, 1963.

Foroozan, P., and Trier, J. S.: Mucosa in the small intestine in pernicious anemia. New Eng. J. Med., *277*:553, 1967.

Marcus, J. R., and Cohen, G.: The riddle of the dangerous bean. Harper's Magazine, June, 1967, p. 98.

Patwardhan, V. N.: Nutritional anemias — WHO Research Program. Am. J. Clin. Nutr., *19*:63, 1966.

Streiff, R. R., and Little, A. B.: Folic acid deficiency in pregnancy. New Eng. J. Med., *276*:776, 1967.

Vitale, J. J.: Present knowledge of folacin. Nutr. Rev., *24*:289, 1966.

Wilson, T. H.: Intrinsic factor and B_{12} absorption. Nutr. Rev., *23*:33, 1965.

For further references see Biobliography in Part Four.

CHAPTER 32

Diseases of the Musculoskeletal and the Nervous Systems

Arthritis • Osteoporosis • Muscular Dystrophy • Collagen Diseases • Epilepsy • Ménière's Syndrome • Multiple Sclerosis • Myasthenia Gravis • Rehabilitation of the Paralyzed Patient • Rehabilitation of the Handicapped Homemaker • Food and Mental Illness

DISEASES OF THE MUSCULOSKELETAL SYSTEM

Arthritis

Arthritis is an inflammatory process of unknown etiology which involves the joints. Perhaps because of its chronicity and its accompanying discomfort and pain, many arthritics become the victims of food faddists, self-appointed "arthritis experts" or quacks, who advocate quick and miraculous cures with bizarre diet plans. At present there is no known cause or cure for arthritis, whether of dietary or other origin.

There are two major classifications of arthritis, which, however, are unrelated. **Osteoarthritis** or degenerative arthritis occurs in the older age group, and more frequently in women than in men. It is thought to be a natural accompaniment of aging. The disease is due to the wearing down of articular cartilage in the joints, usually those which are weight bearing such as the spine and the knees. The stiffness of the joints is very uncomfortable and often painful. For this reason activity may be curtailed, and there is a tendency to overweight in this group of patients, placing additional strain on the affected joints.

The nutritional requirements for the older age individual as described in Chapter 15 are equally important for the person with arthritis. Sufficient protein, calcium, iron and the vitamins are needed to maintain good health. Only the caloric needs are somewhat reduced, since activity is lessened.

The overweight arthritic will benefit from a further decrease in calories. Sometimes the omission of sugar, desserts, fried foods, mayonnaise and oil dressings, or just taking smaller portions of the accustomed foods, will accomplish this purpose. For a more controlled reduction regimen see Chapter 21. As his weight approaches the normal range for his height and build, the patient with osteoarthritis may well experience some relief from his discomfort and pain, and achieve an increase in activity.

Rheumatoid arthritis occurs more frequently than osteoarthritis. It may be seen in children, but usually appears between the ages of 25 to 50. It is three times more common in women than in men. The disease is due to an inflammatory process of the synovium or lining of the joints, accompanied by swelling and eventual deformity. It is a disfiguring, debilitating and chronic disease, marked by exacerbations and remissions. There is thought to be an emotional component which influences the course of the disease.

In contrast with the osteoarthritic, the patient with rheumatoid arthritis is frequently underweight, and the need for a food intake adequate in all nutrients, with additional calories, is obvious. The Four Food Groups (Chap. 10) should be included in liberal supply. Additional calories may be provided by between-meal feedings. Some suggestions will be found in Chapter 36.

Rheumatoid arthritis may be treated with the injection of steroids into the affected joints, or by the oral administration of streoids. However, with long-continued use of oral therapy, there may be disruption of sodium metabolism and edema; loss of calcium from the bones and eventual osteoporosis;[1] or an increase in hydrochloric acid content of the gastric juice, resulting in peptic ulcer. Should any of these occur, a diet restricted in sodium as described in Chapter 24, or the convalescent gastric ulcer diet described in Chapter 26, may be ordered. Calcium loss may be treated with calcium supplements, although an adequate intake of milk and cheese are also important.

Good results with surgery of the involved joints have also been reported.

Gout may produce a condition resembling arthritis which sometimes results in a permanent deformity or crippling of the

---

[1] Whedon, G. O., *et al.*: Arth. and Rheum., 4:445, 1961.

joints. Gout is at present the only form of joint disease that has been proved to be caused by an error in metabolism, and which can be controlled by medication. See Chapter 33 for the dietary regimen.

Other Considerations

The discomfort and the deformities accompanying the arthritides often cause loss of appetite and, thus, poor nutrition. Every means should be used to provide attractive as well as nourishing meals for these patients. Food should be placed so that it can be reached easily. Meats and other firm foods should be cut into bite sized portions, or ground so that they can be eaten with a spoon if necessary. Plastic, lightweight utensils are handled more easily by the crippled person than heavier silverware and china. Especially designed eating utensils such as those pictured on pages 429 and 430 (Figs. 32–1 and 32–2) may prove to be helpful.

The appetite and energy of the arthritic patient may be poor on arising. It will improve after medication begins to take effect, but again diminish by the end of the day, when most chronically ill patients are tired. Meals should be planned to provide as much of the daily food needs during the times of day when the patient is most comfortable. Some patients may manage better when their diets are divided into 6 meals.

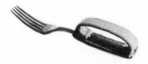

Fig. 32–1. Self-help devices for use in eating. When grasp is entirely absent, an elastic webbing cuff may be made to fit over the metacarpals of the hand. A leather strip that has been doubled and stitched to form a pocket is attached to the palmar side of the cuff. A spoon or a fork may be inserted into this pocket. (The Institute of Physical Medicine and Rehabilitation, New York University—Bellevue Medical Center. From Morrissey and Zimmerman: Helps for the handicapped, Am. J. Nursing, 53:454, 1953)

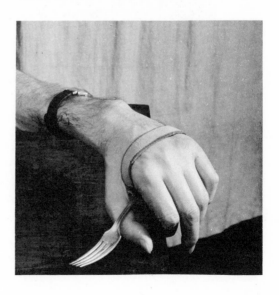

However, if the appetite is poor, the between-meal feedings should be limited to a bedtime snack.

If movement is greatly limited or painful, arthritic patients may neglect to eat properly, especially when they are responsible for their own meal planning and food purchasing and preparation. Along with other nutrition information, the nurse and the dietitian can assist such patients with suggestions for easily prepared foods and by referring them for help in organizing an efficient kitchen.[2] Such resources may be found in the rehabilitation center of a hospital, in public health agencies and industrial clinics, and from the extension services of many state universities.

The services provided for handicapped homemakers by some local chapters of the

American Heart Association will also be found helpful by the housewife with arthritis.

Osteoporosis

Osteoporosis is a disease entity of unknown etiology characterized by demineralization of the bone. It occurs in the later decades of life and is much more common in women than in men. It is responsible for the loss in height frequently seen in older men and women. There may be back pain due to compression or fracture of the weight-bearing lumbar vertebrae. The frequency with which older women sustain hip fractures compared with men is thought to be due to the greater incidence of osteoporosis in women.

The etiology of the disease has been ascribed to the changes in gonadal hormone balance in women after the menopause. The inadequacy of the calcium intake in the diet over many years is also thought to

[2] Beltsville Energy Saving Kitchen, Design 2, U. S. Department of Agriculture Leaflet No. 463, Nov. 1959.

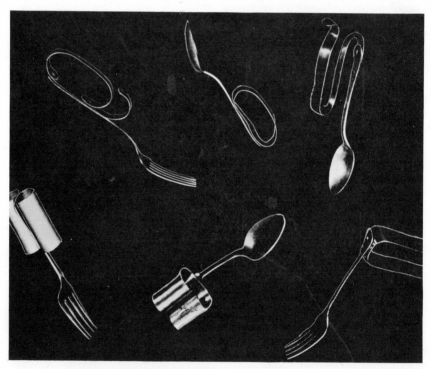

Fig. 32–2. Self-help devices for use in eating. Feeding utensils may be bent or shaped or have metal strips attached to fit the needs of an individual patient. (The Institute of Physical Medicine and Rehabilitation, New York University—Bellevue Medical Center. From Morrissey and Zimmerman: Helps for the handicapped, Am. J. Nursing, 53:454, 1953)

be a factor, and the administration of large quantities of calcium does on occasion reverse the negative calcium balance, but does not necessarily result in the remineralization of bone.[3] Vitamin D, which aids in the absorption of calcium from the intestinal tract, has been used in the treatment of osteoporosis in an attempt to correct the negative calcium balance.

Heaney[4] states that essential to the understanding of osteoporosis is the recognition that bone formation and bone resorption (calcium deposition in and calcium loss from the bone) for the maintenance of adequate calcium levels in the blood are part of the normal homeostatic process, regulated by parathyroid activity. The homeostatic stimuli similarly affect the absorption of calcium from the intestinal tract and the reabsorption or loss of calcium in the kidney tubule. Thus the degree of parathyroid activity and the consequent bone resorption will depend on how well intestinal absorption balances excretory loss. Osteoporosis will result whenever there is an imbalance between internal (bone) and external (intestine, kidney) response to homeostatic stimuli, and bone is forced to provide calcium. Although this concept of the development of osteoporosis is helpful in understanding the disease process, the factors responsible for the imbalance remain obscure.

There is some evidence that fluoride plays a role in the prevention and treatment of osteoporosis. The administration of fluoride to patients with clinical osteoporosis resulted in subjective improvement in many cases.[5] A large scale study of 1,015 subjects in North Dakota,[6] 300 of them living in an area with high fluoride content of the drinking water (4 to 5.8 ppm) and 715 subjects living in an area with water of low fluoride content (0.15 to 0.30 ppm) gave evidence that the incidence of osteoporosis, reduced bone density and collapsed vertebrae, although present in both men and women over 45 years of age, was substantially higher in the low fluoride areas. (It will be remembered that in the fluoridation of water to prevent tooth caries, the amount of fluoride added to water provides 1 part per million. See Chap. 6.) The limited information obtained on milk and cheese consumption in this study did not indicate that the differences in calcium intake in the two groups was a factor in the findings.

Treatment

Heaney concludes that the use of calcium supplements, gonadal hormones and fluorides are a rational as well as an empirical method for the treatment of osteoporosis.[7] These substances will be prescribed by the physician in the form of medication. In view, however, of the possibility of poor dietary intake of essential nutrients in older people, it is important that the diet be checked for inadequacies. Milk consumption is often limited, and may have been so for many years. Unless there is obvious milk intolerance (see Chap. 27), a pint of milk or the equivalent in cheese should be included daily, not only for its calcium content, but for its contribution of protein and vitamins to the diet. Equally important are meat, vegetables, fruits and enriched bread and cereals as outlined in the Four Food Groups in Chapter 10, and for older people in Chapter 15. The caloric intake of the diet may have to be curtailed if there is overweight, frequently found in the elderly, not only to relieve weight-bearing on the affected bony structures, but also because many of the foods providing mainly calories such as sugars, jellies, candy and fats may be substituted for more nutritious foods (see Chaps. 21 and 37).

Muscular Dystrophy

Muscular dystrophy is a familial disease affecting the muscle fibers, causing progressive muscular weakness. It has its onset most frequently in childhood. Blahd[8] has recently shown that patients with muscular

[3] Hegsted, D. M.: J. Am. Dietet. A., *50*:105, 1967.

[4] Heaney, R. P.: Am. J. Med., *39*:877, 1965.

[5] Bernstein, D. S., *et al.*: J. Clin. Invest., *42*:916, 1963.

[6] ———: J.A.M.A., *198*:499, 1966; Hegsted, D. M.: Op. cit.

[7] Heaney, R. P.: Op. cit.

[8] Blahd, W. H., *et al.*: New Eng. J. Med., *276*: 1349, 1967.

dystrophy have decreased body potassium concentration resulting from replacement of potassium-rich muscle tissue by collagen and fat, both low in potassium. The degree of potassium diminution appears to correlate with the severity of muscle involvement. He has also found that some of the non-dystrophic relatives of these patients, particularly mothers and female siblings, have lowered total body potassium, which may indicate a biochemical trait with genetic implications. For a discussion of the problems of the family of a handicapped child, see the introductory paragraphs under Long-Term Illness in Infants and Children in Chapter 34.

Because deficiency of vitamin E in experimental animals causes a disease similar to muscular dystrophy, it has been postulated that there may be a defect in the utilization of vitamin E by patients with this disease. However, the administration of vitamin E does not alter the course of the disease. The mineral selenium is also involved in protecting experimental animals from muscular dystrophy, but its relationship to muscular dystrophy in man is presently unknown.

Muscular dystrophy is accompanied by a defect in creatine metabolism. Normally creatine is synthetized from glycine in the liver, and sent to the muscles where it is phosphorylated to form creatine phosphate, an important metabolic compound. In muscular dystrophy the muscle is unable to accept creatine, and it is excreted in the urine.

At present there is no specific dietary treatment for muscular dystrophy. Since the disease most often occurs in children, it is important that their food intake provide the needs for growth as well as maintenance. As the disease progresses and muscular weakness increases, some of the suggestions for feeding and utensils described earlier in the chapter may be found helpful.

Collagen Diseases

A group of diseases involving the connective tissue of the body are grouped together under the name of collagen disease. Among these are lupus erythematosus, dermatomyositis, polyarteritis and scleroderma.

They are most often treated with corticotropin (ACTH) or cortisone. Because these hormones normally affect the reabsorption of sodium in the kidney, there may be an increase in such reabsorption when they are given as medication over and above the hormones that the adrenal cortex produces naturally. For this reason a diet restricted in sodium may be ordered during the period of treatment. See Chapter 24 for varieties of sodium-restricted diets. Osteoporosis may also develop with long-continued steroid therapy.[9] See earlier in this chapter.

DISEASES OF THE NERVOUS SYSTEM
Epilepsy

Epilepsy is a disease of the central nervous system. It occurs in both children and adults, although it is more frequent in children. The chief symptom is momentary loss of consciousness in petit mal attacks, so short they may hardly be noticed; or the loss of consciousness may be of longer duration, accompanied by convulsions, as in grand mal attacks. Phenobarbital and anticonvulsant drugs are effective in controlling the incidence of attacks in most patients.

A general, nutritionally adequate diet, avoiding excess amounts of food and fluid at any one meal, is recommended. The spacing of fluids throughout the day will prevent an increase in blood volume, which may precipitate an attack. In adults, alcoholic beverages, and especially beer because it is usually consumed in large quantities, should be avoided.

Recently the ketogenic diet, abandoned for many years because of the difficulty in following it, has been used successfully in young patients with petit mal epilepsy who did not respond to drug therapy. Details of the diet will be found in Chapter 34.

Ménière's Syndrome

Ménière's syndrome comprises a group of symptoms which include dizziness and gastrointestinal disturbances associated with unilateral defects in hearing and in equilibrium. This syndrome is thought to be due

---

[9] Whedon, G. O., *et al.*: Op. cit.

to a swelling of the vestibular apparatus of the ear caused by an allergic response or by a spasm of the blood vessels within the ear.

Conservative treatment usually consists of sedation and tranquilizers to prevent attacks; and diuretics and a sodium-restricted diet to relieve the edema if this is thought to be present. In severe situations surgery is performed, and ultrasonic therapy has been found to be successful. Because of the dizziness, nausea and vomiting accompanying an attack, patients need support and instruction to help them to understand and accept their dietary restrictions. See Chapter 24 for diets restricted in sodium.

Multiple Sclerosis

Multiple sclerosis is a chronic, progressive disease of unknown etiology, affecting the myelinated nerve fibers, and the muscles which they innervate.

The majority of patients are between the ages of 20 and 45. There is no specific treatment, but people with the disease can and often do live as long as the average person, or it may have a rapid course. However, as the muscle and the nerve functions gradually weaken, these patients need supportive measures that will prevent atrophy of the affected muscles and train unaffected muscles for new functions. They also need help in devising ways of independently maintaining the activities of daily living as long as possible. Adequate nutrition plays a vital role in this process, psychologically as well as physiologically.

Periodically a dietary regimen is reported which seems to arrest the course of the disease, but these claims have not so far been substantiated. An association of hyperinsulinism and multiple sclerosis has also been suggested. A mildly decreased carbohydrate intake coupled with the administration of tolbutamide was said to give good results. Any therapy is difficult to evaluate, however, because the disease is punctuated by remissions and exacerbations.[10] At present, a nutritionally adequate diet of simply prepared and easily eaten food is the accepted dietary prescription for patients with multiple sclerosis. As the disease progresses, and the patient has difficulty in swallowing, food should be puréed or liquefied. (See Chap. 29, Radical Surgery of the Mouth and the Neck.) When lifting eating utensils becomes a problem, plastic dishes and spoons will be found useful.

Myasthenia Gravis

Myasthenia gravis is another disease of the nervous system of unknown etiology. In this disease motor impulses flow freely through the nerve pathways until they reach the muscle fibers. At the nerve-muscle junction the impulses are only partially carried across, and poor muscle contraction results. These patients develop great muscular fatigue with only a minimum of motion. Medications help to facilitate conduction at the nerve-muscle junction, but they must be given frequently. With drug therapy some patients may return to as much as 90 per cent of normal muscle function; in others death results in from 5 to 10 years.

In myasthenia gravis there is rapid onset of fatigue with all muscular movement, including chewing and swallowing. Soft, easily masticated foods are essential for these patients. They eat very slowly in order to allow time for the masticating muscles to regain their strength between bites of food. Meals should be served in utensils that will retain the temperature of the food for extended periods of time. Nutritionally concentrated foods should be chosen so that the patient will obtain as much nourishment as possible with a minimum of effort (see Chap. 36). As the disease progresses, nasogastric feedings may be necessary to maintain adequate food intake (see Chap. 29).

REHABILITATION OF THE PARALYZED PATIENT

Injury to the brain or the spinal cord, from accident or disease, may result in some degree of paralysis. This may affect movement from the head to the feet, as well as the peristaltic motion in the gastrointestinal tract and the control of the blad-

[10] Q. and A.: J.A.M.A., *196*:198, 1966; Sawyer, G. T.: J.A.M.A., *174*:170, 1960; Swank, R. L.: J. Am. Dietet. A., *36*:322, 1960; Abrahamson, E. M.: N. Y. State J. Med., *54*:1603, 1954.

der. The site and the severity of the injury
determines the degree and the duration of
the paralysis. Total transverse severance
of the spinal cord at the 5th or the 6th
cervical vertebra causes *quadriplegia*. Patients with this type of injury have lost
motor power in the arms and the legs, all
sensation below the level of the lesion and
control of bladder and bowel functions.
Paraplegia results when the spinal cord is
severed in the lumbar region. These patients have lost motor power and sensation
in the legs, and bladder and bowel control.
The patient with *hemiplegia* has lost motor
power over one side of the body and may
also have lost speech, vision, emotional stability and intellectual faculties.

Advances in rehabilitation medicine are
making it possible for increasing numbers
of patients with brain and spinal cord injuries to survive for extended periods of
time. Such programs are designed to restore the patient to the greatest physical,
emotional, social and economic capacities
which he can achieve within the limits of
his disability. With proper care, training
and community opportunity, many handicapped individuals may return to their
homes and vocations as contributing members of society.

Food and nutrition play an important
role in seven principal areas of this process: (1) The maintenance of life and
nutrition immediately following injury; (2)
dietary measures to encourage normal urinary tract function; (3) the prevention and
the healing of decubitus ulcers; (4) mechanical devices to facilitate eating; (5)
training for bladder and bowel control; (6)
weight control; and (7) adequate food intake during periods of strenuous retraining of muscles.

**Diet Immediately Following Brain and
Spinal Cord Injury.** For the first few days
after injury, the quadriplegic patient should
have nothing by mouth, because there may
be gastrointestinal stasis. During this period
nutrition must be maintained by intravenous feeding (see Chap. 29). As gastric
distension subsides and peristalsis returns,
small amounts of water are given by mouth
followed by small feedings of high protein
foods and fluids. A fluid intake of 3,000

ml. or more may be needed to stimulate
kidney function.

In paraplegia, which involves less peristaltic dysfunction, oral feedings may be
tolerated earlier. In both quadriplegic and
hemiplegic patients, fear of choking may
cause the patient to reject food. The nurse
who is feeding these patients must use considerable skill and encouragement to get
them to eat. A variety of foods of different
textures and consistencies should be offered
to see which are best tolerated by the individual patient. Oral hygiene before and
after meals is important. Once the initial
crisis has passed, the nutritional needs of
each patient should be determined by the
several factors discussed in the following
paragraphs.

**Dietary Measures to Encourage Normal
Urinary Tract Functions.** The effect of immobilization on calcium and nitrogen losses
from bone and muscle tissue has been described in Chapter 18. In the paralyzed patient this may be a contributing factor in
the formation of urinary calculi, particularly if ambulation is delayed. The diet and
other measures for the prevention of calcium kidney stones is described in Chapter 25.

Urinary tract infection as a result of
poor bladder function also occurs frequently in paralyzed patients, and may influence the formation of urinary calculi by
alkalinizing the urine. Antibacterial and
acidifying drugs are used, and sometimes
an acid ash diet is ordered to aid in keeping the urine acid (see Chap. 25 and Table
8, Part Four).

A high fluid intake is of importance in
the prevention and the treatment of both
urinary calculi and infection.

**Prevention and Healing of Decubitus
Ulcers.** Constant pressure on, or irritation
of, any part of the body surface will eventually result in the breakdown of the skin
and its supporting tissues. Sensory impairment further complicates this problem for
the paralyzed patient, since he may not be
aware of irritation and pressure. If prolonged bed-rest, sitting, or the use of braces
is necessary, or if the patient is incontinent,
decubitus ulcers are likely to develop unless adequate precautions are taken. Regu-

lar changes in body position, meticulous skin care, proper fitting of braces and early ambulation all help to prevent skin breakdown. However, none of these measures is likely to be effective unless a highly nutritious diet, high in protein, is included.

The immobile patient may require extra protein, up to 1.5 Gm. per Kg. and an increased amount of ascorbic acid, up to 150 mg. daily, to prevent skin breakdown. If ulceration has occurred and is extensive, an increase in food nutrients, except in calories, becomes even more important.

With the capricious appetite and the manual and swallowing difficulties common to these patients, considerable ingenuity is required to have them accept and eat such large quantities of food. Meat, fish, fowl, eggs, and cheese, in easily masticated form, will provide good quality protein in the diet both at mealtime and as snacks. Milk and high protein beverages (see Chap. 36) should be served frequently. Favorite foods may be fortified by the addition of dry skim milk or eggs. Vitamin, mineral and protein supplements may be needed, by vein if oral intake is poor, to maintain adequate nutrition. The use of nasogastric tube feedings (see Chap. 29) may also be of help if it is not possible for the patient to consume the needed amount of food.

There may be conflict in nutritional needs if there is danger of both kidney stones and skin breakdown. If milk must be limited and cheese and dry skim milk omitted, Protinal* which contains no calcium, may be of help as a partial substitute to maintain high protein levels.

Mechanical Devices to Facilitate Eating. Patients with a limited range of motion in the head, the trunk, the arms, the hands and the fingers often have difficulty in using ordinary eating implements. The ability to feed himself, with a minimum of assistance or none, improves the patient's morale as well as his food intake. Therefore suitable eating utensils must be provided for these patients as soon as is feasible. (See illustrations earlier in this chapter.) Some

manufacturers[11] have devised adaptations of regular knives, spoons, forks, cups, glasses and plates for this purpose. Many patients will need individually designed pieces to fit their unique needs. The return to self-feeding is an important step on the patient's road to independence and should be one of the first goals of a rehabilitation program. At the same time his potential for developing self-feeding skills should be carefully evaluated so that unrealistic goals are not set.

Bladder and Bowel Control. If the patient's injury is one that will eventually permit voluntary emptying of the bladder and the bowel, suitable retraining activities will become a part of the rehabilitation program. When bladder training is in progress, the type and the amount of fluid and the spacing throughout the day must be carefully regulated.

From 2,500 to 3,000 ml. of fluid are permitted. This includes all food fluids as well as water. Carbonated and alcoholic beverages are omitted. Each patient's fluid regimen is individualized, but must be carefully spaced throughout the day. No fluids are permitted between 9 P.M. and 7 A.M. the following morning. The mouth may be moistened during this period if it becomes excessively dry.

When bowel training is in progress, a high residue diet served at regular intervals is desirable. This provides bulky intestinal contents which facilitate defecation. Ample supplies of whole grain breads and cereals, leafy green and raw vegetables, salads and fresh and dried fruits should be included in the patient's daily diet. Any food that seems to cause watery feces, and therefore involuntary, irregular defecation, should be avoided. On the other hand, a large amount of bulk may cause fecal impaction. If there is danger of this, a low residue diet should be instituted (see Chap. 27).

Weight Control. Food often becomes a major problem for the paralyzed patient, from the psychological as well as from the

---

* National Drug Co.

11 Everett and Jennings, 1803 Pontius Ave., Los Angeles, Calif.; Fascole Corp., 229 Fourth Ave., New York, N. Y. 10003.

physiologic viewpoint. The attitude of the patient and his family toward his illness and the resultant changes that must be made in his life's goals often affect his nutrition. He may reject all food no matter how thoughtfully prepared, reflecting his difficulty in accepting his disability. He may become very demanding and unreasonable about his food choices, expressing his frustration and insecurity. These situations are difficult for every one concerned with the patient's care. In order to maintain the patient's nutrition, nasogastric or intravenous feeding may have to be instituted until other rehabilitative measures modify the patient's attitude and understanding.

An equally difficult problem arises when the patient uses food to satisfy his emotional needs by overeating and, in doing so, becomes overweight. Family and friends may unwittingly aid this situation by offering too much or the wrong kinds of food as a means of showing their concern. The resultant obesity, further complicated by the patient's limited activity, may be difficult to control. Therefore, prevention of overweight becomes an important aspect of the patient's nutritional care. A plentiful diet of low calorie foods, with snacks consisting of fruit, broth and other beverages of minimal caloric content, will help to satisfy the patient's craving for food (see Chaps. 21 and 37). Family and friends should be helped to find methods other than bringing high calorie foods to show their affection and concern for the patient.

Diet During Retraining Exercises. Patients with a potential for partial or complete recovery of muscle function engage in considerable physical exercise as part of their rehabilitation program. The goal is to enable the patient to perform the activities of daily living as independently and as adequately as his limitations will permit. Muscle training for vocational goals may also be undertaken. During this time the patient's appetite and his actual need for food increases markedly. If he is on a regular or house diet at this time, he will need larger servings and more substantial snacks than this diet usually provides. However, precaution should be taken that

the patient and his family understand the relationship between his high food intake and intensive exercise. Obesity may result if the high food intake is continued in less active periods of the patient's program.

REHABILITATION OF THE HANDICAPPED HOMEMAKER

All patients handicapped by accident, disease or necessary surgery will need rehabilitative care for varying periods of time. This usually begins in the hospital, the clinic or the rehabilitation center, but it may need to be continued after the patient's discharge to his own home or to a nursing home. Sometimes the home to which the handicapped person is discharged requires adaptation, so that he can live there with a degree of independence. Planning and carrying out these modifications may be an important part of the program for the patient and the family during the time of hospitalization.

Nurses and dietitians should assist all patients and their families in this area of the rehabilitation process, but their help is particularly needed by the handicapped homemaker. Women, who through accident or disease find their role of mother, housewife and home manager threatened, need considerable help. Handicapped men may be able to carry on in a former occupation if it requires only minimal physical activity, or they may be trained to new ones and, in this way, regain their masculine role of family head and provider despite their handicap. However, the woman who has always found satisfaction in her homemaking responsibilities and activities usually finds it very difficult to pass these on to others. She needs the sense of worth and contribution to family life that such tasks provide, even when she may have the financial resources to have others carry them out. Furthermore, the activity provided through homemaking serves a valuable therapeutic purpose, and therefore it should be encouraged from this standpoint.

Unfortunately, most homemaking activities require a wide range of physical motion when performed in the ordinary home with conventional equipment and methods. Therefore, modified equipment and new methods may have to be developed to meet the needs of the handicapped homemaker. They must be in accord with her physical limitations and endurance, and with her psychological motivation to accomplish the activity.

The nurse and the dietitian can prepare the hospitalized woman for this process in a number of ways. Her knowledge of nutrition and family food needs can be determined and additional instruction given if needed. She can be guided in the selection of menus and recipes that will be easy to prepare as well as attractive and nutritious. She can be helped to think through the simplest methods of organizing her home and her work schedule so that her energy is not wasted on extra motion while carrying out routine tasks. The nurse, particularly, through her own knowledge of posture and body mechanics and her routine practice of work simplification principles in her nursing tasks, has much to give the handicapped homemaker. These activities will provide therapy for the long hours of inactivity most handicapped women have to endure during their rehabilitative programs. Anticipation of these activities will also provide motivation for muscle retraining exercises when these are needed.

FOOD AND MENTAL ILLNESS

As indicated in Chapter 18, food represents many things other than physical sustenance to man. What, when, where, how and with whom he will eat is more often determined by his psycho-social orientation at any given moment than by his knowledge of his nutritional needs. During periods of extreme food shortage human beings will eat anything in an attempt to maintain life. However, when food supplies are adequate, the choice of food is more likely to be based on its emotional value than on its nutritional worth. From early infancy food intake is related to various degrees of pleasure or pain, satisfaction or frustration, acceptance or rejection. The emotionally stable individual, although he may possess definite food preferences, usually has only transient periods in which food is used as a vehicle for maintaining psychological equilibrium. During men-

tal illness, food often becomes a tool for displaying psychological abnormalities. Therefore, it is not surprising that unusual eating habits are frequently one of the first observable symptoms in mental illness.

An understanding of the significance of these symptoms and the part that these symptoms play in therapy is important to all nurses and dietitians. Psychiatric patients are no longer isolated in mental institutions. Many general hospitals now have psychiatric services.[12] Mental Health centers have Day Care, Night Care and Halfway Homes. Thus public health nurses and nutritionists, school nurses, school lunch personnel and industrial nurses become involved in the care of the mentally ill, including the nutritional problems of the patient and his family.

Unconscious Meanings of Food

During mental illness the unconscious meanings of food become intensified. If these are not properly taken into consideration, they can disrupt the therapy and the recovery of the patient as well as his nutritional status. Food habits may reflect mental illness in a number of ways. Patients may eat too little, or nothing at all, for many reasons. They may feel that attempts are being made to poison them through food. They may have feelings of unworthiness or guilt, or a wish to die. They may be unable to make decisions of any nature, including what to eat. Fatigue and physical illness, depression, or a desire for attention may also cause them to neglect or refuse food. Patients may overeat for a variety of reasons. Feelings of insecurity may cause them to eat constantly. A fear that others will steal their share of the available food may cause them to eat everything in sight as quickly as possible, or to hoard food. Patients may also overeat to gain attention or status.

Fear of Poisoning

The manner of helping each patient depends on the cause of his difficulty. If a patient fears that attempts are being made

---

[12] Gee, D. A.: J. Am. Dietet, A., *41*:345, 1962.

to poison him, his fears may be allayed by providing him with foods that he can prepare himself. Baked potatoes, eggs in the shell, small boxes of cereals, whole unpeeled fruits, small sealed packets of crackers and cookies, and milk in individual cartons, none of which have to be handled by others before they are eaten, may allay the patient's fears. Allowing him to assist in food preparation and service, so that he can see that all patients and staff are fed from the same food containers, or tasting food in his presence may also give him confidence enough to eat.

Feelings of Guilt

The patient who has feelings of guilt and unworthiness and, therefore, thinks he is not deserving of the reward of food when in the company of others, may improve his food intake when he eats alone. This may also be the solution for the patient who overeats when in a group, believing that others will steal his share of the food. The patient who is unable to make decisions will do best when served one food at a time, with only one eating utensil. A preoccupied patient, or one who is too hyperactive to sit down to a regular table meal, should have sandwiches, fruits and other finger foods provided so that he can consume them easily while he walks around. At the same time he will require frequent servings of fluid to prevent dehydration.

Overeating

Overeating is the most frequent nutritional problem of the mentally ill individual. Supportive therapy to meet his needs through activities other than eating is necessary before weight control, with its benefits to emotional as well as nutritional health, is possible. However, the obese patient should be supplied with easily available low caloric snack foods during therapy. The nurse and the dietitian can guide the patient to the selection of bulky but low calorie salads with a minimum of dressing, clear rather than cream soups, meats without gravy, and fruit for desserts and snacks. (See Chaps. 21 and 37 for low caloric foods.) Many of these patients will need large amounts of food or frequent feedings until their emotional problems have been defined and treated. Placing them on severely restricted diets will only increase their difficulties. Therefore, it is important that the nurse and the dietitian cooperate closely with the therapist when planning diets for obese, mentally ill patients.

Mental Illness and Age Groups

Mental illness occurs in people of all ages. When found in young children who have been deprived of attention and affection, it presents a variety of nutritional problems. These children may not eat when alone, but will usually consume adequate amounts of any type of food when staff members join them at mealtime. If seriously disturbed, their eating habits may require unusual tolerance on the part of nurses and dietitians. Adolescents may act out their resentment to a hostile and authoritarian world by refusing balanced meals in favor of carbonated beverages, coffee and sweets, or by selecting bizarre food combinations. They may also refuse all food until anorexia nervosa (see Chap. 21) becomes a serious problem. Or they may become obese from constant nibbling. Elderly patients, becoming senile, may eat only tea and toast or similar foods unless tactfully catered to.

Effect of Drugs

The chemical approach to the treatment of mental illness influences the role of food in patient care. Drugs are used to calm hyperactive patients and to stimulate depressed and retarded ones. They may affect the appetite and the metabolism so that patients gain excessive weight if careful diet planning is not a part of the therapeutic regimen. Forced feedings may no longer be necessary for these patients. However, with some drugs, the time span between the medication and the period when the patient is receptive to eating varies. This must be considered and properly utilized to benefit the patient nutritionally.

In patients receiving antidepressant drugs which inhibit monoamine oxidase in the body, certain foods naturally high in pressor amines should be avoided. These are cheese of all varieties except cream and cottage cheese; yeast and yeast extracts (Vegex, Bovril); chicken livers, herring and broad beans. Attacks of acute hypertension, headache, flushing and palpitation have been reported in patients receiving antidepressant drugs of this type, on the ingestion of one of these foods, particularly cheese.[13]

Patient-Staff Relationships

The trend toward treatment of mentally ill patients in Day Care and Night Care programs gives added opportunity for the nurse and the dietitian to improve the nutritional status of the patient and his family. It may be necessary to work out plans for home or restaurant meals with such patients. Thus the nurse and the dietitian become involved in total family planning with its obvious opportunities for nutrition teaching. In some hospitals, patients are provided with box lunches to take to work, or patients may prepare their own lunches with the aid of the nurse or the dietary staff. This activity has therapeutic value as well as being important nutritionally.

In all patient relationships the symbolic meaning of breaking bread together is very important. Eating together reduces social distance and connotes mutual respect. When the nurse or the dietitian shares a table with a patient for a meal or a snack, she helps him in many ways. She can guide his food choices and encourage the intake of appropriate foods. She can observe the patient's reactions to food and, consequently, discuss them with the therapeutic team. This is important, as reactions to food often give valuable clues to a patient's condition and progress. However, of equal importance is the feeling of acceptance and social worth she gives to the patient by sharing food with him. For the nurse, particularly, this may be the first step toward the establishment of a good therapeutic relationship.

The physical setting in which food is served is especially important to psychiatric patients. Irrational behavior at mealtime may be instigated or intensified by unattractive food served by uncongenial people in an untidy, overcrowded room among unpleasant odors and sounds. Nutritional status as well as physical and emotional health will be improved when patients' meals are served in an attractive setting by tolerant people.

Complexity of the Role of Food in Mental Illness

Because of the complexity of the role of food in the therapy of mentally ill patients, it is necessary for all involved in food preparation and service for these patients to be active and well-informed members of the therapeutic team. As Ross[14] states: "Theirs is the privilege of satisfying the simplest physical and one of the deepest emotional needs of our patients." When this is done sympathetically and intelligently the therapeutic efforts of the other members of the team will be greatly enhanced.

There is no specific diet therapy for mental illness. However, many problems of nutrition may occur in the mentally ill patient. Most psychiatric disorders are the result of extended periods of tension and anxiety, during which proper food intake has been ignored. Therefore it can be assumed that most patients are poorly nourished at the time they initially come for treatment. They may be underweight or obese, and they may have measurable deficiencies from unvaried or inadequate diets. They may also have conditions requiring specific dietary treatment, such as diabetes, peptic ulcer, colitis, cardiovascular or other disease, or they may be pregnant. The general principles of dietary treatment for such specific conditions are discussed elsewhere in this text, but it must be emphasized here that when such diets are adapted for the mentally ill person, they must be extremely well planned. The patient's concept of food as well as his metabolic requirements must be taken into consideration even more

---

[13] Review: Nutr. Rev., 23:326, 1965.

[14] Ross, M.: J. Am. Dietet. A., *40*:318, 1962.

thoroughly than with other patients. As much attention must be given to the modification of the diet to emotional needs as to the metabolic requirements. In fact, if this is not done, recovery is greatly impeded if not impossible.

STUDY QUESTIONS AND ACTIVITIES

1. Make 5 simple suggestions for losing weight to a patient with osteoarthritis who is overweight and inactive because of the disease.

2. Why may sodium have to be restricted in the diet when the adrenal cortex hormones are used in treatment?

3. What may happen to the quantity of gastric juice produced when steroid hormones are given over a longer period of time? To the calcium balance?

4. Write a day's menu for a patient on a 1,000-milligram sodium, convalescent gastric ulcer diet. Is it high enough in calcium?

5. Make out a menu for a high caloric diet for a patient with rheumatoid arthritis who has a poor appetite. Use "easy-to-eat" foods.

6. What type of eating utensils may be substituted for silver and china in the badly crippled arthritic patient?

7. At what time of day does the chronically ill patient have the best appetite? How should this affect the menus planned for him?

8. List 5 ways in which an arthritic patient can save energy when preparing a meal.

9. What type of diet may be used in the treatment of Ménière's syndrome? Why?

10. Make out a menu for a day for a patient with multiple sclerosis who has difficutly chewing and swallowing.

11. How should food be served to a patient with myasthenia gravis? Why?

12. What are some of the problems faced by the parents of a chronically ill child? See Chapter 34.

13. How may calcium kidney stones be prevented in the paralyzed patient? (See Chap. 25.)

14. Make out a menu containing 130 Gm. of protein and 2,500 calories for a day of "easy-to-eat" foods and beverages for a patient who has been admitted with severe decubitus ulcers. Use the Pattern Dietary in Chap. 19.

15. In what way does nutrition play a role in the bladder and the bowel retraining in the rehabilitation program?

16. Why may the paralyzed patient refuse food? Why may he overeat and become overweight?

17. What are some dietary problems encountered in mentally ill patients?

18. What foods would you serve a patient who suspected that attempts were being made to poison him?

19. Why may obesity become a problem in mentally ill patients?

SUPPLEMENTARY READING ON DISEASES OF THE MUSCULOSKELETAL AND THE NERVOUS SYSTEMS

Beltsville Energy Saving Kitchen, Design 2. U. S. Dept. of Agriculture Leaflet No. 463, 1959.

Bernstein, D. S., *et al.*: Prevalence of osteoporosis in high and low fluoride areas in North Dakota. J.A.M.A., *198*:499, 1966.

Chappelle, M. L., and Borsch, R. N.: Use of food in a psychiatric setting. J. Am. Dietet. A., *42*:328, 1963.

Diet and Arthritis. The Arthritis and Rheumatism Foundation, 10 Columbus Circle, New York, N. Y. 10019.

Edit.: Detection of muscular dystrophy. New Eng. J. Med., *276*:1379, 1967.

Fluoride protection against bone loss. J.A.M.A., *200*:31 (adv.), 1967.

Hegsted, D. M.: Nutrition, bone and calcified tissue. J. Am. Dietet. A., *50*:105, 1967.

Howard, M. S.: Energy-saving Kitchen. J. Am. Dietet. A., *39*:201, 1961.

Lamont-Havers, R. W.: Nutrition and the rheumatic diseases. Part I. Arthritis and Gout. Borden's Rev., Vol. 24, No. 1, 1963.

———: Nutrition and the rheumatic diseases. Part II. Collagen diseases. Borden's Rev., Vol. 24, No. 2, 1963.

Lowman, E. W.: Aids to Independence. The Arthritis and Rheumatism Foundation, 10 Columbus Circle, New York, N. Y. 10019.

Lutwak, L., and Whedon, G. D.: Osteoporosis —a disorder of mineral nutrition. Borden's Rev., Vol. 23, No. 4, 1962.

Moser, D.: Nursing care of the myasthenic patient. Am. J. Nursing, *60*:340, 1960.

Quimby, M. A.: Care of the patient with laby-rinthine dysfunction. Am. J. Nursing, *60*: 1780, 1960.

Review: MAO inhibition and toxicity of certain foods. Nutr. Rev., *23*:326, 1965.

Volpe, A., and Kastenbaum, R.: Beer and TLC. Am. J. Nursing, *67*:100, 1967.

Walike, B. C., *et al.*: Rheumatoid arthritis. Am. J. Nursing, *67*:1420, 1967.

Youland, D. M.: Arthritis and nutrition education. J. Am. Dietet. A., *49*:326, 1966.

For further references see Bibliography in Part Four.

CHAPTER 33

Miscellaneous Metabolic Disturbances

Spontaneous Hypoglycemia · Adrenal Cortex Insufficiency ·
Hyperthyroidism · Hypothyroidism · Gout

SPONTANEOUS HYPOGLYCEMIA

Etiology. Spontaneous hypoglycemia is not a clinical entity in itself but a disturbance of carbohydrate metabolism which may be caused by a number of seemingly unrelated factors involving the liver, the pancreas and other organs of the endocrine system, as well as the nervous system. The direct cause is hyperinsulinism, or an overproduction of insulin by the pancreas. This may be a functional disturbance, or it may be due to a tumor of the pancreas, to adrenal cortex insufficiency (see later in this chapter), or it may follow prolonged stress following major surgery. When it occurs in children under 2 years old, it is more likely leucine-induced hypoglycemia, an inborn error of metabolism (see Chap. 34).

Here we shall be concerned with functional hypoglycemia only, that is, hypoglycemia without demonstrable organic disease. Conn[1] states that the individual with functional hypoglycemia tends to be intensive, driving and conscientious, implying that psychosomatic factors may play a part in precipitating an attack.

The symptoms of an attack are almost identical with those produced by an overdose of insulin and are due to a low blood sugar. There is weakness, trembling, sweating and extreme hunger. In severe cases there may be convulsions, hysterical symp-

toms and, eventually, unconsciousness. The attacks do not occur in the fasting state. They are caused by overstimulation of the pancreas resulting in the production of excess insulin, following a meal, particularly one high in quickly digested and absorbed carbohydrate. Abdominal discomfort, which is also characteristic, is sometimes ascribed to peptic ulcer because the symptoms are similar.

Dietary Treatment

The objective of dietary treatment is to prevent a marked rise in the blood sugar which stimulates the islet cells to overproduce insulin. For this reason the individual must avoid the quickly digested sugars, and limit other carbohydrate foods. The more slowly digested proteins and fats may be ingested freely.

The diet should contain from 120 to 150 Gm. of protein, from 75 to 100 Gm. of carbohydrate, and sufficient fat to meet caloric requirements. No candy, sugar, jellies, jams, desserts and soft drinks containing sugar should be eaten. Artificial sweeteners may be substituted for sugar. The low carbohydrate vegetables and fruits (see Chap. 22), and limited quantities of bread, cereal and potatoes should provide the carbohydrate of the diet. A generous serving of meat, fish, fowl, eggs or cheese must be included at each meal. Because milk contains the sugar lactose, it must be limited to a pint a day in the adult. Butter or margarine, cream, bacon, mayonnaise and other

---

[1] Conn, J. W., and Seltzer, H. S.: Am. J. Medicine, *19*:460, 1955.

oil dressing and meat fats will supply the fat needed for calories. It is best to divide the food intake into 5 to 8 meals a day. The patient may find it useful to carry crackers and a cube of cheese with him to control attacks if they are frequent.

ADRENAL CORTEX INSUFFICIENCY

Addison's disease, the medical name for the deficiency or total lack of the hormones of the adrenal cortex, is a disease entity that has been known for many years. To-day it may be produced surgically by abla-tion of the adrenal glands in the treatment of Cushing's syndrome (hyperpituitarism) or in order to delay the growth of some forms of cancer. The syndrome may also occur when the pituitary gland is removed in the treatment of cancer (hypophysec-tomy), so that the adrenal glands atrophy from lack of stimulation. In all of these conditions the physician is able to give the patient replacement therapy for the missing hormones, but, because the regula-tory mechanism is gone, certain symptoms may occur.[2]

The adrenal cortex produces three groups of hormones: the glucocorticoids, which aid in forming glucose from protein and are also insulin antagonists; the electro-corticoids, of which aldosterone is the most important, which maintain sodium-potas-sium balance in the body fluids; and the androgenic hormones, which stimulate the formation of sex hormones, but also affect the synthesis of protein for tissue mainte-nance.

If the patient has true Addison's disease, but in a mild form, he may need only salt tablets to help maintain electrolyte bal-ance. If the disease is somewhat more se-vere, salt tablets and cortisone may be suf-ficient. If the adrenal glands are entirely destroyed, either by surgery or as a result of Addison's disease, there may be symp-toms related to the lack of all three hor-mones.

Dietary Treatment

The most common occurrence in the third group of patients is hypoglycemia due to insufficient glucocorticoid hormones. As has been said earlier, these aid in the syn-thesis of glucose in protein metabolism and are also insulin antagonists. Moreover, the patient who has had an adrenalectomy seems to have an increased sensitivity to the lowering of blood sugar levels.

The hyploglycemic reactions may occur early in the morning, before breakfast, when insulin is still active but there has been no food supply of glucose for 12 hours or more; or 3 to 5 hours following a meal high in carbohydrate which has stim-ulated the production of insulin.[3] The diet should therefore be high in protein, low in carbohydrate, omitting sugar and foods containing sugar and including enough fat to meet caloric needs as described under Spontaneous Hypoglycemia. Meals must be spaced evenly throughout the day, and between meal snacks are needed to pre-vent postprandial hypoglycemia. These pa-tients, in contradistinction to patients with spontaneous hypoglycemia, must have a fairly substantial bed-time feeding, perhaps a sandwich with a meat or cheese filling and a glass of milk, to prevent an early morning hypoglycemic reaction. In the hos-pital, when diagnostic tests may interfere with the regularity of meals, care must be taken that the patient does not go without food for more than 5 hours.

Fatigue, weight loss and muscle weak-ness may also be present due to the ab-sence of androgenic hormones, especially since these are not replaced in the patient with cancer. The high protein diet de-scribed above may also be of help here.

Sodium and potassium imbalance does not usually occur because the electrocorti-coid hormones can be given as replacement therapy.

Occasionally, potassium may have to be restricted in the diet if it is not excreted in sufficient quantity by the kidney. Potas-sium is widely distributed in food (see Table 5 in Part Four), and, if it needs to be restricted, those foods with a particu-larly high potassium content must be omitted or limited.

2 Greenblatt, R. B., and Metts, J. C., Jr.: Am. J. Nursing, *60*:1249, 1960 (Sept.).

3 Reich, B. H., and Ault, L. P.: Am. J. Nursing, *60*:1252, 1960.

Teaching the Patient

In the hospital the nurse should be aware that hypoglycemic reactions may occur, particularly in the newly operated adrenalectomized or hypophysectomized patient, but also in the patient with severe, naturally occurring Addison's disease. She and the dietitian, working together, must teach the patient and his family the importance of the dietary restrictions and regulations. They must especially emphasize the need for the late evening feeding, both in the hospital and at home, to prevent hypoglycemic attacks.

HYPERTHYROIDISM

Etiology. Hyperthyroidism, as the name indicates, is a condition characterized by an excessive secretion of the thyroid gland. It is known also as thyrotoxicosis, Graves' disease or Basedow's disease. The chief symptoms are nervous irritability, fatigue, weakness, rapid pulse, loss of weight and a high basal metabolic rate. The high metabolic rate, of course, accounts for the loss of weight, for it will be remembered that the thyroid gland, through its internal secretion, is probably the chief regulator of energy metabolism. The rate of metabolism is increased from 15 to 20 per cent above normal in mild cases to 75 per cent or more in severe cases. When the metabolic rate is excessive, not only are the nutrients in the body burned too rapidly, but even the tissues are drawn upon as a source of additional fuel. Treatment consists of suppression of the production of thyroxine by drugs or by radioactive iodine; or by excision of the gland.

Dietary Treatment

It is important that extra food be given and that the patient rest to prevent unnecessary expenditure of energy. When the metabolic rate is excessive, it may be necessary to increase the food intake to from 4,000 to 5,000 calories. The high caloric diet (see Chap. 21), therefore, is indicated until normal weight has been reached and the basal metabolic rate has returned to normal levels.

The great increase in calories, if obtained largely from the usual foods in a mixed diet, will also supply the extra protein needed to restore lost tissue protein. Enough milk, at least a quart a day, should be included to offset the greatly increased excretion of calcium and phosphorus in hyperthyroidism. The additional foods will also supply an increase in vitamin intake. Since many of the vitamins, especially those of the B complex, function as parts of metabolic enzymes, the physician may increase the vitamin content of the diet further by the use of supplements to provide for the increased metabolism.

All stimulants such as tea, coffee, alcohol and tobacco are limited or omitted, depending on the doctor's orders.

HYPOTHYROIDISM

Hypothyroidism is marked by a deficient secretion of the thyroid gland. It is also known in its advanced stage as myxedema. It is characterized by a low metabolic rate, ranging from minus 15 per cent to minus 30 per cent or more, and may be said to be the antithesis of hyperthyroidism. Because of the low metabolic rate these patients gain weight rapidly. The treatment for this condition consists of medication in the form of thyroxine and the regulation of the diet, which should be a low caloric diet such as is described in Chapter 21 until normal weight is reached. This condition may be related to iodine deficiency (see Chaps. 6 and 16).

GOUT

Gout is a familial disease of defective purine metabolism, characterized by an increase in blood uric acid levels and the deposition of urate crystals in the soft tissues and in the joints, particularly of the fingers and toes. It is an ancient disease, and it is relatively common today. Very occasionally it appears in children, but the incidence is greatest in men after the age of thirty. It is relatively rare in women.

The nature of the metabolic defect is not known. It is thought that both increased formation of uric acid as well as decreased excretion from the kidney are factors. Normal blood levels of uric acid are from 2.5 to 5 mg. per 100 ml. A level of 6 mg. per cent for men, and of 5.5 mg.

per cent for women is considered as hyper-uricemia (increased uric acid in the blood), and indicative of the presence of gout, although no overt symptoms may be present. It has been found that about one third of individuals with blood uric acid levels of 8 mg. per cent or over will have an attack of gout within the next ten years, following discovery.[4]

The clinical course of gout may best be described as having three stages. The first is hyperuricemia without symptoms, perhaps discovered at a routine physical examination. The second is characterized by an acute and painful attack of gouty arthritis. The attack may subside spontaneously in from 2 days to 2 weeks, but recovery is hastened greatly by the use of uricosuric drugs. There may be a long interval before another attack occurs. Chronic tophaceous gout is the third and most severe form of the disease. Tophi or accumulations of urate crystals are present in and around one or more of the joints, causing destruction of bone and deformity.[5] (See Fig. 33–1.) Kidney stones of urate crystals may also occur.

Gout has been ascribed to the consumption of a "rich" diet, and to alcoholism. The former cause has long been discredited by the fact that most patients showing symptoms of gout have never eaten any other than an ordinary diet. The association of acute gouty attacks with alcoholism, however, has a basis in actual findings. It has been observed that patients placed on a regimen of fasting to induce weight loss have an increase in blood uric acid levels.[6] Attacks of gouty arthritis in a fasting patient has also been reported.[7] In a study of alcoholism and attacks of gout, Maclachlan believes that it is the lack of food intake which so often accompanies a drinking bout that is responsible for the precipitation of an acute gouty attack.[8]

Treatment

The source of uric acid arises from the metabolism of purines, a constituent of nucleoproteins found in all cells. Purines are obtained from ingested food and from the breakdown of body protein. Purines are also synthesized in the liver from

[4] Edit.: Am. J. Publ. Health, 55:353, 1965.

[5] Herman, I. F., and Smith, R. T.: Am. J. Nursing, 64:111, 1964 (Dec.).

[6] Spencer, H., et al.: Am. J. Med., 40:27, 1966.

[7] Drenick, E. J., et al.: J.A.M.A., 187:100, 1964.

[8] Maclachlan, M. J., and Rodnan, G. P.: Am. J. Med., 42:38, 1967.

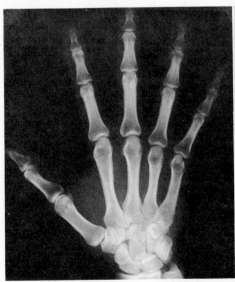 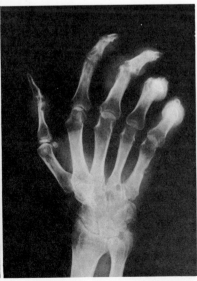

Fig. 33–1. Bones of the hand of a normal person (*left*) and of one with far-advanced gout (*right*), showing marked skeletal changes. (The Department of Radiology, The New York Hospital)

TABLE 33–1. Purine Content of Foods per 100 Grams*

Group I (0–15 mg.)	Group II (50–150 mg.)	Group III (150–800 mg.)
Vegetables	Meats, poultry	Sweetbreads
Fruits	Fish	Anchovies
Milk	Sea food	Sardines
Cheese	Beans, dry	Liver
Eggs	Peas, dry	Kidney
Cereals, bread	Lentils	Meat extracts
Sugars, fats	Spinach	Brains

* Adapted from Turner, D.: Handbook of Diet Therapy, ed. 4, University of Chicago Press, Chicago, 1965.

smaller metabolic fragments. Colchicine, a drug which has been used in the treatment of gout for many years, is thought to inhibit the metabolic reactions by which uric acid is derived from purine compounds. More recently, drugs have been available that facilitate the excretion of uric acid from the kidney. These two drugs help to lower the blood uric acid levels in patients with gout.

Dietary Restrictions. A low purine diet is seldom used routinely today. However, it is probably well for the patient with a raised blood uric acid level to avoid foods very high in purine content, such as liver, kidney, brains and sweetbreads. Patients should also be cautioned about fasting, whether to lose weight or when on an alcoholic spree, as fasting even for one or two days was found to increase the serum uric acid level.[9]

Occasionally a physician will prescribe severe restrictions of purine-containing foods during an acute gouty attack. All cellular tissues contain nucleoproteins from which purines are derived. Some plant foods also give rise to purines, as can be seen in Table 33–1. On a very restricted purine diet, all foods in Groups II and III in Table 33–1 should be omitted, and the diet contain only those foods included in Group I. As soon as the attack subsides, the patient should return to a normal, nutritionally adequate diet, omitting only those foods suggested earlier.

[9] Maclachlan, M. J.: Op. cit.

If the patient with gouty arthritis is overweight, it is important for him to lose weight to avoid strain on the involved joints. However, it should be done slowly so as not to increase the blood uric acid levels, as described above.

STUDY QUESTIONS AND ACTIVITIES

1. Plan a day's menu for a patient who is prone to attacks of spontaneous hypoglycemia. He is on a diet of 125 Gm. of protein, 150 Gm. of fat and 100 Gm. of carbohydrate. What advice would you give him?

2. Plan a day's menu for a woman who has had a hypophysectomy for cancer and who has a tendency to hypoglycemia. Which foods must be omitted, which emphasized? Why is there need for a late evening feeding?

3. A patient with hyperthyroidism has a basal metabolic rate of plus 50. What does this mean? What type of diet will be prescribed for him? Name 5 ways of increasing calories in the normal diet.

4. Why is a low caloric diet indicated in hypothyroidism? Name 5 ways in which to decrease the calories in the ordinary diet.

5. A man weighing 150 lb. has gout and is suffering from an acute attack.

   a. Plan a menu for a day for him from the foods listed in Group I in Table 33–1.

   b. Does this diet adequately meet all the patient's nutritional needs? What nutrient(s) may be low?

   c. Which foods should probably be avoided by all patients with gout?

6. What is thought to be the relationship between alcoholism and a gouty attack?

SUPPLEMENTARY READING IN MISCELLANEOUS METABOLIC DISEASES

Edit: The prevention of gout. Am. J. Publ. Health, 55:353, 1965.
Drenick, E. J., et al.: Prolonged starvation as a treatment for severe obesity. J.A.M.A., 187: 100, 1964.
Greenblatt, R. B., and Metts, J. C., Jr.: Addison's disease. Am. J. Nursing, 60:1249, 1960.
Hamilton, A.: Good news about gout. Today's Health, 45:16, 1967 (Dec.).

Herman, I. F., and Smith, R. T.: Gout and gouty arthritis. Am. J. Nursing, *64*:111, 1964 (Dec.).

Jay, A. N.: Hypoglycemia. Am. J. Nursing, *62*:77, 1962 (Jan.).

Lamont-Havers, R. W.: Nutrition and the rheumatic diseases. Part I. Borden's Rev., Vol. 24, No. 1, Jan.-Mar., 1963.

Reich, B. H., and Ault, L. P.: Nursing care of the patient with Addison's disease. Am. J. Nursing, *60*:1252, 1960.

For further references see Bibliography in Part Four.

CHAPTER 34

Nutrition in Diseases of Infancy and Childhood

Problems of Nutrition in Sick Children • The Child in the Hospital • Acute Illness in Infants • Nutritional Deficiencies in Infants and Children • Emotional Deprivation and Growth Failure • Underweight and Overweight • Long Term Illness in Infants and Children • Family Adjustment • Congenital Anomalies of the Gastrointestinal Tract and Nervous System • Nephrosis • Inborn Errors of Metabolism

PROBLEMS OF NUTRITION IN SICK CHILDREN

When children become ill they tend to regress to an earlier developmental level. This is often the case with eating habits. A baby who has been drinking from a cup will refuse fluids given this way but may accept them eagerly from a bottle. Self-feeding gives way to wanting to be fed. Also, the type of food the sick child will accept often is limited. The wisest response is to let him have his way. When he feels better, he will return quickly to his more recently acquired food practices and will make up, both in quantity and in quality, the nutrients that were missing in his diet during the time he was ill.

Nutrition may become a serious problem in the child who is chronically ill or is suffering from an illness of considerable duration. Not only must enough food be eaten to meet the immediate nutritional needs, but growth and development must also be provided for. If the sick child has a poor appetite, it may be easier for him to eat smaller meals more frequently. Occasional surprises will help him to look forward to mealtimes. A "picnic" lunch or a tea party with mother or friends may stimulate the sick child to eat more than he would otherwise. There may be need of greater variation in the preparation of food. Eggs need not be served as such but may make their appearance in salads, sandwiches and custards. Ice cream and puddings are good substitutes for some of the child's milk. Cereal cooked in milk and served with brown sugar and dates or prunes is high in nutritive value and a pleasant change from plain cooked cereal. Strained vegetables may be added to broth. Canned and strained fruits and ripe bananas may be easier to eat than fresh fruit. Angel food and sponge cake and cookies will add calories. Servings should be small so as not to overwhelm the sick child.

Children who are immobilized with fractures may suffer nitrogen and calcium loss just as adults do in these circumstances (see Chap. 18). It is essential that their protein and calcium intake be kept high by generous servings of meat, fish, poultry, eggs, milk and cheese. If the immobilization is likely to be of long duration, such as that which follows paralytic poliomyelitis, the problem is even more serious, and every effort must be made to maintain good nutrition (see Chap. 20).

The Child in the Hospital

If an infant or a child must be hospitalized, one of the immediate problems may pertain to food. The child is in strange surroundings, among strange people; moreover, he is ill. All the concepts of child feeding discussed in Chapters 13 and 14 are applicable; besides this, the child must be given a great deal of freedom about his food, even to the point of allowing him to refuse it. Some children will eat only bread and butter and drink milk for the first few days in the hospital, as these foods are most reminiscent of home. This may often be the case with children from homes with different national or regional food patterns from those in usage in the hospital. Asking the mother when the child is admitted to the hospital what his food preferences are, and meeting these insofar as possible, will help to bridge the gap between home and hospital. Other children will regress to feeding practices of an earlier age. Demands to be fed or for other types of attention should be met by the nurse with warmth and understanding. If the child is not too ill, he will soon follow the lead of other children in his group and become more self-sufficient.[1]

Many hospitals have daily visiting hours for parents in the late afternoon and the early evening, so that they may feed and play with their children. This has been extended still further by some hospitals, which permit the mother, or both parents, to stay with the child for as much time as

[1] Getty, G., and Hollensworth, M.: Nutrition Today, 2:17, 1967.

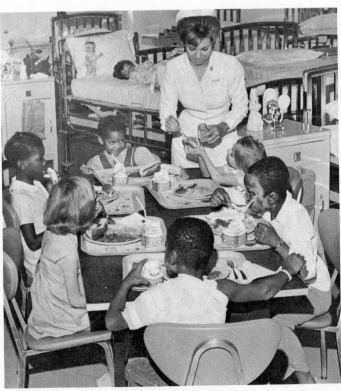

FIG. 34–1. Meals taste better when they are eaten in company with other children in the hospital. (Arkansas Children's Hospital, Little Rock, Arkansas)

they can spare, day or night, for the duration of the child's hospitalization. Not only does this minimize the trauma of separation from the mother, but the child's nutrition is less likely to suffer.

Other ways of helping the child to feel at home in the hospital is to have him eat at a table with other children of his age as soon as this is feasible. Most of all, it is important that mealtime be a happy time, with no pressures about cleaning up plates, drinking all the milk or withholding dessert because some rule about eating habits has not been complied with. During an illness is not the time for a child to have to learn to eat new foods or to acquire new skills in eating unless he does this on his own initiative.

ACUTE ILLNESS IN INFANTS
Diarrhea

Diarrhea may occur in infants and young children for a variety of reasons. It may be due to direct infection of the bowel itself, or to an infection in another part of the body. Or it may be non-specific. It may be caused by disease of the bowel such as the explosive diarrhea which often accompanies one of the disaccharidase deficiencies. Slower in onset, but equally serious is the diarrhea that is symptomatic of celiac disease or cystic fibrosis. The latter are fully discussed under Malabsorption Syndromes in Chapter 27 and later in this chapter for celiac disease in infants. Any diarrhea not responding to the measures described in the following paragraphs, or which is recurrent, should be thoroughly investigated.

Non-specific Diarrhea. A baby digests much larger quantities of food for his weight than an adult, and his digestive system is much more easily upset. Improper care of the formula or other poor sanitary conditions are often the cause of diarrhea in infants. Most such diarrheas are mild and respond to treatment quickly if they are cared for early. For this reason the doctor or the public health nurse should be consulted promptly.

The usual treatment for a mild diarrhea is to give the infant less to eat. Breast feeding may be continued, but the baby may not want the usual amount. If he is on a formula, the doctor will probably dilute it, or prescribe a diluted skim milk formula. Solid foods should be omitted. As the diarrhea subsides, there will be a gradual return to the baby's former diet.

In severe diarrhea with frequent, watery stools, the loss of fluids and electrolytes will cause serious dehydration. Such babies are usually hospitalized. All food by mouth is withheld, and intravenous feedings of water, dextrose and electrolytes are begun. After 24 to 48 hours, water or a mixture of water, glucose and electrolytes may be tried by mouth. If there is no return of diarrhea, a half-and-half mixture of boiled skim milk and water, or a skim milk formula preparation may be given, later increased to skim milk alone, after which the baby is tried on a dilute whole milk formula. Sometimes acidified skim milk is used rather than plain skim milk. These acid milks are available in powdered form. The fine curd and the acidity of the milk are thought to make this type of formula easier to digest by the baby recovering from diarrhea.

When diarrhea occurs in the toddler or the preschool child, food by mouth should be limited to boiled skim milk and dilute fruit and vegetable juices, cooked refined cereals and white bread toast. Scraped raw apple and ripe banana may be beneficial. Strained meats and cottage cheese may be added when the diarrhea begins to subside. As soon as possible the child should return to a normal food intake.

If the diarrhea does not respond or is recurrent, the physician should be consulted immediately.

Dysentery or infectious diarrhea is produced by a specific organism of the dysentery group. Its symptoms, including the presence of blood, pus and mucus in the stools, are more severe than diarrhea. Unless properly diagnosed and treated, it may become recurrent or chronic.

Since the diarrhea is caused by an infection of the intestinal tract itself and may continue for an indefinite time, even when treated with antibiotics, the principal concern is to maintain the hydration and the nutrition of the infant. The progression of fluid and formula for the infant and the diet for the older child, as described under diarrhea, may also be used in dysentery. There may be more setbacks and slower progress, depending on the severity of the infection.

Other Infections

Any infection characterized by fever usually impairs the appetite. It is not necessary to restrict food intake during the acute stages, but the infant or the child should be fed according to his appetite. He should be encouraged to take fluids freely and to return to regular food intake as soon as possible. If the child has a sore throat, it should not be aggravated by fruit juices or salty broth. As the fever subsides, the appetite usually becomes progressively better, and the food intake increases accordingly. If the fever is one of considerable duration, malnutrition may become a problem. Some of the suggestions made at the beginning of this chapter may be found helpful. See also Chapter 20.

NUTRITIONAL DEFICIENCIES

Iron Deficiency Anemia

Iron deficiency anemia may appear in premature infants, in twins, or in infants whose mothers had an inadequate intake of iron during pregnancy. Anemia may also occur in infants and young children who have been kept too long on a diet high in milk and limited in solid foods.[2] Milk, though an excellent food, is seriously deficient in several nutrients, the most notable being iron and ascorbic acid. When the small child drinks more than the needed pint or 1½ pints of milk, there is little room for other foods. The addition of iron-enriched cereal at 2 months and meat at 3 months, plus a wide variety of vegetables and fruits, and a decreasing amount of milk should prevent this type of anemia (see Chap. 13). There has been some consideration given to iron enrichment of milk, and iron-enriched commercial formulas are available. The treatment of this type of iron deficient anemia con-

sists of iron medication and a more liberal diet.

In the past few years it has been observed that some infants and young children with hypochromic, microcytic anemia show blood loss from the intestinal tract. Rasch[3] found a daily fecal loss of 0 to 4.75 ml. in 20 anemic children compared with a fecal loss of 0 to 0.35 ml. of blood in 9 non-anemic infants. In another study Hoag[4] reported a daily fecal blood loss of from 0.25 to 3.82 ml. in infants with anemia. These investigators conclude that protracted blood loss in the amounts observed can adequately explain the development of iron deficient anemia.

More recently Wilson[5] and his co-workers demonstrated intestinal bleeding in three out of five anemic infants, ranging from 0.6 to 3.96 ml. daily, caused by a heat-labile factor in milk. Bleeding ceased or abated when soybean milk or heat-modified cow's milk was substituted for the homogenized milk formula. The nature of the syndrome, the site of the intestinal bleeding and the occurrence of gastrointestinal bleeding as a cause of hypochromic, microcytic anemia in infants have not been determined.

The presence of diarrhea may also be a factor in the development of anemia in infants. Elian *et al.*[6] found a mean daily fecal blood loss of 0.64 ml. in 44 infants, 2 to 17 months of age. In 10 of these infants the average daily fecal loss of blood rose to 1.85 ml. when diarrhea was present.

Infantile Scurvy

That scurvy still occurs in the Western world despite our knowledge about its cause and prevention is shown by the following statistics.

In a survey made by the Committee on Nutrition of the American Academy of Pediatrics of 226 hospitals for the period 1956 to 1960, it was found that 713 infants were admitted for scurvy, or 1 out of every

---

[2] Smith, C. A.: J.A.M.A., *172*:568, 1960.

[3] Rasch, C. A., *et al.*: Am. J. Dis. Child., *100*:627, 1960. (Abst.).

[4] Hoag, M. S., *et al.*: Pediatrics, *27*:199, 1961.

[5] Wilson, J. F., *et al.*: J.A.M.A., *189*:568, 1964.

[6] Elian, E., *et al.*: J. Pediatr., *69*:215, 1966.

3,300 pediatric admissions. The great majority of these were from the South central and Southeastern sections of the United States.[7] In Canada an epidemiologic study revealed 87 cases of infant scurvy for the years 1961 to 1963.[8]

Scurvy may appear in infants due to the mother's lack of knowledge or understanding of proper feeding, to poor economic conditions, or to unavailability of fruit juices high in ascorbic acid. Woodruff[9] reports an increasing incidence of scurvy in a Southern city, where parents had been taught not to give their babies "pot liquor" from vegetables cooked with salt pork or bacon but had failed to substitute the suggested fruit juices.

Canada is meeting the problem of scurvy in infants by permitting the addition of vitamin C to evaporated milk. Nurses and other health workers need to be on guard to be sure that nutrition instruction is understood and followed by the family of the small infant.

Rickets

In the survey of the American Academy of Pediatrics mentioned above, the incidence of rickets in infants admitted to the hospital during the same 5-year period was 843, or 1 in 2,791 pediatric admissions. Although, again, the distribution was greater in the Southeastern part of the United States, large cities throughout the United States also showed considerable incidence.

Undoubtedly these infants did not receive sufficient vitamin D, coupled possibly with a milk intake inadequate for the proper calcification and growth of bone. Again, community health agencies need to be aware that this deficiency disease still occurs and provide both education and help in seeing that adequate food and medication are available.

A rare form of rickets, known as vitamin D resistant, hypophosphatic rickets, is a familial disease.[10] It is not due to deficiency in any of the nutrients needed for

bone formation, but to inability of the kidney tubule to reabsorb phosphate. Since bone consists largely of calcium phosphate, the mineralization of bone is decreased in infants with this disease, with the resultant lesions of rickets and osteomalacia. The problem is a medical rather than a nutritional one, although the disease may be treated with large amounts of vitamin D.

EMOTIONAL DEPRIVATION AND GROWTH FAILURE

When the physician records an infant or child's "failure to thrive," he is dealing with an unknown or unrecognized factor or factors. Many of these are being identified, such as the inborn errors of metabolism discussed later in the chapter.

Other elements besides disease entities may be responsible for a child's failure to thrive. The need for the young infant to relate to the mother or other care-taking person is particularly evident. This was first recognized in foundling and other hospitals, where babies received good physical care, but where, because of inadequate staffing, bottles were "propped" at feeding, and the infants received a minimum of handling, fondling and talking to.[11] These infants failed to thrive, were apathetic and unresponsive, until the cause was recognized and the regimen changed.

This type of deprivation may also be found in the setting of an emotionally disturbed family life. Increasingly in the past few years, reports have appeared in the literature of marked growth failure and bizarre food habits in young children. These children are short in stature to the point of being thought to suffer from dwarfism due to pituitary failure. Powell in one such study of 13 children[12] found they had voracious appetites and were said to eat 2 to 3 times as much as other children, including such items as a whole loaf of bread, a jar of mustard or mayonnaise, or a whole can of luncheon meat. Food was stolen or hidden away. There was also a history of polydipsia, the child asking frequently for water during the night, and

[7] Pediatrics, 29:646, 1962.
[8] Demers, P., *et al.*: Canad. M. A. J., 93:573, 1965.
[9] Woodruff, C. W.: J.A.M.A., 161:448, 1956.
[10] Harrison, H. E.: Am. J. Publ. Health, 56:734, 1966.

[11] Bakwin, H.: Am. J. Dis. Child., 63:30, 1942.
[12] Powell, G. F., *et al.*: New Eng. J. Med., 276: 1271; 276:1279, 1967.

drinking the dishwater, and water from the toilet bowl and from puddles.

On hospitalization Powell[13] found the height of the children to be 30 to 66 per cent of their chronological age. Weight of six of the children was lower than expected for their height; the others were of normal weight for their actual height. All but one of the children were withdrawn, and some had speech impairment. It was found that the commonest defect in six of the eight children tested was a deficiency in ACTH and growth hormone.

The social history disclosed an acutely disturbed home environment. Parents were divorced or separated, or there was marked marital strife. Some fathers were alcoholics, or unfaithful, and had marked tempers. Most spent little time at home with the children. Mothers were somewhat more difficult to evaluate, although immaturity and emotional instability were evident in some.

With a change in environment, the polydipsia and polyphagia and the food stealing pattern disappeared, consistent with improvement in personality and speech patterns. The children became more spontaneous, happier, and less withdrawn. There was a rapid gain in growth, one child growing 8 inches in one year, accompanied by equally rapid weight gains. Growth hormone returned to normal levels in the children tested.

This syndrome, although more striking because of its longer duration and physical expression, is like that described in infants who fail to thrive. Powell concludes[14] that the effect of environment on child development is complex. Short stature may be one of several consequences of a distorted parent-child relationship, and severe, prolonged malnutrition can lead to endocrine imbalance resembling hypopituitarism.

UNDERWEIGHT AND OVERWEIGHT
Underweight

Children vary greatly in their rate of growth. If a child gains weight and grows in height at a regular rate, even though he is somewhat thinner than other children of his height and age, there is no cause for alarm. The child who fails to grow and gain regularly should have his food habits and home environment investigated. Poor housing, inadequate sleeping space, working mothers and poverty may contribute to the child's failure to gain.

The school lunch program, available in most urban areas, can help the child to improve his food habits, and provide him with as much as half of the needed nutrients each day. Under the guidance of the teacher and the school nurse, children and parents may be helped to achieve better nutrition as well as better patterns of rest and sleep for the underweight child.

Anorexia. Occasionally the nurse or the doctor sees a child who suffers from anorexia as a result of the mother's anxiety about his food intake. If the child is otherwise well, reassurance is needed for the mother that a child will eat eventually if tensions are relieved and he is allowed some choice in deciding how much and what he shall eat. Spock[15] suggests serving only the foods the child likes best for the first 2 to 3 months, and omitting all actively disliked foods. For the child who has limited himself to a very few foods this may mean an inadequate diet for a while, but variety of preparation may help to introduce other foods. When the child's appetite has returned to some extent and he begins to look forward to his meals, small quantities of other foods (but never a disliked food) may be tried one at a time. It is always best to serve very small portions and let the child ask for a second helping. Eventually such a child will eat a varied and an adequate diet if the tensions about food intake are not renewed.

Obesity

With the realization that much adult obesity has its origin in childhood and adolescence, efforts are being directed to the control of excessive weight gain during the growing period. However, the same problems that occur in adult obesity are present in the younger age groups. Family patterns of obesity are found in which

---

13 Op. cit.
14 Op. cit.

15 Spock, B.: Baby and Child Care, New York, Duell, 1957.

large food intakes are the expected and accepted norm. There are psychological and emotional factors which play a role in overeating, and the problem of inactivity, a result of the cumbersomeness of the obesity as well as a factor contributing to it, is described frequently in the literature. Bruch[16] warns that we must not look on obesity as "all of one piece," and suggests that there is great need for differential diagnosis of the underlying causes of obesity in each individual.

When overweight in children is due to overeating, uncomplicated by severe emotional disturbances or entrenched family patterns, it is quite possible to help a child or an adolescent return to more normal food habits and weight.

Diet. The calorie restricted diet for a growing child should be calculated carefully so that no essential nutrients, with the

---

[16] Bruch, H.: Am. J. Publ. Health, 48:1349, 1958.

exception of calories, are omitted. For the 10 or 12 year old, the diet should include daily a quart of milk, 1 egg, 1 or 2 servings of lean meat, fish, poultry or other high protein food, 3 to 4 servings of Group A or B vegetables and 2 to 3 servings of fruit (see Exchange Lists in Chapter 22), 2 to 4 servings of bread and cereal, and 1 tablespoon of butter or margarine. Such a diet will contain from 1,500 to 1,600 calories. The use of skim milk for whole milk will reduce the calories by approximately 300. Other adjustments may have to be made, depending on the age of the child and the degree of overweight. Weight loss should not exceed 1 to 2 pounds a week.

Clear broth, gelatin desserts made with artificial sweeteners and a limited amount of non-caloric carbonated beverages may be used as "fill-up" foods. See Chapter 37 for low caloric recipes.

For those boys and girls who are entering the adolescent growth spurt and are not

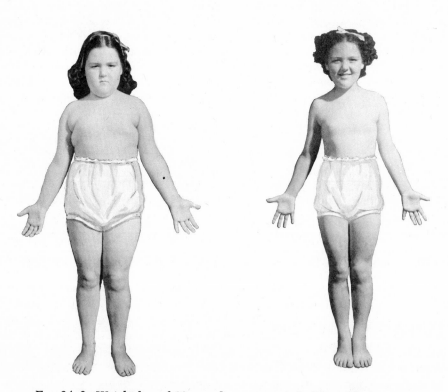

Fig. 34–2. Weight loss of 30 pounds over a period of 7 months in a 10-year-old girl. The personality improvement is at least as striking as the changes in anatomic contour. (Hoffman, R. H.: Obesity in childhood and adolescence, Am. J. Clin. Nutr. 5:1, 1957)

excessively obese, helping them to avoid any gain in weight may be the proper approach to their problem.

Exercise. The obese child or adolescent is frequently one who withdraws from active play rather than participate in it. He should be encouraged to reverse this tendency, not only because it will help to expend some of his stored energy and contribute to weight loss, but also to give him a sense of acceptance and accomplishment in his age group.

Emotional Support. One of the problems which the obese child or adolescent faces is the derogatory and rejecting attitudes often exhibited by playmates, parents and other adults. All who deal with these children should have a supportive approach. If he is on a low caloric diet, the teacher may be of help in seeing that his food in the school lunchroom is as much as possible like that of other children and that teasing is prohibited. The nurse or the dietitian following such a child should give him understanding and encouragement, even when the diet has not been strictly followed, so that he may find his own ways of developing mature and independent behavior in his choices of food. The principles involved in the treatment of obesity are further developed in Chapter 21, Weight Control.

LONG-TERM ILLNESS IN INFANTS AND CHILDREN

Family Adjustment to a Child with a Handicap or Long-Term Illness

In the literature dealing with the diseases of children, and more particularly that dealing with long-term illnesses demanding great readjustment in the family and understanding and often sacrifice by the parents, the need for constructive support is stressed again and again.[17] The financial burden of extra drugs, food and medical bills is often staggering. Other children in the family may suffer because of the time, the energy and the money expended in caring for the ill child. The parents may

have strong feelings of anxiety and guilt at having produced a less than healthy child, and these feelings may communicate themselves to the child, leading to difficult and sometimes bizarre behavior. As the child grows into adolescence, questions will arise in his mind about his future, about marriage, about having to assume his own financial care, and always, about being "different."

These are problems the doctor and the nurse will share with the family. The nurse must keep herself informed of the resources available in the community, and where financial help may be found if it is needed. She must be able to share the family's anxieties, to interpret the doctor's orders for the sick child with specific instructions, and to give the parents confidence in their own resourcefulness to plan and carry out the needed program of care.

Organizations of parents, doctors and other interested individuals, such as the United Cerebral Palsy Association and the National Cystic Fibrosis Research Foundation among others, founded to stimulate research and to promote knowledge of the disease and care of the afflicted child, are often of great help to parents by enabling them to share their anxieties and fears with others facing the same problems, and to channel them into constructive action.

Congenital Anomalies of the Gastrointestinal Tract and Nervous System

Cleft Palate and Lip

Infants born with a cleft palate usually also have a cleft lip. The latter is repaired shortly after birth, but the repair of the palate, usually done in several stages, is postponed for from one to several years if the surgery is to be successful. This leaves the infant for a length of time with a cleft in the roof of the mouth directly connected with the nasal passages. Feeding such a child presents many difficulties.

Babies with a cleft lip and palate cannot suck like other infants. They should be fed from a regular formula bottle with a nipple with an enlarged hole. This allows the formula to flow slowly to the back of the tongue and makes swallowing easier. A baby with an extensive cleft may have to

[17] Korsch, B., and Barnett, H. L.: J. Pediatr., *58:* 707, 1961; Schild, S.: Children, *11:*92, 1964; Mike, E. M.: Am. J. Clin. Nutr., *17:*399, 1965.

be fed with a 10-cc. or a 20-cc. syringe to which a 2-inch piece of sterile rubber tubing has been attached. For very small babies an eye dropper may be used in place of a syringe, or a special Brecht feeder may be of help when the baby is very young. The baby should be held upright when being fed, and burped frequently, as these babies tend to swallow air. Feeding should proceed slowly so as not to tire the baby.

Additional foods should be given as for the normally developing infant, although some adjustments may have to be made. If orange juice irritates the mucous membranes of the mouth and the nose, ascorbic acid will have to be substituted. Strained vegetables may have to be thinned out with milk or broth and given by bottle, or the baby may take them better when thickened with the crumbs of a graham cracker. "Chewy" foods, such as bread crusts, should be introduced as early as possible to aid in developing proper jaw muscles and placement of teeth. Pasty foods, such as peanut butter, cooked cheese dishes, leafy vegetables and creamed foods, all of which may form a part of the diet of the 3 year old, are poorly managed by the child with a cleft palate, as they stick to the roof of the mouth.

Because it takes these children so much longer to eat than normal children, there is a constant danger of malnutrition. The person feeding such a child needs patience and perseverance and, above all, freedom from anxiety so as not to communicate this to the child and impair the feeding process still further. A booklet "Feeding Children with Cleft Lip and Palate"* is available to help parents and public health nurses give care to these children.

Directly following surgical procedures on the cleft palate the most important aspect of feeding is to keep the repaired area clean and free of strain on the suture line. The diet is liquid and semiliquid for as long as 3 weeks (see Chap. 19). Feedings must be given by cup or the side of a spoon, never by nipple or straw.

---

* Available from Division of Crippled Children and Nutrition Services, Delaware State Board of Health, Dover, Del., or from the Division of Health Services, Washington State Department of Health, Olympia, Wash.

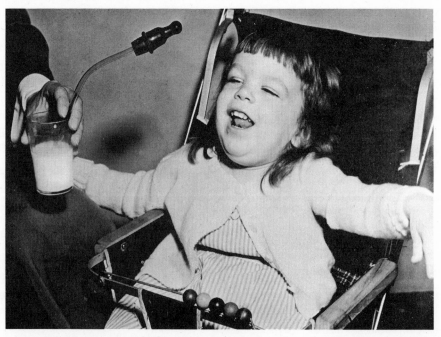

Fig. 34–3. This little girl with cerebral palsy takes her fluids via a nipple attached to a tube. (National Society for Crippled Children and Adults)

When healing has taken place, the child is returned to his regular diet. Those who have carious teeth or poor occlusion may continue to have difficulties in eating until good dental care has overcome this defect.

Cerebral Palsy

Children with cerebral palsy present very special nutrition problems. Some have swallowing difficulties. The constant movement of the child with the athetoid type of palsy increases the need for calories, yet the lack of neuromuscular control may make it difficult for him to drink from a cup or otherwise feed himself. On the other hand, the inactivity of the spastic child may lead to overweight.

The over-all nutrition of the cerebral-palsied child is often poor due to the difficulties in eating and the time required for feeding him or teaching him to feed him-

self. A study by Ruby and Matheny[18] has shown that many cerebral palsied children fall below the height and weight curves of normal children as plotted on the Iowa Growth Charts. Hammond *et al.*[19] in a study of 31 children with cerebral palsy report that the nutrient levels in more than half of the dietaries failed to meet the NRC Allowances, although most of them exceeded the 67 per cent level.

In order to meet the nutritional requirements of these children, the food should be served in as concentrated a form as possible.

Milk puddings, custards, cereals cooked in milk, added butter or margarine on

[18] Ruby, D. O., and Matheny, W. D.: J. Am. Dietet. A., *40*:525, 1962.
[19] Hammond, M. I., *et al.*: J. Am. Dietet. A., 49: 196, 1966.

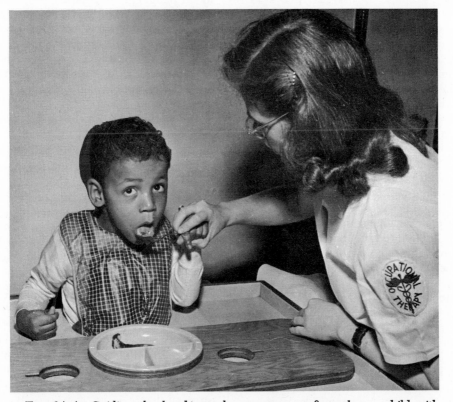

Fig. 34–4. Guiding the hand may be necessary at first when a child with cerebral palsy is learning to feed himself. Mealtime should be quiet and relaxed with all possibilities of excitement eliminated. (National Society for Crippled Children and Adults)

potatoes and bread, and creamed foods add calories and other nutrients without increasing bulk. The addition of dry skim milk to cooked cereals, meat loaf and puddings will increase the child's protein and calcium intake. The substitution of undiluted evaporated milk for the same quantity of whole milk in cooking reduces the amount of liquid that needs to be taken and increases the food value.

Foods that can be eaten in the hand, such as sandwiches, hard-cooked egg cut in quarters, whole vegetables and orange sections (rather than orange juice), will encourage the child to feed himself if his manipulative skills can be developed. Drinking from a plastic tube, as in Figure 34–3, or the use of a cup fitted with a device to reduce the rate of flow of liquid to the child's mouth will help him to take fluids without spilling. Spoons with special handles, easy to grasp, will encourage self-feeding, though it may be necessary to guide the child's hand until he becomes skilled enough to eat by himself. Foods should be those easily eaten with a spoon, such as apple sauce and mashed potatoes, rather than peas or sliced, canned peaches.

The aim for children with cerebral palsy is not only to achieve and maintain good nutrition but to help them to lead as normal a life as possible. The following suggestions may serve as a guide:

1. Strive for an adequate diet based on the same nutritional standards established for normal children.

2. Feed children who can eat only small amounts at a time 5 to 6 times a day.

3. Prepare the child's food as nearly like that of the family as practicable. Help him to feel that he belongs to the family, that he is like, not different from the other members.

4. Allow children to advance at their own rate, but keep offering new foods and experiences.

5. Praise them when they succeed but do not offer sweets as a reward. They decrease the appetite for more nutritious foods, and may cause tooth decay.

Epilepsy

A discussion of epilepsy is included in Chapter 32. The disease is usually controlled with drugs, and few dietary measures except the maintenance of good nutrition are advocated.

Recently the ketogenic diet, abandoned for many years because of its difficulty, has again been used in young patients with petit mal epilepsy who did not respond to drug therapy.[20] The diet was successful in controlling attacks, and had a favorable effect on the restlessness, hypermobility and irritability found in children with convulsive disorders. There was no depression of mental function such as may occur with drugs. Some children previously considered dull or mentally retarded, became alert, bright and sociable when the seizures were controlled by the diet.

There are many drawbacks to the use of the diet, however, and these should be considered before the regimen is attempted. It demands the use of gram scales for the weighing of all food, careful menu planning and rigid control. The diet should not be instituted until the parents are carefully assessed for their emotional stability and their ability to follow directions and accept the restrictions of the diet. Much time must be alotted to instructing them in the details of the diet if it is to be successful.

To produce ketosis, the usual ratio of protein and carbohydrate to fat in the diet must be sharply reversed. Fifty per cent of protein is glucogenic, and it is therefore restricted to 1 Gram to 1.5 Gram per Kg. of body weight, depending on the age of the child. All of the carbohydrate becomes glucose as does 10 per cent of the fat via the glycerol molecule. The remainder of the fat and approximately 50 per cent of the protein are ketogenic. Normally fatty acids are metabolized to carbon dioxide and water. When the ratio of fatty acids to available glucose exceeds 2:1, ketosis occurs. However, the ketogenic-antiketogenic (K-AK) ratio of the diet must be at least 3:1 at the beginning of treatment and maintained at a ratio of 4:1 if it is to be successful.

The method for calculating such a diet to meet the individual child's needs is

[20] Edit.: J.A.M.A., *197*:580, 1966.

TABLE 34–1. Method for Calculating a Ketogenic Diet*

Calorie requirements, rounded to the nearest 100

Age (years)	Cal./Kg. body weight
2–3	100-80
3–5	80-60
5–10	75-55

Protein requirement

1 Gm./Kg. body weight for young children
1.5 Gm./Kg. body weight for older children

To calculate for a 3:1 ratio
1 Gm. fat = 9 Cal. × 3 = 27 Cal.
1 Gm. P + C = 4 Cal. × 1 =   4 Cal.
———
31 Cal.
per unit

To calculate for a 4:1 ratio
1 Gm. fat = 9 Cal. × 4 = 36 Cal.
1 Gm. P + C = 4 Cal. × 1 =   4 Cal.
———
40 Cal.
per unit

Example: 4-year-old child, weighing 18 Kg. × 70 Cal's = 1,260 or 1,300 Calories

For a 3:1 K-AK ratio (31 Cal./unit)
1300 Cal.: 31 Cal. = 42 units
Fat 42 × 3 = 126 Gm.
P + C 42 × 1 = 42 Gm.
P (1 Gm./Kg.) 18 Gm.
C (by difference) 24 Gm.

The diet prescription with a 3:1 K-AK ratio will therefore contain 18 Gm. of protein, 126 Gm. of fat and 24 Gm. of carbohydrate

For a 4:1 K-AK ratio (40 Cal./unit)
1300 Cal.: 40 Cal. = 32.5 units
Fat 32.5 × 4 = 130 Gm.
P + C 32.5 × 1 = 32.5 Gm.
P (1 Gm./Kg.) = 18 Gm.
C (by difference) = 14.5 Gm.

The diet prescription for a 4:1 K-AK ratio will contain 18 Gm. of protein, 130 Gm. of fat and 14.5 Gm. of carbohydrate
See menu on p. 460

*From Mike, E. M.: Practical Guide and Dietary Management of Children with Seizures Using the Ketogenic Diet. Am. J. Clin. Nutr., 17:399, 1965.

given by Mike[21] (see Table 34–1). Her article includes a Table of Food Values, Allowed Foods and many suggestions for using the fats to make the diet as palatable as possible. She warns that the Exchange Lists for diabetic diets are not suitable and should not be used. Table 34–2 shows a menu for an 18-Gm. protein, 130-Gm. fat and 14.5-Gm. carbohydrate diet, with a K-AK ratio of 4:1. It illustrates some of the difficulties presented by a ketogenic diet.

It can readily be seen that milk, due to its carbohydrate content, cannot be used. All protein foods have to be sharply limited. Carbohydrate foods other than fruits and vegetables must be omitted. Butter, heavy cream, mayonnaise and oil form the main part of the diet. The protein, fat and carbohydrate should be equally divided among the 3 meals, and are calculated to the first decimal point. All foods should be eaten at each meal to maintain ketonuria.

The diet is supplemented with an aqueous solution of multiple vitamins; with calcium gluconate or calcium lactate (not as a syrup which contains carbohydrate); and with an iron medication to provide a daily amount of iron.

Hospitalization of the child is necessary to establish the ketosis and allow time for observation and for instruction of the parents. Nothing is given by mouth except 500 to 1,000 ml. of water daily for 24 to 72 hours. Hunger disappears as ketosis develops. When a high degree of ketosis has been achieved, the diet is begun with a

———
[21] Mike, E. M.: Am. J. Clin. Nutr., 17:399, 1965.

TABLE 34–2. Menu for a Ketogenic Diet with a 4:1 K-AK Ratio, Containing 18 Gm. of Protein, 130 Gm. of Fat and 14.5 Gm. of Carbohydrate*

Food	Weight (Gm.)	Protein	Fat	Carbohydrate
Breakfast				
Orange	30	0.3	0.1	3.0
Heavy cream (diluted with water for drinking)	75	1.6	28.1	2.3
Egg, cooked in	25	3.2	2.9	—
Butter	15	—	12.0	—
		5.1	43.1	5.3
Dinner				
Meat, medium fat, cooked in	20	5.6	3.2	—
Butter	15	—	12.0	—
Asparagus	30	.6	—	1.5
Lettuce	20	.4	—	1.0
Mayonnaise	20	.2	16.0	—
Oil (added to mayonn.)	10	—	10.0	—
Cantaloupe	20	.2	—	2.0
		7.0	41.2	4.5
Supper				
Egg, hard cooked	25	3.2	2.9	—
Spinach, cooked in	30	.6	—	1.5
Butter	10	—	8.1	—
Lettuce	20	.4	—	1.0
Mayonnaise	20	.2	16.0	—
Heavy cream, whipped with	50	1.1	18.8	1.5
Apple sauce	10	.1	—	.5
		5.6	45.8	4.5
Totals for the day		17.7	130.1	14.3

* All figures obtained from Mike, E. M.: Practical Guide and Dietary Management of Children with Seizures Using the Ketogenic Diet. Am. J. Clin. Nutr., 17:399, 1965.

3:1 K-AK ratio, then changed to the 4:1 K-AK ratio for the duration of treatment. There may be nausea or vomiting at first, but this disappears. A strongly positive ketonuria should be maintained at all times.

The diet is continued for 1 to 3 years, then a gradual return to a normal diet is made by slowly reducing the fat and increasing the protein and carbohydrate as directed by the physician.

Nutritional Needs of the Mentally Retarded Child

The nutrient needs of the mentally retarded child are generally similar to those of normal children of the same age, size and activity. Exceptions to this are chil-

dren with inborn errors of metabolism such as phenylketonuria and galactosemia who require special diets to prevent or control brain damage, described later in this chapter. Children with athetoid cerebral palsy, who may or may not be retarded mentally, require diets higher in calories than their normal peers because of their constant involuntary movements. This is also discussed earlier in the chapter.

Retarded children may differ from normal children in respect to the kinds of food used to meet their nutrient needs. The age at which they are introduced to solid foods and self-feeding programs, and the manner in which food is served to them may be different from that of the normal child. These aspects of nutritional care must be adjusted in accordance with the retarded child's emotional and psychological age rather than in accordance with his chronologic age.

An understanding of the usual sequence of development of food acceptance and food handling abilities of normal children will assist the parent or the nurse in caring for the mentally retarded child. Most retarded children go through the same developmental sequence as the normal child. However, there will be marked differences in the rate and the timing of this sequence. Educable and trainable children will probably take from 2 to 4 times as long as the normal child to develop independent eating patterns. The nontrainable mentally retarded patient may remain at the infantile level of this process throughout adolescence and adulthood. Thus, the feeding problems of the mentally retarded child are apt to be similar to those of the first 2 years of normal children, but extend over a much longer time span.

The emotional reactions of the parents and siblings to the retarded member of the family may affect the nutritional status and training of the retarded child. Signs of neglect, overfeeding and lack of discipline are frequently seen in retarded children whose families have not been able to accept and work with the problem. This is regrettable, because educable and trainable retarded children can achieve satisfactory eating habits and take pride in this accomplishment.

Other Long-Term Illness

Nephrosis

Nephrosis is a relatively uncommon disorder of unknown etiology, which occurs in young children, the onset being at 2 to 4 years of age. It is characterized by massive loss of albumin in the urine, hypoproteinemia and edema. Hematuria, common in nephritis, is absent or minimal in nephrosis. Treatment with steroid hormones results in diuresis and clinical remission toward the end of 2 weeks in 90 per cent of children. Somewhat later the albuminuria will disappear and serum levels of protein return to normal. Relapse will occur if steroids are withdrawn at this point. Most children will need therapy for 1 to 2 years before a full, sustained remission without therapy is achieved.[22]

The use of such continued corticosteroid therapy may cause a number of undesirable side effects, such as the development of cushingoid features, depression and withdrawal, and poor intellectual performance. More serious is the appearance of osteoporosis, gastrointestinal bleeding, convulsions and growth arrest. In a recent paper Soyka[23] reports on an alternate day administration of steroid therapy which greatly minimized the occurrence of these side effects.

The prognosis in nephrosis is much improved today over the pre-steroid era. Saxena[24] reports an 80 to 90 per cent survival of patients followed for 5 years, and states that complete remission in about 70 per cent of patients can be expected.

Dietary Treatment. The untreated nephrotic child is anorexic, irritable and miserable. The emphasis should be on good general nutrition. Sufficient calories, and palatability and attractiveness of food are the first priority, rather than protein content or too rigid sodium restriction. The diet should be that of the age group of the child, and he should be allowed to eat what he wants of it rather than trying to meet a nutritional standard. When the edema subsides, the appetite will return, and nutritional losses can be made up.

The child with nephrosis typifies the emotional impact of such disease on the family, spoken of at the beginning of this chapter. The physician and nurse must be keenly aware of the need for support and relief of anxiety and guilt for the parents, and help the child achieve as normal a life as possible.

Malabsorption Syndromes

The malabsorption syndromes found in children—Cystic Fibrosis; Disaccharidase Deficiency; Defective Monosaccharide Absorption—are discussed in detail in Chap-

---

[22] Saxena, K. M., and Crawford, J. D.: New Eng. J. Med., *272*:522, 1965.
[23] Soyka, L. F.: Am. J. Dis. Child., *113*:693, 1967.
[24] Op. cit.

ter 27, Diseases of the Intestines. The dietary treatment of Celiac Disease is also included in this chapter. However, the infant or very young child with celiac disease may first be seen in celiac crisis, and subsequently must have his diet adjusted both for the disease and for his age. A description of his treatment as outlined by di Sant'Agnese[25] follows.

CELIAC DISEASE IN VERY YOUNG CHILDREN

If the patient is in celiac crisis on admission, fluid and electrolyte balance are restored by intravenous therapy. Nothing is given by mouth. When the child has improved sufficiently, usually in from 24 to 48 hours, he is placed on a high protein, low fat, no starch (of any kind) diet. Foods permitted are:

Protein milk or boiled skim or whole milk
Sieved or minced liver and beef
Uncreamed cottage cheese
Eggs
Orange, grapefruit or apple juice
Ripe bananas, banana flakes, apple sauce, scraped raw apple
Strained green beans, carrots and squash; tomato juice.

The small child with celiac disease may present a picture of moderate to severe malnutrition. Since the above foods are well tolerated, the total food intake may be quite large and, despite the limitations of the diet, may more than meet the nutritional requirements. However, most physicians prescribe added vitamins and mineral supplements.

In from 1 to 6 months, depending on the rate of recovery and the age of the child, other foods are added gradually, but no wheat, rye, oats, barley or buckwheat is permitted. The exclusion of all cereal grains except corn, rice, soybean flour and wheat starch is no easy matter, especially for the small child. He will want to eat what the other members of the famiy are eating and cannot understand why this is denied him. Neighbors and friends must be warned not to offer cookies or cake, as ingestion of any of the forbidden cereals will cause prompt

return of symptoms. A full discussion of the gluten-free diet and the table listing the Foods Allowed and the Foods to Be Omitted will be found under Celiac Disease in Chapter 27. Recipes for bread, biscuits, cookies and other foods using the permitted flours will be found in Chapter 40.

DIABETES

The dietary treatment of diabetes is discussed in Chapter 22.

CARDIAC DISEASE

The dietary treatment of cardiac disease will be found in Chapter 24.

NEPHRITIS

The dietary treatment of kidney disease, with the exception of Nephrosis which is included in this chapter, will be found in Chapter 25.

ALLERGY

A discussion of allergy in infants and children has been included in Chapter 30.

INBORN ERRORS OF METABOLISM

A number of diseases are known to be due to a specific metabolic defect. Among the best known of these are diabetes and gout. In the last 30 years, as our knowledge of the control of metabolic processes by enzymes has increased, a growing number of diseases due to an inborn error of metabolism (lack of an enzyme) are being identified. This includes diseases of carbohydrate metabolism such as the glycogen storage diseases and galactosemia. An ever-increasing list of amino acid disorders are grouped under the name aminoacidurias. Recently a defect in the metabolism of short-chain fatty acids C:4 and C:6 has been reported.[26] Inborn errors of the metabolism of minerals and vitamins are also known. Vitamin-D-resistant rickets, discussed earlier in the chapter, falls into this category. Many of the defects are of genetic origin as shown by family histories.

The effects of disease due to a metabolic defect may be extremely serious, especially if they occur in newborn infants and young

25 di Sant'Agnese, P. A., and Jones, W. O.: J.A.M.A., *180*:308, 1962.

26 Sidbury, J. B., *et al.*: J. Pediatrics, *70*:8, 1967.

children. Death intervenes in some, because, even when the disease is recognized, there is no known therapy for it. In several diseases of inborn metabolic errors, mental retardation occurs unless the disease is treated promptly. In others the child may live on for a few years but die eventually. And in a few, such as alkaptonuria, an amino acid defect in which the urine becomes dark on standing, the condition is harmless, at least in infancy and childhood, although some pathologic effects become evident by the third decade of life. In the following pages only phenylketonuria and galactosemia, for which dietary treatment has been used successfully for some years, will be discussed in detail. Several other diseases due to inborn metabolic errors will be mentioned briefly. For full discussion the student is referred to the survey articles included in the Supplementary Reading at the end of the chapter, and to the Bibliography in Part Four.

Phenylketonuria

Phenylketonuria is a familial disease inherited through a simple autosomal recessive gene, and is characterized by the presence of phenylpyruvic acid in the urine. Fölling in Norway in 1934 was the first to describe the disease when he discovered phenylpyruvic acid in the urine of two siblings. Affected individuals lack the liver enzyme phenylalanine hydroxylase which converts the amino acid phenylalanine to tyrosine under normal circumstances (see Fig. 34–5). As soon as a newborn infant with phenylketonuria begins to take milk, his serum phenylalanine and phenylpyruvic acid levels will rise. Later these substances will be excreted in the urine.

If the disease goes untreated, about 90 per cent of individuals will develop severe mental retardation. They also usually show neurological disturbances such as irritability, hyperactivity and convulsive seizures. Because tyrosine is involved in the formation of melanin pigments in the body (see Fig. 34–5), these patients are often blond, fair skinned and blue eyed, even when other family members are of darker coloration. It is estimated that from one half to 1 per cent of all patients in institutions for the mentally retarded are phenylketonurics. The continued high level of phenylalanine and its metabolites in the blood is believed in some way to be responsibe for the cerebral damage.

Treatment of the disease was delayed for many years because there was no known method for limiting phenylalanine in the diet. All foods except oils and sugars con-

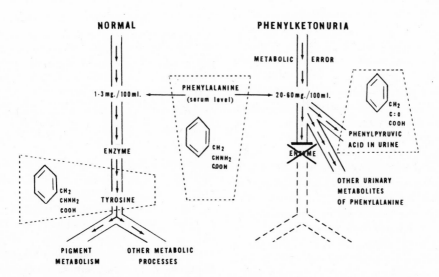

FIG. 34–5. The pathway of phenylalanine metabolism, normally and in phenylketonuria. (Phenylketonuria. Children's Bureau Publ. No. 388, 1965. Department of Health, Education and Welfare)

tain protein. Since all proteins are estimated to contain from 4 to 6 per cent of phenylalanine, the diet is an extremely restricted one. With the development of a satisfactory low-phenylalanine diet described later in the chapter, it has been possible for these children to grow normally both mentally and physically if the diet is started in the first few months of life. Therefore dietary treatment is recommended for all phenylketonurics early in infancy. When the disease is discovered later, dietary treatment is not effective in preventing mental retardation, although the behavior of the child appears to improve with such treatment.

In order to prevent the mental retardation caused by phenylketonuria, a procedure for screening of newborn infants by a simple blood test in the first few days of life, after feeding has begun, has been adopted by law in many states. At present 32 states have compulsory screening programs for all newborn infants, and 5 other states offer this service but have not made it mandatory.

It has become evident, however, that not all infants with an increased serum level of phenylalanine and excretion of phenylpyruvic acid in the urine are true phenylketonurics. Because these infants showed up in the screening process as presumed to have the disease, they were placed on a low-phenylalanine diet, in some instances with disastrous results.[27] It is also known that some adults with phenylketonuria are of normal intelligence and have none of the other symptoms associated with the disease.

In a summary by Berry and Wright[28] of a conference on the treatment of phenylketonuria, 3 types of the syndrome are described. True phenylketonuria is characterized by a rapid rise in serum phenylalanine and the appearance of phenylpyruvic acid in the urine. A second group, including about 25 per cent of low weight and some normal weight infants, is thought to have delayed maturation of the enzyme systems involved in the metabolism of

phenylalanine and tyrosine. They have increased levels of both amino acids in the blood, but these become normal on the administration of vitamin C. A third group is less clearly defined. The rise in serum phenylalanine levels is slow and may remain elevated for some time, but at lower levels than in true phenylketonuria.

For these reasons a caution is sounded against the uncritical application of a low-phenylalanine diet to all infants with an increase in serum phenylalanine. The Committee on Fetus and Newborn of the American Academy of Pediatrics recommends a blood test for elevated serum phenylalanine for all infants 24 hours after the onset of milk feeding, followed by a second blood test at 4 to 6 weeks. The latter will detect infants with borderline serum phenylalanine concentrations who do not have phenylketonuria, and confirm those who do. The Committee advises particular attention to an infant in a family where another member is known to have phenylketonuria. It also recommends that the blood samples be sent to a large central facility with experience in testing and interpreting phenylalanine blood levels.[29]

Dietary Treatment

Phenylalanine is an essential amino acid which the body needs for growth and maintenance. In the phenylketonuric child the diet must provide all the essentials for good nutrition, while the phenylalanine content of the diet must be so limited that it will provide only the minimal amount needed without raising the blood levels above normal. As has already been said, all proteins, from whatever source, contain from 4 to 6 per cent of phenylalanine, and this makes the diet an extremely restricted one. See Table 4, Part Four.

If mental retardation is to be prevented, the disease must be found and treated in early infancy. The first need, therefore, is for a formula that contains only minimal amounts of phenylalanine and can continue to be used as the main source of protein in the diet.

[27] Rouse, B. M.: J. Pediat., *69*:246, 1966.
[28] Berry, H. K., and Wright, S.: J. Pediat., *70*:142, 1967.

[29] Pediatrics, *35*:499, 1965, Part 1.

Lofenalac,* derived from casein hydrolysate, is such a formula. By filtering the hydrolysate through charcoal, all but a very small amount of phenylalanine is removed. This process also removes the other two aromatic amino acids, tryptophan and tyrosine, which are restored to the formula after filtering. Fat, carbohydrate and certain minerals and vitamins are added to the basic amino acid powder to make Lofenalac a complete formula with the exception of phenylalanine. One measure (tablespoon) of Lofenalac added to 60 ml. (2 ounces) of water provides 1½ Gm. of protein and 7½ mg. of phenylalanine, and yields 20 calories to the ounce. It has almost the same appearance and consistency as milk, but a somewhat different flavor, and most infants accept it without difficulty. It is used as the main source of protein throughout the years of treatment.

In order to provide the limited but essential amount of phenylalanine needed for growth and maintenance of the infant with phenylketonuria, it may become necessary to supplement the formula with small quantities of additional protein. These requirements will vary with the individual infant, and will change as he grows older. For the young infant the supplementation would be made by adding a small amount of milk to the formula.

When the baby would normally begin to eat solid foods, fruits and vegetables containing no more than 1 per cent of protein are substituted for or added to the small amounts of milk. The physician decides on the basis of the infant's blood level of phenylalanine and on his progress how much phenylalanine should supplement that present in the amount of formula being given.

Exchange Lists for the Low-Phenylalanine Diet, Tables 34–3, and 34–4, show the foods and quantities used, grouped in 15- and 30-milligram equivalents. Some examples of menus for various ages will be found on p. 470, Table 34–5. From these menus it can be seen that the bulk of protein, calories and other nutrients will continue to be provided by the formula and from foods of very low protein content.

* Mead Johnson Laboratories, Evansville, Indiana.

TABLE 34–3. Average Nutrient Content of Serving Lists*

List	Phenyl-alanine mg.	Protein Gm.	Calories
Vegetables	15	0.5	10
Fruits			
Strained and Junior	15	0.6	150
Table and Juices	15	0.6	70
Breads and Cereals	30	0.6	30
Fats	5	0.1	60
Desserts†	30	varies	varies

* From The Phenylalanine Restricted Diet—for Professional Use, 1966. The Bureau of Public Health Nutrition of the California State Department of Public Health.

† Average of dessert recipes in Phenylalanine-Restricted Diet Recipe Book.

A booklet, Phenylketonuria, containing somewhat more limited Exchange Lists, may be obtained from the Children's Bureau.[30] The State of California Health Department has a booklet, The Phenylalanine-Restricted Diet for Professional Use, from which Tables 34–3, 4, and 5 are taken. The latter also has available a Diet Guide for Parents of Children with Phenylketonuria and a Phenylalanine-Restricted Diet Recipe Book.[31] However, the two booklets published by the California State Department of Public Health are not available for distribution outside of California.

One of the problems of the diet is that at present we do not have precise knowledge of the true phenylalanine content of food. Most figures are derived from the empiric formula that 5 per cent of the protein of a given food is phenylalanine. Miller[32] has shown that the phenylalanine content of some fruits and vegetables is considerably lower than this. There will undoubtedly be refinements in the Exchange Lists as figures for phenylalanine content of food by chemical analysis become available.

30 Children's Bureau Publ. 388, 1965, Department of Health, Education and Welfare, Washington 25, D. C.

31 Bureau of Public Health Nutrition, California State Department of Public Health.

32 Miller, G. T., et al.: J. Am. Dietet. A., 46:43, 1965.

TABLE 34–4. Serving Lists for Phenylalanine Restricted Diet*

Food	Amount	Phenylalanine mg.	Protein Gm.	Calories
VEGETABLES				
Each serving as listed contains 15 milligrams of phenylalanine				
Baby and Junior				
Beets........................	7 tbsp.	15	1.1	35
Carrots.......................	7 tbsp.	15	0.7	28
Creamed Spinach..............	1 tbsp.	16	0.4	6
Green Beans...................	2 tbsp.	15	0.3	7
Squash.......................	4 tbsp.	14	0.4	14
Table Vegetables				
Asparagus, cooked..............	1 stalk	12	0.6	4
Beans, green, cooked...........	4 tbsp. (¼ cup)	14	0.6	9
Beans, yellow, wax, cooked......	4 tbsp. (¼ cup)	15	0.6	9
Bean Sprouts, mung, cooked	2 tbsp.	18	0.6	5
Beets, cooked..................	8 tbsp. (½ cup)	14	0.8	34
Beet greens, cooked............	1 tbsp.	14	0.2	3
Broccoli, cooked...............	1 tbsp.	11	0.3	3
Brussels Sprouts, cooked........	1 medium	16	0.6	5
Cabbage, raw, shredded........	8 tbsp. (½ cup)	15	0.7	12
Cabbage, cooked..............	5 tbsp. (⅓ cup)	16	0.8	12
Carrots, raw...................	1/6 large (¼ cup)	16	0.5	16
Carrots, cooked...............	8 tbsp. (½ cup)	17	0.5	23
Cauliflower, cooked............	3 tbsp.	18	0.6	6
Celery, cooked, diced†.........	4 tbsp. (¼ cup)	15	0.4	6
Celery, raw†...................	1–8 inch stalk	16	0.5	7
Chard leaves, cooked...........	2 tbsp.	19	0.6	6
Collards, cooked...............	1 tbsp.	16	0.5	5
Cucumber slices, raw...........	8 slices, ⅛" thick	16	0.7	12
Eggplant, diced, raw...........	3 tbsp.	18	0.4	9
Kale, cooked	2 tbsp.	20	0.5	5
Lettuce†......................	3 small leaves	13	0.4	5
Mushrooms, cooked†............	2 tbsp.	14	0.4	35
Mushrooms, fresh†..............	2 small	16	0.5	3
Mustard greens, cooked.........	2 tbsp.	18	0.6	6
Okra, cooked†.................	2–3" pods	13	0.4	7
Onion, raw, chopped...........	5 tbsp. (⅓ cup)	14	0.5	20
Onion, cooked.................	4 tbsp. (¼ cup)	14	0.5	19
Onion, young scallion...........	5–5" long	14	0.5	23
Parsley, raw, chopped†.........	3 tbsp.	13	0.4	5
Parsnips, cooked, diced†........	3 tbsp.	13	0.3	18
Peppers, raw, chopped†........	4 tbsp.	13	0.4	12
Pickles, Dill...................	8 slices–⅛" thick	16	0.7	12
Pumpkin, cooked...............	4 tbsp. (¼ cup)	14	0.5	16
Radishes, red, small†...........	4	13	0.4	8
Rutabagas, cooked.............	2 tbsp.	16	0.3	10
Soups				
Beef broth (Campbell's condensed).	1 tbsp.	14	0.5	3
Celery (Campbell's condensed)....	2 tbsp.	18	0.4	19
Minestrone (Campbell's condensed).	1 tbsp.	17	1.5	25
Mushroom (Campbell's condensed).	1 tbsp.	11	0.2	17
Onion (Campbell's condensed).....	1 tbsp.	14	0.6	8
Tomato (Campbell's condensed)....	1 tbsp.	11	0.2	11
Vegetarian Veg. Soup (Campbell's condensed)..................	1½ tbsp.	17	0.4	14
Spinach, cooked.................	1 tbsp.	15	0.4	3
Squash, summer, cooked...........	8 tbsp. (½ cup)	16	0.6	16

*From The Phenylalanine-Restricted Diet—for Professional Use, 1966. The Bureau of Public Health Nutrition of the California State Department of Public Health.

† Phenylalanine calculated as 3.3 per cent of total protein.

TABLE 34–4 (Continued)

Food	Amount	Phenylalanine mg.	Protein Gm.	Calories
VEGETABLES (Continued)				
Squash, winter, cooked..............	3 tbsp.	16	0.6	14
Tomato, raw......................	½ small	14	0.5	10
Tomato, cooked...................	4 tbsp. (¼ cup)	15	0.6	10
Tomato juice......................	4 tbsp. (¼ cup)	17	0.6	12
Tomato catsup....................	2 tbsp.	17	0.6	34
Turnip Greens, cooked.............	1 tbsp.	18	0.4	4
Turnips, diced, cooked.............	5 tbsp. (⅓ cup)	16	0.4	12
FRUITS				
Each serving as listed contains 15 milligrams of phenylalanine				
Baby and Junior				
Applesauce and apricots.........	16 tbsp. (1 cup)	15	0.6	205
Applesauce and pineapple.......	16 tbsp. (1 cup)	11	0.5	176
Apricots with tapioca............	16 tbsp. (1 cup)	16	0.6	187
Bananas........................	8 tbsp. (½ cup)	14	0.6	97
Bananas and pineapple..........	16 tbsp. (1 cup)	18	0.6	187
Peaches........................	10 tbsp.	15	0.7	124
Pears..........................	12 tbsp. (¾ cup)	16	0.5	106
Pears and pineapple............	16 tbsp. (1 cup)	17	1.0	166
Plums with tapioca..............	12 tbsp. (¾ cup)	16	0.5	163
Prunes with tapioca.............	12 tbsp. (¾ cup)	16	0.5	152
Fruit Juices				
Apricot nectar..................	6 oz. (¾ cup)	14	0.6	102
Cranberry juice.................	12 oz. (1½ cup)	15	0.6	39
Grape juice.....................	4 oz. (½ cup)	14	0.5	80
Grapefruit juice................	8 oz. (1 cup)	16	1.2	104
Orange juice....................	6 oz. (¾ cup)	16	1.2	84
Peach nectar....................	5 oz. (⅔ cup)	15	0.5	75
Pineapple juice.................	6 oz. (¾ cup)	16	0.6	90
Prune juice.....................	4 oz. (½ cup)	16	0.5	84
Table Fruits				
Apple, raw.....................	4 small 2½″ diam.	16	0.8	176
Applesauce.....................	16 tbsp. (1 cup)	12	0.6	192
Apricots, raw...................	1 medium	12	0.5	25
Apricots, canned................	2 medium 2 tbsp. syrup	14	0.6	80
Avocado, cubed or mashed†......	5 tbsp. (⅓ cup)	16	0.6	80
Banana, raw, sliced.............	4 tbsp. (¼ cup)	15	0.4	32
Blackberries, raw†.............	5 tbsp. (⅓ cup)	14	0.6	25
Blackberries, canned, in syrup†....	5 tbsp. (⅓ cup)	13	0.5	55
Blueberries, raw or frozen†.......	12 tbsp. (¾ cup)	16	0.6	60
Blueberries, canned, in syrup†.....	10 tbsp.	16	0.6	140
Boysenberries, frozen, sweetened†.	8 tbsp. (½ cup)	16	0.6	72
Cantaloupe.....................	5 tbsp. (⅓ cup)	16	0.4	15
Cherries, sweet, canned, in syrup†..	8 tbsp. (½ cup)	16	0.6	104
Dates, pitted, chopped...........	3 tbsp.	18	0.7	96
Figs, raw†.....................	1 large	18	0.7	40
Figs, canned, in syrup†..........	2 figs 4 tsp. syrup	16	0.6	90
Figs, dried†....................	1 small	16	0.6	40
Fruit cocktail†.................	12 tbsp. (¾ cup)	16	0.6	120
Grapes, American type..........	8 grapes	14	0.5	24
Grapes, American slipskin........	5 tbsp. (⅓ cup)	16	0.6	25
Grapes, Thompson seedless.......	8 tbsp. (½ cup)	13	0.8	64
Guava, raw†..................	½ medium	13	0.5	35
Honeydew melon†.............	¼ small 5″ melon	13	0.5	32
Mango, raw†.................	1 small	18	0.7	66

† Phenylalanine calculated as 2.6 per cent of total protein.

TABLE 34-4 (Continued)

Food	Amount	Phenylalanine mg.	Protein Gm.	Calories
FRUITS (Continued)				
Table Fruits (Continued)				
Nectarines, raw..................	1–2" high, 2" diam.	15	0.4	45
Oranges, raw...................	1 medium 3" diam. or ⅔ cup sections	15	1.1	60
Papayas, raw†..................	¼ med. or ½ cup	14	0.6	36
Peaches, raw...................	1 medium	15	0.5	46
Peaches, canned, in syrup.......	2 medium halves	18	0.6	88
Pears, raw.....................	1–3" × 2½"	14	1.3	100
Pears, canned, in syrup.........	2 med. halves 2 tbsp. syrup	14	1.3	78
Pineapple, raw†................	16 tbsp. (1 cup)	16	0.6	80
Pineapple, canned, in syrup†......	2 small slices	13	0.5	93
Plums, raw.....................	½–2" plum	12	0.3	15
Plums, canned, in syrup..........	3–2 tbsp. syrup	16	0.5	91
Prunes, dried..................	2 large	14	0.4	54
Raisins, dried seedless..........	2 tbsp.	14	0.5	54
Raspberries, raw†..............	5 tbsp. (⅓ cup)	13	0.5	25
Raspberries, canned, in syrup†....	6 tbsp.	14	0.5	78
Strawberries, raw†.............	8 large	16	0.6	32
Strawberries, frozen†...........	6 tbsp.	14	0.5	108
Tangerines....................	1½ large	15	1.2	66
Watermelon†..................	½ cup cubes	13	0.5	28
BREADS AND CEREALS				
Each serving as listed contains 30 milligrams of phenylalanine				
Baby and Junior				
Cereals, ready to serve				
Barley.....................	3 tbsp.	32	0.8	24
Oatmeal....................	2 tbsp.	34	0.8	16
Rice.......................	5 tbsp. (⅓ cup)	30	0.6	40
Wheat.....................	2 tbsp.	30	0.6	17
Creamed corn................	3 tbsp.	30	0.5	27
Sweet Potatoes (Gerber's).......	3 tbsp.	32	0.5	31
Table Foods				
Cereals, cooked				
Cornmeal...................	4 tbsp. (¼ cup)	29	0.6	29
Cream of rice...............	4 tbsp. (¼ cup)	35	0.7	34
Cream of wheat..............	2 tbsp.	27	0.6	16
Farina.....................	2 tbsp.	25	0.5	18
Malt-o-meal.................	2 tbsp.	27	0.5	17
Oatmeal....................	2 tbsp.	32	0.7	18
Pettijohns...................	2 tbsp.	24	0.5	19
Ralstons....................	2 tbsp.	34	0.7	18
Rice, brown or white..........	4 tbsp. (¼ cup)	35	0.7	34
Wheatena...................	2 tbsp.	27	0.5	19
Cereals, ready to serve				
Alpha bits..................	4 tbsp. (¼ cup)	32	0.6	28
Cheerios	3 tbsp.	32	0.6	20
Corn Chex..................	4 tbsp. (¼ cup)	29	0.6	32
Cornfetti...................	5 tbsp. (⅓ cup)	31	0.6	46
Cornflakes..................	5 tbsp. (⅓ cup)	29	0.6	30
Crispy Critters..............	4 tbsp. (¼ cup)	30	0.6	28
Kix........................	5 tbsp. (⅓ cup)	31	0.6	31
Krumbles...................	3 tbsp.	32	0.7	26
Rice Chex..................	6 tbsp.	32	0.7	49
Rice flakes.................	5 tbsp. (⅓ cup)	33	0.6	32

† Phenylalanine calculated as 2.6 per cent of total protein.

TABLE 34–4 (Continued)

Food	Amount	Phenylalanine mg.	Protein Gm.	Calories
BREADS AND CEREALS *(Continued)*				
Table Foods (Continued)				
Rice Krispies...............	6 tbsp.	30	0.6	40
Rice, puffed.................	12 tbsp. (¾ cup)	30	0.6	38
Sugar Crisp puffed wheat......	4 tbsp. (¼ cup)	30	0.6	46
Sugar sparkled flakes.........	5 tbsp. (⅓ cup)	29	0.6	55
Wheat Chex................	10 biscuits	30	0.6	22
Wheaties...................	3 tbsp.	26	0.5	20
Wheat, puffed..............	6 tbsp.	30	0.6	16
Crackers				
Barnum Animal.............	5	30	0.6	45
Graham (65/lb.).............	1	26	0.5	30
Ritz (no cheese).............	2	24	0.5	34
Saltines (140/lb.).............	2	29	0.6	28
Soda (63/lb.)...............	1	36	0.7	30
Wheat thins (248/lb.)........	5	30	0.6	45
Corn, cooked.................	2 tbsp.	32	0.7	17
Hominy......................	2 tbsp.	32	0.7	17
Macaroni, cooked..............	1½ tbsp.	31	0.7	20
Noodles, cooked..............	3 tbsp.	32	0.7	20
Popcorn, popped..............	5 tbsp. (⅓ cup)	31	0.6	17
Potato chips..................	4–2″ diam.	30	0.6	44
Potato, Irish, cooked............	3 tbsp.	33	0.8	31
Spaghetti, cooked..............	1 tbsp.	24	0.5	14
Sweet potato, cooked..........	2 tbsp.	25	0.4	31
Tortilla, corn..................	1½–6″ diam.	30	0.8	31

FATS

Each serving as listed contains 5 milligrams of phenylalanine

Food	Amount	Phenylalanine mg.	Protein Gm.	Calories
Butter..........................	1 tbsp.	5	0.1	100
French dressing, commercial.........	1 tbsp.	5	0.1	59
Margarine......................	1 tbsp.	5	0.1	100
Mayonnaise, commercial...........	½ tbsp.	5	0.1	30
Olives, green or ripe.............	1 medium	5	0.1	12

DESSERTS

Each serving as listed contains 30 milligrams of phenylalanine

Food	Amount
Cake†...	1/12 of cake
Cookies–Rice flour†..	2
Corn starch†..	2
Cookies, Arrowroot...	1½
Ice Cream–Chocolate†...	⅔ cup
Pineapple†..	⅔ cup
Strawberry†..	⅔ cup
Jello..	⅓ cup
Puddings†..	½ cup
Sauce, Hershey...	2 tbsp.
Wafers, sugar, Nabisco..	5

† Low phenylalanine recipes—in Phenylalanine-Restricted Diet Recipe Book.

TABLE 34–4 (Continued)

FREE FOODS

Contain little or no phenylalanine.
May be used as desired.

Apple juice
Beverages, carbonated
Gingerbread†
Guava Butter
Candy
  Butterscotch
  Cream Mints
  Fondant
  Gum drops
  Hard
  Jelly beans
  Lollipops
Cherries, Maraschino
Fruit ices (if no more than ½ cup used daily)
Cornstarch
Jell-quik

Jellies
Kool-ade
Lemonade
Molasses
Oil
Pepper, black, ground
Popsicles, with artificial fruit flavor
Rich's Topping
Salt
Shortening, vegetable
Soy sauce
Sugar, brown, white, or confectioner's
Syrups, corn or maple
Tang
Tapioca

† Special recipe must be used—In Phenylalanine-Restricted Diet Recipe Book.

TABLE 34–5. Meal Patterns for Restricted Phenylalanine Diets for Different Age Infants and Children*

Age	Breakfast	Dinner	Mid-Afternoon	Supper	Bedtime
7 Months	6 T. Baby Oatmeal 8 oz. Formula	7 T. Jr. Carrots 8 oz. Formula		2 T. Jr. Green Beans 12 T. Jr. Peaches 8 oz. Formula	8 oz. Formula
1 Year	¾ cup (2 serv.) Rice Krispies 6 oz. Orange Juice ¼ cup Sliced Banana 4 oz. Formula	3 T. Mashed Potatoes, no Milk, no Butter 8 T. Cooked Carrots 2 Small Slices Canned Pineapple 6 oz. Formula	2 Saltines 8 oz. Formula	8 T. (½ cup) Cooked Green Beans 1 Small Raw Tomato with ½ T. Mayonnaise 2 Halves Canned Peaches 6 oz. Formula	
4 Years	¾ cup (2 serv.) Puffed Wheat 6 oz. Orange Juice ¼ cup Sliced Banana 8 oz. Formula	2 T. Cooked Corn 8 T. Cooked Summer Squash 1 Small Tomato ½ cup Watermelon Cubes 8 oz. Formula		2 T. Mashed Yams 1 cup Applesauce 3 T. Cooked Cauliflower 5 T. Shredded Raw Cabbage with ½ T. Mayonnaise 8 oz. Formula	

*From The Phenylalanine-Restricted Diet—for Professional Use, 1966. The Bureau of Public Health Nutrition of the California State Department of Public Health.

Maintenance of Treatment. If treatment is to be successful, the diet must be adjusted so that serum phenylalanine levels are maintained within 3 to 8 mg. per ml.[33] and the child grows and develops normally. When the serum phenylalanine falls below this level, symptoms of lethargy, refusal to eat and fever occur. The low serum phenylalanine may cause a breakdown of body protein, with a rapid rise of serum phenylalanine above safe levels. If treatment is not promptly instituted, feeding difficulties, failure to thrive and other symptoms of untreated phenylketonuria appear.[34] Frequent monitoring of serum phenylalanine levels and urinary excretion of phenylpyruvic acid is therefore necessary for adequate treatment.

It becomes evident that cooperation and understanding of the parents, and indeed of the whole family, is essential if this difficult regimen is to be successful. Umbarger[35] recommends that treatment be on an outpatient basis from the start, rather than begun in the hospital, in order to involve the parents from the outset in the planning for the infant. It is also strongly recommended that the phenylketonuric child be followed at a center which can provide the services of physician, nutritionist, social worker, public health nurse, and experienced laboratory facilities. The frequent monitoring of blood serum phenylalanine levels and urinary excretion of phenylpyruvic acid, and the necessary adjustment of the diet can thus be accomplished quickly and with least danger to the child.

Duration of Treatment. At present there is no agreement on the length of time the diet must be continued. Dietary control varies as the infant becomes mobile, and maintaining the diet becomes more difficult. O'Flynn states that the brain has reached 90 per cent of adult size at the age of 5 years.[36] There is some indication that children taken off the diet at 5 to 6 years of age progress normally both mentally and physically. Since treatment with the low-phenylalanine diet began less than 10 years ago, it will take a few more years before the age at which the diet can safely be discontinued can be established with certainty.

Galactosemia

Galactosemia is an inherited disorder of carbohydrate metabolism. It is characterized by an inability to convert galactose to glucose in the liver, due to the absence of the enzyme galactose-1-phosphate uridyl transferase. In this disorder an intermediary product of galactose metabolism, galactose-1-phosphate, accumulates in the blood and is thought to be responsible for the symptoms. Some galactose spills into the urine. Unless the disease is recognized and treated promptly, death may ensue. However, in this disorder, as in phenylketonuria, there are adults with elevated galactose-1-phosphate in the blood who have no other signs of the disease.

At present there is no routine screening for the presence of galactosemia in newborns. The Committee on Fetus and Newborn of the American Academy of Pediatrics, however, recommend that the urine of every newborn be tested for reducing substances on the day of discharge from the hospital, after feeding has been started, and that cord blood of newborn siblings of families of known galactosemics be tested for activity of the enzyme involved in this disorder.

In the majority of patients symptoms develop in early infancy. These include jaundice, enlargement of the liver, digestive disturbances and failure to grow and thrive. If the infant survives, cataracts may develop and mental and physical growth is retarded.

Dietary Treatment

Treatment is directed toward rigid exclusion of galactose from the diet. Since galactose is a component of lactose, the sugar found in milk, milk and all foods containing milk must be omitted.

---

[33] Statement on Treatment of Phenylketonuria. Committee on the Handicapped Child, American Academy of Pediatrics, Pediatrics, *35*:501, 1965.
[34] Umbarger, B., and Berry, H. K.: J.A.M.A., *193*: 784, 1965.
[35] Ibid.
[36] O'Flynn, M. E.: Am. J. Nursing, 67:1658, 1967.

In place of milk, the protein hydrolysate Nutramigen* is a satisfactory substitute, or a meat base formula† may be used. These have been fortified with minerals and vitamins, but the physician will wish to check the infant's needs and supplement them as necessary. Small babies accept these substitute feedings well, but parents sometimes have to be helped to see their necessity as a milk replacement, especially as the child gets older.

Soybean "milks" should probably not be used. Soybeans as well as lima beans and peas contain a complex carbohydrate, stachyose, which consists largely of galactose. It is not known if this is released during digestion. Until further information is available, foods containing stachyose had better be omitted.

The small infant will be placed by the physician on the appropriate amount of Nutramigen or meat base formula. As he grows and develops, fruit, vegetables, cereals, meat and eggs should be added as outlined in Chapter 13. Most baby foods are milk-free, but the mother must check labels carefully. "Baby dinners" and soups and puddings usually contain milk in some form. (Gerber's Baby Food Company has a table of their products with the ingredients listed for each.)

As the child grows older, he will eat more foods from the family table. All foods known to contain milk must be omitted by the galactosemic child. Some foods have milk solids added, usually dry skim milk. Among these are most breads (except Vienna bread), pastries, cookies, cake, crackers, prepared mixes, butter and margarine. Some cereals, notably Total, Special K and Instant Cream of Wheat, have milk solids added. Cream and cheese of all kinds contain lactose. Brain tissue contains a compound containing galactose and brains must be omitted. Any food containing lactose as such must be excluded. It is a good thing to learn to check labels for the addition of milk, milk solids, lactose, galactose, whey or curds, as well as any of the foods mentioned above, such as bread or crackers as a stuffing or breading. Unfortunately, under our present labeling laws, not all foods are labeled. If the mother is not sure of the contents, the food should be omitted. An excellent booklet, Nutritional Management of Galactosemia, which contains food lists and recipes, is available from the Mead Johnson Laboratories, Evansville, Indiana. Another occasional source of lactose is a medication in which lactose is used as a filler. No medication, drug or home remedy should be used without consulting the doctor.

If all sources of galactose are removed from the diet, most of the physical signs of the disease, with the possible exception of cataracts and brain damage, will disappear. If the diet is instituted within the first few weeks of life, there is an excellent chance that all symptoms and disabilities will be prevented.

Leucine-Induced Hypoglycemia

Hypoglycemic reactions in infants induced by the amino acid leucine is another inborn error of metabolism of familial origin. It may be manifested from birth, or it may appear later in the first year of life. The symptoms are precipitated by a high-protein meal or a fasting state. They are, in the early stages, irritability and twitching movements of the extremities, and, if the disease is not treated, hypoglycemic convulsions, with blood sugar levels as low as 25 mg. per cent. Eventually failure to thrive and mental and psychomotor retardation occur. Control of the hypoglycemia as early as possible is therefore imperative.

A dietary regimen consisting of leucine restriction and postprandial carbohydrate feedings has been devised by Roth and Segal.[37] Leucine restriction is achieved by limitation of dietary protein, including only sufficient amounts to meet the minimal requirements for growth. Lists of foods to be omitted and those allowed are given, and a series of menus calculated for leucine content are included. The menus and the times for the administration of sugar must be followed exactly if the diet is to be

---

* Mead Johnson and Co., Evansville, Ind.
† Gerber Products Co., Fremont, Mich.

[37] Roth, H., and Segal, H.: Pediatrics, 34:831, 1964.

effective. The diet has been used by these investigators and by others,[38] with good results. Hypoglycemia and the attendant symptoms were controlled, and the children have developed normally. Fortunately, the disease appears to be self-limiting, and by the time the child is 5 to 6 years old he is able to tolerate a normal diet.

Despite numerous studies, the disorder remains a poorly defined entity. No abnormality in the metabolism of leucine has been found, but the evidence suggests that in these patients leucine stimulates an excessive release of insulin from the pancreas. It is estimated that 60 per cent of hypoglycemia found in infants is due to leucine sensitivity.

Maple Syrup Urine Disease

This disease, an inborn error of metabolism, is so called because of the odor of maple syrup of the urine. Infants with this disease cannot metabolize the 3-branched chain amino acids—leucine, isoleucine and valine. The symptoms develop a few days after birth, and babies die with severe neurologic symptoms and high levels of the unmetabolized amino acids in the body fluids. Several children with this disease are being treated with some success with a mixture of amino acids, omitting those that are not tolerated, and small additions of natural foods.[39]

Histidinemia

Histidinemia is an inborn error of the metabolism of the amino acid histidine due to a deficiency of the enzyme histidase. High levels of histidine are found in the blood and urine. Clinical symptoms are manifested in speech disorders, both of articulation and in language, though not in all of the patients known to have this disease. There is mental retardation in some patients, though again not in all. A diet restricted in protein was not effective in lowering histidine in the blood or urine.

There is no specific therapy recommended at this time.[40]

STUDY QUESTIONS AND ACTIVITIES

1. What may the mother or the nurse expect of a child's food habits when he is ill?

2. Name some of the nutritional problems in chronic illness or in illness of more than short duration in children. How may we try to meet these?

3. How can a child be helped to adjust to eating his food in the hospital?

4. What are some of the causes of diarrhea and dysentery? What dietary measures are indicated for each?

5. What is a common cause of nutritional anemia in young children? How may it be prevented?

6. What other causes of iron-deficient anemia in young infants have been reported?

7. Is scurvy still a problem in the United States and Canada? What may happen when the food pattern of a family is changed? What is the nurse's responsibility?

8. Is rickets still a problem in the United States? Where may it occur?

9. What is meant by the term "failure to thrive"? What are some possible causes?

10. What effect may emotional deprivation have on the food habits and nutritional status in children?

11. List some of the causes of underweight in children. How may the nurse help to correct these?

12. How should anorexia in a small child be treated when no disease is present?

13. Why should obesity in the child be treated promptly? Which foods must be included in a restricted calorie diet to keep it adequate for the nutritional needs of the obese child?

14. What should be the relationship between the obese child and the person treating him?

15. What are some of the problems faced by the parents of a handicapped child or one with long-term illness? How may the nurse be of help?

[38] Snyder, R. D., and Robinson, A.: Am. J. Dis. Child., *113*:566, 1967.

[39] Snyderman, S. E.: Am. J. Dis. Child., *113*:68, 1967.

[40] Ghadimi, H.: Am. J. Dis. Child., *113*:83, 1967.

16. How may the nutritional problems of the child with cleft palate be met? What are some of the difficulties?

17. What nutritional problems are common to the child with cerebral palsy? How may some of these be met?

18. When may a ketogenic diet be ordered for epilepsy? How is a condition of ketosis established and maintained?

19. What are some of the difficulties inherent in this diet?

20. What problems will the family with a mentally deficient child encounter? How can the nurse be of help?

21. Why do many physicians permit the child with nephrosis to eat what he wishes? What becomes obvious in such children when the edema subsides?

22. Make out a menu for a day for a 2-year-old child with celiac disease on a no starch, high protein, moderate fat diet, using the foods allowed early in the treatment of the disease.

23. Plan a day's diet for a 5-year-old child with celiac disease on a gluten-free diet. See Chapter 27.

24. Why should calories and protein be increased in the diet of a child with cystic fibrosis? See Chapter 27.

25. Name the 3 methods of dietary restriction used in diabetes, and give the reason for the use of each in the treatment of the child with diabetes. See Chapter 22.

26. Using the Tables for Sodium Restricted Diets in Chapter 24, make out a menu for a 4-year-old child, containing 250 mg. of sodium.

27. Plan a menu containing 60 Gm. of protein for a 12-year-old boy with chronic glomerulonephritis. There is no sodium or potassium restriction. See Chapter 25.

28. List the foods on an elimination diet suitable for a small child suspected of having a food allergy. Is it adequate for his nutritional needs? See Chapter 30.

29. Which milk substitutes may be used for the child with a milk allergy? Are these nutritionally equal to milk? See Chapter 30.

30. What is the metabolic defect in phenylketonuria? Why is it important that it be treated early?

31. How must the diet be restricted? What is the importance of frequent monitoring of blood phenylalanine levels?

32. What is the composition of Lofenalac?

33. List some of the problems that may be encountered in maintaining the phenylalanine-restricted diet in a 3-year-old child.

34. What is galactosemia? Why must milk be omitted from the diet? What may be substituted in the young infant?

35. Name 10 foods which contain hidden sources of lactose. Why must medications be carefully scrutinized?

SUPPLEMENTARY READING IN DISEASES OF CHILDREN

See also Supplementary Readings and Bibliography under chapters dealing with some of the above diseases.

Hospitalization of Sick Children

Erickson, F.: When 6 to 12 year olds are ill. Nursing Outlook, *13*:48, 1965 (July).

Fagin, C. M.: Why not involve parents when children are hospitalized? Am. J. Nursing, *62*:78, 1962 (June).

Getty, G., and Hollensworth, M.: Through a child's eye seeing. Nutrition Today, *2*:17, 1967 (Florida Citrus Commission).

Iron Deficiency Anemia
(See also Chaps. 13 and 16)

Haughton, J. G.: Nutritional anemia of infancy and childhood. Am. J. Publ. Health, *53*:1121, 1963.

Smith, C. A.: Overuse of milk in the diets of infants and children. J.A.M.A., *172*:567, 1960.

Wilson, J. F., *et al.*: Milk-induced gastrointestinal bleeding in infants with hypochromic microcytic anemia. J.A.M.A., *189*:568, 1964.

Scurvy; Rickets
(See also Chaps. 13 and 16)

Committee on Nutrition, American Academy of Pediatrics: Infantile scurvy and nutritional rickets in the U. S. Pediatrics, *29*:646, 1962.

Youmans, J. B.: The changing face of nutritional disease in America. J.A.M.A., *189*:672, 1964.

Failure to Thrive; Emotional Deprivation

Bakwin, H.: Emotional deprivation in infants. J. Pediat., *35*:512, 1949.

———: Loneliness in infants. Am. J. Dis. Child., *63*:30, 1942.

Leonard, M. F., *et al.:* Failure to thrive in infants. Am. J. Dis. Child., *111*:600, 1966.

Silver, H. K., and Finkelstein, M.: Deprivation dwarfism, J. Pediat., *70*:317, 1967.

Obesity
(See also Chapter 21)

Gallagher, J. R.: Weight control in adolescence. J. Am. Dietet. A., *40*:519, 1962.

Wilkes, E. T.: Chubby children need your help. Today's Health, *40*:36, 1962 (May).

Wright, F. H.: Preventing obesity in childhood. J. Am. Dietet. A., *40*:516, 1962.

Families of Handicapped Children

Andersen, D. H.: Cystic fibrosis and family stress. Children, 7:9, 1960 (Jan.-Feb.).

Dittman, L. L.: The mentally retarded child at home: a manual for parents. U. S. Dept. Health, Education and Welfare, Children's Bureau Publ. No. 374, 1959.

Korsch, B., and Barnett, H. L.: Pediatric discussions with parent groups. J. Pediat., *58*: 707, 1961.

Umbarger, B.: Phenylketonuria—treating the disease and feeding the child. Am. J. Dis. Child., *100*:908, 1960.

Cleft Palate

Atkinson, H. C.: Care of the child with cleft lip and palate. Am. J. Nursing, *67*:1889, 1967.

Feeding Children with Cleft Lip and Palate. Washington State Department of Health, Olympia, Washington, 1966.

Zickefoose, M.: Feeding the child with a cleft palate. J. Am. Dietet. A., *36*:129, 1960.

Zickefoose, M., and Frey, P. W.: Helping the disabled person to help himself to good nutrition. Hospitals, *37*:91, 1963.

Cerebral Palsy

Hammond, M. I., *et al.:* A nutritional study of cerebral palsied children. J. Am. Dietet. A., *49*:196, 1966.

Ruby, D. O., and Matheny, W. D.: Comments on growth of cerebral palsied children. J. Am. Dietet. A., *40*:525, 1962.

Epilepsy

Mike, E. M.: Practical guide and dietary management of children with seizures using the ketogenic diet. Am. J. Clin. Nutr., *17*:399, 1965.

Mentally Retarded Children

Adair, R.: Home care and feeding of a mentally retarded child. J. Am. Dietet. A., *36*:133, 1960.

Dittmann, L. L.: The nurse in home training programs for the retarded child. U. S. Dept. of Health, Education and Welfare, Children's Bureau, 1961.

Hall, E. J., and Johnson, G. C.: They turn to nurses. Am. J. Nursing, *61*:60, 1961.

Nephrosis

Saxena, K. M., and Crawford, J. D.: The treatment of nephrosis. New Eng. J. Med., *272*: 522, 1965.

Soyka, L. F.: Treatment of the nephrotic syndrome in childhood. Am. J. Dis. Child., *113*: 693, 1967.

Malabsorption Syndromes
(See also Chap. 27)

di Sant'Agnese, P. A., and Jones, W. O.: The celiac syndrome in pediatrics. J.A.M.A., *180*: 308, 1962.

Schwab, L., *et al.:* Cystic fibrosis. Am. J. Nursing, *63*:62, 1963 (Feb.).

Diabetes
(See also Chap. 22)

Etzwiler, D. D., and Sines, L. K.: Juvenile diabetes and its management. J.A.M.A., *181*: 304, 1962.

Hamwi, G. J.: Treatment of diabetes. J.A.M.A., *181*:124, 1962.

Hooker, A. D.: Camping and the diabetic child. J. Am. Dietet. A., *37*:143, 1960.

Moore, M. L.: Diabetes in children. Am. J. Nursing, *67*:104, 1967.

Inborn Errors—General

Berry, H. K.: Inborn errors of metabolism. J. Am. Dietet. A., *49*:401, 1966.

Phenylketonuria

Composition of Lofenalac. J. Am. Dietet. A., *52*:48, 1968.

O'Flynn, M. E.: Diet therapy in phenylketonuria: how long should it continue? Am. J. Nursing, *67*:1658, 1967.

Phenylketonuria. Children's Bureau Publication 388, Dept. Health, Education and Welfare, 1965, Washington, D. C.

The Phenylalanine-Restricted Diet (for professional use). Bureau of Public Health Nutrition, California State Dept. of Public Health, Berkeley, Calif. (Available only to California residents.)

Umbarger, B. J.: Phenylketonuria: dietary treatment. Am. J. Nursing, *64*:96, 1964 (Jan.).

Galactosemia

Galactose-free diet—Parents' Guide. California State Department of Public Health, Berkeley, Calif. (Available only to California residents.)

Koch, R., *et al.*: Nutrition in the treatment of galactosemia. J. Am. Dietet. A., 43:216, 1963.

Nutritional Management of Galactosemia. Mead Johnson Laboratories, Evansville, Indiana.

Maple Syrup Urine Disease

Review: Dietary treatment of maple sugar urine disease. Nutr. Rev., 23:260, 1965.

For further references see Bibliography in Part Four.

PART THREE
Modification of Food for Therapeutic Diets

Part Three deals with food preparation and selection and with the modification of these for therapeutic diets. Although the nurse today is not often required to prepare food for an individual patient, her role as a teacher and an interpreter of good health practices demands that she have a sound knowledge of food as it appears on the family table. Whether she works at the bedside or in the community as a public health, school or industrial nurse—in fact, in all areas where she functions—she is expected to have reliable information on many matters which deal with the maintenance of health and the treatment of disease. Not the least of these pertains to food and its preparation.

The nurse should know something of the variety of available foods and of how these may contribute to a pleasing and palatable menu. A knowledge of the effect of methods of preservation and of cooking processes on the retention or the destruction of food nutrients will help her to interpret these data to the public. An appreciation of which ingredients a recipe is likely to contain will aid her in knowing whether or not such a food is permissible on a given therapeutic diet. Lastly, if the nurse can make practical suggestions for making a therapeutic diet more palatable and, therefore, more acceptable, it is more likely to be followed. Part Three has been written to help her obtain some of this information by supplying basic recipes and reliable references, and by providing some ideas for adapting these to the more commonly used therapeutic diets.

CHAPTER 35

Basic Food Selection and Preparation

Menu Planning • Directions for Following a Recipe • Utensils and Measurements • Terms Used in Recipes • Selection and Preparation of Foods

MENU PLANNING

Adequate and attractive menus for a day or, preferably, for several days can be planned very easily around the Daily Food Guide which was discussed in Chapter 10. However, food selection in a broad sense covers more than the choice of an adequate amount of a variety of foods; it includes planning good meals which not only will be adequate nutritionally, but will be satisfying to the eye, the appetite and the taste.

Family meals as well as those planned for the ill or the convalescent patient, may include 3, 4 or 5 meals a day, depending on custom and cultural patterns. However, there should be no omission of breakfast. It need not be a large meal, but it should include some of the essentials for the day, including a protein food, such as milk, egg or some form of meat. The main meal of the day may be served at noon or in the evening, to suit convenience and preference. If the family is in the habit of eating a late evening snack, it should be considered in the planning of the menus, both to ensure the total adequacy of the diet and, particularly, to prevent an excess of calories.

The preparation of each meal depends first of all on having all ingredients on hand. Therefore systematic menu planning and marketing, as discussed in Chapter 10, are a prerequisite. Whoever is responsible for preparing the meals needs to be familiar with basic recipes and the time required for their preparation, in order to have all the foods for a meal ready for service at the same time.

USE OF RECIPES

A recipe is a formula for the preparation of a specific food. The ingredients have been found by experiment to produce desirable results when combined according to directions. The beginning cook should follow a recipe exactly as given. As she gains experience, she will realize that those ingredients which determine shape, texture, consistency and tenderness of a mixture cannot be varied from the proportions given in the recipe without changing the basic characteristics of the product. However, flavoring agents may be varied according to the preference of a family or individual. Thus a basic French dressing may have herbs or spices added to give variety; and nutmeg may be sprinkled or omitted on the top of a baked custard according to taste. Some of the suggestions for flavoring specific foods found in Chapter 39, Foods for Sodium Restricted Diets, will add interest and variety to the ordinary menu also, but quantities may have to be reduced with the addition of salt.

To increase a recipe, best results are obtained when not more than a double recipe is prepared. If a greater quantity is needed, it is better to make the product twice. To

GENERAL DIRECTIONS FOR FOLLOWING A RECIPE

1. Select tested recipes from reliable sources, and read them carefully.

2. Turn on the oven to the correct temperature if the product is to be baked or roasted, so that the oven will be at the desired heat when the mixture is ready for cooking.

3. Check supplies and collect the necessary ingredients in one work area.

4. Collect the needed mixing, measuring and cooking equipment in one work area.

5. If baking or roasting, prepare the pan for the product, using the size indicated in the recipe for best results.

6. Check to see if there is anything that should be done to ingredients before adding them to the mixture, such as melting fat or chocolate, beating egg whites or sifting dry ingredients together.

7. Use level measurements, measure exactly—dry ingredients first, then liquids, if possible, to save washing of extra utensils.

8. Combine the ingredients, following the procedure given in the recipe.

9. Bake or cook exactly as directed. Follow cooking times and temperatures given, testing for done-ness as directed. Thermometers for roasting, deep-fat frying and candy making will be found helpful.

10. Handle finished product as directed, such as removing from pans, molding, chilling, etc.; to cool or chill before serving; or to serve at once.

reduce a recipe, choose one in which the ingredients may be divided easily. Measure small amounts carefully. The cooking time may be increased for larger and decreased for smaller quantities.

There are many excellent cookbooks available to acquaint the inexperienced person with the ingredients and the methods of preparation of recipes and menus. Some of these are listed at the end of this chapter. In addition, the labels on many canned, frozen and packaged foods give reliable directions. The nutritional value of a recipe and, thus, its use in the diet, whether normal or therapeutic, can be estimated once its ingredients and method of preparation are known.

UTENSILS AND MEASUREMENTS

For accurate measuring the following utensils are essential: an 8-oz. measuring cup divided into fourths and thirds or a set of measuring cups of the above volumes; tablespoons and teaspoons of regulation sizes or, preferably, a set of measuring spoons.

To measure dry material by the cup, fill lightly with a spoon to brim or to indicated cup level. Do not shake the cup to level the materials. This is particularly impor-

tant in the case of flour sifted before measurement. Granulated sugar may be measured easily, but brown sugar should be packed firmly into the cup. Before measuring honey or syrup, rinse the cup with cold water.

Measurement of butter and margarine, when in ¼-lb. sticks, may be made by accurate division. One stick corresponds to the measurement of ½ cup. To measure bulk fat, pack firmly into cup to the desired mark of measurement. Except for pastry, fat should be at room temperature. (An easy way of measuring ½ cup of shortening is to fill the cup to half mark with cold water and add shortening enough to cause water to rise to the 1-cup mark. To measure ¼ cup, fill with cold water to the three-quarter mark.)

To measure dry ingredients by the tablespoon or the teaspoon, fill until heaping and, with the back edge of a knife, level off all that extends above the edge of the spoon. If one half spoonful is desired, divide the contents of the spoon lengthwise and push off one half. If one fourth is wanted, divide the remaining half crosswise of the spoon and push off the portion not desired. If one eighth is desired, divide the remaining one fourth crosswise and push off the portion not needed. If one third of a spoonful is desired, divide the contents of the spoon crosswise into thirds, pushing off the undesired portion.

To measure spoonfuls of liquid dip the spoon into the liquid.

To measure butter or other solid fats, pack solidly into the spoon and level with a knife.

Measurements and Equivalents*

2 tablespoons	=	1 ounce
½ cup	=	1 gill
2 cups	=	1 pint
4 cups	=	1 quart
4 quarts	=	1 gallon
8 quarts	=	1 peck
4 pecks	=	1 bushel
3 teaspoons	=	1 tablespoon
4 tablespoons	=	¼ cup
5⅓ tablespoons	=	⅓ cup
8 tablespoons	=	½ cup
12 tablespoons	=	¾ cup
16 tablespoons	=	1 cup
1 tablespoon liquid	=	½ ounce
1 cup liquid	=	8 ounces
1 cup flour	=	4½ ounces
1 tablespoon flour	=	¼ ounce
1 tablespoon sugar	=	⅖ ounce
1 cup butter	=	8 ounces
1 cup sugar	=	7 ounces

*For additional equivalents see Table 10 in Part Four.

TERMS USED IN RECIPES

Baste: to pour liquid over the surface of food which is being baked or roasted.

Blanch: to let food stand in hot water 3 to 5 minutes to loosen skin, remove strong flavors, or set color.

Cream: to soften shortening and to blend with sugar by rubbing with a wooden spoon or in an electric mixer.

Cut in: to blend shortening with flour with pastry blender or two knives.

Dice: to cut in small square pieces.

Fold: to add whipped cream or beaten egg whites with a careful folding motion.

Mince: to cut or to chop fine.

Pan-broil: to cook in a heated pan or on a griddle with little or no added fat.

Pan-fry: to cook in shallow pan with just enough added fat to prevent sticking and aid browning.

Parboil: to boil food in water until it is partially cooked.

Purée: to press food through a sieve.

Sauté: to cook in a small amount of fat.

Scald: to heat milk until bubbles appear around the edge.

Sear: to brown quickly over direct heat or in oven.

Shred: to cut or to tear in thin strips.

Simmer or **stew:** to cook in liquid just below boiling point.

Steep: to let stand in hot liquid below boiling point.

SELECTION AND PREPARATION OF FOODS

In the following sections of this chapter, food groups as they appear on the menu are discussed briefly. The selection, the availability, the variety and the method of preparation are included for each group, and a few representative recipes are given. This material forms the groundwork on which the discussion of food for therapeutic diets is based in the succeeding chapters.

However, it is hoped that the student will have available to her a choice of cookbooks, for both normal and therapeutic diets, to encourage her to be imaginative and stimulating in the teaching of her patients.

BEVERAGES

In the opinion of most persons, a meal is incomplete without a beverage, which in its simplest form may be a glass of cold water, chilled with ice if desired.

Hot Beverages

Coffee and tea have no food value unless served with cream and sugar. Cocoa in itself will increase the food value of the milk which is used in its preparation. Coffee, tea and cocoa are stimulants. All contain caffeine, and cocoa also contains theobromine. This quality may be an asset, especially at breakfast time. The heat of a beverage itself may be mildly stimulating. Thus a cup of hot broth may be more acceptable to the debilitated patient than a glass of cold fruit juice.

Hot beverages should be hot when they reach the patient and cold beverages cold.

The former is particularly important, as a lukewarm cup of a beverage which is supposed to be hot may ruin the enjoyment of what otherwise would be a good meal.

Cold Beverages

Cold beverages may be used with meals or between meals. They are more appetizing when chilled, but care should be used in serving an iced beverage to a bedfast patient as it may cause distention.

Fruit juices, freshly squeezed, and canned or diluted frozen concentrates are general favorites. Eggs may be combined with milk, sweetened and flavored for a variety of so-called eggnogs. (See p. 484 for reservations about the use of raw eggs.) Milk in its usual form, or as buttermilk, is a basic beverage. Malted milks of various flavors may be used. Evaporated milk shaken with fruit juices and cracked ice is useful for the patient who does not like fresh milk. Dry skim milk may be incorporated into beverages when it is desirable to restrict calories or fat or to increase protein or calcium content.

Carbonated water, ginger ale and cola drinks, the last often used in the South and mildly stimulating, are refreshing.

Iced tea, coffee and cocoa may be used between or with meals. The choice of beverage will depend largely on whether it is given for its food value or merely as refreshment.

Alcoholic Beverages

Alcohol is the product of fermentation of sugar: sugars found in such foodstuffs as fruits or sugar produced from starch by a malting process. Alcoholic beverages are of two types: those which are produced by fermentation only, such as ale, beer and most wines; and those which are distilled to yield a distillate with a higher percentage of alcohol than can be secured by fermentation only. In alcoholic beverages, the alcoholic concentrations are often increased by fortification or rectification, i.e., by the addition of alcohol or strong alcoholic distillates (neutral spirits). By such procedures the alcoholic content of wines which are not distilled may be as high as from 20 to 24 per cent.

Since Federal, and sometimes state, taxes are based on the alcoholic content, the exact amount must be stated on the label of a retail product of a given manufacturer. It may be stated as percentage of alcohol: e.g., muscatel, 20 per cent, or as "proof alcohol" content. By this latter method 50 per cent alcohol is called 100 proof, and a whisky labeled "90 proof" would contain 45 per cent of pure alcohol.

Sherry or port wine may be prescribed as appetizers. Liquors with a high alcohol content such as whisky or gin may be prescribed when it is essential to dilate blood vessels, as in some types of vascular disease. Alcohol yields 7 calories per gram. It should be used sparingly when calories are restricted in the diet. See Table 7 in Part Four for caloric content of alcoholic beverages.

General Rules and Recipes for Beverages
Coffee

Coffee is cherished for its particular flavor and aroma. For the best results, it should be prepared just below the boiling point to obtain the greatest amount of flavoring substances with a minimal extraction of tannin, which has a bitter flavor. For the same reason coffee should be "held" below the boiling point when it is not to be served immediately.

The method of preparation will determine the coarseness or the fineness of the grind of coffee to be used. In general 1 rounded tablespoon of coffee is used for each large cup of coffee to be served, plus one added tablespoon "for the pot." Some coffee firms supply a coffee measure which may be used.

Boiled or Steeped. Measure coffee and mix it with a small amount of water and some broken eggshells. Pour the required amount of freshly boiling water on the coffee and let it come to a boil. Settle with a little cold water, and set aside to steep for 3 to 5 minutes.

Percolated. Pour required amount of cold water into the coffee pot, measure coffee into percolator basket and set over heat. As soon as coffee begins to bubble, turn down heat and allow to percolate gently for several minutes. Do not overpercolate. Remove basket containing grounds before serving. If an electric percolator is used, it will automatically hold the finished product at the right temperature.

Drip Method. Heat the coffee pot by rinsing with boiling water. Adjust the basket over lower section and measure coffee into it. Adjust upper section of pot, and add measured amount of boiling water. Place over low heat. When coffee has finished dripping, remove upper sections and place cover on lower pot.

Instant Coffee

Soluble powdered coffee dissolves instantly in water which has just come to the boil. The proportions are 1 rounded teaspoon to a cup. It is most flavorful when started in cold water, brought to a boil and allowed to simmer 2 to 3 minutes before serving.

Decaffeinated Coffee

Both regular grinds and instant coffees are available in decaffeinated form. They may be prepared by any of the foregoing methods.

Iced Coffee

Prepare coffee by any of the above methods, using a double proportion of coffee to water, then pour over chopped ice in a tall glass. Add more ice, if necessary, and serve at once with powdered sugar and plain or whipped cream. Iced coffee made with half milk, half coffee (café au lait) is also delicious.

Tea

Tea is available in many varieties, depending on where it is grown, and the degree of oxidation to which the leaves have been subjected after they are harvested. To obtain the best flavor and aroma, and to avoid bitterness due to its tannin content, tea should be steeped at a temperature between 180° and 212° F. for 3 to 5 minutes and serve at once.

Steeped Tea

The proportion of 1 teaspoon of tea or 1 tea ball to 1 cup water is generally used.

Heat the teapot by pouring boiling water into it a few minutes before it is needed. Empty; put tea into the pot. Pour over it water that has just come to a boil and let stand for from 3 to 5 minutes, then serve with lemon, sugar and cream or milk, as preferred.

Instant Tea

Instant tea, which can be made quickly, is now available. It is popular in the preparation of iced tea. Follow the directions on the package.

Iced Tea

Follow directions for making tea, using 2 teaspoons tea to each cup boiling water. After tea has steeped, pour over chopped ice in a tall glass. Add more ice, if necessary, and serve at once with quartered lemon and powdered sugar. The glass may be filled to half its depth with tea, to which, after it has chilled, ginger ale may be added.

Cocoa and Chocolate

Chocolate retains some of the cocoa butter of the cocoa bean, and therefore has a fairly high fat content. It is generally sold in ½-pound cakes, divided into 1-ounce squares. Cocoa has much of the fat removed. It is usually sold in ½-pound or pound tins. Instant cocoa, a mixture of cocoa, sugar and flavoring is also available. Some brands also contain dry milk solids, and may have added vitamins and iron.

Cocoa

Ingredients:
- 2 teaspoons cocoa
- ⅓ cup cold water
- ¾ cup milk
- 1-2 teaspoons sugar

Procedure: Mix cocoa and water, stir over low heat until smooth. Boil 1 minute. Add milk and sugar, heat and beat until foamy with a rotary egg beater to prevent the formation of a scum. If preferred, 2 to 3 tablespoons cocoa syrup may be stirred into 1 cup hot milk.

A drop of vanilla may be added for extra flavor, and a topping of whipped cream or other topping, or a marshmallow (which children often prefer) may be added just before serving. Yield: 1 serving.

Chocolate

Follow directions for cocoa, substituting ½ square unsweetened chocolate cut in small pieces for the cocoa.

Instant Cocoa

The instant cocoa mix dissolves easily and may be used for either hot or cold beverages. Follow directions on the label.

Iced Mocha

This is most easily prepared by stirring a teaspoon of dry instant coffee into a small amount of boiling water and adding it to a glass of instant cocoa prepared with cold milk. Chill and serve in a tall glass with whipped cream or other topping.

Fruit Beverages

A beverage made from fresh fruit is pleasant, and may be economical where such fruit is easily available. Canned and frozen fruit juices, plain or mixed, can be obtained in great variety in most areas, and are highly acceptable. The canned fruit juices may be served undiluted. The frozen concentrates should be diluted according to directions on the can.

Lemonade

Ingredients:
1½ tablespoons sugar
1 cup water
2 tablespoons lemon juice
Procedure: Combine sugar and water, stir until dissolved. Add lemon juice, strain and pour over cracked ice in a tall glass. Yield: 1 serving.

Mint Fruitade

Ingredients:
1½ cups boiling water
¼ cup sugar
2 mint sprigs, crushed
½ cup pineapple or grapefruit juice
Juice of 1 lemon
Procedure: Boil water and sugar 3 minutes, add crushed mint. (If fresh mint is not obtainable, use 2 tablespoons dried spearmint.) Let stand from 5 to 10 minutes, strain and add fruit juices. Pour over cracked ice in a tall glass. Yield: 2 servings.

Fruit Yoghurt Beverage

Ingredients:
1 cup yoghurt
½ can (6 ounce) frozen grape or
 orange concentrate
Procedure: Beat yoghurt with the frozen juice concentrate until blended. Serve in tall parfait glasses or sherbet glasses. Yield: 2 servings.

Milk Shake (Basic Recipe)

Ingredients:	*(1 serving)*	*(4 servings)*
milk,*	1 cup	4 cups
sugar,	2 tablespoons	½ cup
vanilla,	½ teaspoon	1 teaspoon

*Milk may be:
1 cup whole fresh milk
½ cup evaporated milk plus ½ cup water
3 to 6 tablespoons skim milk powder plus ¾ cup water
3 to 6 tablespoons whole milk powder plus ¾ cup water
2 to 4 tablespoons high protein powder plus ¾ cup water

Procedure: Mix sugar, milk and vanilla in a shaker or a tightly covered jar. Add shaved ice, fasten cover tightly and shake well. When milk is frothy, strain into tall glass and serve at once.

Variations in Basic Recipe for Milk Shake (1 serving)
Chocolate: Add 1 or 2 tablespoons chocolate syrup before shaking.
Coffee: Add 1 or 2 teaspoons instant coffee before shaking.
Mocha: Add 1 tablespoon chocolate syrup and 1 teaspoon instant coffee before shaking.
Molasses: Add 2 tablespoons molasses before shaking.
Maple: Add 2 tablespoons maple syrup, omit sugar, before shaking.
Banana: Beat sliced banana until smooth with a fork, add before shaking.
Spiced: Use cinnamon, nutmeg, allspice or almond flavoring in place of vanila.
See also Ice Cream Beverages in Chapter 36.

Milk-and-Egg Beverages

The recent finding that raw eggs may carry the salmonella organism (see Chap. 17) makes the serving of milk and egg beverages questionable, particularly to old or debilitated patients and to children. Since the organism is not destroyed by freezing, frozen eggs may also be contaminated by salmonella.

Dried and powdered eggs, if they have been properly pasteurized, should be free of the organism. However, these are available only in quantity, suitable for institutions or in the home if there is someone for whom egg-milk beverages form a fairly large part of his nourishment.

Recently an instant egg-nog preparation containing pasteurized egg yolk solids has appeared in the retail market. It can be combined with evaporated, whole or skim milk, depending on the calories and richness desired. For variation of the basic recipe, 1 tablespoon brandy, cocoa syrup or molasses may be added.

SOUPS

Today one may take advantage of a wide variety of canned, frozen and dehydrated soups of excellent quality and flavor, available in most markets. The bouillon cubes and powders with a meatlike flavor and condensed meat extract are also useful when a quickly prepared hot liquid is desirable. For all of these the directions on the label should be followed in preparation.

A clear bouillon has little nutritive value, but may stimulate the appetite. Served with a thin slice of lemon and a bit of minced parsley, it is an attractive first part of a meal, or it may supply fluid and salt for the patient on a liquid diet.

Canned, frozen and dehydrated soups vary in nutritive value depending on their content. The addition of a pinch of soup herb mixture or a bit of bay leaf to a vegetable soup, or the mixing of two soups such as tomato and cream of celery will add further variety in flavor and interest.

Cream soups may on occasion be made at home. They should always be thin and delicately flavored. The amount of flour used for the cream sauce will depend on the vegetable with which it is to be used. For example, a potato cream soup will need the lesser amount of flour as given in the recipe below, whereas spinach, being a watery vegetable, will need the slightly larger amount. In all cases the soup should taste of the vegetable with which it is combined and not of the cream sauce.

Recipes
Basic Cream Sauce for Soup

Ingredients:
1 tablespoon butter
1 to 2 teaspoons flour
¼ teaspoon salt
Dash pepper
¾ cup milk

Procedure: Melt butter in small saucepan, stir in flour and seasonings. Stir in milk gradually and continue stirring over low heat until sauce thickens and boils. Yield: Approximately ¾ cup sauce.

Vegetable Purée for Cream Soup

Cooked vegetables such as celery, asparagus, peas, potato, onions, corn or spinach are suitable for cream soup. They may be strained through a coarse sieve or a food mill, or a blender may be used if one is available. Some of the water in which the

vegetable has been cooked should be reserved and used for flavor or for thinning out if needed. Canned strained "baby" vegetables may also be used, and are a time saver. They are very bland and may need some extra seasoning.

General Recipe for Cream Soup

Ingredients:
½ cup vegetable purée
¾ cup basic cream sauce
Seasonings

Procedure: Prepare purée. Make cream sauce, add purée and mix well. Add salt and pepper to taste, and reheat. See suggestions for garnishing given below. Yield: 1 to 2 servings.

Flavoring and Garnishes

For added flavor, vegetables such as potato or peas may be cooked with some onion or celery or both. A bit of chopped chives may be added to potato soup just before serving. A few asparagus tips added to the cream soup, minced parsley or watercress to celery soup, 2 or 3 small onion rings and a dash of paprika to onion soup or a bit of minced, cooked bacon to pea soup add variety and interest.

CEREAL PRODUCTS

In the United States, cereal products usually appear at all three meals, and often as snacks between meals. They may be in the form of breakfast foods, breads, cakes and pastries, rice and macaroni products, or as thickening agents in puddings, gravies and sauces. The caloric contribution of cereals is considered to be one of their greatest assets, but they also add to the protein, vitamin and mineral content of the menu.

Effect of Cooking

Before starch can be used readily by the body, the outer membrane must be broken, either by grinding or cooking. By the application of heat and moisture the outer cellulose envelope is ruptured, and the moisture permeates the starch granules themselves. Starch granules have an affinity for water, absorbing it as a sponge, and increasing greatly in volume. (Fig. 35–1). This occurs slowly at room temperature, rapidly at boiling temperature. Thus, a spoonful of dry cornstarch or flour dropped into cold water may be stirred to a smooth paste, but when dropped into boiling water it forms a lump because the outer grains swell so rapidly that they form a jacket around the others. After rupture of the cellulose wall by cooking, the starch is in a form that can be acted on more easily by digestive enzymes (Fig. 35–2).

Cooking alone may carry the breakdown of starch to the dextrin stage, if continued long enough. Starch granules break down most rapidly when moisture is present. Long application of dry heat, such as in baking or toasting, will also change starch to soluble dextrins. The palatable flavor of the brown crust of rolls or bread or the brown part of toast or of toasted cereals is due partly to forms of dextrin.

Breakfast Cereals

Ready-to-eat and cooked cereals are commonly served at breakfast, and may also be used at supper for small children. The occasional addition of raisins, dates or other fruit to a cooked cereal is good practice.

So far as food value is concerned, it makes little difference whether a hot cereal or a ready-to-eat cereal from the same type of grain is used. An ounce of one in dried form, whether it is cooked at home or made ready for consumption at the factory, will equal an ounce of another. However the cost per portion of ready-to-eat cereal is considerably higher than that of a cooked cereal.

Preparation

Ready-to-eat cereals, usually packed in cartons lined or covered with waxed paper, need no home preparation.

Porridge-type cereals such as oatmeal, ground-wheat products and cornmeal need a certain amount of cooking with water. Most cereals of this type are precooked under pressure at the factory and, therefore, need only short cooking in the home. This may be done over direct heat, with occasional stirring. Follow directions for preparation given on the box.

For cereals needing a longer cooking time and for cereals cooked in milk, it is best to use a double boiler to prevent scorching.

Thin cereal gruels are soothing for the patient with minor gastrointestinal ailments.

Recipes

Oatmeal or Barley Gruel

Ingredients:
  ¼ cup rolled oats or whole barley
  ¼ teaspoon salt
  1½ cups boiling water

Procedure: Add cereal to vigorously boiling salted water, stirring constantly. Turn down heat and simmer gently for one hour. Add more water if necessary. Strain and serve the liquid plain or with cream. Yield: 2 servings.

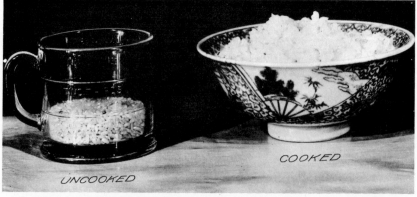

Fig. 35–1. Equal amounts of rice, cooked and uncooked, showing difference in volume. (Institute of Home Economics, U. S. Department of Agriculture)

Thin Cereal Gruel

Ingredients:

 2 tablespoons cream of wheat or
   cream of rice

 1/8 teaspoon salt

 1½ cups water

Procedure: Add cereal to boiling salted water, stirring constantly. Turn down heat and simmer gently for half an hour. Add more water if needed. Serve plain or with cream. Yield: 2 servings.

Breads, Cakes and Pastries

Breads. Whether home-prepared or purchased, breads, rolls, muffins, waffles and similar items are made from enriched flour in most sections of this country. The addition of egg and milk, and sometimes sugar, increases their nutritive value. The wide variety available at moderate cost, and the satiety and adaptability of these foods make them a popular item in the menu.

Cakes and pastries are most often used as dessert or for snacks. Their caloric value is high because of the content of sugar and fat.

Macaroni Products

Macaroni, spaghetti and noodles are grouped as alimentary pastes or "pasta," but they are actually cereal products. A special form of hard wheat is used in their manufacture. From the same paste, macaroni, spaghetti and the even thinner vermicelli are produced. For noodles there is an addition of eggs. Most of these products are fortified with vitamins and minerals. Macaroni products need only a small amount of cooking in boiling salted water to make them tender; they should not be overcooked. They are generally used in combination with a highly seasoned sauce. Grated cheese is usually considered a necessary accessory. While these products are sometimes used as an accompaniment to meat, they may form the main dish of a meal in which a small amount of meat may, or may not, be used. Vermicelli is generally used as an addition to a meat soup, to which it gives body and food value.

Other Grains

Rice, corn meal or hominy and buckwheat grits are used largely in the South and in other areas by certain national groups as accompaniments to meat and as a foundation for main dishes. Examples are Southern spoon bread, hominy pudding, Italian polenta and gnocchi, the Russian kasha or buckwheat grits and the general use of rice by all Orientals.

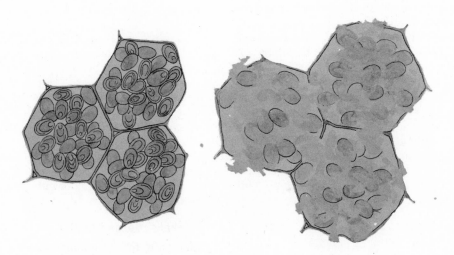

FIG. 35–2. Potato cells, showing starch grains as they appear raw and after cooking. Note the softened appearance and rupture of both cell walls and starch granules. (Broadhurst, Jean: Bacteria in Relation to Man. Philadelphia, J. B. Lippincott)

MEAT AND POULTRY
Effect of Heat on Protein

Protein foods are coagulated by heat. Low-temperature cooking produces a tender product, while high temperatures tend to cause toughening. This is best illustrated in egg cookery, in that an egg cooked below the boiling point is more tender than a "boiled" egg. For baking or roasting meat cookery experts recommend temperatures between 300° and 325° F. to get the best results for more tender meat as well as to lessen shrinkage.

Meat

Under the general term *meat,* poultry is included with beef, veal, lamb and pork. Some form of meat should be served at least once a day unless there is a specific reason for its exclusion from the diet. The importance of the careful handling and refrigeration of meat cannot be overestimated, for very high bacterial counts have been reported for such meat products as sausages and hamburger, where the meat was carelessly handled (soiled hands, dirty meat grinder, etc.) and was allowed to stand at room temperature (see Chap. 17).

Frozen meats are available in packaged form. Although they may be cooked while still frozen, it is generally preferable to allow them to thaw slowly on the shelf of the refrigerator or quickly at room temperature. If not to be used the day of purchase, frozen meat should be stored in freezing compartment of the refrigerator.

Meat in general should be stored, loosely covered with paper, in the refrigerator as soon as it comes from the market. Ground meat and organs such as liver and kidneys, which are highly perishable, should be put in the freezing compartment if not to be used within a few hours. Cooked meat is less subject to spoilage than raw meat, but leftovers should be used within a reasonable time.

Preparation

All cuts of meat, including the inexpensive ones, provide acceptable main dishes when they are properly prepared. The use of moderate temperatures and the selection of the correct method of cooking for each cut of meat is essential. Dry heat (oven roasting, oven broiling, pan broiling and pan frying) should be used only with the tender and therefore usually the more expensive cuts of meat. Moist heat (braising, pot roasting, stewing) and the use of meat tenderizers make the less tender and less expensive cuts almost equally acceptable.

No additional moisture or fat is required for oven roasting and oven broiling. The use of low oven temperatures, checked by an oven thermometer, for roasting prevents overcooking and the shrinkage in size and the loss of vitamins and of palatability that occur with high temperature cooking. When the more tender cuts are pan fried or pan broiled, a small amount of fat is needed to guard against adherence to the frying pan. Some types of utensils are now made to be used without added fat; or a nonfat spray preparation may be used with regular utensils for the individual who is restricting fat in his diet.

In moist heat cookery such as braising, pot roasting or stewing, the addition of an acid—either vinegar or lemon or tomato juice—to the liquid used in cooking increases the tenderizing effect of this method.

Fresh pork should be cooked until every vestige of pink coloring of the flesh has disappeared, to prevent infection with *Trichina spiralis.* Of all food animals, only pigs or hogs are susceptible to trichinosis infection, which may be passed on to humans if sufficient heat is not applied to kill any parasites present. Present methods of slaughtering and handling do not ensure against infection. Thus thorough cooking of all pork products in the home kitchen is essential.

The Meat Cookery Guide presented on page 489 suggests the most desirable cooking methods for a variety of cuts and types of meat.

Chickens, Geese, Ducks and Turkeys

These are the common domestic birds used as food, although chickens are the most plentiful among fowls. Capons (male birds castrated at an early age) are highly prized for their fine flavor and large pro-

MEAT COOKERY GUIDE

COOKING METHODS	BEEF CUTS	VEAL CUTS	PORK CUTS	LAMB CUTS	VARIETY MEATS
ROASTING	Standing Rib Rolled Rib Sirloin Chuck Ribs (high quality) Rump (high quality) Loaf	Rolled Shoulder Cushion Shoulder Arm Roast Blade Roast Rib Loin Rump Leg	Loin Rolled Shoulder Cushion Shoulder Fresh Ham (pork leg) Smoked Picnic Smoked Shoulder Butt Smoked Ham Sausages Sliced Salt Pork	Cushion Shoulder Rolled Shoulder Breast with Pocket Rolled Breast Rack Leg	Liver (beef-veal- pork-lamb)
BROILING and PAN-BROILING	Rib Steaks Club Steaks T-Bone Steaks Porterhouse Steaks Sirloin Steaks Chuck Steaks (high quality) Rump Steaks (high quality) Patties	Veal is not broiled or pan-broiled	Fresh pork is not broiled or pan- broiled Smoked Ham Slices Sliced Bacon Sliced Canadian- style Bacon Smoked Shoulder Butt Slices	Rib Chops Loin Chops Shoulder (arm or blade) Leg Steaks Patties Choplets (from breast stuffed with ground lamb)	Liver (veal-lamb) Kidney (lamb) Sweetbreads (beef-veal- lamb)
FRYING	Thin Steaks (tender or pounded) Patties	Chops Cutlets Steaks Patties	Sausage Sliced Salt Pork	Thin Chops or Thin Steaks	Liver (all kinds if cut thin) Tripe (after pre- cooking in water) Sweetbreads Brains
BRAISING	Chuck (arm or blade) Rump Round Heel of Round Brisket Plate Short Ribs Flank Shanks Ox-joints	Breast Rib Chops Loin Chops Shoulder Chops Cutlets Patties	Rib Chops Loin Chops Shoulder Chops or Steaks Fresh Ham Slices	Breast Neck Slices Shanks Riblets Shoulder (arm or blade)	Liver (beef-pork) Kidney (beef-veal- pork) Heart (beef-veal- pork-lamb) Tripe (beef) Sweetbreads (beef-veal-lamb)
COOKING IN LIQUID (Stews and Large Cuts)	Neck Shank Plate Brisket Flank Heel of Round Ox-joints Corned Beef	Neck Shoulder Shanks Flank	Hocks Shanks Feet Backbones Neck Bones Spareribs Smoked Picnic Smoked Shoulder Butt Smoked Ham Shanks Smoked Spareribs Smoked Hocks	Neck Steaks Shoulder Breast	Kidney (beef- veal-pork-lamb) Heart (beef-veal- pork-lamb) Tongue (beef- veal-pork-lamb) Tripe (beef) Sweetbreads (for precooking) Brains (for pre- cooking)

portion of light meat. Guinea hen, squab, partridges and other game are luxuries, used when obtainable.

The quality of poultry has been standardized to a great extent by modern methods of breeding, care and feeding. The birds come to market in both fresh-killed and frozen form. As poultry is as perishable as meat in general, it should be given the same care after it reaches the home kitchen.

Chickens, the most commonly used type of poultry, are known by various terms which indicate size and, to some extent, tenderness. This is shown in the accompanying chart:

Squab .... ¾-1¼ lbs.

Broiler .... 1¼-2½ lbs.

Fryer .... 2½-3½ lbs.

Roaster .... 3 lbs. or over

Fowl .... 4 lbs. or over

Preparation

Broilers and fryers, split for cooking, and larger chickens and fowl, packaged and entirely ready for cooking, may be purchased in most areas. They are available as fresh, fresh-frozen or frozen. Frozen fowl that has been held for some time may have lost some of its flavor.

Chickens and turkeys may carry the salmonella organism within the body cavity or on the skin. The tight packaging often used for poultry results in a moist surface which enhances bacterial growth. Loosening the wrapping tends to dry the moisture and reduces the possibility of spoilage. All poultry should be thoroughly washed and dried before cooking.

Proper cooking which develops and holds the delicate flavor of the meat is important in preparing chicken. Young chicken may be broiled or pan-fried in a small amount of fat. Older birds should be roasted or simmered, and serve sliced, hot or cold; boiled chicken may be used for fricassée or creamed chicken. A very palatable broth can be made from the bones of roast chicken or turkey.

Recipes

Broiled Lamb Chops

Ingredients:
 2 lamb chops, ¾ to 1 inch thick
  Salt and pepper

Procedure: Slash fat edge around chops to prevent curling during cooking. Place on rack in broiler pan in preheated oven about 2 inches from heat. Brown on one side, season with salt and pepper, turn and finish cooking on second side. Season. Chops 1 inch thick require 12 to 15 minutes of cooking, depending on desired degree of doneness. Yield: 1 to 2 servings.

Pan-broiled Steak

Ingredients:
 ½ to 1 pound club steak
  Salt and pepper

Procedure: Trim excess fat from the meat if necessary. Heat a heavy frying pan and rub lightly with a small piece of fat cut from the meat. Sear the meat on one side and season with salt and pepper, then sear the second side and season. Turn down the heat somewhat and cook to desired doneness, turning meat occasionally. Do not add water and do not cover. Yield: 1 to 3 servings.

Braised Pork Chops

Ingredients:
 2 pork chops
  Salt and pepper

Procedure: Cut a small strip of fat from the edge of the pork chops, and heat in a skillet until some of the fat has liquefied but is not smoking. Brown the chops on both sides, and season with salt and pepper. Add ¼ cup of water, cover, lower the heat and simmer until chops are thoroughly cooked, turning them once or twice. The length of time will depend on the thickness of the chops. Additional water may be needed to keep them from drying out. All the water may be cooked away, leaving the chops nicely browned, or a small amount may be reserved for gravy. Yield: 1 to 2 servings.

Meat Loaf

Ingredients:
 ½ cup milk
 2 tablespoons fat
 2 tablespoons flour
 1½ teaspoon salt°
 ½ teaspoon pepper
 1 pound ground beef
 1 cup soft bread crumbs
 1 tablespoon minced onion
 2 strips bacon
 2 bay leaves

Procedure: Melt the fat, stir in the flour, salt and pepper and mix until smooth. Add the milk and stir over low heat until thickened. Add to the ground meat, bread crumbs and onions; mix thoroughly with wet hands. Shape the mixture into two oval loaves and place on rack in roasting pan, or put into loaf pan. Cover with bacon and insert bay leaves. Bake in moderate oven (375° F.) for 1 hour. Yield: 4 to 6 servings.

° Substitute ½ teaspoon flavor salt, ¼ teaspoon garlic salt and 1 teaspoon Accent (monosodium glutamate) for 1 teaspoon of the salt.

Liver and Sausage Ring

Ingredients:
 1 lb. liver (beef, calves', pork or lamb)
 1 lb. pork sausage meat
 2 tablespoons chili sauce
 2 tablespoons horseradish
 1 tablespoon grated onion
 2 beaten eggs
 2 cups dry bread crumbs
 1 cup water

Procedure: Cover liver with hot water. Cover and simmer 5 minutes. Drain and put through food grinder, using fine plate. Add the remaining ingredients and mix thoroughly. Fill greased 8½-inch ring mold. Bake in moderate oven (350° F.) 1 hour. Serve with chili sauce. Yield: 8 servings.

Goulash

Ingredients:
- 1 lb. stewing beef
- ½ lb. lean pork
- 3 tablespoons bacon fat
- 3 tablespoons minced onion
- 1 cup canned tomatoes
- 1 teaspoon salt
- ⅛ teaspoon pepper
- 3 medium-sized potatoes, pared and cut in cubes

Procedure: Cut meat in 1-inch cubes. Heat bacon fat in heavy frying pan, add onion and meat and sauté until onions and meat are brown. Add tomatoes, salt and pepper, and mix well. Cover and let simmer slowly 1 hour. Uncover, add potatoes, cover and cook until potatoes are tender. Add a little water and more salt if necessary. Yield: 4 to 5 servings.

Broiled Chicken

Ingredients:
- 1 1½- to 2-pound broiler, split lengthwise
  Salt and pepper
  Butter or margarine, melted

Procedure: Brush chicken all over with melted fat. (French dressing may be used to add flavor.) Season with salt and pepper. Flatten chicken on rack in broiler pan, skin side down, and place in a preheated broiler 8 inches from the heat. Broil slowly for 15 to 20 minutes, basting as necessary. Turn chicken skin side up and broil another 15 to 20 minutes. Chicken should be brown, crisp and tender. Serve, skin side up. Yield: 2 to 4 servings.

Fried Chicken

Ingredients:
- 1 2- to 2½-pound broiler or fryer
- ¼ cup flour
- 1 teaspoon paprika
- 1 teaspoon salt
- ⅛ teaspoon pepper
  Hydrogenated fat or salad oil

Procedure: Have chicken cut up into pieces for serving. Mix flour and seasoning in a clean paper bag. Drop each piece of chicken into bag, shaking it until it is thoroughly coated with seasoned flour. Heat a ½-inch layer of fat in a heavy skillet until hot but not smoking. Place chicken pieces in the skillet and cook for 20 minutes, turn as necessary for even browning. When all pieces are a light brown, reduce heat to low, cover tightly and cook until poultry is tender, 20 to 40 minutes. When chicken is almost done, remove cover to recrisp it. Drain off excess fat before serving. Yield: 4 servings.

FISH AND SHELLFISH

Fish is offered on the market today in many forms. It is usually available fresh, frozen, canned or dried in whole, steak or fillet form. Shellfish such as oysters, clams, mussels, scallops, lobster, crab and shrimp are popular foods for appetizers, snacks and salads as well as for main dishes.

Preparation

All fish should be stored in a covered utensil in the refrigerator. Frozen fish should not be defrosted until just before it is to be used. Canned fish should be stored in a dry, cool place, and the cans should not be opened until just before the fish is to be used. Quantities of fish are still prepared for shipping by the oldest methods of food preservation—drying, smoking, salting and pickling. With such methods fish will keep in good condition a long time.

The general rule for cooking fish may be summed up in one sentence: short cooking just before serving is most important. This rule is particularly applicable in the case of broiled and pan-broiled fish, which after cooking dries out quickly. The test for cooking is simple. When tried with a fork, the flesh should flake. Sliced or quartered lemon is the chosen garnish for fish for both appearance and flavor.

Two basic methods for the cooking of fish are given below. See also Suggestions for Cooking Fresh Fish on page 492.

Recipes

Fish, Baked Fillets

Wash fish fillet and wipe with cloth. Dip in milk, sprinkle with salt and roll in fine, dry bread crumbs or rolled cornflakes. Place in a small, greased baking pan, sprinkle with melted butter or salad oil and bake in a very hot oven (500° F.) 10 minutes or until well browned. Serve with tartare sauce in a lettuce cup, if desired, and lemon quarter.

Tartare sauce: Mix 1 teaspoon finely minced olives or pickles and a few drops onion juice with 1 tablespoon mayonnaise.

Broiled Fish

Wash fish thoroughly, wipe with cloth. Brush with melted butter or salad oil, sprinkle with salt

SUGGESTIONS FOR COOKING FRESH FISH

Kind of Fish	Preparation at Market	Methods of Cooking	Sauce or Garnish
Bass, black	Split	Broil	Lemon
Bass, sea	Split* Whole	Broil Stuff and bake	Lemon Tomato sauce
Bluefish	Split Whole	Broil, bake, plank Stuff and bake	Sliced tomatoes Sliced pickles Parsley sauce
Cod, small large	Whole Steaks*	Stuff and bake Broil, bake	Anchovy sauce Melted butter Lemon sprinkled with paprika
Flounder	Fillets*	Bake	Lemon, parsley
Haddock, small large large	Whole Fillets* Steaks*	Stuff and bake Bake Bake, broil	Mock Hollandaise sauce Grilled tomatoes Tartare sauce
Halibut	Steaks* Thick slice*	Broil, bake, pan-fry Steam	Cucumber sauce Hollandaise sauce
Mackerel	Split*	Broil, bake	Sliced cucumbers
Pompano	Split Fillets*	Broil, plank Bake	Melted butter Minced parsley Lemon, parsley
Salmon	Steaks* Thick slice*	Broil Steam	Sliced cucumbers Egg sauce
Scrod	Split*	Broil	Melted butter Pepper relish
Shad	Split	Bake, plank	Lemon Radishes
Shad roe*		Parboil, then bake	Bacon Lemon
Smelts	Whole*	Broil, bake, pan-fry	Tartare sauce
Sole	Fillets*	Broil, bake	Melted butter Grilled tomatoes
Snapper, red	Split	Bake, broil, plank	Sliced cucumbers
Swordfish	Steaks*	Broil, pan-fry	Cucumber sauce
Trout, lake and sea	Split	Broil, bake	Melted butter Minced parsley
Tuna, fresh	Steak* Thick piece*	Bake, broil Steam	Lemon sprinkled with paprika Hollandaise sauce
Weakfish	Split*	Broil, bake	Sliced tomatoes
Whitefish	Split Whole	Broil, bake, plank Stuff and bake	Lemon Parsley sauce

*Especially adapted to service in small family.
From Heseltine, M., and Dow, U. M.: *The Basic Cookbook*, ed. 5. Boston, Houghton Mifflin Co., 1967.

and pepper. Place skin side down on well-greased broiler rack, broil 2 inches from heat for 10 to 15 minutes (until brown). The flesh should flake when tried with a fork. Serve with melted butter and sliced lemon. Allow 1 small fish or ⅓ lb. fish fillet for each serving.

EGGS

Eggs are an excellent protein food with nutritive values similar to meat. When eggs are plentiful and therefore cheap, they are an economical source of protein. They may appear in the menu in a variety of ways, not only in their native form but as a constituent of custards, puddings and cakes. They may be served plain at breakfast, as an omelet or a souffle at luncheon, and they make a tasty sandwich filling.

The U. S. Department of Agriculture has established four grades of eggs, depending on quality and size. The label on the carton of U. S. graded eggs gives the grade and the date the grading was done. Grades AA or A should be bought when eggs are to be served in their simple form or when they are to be used for a meringue or as a leavening agent such as in sponge cake. Grade B eggs may be used in cakes and for other general cooking purposes. Medium size eggs are often a more economical buy than Extra Large or Large eggs. Brown and white eggs are of equal nutritive value.

Preparation

As soon as eggs come from the market they should be placed in the refrigerator. Good-quality eggs have clean shells and should not be washed before storage, as washing removes the natural protective coating. Eggs should remain in the refrigerator until just before they are to be cooked, except when they are to form an ingredient of a cake, in which case they will blend better with the batter if they have been allowed to come to room temperature.

Low temperature and short cooking are desirable for most egg dishes, as the texture will be more delicate and tender under these conditions. For this reason, soft-cooked eggs generally are coddled by being allowed to stand covered in water that has been brought to the boiling point. Hard-cooked eggs, prepared by boiling, have a firmer texture and are easier to slice or to stuff.

When they are part of a meal, eggs should be prepared just before they are to be served. Coddled eggs in their shells should be opened just before they are to be eaten.

Recipes

Coddled Eggs

Place 2 cups boiling water in small saucepan and bring again to boiling point. Place 1 or 2 eggs in water. If eggs are not entirely covered, add more boiling water. Remove from heat, cover and let stand where water will remain hot from 6 to 10 minutes, according to degree of firmness preferred. An allowance of about twice as much time as for boiled eggs must be made for coddled eggs. A 3-minute boiled egg will be about the same firmness as one coddled for 6 minutes. If eggs are taken directly out of the refrigerator, allow 1 extra minute for coddling.

Hard-Cooked Eggs

Place eggs in saucepan and add cold water to cover entirely. Bring water to boiling point and simmer 15 minutes. Drain and cover eggs with cold water. When thoroughly cold remove shell and slice or stuff. Eggs may be hard cooked by following the recipe for coddled eggs but allowing the eggs to stand 45 minutes.

Poached Eggs

Place boiling water to the depth of 1 inch in a skillet. Add dash of salt. Break each egg into saucer; slip egg into boiling water. Remove from heat, cover, let stand about 5 minutes (until eggs are firm). Remove from water with slotted spoon, allowing water to drain from eggs, and serve on hot buttered toast.

Eggs Poached in Milk

Follow preceding directions for poached eggs, substituting hot milk for water. Serve eggs on toast and pour hot milk over them.

Eggs Poached in Butter

Place 1 teaspoon butter in a small frying pan and melt over low heat. Break each egg into saucer and slip into frying pan. Remove from heat, cover, let stand about 5 minutes (until eggs are firm). If a harder egg is desired, let stand over low heat 1 more minute.

Poached Egg with Cheese Sauce

Ingredients:
- ⅛ lb. grated cheese (½ cup)
- 2 tablespoons evaporated milk
- 1 slice toast
- 1 egg, poached
- Salt and pepper to taste

Procedure: Melt the cheese over hot water. Add the milk gradually, stirring constantly. Add seasonings. Pour hot cheese sauce on toast, top with the poached egg.

Scrambled Eggs

Ingredients:
- 2 eggs
- 2 tablespoons milk or cream
- ¼ teaspoon salt
- Dash pepper
- 1 tablespoon butter

Procedure: Beat eggs just enough to mix yolks and whites, stir in milk or cream and seasonings. Melt butter in small frying pan and add egg mixture. Stir over low heat as eggs become firm. Stir only enough to prevent eggs sticking to pan. Serve at once. Yield: 1 serving.

Scrambled eggs may also be prepared over hot water in a double boiler. They will take longer to cook and need not be stirred as frequently. They will be very delicate and tender when done.

Shirred Eggs

Butter an individual baking dish and line with soft buttered and seasoned bread crumbs. Break 1 or 2 eggs carefully into dish and sprinkle with salt and pepper. Add 1 tablespoon cream, cover with buttered soft bread crumbs and bake in moderate oven (375° F.) about 15 minutes (until eggs are firm). Yield: 1 serving.

Plain Omelet

Ingredients:
- 2 eggs
- ¼ teaspoon salt
- Dash pepper
- 2 tablespoons water
- 1 tablespoon butter

Procedure: Beat eggs until well blended. Add seasonings and liquid. Melt butter in small frying pan and add egg mixture. Place over medium heat and lift edges of omelet as it cooks. Tip frying pan to allow liquid to run under the firm portion. Shake over heat until slightly brown and fold with spatula from handle of frying pan to outer edge. Slip onto a hot plate and garnish with parsley. Yield: 1 serving.

CHEESE

The general term *cheese* is applied to any product made from the concentrated curd of milk.

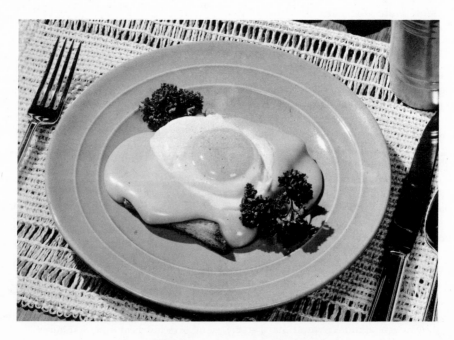

Fig. 35–3. Poached egg with cheese sauce.

Cheddar or American cheese, often called hard cheese, is made from whole milk and has relatively the same food value as whole milk.

Cottage cheese, made from pasteurized skim milk, is next in order of consumption to Cheddar cheese. Because of the absence of cream, the caloric value is much lower than that of Cheddar unless extra cream is added to the finished product. Then it is sold as "creamed" cottage cheese. A considerable amount of the calcium is lost in the process of manufacture, and it is not as good a source of this mineral as milk and hard cheese. Most of the vitamin A is also removed.

Cream cheese, which, like cottage cheese is not ripened and is, therefore, also a perishable product, is made from whole milk with a certain amount of cream added, which gives it a higher caloric value.

Other Cheeses. Many other varieties of cheese are available in today's markets. They may be imported as the specialties of other countries, or made domestically. They most often form an accessory to a meal rather than as a staple part of it.

Cheese mixed with other ingredients is another variation in common use, served on crackers or as a sandwich spread.

Place in the Menu

The increased availability of variations of the Cheddar type of cheese, sold by the package, by the pound and in spread form, each with its own distinctive name and flavor, has stimulated the use of cheese on the table. Cottage and cream cheese, especially the former, are also used largely, often with green salads or as a stuffing for celery. Cottage cheese has some use also as an ingredient of a few cooked dishes.

Both because they are expensive and because most of them have such distinctive flavor, the fine "luxury" types of cheese are reserved as a general rule for serving after meals, although occasionally they appear with salad. For a special salad dressing, Roquefort or blue cheese is a favorite ingredient.

Preparation

When cheese is used in cooking it is usually grated or finely flaked, or cut into small pieces. For top-of-stove cooking, it is generally best to use a double boiler and to cook the cheese over hot water. For baked cheese dishes, a low temperature is generally used, and sometimes directions call for placing the dish containing the cheese mixture in a pan of hot water.

When a high temperature is used, as for instance in toasting an open cheese sandwich under the broiler, the cooking period should be short. The texture of cheese will toughen when it is overcooked by any method.

Recipes

Cheese Souffle

Ingredients:
   2 tablespoons butter or margarine
   2 tablespoons flour
  1/4 teaspoon salt
  1/2 cup milk
  1/4 pound (1 cup) Cheddar cheese, grated
   2 egg yolks
   2 egg whites, stiffly beaten

Procedure: Melt butter or margarine in a small saucepan. Stir in flour and salt. When smooth, stir in milk gradually. Continue stirring until sauce thickens and boils. Remove from heat, add cheese and stir until melted. Stir in egg yolks one at a time, beating after each addition. Fold into the stiffly beaten egg whites. Pour into greased 1-pint casserole and bake in slow oven (300° F.) 1 hour or in moderately hot oven (425° F.) 25 minutes. Yield: 2 generous servings.

Macaroni and Cheese

Ingredients:
  1/4 pound macaroni
   4 tablespoons butter or margarine
   4 tablespoons flour
   1 teaspoon salt
   2 cups milk
   1 to 1½ cups grated or cubed cheese
  1/2 tablespoon butter or margarine
  1/2 cup buttered crumbs

Procedure: Cook macaroni in large amount of boiling, salted water until tender. Drain and place in casserole. Melt butter or margarine in top of double boiler, add flour and salt and mix till smooth. Add milk and cook over low heat until thickened, stirring constantly. Place over boiling water, add cheese and stir until melted. Melt 1/2 tablespoon butter or margarine and mix with 1/2 cup of dry bread crumbs. Pour cheese sauce over macaroni in casserole, cover with buttered bread crumbs and bake in moderate oven (375° F.) until thoroughly heated and crumbs are brown. Yield: 4 servings.

Welsh Rarebit

Ingredients:
> 1 tablespoon butter
> 1 tablespoon flour
> ¼ teaspoon dry mustard
> ¼ teaspoon salt
> Few grains pepper
> 1 cup milk
> ¼ to ½ pound Cheddar type cheese
> 4 slices thin, dry toast

Procedure: Melt butter in top of double boiler over direct heat, add flour and seasonings and stir till smooth. Add milk and cook over low heat until thickened, stirring constantly. Place over hot water, add the cheese cut into small pieces, and stir till cheese has melted and sauce is smooth. Pour over toast and serve at once. Yield: 3 to 4 servings.

VEGETABLES

Under the term *vegetables* are grouped foods representing practically every part of edible plants—leaves, stems, seeds and seed pods, flowers, roots, tubers and fruits.

In addition to their nutritive quality, vegetables are valued because of the variety they give to the diet through texture, flavor, odor and color.

A well-planned menu will include potatoes and at least two additional servings of vegetables each day. Dark green or yellow vegetables are particularly important for their nutrient content, and may be served raw as relishes or salads as well as cooked in a variety of different ways.

Preparation

The care of vegetables in the home kitchen, for use in either raw or cooked form, is important. The length of time during which they will keep in good condition depends on the type and the facilities for storage. Root crops, such as turnips, potatoes, carrots and beets, lose their ascorbic acid content slowly, but preferably they should be kept in a dark, dry, cool place. All other fresh vegetables such as salad greens, celery, carrots, cucumbers, green and lima beans, peas, corn, eggplant, broccoli, cauliflower, parsley, radishes and tomatoes should be refrigerated to prevent deterioration in quality and loss of vitamins.

Vegetables should be washed thoroughly to remove soil and traces of spray. Root vegetables should be scrubbed; asparagus, spinach and other greens should be washed under running water to remove sand. Vegetables such as potatoes and carrots should not be pared or scraped until just before they are to be used. Peas and beans should not be shelled or corn husked until just before they are to be cooked. Outer leaves of cauliflower and cabbage should not be removed until just before they are to be used. A larger loss of vitamins occurs when vegetables are cut in small pieces. Grated carrots, for instance, lose vitamins more quickly than the sliced vegetable.

All vegetables should be cooked as short a time as possible, as long cooking destroys vitamins and changes flavor, color and texture. The use of baking soda in the cooking of green vegetables is not recommended because an alkali such as soda hastens the destruction of the B vitamins and ascorbic acid.

Only a small amount of water should be used for boiling most vegetables. There will be little evaporation if the utensil is tightly covered and if the cooking is done over low heat. See the accompanying chart for General Rules for Boiling Vegetables.

Although boiling vegetables is the most common practice, other methods of preparation can be used to add interest and palatability to everyday meals. Potatoes, winter squash, onions and tomatoes are especially attractive and flavorful when baked in the oven. Sautéeing or frying such vegetables as eggplant, summer squash, parsnips, mushrooms or peppers may add special appeal to a meal. Steaming spinach and cabbage helps to retain the natural flavor and texture as well as the nutritive value of these products. There are numerous popular vegetable combinations: two or more vegetables cooked together, or vegetables combined with protein foods such as eggs, cheese, meat or fish, with sauces or garnishes. Imagination on the part of the homemaker will often bring about enthusiastic acceptance of vegetables where only mere tolerance existed.

General Rules for Boiling Vegetables

1. Use only enough water barely to cover the vegetables. (Exceptions to this rule are noted by an asterisk.) Spinach and other tender greens need no water.

2. Bring water to boiling point and add salt before vegetable is added.

3. Cover tightly and cook over low heat only until vegetables are tender.

4. Use any remaining liquid of mild-flavored vegetables for soup or sauce.

5. Vegetables may be baked in tightly covered casseroles when the oven is being used for some other purpose. The time of cooking will be about one and a half times again as long as for boiling.

6. Variations from the general rules:

Whole artichokes, beets, the cabbage family, onions, parsnips, turnips, potatoes and corn on the cob should be cooked in water to cover, and the water discarded. Keeping the pot tightly covered will prevent spreading the strong cooking odors of some of these vegetables through the house.

Stalks of asparagus and broccoli may be laid side by side in a skillet with one inch of water, or tied and placed upright in the top of a tall double boiler with 1 to 2 inches of water. The skillet or pot should be tightly covered.

7. When a pressure saucepan is to be used, the time chart provided with the utensil should be followed exactly for best results.

Timetable for Boiling

As vegetables differ in texture according to maturity, directions for cooking time can only be approximate.

Vegetable	Minutes	Vegetable	Minutes
Artichokes		Dandelion greens	10–20
American or Jerusalem	15–20	Eggplant	10–15
French or Globe*	20–30	Kohlrabi	20–30
Asparagus*	15–20	Mushrooms	7–10
Beans		Okra	20–25
String	15–30	Onions*	20–40
Lima	20–30	Parsnips*	30–50
Beets*	20–60	Peas	8–15
Beet greens	10–20	Potatoes*	
Broccoli*	15–25	White	20–30
Brussels sprouts*	10–20	Sweet	20–30
Cabbage*	5–10	Spinach	6–10
Carrots	15–30	Squash	
Cauliflower*	10–30	Summer	10–20
Celery	10–15	Winter	20–30
Corn*	5–10	Turnips*	15–60
Cucumbers	10–15		

* See General Rules for Cooking, No. 6, above.

Canned and Frozen Vegetables

Canned vegetables provide out-of-season products which contribute practically the same food value as cooked fresh vegetables. The scientific methods used for the preservation of perishable foods guarantee that the products will be safe and wholesome.

Quick-frozen vegetables are equal or superior in food value to fresh vegetables other than those freshly picked from the garden. Directions for preparation will be found on each package.

Dehydrated and Freeze-Dried Vegetables

Dehydration by some means is the oldest known method of preserving food and was used extensively for vegetables until modern methods of canning and freezing became popular. The new version of dehydration is that of freezing before drying, thus retaining the texture and the fresh appearance of the product when it is reconstituted. Freeze-dried foods are rehydrated quickly. For instance, mashed potatoes need only the addition of boiling water and milk to be ready for serving. Directions for preparation accompany each of the available freeze-dried foods. It needs to be remembered that these products are considerably more expensive than home-prepared foods.

SALADS AND RELISHES

A salad may be served in place of a cooked vegetable or as an extra vegetable at a meal, or it may form the main course. Through different combinations of salad greens, of fruits or vegetables, of eggs, chicken, fish or cheese, or by serving them in jellied form a great variety of flavor and attractiveness can be achieved. Different dressings will also add variety and interest.

Preparation

Salad greens should be separated and thoroughly washed under cold running water and allowed to drain or be dried with a clean towel. Placing them in a plastic bag in the refrigerator will help to keep them crisp. Salads should be prepared for serving just before the meal and the dressing added at the last moment.

The following standards will be helpful in preparing salads. The first 3 standards apply to relishes also:

1. They should be cold and crisp.
2. They should be attractive to the eye.
3. They should be simple rather than elaborate.
4. They should have a dressing which is well but moderately seasoned.

Salad Dressings

French dressing is the simplest and the most widely used of all salad dressings. By varying the basic ingredients and by adding special seasonings, it may be adapted for use with a wide range of salads. Mayonnaise, another commonly used dressing, is more easily bought in the market than prepared at home. It sepa-

rates on freezing and should not be stored in the coldest part of the refrigerator.

Relishes

Relishes may be used in place of or in addition to a salad at a meal.

Celery, radishes and carrot strips are the relishes most used. Scallions, flowerets of raw cauliflower, strips of young turnip and green pepper and thin wedges of cucumber may also be used. The hearts of celery are generally chosen, although the outer stalks of the green Pascal celery are tender enough to be acceptable. Cut stalks of celery may be stuffed with a flavored cottage or cream cheese or with a blend of a highly flavored cheese with cream or cottage cheese.

All vegetables should be washed carefully and trimmed. Carrots should be scraped before being sliced into thin strips. Although it is customary to crisp these vegetables for half an hour or more in iced, salted water, some of the nutrients may be lost.

Recipes

French Dressing

Ingredients:
    ½ teaspoon salt
    ⅛ teaspoon pepper
    ½ teaspoon sugar
    ½ teaspoon dry mustard
    ½ teaspoon paprika
    2 tablespoons vinegar
    ⅓ cup salad oil

Procedure: Place all ingredients in a jar or in a bottle with a lip. Store in refrigerator. Shortly before serving, shake vigorously until the oil and vinegar blend to form a thick emulsion. Yield: ½ cup.

Variations: Add herbs or other seasonings singly or in combination; catsup, chili sauce or piccalilly; crumble Roquefort or blue cheese and add; or substitute grapefruit juice for vinegar and omit mustard for a fruit salad.

Tossed Salad

Place lettuce of one or more varieties, torn into bite-size pieces, into a salad bowl. Add one or more of the following: tomatoes, cut in quarters, sliced cucumbers, onion rings, green pepper rings, diced celery, carrot strips, radish circles; or whole, cooked string beans, or sliced pickled beets; or grapefruit sections and avocado slices. Toss with French dressing just before serving.

Tomato Aspic

Ingredients:

1 tablespoon gelatin
2 cups tomato juice
½ teaspoon salt
Few grains pepper
1 slice onion, chopped
2 ribs celery and leaves, chopped
½ bay leaf
Lettuce

Procedure: Mix ⅓ cup tomato juice with the gelatin; let stand for 5 minutes or more. Heat the remainder of the tomato juice with the seasonings. Dissolve the gelatin in the boiling juice; strain. Pour into individual molds or into a ring mold; chill until firm. Unmold by dipping into hot water; serve on lettuce with mayonnaise dressing. Yield: 6 servings.

Crabmeat Salad

Ingredients:

1 cup canned crabmeat
1 cup diced celery
French dressing
Lettuce
Mayonnaise dressing
1 hard-cooked egg, quartered
1 tablespoon minced parsley

Procedure: Remove membranes from crabmeat and flake; mix crabmeat and celery. Moisten with French dressing and let stand in refrigerator ½ hour or more. Arrange in individual mounds in cup-shaped lettuce leaves; garnish with mayonnaise, egg and parsley. Yield: 3 to 4 servings.

FRUITS

Fruits make a strong appeal to the appetite through the senses of sight, smell and taste. Shape, color, delightful aroma and delicious flavor all contribute to popularizing this group of foods and makes it easy to find a place for them on the menu. The custom of serving fruits twice a day, for breakfast and at some other meal, is good nutrition practice.

Fruit Juices. Orange juice is the longtime favorite of all fruit juices, especially for breakfast, but many other types of fruit juices are popular today and are available both canned and frozen.

Frozen juice concentrates should be stored in the freezing compartment of the refrigerator and should be diluted according to the directions on the can. One fourth of a standard 6-oz. can, enough for one serving, may be diluted and used, and the remainder of the still frozen contents returned to the freezing compartment for future use. Most of the frozen fruit juices will retain good flavor and vitamin content up to 24 hours after reconstituting.

A wide variety of canned fruit juices is also available. Their flavor has been greatly improved by modern methods of food technology. The label on the can will tell whether the juice has been canned with or without added sugar. Some canned fruit juices have been fortified with ascorbic acid.

Stewed, Canned and Cooked Fruits. Dried fruits should be prepared according to the directions on the package, or they may be purchased already prepared. Canned fruits, prepared with heavy or medium syrup or without added sugar, are available, and may be served in the syrup or drained for use in salads. Cooked fruits are usually stewed or baked. For baked apples or apple sauce, a dash of cinnamon or nutmeg may be added for interest.

Frozen Fruits should be stored in the freezing compartment unless they are to be used within a few hours. Some fruits thaw more rapidly than others. One should make sure that fruits are thoroughly thawed before they are served.

Preparation

Most fresh fruits may be eaten raw. Fruits such as apples, pears, peaches, plums, grapes and cherries should be washed thoroughly to remove any traces of insecticide spray residue. If fruits are just ripe enough to eat, they should be refrigerated, except bananas, which should be kept at cool room temperature. Green or unripe fruits should be allowed to ripen at room temperature. Berries should be refrigerated and washed just before serving. Strawberries should be washed before being hulled. Peaches, pears and apples may be served whole or peeled and sliced or sectioned. They, and bananas, should be peeled or sliced just before serving or they will discolor due to oxidation. Sprinkling or dipping them in lemon juice or ascorbic acid solution or adding sugar at the time of slicing will prevent discoloration.

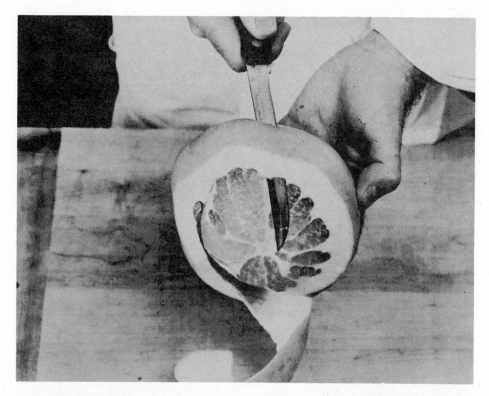

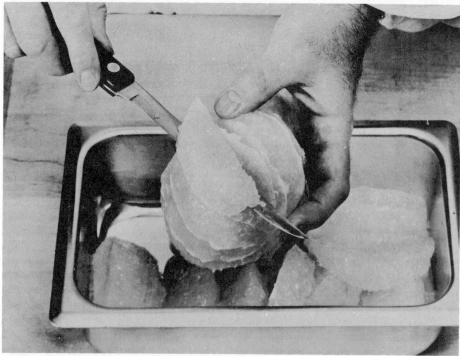

Fig. 35–4. Preparation of grapefruit sections used for salad. Step 1. Cut off peel round and round, spiral fashion, in a sawing motion, cutting directly into the flesh. Step 2. Gently cut down both sides of the membrane with a sharp knife. Remove section by section, holding fruit over bowl to retain juice. (Florida Citrus Commission)

Melons should be tested for ripeness by feeling the "softness" of the stem end, or by the sound it makes, rather dull and thick, when slapped. The safest method, however, may be to ask the fruit or vegetable man to choose one that is ripe. Melons should be washed and chilled in the refrigerator before serving. Cantaloupe and medium sized melons are served in halves or wedges after the seeds are carefully removed. Watermelon is served in inch or 1½ inch slices or, if small, in half of a lengthwise wedge. Cut portions of left-over melon should be wrapped tightly in waxed paper so that their flavor will not permeate other foods in the refrigerator.

Pineapple may be kept at room temperature unless it is very ripe. The easiest method of preparation is to cut the fruit in thick slices or wedges, pare each piece and remove the "eyes," then cut it into bite-size pieces. Sugar or other sweetening is usually needed. The flavor is improved by adding the sugar an hour beforehand and letting the mixture stand. In Hawaii and Puerto Rico, where garden ripe pineapple is available, no sweetening is needed.

Fresh pineapple should not be used with gelatin, as it contains a proteolytic enzyme which "digests" the gelatin and keeps it from setting. The enzyme is usually destroyed in canned fruit or juice.

Of the citrus fruits, oranges and grapefruit are usually preferred for breakfast and are available almost throughout the year. Lemons and limes are most often used as garnish, for seasoning of sauces or as flavoring for cold drinks. Tangerines, kumquats and other special types of citrus fruit may be used as snack foods. When large oranges or grapefruit are cut in half for serving, the segments should be loosened with a curved knife made for the purpose. It should be run between the pulp and the fiber membranes, although the fiber partitions should never be cut. Oranges and grapefruit may also be served in sections by themselves or in combination with other fruits in a fruit plate or salad. They should be peeled with a sharp or serrated knife, round and round, directly into the flesh, and the sections between the membranes removed with a sharp knife. (See Fig. 35–4.)

DESSERTS

Desserts serve several functions in the menu. Perhaps the first is the satisfaction that most people feel in having an attractive sweet at the end of a meal. At the same time, a dessert may supply needed nutrients, either in the form of calories and protein as in milk and egg desserts, or as minerals and vitamins when fruit is the choice.

Desserts fall into several categories, some of which may overlap. For instance, simple combinations of milk and eggs are known as custard. When the same ingredients are thickened with a cereal such as rice or cornstarch, they are called pudding. When gelatin is used for thickening, they are usually known as jelly or gelatin dessert.

Frozen desserts such as ice cream are valuable because they are both refreshing and nourishing. Good quality ices and ice cream are commonly available in most markets. They should be kept in the freezing compartment of the refrigerator until they are used.

Pies and cake are high caloric desserts traditional in the North American dietary. They may be obtained, prepared, in a wide variety in the market. They are considered best, however, when prepared at home, either directly from a recipe or from one of the many packaged mixes available.

Preparation

For the principles underlying the preparation of custard and pudding see the discussion earlier in this chapter under Eggs and Cereals. In the preparation of gelatin desserts, the unflavored gelatin should be softened in cold liquid, then dissolved in hot liquid or over hot water. Flavored gelatin should be prepared according to the directions on the package. Gelatin desserts are usually poured into a wet mold and cooled before being placed in the refrigerator. In small molds the jelly will set completely in about two hours. To unmold gelatin, set the mold in lukewarm water for ½ minute. Loosen the edge with a pointed knife, place serving dish over the mold and invert, shaking gently.

Packaged pudding, custard and gelatin desserts are available. They come in a variety of flavors and call for the addition of milk or water, and sometimes a short cooking period. Many of them compare favorably with desserts prepared by a home recipe.

Recipes

Baked Custard

Ingredients:
- 2 cups milk, scalded
- 3 eggs
- ¼ to ½ cup sugar
- Few grains salt
- ½ teaspoon vanilla *or* sprinkling of nutmeg

Procedure: Beat the eggs slightly; beat in the sugar, salt and vanilla; stir in the hot milk; pour into individual molds of oven glassware or earthenware. Set the molds into a pan; pour in hot water nearly to the top of the molds. Bake in a moderate oven (350° F.) for about 45 minutes. The custard is done when a knife, inserted in the center, comes out clean. Yield: 6 servings.

Indian Pudding

Ingredients:
- 2 cups scalded milk
- 2 tablespoons cornmeal
- 2 to 3 tablespoons molasses
- 3 to 4 tablespoons sugar
- ½ teaspoon salt
- ½ teaspoon ginger

Procedure: Pour milk slowly over cornmeal and cook in double boiler 20 minutes. Add remaining ingredients. Pour into oiled baking dish; bake at 300° F. for 2 hours. Serve warm with ice cream or hard sauce. Yield: 3 to 4 servings.

Fruit Gelatin

Ingredients:
- 1 tablespoon gelatin
- ½ cup cold water
- ¼ to ⅓ cup sugar
- ¾ cup juice, drained from fruit
- ¼ cup lemon juice
- ⅔ cup diced mixed fruits

Procedure: Place gelatin in top of double boiler; add ½ cup cold water; let stand for 5 to 10 minutes until gelatin has absorbed the water. Stir over boiling water until gelatin has dissolved. Add the sugar and stir until it has dissolved. Remove from stove; add the fruit juice and the lemon juice. Cool until the jelly is the consistency of an unbeaten egg white. Stir in the fruit and pour into individual molds rinsed in cold water; or the mixture may be put directly into serving dishes. Chill for 2 to 4 hours. Serve plain or with whipped cream or other topping. Yield: 4 servings.

NOTE: Fresh pineapple should not be used or the gelatin will not set.

True Sponge Cake

Ingredients:
- 3 eggs
- ⅓ cup sugar
- ⅓ cup flour
- Pinch salt
- ½ tablespoon lemon juice
- ½ teaspoon grated rind of 1 lemon

Procedure: Sift sugar, flour and salt together. Separate egg whites from yolks and place whites in large bowl. Beat yolks with lemon juice and rind. With a rotary beater, beat egg whites until they peak but are not dry. Alternately fold in the flour and egg yolk mixtures. Pour into ungreased loaf pan 8½ × 4½ × 2¾ inches. Bake in a slow oven (325° F.) for about an hour. Invert on wire rack and allow to cool. Remove from pan by running the blade of a spatula around the edge.

Junket

Ingredients:
- ½ junket tablet
- ½ tablespoon cold water
- 1 cup milk
- 1 tablespoon sugar
- ¼ teaspoon vanilla

Procedure: Crush junket tablet and dissolve in cold water. Heat milk until lukewarm. Add sugar and vanilla, stir until dissolved. Stir in dissolved junket and pour at once into individual serving dishes. Let stand in a warm place until set. Chill and serve with a bright red jelly or whipped cream. Junket custards are now available in package form. Yield: 2 servings.

STUDY QUESTIONS AND ACTIVITIES

1. Why should the nurse know something of food preparation?

2. Why is it important to plan menus for the whole day or, preferably, for 2 to 3 days at a time?

3. What are some of the recommended steps in following a recipe in order to obtain a successful product?

4. Give the equivalent measurements for the following: 1 cup equals _____ tablespoons; 1 cup equals _____ ounces; 1 tablespoon equals _____ teaspoons. Why should all measurements be level?

5. Define oven-broiling; pan-frying; basting; braising; searing.

6. Give directions for making tea; a chocolate milk shake.

7. Why is the use of raw eggs not recommended by public health authorities?

8. When would you use a clear soup in the diet? When a cream soup?

9. Discuss the uses of cereal products in meal planning.

10. How should the less expensive or less tender cuts of meat be prepared?

11. Look at the recipe for Liver and Sausage Ring. To which groups of patients could this be recommended? Why should it not be suggested to Jewish patients?

12. Give the general rule for cooking fish. What is the test for doneness?

13. What precautions should be used in regard to temperature in cooking protein foods? Why? Why is this especially important in the cooking of eggs and cheese?

14. How may the vitamin content of vegetables be preserved in cooking?

15. Why is a salad a good addition to the menu?

16. List three ways in which fruit may be included in the menu.

17. What precautions should be taken in the preparation of fresh, raw fruits and relishes so that they will be fresh and crisp?

18. What place do desserts have in the menu? What types are most nutritious and digestible?

SUPPLEMENTARY REFERENCES ON FOOD SELECTION AND PREPARATION
General

General Foods: The General Foods Kitchen Cook Book. New York, Random House, 1959.

General Mills: Betty Crocker's New Good and Easy Cook Book. N. Y., Golden, 1962.

————: Betty Crocker's New Picture Cook Book. New York, McGraw-Hill, 1961.

Heseltine, M., and Dow, U.: The Basic Cook Book. ed. 5. Boston, Houghton, Mifflin, 1967.

Hughes, O.: Introductory Foods. Ed. 4, New York, Macmillan, 1962.

McWilliams, M.: Food Fundamentals. New York, Wiley, 1966.

Niles, K. B.: Food Preparation Recipes. New York, Wiley, 1955.

Rombauer, I. S., and Becker, M. R.: Joy of Cooking. New York, Bobbs Merrill, 1962.

Vail, G. E., Griswold, R. M., Justin, M. M., and Rust, L. O.: Foods—An Introductory College Course. Boston, Houghton Mifflin, 1967.

International

Dooley, E. B. K.: Puerto Rican Cook Book. Richmond, Va., Dietz, 1948.

London, A., and Bishov, B.: The Complete American Jewish Cookbook. New York, World, 1952.

Small, M.: The World's Best Recipes. New York, Pocket Books, 1957.

United Nations Association of the United States: Cookbook of the United Nations. New York, Wiley.

Waldo, M.: The Complete Book of Oriental Cooking. New York, Bantam, 1960.

————: The Round the World Cook Book. Garden City, L. I., N. Y., Doubleday, 1954.

CHAPTER 36

Foods With Increased Nutritive Value

Foods Increased in Protein • *Foods Increased in Calories*

Throughout Part Two reference has been made to the use of foods with increased nutritive value, particularly of protein and calories. Methods for increasing protein and calories, most of which also contribute other nutrients to the diet, are discussed in this chapter.

FOODS INCREASED IN PROTEIN

High protein diets may be prescribed for patients prior to or following surgery, during convalescence from wasting or infectious disease, and at other times when food intake or utilization has been poor and when growth and repair of body tissue is essential. The normal diet provides between 60 and 70 Gm. of protein a day (see Pattern Dietary in Chap. 19). High protein diets should contain from 100 to 150 Gm. of protein, depending on the age and the condition of the patient. In severe burns the need for dietary protein may be even higher.

Many patients requiring a high protein diet have a poor appetite and a limited capacity for food; therefore care must be taken in planning the menu so that the desired amount of additional protein will be eaten. Foods such as dry skim milk powder and eggs and cheese, which can be added to regular foods without increasing the bulk, are particularly helpful. Between-meal snacks based on milk, and desserts made with milk and eggs are also useful. Because ill people often do not tolerate very sweet flavors, excessive sweetness in drinks and desserts should be avoided.

The use of raw eggs for beverages is discouraged because they may carry salmonella organisms. (See Chaps. 17 and 35.) A pasteurized eggnog mixture is available in the retail market, and its use in place of raw eggs is recommended.

When a high protein diet is needed for the patient at home, several easily available and inexpensive foods can be added to regular recipes and menus to accomplish this goal. Some good sources of protein suitable for this purpose are listed in Table 36–1. By using moderate amounts of these foods, in addition to the recommended daily servings of meat, fish, poultry, eggs and milk, the protein intake can be measurably increased without much added expense, effort or disruption of regular family meal preparation and service. There are psychological advantages in having a patient on a modified diet eat foods similar to those on the regular family menu. The person preparing the meals will find it convenient and economical to adopt some of the following methods for increasing the protein in the diet, as it eliminates the necessity of preparing separate meals for the family member needing the high protein diet.

DRY SKIM MILK POWDER

Dry skim milk powder offers many possibilities for increasing the protein content of a recipe without changing its flavor, texture or appearance. Two tablespoons of this powder adds an average of 6 Gm. of protein and 52 calories to any serving of food

TABLE 36–1. Protein and Caloric Content of Foods Useful for High Protein Diets

Food	Amount	Protein (Gm.)	Calories
Powdered skim milk..........	1 T. (7.5 Gm.)	3	26
Evaporated milk.............	½ C. (100 Gm.)	7	138
Whole milk.................	1 C. (244 Gm.)	8.5	166
Skim milk, fluid.............	1 C. (246 Gm.)	8.6	87
Cottage cheese.............	1 oz. (30 Gm.)	6	27
Cream cheese..............	1 oz. (30 Gm.)	3	106
Hard cheese...............	1 oz. (30 Gm.)	7	113
Whole egg*...............	1 (50 Gm.)	7	81
Peanut butter..............	1 T. (16 Gm.)	4	92
Ice cream.................	3½ oz. (62 Gm.)	3	129
Walnuts..................	1 T. (8 Gm.)	1	49

Figures from Table 1 in Part Four.

* See warning on the use of raw eggs.

to which it is added, at minimum cost. This can be used in addition to the regular amount of milk used in the recipe or served with the food, in any of the following ways.

At breakfast, add to:

1. Hot cereal. Hot cereal may be cooked in milk instead of water to increase the protein content.

2. Scrambled eggs or omelet.

3. Cocoa or milk used as a beverage, or in eggnog.

At luncheon or dinner, add to:

1. Canned, frozen, concentrated, dehydrated or homemade cream soup, fish or vegetable chowder.

2. Hamburger, lamb or other ground meat patty, croquettes and fish cakes.

3. Sandwich filling such as egg salad, deviled ham, cream or cottage cheese, peanut butter, ground meat or fish, mixed with mayonnaise.

4. Creamed and casserole dishes, using prepared or homemade cream of mushroom, celery, chicken or cheese soup combined with cooked, flaked fish, meat, poultry, hard cooked eggs or vegetables and served on toast, rusks, crackers, mashed or baked potatoes. Further to increase protein and calories, condensed canned cream soup may be diluted with a can of milk plus extra dry skim milk, or undiluted evaporated milk may be used.

5. Mashed and creamed potatoes; or scalloped potatoes, onions, cauliflower, corn, peas, lima or shell beans.

6. Egg, meat, fish or vegetable salad, either sprinkled in during mixing, or added to the dressing.

In beverages and desserts, add to:

1. Eggnog, milkshake, frappe, float, cocoa.

2. Homemade puddings.

Whole Recipes

For greater convenience, 4 to 6 tablespoons of dry skim milk powder can be added to an entire recipe, homemade or packaged, for:

1. Muffins, cornbread, pancakes, waffles, rolls and breads.

2. Cake, cookies, gingerbread, cookie bars and some candies.

3. Cream pie and cake fillings.

4. Cream sauce and poultry gravy.

5. Ice cream, sherbet, frozen desserts.

6. Fruit cobblers, bread or rice pudding, steam pudding.

7. Gelatin desserts.

CHEESE

Cheese offers another method for increasing the protein content of the diet, but it is not as easily incorporated into recipes and menus as powdered skim milk because of its distinctive flavor. However, if the individual likes cheese, some of the following methods can be used.

At breakfast, cheese can be

1. Used for a spread on toast and muffins.

2. Sprinkled over scrambled, fried or poached eggs or omelet.

3. Spread on English muffins or rusks and put under broiler.

4. Melted for a sauce for toast and poached eggs.

At luncheon or dinner, and for snacks

1. Shredded or grated cheese can be added to hot soups, casseroles or creamed dishes, tossed or gelatin salads, vegetable, fish or meat salads and sandwiches.

2. Cottage or cream cheese can be used for topping for fruit salads and desserts, as a spread for crackers served with soups and salads, and as a base for sandwich fillings.

3. Soft cheeses can be used as a base for salad dressing, and grated or shredded hard cheese can be added to French type dressing.

4. Cheese sauce can be served with hot vegetables and fish.

5. Hard or processed cheese can be grilled with meat patties.

6. Cheese and fresh fruit provide an interesting dessert.

EGGS

Eggs in any form add protein to the diet. For the person who likes eggs, they may be served in any of the usual forms. In addition hard-cooked eggs may be sliced or diced and added to tossed and vegetable salads, made into sandwich fillings, added to creamed and casserole dishes, and shredded or crumbled into sauces for vegetables and fish.

For the patient who is less fond of eggs, an egg or two tablespoons of a pasteurized eggnog mixture may be added to a flavored milk drink such as banana, molasses or chocolate milk shakes.

PEANUT BUTTER

Peanut butter is an inexpensive food that yields 4 Gm. of protein per tablespoon. Most cookbooks give a variety of ways for using it in sandwich fillings, shortening in cakes, cookies, cookie bars, hot breads,

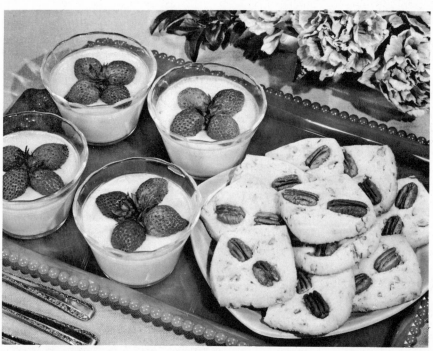

Fig. 36–1. Protein may be increased by the use of extra dried skim milk in desserts and cookies.

frostings and candy. It can be used as a spread on hot toast. Bananas sliced lengthwise, spread with peanut butter and rolled in chopped peanuts make an interesting addition to fruit salads.

NUTS

Nuts yield 1 to 2 Gm. of protein per tablespoon and add texture and flavor to salads, desserts, sandwiches, casserole and creamed dishes. They make good "nibbling" foods.

Recipes With Increased Protein

The recipes which follow may be used for the patient on a high protein diet, either in the hospital or at home. They will be found particularly useful to supplement the diet of those patients who have difficulty in consuming sufficient food from the hospital or family menu. If a high protein tube feeding is required, see Chapter 29. Some of the recipes may be made low in sodium by substituting Protinal (National Drug Co., Philadelphia, Pa.) and low sodium milk for dry skim milk powder and regular milk. Check Table 5 in Part Four for sodium content of foods.

High Protein Beverages with a Milk Base
Basic Recipe—Eggnog:

Ingredients: (1 serving)	(4 servings)
*Egg, 1	4
Milk, whole fluid, ¾ cup	3 cups
Dry skim milk, 2 tablespoons	½ cup
Sugar, 1 tablespoon	¼ cup
Salt, pinch	¼ teaspoon
Flavoring, ½ teaspoon	1 teaspoon

Procedure: Beat egg thoroughly, add salt and sugar and beat until dissolved. Stir in milk and flavoring and mix well. Or put all ingredients in an electric blender and mix until smooth, using lowest speed. Serve chilled in attractive glass.

* Or substitute 2 heaping tablespoons eggnog preparation for one egg and omit sugar.

Variations in Basic Recipe for Eggnog (for 1 serving).

Chocolate: Use 1 tablespoon cocoa and ½ teaspoon vanilla for flavoring.

Coffee: Add 1 or 2 teaspoons instant coffee with sugar.

Molasses: Use 2 tablespoons molasses in place of sugar.

Brandy: Add 1 tablespoon brandy, sprinkle with nutmeg.

Maple: Use 2 tablespoons maple syrup in place of sugar or add Mapleine flavoring to taste.

Banana: Beat sliced banana until smooth with a fork, add to egg mixture with ½ teaspoon vanilla; or use blender if one is available.

Malted milk: Use 4 tablespoons malted milk powder and ¾ cup hot water in place of milk. Reduce sugar in basic recipe.

Protinal: Use ¼ cup Protinal in place of sugar and salt, flavor with chocolate syrup to taste.

Spiced: Use cinnamon, nutmeg, allspice or almond or vanilla to taste.

Low sodium: Omit egg and salt. Use low sodium milk. Substitute ¼ cup Protinal for dry skim milk.

Tomato Juice and Meat Cocktail

Ingredients:	
Tomato juice, chilled	2 cups
Baby strained meat, any variety	1 can
Lemon juice	2 teaspoons
Salt and pepper to taste	

Procedure: Blend well together and serve cold, or serve heated as a soup. Yield: 2 servings.

Tomato Juice Appetizer

Ingredients: (1 serving)	(4 servings)
Tomato juice, ⅓ cup	1⅓ cup
Water, ½ cup	2 cups
Onion juice, few drops	½ teaspoon
Lemon juice, few drops	½ teaspoon
Salt, ⅛ teaspoon	½ teaspoon
Skim milk powder, 3 tablespoons	¾ cup

Procedure: Combine tomato juice, water and seasonings in a saucepan. A few drops of Tabasco sauce may be added if desired. Add milk powder and beat until smooth. Heat quickly until just hot and serve. Avoid overheating.

Protinal Powder Sand Tarts

Ingredients:
  1 cup Protinal Powder
  ¼ cup butter or margarine
  ½ cup sugar
  1 egg

Procedure: Cream Protinal Powder with shortening. Add sugar and mix well. Beat the egg and add, mixing batter thoroughly. Drop by teaspoonful on a lightly greased cookie sheet. Bake in a slow oven (300° F.) for about 20 minutes or until the edges are golden brown. If desired, brush each cookie with white of egg and sprinkle with half-and-half mixture of cinnamon and sugar before baking.

TABLE 36–2. Composition and Caloric Content of Foods Useful for High Caloric Diets

Food	Amount	Protein (Gm.)	Fat (Gm.)	CHO (Gm.)	Calories
Light cream...........	1 T. (15 Gm.)	..	3	1	30
Heavy cream.........	1 T. (15 Gm.)	..	5	1	49
Butter or margarine....	1 T. (14 Gm.)	..	11	..	100
Vegetable oil.........	1 T. (14 Gm.)	..	14	..	124
Whole egg*..........	1 (50 Gm.)	7	6	..	81
Peanut butter.........	1 T. (16 Gm.)	4	8	3	92
Mayonnaise...........	1 T. (13 Gm.)	..	10	..	92
Ice cream............	3½ fl. oz. (62 Gm.)	3	8	13	129
Bread...............	1 slice (23 Gm.)	2	1	12	63
Oatmeal.............	⅔ C. cooked (100 Gm.)	2	1	11	63
Sugar, granulated.....	1 T. (12 Gm.)	..	..	12	48
Lactose..............	1 T. (8 Gm.)	..	..	8	32
Syrup...............	1 T. (20 Gm.)	..	..	15	57
Molasses.............	1 T. (20 Gm.)	..	..	12	48
Honey...............	1 T. (21 Gm.)	..	..	17	62
Jam, jelly............	1 T. (20 Gm.)	..	..	14	55

Figures from Table 1 in Part Four.
* See warning on the use of raw eggs.

Fruit Sherbet

Ingredients:
    1 package fruit gelatin dessert powder
  1½ cups sugar
    2 cups boiling water
   ⅓ cups lemon juice
    1 tablespoon grated lemon rind
    3 cups cold water
    2 cups dry milk powder

Procedure: Mix dessert powder and sugar, add boiling water and stir until dissolved. Cool. Add lemon juice and rind. Put 3 cups cold water into a large bowl, add the milk powder and beat until smooth. Stir into cooled gelatin mixture. Freeze. Yield: 10 servings.

FOODS INCREASED IN CALORIES

The high caloric diet is ordered for patients who are underweight as a result of disease or who, for other reasons, have been unable to obtain or eat sufficient food to meet their energy needs. Since fats yield 9 calories per gram, they should be included in the high caloric diet over and above the quantity usually taken. However, fat has a high satiety value, and, if the patient has a poor appetite, a high fat intake may depress it still further. Carbohydrate foods are usually better tolerated, but sugar, with its sweet taste, may also not be acceptable to the patient with a poor appetite or a limited capacity for food. Therefore, foods for the high caloric

diet must be chosen carefully and adapted to the patient's needs and circumstances.

Best results are obtained if the patient is served 5 or 6 small meals during the day rather than 3 regular meals. Attractive dishes and mealtime companionship will also help to increase the desire for and enjoyment of food. Table 36–2 gives the composition and the caloric value of some foods which will aid in increasing the caloric content of the diet.

CREAM

Either light (20%) or heavy (35%) cream may be used in place of, or mixed half and half with, milk in making beverages, soups, chowders and sauces. It may also be served with hot or cold cereals, fruits and pudding desserts. Whipped cream can be used as a topping for cocoa, coffee, desserts and cold or hot soups. Cream may be used alone or mixed with mayonnaise as dressing for fruit salads and as an ingredient in desserts. Commercially soured cream may also be used for topping on soups, salads, fruits and desserts, and as an ingredient in salad dressings, sauces and in dips and spreads for snacks and sandwiches.

BUTTER AND MARGARINE

In addition to their regular use as spreads for bread, pancakes and vegetables, and for frying and shortening, butter or margarine can be added to hot soups, chowders and hot cereals. Extra butter or margarine may be added to broiled foods. Using both butter or margarine and mayonnaise on sandwiches will help to increase the caloric content.

SUGAR, SYRUP, JELLY

These are available in several forms and are a good source of carbohydrate calories in the diet. All sugars have the same caloric value, but differ in weight and in degree of sweetness. Lactose is less sweet than corn syrup, and corn syrup is not as sweet as granulated sugar. Lactose may be used to provide calories for the very ill patient who cannot tolerate the sweetness of table sugar. In the following recipes 3 tablespoons of lactose may be substituted for 1 tablespoon of table sugar. Corn syrup, although somewhat sweeter than lactose, is less sweet than granulated sugar. Two tablespoons of corn syrup may be substituted for one of sugar.

Molasses, corn and maple syrup may be served on griddle cakes and waffles or added to milk beverages. Honey, although very sweet, may be enjoyed as a spread for bread, griddle cakes and waffles. Brown sugar is a pleasant variant for granulated sugar on cereal. Jams and jellies not only serve as a spread for bread, but can be added to puddings for color and flavor, and, heated, serve as a sauce.

BREADS, CAKES, COOKIES, DESSERTS

If the patient's appetite warrants it, an additional slice of bread at a meal, accompanied by butter and jelly, is an easy way to increase calories. Likewise, a cookie or a small piece of cake may be served with dessert. As stated earlier, cream used either in the preparation of a dessert or as a topping adds calories without adding bulk.

Recipes for High Caloric Foods

The recipes which follow are designed to add calories to the normal diet. They will also add other needed nutrients, depending on their ingredients. Some of the high protein recipes found earlier in the chapter may also be suitable for high caloric diets.

High Caloric Beverages with an Ice Cream Base: Basic Recipe

Ingredients: (1 serving)   *(4 servings)*
  Ice cream, ½ cup   2 cups
  Carbonated beverage, ¾ cup   3 cups

Procedure: Put ice cream in tall glass and pour half the carbonated beverage over it. Stir till well mixed, then add remainder of fluid and serve at once.

Variations: Many flavor combinations are possible using a variety of ice creams and carbonated beverages.

High Caloric Beverages with a Fruit Base: Basic Recipe

Ingredients: (1 serving)   *(4 servings)*
  Fruit juice,* ¾ cup   3 cups
  Sugar, 1 tablespoon   ¼ cup
  Lactose, 3 tablespoons   ¾ cup
  Lemon juice, 1 tablespoon   ¼ cup

Procedure: Combine all ingredients and mix thoroughly until sugar is dissolved. Chill before serving, or pour over cracked ice, strain. Serve with a sprig of fresh mint or a thin lemon slice garnish.

* Fresh, frozen reconstituted, or canned orange, pineapple, grape, tomato, prune, apple or mixed fruit juices are suitable.

Corn Syrup Lemonade

Ingredients: (1 serving)   *(4 servings)*
  Corn syrup, ¼ cup   1 cup
  Lemon juice, 3 tablespoons   ¾ cup
  Water, ¾ cup   3 cups

Procedure: Mix corn syrup with lemon juice until thoroughly blended. Add water and chill. Serve with a sprig of mint.

NOTE: This recipe is particularly suitable for raising calories on a low protein diet.

High Caloric Eggnog

Ingredients:
  1 egg*
  1 tablespoon sugar
  3 tablespoons lactose
  ¾ cup milk
  2 tablespoons cream
  ½ teaspoon vanilla

Procedure: Beat egg and add sugar and lactose. Combine with milk, cream and vanilla. Mix thoroughly, chill and serve. Yield: 1 serving.

* Two tablespoons pasteurized eggnog mixture may be substituted for one egg and 1 tablespoon sugar.

High Caloric Cereal Gruel

Ingredients:
    2 tablespoons farina or oatmeal
    ¼ teaspoon salt
    1 cup water
    2 tablespoons lactose
    ¼ cup cream
        Sugar or additional salt to taste

Procedure: Add farina or oatmeal slowly to boiling, salted water and simmer for 15 minutes, adding water as necessary to maintain volume. Strain the liquid into another pan; add lactose and cream, and sugar and salt to taste; reheat and serve. Yield: 1 to 2 servings.

Pineapple Cream

Ingredients:
    ½ cup boiled rice
    2 tablespoons crushed pineapple
    ¼ cup heavy cream

Procedure: Combine rice with crushed pineapple. Whip cream and fold into rice mixture. Serve in sherbet glass. Yield: 1 liberal serving or 2 small servings.

High Caloric Custard

Ingredients:
    2 tablespoons sugar
    4 tablespoons lactose
    1 cup light cream
    1 egg
    ⅛ teaspoon salt
    ¼ teaspoon vanilla
        Nutmeg

Procedure: Add sugar and lactose to cream; warm to dissolve the sugars. Beat egg, add salt and vanilla; stir in cream mixture. Pour into custard cups and sprinkle with nutmeg. Place in pan of hot water. Bake in moderate oven (375° F.) until set, about 35 minutes. The custard is cooked when mixture does not adhere to knife when inserted. Cool quickly by placing cups in cold water. Yield: 2 servings.

Bavarian Cream

Ingredients:
    1 cup milk
    ½ tablespoon unflavored gelatin
    2 tablespoons cold water
    1 egg, separated
    2 tablespoons sugar
        Dash salt
    ½ teaspoon vanilla extract
    ¼ cup whipped cream

Procedure: Scald milk. Soften gelatin in cold water and dissolve with scalded milk. Beat egg yolk with sugar and salt, stir the hot mixture into this. Place in small double boiler and stir over hot water until mixture thickens slightly. Add vanilla extract and chill until mixture begins to set. Fold in whipped cream and pour into sherbet glasses. Serve with sweetened crushed fruit. Yield: 3 servings.

Mocha Bavarian Cream

Procedure: Follow directions for Bavarian Cream. Add 1 teaspoon instant coffee and 1 tablespoon instant cocoa to hot milk and mix well before adding to gelatin. Increase sugar to 3 tablespoons. Undiluted evaporated milk may be substituted for the milk. Serve with whipped cream or other topping.

STUDY QUESTIONS AND ACTIVITIES

1. List 10 foods to which dry skim milk may be added to increase the protein content. Approximately how much should be added per serving?

2. How many grams of protein do 2 level tablespoons of dry skim milk contain?

3. List 5 ways in which cheese may be added to a food to increase its protein content.

4. What other protein foods are suitable as additions to high protein diets?

5. How can high protein beverages be made low in sodium?

6. What foods may be used to increase the calories in the diet?

7. Why may large quantities of fat be contraindicated in the high caloric diet?

8. Why should sugar not be used in large quantities in a high caloric diet? What sugar is less sweet than granulated sugar?

SUPPLEMENTARY READING FOR FOODS WITH INCREASED NUTRITIVE VALUE

Church, R. E.: Mary Meade's Magic Recipes for the Electric Blender. Rev. Ed. Indianapolis, Bobbs-Merrill, 1965.

Rollin, B., and Rosenfeld, L.: The Non-Drinker's Drinkbook. Garden City, N. Y., Doubleday, 1965.

Seifrit, E.: The high caloric diet, Am. J. Clin. Nutr., *12*:66, 1963.

CHAPTER 37

Foods for Low Caloric and Diabetic Diets

The discussion of food preparation for these two therapeutic regimens has been placed together, since what is said about one is often applicable to both. Many diabetics, particularly those over 40 years of age, are overweight. The loss of excess weight in this age group may be all that is needed to control their diabetes. On the other hand, diabetic patients who are on a weighed diet regimen (see Chap. 22) should probably not use the recipes under Low Caloric Diets, unless permitted by the physician.

FOODS FOR LOW CALORIC DIETS

As indicated in Chapter 21, it is essential that low calorie diets be adequate in all nutrients, but at a caloric level low enough to encourage weight loss. The diet should include a variety of readily available foods and provide enough substance to be satisfying. Methods of cooking meat, fish, poultry, eggs and vegetables, and the sauces and dressings used with desserts and salads are discussed, as they affect the total caloric level of a menu. The recipes which follow are examples of ways in which calories can be reduced in the menu without decreasing the other essential nutrients or the taste appeal. Sparing the calories behind the scenes, that is, in the buying and the method of preparation, makes it easier for the dieter to follow instructions.

FOOD SELECTION AND COOKING METHODS FOR LOW CALORIC DIETS
Soups

Soups made from meat stock, strained, cooled and skimmed, canned bouillon or consommé, and broth made with bouillon

cubes have little or no caloric value. This also is true when these products are jellied or bought in the form of "madrilene." Clam juice also lacks calories. Any of these clear soups may be flavored with tomato juice and savory seasonings and served in liquid form or jellied.

Tomato juice, served plain or seasoned and without dilution, will still have a low caloric content, as it will when it is made into aspic with plain gelatin. In this same class is a vegetable soup when made with either a stock or tomato juice.

Meats

Meats for low caloric diets should be from the lean cuts, and the visible fat should be trimmed off before cooking.

Roasting and broiling are the easiest methods to use for cooking meat when calories must be limited. Roasting should be done on a rack, as, in this way, most of the fat will drip into the bottom of the pan. Extra fat may be trimmed after the meat is sliced and before it is served. Broiling is, of course, always done on a rack. However, pan-broiling calls for a skillet. Sprinkle skillet surface with salt by means of a shaker. In the case of veal, rub surface lightly with fat before adding salt. If fat accumulates in the pan, it should be poured off during the cooking. When cooking has been completed, the meat should be placed on a paper towel and turned so that extra fat will be absorbed before it is served. For hamburger patties, lean beef should be ground especially, as normal hamburger contains a comparatively large amount of fat.

Braising, pot roasting or stewing are methods used for less tender cuts of meat. The meat should be browned according to directions for broiling, after which liquid is added. A stew for which the meat is cut in pieces calls for the same initial preparation. If fat accumulates in the liquid during the long cooking, the meat should be drained, the liquid chilled and the hardened fat skimmed. The meat then may be reheated in the remaining liquid.

Leftover cooked meat may be combined with vegetables and a well-seasoned gelatin mixture. See jellied fish salad on recipe pages.

The addition of herbs and spices to meats, poultry, fish and vegetables adds to their flavor and acceptability. See Chapter 39 for suggestions.

Fish

The best methods for cooking fish for a low caloric diet are "poaching" (simmering gently in water in a covered utensil) and baking in greased foil. Fish also may be broiled on a greased broiler rack if the fish is sprinkled lightly with milk or tomato juice. If a Teflon pan is available, fish may be fried with almost no fat. Poached fish (see above) may be used to advantage in a jellied salad. "Dietetic Tuna" packed in brine is useful in a low caloric diet.

Vegetables

Special care must be taken in cooking vegetables so as to retain all their natural flavors (see Chap. 35). They must be particularly well seasoned, as the use of butter and margarine as a dressing must be limited. Minced parsley, chives or sweet onion, minced celery or green pepper often is a welcome addition. Tomatoes may be used in combination with some vegetables.

Salads

Salads have a valuable place in a reducing diet. Such large portions of vegetables and fruit salads may be used that a limited meal will appear to be more satisfying as well as actually be so. The occasional use of an "aspic base" for fruits or vegetables, or a combination of both, lends variety.

Cottage cheese also may be put to good use in salads. Although salad oil in dressings must be avoided or limited in amount, there are a number of savory dressings that can be prepared without its use. Low caloric salad dressings in a variety of flavors are available commercially.

Desserts

In a reducing diet, fresh fruits are the usual choice for dessert. Frozen fruits are packed in a syrup, but this is very light. Water packed, canned fruits contain no added sugar.

When milk is a dessert ingredient, fresh or reconstituted dry skim milk may be used. Baked custard may be made with skim milk and an artificial sweetener. Low caloric, flavored gelatin desserts containing an artificial sweetener are readily available in the grocery store.

Beverages

Coffee and tea to which neither sugar or milk or cream are added have no food value. Non-caloric carbonated beverages, pleasant on a hot summer's day, are available in the markets.

Artificial Sweeteners

Artificial sweeteners are in common use today as calorie sparers. They are also used by those who must curtail sugar intake for other reasons. These sweeteners are organic compounds which taste sweet but have no food value. The common ones in use are saccharin and the cyclamates (either the sodium or the calcium salts, sold under the name of Sucaryl, Sweeta and other brand names). Saccharin has about 300 times and the cyclamates 30 times the sweetening power of cane sugar. Both types are available in tablet, powder and liquid form.

There is no evidence that the use of the non-caloric sweeteners is hazardous to health. Actually, most persons who use them make only a partial substitution for sugars, because real sugar is necessary in certain baked products for texture and tenderness. They have a large use, however, in certain bottled beverages that supply flavor without extra calories.

When non-nutritive sweeteners are used in cooking, it is well to recognize that saccharin may give a bitter flavor, especially after heating, whereas the cyclamates do not seem to have this disadvantage. Experience teaches a person how much of either type to use, and equivalents are suggested on the labels. Suitable quantities are suggested in the low caloric and diabetic recipes given in this chapter.

Recipes for Low Caloric Diets
Soups

Jellied Consommé

Ingredients:
> 1 tablespoon unflavored gelatin
> 2 cups well-seasoned soup stock or consommé
> Sliced lemon
> Minced parsley

Procedure: Soften gelatin in ¼ cup stock. Heat remainder of stock and stir into gelatin. Chill. When set, beat lightly with a fork and serve in soup cups. Serve each with slice of lemon dipped in parsley. Yield: 3 or 4 servings.

Tomato Madrilene

Procedure: Follow directions for jellied consommé (above), substituting 1 cup tomato juice cocktail for 1 cup stock or consommé. If a highly seasoned madrilene is desired, add Worcestershire sauce and Tabasco to taste. Serve sprinkled with finely cut Pascal celery or green pepper. Place wedge of lemon on side of plate.

Chinese Egg Soup

Ingredients:
> 2 cups clear, seasoned broth (chicken or meat)
> 1 egg, beaten
> 1 teaspoon chopped parsley (fresh or dry)

Procedure: Heat broth; while boiling, pour in beaten egg slowly, stirring constantly. Add parsley and serve. Yield: 2 servings.

Meat and Fish

Meat Loaf

Ingredients:
> 1 lb. ground lean meat
> ⅓ cup soft bread crumbs
> 3 tablespoons finely cut onions
> ⅓ cup drained, canned tomatoes
> ½ cup dry skim milk powder
> Salt and pepper to taste

Procedure: Mix ingredients thoroughly. Shape into loaf and place into greased shallow baking pan. Bake in oven at 350° F. for 40 minutes or until brown. Yield: 4 servings.

Hamburgers

Procedure: Shape above meat mixture into 8 flat patties. Place on broiler pan about 4 inches from heat. Broil slowly until brown, about 5 minutes on each side. Yield: 4 servings.

Baked Fish in Foil

Procedure: Grease pieces of foil about 3 times the size of fish fillet. Season fillet. Place on foil and fold over fillet. Press edges together to seal tightly. Bake in hot oven (450° F.) about 25 minutes.

Jellied Fish Salad

Ingredients:
> 1 tablespoon unflavored gelatin
> ¼ cup cold water
> 1½ cups boiling water
> ½ teaspoon salt
> 1 drop Sucaryl solution
> 3 tablespoons vinegar
> 1 8-ounce can tuna fish, flaked; brine or dietetic
> 2 tablespoons sweet, minced pickle or pepper relish
> ¼ green pepper, minced
> ½ small onion, minced
> 1 cup celery, minced

Procedure: Soften gelatin in ¼ cup cold water. Add boiling water, salt and Sucaryl, and stir until gelatin is dissolved. Add vinegar. Chill When jelly is nearly set, stir in flaked fish, pickles or relish and minced vegetables. Pour into mold and chill until firm. Unmold and garnish with salad greens. Serve with low caloric dressing. Yield: 4 servings.

NOTE: 1 cup canned shellfish or diced cooked meat or chicken may be substituted for the tuna fish.

Cucumber Boat

Ingredients:
> ¼ cup flaked fish, shrimp or crabmeat
> ¼ cup chopped celery or green pepper
> Low caloric dressing
> Salt

Procedure: Mix fish, vegetable and dressing. Add salt to taste. Peel cucumber, cut lengthwise in half and scoop out center. Fill with fish mixture. Garnish with strip of pimiento or sprig of parsley. Yield: 2 servings.

Egg

Fluffy Omelet

Ingredients:
> 3 tablespoons dry skim milk powder
> 2 egg whites
> 2 egg yolks

2 tablespoons water
½ teaspoon salt
Few grains pepper
½ teaspoon butter or margarine
¼ cup strained canned tomatoes or
1 tablespoon minced parsley

Procedure: Beat dry skim milk powder with egg whites until mixture stands in moist, stiff peaks. In another bowl beat the egg yolks, water, salt and pepper until lemon colored. Fold into egg white mixture. Melt butter or margarine in hot skillet and pour egg mixture into skillet. Cook over very low heat about 2 minutes or until bottom is light brown. Put skillet in previously heated oven at 350° F. Bake about 10 minutes or until top is brown. Remove from oven and cut about ½ inch deep across the omelet, dividing it in half. Spread one half of omelet with strained, canned tomatoes or with minced parsley, or with a mixture of both. Fold over the other half, lift from skillet to warm plate and serve at once. Yield: 2 servings.

Dressings

Zero Salad Dressing

Ingredients:
½ cup tomato juice
2 tablespoons lemon juice or vinegar
1 tablespoon onion, finely chopped
Salt and pepper
Chopped parsley or green pepper, horse-radish or mustard, etc., may be added, if desired.

Procedure: Combine ingredients in a jar with a tightly fitted top. Shake well before using.

Buttermilk or Yoghurt Dressing

Ingredients:
1 cup buttermilk or yoghurt
1 tablespoon minced onion
1 tablespoon minced green pepper
1 tablespoon minced celery
1 tablespoon catsup
1 tablespoon herb vinegar
Salt to taste

Procedure: Mix ingredients thoroughly and let stand 1 hour or more to ripen flavor. A peeled clove of garlic may be placed in the dressing and removed before dressing is used. The use of yoghurt produces a thicker dressing. Yield: About 1 cup.

Desserts

Gelatin Blancmange

Ingredients:
1 tablespoon unflavored gelatin
¼ cup cold skim milk
2 teaspoons Sucaryl solution
½ teaspoon salt

1½ cups scalded skim milk
1 teaspoon almond or mint extract

Procedure: Soak gelatin in cold milk 5 minutes. Add Sucaryl and salt to scalded milk and stir until thoroughly dissolved. Add to softened gelatin and stir until thoroughly dissolved. Chill until as thick as unbeaten egg white. Add flavoring and beat until frothy. Pour into serving dish or mold and chill until set. Unmold and garnish with a maraschino cherry or with mint leaves. Yield: 4 servings.

Spiced Apple Compote

Ingredients:
6 cooking apples with a firm texture
2 cups water or apple juice
3 tablespoons cornstarch
2 teaspoons Sucaryl solution
½ teaspoon cinnamon
¼ teaspoon nutmeg
¼ teaspoon salt

Procedure: Peel, quarter and core the apples and place in custard cups or in casserole. Mix cornstarch, cinnamon, nutmeg and salt with ½ cup of water or apple juice until smooth. Bring the remainder of the liquid to a boil, add the cornstarch mixture and sweetening, stirring constantly until thickened. Pour over apples and bake in oven at 350° F. until apples are soft but not mushy, about 30 minutes. Serve plain or with a low caloric topping. Yield: 6 servings.

Fruit Gelatin

Ingredients:
1 tablespoon unflavored gelatin
¼ cup cold water
1 1-lb. can of dietetic fruit salad or
   fruit cocktail
Water, ginger ale or noncaloric beverage
2 tablespoons lemon juice
2 teaspoons Sucaryl solution
Artificial coloring if desired

Procedure: Soften gelatin in cold water and dissolve over boiling water. Remove from heat. Drain fruit and measure juice; add enough water, ginger ale or noncaloric beverage to make 1½ cups. To this add lemon juice, Sucaryl and artificial coloring if desired. Stir in dissolved gelatin mixture and chill until partially thickened. Place fruit in 6 molds or sherbet glasses, and add thickened gelatin mixture. Chill until firm. Serve with a low caloric topping. Yield: 6 servings.

Variations: This recipe may be made with fresh or frozen melon balls combined with ginger ale; grapes with grape-flavored non-caloric beverage; black cherries, either fresh or canned, with black cherry flavored non-caloric beverage; and many other combinations.

FOODS FOR DIABETIC DIETS

There are a number of foods which contain little or no protein, fat or carbohydrate that may be used freely on the diabetic diet. Black coffee, tea, bouillon and clear broth are in this group. A number of vegetables (see Vegetable Exchanges—Group A—in Chap. 22) up to 1 cup a day may be included without counting them in the diet. These foods, besides being served hot as part of the menu, can be used as between-meal snacks or made into soups or salads. The use of Zero Dressing for salads will enhance their flavor and acceptability. Spices and herbs may also be added to diabetic diets as to others, to give variety and interest. See Chapter 39 for suggestions.

Non-caloric artificial sweeteners, described earlier in this chapter, are imperative for the diabetic individual who likes sweet foods, for whom sugars, syrups and jams and jellies are forbidden. They can be used not only for coffee and tea, but to sweeten a number of other foods as shown in some of the accompanying recipes.

These sweeteners are also used in the manufacture of non-caloric carbonated beverages.

Diabetic patients sometimes ask about the use of foods specially prepared for the diabetic, such as candies, cookies and desserts. Many of these may be found in today's supermarkets or in the so-called "health stores." However, these foods are more expensive than ordinary foods, because the demand for them is not as great. The use of water-packed or juice-packed fruits is perhaps the most common.

Diabetes is often accompanied by overweight. Suggestions for food purchasing and preparation described under Low Caloric Diets earlier in this chapter should also be followed by the diabetic who is overweight.

As discussed in Chapter 22, there are three methods in use in the dietary treatment of diabetes. When the patient is following the dietary plan based on Meal Planning and Exchange Lists, described in Chapter 22, the following recipes will be helpful, as they demonstrate how "mixed" dishes can be included on this regimen.

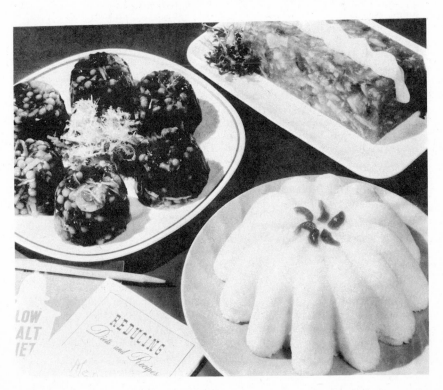

FIG. 37–1. Gelatin is a good stretcher for low caloric foods in salads, entrées and desserts.

Some of the recipes found under Low Caloric Diets in this chapter, particularly those which include artificial sweeteners, are also suitable for the diabetic patient if the other ingredients are permitted.

Recipes for Diabetic Diets
Soups

Vegetable Soup

(1 serving equals 1 vegetable from List 2B)
  Ingredients:
  1 cup meat stock or bouillon cube and
      1 cup water
  ½ cup mixed vegetables: carrots, peas
  ½ small onion, chopped
  ¼ cup cabbage, shredded
  1 stalk celery, diced
  ¼ cup tomato juice
      Salt and pepper
Procedure: Prepare vegetables and add to broth. Boil together until vegetables are just tender, about 20 minutes.

Green Pea Soup

(1 serving equals ½ Milk Exchange, 1 Bread Exchange and 1 serving vegetable from List 2B. If bacon is used, add 1 Fat Exchange)
  Ingredients:
  ½ cup peas, cooked, canned or
      infant, strained
  ½ cup beef broth or bouillon
  ½ cup milk
      Salt and pepper to taste
  1 slice bread, toasted
Procedure: Purée cooked or canned peas in a blender. Heat the milk and add it to the hot broth. Stir in the strained peas and reheat. Season to taste. Cut the toasted bread in cubes and use as croutons in soup. One strip of bacon may be fried, diced and added to the soup. Yield: 1 serving.

Meat, Fish and Cheese

Meat Stew

(1 serving equals 2 or 3 Meat Exchanges and 1 Bread Exchange and 1 serving vegetable from List 2B and 1 Fat Exchange)
  Ingredients:
  1 teaspoon fat
  ½ cup mixed vegetables, list 2B
      (carrots, peas, onions)
  2 or 3 oz. meat, cubed
  1 small potato
      Salt and pepper to taste
Procedure: Brown meat in fat. Add 1 cup water, salt, pepper and a few celery leaves for seasoning. Simmer slowly until meat is tender.

Add ½ cup vegetables, List 2B, and any additional vegetables from List 2A, if desired. Cut potato into quarters and add. Cook for 30 minutes or until vegetables are done.

Baked Chicken and Rice

(1 serving equals 1 Bread Exchange and 1 or 2 Meat Exchanges)
  Ingredients:
  ½ cup cooked rice
  ¼ or ½ cup diced chicken (1 or 2 ozs.)
  ¼ cup clear broth
      Salt and pepper
      Chopped parsley, onions, celery, mushrooms, green pepper, pimiento or tomatoes may be added for variety, if desired.
Procedure: Combine the above ingredients and place in small casserole. Bake in moderate oven (350° F.) until brown.

Noodles or spaghetti may be used in place of rice. For the chicken, any type of meat or fish, such as lamb, ham, tuna or shrimp, may be substituted.

Fish Chowder

(1 serving equals 1 Fat Exchange and 1 Bread Exchange and 1 or 2 Meat Exchanges and 1 cup milk)
  Ingredients:
  1 teaspoon fat
  ½ small onion, chopped
  1 small potato, sliced
  ¼ or ½ cup cooked fish (1 or 2 ozs.)
  1 cup milk
      Salt and pepper
Procedure: Cook fish in salted water. Melt fat in saucepan, brown the onion. Add cooked fish, sliced potato, ½ cup water in which fish was cooked. Cover and cook for 15 minutes until potatoes are tender. Add milk and seasonings.

Cheese Fondue

(1 serving equals 1 Bread Exchange and 2 Meat Exchanges and 1 cup milk)
  Ingredients:
  1 egg
  1 cup milk
  1 slice bread, cubed
  ¼ cup cheese, diced (1 oz.)
      Salt, pepper, chopped parsley and onion
Procedure: Beat the egg, add milk, bread, cheese and seasoning. Bake in a moderate oven (350° F.) until firm in the center, about 20 or 30 minutes.

In place of cheese, ¼ cup (1 oz.) of chopped ham, chicken, tuna fish or salmon may be used.

Italian Spaghetti

(1 serving equals 1 or 2 Meat Exchanges and 1 or 2 Bread Exchanges and 1 Fat Exchange)

Ingredients:

   ½ cup cooked spaghetti
   1 teaspoon fat
   ½ small onion, chopped
   1 or 2 ozs. ground meat
   2 tablespoons tomato paste
   ¼ cup water
   Salt, pepper
   ½ cup tomatoes

Procedure: Brown the onion and ground meat in the fat. Add the tomato paste, water, tomatoes and seasonings. Allow to simmer gently 1 hour or more. If needed, add more water. Serve on ½ or 1 cup cooked spaghetti. One or 2 teaspoons grated cheese may be used.

Macaroni and Cheese

(1 serving equals 1 Bread Exchange and 1 or 2 Meat Exchanges and ¼ cup milk)

Ingredients:

   ¼ cup milk
   ¼ or ½ cup diced cheese (1 or 2 ozs.)
   ½ cup cooked macaroni
   Salt, pepper, dash of mustard

Procedure: Cook cheese and milk together in double boiler until smooth. Add macaroni and mix well. Bake in moderate oven (350° F.) about 20 minutes or until brown.

In place of macaroni, ½ cup cooked rice, noodles or spaghetti may be used.

Vegetables and Salads

Sweet-Sour German Cabbage

(1 serving equals 1 cup of "A" Vegetable Exchange, 1 Fat Exchange)

Ingredients:

   2 tablespoons butter or margarine
   6 cups raw, shredded red cabbage, washed and drained
   1 medium onion, sliced in rings
   ¼ cup water
   ½ cup vinegar
   1 teaspoon Sucaryl solution

Procedure: Melt butter in a large saucepan. Add cabbage (use only water which still clings to leaves). Cook covered over low heat until tender, stirring occasionally to prevent sticking. Add onion rings, water, vinegar and Sucaryl. Cover and cook about 10 minutes longer. Yield: 6 servings.

Orange Glazed Beets

(1 serving equals 1 "B" Vegetable Exchange, 1 Fat Exchange)

Ingredients:

   2 tablespoons butter or margarine
   2 teaspoons cornstarch
   ¼ teaspoon salt
   1 tablespoon Sucaryl solution
   1 teaspoon cider vinegar
   2 teaspoons grated orange rind
   ½ cup orange juice
   3 cups cooked sliced beets (1½ pounds)

Procedure: Melt butter in saucepan. Blend in cornstarch and salt. Add Sucaryl, vinegar, orange rind and juice. Cook over medium heat until smooth and thick, stirring constantly. Add beets and simmer over low heat about 10 minutes until heated through. Yield: 6 servings.

Mixed Vegetable Salad

(May be used up to 1 cup)

Ingredients:

Any combination of vegetables from List 2A may be used, such as:

1. Lettuce, cucumber, celery, green pepper
2. Chicory, tomato, radish
3. Lettuce, parsley, raw cauliflower, tomato
4. Escarole, tomato, cucumber
5. Cabbage, celery, green pepper
6. Lettuce, watercress, cucumber
7. Lettuce, raw spinach, radish

Procedure: Salad may be combined with Zero salad dressing, French dressing or mayonnaise, depending upon fat allowed in the meal plan.

Zero Salad Dressing

See under Low Caloric Recipes.

Potato Salad I

(1 serving equals 1 Bread Exchange)

Ingredients:

   ½ cup cooked potato, diced
   1 or 2 tablespoons Zero salad dressing
   Salt, pepper, chopped onion, celery, parsley, green pepper, as desired.

Procedure: Combine ingredients and serve.

Potato Salad II

(1 serving equals 1 Fat Exchange and 1 Bread Exchange)

Ingredients:

Use recipe for Potato Salad I except that 1 teaspoon of mayonnaise may be used in place of Zero salad dressing.

Potato Salad III

(1 serving equals 1 Bread Exchange and 1 Meat Exchange and 1 Fat Exchange, if desired)

Ingredients:

1 hard-cooked egg, sliced, may be added to recipe for Potato Salad I or II
¼ cup (1 oz.) diced ham, bologna or frankfurter or 5 small shrimps may be used in place of egg.

Fruit and Cheese Salad

(1 serving equals 1 Fruit Exchange, 1 Meat Exchange and ½ cup List 2A vegetables)

Ingredients:

2 dried prunes, cooked without sugar
3 medium slices tomato
3 level tablespoons cottage cheese
2 lettuce leaves

Procedure: Place the three slices of tomato on lettuce leaves. Top with cottage cheese. Place pitted prunes on the side. Garnish with chopped chives, watercress or parsley. Serve with Zero dressing. Yield: 1 serving.

Jellied Spring Vegetable Salad

(Need not be calculated as Exchanges)

Ingredients:

1 tablespoon unflavored gelatin
¼ cup cold water
2 cups boiling water
½ teaspoon salt
¼ cup lime juice
2 teaspoons Sucaryl solution
Few drops green food coloring
1 cup diced, peeled cucumber
1 cup sliced radishes
¼ cup sliced scallions

Procedure: Soften gelatin in cold water; dissolve in boiling water. Add salt, lime juice, Sucaryl and coloring. Chill until mixture begins to thicken. Fold in remaining ingredients. Chill until set in a 5-cup mold. Yield: 8 servings.

Cranberry-Orange Relish

(serve with turkey or chicken)
(1 serving equals ½ Fruit Exchange)

Ingredients:

2 cups cranberries
1 orange
2 tablespoons Sucaryl solution

Procedure: Wash and sort cranberries. Remove seeds from orange. Put both through the fine blade of a food chopper. Blend in the Sucaryl. Chill well before serving. Yield: 8 servings.

Desserts

Baked Custard

(1 serving equals ½ cup milk and 1 Meat Exchange)

Ingredients:

1 egg
½ cup milk
Few grains salt
¼ teaspoon (scant) vanilla
⅛ teaspoon Sucaryl solution
Sprinkle of nutmeg

Procedure: Beat the egg slightly; stir in milk, salt, Sucaryl solution and vanilla. Pour into a custard cup and sprinkle with nutmeg. Set in pan of hot water and bake in a moderate oven (350° F.) for about 45 minutes. (Other flavors such as almond, lemon, orange or maple may be used in place of vanilla.)

Fresh Fruit Cup

(1 serving equals 1 Fruit Exchange)

Any fruits in List 3 may be combined to make a fruit cup. One half cup of mixed fruits equals 1 serving. Example:

Orange, grapefruit, pineapple
Apple, grapefruit, strawberries
Peach, orange, blackberries
Grapes, orange, melon
Melon, grapefruit, banana

Chocolate-Nut Brownies

(1 Brownie equals ½ Bread Exchange, 2 Fat Exchanges)

Ingredients:

1 square unsweetened chocolate
⅓ cup butter
2 tablespoons Sucaryl solution
2 teaspoons vanilla
2 eggs, beaten
1 cup sifted cake flour
½ teaspoon salt
½ teaspoon baking soda
¾ cup chopped walnuts

Procedure: Melt the unsweetened chocolate and butter in a saucepan over low heat. Remove from heat. Add Sucaryl, vanilla and the beaten eggs. Stir until well blended. Add sifted cake flour, salt and baking soda. Mix until blended. Stir in the chopped walnuts. Pour into a greased 8-inch square pan. Level batter in pan. Bake in a slow oven (325° F.) 20 minutes. Cool. Cut into bars. Yield: 16 2″ × 2″ squares.

Orange-Marmalade Nut Bread

(1 slice equals 1 Bread Exchange, 1 Fat Exchange)

Ingredients:

2 cups sifted flour
1½ teaspoons baking powder
½ teaspoon baking soda
¼ teaspoon salt
⅓ cup skim milk
1 egg
2 tablespoons melted butter
1 tablespoon Sucaryl solution
½ cup dietetic orange marmalade
¼ cup chopped walnuts

Procedure: Combine flour, baking powder, soda, and salt in a mixing bowl. Combine skim milk, egg, butter, Sucaryl; add to flour mixture.

Stir only until all flour is dampened. Fold in marmalade and chopped nuts, mixing as little as possible. Spoon batter into lightly greased, 9 × 5 × 3-inch loaf pan. Bake in moderate oven (350° F.) for 1 hour and 40 minutes. Cool before slicing. Yield: 12 slices.

Beverages

Lemonade

(Need not be calculated as Exchanges)

Put ¼ teaspoon Sucaryl or 2 tablets in 2 tablespoons fresh, strained lemon juice; add enough water to make 8 ounces. Add ice as desired, garnish with slice of lemon.

Cocoa

(1 serving equals ¾ cup skim milk. *Note to diabetics:* No more than 1 serving of cocoa should be consumed in 1 day unless carbohydrate in cocoa is calculated.)

Ingredients:
3 tablespoons cocoa
1½ teaspoons Sucaryl solution
3 cups skim milk

Procedure: Place cocoa in top of double boiler. Combine Sucaryl solution with ¼ cup of the milk and blend with cocoa to make a smooth paste. Gradually add the remaining milk and heat thoroughly over boiling water. Add salt or cinnamon to taste. Yield: 4 servings.

STUDY QUESTIONS AND ACTIVITIES

1. What soups contain only negligible calories and may be served freely on low caloric and diabetic diets?

2. Give some variations of these soups which will change flavor or appearance without appreciably increasing the calories.

3. How should tender cuts of meat be cooked for low-caloric diets?

4. How should hamburger be bought for low caloric diets?

5. When braising, stewing or potroasting less tender cuts of meat, how should the cooking liquid be treated if the fat must be removed?

6. How should fish be cooked for the low caloric diet?

7. List some of the herbs and other additions which may be used to flavor vegetables.

8. What substances are used as artificial sweeteners? Do they have any caloric value? Which is better for cooking purposes?

9. What are the ingredients for Zero salad dressing? Why is it called "zero" dressing?

10. What would you tell a patient who asked about the use of specially prepared diabetic foods?

11. What does the booklet Meal Planning and Exchange Lists contain? How is it used by the diabetic patient? Can it be used equally well by the person on a low caloric diet?

SUPPLEMENTARY SOURCES OF FOODS AND RECIPES FOR LOW CALORIC AND DIABETIC DIETS
Low Caloric

Kain, I. J., and Gibson, M. B.: Stay Slim For Life. Garden City, Doubleday, 1966.

Maddox, G.: The Safe and Sane Way to Reduce. New York, Random House, 1960.

Small, M.: The Low Calorie Diet. New York, Pocket Books, 1954.

Diabetic

Behrman, Des. M.: A Cookbook for Diabetics. The American Diabetes Association, 18 East 48th Street, New York, N. Y. 10017 ($1.00)

Maddox, G.: Cookbook for Diabetics. (Canadian Dietetic A.) New York, Taplinger, 1966.

Meal Planning and Exchange Lists. The American Dietetic Association, 620 N. Michigan Avenue, Chicago, Ill. 60611 (25 cents)

West, B. M.: Diabetic Menus, Meals and Recipes, New York, Doubleday, 1959.

Commercial booklets: Abbott Laboratories, North Chicago, Ill. Sucaryl recipe booklets.

CHAPTER **38**

Foods for Fat-Controlled and Fat-Restricted Diets

In the treatment of atherosclerosis (See Chap. 23) the diet may be modified in total fat, the kind of fat (saturated vs. polyunsaturated fatty acids), cholesterol, or, if the patient is overweight his diet may also be restricted in calories. The total fat may also be reduced in diseases of the gallbladder.

Food sources of fat are given in Chapter 3. Obvious sources such as butter, margarine, cream, oils, cooking fats and the visible fat on meat and poultry are easy to recognize. There are many "hidden" sources of fat such as the fat in homogenized milk, eggs, cheese, ice cream, nuts, avocado and olives; in special breads and pastries, cake (except angel food and lady fingers), cookies and doughnuts; and the invisible fat in meat, fish and poultry. All of these sources of fat in foods must be taken into consideration when a diet prescription indicates either an amount or type of fat.

FOODS FOR FAT-CONTROLLED DIETS

Planning the Fat-Controlled Pattern Dietary is described is Chapter 23. Meat selection and preparation are extremely important. Only lean cuts of the meats listed in Table 23–3 should be purchased. Methods for cooking meat to eliminate the fat from the inner or the marbled parts are described in Chapter 37, pages 511–512. Figure 38–1 shows separate fat and marbling in several varieties of meat. The skin of poultry is not eaten because of its high fat content.

Meat drippings can be chilled and the fat removed before they are used for gravy. The same applies when making meat stews.

Packaged, canned and frozen prepared foods and frozen dinners cannot be used because the fat content is not known. Pies, biscuits and muffins can be used if made with corn, cottonseed, safflower and soy bean oils, special margarines or shortening.

Corn, cottonseed, safflower, and soybean oils, and mayonnaise and French dressings made with these oils, are readily available in our markets. Also, the special margarines which list liquid oil as the first ingredient are readily available.

USING VEGETABLE OILS IN COOKING

The homemaker may find it difficult to use oil in place of solid fats in food preparation. The suggestions and recipes which follow may be helpful in making this change.

Meats, fish and poultry may be marinated for several hours in a mixture of oil, vinegar or lemon juice, salt and pepper, before broiling or roasting. Wine, if permitted by the physician, may be used in the marinade in place of vinegar.

Vegetables may be cooked with little or no water by placing 1 to 2 tablespoons of oil per serving in a skillet with a tight cover, adding the vegetables and salt and cooking over very low heat, stirring occasionally until done. A small amount of water may be added if needed.

Vegetables cooked in water may be seasoned with a mixture of oil, vinegar or lemon juice, and herbs.

Oil may be used in pan-frying or oven-roasting of meat, fish and poultry, and vegetables such as potato and eggplant.

Gravy may be made from a bouillon cube or crystals, flour, seasonings and oil. Oil can also be used in place of other fat in making a white sauce (using skim milk) for cream soups and scalloped dishes. French dressings and homemade or commercial mayonnaise may be used for salads.

Oil may be used in the making of hot breads, pastry and cake in place of the usual fats. See recipes later in this chapter.

Recipes for Fat-Controlled Diets

Dressings and Sauces

Basic French Dressing (for salads or marinade)

Ingredients:
⅔ cup vegetable oil
⅓ cup vinegar, lemon juice or half and half
1 teaspoon salt
½ teaspoon pepper
½ teaspoon sugar
¼ teaspoon paprika

Procedure: Combine ingredients in jar with tight cover and shake well. Vary seasonings to taste with dry mustard, minced onion, garlic, etc.

Fruit Salad Dressing: Use half lemon, half orange juice in place of vinegar and add 1 teaspoon grated orange peel. Yield: 1 cup. 1 tablespoon = 2 teaspoons oil.

Seasoned Dressing or Marinade

Ingredients:
⅓ cup tomato sauce
⅓ cup vegetable oil
¼ cup vinegar
1 teaspoon salt
¼ teaspoon pepper
½ teaspoon oregano
½ teaspoon dry mustard
¼ teaspoon soy sauce

Procedure: Combine all ingredients and shake well. Yield: 1 cup. 1 tablespoon = 1 teaspoon oil.

Variations:

Chive Dressing: Add 2 tablespoons finely chopped chives or scallions to the above.

Onion Dressing: To the basic recipe add 1 tablespoon chopped onion, a dash of Tabasco. Shake well.

Quick Hollandaise Sauce

Ingredients:
½ cup mayonnaise

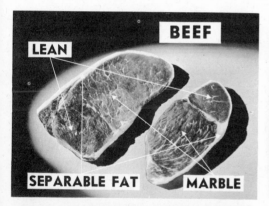

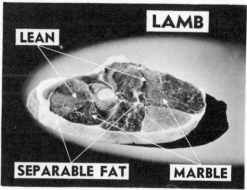

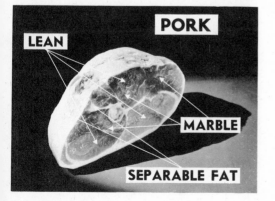

Fig. 38–1. Separable fat and marbling in several varieties of meat. (National Live Stock and Meat Board)

2 tablespoons hot water
1 teaspoon lemon juice

Procedure: In a double boiler add hot water to the mayonnaise. Stir until blended and heated through. Add lemon juice, stirring constantly. Serve with vegetables. Yield: about ½ cup. 1½ teaspoons = 1 teaspoon oil.

Creole Sauce

Ingredients:
  2 tablespoons chopped onion
  2 tablespoons chopped green pepper
  ¼ cup sliced mushrooms
  3 tablespoons vegetable oil
  2 cups stewed or fresh tomatoes
  ½ teaspoon salt
    Dash pepper
    Few drops of Tabasco Sauce (optional)
  ½ teaspoon basil (optional)

Procedure: Cook onion, green pepper and sliced mushrooms in oil over low heat for about 5 minutes. Add tomatoes and seasonings and simmer until sauce is thick, about 30 minutes. ¼ cup sauce = 2 teaspoons oil.

Meat, Fish, Fowl

Seafood Creole

Add cooked fish, shrimp, lobster or crabmeat to creole sauce and heat thoroughly. Serve on rice. Or pour sauce over broiled or baked fish.

Spanish Chicken

Brown chicken pieces lightly in vegetable oil. Add creole sauce, cover pan and cook slowly until chicken is tender, about 40 to 60 minutes. Or place uncooked chicken and sauce in baking dish and bake at 350° F. for about 1 hour, basting occasionally. For fat-controlled diet, skin should be removed from chicken.

Veal Casserole

Have lean veal cut in cubes. Brown in pan or under broiler. Combine with creole sauce, cover and cook gently on top of stove about 1 hour, or bake in oven at 350° F.

Fish Skillet

Ingredients:
  1 pound fish fillets or steaks (fresh or frozen, partially thawed)
  3 tablespoons vegetable oil
  1 chopped onion
  3 tablespoons chopped green pepper
  2 tablespoons chopped parsley
  2 medium tomatoes, cut in pieces, or one 8-ounce can tomatoes
  ½ cup water or tomato juice
  ½ teaspoon salt

½ teaspoon basil or oregano
  Dash pepper

Procedure: Heat oil in skillet. Add chopped vegetables and cook until onion is golden, about 5 minutes. Add tomatoes, water or tomato juice and seasonings; cook until tomatoes are soft. Add fish. Cover and cook gently about 10 minutes or until fish is done. Yield: 4 servings. 1 serving = 2 teaspoons oil.

Lemon Baked Chicken

Ingredients:
  1 frying chicken (2½ to 3 pounds) cut in serving pieces
  3 tablespoons vegetable oil
  3 tablespoons fresh lemon juice
  1 crushed clove garlic
  ½ teaspoon salt
    Dash pepper
    Chopped parsley

Procedure: Arrange chicken in shallow casserole or baking dish. Mix all other ingredients and pour over chicken. Cover and bake at 350° F. until tender, about 45 to 50 minutes. Uncover casserole the last 10 minutes to allow chicken to brown. Before serving sprinkle with chopped parsley. For fat-controlled diet, skin should be removed from chicken. Yield: 4 servings. 1 serving = 2 teaspoons oil.

Vegetables

Pan Crisped Potatoes

Ingredients:
  4 to 6 medium potatoes
  ½ teaspoon salt
  ½ teaspoon seasoned salt
    Dash pepper
    Sprinkle paprika
    Vegetable oil

Procedure: Scrub potatoes and cook in as little boiling salted water as possible. Cover and boil till tender. Drain and cool. Remove skins and slice potatoes lengthwise into eighths. Cover bottom of a large heavy skillet with ⅛ inch vegetable oil and heat. Add potato segments. Sprinkle with salts, pepper and paprika. Cook over medium heat for 15 to 20 minutes, shaking pan frequently and turning potatoes with a spatula so they will get brown and crusty all over. Yield: 4 to 6 servings.

Rice and Noodle Pilaf

Ingredients:
  3 tablespoons vegetable oil
  3 ounces fine noodles or vermicelli, uncooked
  1½ cups "converted" rice, uncooked

3 cups chicken broth, fresh or made from
  bouillon cubes
Salt and pepper

Procedure: Heat vegetable oil in large skillet
and add noodles, turning them frequently.
When they are crisp and brown, add rice, pepper and 2 cups of the broth. The amount of salt
needed will depend on the saltiness of the broth.
Cover skillet and cook over low flame 10 minutes. Add remaining broth, taste and correct
seasoning. Cook, covered, until all liquid is absorbed and the rice is soft and fluffy, about 25
minutes in all. Yield: 4 servings. 1 serving =
2 teaspoons oil.

Glazed Carrots or Onions

Ingredients:
  6 long carrots or 12 to 15 small white
    onions
  2 tablespoons oil
  2 tablespoons sugar, white or brown
  2 tablespoons lemon juice
  1 tablespoon chopped parsley

Procedure: Clean vegetables and cook in boiling, salted water until almost done. Do not cook
too soft. Drain. In medium sized skillet heat
oil, add sugar, lemon juice and parsley and cook
over low flame until mixture bubbles. Add vegetables and cook slowly until browned. Turn
vegetables often, so that glaze will be even.
Yield: 4 servings. 1 serving = 1½ teaspoons oil.

Vegetables Polonaise

Ingredients:
  ½ cup fine bread crumbs
  2 tablespoons vegetable oil
  1 teaspoon chopped parsley

Procedure: Brown the bread crumbs in the
heated oil, cooking over slow fire. Add 1 teaspoon chopped parsley and mix well. Sprinkle
over cooked vegetable in serving dish. Good for
asparagus, cauliflower and broccoli.

Pastry, Breads and Cake

Pastry Shell

Ingredients:
  1 cup sifted flour
  ¾ teaspoon salt
  ¾ teaspoon sugar (optional)
  ¼ cup vegetable oil
  2¼ tablespoons ice water or skim milk

Procedure: Sift together flour, sugar and salt.
Combine vegetable oil and ice water in measuring cup. Beat with fork until creamy. To avoid
oil separation, immediately pour *all at once* over
flour mixture. Toss and mix with fork. Form
into ball. The dough will be moist. Shape into
flat round. Roll out dough between two 12-inch
squares of wax paper. (Paper will not slip if

table is wiped with damp cloth.) Roll out until
dough forms circle, reaching edges of paper.
Remove top sheet of wax paper; invert dough
over pie pan; peel off bottom paper. Fit pastry
into pan, fold edge and flute. Prick entire surface of crust. Bake in hot oven (475° F.) 10 to
12 minutes.

For two crust pie, double the recipe and
divide into two balls.

NOTE: Always prepare pastry just before
ready to use. Do not store.

Muffins

Ingredients:
  2 cups sifted all-purpose flour
  2¼ teaspoons baking powder
  ½ teaspoon salt
  ¼ cup sugar
  1 egg, beaten
  1 cup skim milk
  ¼ cup vegetable oil or special margarine
    or shortening, melted

Procedure: Heat oven to 400° F. (hot).
Lightly oil muffin pans. Sift dry ingredients together. Combine egg, milk and vegetable oil.
Stir quickly into flour mixture until dry ingredients are just dampened and batter has lumpy
appearance. Fill muffin pans ⅔ full. Bake 20
minutes. Serve hot. Yield: 12 muffins. 1 muffin
= 1 teaspoon oil or fat.

Variations: ½ cup raisins, dates, chopped
apple, dried apricots or sliced raw cranberries,
or 2 tablespoons grated orange rind may be
added to the mixture.

Biscuits

Ingredients:
  2 cups sifted flour
  3 teaspoons baking powder
  1 teaspoon salt
  ⅓ cup vegetable oil or special margarine or
    shortening, melted
  ⅔ cup skim milk

Procedure: Mix and sift dry ingredients together. Combine oil and milk. Pour all at once
over entire surface of flour mixture. Mix with
fork to make a soft dough. Shape lightly with
hands to make a round ball. Place on wax paper
and knead lightly ten times or until smooth. Pat
out to ½ inch thickness or roll between 2
squares of wax paper (about 12 inches square).
Remove top sheet of paper; cut biscuits with
unfloured 2-inch biscuit cutter. Place biscuits
on ungreased cookie sheet. Bake on hot oven
(450° F.) 12 to 15 minutes. Yield: 12 biscuits.
1 biscuit = 1 teaspoon oil or fat.

NOTE: For soft biscuits place biscuits close
together with sides touching. For crusty biscuits place well apart.

Yellow Chiffon Cake

Ingredients:

    2 eggs, separated
    1½ cups sugar
    2¼ cups sifted cake flour
    3 teaspoons baking powder
    1 teaspoon salt
    ⅓ cup vegetable oil
    1 cup skim milk
    1½ teaspoons vanilla

Procedure: Heat oven to 350° F. Lightly oil and dust with flour 2 round layer pans, 8 × 1½ inches deep or 9 × 1½ inches deep; or use 1 oblong pan, 13 × 9 × 2 inches. Beat egg whites until frothy. Gradually beat in ½ cup of sugar. Continue beating until very stiff and glossy. Sift rest of sugar, flour, baking powder, salt into another bowl. Add oil, half the milk, vanilla. Beat 1 minute medium speed on mixer, or 150 vigorous strokes by hand. Scrape sides and bottom of the bowl constantly. Add remaining milk, egg yolks, then beat 1 minute more, scraping the sides of the bowl constantly. Fold in egg white mixture. Pour into prepared pans. Bake layers 30 to 35 minutes. Oblong should be baked 40 to 45 minutes. After cooling, fill with jelly, preserves or lemon cornstarch filling. Frost with plain confectioner's sugar frosting.

NOTE: Do not use in diets restricted to 350 mg. cholesterol or less.

Sugar Cookies

Ingredients:

    2 cups all-purpose flour, sifted
    2 teaspoons baking powder
    ½ teaspoon salt
    ¼ teaspoon nutmeg
    2 eggs
    ⅔ cup vegetable oil
    1 teaspoon vanilla
    ¾ cup sugar

Procedure: Preheat oven to 400° F. (hot). Sift together flour, baking powder, salt and nutmeg. In a large bowl beat eggs. Stir in oil and vanilla. Blend in sugar. Stir flour mixture into egg mixture. Drop by teaspoonfuls 2 inches apart on an ungreased cookie sheet. Flatten each cookie with oiled glass dipped in sugar. Bake 8 to 10 minutes until a delicate brown. Remove immediately from baking sheet. Yield: about 60 cookies.

FOODS FOR FAT-RESTRICTED DIETS

Depending on the degree of fat reduction prescribed, visible fats are limited or entirely omitted in the fat-restricted diet. Skim milk is used and eggs (if tolerated) are limited. Meat, fish and poultry should be lean. See Table 1, Part Four, for fat content of food. The use of fat in food preparation is restricted. (See Chapter 37, Low Calorie Diets.) If tolerated, herbs, spices and other flavorings are important in fat-restricted diets, since we normally depend on fat for flavoring (See Chap. 39).

Packaged, canned and prepared foods such as frozen dinners, canned and frozen cream soups, meat stews and gravies, and cake and other mixes are not used because the fat content is not known and may be high.

Calories will be low, particularly in the severely fat-restricted diet (10% of calories from fat), and foods high in carbohydrate will be used to make up sufficient calories. Foods such as breads, cereals, potatoes, macaroni, sugar, honey jellies, and desserts made without fats, milk, and eggs can be used. If the diet is also restricted in cholesterol eggs will be omitted.

The following recipes are suggested for use by the patient on a fat-restricted diet.

Recipes for Fat-Restricted Diets

Vegetable Chowder with Milk

Ingredients:

    2 slices onion
    1 small stalk celery
    1 small carrot
    1 cup skim milk
    Salt
    Paprika
    Chives or parsley

Procedure: Peel, slice and chop onion. Chop celery. Scrape and chop carrot. Combine with small amount of water and cook until tender. Stir in milk slowly and reheat. Season to taste and serve sprinkled with minced chives or parsley. Yield: 1 serving.

Herb Flavored Meat Loaf

Ingredients:

    ½ cup soft bread crumbs
    ½ cup skim milk
    1 pound lean ground beef round
    1 egg, slightly beaten
    2 tablespoons grated onion
    2 tablespoons parsley, finely chopped
    1 clove garlic, finely chopped
    1 teaspoon salt
    ¼ teaspoon oregano
    ⅛ teaspoon rosemary

¼ teaspoon basil
½ teaspoon paprika
¼ teaspoon pepper

Procedure: Soak bread crumbs in milk. Combine all ingredients and mix thoroughly. Make into a loaf in loaf pan. Bake for 1 hour in a moderate oven (350° F.). Serve hot or cold. When cold, can be sliced thin for cold buffet. Yield: 4 servings.

Swedish Meat Cakes

Ingredients:
¾ pound lean ground beef round
1 egg
¼ cup cooked carrots
¼ cup cooked turnips
2 tablespoons grated onion
1 tablespoon chopped capers
1 teaspoon horseradish
1 teaspoon salt
⅛ teaspoon pepper

Procedure: Combine ground meat and egg. Mix well. Mash cooked carrots and turnips. Blend with the meat, add other ingredients and mix well with hands. Shape into 4 large patties. Chill thoroughly in refrigerator for at least 30 minutes. Preheat broiler and broil meat cakes until brown on both sides. Yield: 4 servings.

Peppers Stuffed with Beef and Wild Rice (or white rice)

Ingredients:
6 green peppers
2 cups cooked wild rice (or white rice)
¼ teaspoon salt
¼ pound chopped lean beef
   (or lean leftovers)

Procedure: Cut tops off peppers and remove seeds. Mix rice, salt and meat. Add small amount of water if rice is very dry. Fill peppers and place in baking dish. Surround peppers with a small amount of hot water. Bake in moderate oven (350° F.) until peppers are tender. Yield: 6 servings.

Hungarian Goulash

Ingredients:
2 pounds top round of beef, cut into 1-inch squares (trim off all fat)
1 cup canned consommé
1 cup tomato juice
½ medium size green pepper, diced
2 cloves garlic
1 teaspoon paprika
½ teaspoon salt
½ teaspoon pepper
1 bay leaf
3 medium carrots cut in 1-inch lengths

Procedure: Use large iron pot and put in all ingredients except carrots. Cover and simmer for 2½ hours. Add the carrots and simmer another 30 minutes. If necessary add a little more consommé or tomato juice. Yield: 6 servings.

Perfect Baked Potatoes

Ingredients:
1 baking potato
3 tablespoons cottage cheese
½ tablespoon chopped chives

Procedure: Wash and dry potato. Bake at 375° F. one hour, or until done. Remove slice from top, or make a quarter cut and open potato. Combine cottage cheese with chopped chives, flavor generously with salt and pepper and pile on top of potato.

Transparent Salad Dressing

Ingredients:
¼ cup sugar
½ teaspoon salt
½ teaspoon dry mustard
1 tablespoon cornstarch
⅓ cup vinegar
⅔ cup water
1 tablespoon minced onion

Procedure: Mix all ingredients in a saucepan and stir over heat until mixture boils. Continue to stir 1 to 2 minutes longer. Chill before using. Yield: 1 cup. This is good with tomato salad and mixed vegetable salads.

STUDY QUESTIONS AND ACTIVITIES

1. Name 10 food sources of fat. Which of these would be called visible fats? Which are "hidden" sources?

2. Why should prepared packaged, canned and frozen foods not be used by the patient on a fat-restricted or fat-controlled diet?

3. What foods should be increased in the diet if fat is severely restricted? Why?

4. What can be used for a topping for baked potato if the fat must be kept low?

5. Look under the recipes for low-caloric diets and high protein diets. Which of these can be used for the fat-restricted and the fat-controlled diets also?

6. Why is the use of herbs and spices important on the severely fat-restricted diet? Name some which can be used.

7. List the foods containing largely saturated fat.

8. Name some of the cuts of meat suitable for a fat-restricted and a fat-controlled diet.

9. How should meat be trimmed for these diets? How should it be cooked?

10. How may fat be removed from soups and gravies?

11. List 4 oils which are polyunsaturated. Name some of the ways in which oils may be used to replace solid fats.

12. What is a marinade? How may it be used?

SUPPLEMENTARY SOURCES OF FOODS AND RECIPES FOR FAT-RESTRICTED AND FAT-CONTROLLED DIETS

Payne, A. S., and Callahan, D.: The Fat and Sodium Control Cookbook. Ed. 3. Boston, Little, Brown, & Co., 1965.

Planning Fat-Controlled Meals at 1,200 and 1,800 Calories, Rev. 1966. Available from local Heart Associations or from the American Heart Association, 44 East 23rd St., New York, N. Y.

CHAPTER 39

Foods for Sodium-Restricted Diets

When the physician has prescribed a sodium-restricted diet, salt as a seasoning must be avoided completely. This applies not only to cooking and its use on the table, unless a small amount has been specifically allowed, but also to the omission of foods which are high in sodium content and to prepared foods to which salt or sodium has been added in the processing.

In Chapter 24 will be found the discussion of varying degrees of sodium restriction in the diet, and the foods and the quantities which may be included or must be omitted. Here we shall emphasize the availability of low sodium foods and some of the methods of preparation which will help to minimize the flat taste of food prepared without salt. If the nurse or the dietitian can convey some of these concepts to the patient, he may accept and follow his diet more happily.

FOODS FOR THE SODIUM-RESTRICTED DIET

Milk. Ordinary milk may be used up to one pint a day on most sodium-restricted diets. When sodium must be severely restricted, or when it is desirable to increase the milk in the diet, low sodium milk is available in fresh fluid and canned forms, and in powdered whole (Lonalac)* and powdered skim (Cellu)† form. The fresh fluid and the canned low sodium milks are more desirable in taste and are cheaper than the dried forms. Any of them may be substituted for regular milk as a beverage or a recipe ingredient.

* Mead Johnson and Co., Evansville, Ind.
† Dietetic Cellu Foods, Chicago Dietetic Supply House, Chicago, Ill. 60612.

Meats, Poultry, Fish. All fresh and frozen meat and poultry, and dietetic low sodium canned tuna and salmon may be used. Fresh fish should be thoroughly rinsed in water, for it is sometimes kept in a salt solution on the fishing boats. Frozen fish fillets are frozen in brine and should never be used.

The use of a marinade consisting of oil, lemon juice or vinegar and pepper to flavor and season meat or poultry before it is cooked will add to its palatability. Herbs and spices used in cooking may also help to hide the lack of salt. See recipe section in this chapter.

Vegetables. Fortunately, a number of vegetables are low in sodium, and their use adds variety to restricted meals. As no salt can be used in cooking, every care must be taken to preserve the natural fresh flavor. They should be of the best quality when purchased and should be cooked in as small an amount of water as possible.

The flavor of vegetables cooked without salt can be greatly improved by the use of spices and herbs as suggested later in the chapter. A pinch of sugar or a dash of nutmeg may also lend variety. They may be seasoned before serving with unsalted butter or margarine to which a small amount of lemon juice or vinegar or some grated lemon or orange peel has been added, or with an herb butter.

The following list of vegetables, fresh, dried and those canned or frozen without added salt, may be used:

Asparagus
Beans, green, wax, dried lima or navy
Broccoli
Brussels sprouts

Cabbage
Cauliflower
Chicory
Corn
Cucumber
Eggplant
Endive
Escarole
Lentils
Lettuce
Mushrooms
Okra
Onions
Parsnips
Peas, fresh; split green or yellow; cowpeas
Peppers, green or red
Potato, white or sweet
Pumpkin
Radishes
Rutabagas (yellow turnip)
Squash, all varieties
Tomatoes
Tomato juice (low sodium only)
Turnip greens

The vegetables listed below are high in natural sodium content. They must be omitted on all but the Mild Sodium-Restricted Diet. Sauerkraut should *never* be used.

Artichokes
Beet greens
Beets
Carrots
Celery
Chard, Swiss
Collards
Dandelion greens
Hominy
Kale
Lima beans, frozen
Mustard greens
Peas, frozen
Sauerkraut
Spinach
Turnips, white

Fruits. Fruits are very low in sodium content. In the sodium-restricted diet they will be used mainly as dessert, but they will also add variety as accompaniments to the main meal or to give flavor to meat dishes. An example is the serving of apple sauce with pork.

Breads, Quickbreads and Cereals. Low sodium bread is available in many areas, either at a bakery or in the supermarket. It may be made at home from a regular yeast recipe, omitting the salt and using unsalted fat. Adding some grated lemon or orange rind to the yeast dough provides an interesting flavor. If the bread is stored, tightly wrapped, in the refrigerator, it will stay fresh for a considerable time. Also, it may be sliced and frozen and used as needed. An extra loaf may be kept in the freezing compartment for future use.

Quickbreads, cake and cookies may be made from regular recipes by substituting a sodium-free baking powder for regular baking powder, omitting the salt and using oil or an unsalted shortening. A low sodium baking powder is available (Cellu), or it may be compounded by the local druggist from the following formula:

Potassium bicarbonate ...	39.8 Gm.
Cornstarch	28.0 Gm.
Tartaric acid	7.5 Gm.
Potassium bitartrate	56.1 Gm.

Substitute 1½ teaspoons of this low sodium baking powder for 1 teaspoon regular baking powder. Cellu baking powder may be substituted equally for regular baking powder.

Packaged bread, cake, cookie and pudding mixes and self-rising flour should not be used.

The following cereal products may be served plain or cooked, or as an ingredient in a recipe, as they are processed without added salt or sodium compounds. No salt should be added in the preparation, of course.

Farina, unsalted
Hominy grits
Oatmeal
Rolled wheat
Wheat meal
Puffed rice
Puffed wheat
Shredded wheat
Macaroni
Noodles
Spaghetti
Barley
Rice
Unsalted popcorn
Flour

Other cereal products should not be used unless the information on the label gives definite proof that the sodium content is no higher than 6 mg. per 100 Gm. of cereal. (See Chap. 24 for labeling laws.)

The addition of some dried fruit or small amounts of some of the "sweet" spices to hot cereal will give an agreeable flavor and help to overcome the "flat" taste of unsalted food.

Fats and Oils. Sweet and unsalted butter and unsalted margarine are readily available and can be used as a spread or as ingredients in a recipe. Oils and most solid shortenings may be used in recipes requiring liquid or solid fats. Labels should be checked for the addition of salt to solid shortenings.

Spices and Herbs to Flavor Unsalted Foods

Meats, vegetables and salads may be made more palatable with the use of spices and herbs. Fortunately, many of these are low in sodium content. (See Table later in the chapter.) However, they must be used with a light hand, and, if several spices or herbs are used together in a recipe, each small quantity should be carefully measured. About ¼ teaspoon of dried herb is sufficient for a dish serving 4 people. If fresh herbs are used ¾ to 1 teaspoon is usually enough. More can always be added, but, once added, none can be taken away. Overcooking should also be avoided to save fine flavors and aroma.

Certain herbs have been found to blend or contrast better than others with various foods. The following suggestions may be found useful.

Beef. FOR STEAKS AND ROASTS. Season with pepper and mustard, sage, marjoram or thyme before cooking. *Or* after cooking, top with herb butter flavored with garlic, parsley, thyme, dill or marjoram and a little lemon juice.

FOR HAMBURGER, MEAT LOAF OR STEWS: add browned onion or mushrooms, chopped green pepper, chopped tomato, or one of the herbs above before cooking. A single stalk of celery or a bay leaf may be added to a pot of stew.

Lamb. FOR ROASTS OR CHOPS: season with curry, garlic, mint, onion, parsley, rosemary, thyme or marjoram. *Or* use herb butter on chops after cooking.

Liver. Use any herb butter, or parsley, onion or chives.

Pork. FOR CHOPS AND ROASTS: rub with garlic, marjoram or lemon juice before cooking. *Or* cook with apples or apple sauce, onion or sage.

Veal. FOR ROASTS AND CUTLETS: try summer savory and chervil, or basil and marjoram. *Or* season with bay leaf, curry, garlic, ginger, mushrooms, oregano or paprika.

Poultry. Choose one or more of these: fresh or dried leaves of celery, basil, marjoram, parsley, rosemary, summer savory, sage or thyme for the many dishes prepared from chicken, turkey or other poultry. Stuffing for poultry may be made with low sodium bread and unsalted butter or margarine.

Fish. Try lemon, garlic, dill or mustard butter on broiled or fried fish. Finely chopped dill, basil or tarragon leaves, or paprika add color and accent.

For boiled fish and chowders, chopped basil leaves, dill, or a dash of powdered thyme is the "right" flavor for some.

Eggs. Add finely minced chives or parsley, or a dash of curry to deviled, creamed or scrambled eggs for special accent.

Enhance omelets by adding one or more of the fine herbs—basil, marjoram, rosemary, tarragon or thyme. Finely chopped onion, green pepper or tomato are favorites for other egg mixtures. Salt-free mayonnaise may be used for egg salads or sandwiches.

Vegetables. Season these delicately for best results.

ASPARAGUS: Season with chives, lemon, caraway or herb butter.

CAULIFLOWER: Add nutmeg, herb butter.

CORN: Use chives, parsley, green pepper, onion or tomato.

PEAS: Use chives, mint, parsley, chervil or onion.

POTATOES: Parsley, chives, dill, onion, rosemary or mace may be added.

GREEN BEANS: Add onion, chives, scallion, dill, marjoram, nutmeg, rosemary or lemon.

Seasonings, Extracts, Herbs and Spices

Low in Sodium May Be Used Freely		High in Sodium Do NOT Use
Allspice	Meat tenderizers, low-sodium dietetic	Bouillon cubes, regular
Almond extract	Mint	Catsup
Anise seed	Mustard, dry, or mustard seed	Celery flakes, seed, salt
Basil	Nutmeg	Chili sauce
Bay leaf	Onion, onion juice, or onion powder	Cyclamate, sodium (sugar substitute)
Bouillon cube, low-sodium dietetic if less than 5 mg. of sodium per cube	Orange extract	Garlic salt
Caraway seed	Oregano	Horseradish, prepared with salt
Cardamon	Paprika	Meat extracts
Catsup, low sodium dietetic	Parsley	Meat sauces
Chili powder	Pepper, fresh green or red	Meat tenderizers
Chives	Pepper, black, red, or white	Monosodium glutamate
Cinnamon	Peppermint extract	Mustard, prepared
Cloves	Pimiento peppers for garnish	Olives
Cocoa (1 to 2 teaspoons)	Poppy seed	Onion salt
Coconut	Poultry seasoning	Parsley flakes
Cumin	Purslane	Pickles
Curry	Rosemary	Relishes
Cyclamate, calcium (sugar substitute)	Saccharin, calcium (sugar substitute)	Saccharin, sodium (sugar substitute)
Dill	Saffron	SALT
Fennel	Sage	Salt substitutes, unless recommended by the physician
Garlic, garlic juice, or garlic powder	Salt substitutes, if recommended by the physician	Soy sauce
Ginger	Savory	Tomato paste
Horseradish root or horseradish prepared without salt	Sesame seeds	Worcestershire sauce
Juniper	Sorrel	
Lemon juice or extract	Sugar	
Mace	Tarragon	
Maple extract	Thyme	
Marjoram	Turmeric	
Meat extract, low-sodium dietetic	Vanilla extract	
	Vinegar	
	Wine if allowed	
	Walnut extract	

Adapted from "Your 1,000 milligram Sodium Diet," The American Heart Association, New York, N. Y. 10010

SQUASH: Try lemon, ginger, mace, basil or chives.

TOMATOES: Use garlic, onion, parsley, basil or sage.

There are many other herbs and spices which will suggest themselves. The addition of oregano, dry mustard, leeks, chili powder, poultry seasoning, mint, sage, curry, cloves or mace will aid in giving variety of flavor and interest to many foods. The housewife who learns to experiment with these may find that the loss of salt as a flavor becomes greatly minimized.

A number of seasonings are either high in natural sodium or else have salt added in their preparation. These should never be used on the salt-restricted diet. The table on this page shows those seasonings that may be used freely, and those which must be omitted.

Salt Substitutes

A number of "salt substitutes" which owe their flavor to mineral salts other than sodium chloride are available. The most acceptable of these has a number of spices added as well. They are often a welcome addition to recipes for main dishes and soups. Salt substitutes should not be used without permission of the physician.

Dietetic Canned or Prepared Foods; Sweetenings

A variety of low sodium vegetables, desserts, crackers, cookies, salad dressings, chicken, fish and even low sodium cheddar cheese are available and may be found at supermarkets or at "health food" stores. They are usually more expensive than the regular varieties, but they do provide a convenience. Since the contents of all dietetic foods must be listed on the label of the container, the label should be checked for sodium content. It should be emphasized that high sodium vegetables (see list earlier in the chapter) should not be used even when they are dietetically packed, as they contain the same quantity of sodium as if they were fresh.

Calcium cyclamate and calcium saccharin, useful for sweetening for the patient who must restrict both calories and sodium, may be obtained at most drugstores.

Recipes for Sodium-Restricted Diets
Dressings, Sauces and Spreads

Lemon and Herb Butter (basic recipe)

Ingredients:
  1½ teaspoons boiling water
  2 tablespoons sweet butter, softened
  1 tablespoon fresh lemon juice

Procedure: Add boiling water to softened butter. Mix well. Add lemon juice and whip mixture until smooth and creamy. Makes enough for 2 cups of vegetables.

Variations—to basic mix add:
  1. 1 tablespoon chopped fresh parsley for sandwich spread; also fine for meats and vegetables.
  2. 1 tablespoon chopped fresh herbs or 1½ teaspoons approved dried herbs; use on meats and vegetables; vary amounts to individual taste.
  3. 1 tablespoon grated onion or chopped chives; excellent on baked potato; try also on green beans and squash.
  4. ½ teaspoon dry mustard and ¼ teaspoon marjoram; very good on steamed cabbage.
  5. ½ teaspoon nutmeg; good on cooked green beans or zucchini; or on baked potato.
  6. 1 teaspoon poppy seed, dash of marjoram and paprika; good on asparagus, onions and cauliflower.

Transparent Salad Dressing

See recipe in Chapter 38. Omit salt.

French Dressing

Ingredients:
  ⅜ cup salad oil
  ½ teaspoon paprika
  ⅛ teaspoon dry mustard
  ½ teaspoon sugar
  2 tablespoons vinegar
  2 tablespoons lemon juice

Procedure: Place all ingredients in bowl and chill thoroughly. Just before serving, beat vigorously with fork until well blended. Yield: ½ cup.

Variations:
  1. Substitute grapefruit juice for the vinegar.
  2. Add ¼ cup strained fresh tomato pulp or unsalted tomato juice.
  3. Add peeled clove of garlic before chilling. Remove garlic before serving.
  4. Add dash of Tabasco* to taste.

* Tabasco sauce contains 400 to 500 mg. of sodium per 100 cc. The quantity used in a recipe is so small, however, that its contribution to the total sodium content of a dish is negligible.

Marinade for Meat, Poultry or Fish

1. Use French Dressing or one of its variations above; omit sugar from recipe.
2. To unsalted French Dressing add: chopped onion, chopped green pepper, and/or chopped tomato pulp, or a variety of herbs. (See earlier in chapter.) Allow meat to stand in marinade for an hour or more before cooking; baste with marinade during cooking.

Creole Sauce

See recipe in Chapter 38 for Creole Sauce and directions for using. Omit salt.

Mustard Sauce for Fish

Ingredients:
  1 tablespoon minced onion
  2 tablespoons salad oil
  2 tablespoons flour
  1 cup strained unsalted fish stock
  ½ teaspoon dry mustard
  ¼ teaspoon black pepper
  2 tablespoons sherry (optional)

Procedure: Sauté onion in oil until golden. Blend in flour and gradually stir in the fish stock mixed with mustard and pepper. Simmer, stirring, until thick and smooth. Stir in sherry. Serve over unsalted poached or boiled fish. Yield: 1 cup.

Variations: Add to sauce 1 tablespoon chopped, hard cooked egg yolk and 1 teaspoon minced parsley. *Or* add a tablespoon minced chives or a tablespoon minced parsley.

Meat, Fish and Fowl

Savory Steak

Ingredients:

- 1 flank steak
  Flour
  Pepper
- 3 tablespoons unsalted fat
- 2 onions, peeled and sliced
- 1 small green pepper, seeded and sliced
- 1 bay leaf
- 3 cloves
- 2 cups unsalted tomatoes
- 1 teaspoon sugar

Procedure: Score steak and pound in the flour and the pepper. Heat shortening in skillet and brown meat on both sides. Add remaining ingredients, cover and let simmer 1½ to 2 hours until meat is tender. Yield: 4 to 5 servings.

or: A stuffing of low sodium bread and unsalted butter or margarine may be made. After browning, spread the stuffing on the steak, roll it and fasten with string or skewers. Then proceed as above.

Herb-Flavored Meat Loaf

See recipe in Chapter 38. Use unsalted soft bread crumbs and either whole or skim milk. Omit salt.

Brown Beef Stew

Ingredients:

- 2 lbs. lean beef (boned chuck, round or rump)
- 1 teaspoon paprika
- ⅛ teaspoon pepper
- 3 tablespoons flour
- 3 tablespoons salad oil or unsalted butter
- 3 cups water
- 1 bay leaf
- 2 drops Tabasco
- 4 cloves
- 12 small white onions, peeled
- ½ pound green beans, cut in short lengths
- 3 medium potatoes, peeled and halved

Procedure: Have beef cut in 1½-inch pieces. Blend together paprika, pepper and flour. Roll pieces of meat in flour mixture. Melt fat in heavy kettle. Add meat and brown on all sides. Add water, bay leaf, Tabasco and cloves. Cover and simmer 2 to 2½ hours until meat is almost tender. Add onions, green beans and potatoes. Cover and cook until vegetables are tender. Yield: 6 to 8 servings.

Chicken Tabasco

Ingredients:

- 1 2-lb. dressed broiler
- ½ lime or lemon
- 2 tablespoons melted unsalted butter
  Dash of Tabasco
- 1 teaspoon sugar
  Chopped parsley

Procedure: Clean and wipe chicken dry. Rub surface of chicken with the cut lime or lemon, squeezing to keep the juice flowing. Combine melted butter and Tabasco and brush chicken with the mixture. Sprinkle lightly with sugar. Place in broiler pan, skin side down. Broil for 10 minutes as far from the heat as possible. Raise chicken to 4 inches from heat and turn occasionally to ensure even browning. Allow about 35 minutes' total cooking for broiler of this size. To serve, sprinkle with chopped parsley. Yield: 2 servings.

Curried Tuna Fish

Ingredients:

- 3 tablespoons unsalted butter or other unsalted shortening
- 3 tablespoons flour
- 2 cups milk
- 1 tablespoon lemon juice
- 1-2 teaspoons curry
- 1 can low sodium "dietetic" tuna

Procedure: Melt butter or other shortening in double boiler or over low direct heat. Stir in flour. Stir in milk and continue stirring until sauce thickens. Add lemon juice and curry. Add tuna, flaked but not drained, and reheat. Serve over rice cooked without salt. Yield: 4 to 5 servings.

Vegetables

Scalloped Potatoes

Ingredients:

- 4 medium potatoes
- 2 tablespoons unsalted butter
- 2 tablespoons flour
- 1 to 2 tablespoons minced onion
  Pepper
- 2 cups milk (approx.)

Procedure: Pare potatoes and cut in thin, crosswise slices. Reserve enough potatoes for a top layer. Place half the potatoes in a buttered baking dish (use unsalted butter). Cover with half the fat cut into tiny bits or melted. Sprinkle with half the flour, onion and pepper. Repeat. Top casserole with remaining potatoes. Pour in milk until it can be seen between pieces of potatoes. Cover and bake in moderate oven (350° F.) for ½ hour. Uncover and bake for 1 hour longer or until tender and brown on top. Yield: 4 servings.

NOTE: If it is desired to lower the sodium content still more, use low sodium instead of regular milk.

Sweet Potato and Apple Casserole

Ingredients:

1 large sweet potato, boiled, unsalted
½ cup applesauce
Sugar
Cinnamon

Procedure: Place in buttered casserole alternate layers of sliced sweet potato and applesauce. Top with sugar and cinnamon and heat in moderate oven (350° F.) until hot. Serve immediately. Yield: 1 to 2 servings.

Sweet and Sour Wax Beans

Ingredients:

1 pound yellow wax beans or 1 package frozen
2 tablespoons unsalted butter or margarine
1 tablespoon chopped onion
1 tablespoon flour
2 tablespoons brown sugar
2 tablespoons vinegar
Paprika

Procedure: Cook beans until just tender in boiling water. Reserve cooking water; make up to 1 cup with boiling water if necessary. Brown onion in butter or margarine, stir in flour, add bean liquid and cook until smooth and thick. Add sugar and vinegar and cook 2 minutes longer. Add cooked beans and reheat. Serve with paprika. Yield: 4 servings.

Tomato Aspic

Ingredients:

2 cups unsalted tomato juice
1 bay leaf
4 whole cloves
1 slice onion
6 peppercorns
1 tablespoon unflavored gelatin
1 tablespoon lemon juice

Procedure: Measure 1½ cups tomato juice into saucepan. Add bay leaf, cloves, onion and peppercorns. Bring to a boil and simmer 10 minutes. Strain. Soften gelatin in remaining ½ cup tomato juice and dissolve in hot tomato juice. Add lemon juice. Pour into mold and chill until firm; serve as a basis for a salad. Or break up with fork before placing in soup cups. Yield: 4 servings.

Breads and Desserts

Bread

Ingredients:

¾ cup milk
1½ teaspoons sugar
2 tablespoons unsalted shortening
½ package of cake yeast, active dry or compressed
¼ cup water (warm for dry, lukewarm for compressed)
2½ to 3 cups sifted all-purpose flour

Procedure: Scald milk. Stir in sugar and shortening and set aside to cool until lukewarm. Sprinkle yeast over water and stir until dissolved. Stir into milk mixture. Add half the flour and stir in well. Add remaining flour, stirring to make a stiff dough. On lightly floured board, knead dough until smooth. Place in lightly greased bowl and turn over once to grease all sides. Cover with towel and let rise in warm place (80 to 85° F.) until double in bulk. Remove from bowl and knead again until smooth. Shape into loaf and place in well-greased 9 × 5 × 3-inch loaf pan. Cover with towel and let rise again in warm place until double in bulk. Bake in moderate oven (350° F.) about 1 hour, or until done. Yield: About 20 slices.

Cinnamon Toast

Procedure: Mix cinnamon with granulated sugar, using a mixture of 2 teaspoons cinnamon and ½ cup sugar. Sprinkle this mixture generously over hot unsalted buttered toast made from unsalted bread, and serve hot.

Variations:

1. Use 2 teaspoons cinnamon with ½ cup brown sugar.

2. Use a mixture of 1 tablespoon orange juice and 1 tablespoon grated orange rind with ½ cup sugar.

Thumb Cookies

Ingredients:

1 teaspoon vanilla
¼ teaspoon lemon extract
½ cup unsalted butter or margarine
¼ cup sugar
1 egg yolk, unbeaten
1 cup all-purpose flour, sifted
Raspberry jam

Procedure: Cream vanilla and lemon extract into the fat, add sugar gradually, then beat egg into the mixture thoroughly. Put flour in all at once, stir to a thick dough. Shape the dough into small balls, using about 1 teaspoon of the mixture each time. Put on an ungreased cookie sheet. Make a dent in each ball with floured thumb. Place a small amount of raspberry jam in each dent. Bake cookies about 15 minutes at 400° F. Makes about 24 cookies.

Fruit Cobbler

Ingredients:

¼ cup softened unsalted butter
1 cup sugar
¾ cup sifted all-purpose flour
4 cups sliced apples or 2 cups canned or
     cooked fruit
¼ cup water
1 teaspoon cinnamon

Procedure: Heat oven to 350° F. Grease 10 × 6 × 1½-inch baking dish. Cream butter and sugar together. Blend in flour, mixing well. Place fruit in baking dish. Sprinkle with water and cinnamon. Spread flour mixture on top of fruit. Bake in moderate oven (350° F.) 40 to 45 minutes. Serve warm with or without lemon or spicy sauce. Yield: 6 servings.

Lemon Sauce

Ingredients:

1 tablespoon cornstarch
½ cup sugar
1 cup boiling water
1 tablespoon butter
    Grated rind of ½ lemon
¼ cup lemon juice

Procedure: Mix cornstarch and sugar in a saucepan; stir in the boiling water. Stir over direct heat until the mixture boils. Add butter, lemon rind and lemon juice. Yield: 4 to 6 servings.

Spicy Sauce

Mix ½ teaspoon cinnamon, ¼ teaspoon nutmeg and ¼ teaspoon cloves with 1 tablespoon vinegar; add to Lemon Sauce.

Puffed Rice Balls

Ingredients:

1 cup sugar
½ cup water
2 teaspoons lemon juice
3 cups puffed rice

Procedure: Boil the sugar, water and lemon juice to the hard-ball stage (265° F.). Pour the syrup very quickly over the puffed rice in a bowl. Make into small balls, allowing to cool on waxed paper.

STUDY QUESTIONS AND ACTIVITIES

1. What varieties of low sodium milk are available in your community? Which is least expensive? Have you tasted any of these? Is there a difference?

2. Can sodium-free baking powder be bought in your community? Where? How much sodium-free baking powder should be substituted for one teaspoon regular baking powder in a recipe?

3. What must be omitted, what substituted to make a regular recipe for biscuits, cake or cookies suitable for the sodium-restricted diet?

4. What is a marinade? How may it be used?

5. List 5 ways in which herbs or spices may be added to foods to make them more palatable.

6. Give the ingredients and directions for making an herb butter. How can it be varied?

7. Try to list *all* the seasonings and spices which should *never* be used by the patient on a sodium-restricted diet. You may use groupings such as bouillon cubes and meat sauces.

8. Have you tasted salt substitutes? What elements may be used in place of sodium? Which salt substitute tastes better to you? Is it available in your community? What should you tell a patient who asks about salt substitutes?

SUPPLEMENTARY SOURCES OF FOODS AND RECIPES FOR SODIUM-RESTRICTED DIETS

American Spice Trade Association, Institutional Department, Empire State Building, New York, N. Y. 10001.

Bagg, E. W.: Cooking Without a Grain of Salt. Garden City, N. Y., Doubleday, 1964.

Field, F.: Gourmet Cooking for Cardiac Diets. Collier Books, 1962 (paperback).

Flavorsome Cooking Without Salt. Division of Cancer and Chronic Disease, Massachusetts Department of Public Health, Boston.

Hasker, R. R.: The Cook Book for Low Sodium Diets. Rev. Ed. Massachusetts Heart Assn., Inc., 636 Beacon Street, Boston 15.

Payne, A. S., and Callahan, D.: The Fat and Sodium Control Cookbook. Ed. 3. Boston, Little, Brown & Co., 1965.

Your 500 milligram Sodium Diet; Your 1,000 milligram Sodium Diet; Your Mild Sodium Restricted Diet. Available from your local Heart Association or through the American Heart Association, 44 East 23rd Street, New York, N. Y. 10010.

CHAPTER 40

Foods for Gluten-Free Diets

On the gluten-free diet wheat, rye, oats, barley and buckwheat must be omitted as discussed in Chapters 27 and 34. Since wheat in particular is used widely in a variety of ways in the North American and the European diets, its exclusion presents considerable difficulty for the homemaker. The list of foods allowed and to be omitted on the gluten-free diet, found in Chapter 27, illustrates the extent of the problem.

CEREAL GRAINS AND FLOURS ON THE GLUTEN-FREE DIET

In place of the excluded cereal grains, corn flour, cornmeal, rice, rice flour, soy flour and gluten-free wheat starch[1] may be used freely as well as potato flour, cornstarch and lima bean flour. Later in the chapter a number of recipes will be found using these flours.

The great problem of the patient with celiac disease is to find an acceptable bread or bread mix. Two recipes for bread are included in this chapter, but the patient may find a commercial gluten-free bread mix more satisfactory. Some of these presently available are:

Cellu Gluten Free Bread Mix, containing largely gluten-free wheat starch. The Chicago Dietetic Supply House, Inc., 1750 West van Buren Street, Chicago, Ill. 60612.

Rice Bread Mix, Lima-Potato Bread Mix and Lima-Soya Bread Mix. Giusto Specialty Foods, Inc., 420 Fulton St., San Francisco 2, Calif.

Unimix — Gluten-free Bread Mix. Scientific Development Committee, University of Toronto, Toronto, Ontario, Canada.

---

[1] Cellu Products, Chicago Dietetic Supply House, Inc., 1750 W. van Buren St., Chicago, Ill. 60612.

These and other gluten-free bread mixes may be obtainable at the local "health food" store. However, such a mix (other than those listed above) should be checked carefully for contents, to be sure that none of the forbidden cereals has been included.

Since the gluten-free bread will probably be used only by the member of the family with celiac disease, it is important to keep it fresh as long as possible. The loaf may be sliced after baking, wrapped carefully and frozen, removing and defrosting the slices as needed. Toasting the bread will make it more palatable.

Some of the problems in baking with flours other than wheat are discussed in Chapter 41. In some recipes rice, potato, corn and soya flours and gluten-free wheat starch may be substituted for regular wheat flour. The quantities will vary somewhat depending on the type of flour used. The following will serve as a guide.

Substitutions for 1 Cup Wheat Flour

1 cup corn flour
¾ cup cornmeal (coarse)
1 cup (scant) cornmeal (fine)
⅝ cup potato starch (10 tablespoons)
⅞ cup rice flour
1 cup soy flour plus ¾ cup potato starch flour

The fine flours are best when used with milk and eggs in a recipe. The coarse flours are best combined with one of the fine flours. The coarse flours may give a grainy taste to the baked product. Rice flour may be brought to a boil in the amount of the allowed liquid, cooled and added to the remainder of the recipe.

When no baking powder is included in the recipe, the mixed ingredients may be put in the refrigerator for a half hour or so before baking to eliminate the grainy taste.

For the thickening of sauces, cream soups and gravies, potato and cornstarch will be found satisfactory, but only half the quantity of the thickening agent called for in the recipe should be used.

Recipes for Gluten-Free Diets

Breads

Rice or Wheat Starch Bread I

Ingredients:
- 1 cup unsifted rice flour *or* 1¼ cup gluten-free wheat starch
- ½ teaspoon salt
- 3 teaspoons baking powder
- 4 tablespoons vegetable shortening
- 4 tablespoons sugar
- 2 egg yolks
- ½ cup milk
- 2 egg whites, well beaten

Procedure: Measure flour, baking powder and salt. Combine and sift. Cream softened shortening; then cream with sugar until well blended. Stir in unbeaten egg yolks. Add flour alternately with the milk, beating after each addition. Fold in the well-beaten egg whites. Spread batter into well-greased loaf pan (8 × 4 × 3 inches). Bake in preheated slow oven (325° F.) about 45 minutes until crumb is dry when tested with toothpick. If a browner loaf is desired, temperature may be raised to 450° F. for the last 5 minutes of baking. Remove bread from oven. Let stand 5 minutes. Loosen loaf with spatula and turn out on rack. Cool before slicing. Yield: 1 loaf.

Variations: For variety of texture and flavor a medium ripe mashed banana or ½ cup fluffy mashed potato may be folded into the batter before folding in the egg whites.

Wheat Starch Bread II

Ingredients:
- 1 cup gluten-free wheat starch
- 1 tablespoon sugar
- 2 teaspoons baking powder
- ⅓ teaspoon soda
- ½ teaspoon salt
- 1 beaten egg
- ¼ cup cottage cheese
- 2 tablespoons melted butter
- ½ cup buttermilk

Procedure: Place dry ingredients into a mixing bowl and combine thoroughly. In another bowl place beaten egg, cottage cheese (small curd type), melted butter and buttermilk and beat thoroughly. Add this mixture to the dry ingredients and stir until well blended (do not overstir). Pour into well greased 7½-inch pie tin and bake in a preheated 350° F. oven for about 25 minutes.

NOTE: This recipe may be made into cake or other types of bread by modification of ingredient content. Use more sugar for cake; ½ cup shredded pineapple with juice in place of the buttermilk; flavor with grated orange or lemon rind; add ⅓ cup fresh blueberries.

Rice Flour Muffins

Ingredients:
- 1 cup unsifted rice flour
- 3 teaspoons baking powder
- ½ teaspoon salt
- ¼ cup vegetable shortening
- ¼ cup sugar
- 2 egg yolks
- ¾ cup milk
- 2 egg whites
- ½ teaspoon vanilla, lemon or almond flavoring

Procedure: Measure rice flour, baking powder, salt and sift together twice. Cream softened shortening, add sugar and cream together. Stir in egg yolks. Add flour mixture alternately with milk, beating after each addition. Fold in well beaten (but not dry) egg whites and flavoring. Spoon into a well-greased muffin tin. Bake 30 minutes in a 325° F. (moderate oven) or until lightly browned. Yield: 6 muffins.

Wheat Starch Muffins

Ingredients:
- 1½ cups gluten-free wheat starch
- 2 teaspoons baking powder
- 3 tablespoons sugar
- ½ teaspoon salt
- 4 tablespoons melted shortening
- 1 egg
- ½ cup milk

Procedure: Sift the dry ingredients into a mixing bowl. Add shortening, the egg slightly beaten and the milk. Mix just until well blended. Pour into well oiled muffin tins and bake about 25 minutes in a 375° F. oven. A combination of wheat starch and rice flour or wheat starch and soy bean flour can be used. With rice, increase the milk about 1 tablespoon per cup of flour.

Rice Flour Baking Powder Biscuits

Ingredients:
- 1¾ cups rice flour
- ¼ teaspoon salt
- 2 teaspoons baking powder
- 3 tablespoons shortening
- 3 tablespoons milk or water

Procedure: Sift dry ingredients. Cut in shortening using two knives. Add liquid. Roll to about ½ inch thickness, shape with cutter. Bake about 15 minutes at 400° F.

Variation: Dip a cube of sugar in orange juice and then press into the biscuit before baking. *Or* roll the biscuit dough into a rectangular shape, sprinkle with brown sugar and cinnamon, add raisins or nuts. Roll as for cinnamon rolls, slice into ¼ inch pieces, place on baking sheet and bake the same as biscuits.

Wheat Starch Baking Powder Biscuits

Ingredients:
1 cup gluten-free wheat starch
2 teaspoons baking powder
¼ teaspoon salt
1 teaspoon sugar
2 tablespoons shortening
¼ cup milk

Procedure: Sift wheat starch, baking powder, sugar and salt into a bowl. Add the shortening and blend with a fork. Add the milk, enough to make a dough. Place on floured board, roll ½ inch thick; cut. Bake in 450° F. oven about 20 minutes. A combination of wheat starch and rice flour can be used, or a combination of the wheat starch and soy flour is good. The rice flour requires slightly more liquid to handle, approximately 1 tablespoon.

Rice and Corn Bread

Ingredients:
⅞ cup rice flour
¼ cup sugar
4 teaspoons baking powder
¾ teaspoon salt
1 cup yellow cornmeal
2 eggs
¼ cup shortening
1 cup milk

Procedure: Sift flour with sugar, baking powder and salt. Stir in the cornmeal. Add eggs to softened shortening and beat. Add milk and add liquid mixture to dry ingredients. Beat about 1 minute. Pour into greased, hot pan, 9 × 9 inches. Bake at 425° F. for 20 minutes. Good when cold, crisped under a broiler.

Pastry, Cookies and Cake

Pie Crust

Ingredients:
1 cup rice flour
1 cup wheat starch
½ cup shortening
1 teaspoon salt

Procedure: Mix rice flour and wheat starch together. Cut in shortening. Add salt. Pat into pie plate and fill with a fruit filling. Bake in a hot oven (400° F.) until slightly brown.

Rice Flour Cookies

Ingredients:
¼ lb. butter or margarine
¼ cup sugar
1 egg yolk
½ teaspoon vanilla
1 cup rice flour
¼ teaspoon salt

Procedure: Mix butter, sugar and egg yolk well; add vanilla and flour mixed with salt to make a soft dough. Divide dough into small balls the size of a walnut. Place on greased cookie sheet. Press center with thumb and place dab of jelly in the depression. Bake at 350° F. until brown.

Rice Flour Brownies

Ingredients:
2 squares unsweetened chocolate (2 oz.)
⅓ cup shortening (margarine)
1 cup sugar
2 eggs
⅔ cup rice flour, sifted twice before measuring
½ teaspoon baking powder
½ teaspoon salt

Procedure: Melt chocolate and shortening in a double boiler over hot water. Remove pan from hot water and beat in sugar and eggs. Sift rice flour, baking powder and salt together and stir into chocolate mixture. Spread into a greased 8-inch-square pan. Allow mixture to stand ½ hour before baking. Bake in a 350° F. moderate oven for 30 to 35 minutes. A slight imprint is left when the top is touched. Cool slightly; cut into squares. Yield: 16 2-inch squares.

Ginger Cookies

Ingredients:
2¼ cups rice flour
2 teaspoons soda
¼ teaspoon salt
½ teaspoon cloves
1 teaspoon ginger
1 teaspoon cinnamon
¾ cup shortening
1 cup brown sugar
1 egg
¼ cup molasses

Procedure: Sift dry ingredients except sugar together. Cream shortening with brown sugar, add egg and molasses. Add dry ingredients and mix. Chill dough in refrigerator for 30 minutes. Roll into small balls, dip the top in sugar, flatten with fork on greased cookie sheet. Bake at 375° F. for about 10 minutes.

Date Drop Cookies

Ingredients:
    ¾ cup shortening
    1 cup sugar
    2 eggs
    1 tablespoon grated orange rind
    2¼ cups rice flour
    1 teaspoon salt
    ½ teaspoon soda
    ⅓ cup orange juice
    1 cup dates

Procedure: Cream shortening and sugar. Beat eggs and rind. Sift flour, salt and soda. Blend into creamed mixture with orange juice. Stir in chopped or ground dates. Drop by spoonfuls onto greased cookie sheet. Sprinkle with mixture of sugar, cinnamon and cloves. Bake at 400° F. for about 12 minutes.

Apple Upside Down Cake

Ingredients:
    Brown sugar
    Butter
    Peeled, sliced apples
    Cinnamon
Batter:
    ⅞ cup rice flour
    1 teaspoon baking powder
    ½ cup sugar
    ¼ teaspoon salt
    1 beaten egg
    ¼ cup melted butter
    ¼ cup milk

Procedure: Into buttered baking dish sprinkle brown sugar, enough to cover bottom, dot with butter and cover with a layer of sliced apples. Sprinkle with sugar and cinnamon.

Batter: Sift dry ingredients, add beaten egg, melted butter and milk. Beat until smooth and pour over apple mixture. Bake at 350° F. for about an hour. Serve upside down on platter with whipped cream.

Cheese Cake Without Crust

Ingredients:
    1 pound pot cheese, strained through a
        ricer
    ⅓ cup sugar
    2 eggs
    1 teaspoon vanilla
    Sour cream
    Sugar
    Cinnamon

Procedure: Mix first four ingredients thoroughly and fit into a greased, 6-inch pie plate. Bake in oven at 350° F. for 40 minutes. Cool for half an hour, then spread with sour cream and sprinkle with cinnamon and sugar.

Potato Starch Sponge Cake

Ingredients:
    7 eggs
    1½ cups sugar, sifted
        Grated rind of ½ lemon
        Juice of ½ lemon
    ¾ cup potato starch, sifted twice with a
        dash of salt

Procedure: Separate 6 eggs. Beat 6 yolks and one whole egg together until frothy. Gradually add sifted sugar, lemon juice and grated rind, beating constantly until thick and lemon colored. (If using an electric mixer, use low speed for 5 minutes.)

Gradually add sifted potato starch, folding in by hand with a spatula. Beat 6 egg whites stiff, but not dry, then gently fold into the above mixture. Pour entire mixture into ungreased regulation tube cake pan. Bake at 350° F. for about 50 to 55 minutes.

This cake will keep at least a week if wrapped in foil and kept in refrigerator.

STUDY QUESTIONS AND ACTIVITIES

1. What cereals must be omitted on the gluten-free diet? What problems does this create?

2. Name 20 foods which contain one or more of the excluded cereals. Which of these are "hidden" in the food?

3. What should the patient on a gluten-free diet be told about labeling laws? (See Chap. 41.)

4. Which cereals and starches may be used freely on a gluten-free diet?

5. Have you tried any of the gluten-free recipes? What can you tell your patient about them?

6. How can the grainy taste of rice flour be avoided in baked foods?

7. What can you tell a patient about gluten-free bread mixes? Are any of these available in your community?

8. How can a gluten-free bread be kept fresh for as long as possible?

9. How may sauces and gravies be thickened for the gluten-free diet? What warning should be given about quantities?

SUPPLEMENTARY SOURCES OF FOODS AND RECIPES FOR GLUTEN-FREE DIETS

How to eat well on a gluten-free diet. Today's Health, *43*:38, 1965 (Oct.).

Low Gluten Diet with Tested Recipes. $1.00. Arthur B. French, Clinical Research Unit, University Hospital, Ann Arbor, Mich. 48104.

Nutrition Division, Department of Health and Welfare, Ottawa, Ontario, Canada.

Sleisenger, M. H., *et al.:* A Wheat, Rye and Oat Free Diet. American Dietetic Association, 620 North Michigan Avenue, Chicago, Ill. 60611.

Wood, M. N.: Gourmet Food on a Wheat-Free Diet. Springfield, Ill., Charles C Thomas, 1967.

CHAPTER 41

Foods for Allergy Diets

A discussion of allergy will be found in Chapters 30 and 34. The preparation of food for a patient with allergy may be a real problem, especially when the more common foods produce allergic symptoms. It is not too difficult to eliminate fish, shellfish and certain vegetables and fruits, but when the offender is wheat, milk or eggs, or a combination of these, all of which are used in the preparation of everyday meals, meal planning and preparation demand constant watchfulness.

Today the homemaker buys many foods which she formerly prepared herself, such as mayonnaise, packaged mixes, and so on. For this reason it is not always recognized what the ingredients in a given food combination are likely to be. Although many foods are labeled as to their contents by law, many others fall under the "standards of identity" clause. (See Chap. 17.) This provides that certain ingredients must be present in at least minimum quantities, but that others may be added, and that the product need not be labeled. Therefore, it is best not to use packaged or prepared foods of any kind unless the container is labeled.

Wheat. If the allergy is to wheat alone, the list of foods allowed and those to be omitted under the Gluten-Free Diet in Chapter 27 will be found of help. Besides wheat, this list omits the use of rye, oats, barley and buckwheat, which does not need to be taken into consideration by the person allergic to wheat only. However, rye bread as purchased may be made from a mixture of wheat and rye flours, and a pancake mix may contain both buckwheat and wheat flours. For this reason it is safest to use only single flours or mixtures of single flours in the preparation of breads, cakes and cookies.

A number of flours can be used to make acceptable bread and baked products. Some of these may be found on the grocery shelves, but others will have to be purchased in a "health food" store. Rye, barley, potato, rice and soy flours, and cornmeal and oatmeal may be used singly or in combination in a recipe. However, most of them should not be used in equivalent quantities as wheat flour. The following table of substitutions and combinations may be used to alter a recipe containing wheat flour.

Substitutes for 1 Cup of Wheat Flour

½ cup barley flour
1 cup corn flour
¾ cup cornmeal (coarse)
1 scant cup cornmeal (fine)
⅝ cup potato starch
⅞ cup rice flour
1¼ cups rye flour
1 cup rye meal
1⅓ cups ground rolled oats

Combinations of Flour Equal to 1 Cup Wheat Flour

1.	rye flour	½ cup
	potato flour	½ cup
2.	rye flour	⅔ cup
	potato flour	⅓ cup
3.	rice flour	⅝ cup (10 tablespoons)
	rye flour	⅓ cup
4.	soy flour	1 cup
	potato starch	¾ cup

540

The coarse flours such as cornmeal, rice and soy flour need not be sifted before measuring. When a combination of flours is used, care must be taken that they are thoroughly mixed. When coarse flours are used, increasing the amount of baking powder to 2½ teaspoons per cup of flour will improve the product. The texture of foods made with coarse flours is sometimes grainy. This may be remedied when using rice flour by bringing it to a boil with the amount of liquid allowed, cooling it, then mixing it with the remainder of the ingredients.

In baking with flours other than wheat, long slow baking is advisable—especially so if eggs and milk also must be omitted. Most muffins and biscuits have better texture when made in small sizes.

Rice flakes and cornflakes, rolled fine, make an excellent breading for chicken, meat or fish patties, and for topping in place of bread crumbs. Potato flour or cornstarch may be used for thickening cream sauces or gravies, but the quantity called for in the recipe should be cut in half.

Milk. Some patients sensitive to whole fluid milk may be able to use it after it has been boiled, or in dried or evaporated form, since heating may denature the offending protein so that it no longer causes a reaction. The physician's advice should be followed in this respect. If cow's milk is not tolerated in any form, one of the soybean "milks" may be substituted and used on cereals and in puddings. However, the flavor is not that of milk, but it may be disguised somewhat by the use of brown sugar instead of white.

Both butter and margarine contain dry milk solids. The patient with a severe milk allergy should omit both fats. Oil and hydrogenated cooking fats may be substituted for other fat in a recipe, and, in a few recipes such as puddings, water in combination with a fruit may be substituted for milk.

Most commercial bread, except Vienna bread, has dried milk solids added. Cakes, pastries, cookies and other baked goods need to be checked carefully for the addition of milk, and it is probably safer to use home-baked varieties.

Eggs. Whole egg is used in the preparation of many foods, and, again, commercially prepared cake, pastries and cookies are best omitted. Egg white is used for glazing pretzels and in the manufacture of marshmallows and meringues. Ice creams usually contain eggs. Dried egg white is an ingredient of some baking powders. Careful reading of labels and the omission of food of which the composition is not known are essential for the patient allergic to eggs.

In batter and dough recipes an additional teaspoon of baking powder should be used for each egg omitted from the recipe.

Recipes for Wheat-, Milk- and Egg-Free Diets

A patient may be allergic to any one of the three foods discussed above, to a combination of two of them or to all three. In the following recipes, the letters W-M-E denote the absence of wheat, milk and eggs, according to the initials used.

Rye Bread (W-M-E)

Ingredients:
  1½ cakes compressed yeast *or*
       2 tablespoons active dry yeast
  1⅓ cups water
  2 teaspoons salt
  3 tablespoons sugar
  4 tablespoons fat
  5 cups rye flour

Procedure: Soften yeast in ⅓ cup lukewarm water. Add 1 teaspoon sugar. Measure remaining water, salt, sugar and softened fat into a bowl; add dissolved yeast mixture. Pour half of flour into this liquid mixture and beat until well blended. Add remaining flour; knead on floured board until dough is smooth and will spring back when pressed lightly with finger (about 200 strokes).

Place in well oiled bowl. Let rise until double in bulk (about 1 hour) at 80° F. Knead about 100 times and place in two small loaf pans which have been greased only on the bottom.

Let rise again until double in bulk (about 30 minutes) at 80° F. Bake at 425° F. for 10 to 15 minutes until brown; then at 350° F. for 25 to 35 minutes until done. Yield: 2 small loaves.

Rolled Oats Biscuits (W-M-E)

Ingredients:
  2 cups finely ground rolled oats
  1 teaspoon salt

3 teaspoons baking powder
3 tablespoons shortening
$\frac{3}{8}$ to $\frac{1}{2}$ cup water

Procedure: Mix ground oats thoroughly with salt and baking powder. Cut in or rub in shortening until mixture is as fine as coarse corn meal. Stir in enough water to make a stiff dough. Pat out and cut into rounds. For a drop biscuit, add more water and drop by tablespoonfuls on baking sheet. Bake in hot oven (450° F.) from 10 to 12 minutes. Yield: 12 small biscuits.

NOTE: 1 cup light-rye flour may replace 1 cup ground rolled oats.

Cornmeal and Rye Muffins (W-M-E)

Ingredients:
$\frac{1}{2}$ cup cornmeal
$\frac{1}{2}$ cup rye flour
$2\frac{1}{2}$ teaspoons baking powder
2 tablespoons sugar
1 teaspoon salt
2 tablespoons raisins
1 tablespoon fat, melted
$\frac{1}{2}$ cup water

Procedure: Sift dry ingredients together. Add raisins. Combine fat and water. Add to dry ingredients. Stir only enough to mix ingredients slightly. Batter will be lumpy. Fill greased muffin pans $\frac{2}{3}$ full. Bake at 400° F. for about 30 minutes. Yield: 6 muffins.

Oatmeal and Rice Muffins (W-M-E)

Ingredients:
3 tablespoons ground oatmeal
$\frac{3}{4}$ cup rice flour
1 tablespoon baking powder
$\frac{1}{2}$ teaspoon salt
$\frac{1}{2}$ cup water (or enough to make a
thin batter)
1 tablespoon fat, melted
3 tablespoons raisins

Procedure: Grind oatmeal using a medium coarse blade. Sift rice flour, baking powder and salt together; mix with ground oatmeal. Combine water with fat. Add liquid to dry ingredients and stir just enough to dampen flour mixture; add raisins. Fill greased muffin pans $\frac{2}{3}$ full. Bake at 400° F. about 30 minutes. Yield: 6 muffins.

Old-fashioned Johnnycakes (W-M-E)

Ingredients:
1 tablespoon bacon drippings
$\frac{1}{2}$ cup boiling water
$\frac{1}{2}$ cup cornmeal
$\frac{1}{2}$ teaspoon salt
1 tablespoon sugar

Procedure: Add shortening to boiling water. Stir in cornmeal, salt and sugar and stir over low heat until mixture thickens. Drop by tablespoonfuls on preheated well-greased griddle and bake until lightly browned on both sides. Lower heat under griddle and bake 5 minutes more, turning often. Yield: 6 to 8 cakes.

Steamed Brown Bread (W-M-E)

Ingredients:
1 cup rye flour
1 cup cornmeal
$\frac{1}{4}$ teaspoon baking soda
1 teaspoon salt
1 cup quick oatmeal
$\frac{3}{4}$ cup molasses
1 cup water

Procedure: Sift rye flour, cornmeal, soda and salt together. Add oatmeal and mix. Add molasses and water. Mix. Fill greased molds not more than $\frac{2}{3}$ full. Cover tightly with greased lid. Steam $3\frac{1}{2}$ hours. Remove covers and dry in oven 15 minutes. Bread may be baked at 375° F. about 1 hour. Yield: 3 loaves using 10 oz. cans.

Rice Stuffing (W-M-E)

Ingredients:
$\frac{1}{3}$ cup rice
$\frac{1}{2}$ teaspoon salt
3 cups boiling water
$\frac{1}{2}$ cup diced celery
$\frac{1}{4}$ cup diced onion
$\frac{1}{3}$ cup fat
$5\frac{1}{2}$ cups (1 package) crisp rice cereal
2 tablespoons minced parsley
1 tablespoon poultry seasoning
$\frac{1}{2}$ teaspoon salt
$\frac{1}{2}$ cup stock or water

Procedure: Wash rice thoroughly in a sieve and drain well. Add rice to boiling salted water slowly so that water continues to bubble. Boil rapidly 15 to 20 minutes until rice is tender. Drain in sieve. Brown celery and onion in fat. Stir in rice and mix well. Crush Rice Krispies into coarse crumbs. Add parsley, seasonings and stock. Combine with rice and mix thoroughly. Yield: $3\frac{1}{2}$ cups stuffing.

NOTE: Stuffing may be baked in a covered casserole in moderate oven (375° F.) for 25 minutes.

Apple Strudel (W-M-E)

Ingredients:
5 cups cornflakes
3 cups sliced apples
$\frac{3}{4}$ cup sugar, granulated or brown
Cinnamon
3 tablespoons vegetable oil

Procedure: Put layer of cornflakes in greased 1½-quart casserole. Cover with layer of apples. Add half the sugar, sprinkle with cinnamon and dot with one third of the oil. Add another layer of cornflakes, remaining apples and sugar. Sprinkle with cinnamon and dot with more oil. Put a layer of cornflakes on top, dot with remaining oil and sprinkle with a little sugar. Cover casserole and bake in moderate oven (375° F.) about 35 minutes, or until apples are soft. Serve hot or cold with cream. Yield: 6 servings.

NOTE: Add about 2 tablespoons water to strudel before baking if apples are not juicy. Sprinkle few drops lemon juice over apples if they are not tart.

Spice Cake (W-M-E)

Ingredients:

    1 cup brown sugar
    1¼ cup water
    1 cup raisins, seedless
    2 ounces citron, cut fine
    ⅓ cup fat
    ½ teaspoon salt
    1 teaspoon nutmeg
    1 teaspoon cinnamon
    4 teaspoons baking powder
    1 cup cornmeal, fine
    1 cup rye flour

Procedure: Boil sugar, water, fruit, fat and salt together for 3 minutes. When cool add to sifted dry ingredients. Mix thoroughly. Bake in a greased loaf pan at 375° F. for about 45 minutes. Yield: 1 loaf cake.

Soy Cookies (W-M-E)*

Ingredients:

    3 tablespoons fat, melted, or oil
    ⅓ cup sugar
    ½ teaspoon vanilla or lemon extract
    1 cup soy flour
    2 teaspoons baking powder
    ¼ teaspoon salt
    4 tablespoons water

Procedure: Mix fat and sugar; add flavoring. Sift dry ingredients together three times; add to fat and sugar; add water. Mix. Form into a roll; chill for 1 to 2 hours. Cut into as thin slices as possible and bake on a well greased cookie sheet. Bake at 325° F. about 15 minutes. Yield: 20 cookies.

Variations:

1. Drop cookies may be prepared from this recipe, and it is not necessary to chill the dough. Form dough into balls. Place on greased cookie sheet. Press each cookie with tines of fork, add ½ teaspoon jelly to each.

2. ½ cup finely diced dates may be added to above recipe.

* Soy flour is naturally moist, and only a small amount of liquid is needed in a recipe.

Rice and Barley Flour Muffins (W-E)

Ingredients:

    ⅓ cup rice flour
    ⅔ cup barley flour
    3 teaspoons baking powder
    2 tablespoons sugar
    ¼ teaspoon salt
    ¾ cup milk
    1 tablespoon fat, melted

Procedure: Mix and sift dry ingredients together. Add liquid and melted fat. Stir only enough to combine. Fill greased muffin tins ⅔ full. Bake at 400° F. for about 35 minutes. Yield: 5 muffins.

Plain Cake (W-E)

Ingredients:

    1 cup barley flour
    3 teaspoons baking powder
    ¼ teaspoon salt
    4 tablespoons fat
    ½ cup sugar
    ½ cup plus 1 tablespoon milk
    ½ teaspoon vanilla

Procedure: Sift dry ingredients together. Cream fat, add sugar, mix well. Add liquid, dry ingredients and vanilla. Bake in greased pan (9″ × 9″ × 2″) or muffin pans at 375° F. for 25 to 30 minutes. Yield: 1 layer cake or 6 cup cakes.

Variations: Barley, rye, rice or a combination of these flours may be used.

Quick Chocolate Drops (W-E)

Ingredients:

    2 squares chocolate, melted
    1⅓ cups (14½-oz. can) sweetened
        condensed milk
    2 cups chopped nut meats or 3 cups
        shredded coconut

Procedure: Blend melted chocolate with condensed milk. Stir in chopped nut meats or coconut and mix well. Drop by teaspoonfuls on greased baking sheet and bake in moderate oven (350° F.) from 15 to 20 minutes. Yield: 4 dozen cookies 1 inch in diameter.

NOTE: This recipe may be halved if there is some other use for the condensed milk. These cookies keep indefinitely, however, and it may be more practical to make up the entire recipe.

Pineapple Rye Muffins (W-M)

Ingredients:

1½ cups rye flour
½ teaspoon salt
4 tablespoons sugar
5 teaspoons baking powder
4 tablespoons crushed pineapple, drained
1 egg
½ cup water
4 tablespoons fat, melted

Procedure: Sift dry ingredients; add drained crushed pineapple. Combine beaten egg, water, and melted fat. Add to dry ingredients; stir only enough to combine. (Mixture will have a lumpy appearance.) Fill greased muffin pans ⅔ full, handling the batter as little as possible. Bake at 400° F. for about 35 minutes. Yield: 12 muffins.

Butterscotch Wafers (W-M)

Ingredients:

½ cup unsifted rye flour
¾ teaspoon baking powder
¼ teaspoon salt
¼ cup shortening
1 cup brown sugar, firmly packed
1 egg, well beaten
¾ cup chopped nut meats

Procedure: Mix flour, baking powder and salt. Melt shortening, stir in sugar and mix well. Remove from heat and stir in well-beaten egg. Stir in sifted dry ingredients to which nut meats have been added. Drop by ½ teaspoonfuls on greased baking sheet and bake in slow oven (325° F.) about 15 minutes. Cool slightly, then remove carefully with a thin knife or spatula. If cookies harden on sheet, return to the oven for a few minutes. Yield: about 3½ dozen cookies 2 inches in diameter.

Bacon Muffins (W-E)

Ingredients:

1½ cups rye flour
5 teaspoons baking powder
½ teaspoon salt
¼ cup sugar
2 slices bacon, cooked
1 cup milk
2 tablespoons fat, melted

Procedure: Mix and sift dry ingredients together. Add chopped bacon to flour. Add liquid and melted fat and stir only enough to combine. Fill greased muffin tins ⅔ full. Bake at 400° F. for about 35 minutes. Yield: 8 muffins.

White Bread (M-E)

Ingredients:

2 cups lukewarm potato water (water in which potatoes have been cooked)
2 tablespoons fat
2 tablespoons sugar
2 teaspoons salt
1 cake yeast
2 tablespoons lukewarm water
6 cups white flour (approximately)

Procedure: Combine lukewarm potato water, fat, sugar and salt. Soften yeast in 2 tablespoons water; add to above mixture. Add about 5 or 6 cups white flour, enough to make a stiff dough. Mix thoroughly. Turn on floured board and knead about 10 minutes until smooth and satiny. Place dough in warm greased bowl, brush surface lightly with melted shortening, cover and let rise 2 hours. Punch dough down thoroughly in bowl, cover and let rise about ½ hour, or until doubled in bulk. Turn out on floured board. Divide into 2 equal parts. Place in 2 greased loaf pans, brush top with melted shortening, cover and let rise 1 hour. Bake in hot oven (400° F.) for 40 to 45 minutes. Yield: 2 loaves.

Spice and Raisin Cake (M-E)

Ingredients:

1 cup water
2 cups raisins
1 cup brown sugar
⅓ cup fat
½ teaspoon salt
½ teaspoon cinnamon
½ teaspoon allspice
⅛ teaspoon nutmeg
2 cups cake flour
1 teaspoon baking powder
1 teaspoon soda
1 cup nuts, finely cut

Procedure: Boil water, raisins, sugar, fat, salt and spices for 3 minutes. Cool. Sift flour, baking powder and soda. Stir flour mixture gradually into other ingredients. Beat until batter is smooth. Add nuts. Bake in a greased 9-inch tube pan at 325° F. for about 1 hour. Yield: 1 9-inch cake.

See Chapter 40 for some Wheat-Free recipes. Recipes containing gluten-free wheat starch should not be used.

STUDY QUESTIONS AND ACTIVITIES

1. Why it it important for the patient with an allergy to check the labels of prepared packaged foods?

2. What is meant by the term "standard of identity"? See if you can find some unlabeled foods in your local grocery store or supermarket. Should any of these probably be omitted by the patient who is allergic to wheat, milk and eggs?

3. Name 10 foods (other than bakery goods) which contain wheat flour.

4. How many of these might also contain milk? Eggs?

5. List some of the flours which may be substituted for wheat flour.

6. What should the patient who is allergic to milk be told about breads, butter and margarine?

7. Name 3 foods or mixtures containing egg white which might not be suspected.

Look up a can of baking powder. Does it contain egg white?

SUPPLEMENTARY SOURCES OF FOODS AND RECIPES FOR ALLERGY DIETS

Allergy Recipes, American Dietetic Association, 620 N. Michigan Avenue, Chicago, Ill. 60611 (50 cents)

Commercial sources: Cellu Products, The Chicago Dietetic Supply House, 1750 W. van Buren St., Chicago, Ill. 60612.

PART FOUR
Tabular Material and Bibliography

EXPLANATION OF TABLES

Table 1. Composition of Foods Edible Portions in Common Measures

This table of food values gives proximate composition and mineral and vitamin content of most foods in common use in the United States. It includes processed and prepared foods where such foods would not be consumed in the natural state. The foods have been arranged alphabetically for convenience. The values for 100-Gm. portions are given for all natural foods, but for some processed foods the common unit of package or can is given where a 100-Gm. portion would seldom be used.

Most of the values are taken from the second edition of Handbook No. 8[6] and a few values from other sources.[1,2,3,4,5]

Reliability of Data

Research in food values has demonstrated repeatedly that the composition of foods is variable, due to differences in variety, soil and climate in which grown, the method of handling, and the sampling and the analyzing. The values given are usually averages of several determinations on a variety of samples and frequently include a wide range of values; therefore, it seems unnecessary to retain decimals where they are of questionable significance. Thus the values for calories and for grams of protein, fat, carbohydrate and water are given in whole numbers, and fiber is carried to one decimal place only.

Minerals and vitamins are all measured in milligrams (mg.), except for vitamin A, which is still usually given in International Units (I.U.). In order to be consistent in the use of mg., it is necessary to use decimals for measuring the B complex vitamins because they are present in such small amounts.

The common measures for 100-Gm. or other quantities commonly used are only approximate. For instance, 100 Gm. of most liquids would measure about ⅖ of a cup. Since this is not a convenient fraction for measuring, the designation *½ cup scant* has been used. This would mean about 1½ tbsp. less than ½ cup.

The individual nutrients in foods have been determined by many different laboratories and the data assembled by the Department of Agriculture or other agencies.

Food Energy

In this 15th edition of the text, as in the previous edition and in all recent government publications, calorie values have been calculated by using specific factors for individual foods, taking into consideration the digestibility and the physiologic value of nutrients. It is still possible to estimate caloric value of a food by applying the factors 4, 9 and 4 calories per gram of protein, fat and carbohydrate, respectively, but the values will be slightly different from those calculated by the more accurate method mentioned.

Niacin Values

The values for niacin are for the preformed niacin present in the food. Since niacin may be formed in the body from tryptophan in food protein, the total niacin equivalent will be larger than the figure given in most cases. "The average diet in the United States, which contains a generous amount of protein, provides enough tryptophan to increase the niacin value by about a third."[5]

Tables 3 and 4

Tables 3 and 4 are entirely new. The fatty acid and cholesterol content of common foods includes the saturated and polyunsaturated acid linoleic, the most significant for dietary planning. Values are taken from Handbook No. 8[6] and from Hardinge and Crooks.[3] The amino acid content of selected foods are listed in an order convenient for dietitians dealing with inborn errors of metabolism. The values are given in micrograms rather than milligrams to avoid the use of decimals.

Table 5

Table 5 gives sodium, potassium and magnesium content of foods. Copper values are omitted because the values given in the literature are conflicting and incomplete. References to pertinent articles are given at the end of Table 5.

Signs and Symbols Used

An asterisk in the table indicates an item for which the composition has been calculated from a recipe.

Dots (..) show that no basis could be found for imputing a value, although there was some reason to believe that a measurable amount of the constituent might be present.

The designation Tr. (trace) is used to indicate values that would round to zero when calculated to the number of decimal places used in each column.

REFERENCES USED IN COMPILING FOOD TABLES

1. Burger, M., *et al.*: Vitamin, mineral and proximate composition of frozen fruits, juices and vegetables. J. Agr. & Food Chem., 4: 417, 1956.
2. Church, C. E., and Church, H. N.: Food Values of Portions Commonly Used. Ed. 10. Philadelphia, Lippincott, 1966.
3. Hardinge, M. G., and Crooks, H.: J. Am. Dietet. A., 34:1065, 1958.
4. Orr., M. L., and Watt, B. K.: Home Ec. Res. Report No. 4. Washington, U.S.D.A., 1957.
5. Nutrition Value of Foods. Home and Garden Bulletin No. 72. Agricultural Research Service, U.S.D.A., Washington, 1960.
6. Watt, B. K., and Merrill, A. L.: Composition of Foods—Raw, Processed, Prepared. U.S.D.A. Agr. Handbook No. 8 Ed. 2, 1963.

For additional references on food values see Bibliography in Part Four.

TABLE 1. Composition of Foods—Edible Portion

Food and Description	Wt. Gm.	Approximate Measure	Food Energy Cal.	Protein Gm.	Fat Gm.	Carbohydrate Total Gm.	Carbohydrate Fiber Gm.	Water Gm.	Minerals Ca Mg.	Minerals P Mg.	Minerals Fe Mg.	Vitamins Vitamin A I.U.	Vitamins Thiamine Mg.	Vitamins Riboflavin Mg.	Vitamins Niacin Mg.	Vitamins Ascorbic Acid Mg.
Acerola (West Indian cherry) raw	100	1 c.	28	Tr.	Tr.	7	0.4	92	12	11	0.2	..		0.02	0.06	0.4	1,300†
Almonds, dried	100	⅔ c.	598	19	54	20	2.6	5	234	504	4.7	0	0.24	0.92	3.5	Tr.
salted	15	12–15	94	3	9	3	0.4	1	35	75	0.7	0	0.04	0.14	0.5	Tr.
Apples:																
Raw, pared	100	medium	54	Tr.	Tr.	14	0.6	85	6	10	0.3	40	0.03	0.02	0.1	2
Frozen, sliced, sweetened	100	⅔ c.	93	Tr.	Tr.	24	0.7	75	5	6	0.5	20	0.01	0.03	0.2	7
Apple Betty*	100	½ c. scant	151	2	4	30	0.5	64	18	22	0.6	100	0.06	0.04	0.4	1
Apple juice, bottled or canned	100	½ c. scant	47	Tr.	0	12	0.1	88	6	9	0.6	..	0.01	0.02	0.1	1
	250	1 c.	120	Tr.	0	30	..	220	15	22	1.5	..	0.03	0.05	0.3	3
Apple sauce, canned:																
Unsweetened	100	½ c. scant	41	Tr.	Tr.	11	0.6	88	4	5	0.5	40	0.02	0.01	Tr.	1
Sweetened	100	½ c. scant	91	Tr.	Tr.	24	0.5	76	4	5	0.5	40	0.02	0.01	Tr.	1
Apricots:																
Raw	100	3 medium	51	1	Tr.	13	0.6	85	17	23	0.5	2,700	0.03	0.04	0.6	10
Canned:																
Solids and liquid water pack	100	½ c. scant	38	1	Tr.	10	0.4	89	12	16	0.3	1,830	0.02	0.02	0.4	4
Syrup pack (heavy syrup)	100	½ c. scant	86	1	Tr.	22	0.4	77	11	15	0.3	1,740	0.02	0.02	0.4	4
Dried, sulfured uncooked	100	20 large or 30 small halves	260	5	Tr.	67	3.0	25	67	108	5.5	10,900	0.01	0.16	3.3	12
Cooked, sweetened fruit and liquid*	100	⅓ c.	122	1	Tr.	31	0.9	66	19	31	1.6	2,600	Tr.	0.04	0.9	2
Frozen, sweetened	100	½ c.	98	1	Tr.	25	0.6	73	10	19	0.9	1,680	0.02	0.04	0.8	28‡

Tr. (trace) is used to indicate values that would round to zero with the number of decimal places carried in this table. Thus Tr. means 0.4 Gm. or less of protein, fat, carbohydrate or water.

*Values are calculated from a recipe.
†Value for fully ripe fruit. Av. for firm ripe is 1,900; Av. for partially ripe is 2,500.
‡Varying amounts of ascorbic acid are added in processing.

TABLE 1. Composition of Foods—Edible Portion (Continued)

Food and Description	Wt. Gm.	Approximate Measure	Food Energy Cal.	Protein Gm.	Fat Gm.	Carbohydrate Total Gm.	Carbohydrate Fiber Gm.	Water Gm.	Minerals Ca Mg.	Minerals P Mg.	Minerals Fe Mg.	Vitamins Vitamin A I.U.	Vitamins Thiamine Mg.	Vitamins Riboflavin Mg.	Vitamins Niacin Mg.	Vitamins Ascorbic Acid Mg.
Asparagus:																
Fresh, cooked	100	6–7 spears	20	2	Tr.	4	0.7	94	21	50	0.6	900	0.16	0.18	1.4	26
Frozen, cooked	100	6–7 spears	22	3	Tr.	4	0.8	92	22	67	1.1	780	0.16	0.14	1.1	26
Canned:																
Green, drained, solids	100	½ c. cut or 6–7 spears	21	2	Tr.	3	0.8	93	19	53	1.9	800	0.06	0.10	0.8	15
Avocados, raw commercial varieties	100	½ peeled	167	2	16	6	1.6	74	10	42	0.6	290	0.11	0.20	1.6	14
Baby Foods:																
Cereals, pre-cooked:																
Mixed, dry, with added nutrients	100	3½ ozs.	368	15	3	71	1.1	7	820	741	56.4	..	3.15	1.35	22.3	0
Dessert:																
Custard pudding	100	3½ ozs.	100	2	2	19	0.2	77	64	62	0.3	100	0.02	0.12	0.1	1
Fruits:																
Apple sauce	100	3½ ozs.	72	Tr.	Tr.	19	0.5	81	4	7	0.4	40	0.01	0.02	0.1	Tr.
Apple sauce and apricot	100	3½ ozs.	86	Tr.	Tr.	23	0.5	77	4	14	0.3	600	0.01	0.02	0.1	2
Apricot, pineapple, and/or orange with tapioca	100	3½ ozs.	84	Tr.	Tr.	22	0.2	78	15	9	0.4	450	0.02	0.01	0.2	4
Peaches	100	3½ ozs.	81	1	Tr.	21	0.5	78	6	14	0.3	500	0.01	0.02	0.7	3
Pears	100	3½ ozs.	66	Tr.	Tr.	17	1.0	82	7	8	0.2	30	0.02	0.02	0.2	2
Prunes with tapioca	100	3½ ozs.	86	Tr.	Tr.	22	0.3	77	7	21	0.9	400	0.02	0.06	0.4	4
Meats, Poultry and Eggs:																
Beef, strained	100	3½ ozs.	99	15	4	0	0	80	8	127	2.0	..	0.01	0.16	3.5	0
junior	100	3½ ozs.	118	19	4	0	0	76	8	163	2.5	..	0.02	0.20	4.3	0
Beef heart	100	3½ ozs.	93	14	4	Tr.	0	81	5	155	3.7	..	0.06	0.62	3.6	0
Chicken	100	3½ ozs.	127	14	8	0	0	77	..	129	1.9	..	0.02	0.16	3.5	0
Egg yolk, strained	100	3½ ozs.	210	10	18	Tr.	0	70	81	256	3.0	1,900	0.12	0.22	Tr.	Tr.

Food	g	Measure													
Lamb, strained	100	3½ ozs.	107	15	5	0	79	9	124	2.1	..	0.02	0.17	3.3	..
junior	100	3½ ozs.	121	18	5	0	76	13	156	2.7	..	0.02	0.21	4.1	..
Liver, strained	100	3½ ozs.	97	14	3	2	80	6	182	5.6	24,000	0.05	2.00	7.6	10
Pork, strained	100	3½ ozs.	118	15	6	0	78	8	130	1.5	..	0.19	0.20	2.7	..
junior	100	3½ ozs.	134	19	6	0	74	8	144	1.2	..	0.23	0.23	2.8	..
Veal, strained	100	3½ ozs.	91	16	3	0	81	10	145	1.7	..	0.03	0.20	4.3	..
junior	100	3½ ozs.	107	19	3	0	77	8	157	1.6	..	0.03	0.22	6.0	..
Vegetables:															
Beans, green	100	3½ ozs.	22	1	Tr.	5	93	33	25	1.1	400	0.02	0.06	0.3	3
Beets	100	3½ ozs.	37	1	Tr.	8	89	18	27	0.7	20	0.02	0.03	0.1	3
Carrots	100	3½ ozs.	29	1	Tr.	7	92	23	21	0.5	13,000	0.02	0.03	0.1	3
Mixed vegetables	100	3½ ozs.	37	2	Tr.	9	89	22	36	0.9	4,700	0.05	0.04	0.6	2
Peas	100	3½ ozs.	54	4	1	9	86	11	63	1.2	500	0.08	0.09	1.2	10
Spinach, creamed	100	3½ ozs.	43	2	Tr.	8	88	64	63	0.6	5,000	0.02	0.13	0.3	6
Squash	100	3½ ozs.	25	1	Tr.	6	92	24	17	0.4	2,400	0.02	0.04	0.3	8
Sweet potatoes	100	3½ ozs.	67	1	Tr.	16	82	16	34	0.4	4,900	0.04	0.03	0.4	8
Tomato soup	100	3½ ozs.	54	2	Tr.	14	83	24	52	0.4	1,000	0.05	0.12	0.7	3
Bacon, broiled or fried	100	12 strips	611	30	52	3	8	14	224	3.3	0	0.51	0.34	5.2	0
	16	2 strips	100	5	8	1	1	2	37	0.5	0	0.08	0.06	0.8	0
Bacon, Canadian, broiled or fried	100	3½ ozs.	277	28	18	Tr.	50	19	218	4.1	0	0.92	0.17	5.0	0
Bananas, raw	100	1 small	85	1	Tr.	22	76	8	26	0.7	190	0.05	0.06	0.7	10
Barley, pearled, light uncooked	100	½ c.	349	8	1	79	11	16	189	2.0	0	0.12	0.05	3.1	?
Beans, common or kidney:															
Red kidney, canned or cooked, solids and liquids	100	½ c. scant	90	6	Tr.	16	76	29	109	1.8	0	0.05	0.04	0.6	..
Canned, baked:															
Pork and molasses	100	½ c. scant	150	6	5	21	66	63	114	2.3	..	0.06	0.04	0.5	..
Pork and tomato sauce	100	½ c. scant	122	6	3	19	71	54	92	1.8	130	0.08	0.03	0.6	2
Beans, Lima:															
Fresh, cooked	100	⅔ c.	111	8	Tr.	20	71	47	121	2.5	280	0.18	0.10	1.3	17
Frozen, cooked	100	⅔ c.	99	6	Tr.	19	74	20	90	1.7	230	0.07	0.05	1.0	17
Canned, drained solids	100	½ c. scant	96	5	Tr.	18	75	28	70	2.4	190	0.03	0.05	0.5	6

TABLE 1. Composition of Foods—Edible Portion (Continued)

Food and Description	Wt. Gm.	Approximate Measure	Food Energy Cal.	Protein Gm.	Fat Gm.	Carbohydrate Total Gm.	Carbohydrate Fiber Gm.	Water Gm.	Minerals Ca Mg.	Minerals P Mg.	Minerals Fe Mg.	Vitamins Vitamin A I.U.	Vitamins Thiamine Mg.	Vitamins Riboflavin Mg.	Vitamins Niacin Mg.	Vitamins Ascorbic Acid Mg.
Beans:																
Snap green:																
Cooked, fresh or frozen	100	3/4 c.	25	2	Tr.	5	1.0	92	50	37	0.6	540	0.07	0.09	0.5	12
Canned, drained solids	100	3/4 c.	24	1	Tr.	5	1.0	92	45	25	1.5	470	0.03	0.05	0.3	4
Wax or yellow:																
Canned, drained solids	100	1/2 c.	22	1	Tr.	5	1.0	93	50	37	0.6	230	0.07	0.09	0.5	13
Bean Sprouts, mung, raw	100	1 c.	35	4	Tr.	7	0.7	89	19	64	1.3	20	0.13	0.13	0.8	19
Beef, trimmed to retail basis, cooked:																
Cuts, braised, simmered or pot-roasted:																
Lean and fat	100	3½ ozs.	289	27	19	0	0	53	12	134	3.4	30	0.05	0.21	4.2	0
Lean only (from above serving)	85	3 ozs.	165	26	6	0	0	52	12	128	3.2	10	0.05	0.19	3.2	0
Hamburger, broiled:																
Market ground	100	3½ ozs. or 2 patties	286	25	20	0	0	54	11	194	3.2	40	0.09	0.21	5.4	0
Ground lean	100		219	27	11	0	0	60	12	230	3.5	20	0.09	0.23	6.0	0
	50	1 patty	109	14	6	0	0	30	6	115	1.8	10	0.05	0.12	3.0	0
Roast, oven-cooked no water added																
Relatively fat such as rib:																
Lean and fat	100	3½ ozs.	417	21	36	0	0	42	9	175	2.7	70	0.06	0.16	3.8	0
Lean only (from above serving)	63	2.2 ozs.	135	18	6	0	0	38	7	153	2.3	12	0.04	0.14	3.3	0
Relatively lean such as round:																
Lean and fat	100	3½ ozs.	317	25	23	0	0	51	11	207	3.1	40	0.06	0.19	4.5	0
Lean only (from above serving)	76	2.8 ozs.	145	23	5	0	0	47	10	186	2.8	7	0.06	0.17	4.0	0
Steak, broiled																
Relatively fat such as sirloin:																
Lean and fat	100	3½ ozs.	387	23	32	0	0	44	10	191	2.9	50	0.06	0.18	4.7	0
Lean only (from above serving)	66	2.3 ozs.	136	21	5	0	0	39	8	173	2.6	7	0.06	0.17	4.2	0

Relatively lean such as round:															
Lean and fat............	100	3½ ozs.	261	29	15	0	0	55	12	250	3.5	30	0.08	0.22	5.6	0
Lean only (from above serving)............	81	2.9 ozs.	152	25	5	0	0	50	11	218	3.0	8	0.07	0.19	4.9	0
Beef, canned:															
Corned beef............	100	3½ ozs.	185	26	8	0	0	62	21	110	4.5	..	0.02	0.25	3.5	0
Corned beef hash............	100	3½ ozs.	181	9	11	11	1	67	13	67	2.0	..	0.01	0.09	2.1	..
Beef, dried or chipped............	100	3½ ozs.	203	34	6	0	0	48	20	404	5.1	0	0.07	0.32	3.8	0
cooked, creamed............	100	3½ ozs.—	154	8	10	7	0	72	105	140	0.8	360	0.06	0.19	2.6	Tr.
Beef and vegetable stew canned............	100	½ c.	79	6	3	7	0.3	83	12	45	0.9	970	0.03	0.05	1.0	3
Beets, cooked, drained............	100	½ c.	32	1	Tr.	7	0.8	91	14	23	0.5	20	0.03	0.04	0.3	6
canned, solids............	100	½ c.	37	1	Tr.	9	0.8	90	19	18	0.7	20	0.01	0.03	0.1	3
Beet greens, cooked............	100	⅔ c.	18	2	Tr.	3	1.1	94	99†	25	1.9	5,100	0.07	0.15	0.3	15
Beverages, carbonated:															
Ginger ale............	100	3½ ozs.	31	..	..	8	..	92	..	..	..	..	..	..	..	..
Other, including cola type............	100	3½ ozs.	40	..	..	10	..	90	..	..	..	..	..	..	..	..
Biscuits, baking powder, made with enriched flour*............	100	3 biscuits 2-in. diam.	369	7	17	46	0.2	27	121	175	1.6	Tr.	0.21	0.21	1.8	Tr.
Blackberries: including dewberries, boysenberries															
Raw............	100	⅔ c.	58	1	1	13	4.2	85	32	19	0.9	200	0.03	0.04	0.4	21
Canned, solids and liquids:															
Water pack............	100	½ c. scant	40	1	1	9	2.8	89	22	13	0.6	140	0.02	0.02	0.2	7
Syrup pack............	100	½ c. scant	91	1	1	22	2.6	76	21	12	0.6	130	0.01	0.02	0.2	7
Blueberries:															
Raw............	100	⅔ c.	62	1	1	15	1.5	83	15	13	1.0	100	0.03	0.06	0.5	14
Frozen without sugar............	100	⅔ c.	55	1	Tr.	14	1.5	85	10	13	0.8	70	0.03	0.06	0.5	7
Canned, solids and liquid:															
Water pack............	100	½ c. scant	39	Tr.	Tr.	10	1.0	89	10	9	0.7	40	0.01	0.01	0.2	7
Syrup pack............	100	½ c. scant	101	Tr.	Tr.	26	1.0	73	9	8	0.6	40	0.01	0.01	0.2	6
Bouillon cubes............	100	25 cubes	120	20	3	5	0	4	..	..	..	..	..	..	..	..
	4	1 cube	2	Tr.	Tr.	Tr.	0	Tr.	..	..	..	..	..	..	..	..

*Values are calculated from a recipe.

†Calcium may not be available because of the presence of oxalic acid.

TABLE 1. Composition of Foods—Edible Portion (Continued)

Food and Description	Wt. Gm.	Approximate Measure	Food Energy Cal.	Protein Gm.	Fat Gm.	Carbohydrate Total Gm.	Carbohydrate Fiber Gm.	Water Gm.	Ca Mg.	P Mg.	Fe Mg.	Vitamin A I.U.	Thiamine Mg.	Riboflavin Mg.	Niacin Mg.	Ascorbic Acid Mg.
Brains, all kinds, raw........	100	3½ ozs.	125	10	9	1	0	79	10	312	2.4	0	0.23	0.26	4.4	18
Bran (breakfast cereal, almost wholly bran)........	28	1 oz.	95	3	1	21	2.0	1	24	350	2.9	0	0.11	0.09	5.0	0
Bran flakes (40 per cent bran) with added thiamine........	100	2½ c.	303	10	2	81	3.6	3	71	495	4.4	0	0.40	0.17	6.2	0
	28	¾ c. 1 oz.	85	3	1	23	1.0	1	20	138	1.2	0	0.11	0.05	1.7	0
Bran flakes with raisins added thiamine........	100	2 c.	287	8	1	79	3.0	7	56	396	4.0	..	0.32	0.13	5.3	0
Brazil nuts, shelled........	100	⅔ c.	654	14	67	11	3.1	5	186	693	3.4	Tr.	0.96	0.12	1.6	0
Breads:*																
Boston brown bread made with degermed corn meal, enriched........	100	2 sl. 3 x ¾ in.	211	6	1	46	0.7	45	90	160	1.9	..	0.11	0.06	1.2	0
Cracked wheat bread made with enriched flour........	100	4 sl.	263	9	2	52	0.5	35	88	128	1.1	0	0.12	0.09	1.3	Tr.
	23	1 sl.	60	2	Tr.	12	0.1	8	20	29	0.3	0	0.03	0.02	0.3	Tr.
French or Vienna breads, unenriched........	100	3½ ozs.	290	9	3	55	0.2	31	43	85	0.7	0	0.08	0.08	0.8	Tr.
enriched........	100	3½ ozs.	290	9	3	55	0.2	31	43	85	2.2	0	0.28	0.22	2.5	Tr.
Italian bread:																
unenriched........	100	3½ ozs.	276	9	1	56	0.2	32	17	77	0.7	0	0.09	0.06	0.8	0
enriched........	100	3½ ozs.	276	9	1	56	0.2	32	17	77	2.2	0	0.29	0.20	2.6	0
Raisin bread........	100	4 sl.	262	7	3	54	0.2	35	71	87	1.3	Tr.	0.05	0.09	0.7	Tr.
	23	1 sl.	60	2	1	13	Tr.	7	16	20	0.3	Tr.	0.01	0.02	0.2	0
Rye bread, American (⅓ rye, ⅔ wheat flour)........	100	4 sl.	243	9	1	52	0.4	36	75	147	1.6	0	0.18	0.07	1.4	0
	23	1 sl.	56	2	Tr.	12	0.1	9	17	34	0.4	0	0.04	0.02	0.3	0
White bread, unenriched, 4 per cent nonfat dry milk...	100	4 sl.	270	9	3	51	0.2	36	84	97	0.7	Tr.	0.07	0.09	1.1	Tr.
	23	1 sl.	62	2	1	12	Tr.	8	19	22	0.2	Tr.	0.02	0.02	0.3	Tr.

Food	Wt. (g)	Measure	Food energy (Cal.)	Protein (g)	Fat (g)	Carbohydrate (g)	Fiber (g)	Water (%)	Calcium (mg)	Phosphorus (mg)	Iron (mg)	Vit. A (I.U.)	Thiamine (mg)	Riboflavin (mg)	Niacin (mg)	Ascorbic acid (mg)
White bread, enriched:																
1–2 per cent nonfat dry milk.	100	4 sl.	269	9	3	50	0.2	36	70	87	2.4	Tr.	0.25	0.17	2.3	Tr.
	23	1 sl.	62	2	1	12	0.1	9	16	20	0.6	Tr.	0.06	0.04	0.5	Tr.
3–4 per cent nonfat dry milk†.	100	4 sl.	270	9	3	50	0.2	36	84	97	2.5	Tr.	0.25	0.21	2.4	Tr.
	23	1 sl.	62	2	1	12	0.1	9	19	22	0.6	Tr.	0.06	0.05	0.6	Tr.
5–6 per cent nonfat dry milk.	100	4 sl.	275	9	4	50	0.2	35	96	102	2.5	Tr.	0.27	0.20	2.4	Tr.
	23	1 sl.	63	2	1	12	0.1	9	22	24	0.6	Tr.	0.06	0.05	0.6	Tr.
Whole wheat, graham, entire wheat bread, 2 per cent dry milk.	100	4 sl.	243	10	3	48	1.6	37	99	228	2.3	Tr.	0.26	0.12	2.8	Tr.
	23	1 sl.	56	2	1	11	0.4	9	23	53	0.6	Tr.	0.06	0.03	0.6	Tr.
Bread crumbs, dry.	100	1 c.	392	13	5	73	0.3	7	122	141	3.6	Tr.	0.22	0.30	3.5	Tr.
Breakfast foods. See individual grain, as corn, oatmeal, etc.																
Broccoli, flower stalks, fresh or frozen	100	⅔ c.	32	4	Tr.	6	1.5	89	103	78	1.1	2,500	0.10	0.23	0.9	113
cooked	100	⅔ c.	26	3	Tr.	5	1.5	91	88	62	0.8	2,500	0.09	0.20	0.8	90
Brussels sprouts, fresh or frozen, cooked	100	¾ c.	36	4	Tr.	6	1.6	88	32	72	1.1	520	0.08	0.14	0.8	87
Buckwheat flour, light.	100	1 c. sifted	347	6	1	80	0.5	12	11	88	1.0	0	0.08	0.04	0.4	0
Bun, hamburger. See Rolls.																
Butter.	100	½ c. scant	716	1	81	Tr.	0	16	20	16	0	3,300‡	..	..	..	0
	14	1 tbsp.	100	Tr.	11	Tr.	0	2	3	2	0	460‡	..	..	..	0
Buttermilk, cultured (made from skim milk).	100	½ c. scant	36	4	Tr.	5	0	91	121	95	Tr.	Tr.	0.04	0.18	0.1	1
Cabbage:																
Raw	100	wedge 3½ x 4½ in.	24	1	Tr.	5	0.8	92	49	29	0.4	130	0.05	0.05	0.3	47§
Cooked (short time)	100	1⅔ c.	20	1	Tr.	4	0.8	94	44	20	0.3	130	0.04	0.04	0.3	33
Cabbage, celery or Chinese, raw	100	1 c., 1-in. pieces	14	1	Tr.	3	0.6	95	43	40	0.6	150	0.05	0.04	0.6	25

*Values are calculated from a recipe.
†When the amount of nonfat milk solids in commercial bread is unknown, use bread with 3 to 4 per cent nonfat milk solids.
‡Year-round average.
§Freshly harvested av. 51 Mg.; stored av. 42 Mg.

TABLE 1. Composition of Foods—Edible Portion (Continued)

Food and Description	Wt. Gm.	Approximate Measure	Food Energy Cal.	Protein Gm.	Fat Gm.	Carbohydrate Total Gm.	Carbohydrate Fiber Gm.	Water Gm.	Minerals Ca Mg.	Minerals P Mg.	Minerals Fe Mg.	Vitamins Vitamin A I.U.	Vitamins Thiamine Mg.	Vitamins Riboflavin Mg.	Vitamins Niacin Mg.	Vitamins Ascorbic Acid Mg.
Cakes: home recipes:																
Chocolate (devil's food with icing)...............	100	1 piece	369	4	16	56	0.3	22	70	131	1.0	160	0.02	0.10	0.2	Tr.
Fruit cake, dark type............	100	3 pieces	379	5	15	60	0.6	18	72	113	2.6	120	0.13	0.14	0.8	Tr.
Plain or cup cake, no icing......	100	2 cupcakes	364	5	14	56	0.1	25	64	102	0.4	170	0.02	0.09	0.2	Tr.
Sponge cake............	100	2 pieces	297	8	6	54	0	32	30	112	1.2	450	0.05	0.14	0.2	Tr.
Cakes: made from mixes:																
Angel food............	100	2 pieces	259	6	Tr.	59	Tr.	34	95	119	0.3	0	Tr.	0.11	0.1	0
Coffee cake............	100	2 pieces	322	6	10	52	0.1	30	61	174	1.6	160	0.18	0.16	1.4	Tr.
Yellow cake, chocolate icing....	100	3-in. piece	337	4	11	58	0.2	26	91	182	0.6	140	0.02	0.08	0.2	Tr.
Cake icing, mix:																
Chocolate fudge............	100	3½ ozs.	378	2	14	67	0.5	15	16	66	1.0	270	0.01	0.04	0.2	0
Candy:																
Candied or glacé peel—lemon, orange or grapefruit peel............	100	3½ ozs.	316	Tr.	Tr.	81	..	17	..	..	..	40	..	..	..	..
Butterscotch............	28	1 oz.	111	..	1	26	0	..	5	2	0.4	..	0	0	0	0
Caramels, plain............	28	1 oz.	109	1	3	27	0.1	2	42	34	0.4	3	0.01	0.05	0.1	Tr.
Chocolate, plain, milk............	28	1 oz.	146	2	9	16	0.1	Tr.	64	65	0.3	75	0.02	0.10	0.1	Tr.
Chocolate, milk with almonds...	28	1 oz.	150	3	10	14	0.2	Tr.	64	76	0.4	64	0.02	0.11	0.2	Tr.
Chocolate covered peanuts...	28	1 oz.	157	4	12	11	0.3	Tr.	32	84	0.4	Tr.	0.10	0.05	2.4	Tr.
Fudge, plain chocolate............	28	1 oz.	112	1	3	21	Tr.	2	22	24	0.3	Tr.	0.01	0.03	0.1	Tr.
Hard candy............	28	1 oz.	108	0	Tr.	27	0	5	7	2	0.7	0	0	0	0	0
Marshmallows............	28	1 oz.	85	1	Tr.	22	0	..	5	2	0.4	0	0	0	0	0
Peanut bar............	28	1 oz.	144	5	9	13	0.3	Tr.	12	74	0.5	0	0.12	0.02	2.6	0
Peanut brittle............	28	1 oz.	118	2	3	22	0.1	Tr.	10	28	0.6	0	0.04	0.01	0.9	0
Cantaloupe, raw netted type....	100	⅛ melon, 5 in. diam.	30	1	Tr.	8	0.3	91	14	16	0.4	3,400	0.04	0.03	0.6	33

Food	Wt. (g)	Measure													
Carrots:															
Raw	100	2 carrots, 5½ x 1 in. or 1 c. grated	42	1	Tr.	10	1.0	88	37	36	0.7	11,000	0.06	0.05	0.6	8
Cooked, drained	100	2/3 c.	31	1	Tr.	7	1.0	92	33	31	0.6	10,500	0.05	0.05	0.5	6
Canned: Drained solids	100	2/3 c.	30	1	Tr.	7	0.8	92	30	22	0.7	15,000	0.02	0.03	0.4	2
Cashew nuts, roasted or cooked	100	3½ ozs.	561	17	46	29	1.4	5	38	373	3.8	100	0.43	0.25	1.8	0
	28	1 oz.	168	5	14	9	0.4	1	11	112	1.1	30	0.13	0.08	0.5	0
Cauliflower:															
Raw	100	1 c. flower buds	27	3	Tr.	5	0.9	91	25	56	1.1	60	0.11	0.10	0.7	78
Cooked, drained	100	1 c. scant	22	2	Tr.	4	0.9	93	21	42	0.7	60	0.09	0.08	0.6	55
Frozen, raw	100	1 c. scant	22	2	Tr.	4	0.8	93	19	42	0.6	30	0.06	0.06	0.5	56
Celery, bleached:															
Raw	100	2 large stalks or 1 c. diced	17	1	Tr.	4	0.6	94	39	28	0.3	240	0.03	0.03	0.3	9
Cooked	100	3/4 c. diced	14	1	Tr.	3	0.6	95	31	22	0.2	230	0.02	0.03	0.3	6
Chard, leaves and stalks, cooked	100	2/3 c.	18	2	Tr.	3	0.7	94	73†	24	1.8	5,400	0.04	0.11	0.4	16
Cheeses:															
Blue mold, or Roquefort	100	3½ ozs.	368	22	31	2	0	40	315	339	0.5	1,240	0.03	0.61	1.2	0
	28	1 oz.	110	6	9	1	0	11	88	95	0.1	343	0.01	0.18	0.4	0
Camembert	100	3½ ozs.	299	18	25	2	0	52	105	184	0.5	1,010	0.04	0.75	0.8	0
	28	1 oz.	84	5	7	1	0	15	29	52	0.2	282	0.01	0.22	0.2	0
Cheddar, American, regular	100	3½ ozs.	398	25	32	2	0	37	750	478	1.0	2,310	0.03	0.46	0.1	0
	28	1 oz.	120	7	9	1	0	10	210	134	0.3	650	0.01	0.14	Tr.	0
Cheddar, American, processed	100	3½ ozs.	370	23	30	2	0	40	697	771	0.9	1,220	0.02	0.41	Tr.	0
	28	1 oz.	107	6	8	1	0	11	195	218	0.3	340	0.01	0.11	Tr.	0
Cottage, from skim milk creamed	100	3½ ozs.	106	14	4	3	0	78	94	152	0.3	170	0.03	0.25	0.1	0
	28	1 oz.	30	4	1	1	0	23	28	43	0.1	48	0.01	0.07	Tr.	0
Cream cheese	100	3½ ozs.	374	8	38	2	0	51	62	95	0.2	1,540	0.02	0.24	0.1	0
	28	1 oz.	113	2	10	1	0	14	17	27	0.1	430	0.01	0.07	Tr.	0
Parmesan	100	3½ ozs.	393	36	26	3	0	30	1,140	781	0.4	1,060	0.02	0.73	0.2	0
	28	1 oz.	110	11	8	1	0	9	312	218	0.1	296	0.01	0.20	0.1	0
Pimiento, American, processed	100	3½ ozs.	371	23	30	2	Tr.	40	..	..	..	..	..	..	..	..
	28	1 oz.	103	6	8	1	Tr.	11	..	..	..	..	..	..	..	0
Swiss, processed	100	3½ ozs.	355	26	27	2	0	40	887	867	0.9	1,100	0.01	0.40	0.1	0
	28	1 oz.	99	7	8	1	0	11	245	240	0.3	310	Tr.	0.11	Tr.	0

†Calcium may not be available because of the presence of oxalic acid.

TABLE 1. Composition of Foods—Edible Portion (Continued)

Food and Description	Wt. Gm.	Approximate Measure	Food Energy Cal.	Protein Gm.	Fat Gm.	Carbohydrate Total Gm.	Fiber Gm.	Water Gm.	Minerals Ca Mg.	P Mg.	Fe Mg.	Vitamins Vitamin A I.U.	Thiamine Mg.	Riboflavin Mg.	Niacin Mg.	Ascorbic Acid Mg.
Cherries:																
Sour, red, raw..........	100	1 c. whole or pitted	58	1	Tr.	14	0.2	84	22	19	0.4	1,000	0.05	0.06	0.4	10
Sweet, raw........	100	⅔ c. pitted	70	1	Tr.	17	0.4	80	22	19	0.4	110	0.05	0.06	0.4	10
Red, sour, canned, heavy syrup.	100	½ c. scant	89	1	Tr.	23	0.1	76	14	12	0.3	650	0.03	0.02	0.2	5
Maraschino	100	½ c. scant	116	Tr.	Tr.	29	0.3	70	..	..	..	..	..	..	..	..
Chicken, cooked																
Light meat...........	100	3½ ozs.	166	32	3	0	0	64	11	265	1.3	60	0.04	0.10	11.6	0
no skin, roasted, fried.......	100	3½ ozs.	197	32	6	1	0	60	12	280	1.3	50	0.05	0.25	12.9	0
Dark meat........	100	3½ ozs.	176	28	6	0	0	64	13	229	1.7	150	0.07	0.23	5.6	0
no skin, roasted, fried.......	100	3½ ozs.	220	30	9	2	0	58	14	225	1.8	130	0.07	0.45	6.8	0
Canned, boneless.........	100	3½ ozs.	198	22	12	0	0	65	21	247	1.5	230	0.04	0.12	4.4	4
Chickpeas or garbanzos, dry, whole seed, raw...........	100	½ c.	360	21	5	61	5.3	11	150	331	6.9	50	0.31	0.15	2.0	..
Chili sauce.............	100	½ c. scant	104	3	Tr.	25	0.7	68	20	52	0.8	1,400	0.09	0.07	1.6	..
	17	1 tbsp.	18	1	Tr.	4	0.1	11	3	9	0.1	238	0.02	0.01	0.3	..
Chocolate:																
Bitter or unsweetened...........	100	3½ ozs.	505	11	53	29	2.5	2	78‖	384	6.7	60	0.05	0.24	1.5	0
	28	1 oz. square	142	3	15	8	0.8	1	23‖	116	2.0	18	0.01	0.07	0.5	0
Bittersweet........	100	3½ ozs.	477	8	40	47	1.8	2	58‖	284	5.0	40	0.03	0.17	1.0	0
	28	1 oz.	143	2	12	14	0.5	1	17‖	85	1.5	12	0.01	0.05	0.3	0
Chocolate syrup, thin type........	100	⅓ c.	245	2	2	63	0.6	32	17‖	92	1.6	Tr.	0.02	0.07	0.4	0
	20	1 tbsp.	49	Tr.	Tr.	13	0.1	6	3‖	18	0.3	Tr.	Tr.	0.01	0.1	0
Clams, long and round:																
Raw, meat only.............	100	3½ ozs.	76	13	2	2	..	82	69	162	6.1	100	0.10	0.18	1.3	10
Canned, solids and liquid......	100	3½ ozs.	52	8	1	3	..	86	55	137	4.1	..	0.01	0.10	1.1	..
Cocoa beverage, made with all milk*........	100	½ c. scant	95	4	5	11	0.1	79	119	114	0.4	160	0.04	0.19	0.2	1
	250	1 c.	236	10	12	27	0.3	198	298	285	1.0	400	0.10	0.46	0.5	3

Food	Amount (g)	Measure													
Coconut:															
Fresh, meat	100	1 c. shredded	346	4	35	9	4.0	51	13	95	1.7	0	0.05	0.02	0.5	3
Dried, shredded (sweetened)	100	3½ ozs.	548	4	39	53	4.1	3	16	112	2.0	0	0.04	0.03	0.4	0
Coleslaw, French dressing	100	¾ c.	95	1	7	8	0.7	84	42	26	0.4	110	0.04	0.04	0.3	29
Collards: leaves only															
Cooked (boiled in small amount of water)	100	½ c.	33	4	1	5	1.0	90	188	52	0.8	7,800	0.11	0.20	1.2	76
Cookies:*															
Assorted, commercial	25	1 cookie	120	1	5	18	Tr.	1	9	41	0.2	20	0.01	0.01	0.1	Tr.
Brownie with nuts	50	1 bar	242	3	16	25	0.5	5	20	74	1.0	100	0.10	0.06	0.4	Tr.
Chocolate chip	25	3 small	129	1	8	15	0.1	1	8	25	0.5	28	0.03	0.03	0.2	Tr.
Macaroons, coconut	20	1 cookie	95	1	5	13	0.4	1	5	17	0.2	0	0.01	0.03	0.1	0
Oatmeal with raisins	20	1 cookie	90	1	3	15	0.1	1	4	20	0.6	10	0.02	0.02	0.1	Tr.
Sandwich type, commercial	20	1 cookie	99	1	5	14	Tr.	Tr.	5	48	0.1	0	0.01	0.01	0.1	0
Corn, sweet:															
Cooked, fresh on cob	100	1 small ear	91	3	1	21	0.7	74	3	89	0.6	400†	0.11	0.10	1.4	9
Canned: Cream style	100	½ c. scant	82	2	1	20	1.0	76	3	56	0.6	330†	0.03	0.05	1.0	5
Whole kernel	100	½ c. scant	66	2	1	16	0.8	81	4	50	0.4	270†	0.03	0.05	0.9	5
Corn bread or muffins* made with:															
Whole ground corn meal	100	2 muffins, 2¾ in. diam.	215	7	6	35	0.6	49	141	216	1.7	130‡	0.15	0.18	0.8	0
Enriched, degermed corn meal	100	2 muffins, 2¾ in. diam.	219	7	5	37	0.2	49	139	155	1.9	130§	0.17	0.23	1.3	0
Corn Cereals:															
Cornflakes (added thiamine, niacin and iron)	100	4 c.	386	8	Tr.	86	0.6	4	17	45	1.4	0	0.42	0.07	2.1	0
	28	1 c., 1 oz. pkg.	108	2	Tr.	24	0.2	1	5	13	0.4	0	0.12	0.02	0.6	0
Corn, puffed, sweetened	100	4 c.	379	4	Tr.	90	0.3	5	11	28	1.8	0	0.42	0.17	2.1	0
	28	1 oz. package	106	1	Tr.	25	0.1	1	3	8	0.5	0	0.11	0.05	0.6	0
Corn shredded (added thiamine and niacin)	100	2½ c.	389	7	Tr.	87	0.6	3	5	39	2.4	0	0.42	0.18	2.1	0
	28	¾ c., 1 oz. pkg.	109	2	Tr.	25	0.2	1	1	11	0.7	0	0.12	0.05	0.6	0

*Values are calculated from a recipe.

†Vitamin A based on yellow corn: white corn contains only a trace.

‡Based on recipe using white corn meal: if yellow corn meal, the vitamin A value is 330 I. U.

§Based on recipe using white corn meal: if yellow corn meal, the vitamin A value is 250 I. U.

‖Calcium may not be available because of the presence of oxalic acid.

TABLE 1. Composition of Foods—Edible Portion (Continued)

Food and Description	Wt. Gm.	Approximate Measure	Food Energy Cal.	Protein Gm.	Fat Gm.	Carbohydrate Total Gm.	Carbohydrate Fiber Gm.	Water Gm.	Ca Mg.	P Mg.	Fe Mg.	Vitamin A I.U.	Thiamine Mg.	Riboflavin Mg.	Niacin Mg.	Ascorbic Acid Mg.
Corn grits, degermed, white:																
Unenriched, cooked*	100	½ c. scant	51	1	Tr.	11	0.1	87	1	10	0.1	Tr.	0.02	0.01	0.2	0
Enriched, cooked*	100	½ c. scant	51	1	Tr.	11	0.1	87	1	10	0.3	Tr.	0.04	0.03	0.4	0
Corn meal, white or yellow:																
Degermed, unenriched, cooked*	100	½ c. scant	50	1	Tr.	11	0.1	88	1	14	0.2	60†	0.02	0.01	0.1	0
Degermed, enriched, cooked*	100	½ c. scant	50	1	Tr.	11	0.1	88	1	14	0.4	60†	0.06	0.04	0.5	0
Cowpeas, immature seeds, cooked	100	⅔ c.	108	8	1	18	1.8	72	24	146	2.1	350	0.30	0.11	1.4	17
Crabs, Atlantic and Pacific,																
hard shell, steamed	100	3½ ozs.	93	17	2	1	..	79	43	175	0.8	2,170	0.16	0.08	2.8	2
Canned, meat only	100	3½ ozs.	101	17	3	1	..	77	45	182	0.8	..	0.08	0.08	1.9	..
Crackers:																
Graham	14	2 medium	55	1	1	10	0.1	1	3	28	0.3	0	0.04	0.02	0.2	0
Saltines	8	2 crackers	34	1	1	6	Tr.	1	2	7	0.1	0	Tr.	Tr.	0.1	0
Soda, plain or oyster crackers	14	2 crackers	60	1	1	5	..	..	..	..	..	..	..	..	..	..
Ritz type	7	1 cracker	34	1	2	4	..	..	..	..	..	..	..	..	..	..
Cranberries:																
Raw	100	1 c.	46	Tr.	1	11	1.4	88	14	11	0.5	40	0.03	0.02	0.1	11
Juice, cocktail	100	½ c. scant	65	Tr.	Tr.	17	Tr.	83	5	3	0.3	Tr.	0.01	0.01	Tr.	40†
Sauce, sweetened, canned strained	100	½ c. scant	146	Tr.	Tr.	38	0.2	62	6	4	0.2	20	0.01	0.01	Tr.	2
Cream:																
Light, table or coffee	100	½ c. scant	211	3	21	4	0	72	102	80	Tr.	840	0.03	0.15	0.1	1
	15	1 tbsp.	31	Tr.	3	1	0	11	15	12	0	125	Tr.	0.02	Tr.	Tr.
Heavy or whipping	15	1 tbsp.	53	Tr.	6	1	0	8	12	9	0	230	Tr.	0.02	Tr.	Tr.
Cucumbers, raw pared	100	⅓ of 7-8 in. cucumber	14	1	Tr.	3	0.3	96	17	18	0.3	Tr.	0.03	0.04	0.2	11
Currants, red & white, raw	100	1 c.	50	1	Tr.	12	3.4	86	32	23	1.0	120	0.04	0.05	0.1	41
Custard, baked*	100	½ c. scant	115	5	6	11	0	77	112	117	0.4	350	0.04	0.19	0.1	Tr.

Item	Gm.	Measure														
Dandelion greens, raw	100	1 c.	45	3	1	9	1.6	86	187	66	3.1	14,000	0.19	0.26	..	35
cooked	100	½ c.	33	2	1	6	1.3	90	140	42	1.8	11,700	0.13	0.16	..	18
Dates, "fresh" and dried	100	½ c. pitted	274	2	1	73	2.4	23	59	63	3.0	50	0.09	0.10	2.2	0
Doughnuts, cake type made with enriched flour*	100	2 or 3 doughnuts	391	5	19	51	0.1	24	40	190	1.4	80	0.16	0.16	1.2	Tr.
Duck, domestic raw, flesh only	100	3½ ozs.	165	21	8	0	0	69	12	203	1.3	..	0.10	0.12	7.7	..
Eels, raw, American	100	3½ ozs.	233	16	18	0	0	66	18	202	0.7	1,610	0.22	0.36	1.4	..
Eggplant, boiled, drained	100	3½ ozs.	19	1	Tr.	4	0.9	94	11	21	0.6	10	0.05	0.04	0.5	3
Eggs, fresh, stored or frozen: Raw or cooked: Whole	100	2 medium	163	13	12	1	0	74	54	205	2.3	1,180	0.10	0.29	0.1	0
Whole	50	1 medium	81	7	6	Tr.	0	38	27	102	1.2	590	0.05	0.15	Tr.	0
White	100	3 medium	51	11	0	1	0	89	9	15	0.1	0	0	0.27	0.1	0
White	31	1 medium	16	3	0	Tr.	0	27	3	5	Tr.	0	0	0.08	Tr.	0
Yolk	100	6 medium	348	16	31	1	0	51	141	569	5.5	3,400	0.27	0.44	0.1	0
Yolk	17	1 medium	58	3	5	Tr.	0	9	24	96	0.9	580	0.05	0.07	Tr.	0
Cooked, omelet or scrambled*	100	made with 2 small eggs	173	11	13	2	0	73	80	189	1.7	1,080	0.08	0.28	0.1	0
Dried, whole	100	1 c.	592	47	41	4	0	5	187	800	8.7	4,290	0.33	1.20	0.2	0
Endive or escarole, raw	100	3½ ozs.	20	2	Tr.	4	0.9	93	81	54	1.7	3,300	0.07	0.14	0.5	10
Evaporated milk. See milk.																
Farina: quick cooking Unenriched, cooked*	100	½ c. scant	43	1	Tr.	9	0	89	4	13	0.2	0	0.01	0.01	0.1	0
Enriched, cooked	100	½ c. scant	43	1	Tr.	9	0	89	60	13	5.0	0	0.05	0.03	0.4	0
Fats, cooking (vegetable fat or oil)	100	½ c.	884	0	100	0	0	0	0	0	0	0	0	0	0	0
	12.5	1 tbsp.	110	0	13	0	0	0	0	0	0	0	0	0	0	0
Figs: Raw	100	3 small	80	1	Tr.	20	1.2	78	35	22	0.6	80	0.06	0.05	0.4	2
Canned, heavy syrup, solids and liquid	100	3 figs and 2 tbsp. syrup	84	1	Tr.	22	0.7	77	13	13	0.4	30	0.03	0.03	0.2	1
Dried	100	5 figs	274	4	1	69	5.6	23	126	77	3.0	80	0.10	0.10	0.7	0
Filberts or hazelnuts	100		634	13	62	17	3.0	6	209	337	3.4	..	0.46	..	0.9	Tr.

*Values are calculated from a recipe.   †Ascorbic acid added in processing.

TABLE 1. Composition of Foods—Edible Portion (Continued)

Food and Description	Wt. Gm.	Approximate Measure	Food Energy Cal.	Protein Gm.	Fat Gm.	Carbohydrate Total Gm.	Fiber Gm.	Water Gm.	Ca Mg.	P Mg.	Fe Mg.	Vitamin A I.U.	Thiamine Mg.	Riboflavin Mg.	Niacin Mg.	Ascorbic Acid Mg.
Fig Bars	100	4 large	350	4	5	76	1.7	14	69	69	1.3	0	0.02	0.06	0.9	0
	25	1 large	88	1	1	19	0.4	3	17	17	0.3	0	0.01	0.01	0.2	0
Fish:																
Bluefish:																
Baked or broiled	100	3½ ozs.	159	26	5	0	0	68	29	287	0.7	50	0.11	0.10	1.9	..
Fried	100	3½ ozs.	205	23	10	5	0	61	35	257	0.9	..	0.11	0.11	1.8	..
Cod:																
Broiled	100	3½ ozs.	170	29	5	0	0	65	31	274	1.0	180	0.08	0.11	3.0	..
Dried	100	3½ ozs.	375	82	3	0	0	12	..	891	3.6	0	0.08	0.45	10.9	0
Flounder, baked	100	3½ ozs.	202	30	8	0	0	58	23	344	1.4	..	0.07	0.08	2.5	..
Haddock, fried	100	3½ ozs.	165	20	6	6	.0	67	40	247	1.2	..	0.04	0.07	3.2	2
Halibut, broiled	100	3½ ozs.	171	25	7	0	.0	67	16	248	0.8	680	0.05	0.07	8.3	..
Herring:																
Atlantic, raw	100	3½ ozs.	176	17	11	0	0	69	..	256	1.1	110	0.02	0.15	3.6	..
Pacific, raw	100	3½ ozs.	98	18	3	0	0	79	..	225	1.3	100	0.02	0.16	3.5	..
Canned in tomato sauce	100	3½ ozs.	176	16	11	4	0	67	..	243	..	..	..	0.11	3.5	..
Smoked, kippered	100	3½ ozs.	211	22	13	0	0	61	66	254	1.4	30	..	0.28	3.3	..
Mackerel:																
Atlantic, broiled	100	3½ ozs.	236	22	16	0	0	62	6	280	1.2	530	0.15	0.27	7.6	..
Pacific, canned, solids and liquid	100	3½ ozs.	180	21	10	0	0	66	260	288	2.2	30	0.03	0.33	8.8	..
Salmon:																
Cooked, broiled or baked	100	3½ ozs.	182	27	7	0	0	63	..	414	1.2	160	0.16	0.06	9.8	..
Canned: solid & liquid																	
Chinook or King	100	3½ ozs.	210	20	14	0	0	65	154	289	0.9	230	0.03	0.14	7.3	..
Pink or humpback	100	3½ ozs.	141	21	6	0	0	70	196	286	0.8	70	0.03	0.18	8.0	..
Sockeye or red	100	3½ ozs.	171	20	9	0	0	67	259	344	1.2	230	0.04	0.16	7.3	..
Smoked	100	3½ ozs.	176	22	9	0	0	59	14	245	..	..	..	..	..	..
Sardines:																
Atlantic type, canned in oil, drained solids	100	3½ ozs.	203	24	11	0	Tr.	62	437†	499†	2.9	220	0.03	0.20	5.4	..
Pacific type,																	
In brine or mustard	100	3½ ozs.	196	19	12	2	..	64	303	354	5.2	30	0.01	0.30	7.4	..
In tomato sauce	100	3½ ozs.	197	19	12	2	..	64	449	478†	4.1	30	0.01	0.27	5.3	..

Food	Wt. (g)	Measure												
Shad, baked	100	3½ ozs.	201	23	11	0	64	24	313	0.6	30	0.13	0.26	8.6	..
Swordfish, broiled	100	3½ ozs.	174	28	7	0	65	27	275	1.3	2,050	0.04	0.05	10.9	..
Tuna fish, canned in oil drained solids	100	3½ ozs.	197	29	8	0	61	8	234	1.9	80	0.05	0.12	11.9	0
Canned in water solids and liquid	100	3½ ozs.	127	28	1	0	70	16	190	1.6	..	..	0.10	13.3	..
White fish, cooked baked, stuffed	100	3½ ozs.	215	15	14	6	63	..	246	0.5	2,000	0.11	0.11	2.3	Tr.
Frog legs, raw	100	3½ ozs.	73	16	Tr.	0	82	18	147	1.5	0	0.14	0.25	1.2	..
Fruit cocktail, canned, light syrup solids and liquids,	100	½ c. scant	60	Tr.	Tr.	16	84	9	12	0.4	140	0.02	0.01	0.5	2
Gelatin, dry: Plain	100	⅔ c.	335	86	Tr.	0	13	0	0	0	0	0	0	0	0
Gelatin, dry: Plain	10	1 tbsp.	34	9	0	0	1	0	0	0	0	0	0	0	0
Gelatin dessert, ready to serve: Plain	100	½ c. heaping	59	2	0	14	84	0	0	0	0	0	0	0	0
With fruit added	100	½ c. heaping	67	1	Tr.	16	82	6	11	3	110	0.03	0.02	0.2	3
Gingerbread from a mix	100	2 pieces, 2x2x2 in.	276	3	7	51	37	90	100	1.6	Tr.	0.03	0.09	0.8	Tr.
Grapefruit: white Raw, pulp only	100	½ small	41	1	Tr.	11	88	16	16	0.4	80	0.04	0.02	0.2	38
Canned in syrup, solids and liquid	100	½ c. scant	70	1	Tr.	18	81	13	14	0.3	10	0.03	0.02	0.2	30
Grapefruit juice: Fresh or frozen reconstituted	100	½ c. scant	41	1	Tr.	10	90	10	17	0.1	10	0.04	0.02	0.2	38
Canned: Unsweetened	100	½ c. scant	41	1	Tr.	10	89	8	14	0.4	10	0.03	0.02	0.2	34
Sweetened	100	½ c. scant	53	1	Tr.	13	86	8	14	0.4	10	0.03	0.02	0.2	31
Grapefruit-orange juice blend, canned or frozen reconstituted: Unsweetened	100	½ c. scant	43	1	Tr.	10	89	10	15	0.3	100	0.05	0.02	0.2	34
Sweetened	100	½ c. scant	50	1	Tr.	12	87	9	15	0.3	100	0.05	0.02	0.2	34

†Includes skin and bones; if discarded, Ca 54 mg; P319 per 100 Gm.

TABLE 1. Composition of Foods—Edible Portion (Continued)

Food and Description	Wt. Gm.	Approximate Measure	Food Energy Cal.	Protein Gm.	Fat Gm.	Carbohydrate Total Gm.	Carbohydrate Fiber Gm.	Water Gm.	Ca Mg.	P Mg.	Fe Mg.	Vitamin A I.U.	Thiamine Mg.	Riboflavin Mg.	Niacin Mg.	Ascorbic Acid Mg.
Grapes, raw:																
American type (slip skin) as Concord, Delaware, Niagara and Scuppernong	100	1 bunch 3½ x 3 in.	69	1	1	16	0.6	82	16	12	0.4	100	0.05	0.03	0.3	4
European type (adherent skin) as Malaga, muscat, sultanina, Thompson seedless and Tokay	100	⅔ c.	67	1	Tr.	17	0.5	82	12	20	0.4	100	0.05	0.03	0.3	4
Grape juice, bottled, commercial.	100	3½ ozs.	66	Tr.	0	17	..	83	11	12	0.3	..	0.04	0.02	0.2	Tr.
Guavas, common, raw	100	1 large	62	1	1	15	5.5	83	23	42	0.9	280	0.05	0.05	1.2	242†
Heart:																
Beef, lean, braised	100	3½ ozs.	188	31	6	1	0	61	6	181	5.9	30	0.25	1.22	7.6	1
Chicken, cooked	100	3½ ozs.	173	25	7	Tr.	0	67	4	107	3.6	30	0.06	0.92	5.3	4
Pork, cooked	100	3½ ozs.	195	31	7	Tr.	0	61	4	121	4.9	40	0.20	1.72	6.7	1
Honey, strained or extracted	21	1 tbsp.	64	Tr.	0	17	..	4	1	1	0.1	0	Tr.	0.01	Tr.	Tr.
Honeydew melon, raw	100	wedge 1½ x 7 in.	33	1	Tr.	8	0.6	91	14	16	0.4	40	0.05	0.03	0.6	23
Ice cream, plain, 12 per cent fat.	100	¾ c.	207	4	13	21	0	62	123	99	0.1	520	0.04	0.19	0.1	1
	62	1 container	129	3	8	13	0	37	76	61	0.1	320	0.03	0.12	0.1	1
Ice milk	100	⅔ c.	152	5	5	22	0	67	156	124	0.1	210	0.05	0.22	0.1	1
Infant Foods See Baby Foods.																
Jams, marmalades, preserves..	20	1 tbsp.	55	Tr.	Tr.	14	0.2	6	4	2	0.2	Tr.	Tr.	Tr.	Tr.	2‡
Jellies	20	1 tbsp.	50	0	0	14	0	7	4	2	0.3	Tr.	Tr.	Tr.	Tr.	1‡
Kale: leaves only																
Cooked, fresh	100	1 c.	39	5	1	6	..	87	187	58	1.6	8,300	0.10	0.18	1.6	93
Frozen, boiled, drained	100	1 c.	31	3	1	5	0.9	90	121	48	1.0	8,200	0.06	0.15	0.7	38

	Gm.	Measure													
Kidneys, raw:															
Beef	100	3½ ozs.	130	15	7	1	0	76	11	219	7.4	690	0.36	2.55	6.4	15
Lamb	100	3½ ozs.	105	17	3	1	0	78	13	218	7.6	690	0.51	2.42	7.4	15
Pork	100	3½ ozs.	106	16	4	1	0	78	11	218	6.7	130	0.58	1.73	9.8	12
Kohlrabi:															
Raw	100	¾ c. diced	29	2	Tr.	7	1.1	90	41	51	0.5	20	0.06	0.05	0.2	66
Cooked	100	⅔ c.	24	2	Tr.	7	1.1	92	33	41	0.3	20	0.06	0.03	0.2	43
Lamb, trimmed to retail basis, cooked:															
Chop, thick, broiled															
Lean and fat	100	3½ ozs.	359	22	29	0	0	47	9	172	1.3	..	0.12	0.23	5.0	..
Lean only (from above serving)	66	2.4 ozs.	125	19	5	0	0	41	8	145	1.3	..	0.10	0.18	4.1	..
Leg, roasted															
Lean and fat	100	3½ ozs.	266	26	17	0	0	55	11	212	1.8	..	0.15	0.27	5.6	..
Lean only (from above serving)	85	3 ozs.	121	19	4	0	0	41	8	157	1.5	..	0.11	0.20	4.1	..
Shoulder, roasted															
Lean and fat	100	3½ ozs.	338	22	27	0	0	50	10	172	1.2	..	0.13	0.23	4.7	..
Lean only (from above serving)	74	2.7 ozs.	150	20	7	0	0	46	9	162	1.4	..	0.11	0.21	4.3	..
Lard	100	½ c.	902	0	100	0	0	0	0	0	0	0	0	0	0	0
	14	1 tbsp.	126	0	14	0	0	0	0	0	0	0	0	0	0	0
Lemons, peeled fruit	100	1 medium, 2¾ x 2 in.	27	1	Tr.	8	0.4	90	26	16	0.6	20	0.04	0.02	0.1	53
Lemon juice, fresh and canned, unsweetened	100	½ c. scant	24	Tr.	Tr.	8	0	91	7	10	0.2	20	0.03	0.01	0.1	42
Lentils, mature, cooked	100	3½ ozs.	106	8	Tr.	19	1.2	72	25	119	2.1	20	0.07	0.06	0.6	0
Lettuce, crisp, headed	100	¼ head	13	1	Tr.	3	0.6	96	20	22	0.5	330	0.06	0.06	0.3	6
leafy types, Boston, Bibb	100	4 large leaves	14	1	Tr.	3	0.5	95	35	26	2.0	970	0.06	0.06	0.3	8
Limes, peeled fruit	100	2 medium	28	1	Tr.	10	0.5	89	33	18	0.6	10	0.03	0.02	0.2	37
Lime juice, fresh	100	½ c. scant	26	Tr.	0	9	0.2	90	9	11	0.2	10	0.02	0.01	0.1	32

†Variable according to fruit used.

†Range for varietes grown in U. S.—23 to 1160 mg.

[565]

TABLE 1. Composition of Foods—Edible Portion (Continued)

Food and Description	Wt. Gm.	Approximate Measure	Food Energy Cal.	Protein Gm.	Fat Gm.	Carbohydrate Total Gm.	Carbohydrate Fiber Gm.	Water Gm.	Ca Mg.	P Mg.	Fe Mg.	Vitamin A I.U.	Thiamine Mg.	Riboflavin Mg.	Niacin Mg.	Ascorbic Acid Mg.
Liver:																
Beef:																
Raw	100	3½ ozs.	140	20	4	5	0	70	8	352	6.5	43,900	0.25	3.26	13.6	31
Fried	100	3½ ozs.	229	26	11	5	0	56	11	476	8.8	53,400	0.26	4.19	15.6	27
Calf, fried	100	3½ ozs.	261	30	13	4	0	51	13	537	14.2	32,700	0.24	4.17	16.5	37
Chicken, simmered	100	3½ ozs.	165	27	4	3	0	65	11	159	8.5	12,300	0.17	2.69	11.7	16
Lamb, broiled	100	3½ ozs.	261	32	12	3	0	50	16	572	17.9	74,500	0.49	5.11	24.9	36
Pork, fried	100	3½ ozs.	241	30	12	3	0	54	15	539	29.1	14,900	0.34	4.36	22.3	22
Lobster:																
Raw	100	3½ ozs. meat	91	17	2	1	0	79	29	183	0.6	..	0.40	0.05	1.5	..
Canned or cooked	100	3½ ozs.	95	19	2	Tr.	0	77	65	192	0.8	..	0.10	0.07	..	..
Loganberries, raw	100	⅔ c.	62	1	1	15	3.0	83	35	17	1.2	200	0.03	0.04	0.4	24
Luncheon meat:																
Canned, ham or pork	100	3½ oz. slice	294	15	25	1	0	55	9	108	2.2	0	0.31	0.21	3.0	..
Macaroni:																
Unenriched:																
Cooked,* firm	100	⅔ c. elbow type	148	5	1	30	0.1	64	11	65	0.5	0	0.02	0.02	0.4	0
Enriched:																
Cooked,* firm	100	⅔ c. elbow type	148	5	1	30	0.1	64	11	65	1.1	0	0.18	0.10	1.4	0
Macaroni and cheese, baked* made with enriched macaroni	100	½ c.	215	8	11	20	0.1	58	181	161	0.9	430	0.10	0.20	0.9	Tr.
Mangos, raw	100	½ medium	66	1	Tr.	17	0.9	81	10	13	0.4	4,800	0.05	0.05	1.1	35
Margarine, fortified	100	½ c. scant	720	1	81	Tr.	0	16	20	16	0	3,300	..	..	..	0
	14	1 tbsp.	101	Tr.	11	Tr.	0	2	3	2	0	460	..	..	..	0
Marmalades. See Jams,																
citrus	100	½ c. scant	257	1	Tr.	70	0.4	29	35	9	0.6	..	0.02	0.02	0.1	6
	14	1 tbsp.	36	Tr.	Tr.	10	0.1	4	5	1	0.1	..	Tr.	Tr.	Tr.	1

Mayonnaise. See Salad dressings.

Meat. See Beef, Lamb, Pork, Veal.

Food	Wt. (g)	Measure													
Milk, cow:															
Fluid (pasteurized and raw):															
Whole	100	½ c. scant	65	3.5	3.5	5	0	87	118	93	Tr.	140	0.03	0.17	0.1	1
	244	1 c.	160	8.5	8.5	12	0	212	288	226	0.2	350	0.08	0.42	0.2	2
Nonfat (skim)	100	½ c. scant	36	3.6	3.6	5	0	91	121	95	Tr.	Tr.	0.04	0.18	0.1	1
	246	1 c.	88	8.8	8.8	13	0	224	297	234	0.2	Tr.	0.10	0.44	0.2	2
Canned:															
Evaporated (unsweetened)	100	½ c. scant	137	7	8	10	0	74	252	205	0.1	320	0.04	0.34	0.2	1
Condensed (sweetened)	100	⅓ c.	321	8	9	54	0	27	262	206	0.1	360	0.08	0.38	0.2	1
Dried:															
Whole	100	1 c. scant	502	26	28	38	0	2	909	708	0.5	1,130	0.29	1.46	0.7	6
	8	1 tbsp.	40	2	2	3	0	Tr.	72	56	0.1	90	0.02	0.12	0.1	1
Skim, instant	100	1¼ c.	359	36	1	52	0	4	1,293	1,005	0.6	30	0.35	1.78	0.9	7
	8	1 tbsp.	29	3	Tr.	4	0	Tr.	103	80	0.1	2	0.03	0.31	0.1	1
Malted†															
Dry powder	30	1 oz.	115	4	2	20	0	Tr.	81	107	0.6	285	0.09	0.15	‥	0
Beverage with whole milk powder	270	1 c.	281	12	12	32	0	210	364	328	0.8	670	0.17	0.56	‥	2
Chocolate flavored*	100	½ c. scant	76	3	2	11	0	83	108	91	0.2	80	0.04	0.16	0.1	1
made with skim milk	250	1 c.	190	7	6	27	0	207	272	228	0.5	200	0.10	0.40	0.2	2
Milk, goat, fluid	100	½ c. scant	67	3	4	5	0	87	129	106	0.1	160	0.04	0.11	0.3	1
	244	1 c.	164	7	10	12	0	212	315	259	0.2	390	0.10	0.26	0.7	2
Molasses, cane:															
First extraction or light	100	⅓ c.	252	‥	‥	65	‥	24	165	45	4.3	‥	0.07	0.06	0.2	‥
Second extraction or medium	100	⅓ c.	232	‥	‥	60	‥	24	290	69	6.0	‥	‥	0.12	1.2	‥
Third extraction or blackstrap	100	⅓ c.	213	‥	‥	55	‥	24	579	85	11.3	‥	0.12	0.18	2.0	‥
Muffins, made with enriched wheat flour*	100	2 muffins, 3¾-in. diam.	294	8	10	42	0.1	38	104	151	1.6	100	0.17	0.23	1.4	Tr.
Corn, enriched, ungerminated meal	100		314	7	10	48	0.2	33	105	169	1.7	300	0.20	0.23	1.6	Tr.

*Values are calculated from a recipe.

†Based on unfortified products.

TABLE 1. Composition of Foods—Edible Portion (Continued)

Food and Description	Wt. Gm.	Approximate Measure	Food Energy Cal.	Protein Gm.	Fat Gm.	Carbohydrate Total Gm.	Carbohydrate Fiber Gm.	Water Gm.	Minerals Ca Mg.	Minerals P Mg.	Minerals Fe Mg.	Vitamins Vitamin A I.U.	Vitamins Thiamine Mg.	Vitamins Riboflavin Mg.	Vitamins Niacin Mg.	Vitamins Ascorbic Acid Mg.
Mushrooms,																
cultivated, raw	100	½ c.	28	3	Tr.	4	0.8	90	6	116	0.8	Tr.	0.10	0.46	4.2	3
canned, solids and liquid	100	½ c.	17	2	Tr.	2	0.6	93	6	68	0.5	Tr.	0.02	0.25	2.0	2
Muskmelons																
See Cantaloupe.																
Mustard greens:																
Cooked	100	⅔ c.	23	2	Tr.	4	0.9	92	138	32	1.8	5,800	0.08	0.14	0.6	48
Frozen, cooked	100	⅔ c.	20	2	Tr.	3	0.9	93	104	43	1.5	6,000	0.03	0.10	0.4	20
Nectarines, raw	100	1 small	64	1	Tr.	17	0.4	82	4	24	0.5	1,650	..	..	..	3
Noodles (containing egg), enriched, cooked*	100	⅔ c.	125	4	2	23	0.1	70	10	59	0.9	70	0.14	0.08	1.2	0
Oat cereal, ready-to-eat (added vitamins and minerals)	100	4 c.	397	12	6	75	1.1	3	177	408	4.7	0	0.98	0.18	1.9	0
	25	1 c.	100	3	2	19	0.3	1	44	102	1.2	0	0.25	0.04	0.5	0
Oatmeal or rolled oats:																
Cooked*	100	⅔ c.	55	2	1	10	0.2	87	9	57	0.6	0	0.08	0.02	0.1	0
Oils, salad or cooking	100	½ c.	884	0	100	0	0	0	0	0	0	0	0	0	0	0
	14	1 tbsp.	124	0	14	0	0	0	0	0	0	0	0	0	0	0
Okra, cooked	100	9 pods	29	2	Tr.	6	1.0	90	92	41	0.5	490	0.13	0.18	0.9	20
Olives, pickled:																
Green	100	16 olives	116	1	13	1	1.3	78	61	17	1.6	300	..	..	..	..
Ripe, Mission	100	10 olives	184	1	20	3	1.5	73	106	17	1.7	70	Tr.	Tr.	..	..
	20	2 olives	37	Tr.	2	Tr.	0.3	15	21	3	0.3	14	..	..	..	..

Food	Weight (g)	Approximate measure	Food energy (cal.)	Protein (g)	Fat (g)	Carbohydrate (g)	Fiber (g)	Water (%)	Calcium (mg)	Phosphorus (mg)	Iron (mg)	Vit. A (I.U.)	Thiamine (mg)	Riboflavin (mg)	Niacin (mg)	Ascorbic acid (mg)
Onions: Mature: Raw	100	1 onion, 2½-in. diam.	38	2	Tr.	9	0.6	89	27	36	0.5	40	0.03	0.04	0.2	10
Cooked, drained	100	½ c.	29	1	Tr.	7	0.6	92	24	29	0.4	40	0.03	0.03	0.2	7
Young, green, raw bulb and white top	100	12 small, without tops	45	1	Tr.	11	1.8	88	40	39	0.6	Tr.	0.05	0.04	0.4	25
Oranges, all varieties peeled fruit	100	1 small	49	1	Tr.	12	0.6	86	41	20	0.4	200	0.10	0.04	0.4	50‡
Orange juice: Fresh	100	½ c. scant	45	1	Tr.	11	0.1	88	11	17	0.2	200	0.09	0.03	0.4	50‡
Canned, unsweetened	100	½ c. scant	48	1	Tr.	11	0.1	88	10	18	0.4	200	0.07	0.02	0.3	40
Orange juice, concentrate, Frozen: Undiluted	100	3½ ozs.	158	2	Tr.	38	0.2	58	33	55	0.4	710	0.30	0.05	1.2	158
Reconstituted, 3 parts water	100	3½ ozs.	45	1	Tr.	11	Tr.	88	9	16	0.1	200	0.09	0.01	0.3	45
Oysters, meat only, raw Av. Eastern	100	5–8 medium	66	8	2	3	..	85	94	143	5.5	310	0.14	0.18	2.5	..
Oyster stew: 1 part oysters to 3 parts milk by volume	100	½ c. scant	86	5	5	5	..	84	117	109	1.4	280	0.06	0.18	0.7	..
Pancakes (griddlecakes):* Wheat (home recipe), with enriched flour	100	4 cakes, 4 in. diam.	231	7	7	34	0.1	50	101	139	1.3	120	0.17	0.22	1.3	Tr.
Buckwheat, with milk and egg pancake mix	100	4 cakes	200	7	9	24	0.4	58	220	337	1.3	230	0.12	0.16	0.7	Tr.
Papayas, raw	100	½ c., ½ in. cubes	39	1	Tr.	10	0.9	89	20	16	0.3	1,750	0.04	0.04	0.3	56
Parsley, common, raw	3½	1 tbsp. chopped	1	Tr.	0	Tr.	Tr.	3	7†	2	0.2	300	Tr.	0.01	0.1	7
Parsnips, cooked	100	⅔ c.	66	2	1	15	2.0	82	45	62	0.6	30	0.07	0.08	0.1	10

*Values are calculated from a recipe.
‡Year-round average.
†Calcium may not be available because of the presence of oxalic acid.

TABLE 1. Composition of Foods—Edible Portion (Continued)

Food and Description	Wt. Gm.	Approximate Measure	Food Energy Cal.	Protein Gm.	Fat Gm.	Carbohydrate Total Gm.	Carbohydrate Fiber Gm.	Water Gm.	Minerals Ca Mg.	Minerals P Mg.	Minerals Fe Mg.	Vitamins Vitamin A I.U.	Vitamins Thiamine Mg.	Vitamins Riboflavin Mg.	Vitamins Niacin Mg.	Vitamins Ascorbic Acid Mg.
Peaches:																
Raw	100	1 peach, 2½x2 in. diam.	38	1	Tr.	10	0.6	89	8	19	0.5	1,330§	0.02	0.05	1.0	7
Canned, solids and liquid:																
Water pack	100	½ c. scant	31	Tr.	Tr.	8	0.4	91	4	13	0.3	450	0.01	0.03	0.6	3
Syrup pack, heavy	100	½ c. scant	79	Tr.	Tr.	20	0.4	79	4	12	0.3	430	0.01	0.02	0.6	3
Frozen, sliced	100	3½ ozs.	88	Tr.	Tr.	23	0.4	77	4	13	0.5	650	0.01	0.03	0.7	40‡
Dried, sulfured:																
Uncooked	100	⅔ c.	262	3	1	68	3.1	25	48	117	6.0	3,900	0.01	0.19	5.3	18
Cooked, sugar added*	100	4–5 halves 2 tbsp. fluid	119	1	Tr.	31	0.8	67	13	32	1.6	1,070	Tr.	0.05	1.4	2
Peanuts:																
roasted and salted	100	⅔ c.	585	26	50	19	2.4	2	74	401	2.1	0	0.32	0.13	17.2	0
	9	1 tbsp. chopped	52	2	5	2	0.2	Tr.	7	36	0.2	0	0.03	0.01	1.6	0
Peanut butter, made with small am't added fat	100	1 tbsp.	581	28	49	17	1.9	2	63	407	2.0	0	0.13	0.13	15.7	0
	15		87	4	7	3	0.3	Tr.	10	61	0.3	0	0.02	0.02	2.3	0
Pears:																
Raw, including skin	100	1 med. pear, 2½ x 2 in.	61	1	Tr.	15	1.4	83	8	11	0.3	20	0.02	0.04	0.1	4
Canned, solids and liquid:																
Water pack	100	½ c. scant	32	Tr.	Tr.	8	0.7	91	5	7	0.2	Tr.	0.01	0.02	0.1	1
Syrup pack, light	100	2 med. halves	61	Tr.	Tr.	16	0.7	84	5	7	0.2	Tr.	0.01	0.02	0.1	1
Peas, green: Immature:																
Cooked fresh or frozen	100	⅔ c. drained	72	5	Tr.	12	2.0	82	22	93	1.9	610	0.27	0.10	2.0	16
Canned:																
Solids and liquid	100	½ c. scant	66	4	Tr.	13	1.5	83	20	66	1.7	450	0.09	0.05	0.9	9
Drained solids	100	⅔ c.	88	5	1	17	2.3	77	26	76	1.9	690	0.09	0.06	0.8	8
Mature dry seeds, split	100	½ c.	348	24	1	62	1.2	9	33	268	5.1	120	0.74	0.28	3.0	..
Pecans, shelled	100	1 c. halves	687	9	71	15	2.3	3	73	289	2.4	130	0.86	0.13	0.9	2
	7½	1 tbsp. chopped	51	1	5	1	0.2	Tr.	5	22	0.2	10	0.06	0.01	0.1	Tr.

Food	Gm	Measure														
Peppers, green:																
Raw	100	1 large	22	1	Tr.	5	1.4	93	9	22	0.7	420	0.08	0.08	0.5	128
Cooked, boiled and drained	100	1 large or 2 small	18	1	Tr.	4	1.4	95	9	16	0.5	420	0.06	0.07	0.5	96
Persimmons, Japanese, raw	100	1 medium	77	1	Tr.	20	1.6	79	6	26	0.3	2,710	0.03	0.02	Tr.	11
Pickles:																
Dill, cucumber	100	1 large	11	1	Tr.	2	0.5	93	26	21	1.0	100	Tr.	0.02	Tr.	6
Fresh, cucumber (as bread and butter pickles)	100	1/2 c.	73	1	Tr.	18	0.5	79	32	27	1.8	140	Tr.	0.03	Tr.	9
Sour, cucumber or mixed	100	1/2 c.	10	1	Tr.	2	0.5	95	17	15	3.2	100	Tr.	0.02	Tr.	7
Sweet, cucumber or mixed	100	1/2 c.	146	1	Tr.	37	..	61	12	16	1.2	90	Tr.	0.02	Tr.	6
Pies:*		1/6 of 9-in. pie														
Apple	160		410	3	18	61	0.6	76	1	35	0.5	48	0.03	0.03	0.6	2
Blueberry	160		387	4	17	56	1.1	82	18	37	1.0	48	0.03	0.03	0.5	5
Cherry	160		418	4	18	62	0.2	74	22	40	0.5	705	0.03	0.03	0.8	Tr.
Chocolate chiffon	160		525	11	25	70	0.3	53	38	155	1.9	496	0.05	0.16	0.3	0
Custard	150		327	9	17	35	Tr.	87	144	170	0.9	345	0.08	0.24	0.4	0
Mince	160		434	4	18	66	0.6	69	45	61	1.6	Tr.	0.11	0.06	0.6	2
Pecan	160		668	8	37	82	0.8	31	75	165	4.5	256	0.25	0.11	0.5	Tr.
Pumpkin	150		317	6	17	37	0.8	94	76	104	0.8	3,700	0.04	0.15	0.8	Tr.
Pimientos, canned solid and liquid	38	1 medium	10	Tr.	Tr.	2	0.2	35	3	6	0.6	875	0.01	0.02	0.1	36
Pizza:																
Cheese topping	100	1/6 of 14-in. pie	236	12	8	28	0.3	48	221	195	1.0	630	0.06	0.20	1.0	8
Sausage topping	100		234	8	9	30	0.3	51	17	92	1.2	560	0.09	0.12	1.5	9
Pineapple:																
Raw	100	3/4 c. diced or 1 med. slice	52	Tr.	Tr.	14	0.4	85	17	8	0.5	70	0.09	0.03	0.2	17
Canned, solids and liquid in juice	100	1 med. slice	58	Tr.	Tr.	15	0.3	84	16	8	0.4	60	0.10	0.03	0.3	10
in heavy syrup	100	1 med. slice,	74	Tr.	Tr.	19	0.3	80	11	5	0.3	50	0.08	0.02	0.2	7
Frozen, chunks	100	3 1/2 ozs.	86	Tr.	Tr.	22	0.3	77	9	4	0.4	30	0.10	0.03	0.3	8
Pineapple juice, canned unsweetened	100	1/2 c. scant	55	Tr.	Tr.	14	0.1	86	15	9	0.3	50	0.05	0.02	0.2	9
Frozen, reconstituted	100	1/2 c. scant	52	Tr.	Tr.	13	0.1	87	11	8	0.3	10	0.07	0.02	0.2	12

*Values are calculated from a recipe.
§Based on yellow varieties; White types 50 I.U. 100 Gm.
‡Ascorbic acid added in processing.

TABLE 1. Composition of Foods—Edible Portion (Continued)

Food and Description	Wt. Gm.	Approximate Measure	Food Energy Cal.	Protein Gm.	Fat Gm.	Carbohydrate Total Gm.	Carbohydrate Fiber Gm.	Water Gm.	Minerals Ca Mg.	Minerals P Mg.	Minerals Fe Mg.	Vitamins Vitamin A I.U.	Vitamins Thiamine Mg.	Vitamins Riboflavin Mg.	Vitamins Niacin Mg.	Vitamins Ascorbic Acid Mg.
Pine nuts:																
Pignolias................	100	3½ ozs.	552	31	47	12	0.9	6	..		..		0.62	..	..	..
Piñon...................	100	3½ ozs.	635	13	61	21	1.1	3	12	604	5.2	30	1.28	0.23	4.5	Tr.
Pistachio nuts...........	100	3½ ozs.	594	19	54	19	1.9	5	131	500	7.3	230	0.67	..	1.4	0
Plantain, raw, baking banana ...	100	1 small	119	1	Tr.	31	0.4	66	7	30	0.7	..	0.06	0.04	0.6	14
Plums:																
All, excluding prunes, raw.....	100	2 medium	48	1	Tr.	12	0.6	87	12	18	0.5	250	0.03	0.03	0.5	6
Italian prunes, canned, syrup pack, solids and liquid.......	100	½ c. scant or 3 med. prunes	83	Tr.	Tr.	22	0.3	77	9	10	0.9	1,210	0.02	0.02	0.4	2
Popcorn, popped.............	14	1 c.	54	2	1	10	0.3	1	2	39	0.4	0	..	0.02	0.3	0
Pork, fresh, trimmed to retail basis, cooked:																
Chop, thick:																
Lean and fat.............	100	1 large chop	391	25	32	0	0	42	12	268	3.4	0	0.96	0.28	5.6	..
	72	3½ ozs.	195	22	11	0	0	38	9	248	2.7	0	0.82	0.24	4.9	..
Lean only from 1 chop......	100	2.6 ozs.	373	23	31	0	0	45	10	232	2.9	0	0.50	0.23	4.9	..
Roast, loin or shoulder.........	77	3½ ozs.	182	22	10	0	0	44	9	226	2.8	0	0.46	0.22	4.2	..
Lean only from above serving		2.9 ozs.														
Picnic cut simmered																
Lean and fat.............	100	3½ ozs.	374	23	31	0	0	46	10	139	3.0	0	0.54	0.25	4.8	..
Lean only from above serving	74	2.6 ozs.	157	21	7	0	0	45	9	130	2.7	0	0.49	0.22	4.4	..
Pork, smoked ham																
Ham, cooked																
Lean and fat.............	100	3½ ozs.	289	21	22	0	0	54	9	172	2.6	0	0.47	0.18	3.6	..
Lean only from above serving	84	3 ozs.	157	21	7	0	0	52	9	170	2.7	0	0.49	0.19	3.8	..
Ham, canned.............	100	3½ ozs.	193	18	12	1	0	65	11	156	2.7	0	0.53	0.19	3.8	..
**Pork, fat, salted raw..........	100	3½ ozs.	783	4	85	0	0	8	Tr.	Tr.	0.6	0	0.18	0.04	0.9	..

	Gm.	Measure													
Potatoes:															
Baked in skin	100	1 med.	75	93	3	Tr.	21	0.6	9	65	0.7	Tr.	0.10	0.04	1.7	20‡
Boiled, pared before cooking	100	1 med.	83	65	2	Tr.	15	0.5	6	48	0.5	Tr.	0.09	0.03	1.2	16
French fried	100	20 pieces 2 x ½ x ½	45	274	4	13	36	1.0	15	111	1.3	Tr.	0.13	0.08	3.1	21
Fried from raw	100	⅔ c.	47	268	4	14	33	1.0	15	101	1.1	Tr.	0.12	0.07	2.8	19
Hash brown after holding overnight	100	½ c.	54	229	3	12	29	0.8	12	79	0.9	Tr.	0.08	0.05	2.1	9
Mashed, milk and table fat added	100	½ c.	80	94	2	4	12	0.4	24	53	0.4	170	0.08	0.05	1.0	9
Dehydrated Flakes, prep. with water, milk and butter added	100	3½ ozs.	79	93	2	3	15	0.3	31	47	0.3	130	0.04	0.04	0.9	5
Potato chips	20	10 med. or 7 large	1	114	1	8	10	0.1	8	28	0.4	Tr.	0.04	0.02	1.0	3
Potato flour	100	1 c. sifted	8	351	8	1	80	1.6	33	178	17.2	0	0.42	0.14	3.4	19
Pretzels	5	5 small sticks	Tr.	19	Tr.	Tr.	4	Tr.	1	6	Tr.	0	Tr.	Tr.	Tr.	0
Prunes:															
Dried, softenized uncooked	100	⅔ c. medium	28	255	2	Tr.	67	1.6	51	79	3.9	1,600	0.09	0.17	1.6	3
Cooked, no sugar added	100	6 prunes, 2 tbsp. juice	66	119	1	Tr.	31	0.8	24	37	1.8	750	0.03	0.07	0.7	1
Cooked, sugar added	100	6 prunes, 2 tbsp. juice	53	172	1	Tr.	45	0.6	19	30	1.5	600	0.03	0.06	0.6	1
Prune juice, canned	100	½ c. scant	80	77	Tr.	Tr.	19	..	14	20	4.1	..	0.01	0.01	0.4	2
Prune whip*	100	¾ c.	59	148	3	Tr.	37	0.7	26	42	1.8	460	0.04	0.11	0.7	2
Pudding, chocolate*	100	½ c.	66	148	3	5	26	0.2	96	98	0.5	150	0.02	0.14	0.1	Tr.
Pumpkin, canned	100	⅞ c.	90	33	1	1	8	1.2	25	26	0.4	6,400	0.03	0.05	0.6	5
Radishes, raw	40	4 small	37	7	Tr.	Tr.	1	0.1	12	12	0.4	Tr.	0.01	0.01	0.1	10
Raisins, natural dried, seedless (unbleached)	100	⅔ c.	18	289	3	Tr.	77	0.9	62	101	3.5	20	0.11	0.08	0.5	1
	10	1 tbsp.	2	29	Tr.	Tr.	8	0.1	6	10	0.3	Tr.	0.01	0.01	Tr.	Tr.

*Values are calculated from a recipe.

‡Year-round average. Recently dug potatoes contain about 24 mg. of ascorbic acid per 100 Gm. The value is only half as high after 3 months of storage and about one third as high when potatoes have been stored as long as 6 months.

TABLE 1. Composition of Foods—Edible Portion (Continued)

Food and Description	Wt. Gm.	Approximate Measure	Food Energy Cal.	Protein Gm.	Fat Gm.	Carbohydrate Total Gm.	Carbohydrate Fiber Gm.	Water Gm.	Minerals Ca Mg.	Minerals P Mg.	Minerals Fe Mg.	Vitamins Vitamin A I.U.	Vitamins Thiamine Mg.	Vitamins Riboflavin Mg.	Vitamins Niacin Mg.	Vitamins Ascorbic Acid Mg.
Raspberries:																
Black, raw	100	¾ c.	73	2	1	16	5.1	81	30	22	0.9	0	0.03	0.09	0.9	18
Red:																
Raw	100	¾ c.	57	1	1	14	3.0	84	22	22	0.9	130	0.03	0.09	0.9	25
Frozen, sweetened	100	3½ ozs.	98	1	Tr.	25	2.2	74	13	17	0.6	70	0.02	0.06	0.6	21
Rhubarb, stems only:																
Raw	100	¾ c. diced	16	1	Tr.	4	0.7	95	96†	18	0.8	100	0.03	0.07	0.3	9
Cooked, sugar added or canned in syrup*	100	⅓ c.	141	Tr.	Tr.	36	0.6	63	78†	15	0.6	80	0.02	0.05	0.3	6
Rice:																
Brown, cooked	100	⅔ c.	119	3	1	26	0.3	70	12	73	0.5	0	0.09	0.02	1.4	0
White, milled enriched, cooked	100	⅔ c.	109	2	Tr.	24	0.1	73	10	28	0.9‡	0	0.11‡	0.01	1.0†	0
Parboiled, converted, cooked	100	⅔ c.	106	2	Tr.	23	0.1	73	19	57	0.8	0	0.11	0.03	1.2	0
Precooked, instant, cooked	100	⅔ c.	109	2	Tr.	24	0.1	73	3	19	0.8	0	0.13‡	0.01	1.0‡	0
Rice products (added thiamine and niacin):																
Flakes	30	1 c.	118	2	Tr.	26	0.2	1	9	40	0.5	0	0.11	0.02	1.6	0
Krispies	30	1 c.	107	2	Tr.	25	0.1	Tr.	7	33	0.5	0	0.11	0.01	2.0	0
Puffed, presweetened	14	1 c.	55	1	Tr.	12	Tr.	Tr.	6	10	0.3	0	0.05	..	0.6	0
Rice pudding with raisins	100	⅔ c.	146	4	3	27	0.1	66	98	94	0.4	110	0.03	0.14	0.2	Tr.
Rolls:*																
Hard, enriched	35	one roll	109	3	1	21	0.1	9	16	32	0.8†	Tr.	0.09‡	0.08‡	0.9†	Tr.
Plain, enriched (pan roll)	38	average	113	3	2	20	0.1	12	28	32	0.7†	Tr.	0.11‡	0.07‡	0.8†	Tr.
Hamburg bun	30	1 large	89	3	2	16	0.1	10	22	26	0.6†	Tr.	0.08‡	0.05‡	0.7†	Tr.
Sweet roll, enriched	55	average	178	5	4	30	0.3	16	35	57	0.3	0	0.03	0.07	0.6	0
Danish pastry	35	1 small	148	3	8	16	Tr.	8	17	38	0.3	108	0.02	0.05	0.3	Tr.
Rutabagas, boiled, drained	100	⅔ c. diced	35	1	Tr.	8	1.4	91	59	31	0.3	550	0.06	0.06	0.8	26
Rye wafers or "Swedish health bread" or Rye Krisp.	13	2 wafers 1⅛ x 3½ in.	43	2	Tr.	10	0.3	1	6	52	0.6	0	0.04	0.03	0.2	0

Salad dressings:															
French, commercial	½ c.	100	410	1	39	18	0.3	39	11	14	0.4	..	..	..	..
	1 tbsp.	15	61	Tr.	6	3	Tr.	6	2	2	0.1	..	..	..	..
Italian	1 tbsp.	15	83	Tr.	9	1	Tr.	4	2	1	Tr.	..	..	..	..
Mayonnaise, commercial	½ c.	100	718	1	80	2	Tr.	15	18	28	0.5	280	0.02	0.04	..
	1 tbsp.	13	93	Tr.	10	Tr.	Tr.	2	2	4	0.1	36	Tr.	0.01	..
Salad dressing,															
Mayonnaise type	½ c.	100	435	1	42	14	..	41	14	26	0.2	220	0.01	0.03	Tr.
	1 tbsp.	15	65	Tr.	6	2	..	6	2	4	Tr.	33	Tr.	Tr.	Tr.
Homemade, cooked	½ c. scant	100	164	4	10	15	0	68	89	93	0.6	490	0.05	0.16	0.2
	1 tbsp.	17	28	1	2	3	0	12	15	16	0.1	83	0.01	0.03	Tr.
Thousand Island	½ c.	100	502	1	50	15	0.3	32	11	17	0.6	320	0.02	0.03	0.2
	1 tbsp.	15	75	Tr.	8	2	Tr.	5	2	3	0.1	48	Tr.	Tr.	Tr.
Sauerkraut, canned,															
drained solids	⅔ c.	100	18	1	Tr.	4	0.7	93	36	18	0.5	50	0.03	0.04	14
Sausage:															
Bologna	3½ ozs.	100	304	12	28	1	0	56	7	128	1.8	..	0.16	0.22	2.6
Frankfurter, cooked	2 medium	100	309	13	28	2	0	56	7	133	1.9	..	0.16	0.20	2.7
Liver, liverwurst	3½ ozs.	100	307	16	26	2	0	54	9	238	5.4	6,350	0.20	1.30	5.7
Pork, links or bulk, cooked	3½ ozs.	100	476	18	44	0	0	35	7	162	2.4	0	0.79	0.34	3.7
Pork, bulk, canned	3½ ozs.	100	381	18	33	0	0	43	11	210	2.8	0	0.20	0.24	3.0
Vienna sausage, canned	3½ ozs.	100	240	14	20	0	0	63	8	153	2.1	0	0.08	0.13	2.6
Scallops, cooked, steamed	3½ ozs.	100	112	23	1	..	..	73	115	338	3.0	..	..	..	..
Sherbet,* orange	½ c.	100	134	1	1	31	0	67	16	13	0	60	0.01	0.03	Tr.
Shortbread*	2 squares, 1¾ x 1¾ in.	16	81	1	4	10	Tr.	1	2	9	0.1	0	0.01	Tr.	0
Shrimp, French fried	3½ ozs.	100	225	20	11	10	..	57	72	191	2.0	..	0.04	0.08	2.7
Canned, dry pack or drained	3½ ozs.	100	116	24	1	1	..	70	115	263	3.1	60	0.01	0.03	1.8
Soups, canned:‖¶															
prepared to serve															
Bean with pork	2/5 c.§	100	67	3	2	9	0.6	84	25	51	0.9	260	0.05	0.03	0.4
Beef bouillon	2/5 c.	100	13	3	0	1	Tr.	96	Tr.	13	0.2	Tr.	Tr.	0.01	0.5
Celery, cream of	2/5 c.	100	69	3	4	6	0.2	86	81	63	0.3	160	0.02	0.11	0.3

*Values are calculated from a recipe.

†Calcium may not be available because of the presence of oxalic acid.

‡Based on minimum levels of enrichment specified in standard of identity, F.D.A., for iron, thiamine, riboflavin and niacin.

§Usual serving of soups is 1 cup, 2½ times amount given here.

‖All ready-to-serve soups are calculated from equal weights of the condensed soup and water, except cream soup, which is based on equal weights of the condensed soups and milk.

¶Dehydrated soups have about the same nutritive values as canned soups when each is prepared as directed on can or package.

[575]

TABLE 1. Composition of Foods—Edible Portion (Continued)

Food and Description	Wt. Gm.	Approximate Measure	Food Energy Cal.	Protein Gm.	Fat Gm.	Carbohydrate Total Gm.	Carbohydrate Fiber Gm.	Water Gm.	Ca Mg.	P Mg.	Fe Mg.	Vitamin A I.U.	Thiamine Mg.	Riboflavin Mg.	Niacin Mg.	Ascorbic Acid Mg.
Soups†† (Continued)																
Chicken, cream of	100	2/5 c.§	73	3	4	6	0.1	85	70	62	0.2	250	0.02	0.11	0.3	Tr.
Chicken noodle	100	2/5 c.	26	1	1	3	0.1	93	4	15	0.2	20	0.01	0.01	0.3	Tr.
Clam chowder, Manhattan with tomato, no milk	100	2/5 c.	33	1	1	5	0.2	92	14	19	0.4	360	0.01	0.01	0.4	..
Minestrone	100	2/5 c.	43	2	1	6	0.3	90	15	24	0.4	960	0.03	0.02	0.4	..
Mushroom, cream of	100	2/5 c.	88	3	6	7	0.1	83	78	69	0.2	100	0.02	0.14	0.3	Tr.
Onion	100	2/5 c.	27	2	1	2	0.2	93	12	11	0.2	Tr.	Tr.	0.01	Tr.	..
Pea (green), made with water	100	2/5 c.	53	2	1	9	0.4	86	18	46	0.4	140	0.02	0.02	0.4	3
Tomato, with water	100	2/5 c.	36	1	1	6	0.2	91	6	14	0.3	410	0.02	0.02	0.5	5
Made with milk	100	2/5 c.	69	3	3	9	0.2	84	67	62	0.3	480	0.04	0.10	0.5	6
Vegetable beef	100	2/5 c.	32	2	1	4	0.2	92	5	20	0.3	1,100	0.02	0.02	0.4	..
Soups, frozen: prepared																
Clam chowder, N.E. style with milk	100	2/5 c.	86	4	5	7	0.1	83	98	82	0.4	100	0.03	0.12	0.2	Tr.
Shrimp, cream of	100	2/5 c.	99	4	7	6	0.2	82	77	68	0.2	120	0.03	0.11	0.2	Tr.
Soybeans, canned, immature, boiled	100	3½ ozs.	103	9	5	7	1.4	77	67	114	2.8	340	0.06	..	..	2
Soybean flour or grits:																
High fat	100	1 c.	380	41	12	33**	2.2	8	240	650	9.0	..	0.89	0.36	2.3	0
Low fat	100	1 c.	356	43	7	37**	2.5	8	263	634	9.1	80	0.83	0.36	2.6	0
Defatted	100	1 c.	326	47	1	38**	2.3	8	265	655	11.1	40	1.09	0.34	2.6	0
Soybean Products:																
Soybean milk, fluid	100	½ c. scant	33	3	2	2	0	92	21	48	0.8	40	0.08	0.03	0.2	0
Soybean curd (Tofu)	100	3½ ozs.	72	8	4	2	0.1	85	128	126	1.9	0	0.06	0.03	0.1	0
Fermented (Natto)	100	3½ ozs.	167	17	7	12	3.2	63	103	182	3.7	0	0.07	0.05	..	0
Soy sauce	15	1 tbsp.	10	1	Tr.	1	0	10	12	16	0.7	0	Tr.	0.04	0.1	0
Soybean sprouts, cooked boiled, drained	100	1 c.	38	5	1	4	0.8	89	43	50	0.7	80	0.16	0.15	0.7	4

	Wt. (g)	Measure													
Spaghetti:															
Enriched: Cooked* plain	100	⅔ c.	149	5	1	30	61	9	65	1.1	0	0.18	0.10	1.4	0
With tomato and cheese sauce*	100	⅔ c.	104	4	4	15	77	32	54	0.9	430	0.10	0.07	0.9	5
With meat balls in tomato sauce, canned	100	⅔ c.	103	5	4	11	78	21	45	1.3	400	0.06	0.07	0.9	2
Spinach:															
Raw	100	3½ ozs.	26	3	Tr.	4	91	93‖	51	3.1	8,100	0.10	0.20	0.6	51
Cooked	100	½ c. packed	23	3	Tr.	4	91	93‖	38	2.2	8,100	0.07	0.14	0.5	28
Canned: Drained solids	100	½ c. packed	24	3	1	4	91	118‖	26	2.6	8,000	0.02	0.12	0.3	14
Frozen, cooked drained	100	3½ ozs.	23	3	Tr.	4	92	113‖	44	2.1	7,900	0.07	0.15	0.4	19
Squash:															
Summer: Cooked, diced, fresh or frozen	100	½ c.	15	1	Tr.	3	95	25	25	0.4	440	0.05	0.08	0.8	11
Winter: Baked	100	3½ ozs.	63	2	Tr.	15	86	28	48	0.8	4,200	0.05	0.13	0.7	13
Boiled, mashed	100	½ c.	38	2	Tr.	9	89	19	32	0.5	3,500	0.04	0.10	0.4	8
Starch, pure (including arrowroot, corn, etc.)	100	¾ c.	362	Tr.	Tr.	87	12	0	0	0	0	0	0	0	0
	8	1 tbsp.	29	0	0	7	1	0	0	0	0	0	0	0	0
Strawberries:															
Raw	100	⅔ c.	37	1	1	8	90	21	21	1.0	60	0.03	0.07	0.6	59
Frozen, sugar added	100	3½ ozs.	109	1	Tr.	28	71	14	17	0.7	30	0.02	0.06	0.5	53
Sugars:															
Granulated, cane or beet	100	½ c.	385	0	0	100	1	..	..	..	0	0	0	0	0
	12	1 tbsp.	46	0	0	12	..	..	..	..	0	0	0	0	0
Powdered	100	¾ c.	385	0	0	100	..	..	..	..	0	0	0	0	0
Brown	100	½ c.	373	0	0	96	3	88	19	3.4	0	0.01	0.03	0.2	0
Maple	100	3½ ozs.	348	..	..	90	8	143	11	1.4	..	..	..	..	..

*Values are calculated from a recipe.

†All ready-to-serve soups are calculated from equal weights of the condensed soup and water, except cream soup, which is based on equal weights of the condensed soups and milk.

‡Dehydrated soups have about the same nutritive values as canned soups when each is prepared as directed on can or package.

§Usual serving of soups is 1 cup, 2½ times amount given here.

‖Calcium may not be available because of presence of oxalic acid.

**Approximately 40 per cent of this total amount of carbohydrate calculated by difference is sugar, starch and dextrin. The remaining portion is made up of materials thought to be utilized only poorly, if at all, by the body.

TABLE 1. Composition of Foods—Edible Portion (Continued)

Food and Description	Wt. Gm.	Approximate Measure	Food Energy Cal.	Protein Gm.	Fat Gm.	Carbohydrate Total Gm.	Fiber Gm.	Water Gm.	Ca Mg.	P Mg.	Fe Mg.	Vitamin A I.U.	Thiamine Mg.	Riboflavin Mg.	Niacin Mg.	Ascorbic Acid Mg.
Sweet potatoes:																
Baked in skin	100	1 small	141	2	1	33	0.9	64	40	58	0.9	8,100	0.09	0.07	0.7	22
Boiled in skin	100	1 medium	114	2	Tr.	26	0.7	71	32	47	0.7	7,900	0.09	0.06	0.6	17
Candied	100	½ medium	168	1	3	34	0.6	60	37	43	0.9	6,300	0.06	0.04	0.4	10
Canned, vacuum or solid pack	100	½ c.	108	2	Tr.	25	1.0	72	25	41	0.8	7,800	0.05	0.04	0.5	14
Syrup, table blends (chiefly corn syrup)	100	⅓ c.	290	0	0	75	..	24	46	16	4.1	0	0	0	0	0
	20	1 tbsp.	58	0	0	15	..	5	9	3	0.8	0	0	..	..	0
Tangerines (including other Mandarin type oranges)	100	1 medium	46	1	Tr.	11	0.5	87	40	18	0.4	420	0.06	0.02	0.1	31
Tangerine juice, unsweetened:																
Fresh or frozen reconstituted	100	½ c. scant	43	1	Tr.	10	..	89	18	14	0.2	420	0.06	0.02	0.1	31
Canned, unsweetened	100	½ c. scant	43	1	Tr.	10	..	89	18	14	0.2	420	0.06	0.02	0.1	22
Tapioca, cream pudding	100	½ c.	134	5	5	17	0	72	105	109	0.4	290	0.04	0.18	0.1	1
Tomatoes:																
Raw	100	1 small	22	1	Tr.	5	0.5	94	13	27	0.5	900	0.06	0.04	0.7	23
Canned or cooked	100	½ c.	23	1	Tr.	5	0.4	94	6	19	0.5	900	0.05	0.03	0.7	20
Tomato juice, canned	100	½ c. scant	19	1	Tr.	4	0.2	94	7	18	0.9	800	0.05	0.03	0.8	16
Tomato ketchup	17	1 tbsp.	18	Tr.	Tr.	4	0.1	12	4	5	0.1	340	0.02	0.01	0.3	3
Tomato purée, canned	100	½ c. scant	39	2	Tr.	9	0.4	87	13	34	1.7	1,000	0.09	0.05	1.4	33
Tongue beef, canned	100	3½ ozs.	267	19	20	Tr.	0	57	10	180	2.5	0	0.05	0.22	2.5	0
Tortillas	30	1 tortilla	63	2	Tr.	13	0.3	8	35	57	0.3	0	0.03	0.07	0.6	..
Tuna fish. See Fish.																
Turkey, total edible roasted	100	3½ ozs.	263	27	16	0	0	55	..	..	..	Tr.	0.09	0.14	8.0	0
Flesh only, roasted	100	3½ ozs.	190	32	6	0	0	61	8	251	1.8	..	0.05	0.18	7.7	0

Food	Wt. (g)	Measure														
Turnips:																
Raw	100	¾ c. diced	30	1	Tr.	7	0.9	92	39	30	0.5	Tr.	0.04	0.07	0.6	36
Cooked, boiled, drained	100	⅔ c. diced	23	1	Tr.	5	0.9	94	35	24	0.4	Tr.	0.04	0.05	0.3	22
Turnip greens, boiled in small amount of water, short time	100	⅔ c.	20	2	Tr.	4	0.7	93	184	37	1.1	6,300	0.15	0.24	0.6	69
Veal, cooked:																
Cutlet, broiled	100	3½ ozs.	234	26	13	0	0	59	11	225	3.2	..	0.07	0.25	5.4	..
Roast, medium fat, rib, 82 per cent lean	100	3½ ozs.	269	27	17	0	0	55	12	248	3.4	..	0.13	0.31	7.8	..
Stew meat without bone, medium fat, cooked	100	3½ ozs.	303	26	21	0	0	52	12	138	3.3	..	0.05	0.24	4.6	..
Vinegar, distilled	100	½ c. scant	12	0	..	5	0	95	..	..	..	..	..	..	..	..
Waffles, made with enriched flour*, egg and milk	100	2 small waffles, 4½ x 5½ x ½	279	9	10	38	0.1	41	113	173	1.7	330	0.17	0.25	1.3	Tr.
Walnuts, Persian or English	100	1 c. of halves	651	15	64	16	2.1	4	99	380	3.1	30	0.33	0.13	0.9	2
	8	1 tbsp. chopped	52	1	5	1	0.2	Tr.	8	31	0.2	Tr.	0.03	0.01	0.1	Tr.
Watermelons	100	3½ oz. portion	26	1	Tr.	6	0.3	92	7	10	0.5	590	0.03	0.03	0.2	7
Wheat flours:																
Whole (from hard wheat)	100	1 c. scant	333	13	2	71	2.3	12	41	372	3.3	0	0.55	0.12	4.3	0
Self-rising, enriched	100	1 c. scant	352	9	1	74	0.4	12	265	466	2.9†	0	0.44	0.26	3.5	0
Patent:																
All purpose or family flour:																
Unenriched	100	1 c. scant	364	11	1	76	0.3	12	16	87	0.8	0	0.06	0.05	0.9	0
Enriched	100	1 c. scant	364	11	1	76	0.3	12	16	87	2.9†	0	0.44	0.26	3.5	0
Bread flour:																
Unenriched	100	1 c. scant	365	12	1	75	0.3	12	16	95	0.9	0	0.08	0.06	1.0	0
Enriched	100	1 c. scant	365	12	1	75	0.3	12	16	95	2.9†	0	0.44	0.26	3.5	0
Cake or pastry flour	100	1 c. level	364	8	1	79	0.2	12	17	73	0.5	0	0.03	0.03	0.7	0
Wheat products:																
Flakes (added iron, thiamine and niacin)	100	4 c.	354	10	2	81	1.6	4	41	309	4.4	0	0.64	0.14	4.9	0
	35	1 c.	125	4	1	28	0.6	1	..	107	1.5	0	0.22	0.05	1.7	0
Germ, commercially milled	100	3½ ozs., 1 c.	363	27	11	47	2.5	12	72	1,118	9.4	0	2.01	0.68	4.2	0
Germ cereal with added nutrients	28	1 oz.	110	8	3	14	0.5	1	13	310	2.5	0	0.55	0.27	1.5	0

*Values are calculated from a recipe. †Based on the minimum level of enrichment specified under the Food, Drug and Cosmetic Act.

TABLE 1. Composition of Foods—Edible Portion (Continued)

Food and Description	Wt. Gm.	Approximate Measure	Food Energy Cal.	Protein Gm.	Fat Gm.	Carbohydrate Total Gm.	Carbohydrate Fiber Gm.	Water Gm.	Ca Mg.	P Mg.	Fe Mg.	Vitamin A I.U.	Thiamine Mg.	Riboflavin Mg.	Niacin Mg.	Ascorbic Acid Mg.
Wheat Products: (Continued)																
Puffed (added iron, thiamine and niacin)	100	8 c.	363	15	2	79	2.0	3	28	322	4.2	0	0.55	0.23	7.8	0
	12	1 c.	43	2	Tr.	10	0.2	Tr.	3	39	0.5	0	0.07	0.03	0.9	0
Rolled, cooked*	100	½ c. scant	75	2	Tr.	17	0.5	80	8	76	0.7	0	0.07	0.03	0.9	0
Shredded, plain	30	1 large biscuit, 4 x 2¼ in.														
Wheat, whole meal cooked*	100	⅓ c. scant	107	3	1	24	0.7	2	13	117	1.0	0	0.07	0.03	1.3	0
			45	2	Tr.	9	0.3	88	7	52	0.5	0	0.06	0.02	0.6	0
Wheat and malted barley cereal quick cooking, cooked.	100	½ c. scant	65	2	Tr.	13	0.2	84	9	59	0.4	0	0.05	0.01	..	0
White sauce, medium*	100	½ c. scant	162	4	13	9	0	73	115	93	0.2	460	0.04	0.17	0.2	Tr.
Wild rice, parched, raw	100	⅔ c.	353	14	1	75	1.0	9	19	339	..	0	0.45	0.63	6.2	0
Yeast:																
Dried, brewer's	8	1 tbsp.	22	3	Tr.	3	0.1	1	16	141	1.4	0	1.24	0.35	3.0	0
Yoghurt, from partially skimmed milk	100	⅓ c.	50	3	2	5	0	89	120	94	Tr.	70	0.04	0.18	0.1	1
	246	1 c.	123	8	4	13	0	218	295	230	Tr.	170	0.10	0.43	0.2	2

*Values are calculated from a recipe.

TABLE 2. Food Composition Table for Short Method of Dietary Analysis (3rd Revision)*

Food and Approximate Measure	Weight Gm.	Food Energy Cal.	Protein Gm.	Fat Gm.	Carbohydrate Gm.	Calcium mg.	Iron mg.	Vitamin A IU	Thiamine mg.	Riboflavin mg.	Niacin mg.	Ascorbic Acid mg.
Milk, Cheese, Cream; Related Products												
Cheese: blue, cheddar (1 cu. in., 17 Gm.), Cheddar process (1 oz.), Swiss (1 oz.)........	30	105	6	9	1	165	0.2	345	0.01	0.12	trace	0
Cottage (from skim) creamed (½ c.)........	115	120	16	5	3	105	0.4	190	0.04	0.28	0.1	0
Cream: half-and-half (cream and milk) (2 tbsp.)........	30	40	1	4	2	30	trace	145	0.01	0.04	trace	trace
For light whipping add 1 pat butter........												
Milk: whole (3.5% fat) (1 c.)........	245	160	9	9	12	285	0.1	350	0.08	0.42	0.1	2
Fluid, nonfat (skim) and buttermilk (from skim)........	245	90	9	trace	13	300	trace	..	0.10	0.44	0.2	2
Milk beverages, (1 c.) cocoa, chocolate drink made with skim milk. For malted milk add 4 tbsp. half-and-half (270 Gm.)........	245	210	8	8	26	280	0.6	300	0.09	0.43	0.3	trace
Milk desserts, custard (1 c.) 248 Gm., ice cream (8 fl. oz.) 142 Gm.........	..	290	8	17	29	210	0.4	785	0.07	0.34	0.1	1
Cornstarch pudding (248 Gm.), ice milk (1 c.) 187 Gm.....	..	280	9	10	40	290	0.1	390	0.08	0.41	0.3	2
White sauce, med. (½ c.).....	130	215	5	16	12	150	0.2	610	0.06	0.22	0.3	trace
Egg: 1 large.....	50	80	6	6	trace	25	1.2	590	0.06	0.15	trace	0
Meat, Poultry, Fish, Shellfish, Related Products												
Beef, lamb, veal: lean and fat, cooked, inc. corned beef (3 oz.) (all cuts).....	85	245	22	16	0	10	2.9	25	0.06	0.19	4.2	0
Lean only, cooked; dried beef (2+ oz.) (all cuts).....	65	140	20	5	0	10	2.4	10	0.05	0.16	3.4	0
Beef, relatively fat, such as steak and rib, cooked (3 oz.)..	85	350	18	30	0	10	2.4	60	0.05	0.14	3.5	0
Liver: beef, fried (2 oz.).....	55	130	15	6	3	5	5.0	30,280	0.15	2.37	9.4	15
Pork, lean and fat, cooked (3 oz.) (all cuts).....	85	325	20	24	0	10	2.6	0	0.62	0.20	4.2	0
Lean only, cooked (2+ oz.) (all cuts).....	60	150	18	8	0	5	2.2	0	0.57	0.19	3.2	0
Ham, light cure, lean and fat, roasted (3 oz.).....	85	245	18	19	0	10	2.2	0	0.40	0.16	3.1	0
Luncheon meats: bologna (2 sl.), pork sausage, cooked (2 oz.), frankfurter (1), bacon, broiled or fried crisp (3 sl.)......	..	185	9	16	..	5	1.3	..	0.21	0.12	1.7	0
Poultry												
Chicken: flesh only, broiled (3 oz.).....	85	115	20	3	0	10	1.4	80	0.05	0.16	7.4	0
fried (2+ oz.).....	75	170	24	6	1	10	1.6	85	0.05	0.23	8.3	0
Turkey, light and dark, roasted (3 oz.).....	85	160	27	5	0	..	1.5	..	0.03	0.15	6.5	0
Fish and shellfish												
Salmon (3 oz.) (canned).....	85	130	17	5	0	165	0.7	60	0.03	0.16	6.8	0

* From Wilson, Fisher and Fuqua: Principles of Nutrition. New York, Wiley, 1966.

TABLE 2. Food Composition Table for Short Method of Dietary Analysis (3rd Revision) * (Continued)

Food and Approximate Measure	Weight Gm.	Food Energy Cal.	Protein Gm.	Fat Gm.	Carbohydrate Gm.	Calcium mg.	Iron mg.	Vitamin A IU	Thiamine mg.	Riboflavin mg.	Niacin mg.	Ascorbic Acid mg.
Meat, Poultry, Fish, Shellfish, Related Products (Continued)												
Fish sticks, breaded, cooked (3—4)	75	130	13	7	5	10	0.3	..	0.03	0.05	1.2	0
Mackerel, halibut, cooked	85	175	19	10	0	10	0.8	515	0.08	0.15	6.8	0
Bluefish, haddock, herring, perch, shad, cooked (tuna canned in oil, 20 Gm.)	85	160	19	8	2	20	1.0	60	0.06	0.11	4.4	0
Clams, canned; crabmeat, canned; lobster; oyster; raw; scallop; shrimp, canned	85	75	14	1	2	65	2.5	65	0.10	0.08	1.5	0
Mature Dry Beans and Peas, Nuts, Peanuts, Related Products												
Beans: white with pork and tomato, canned (1 c.)	260	320	16	7	50	140	4.7	340	0.20	0.08	1.5	5
Red (128 Gm.), lima (96 Gm.), cowpeas (125 Gm.), cooked (½ c.)	..	125	8	..	25	35	2.5	5	0.13	0.06	0.7	..
Nuts: almonds (12), cashews (8), peanuts (1 tbsp.), peanut butter (1 tbsp.), pecans (12), English walnuts (2 tbsp.), coconut (¼ c.)	15	95	3	8	4	15	0.5	5	0.05	0.04	0.9	..
Vegetables and Vegetable Products												
Asparagus, cooked, cut spears (⅔ c.)	115	25	3	trace	4	25	0.7	1,055	0.19	0.20	1.6	30
Beans: green (½ c.) cooked 60 Gm.; canned 120 Gm.	..	15	1	trace	3	30	0.4	340	0.04	0.06	0.3	8
Lima, immature, cooked (½ c.)	80	90	6	1	16	40	2.0	225	0.14	0.08	1.0	14
Broccoli spears, cooked (⅔ c.)	100	25	3	trace	4	90	0.8	2,500	0.09	0.20	0.8	90
Brussels sprouts, cooked (⅔ c.)	85	30	3	trace	5	30	1.0	450	0.07	0.12	0.7	75
Cabbage (110 Gm.); cauliflower, cooked (80 Gm.); sauerkraut, canned (150 Gm.) (reduce ascorbic acid value by one-third for kraut) (⅔ c.)	..	20	1	trace	4	35	0.5	80	0.05	0.05	0.3	37
Carrots, cooked (⅔ c.)	95	30	1	trace	7	30	0.6	10,145	0.05	0.05	0.5	6
Corn, 1 ear, cooked (140 Gm.); canned (130 Gm.) (½ c.)	..	75	2	trace	18	5	0.4	315	0.06	0.06	1.1	6
Leafy greens: collards (125 Gm.), dandelions (120 Gm.), kale (75 Gm.), mustard (95 Gm.), spinach (120 Gm.), turnip (100 Gm. cooked, 150 Gm. canned) (⅔ c. cooked and canned) (reduce ascorbic acid one-half for canned)	..	30	3	trace	5	175	1.8	8,570	0.11	0.18	0.8	45
Peas, green (½ c.)	80	60	4	1	10	20	1.4	430	0.22	0.09	1.8	16
Potatoes—baked, boiled (100 Gm.), 10 pc. French fried (55 Gm.) (for fried, add 1 tbsp. cooking oil)	..	85	3	trace	30	10	0.7	trace	0.08	0.04	1.5	16
Pumpkin, canned (½ c.)	115	40	1	1	9	30	0.5	7,295	0.03	0.06	0.6	6

Squash, winter, canned (½ c.)	100	65	2	1	16	30	0.8	4,305	0.05	0.14	0.7	14
Sweet potato, canned (½ c.)	110	120	2	..	27	25	0.8	8,500	0.05	0.05	0.7	15
Tomato, 1 raw (⅔ c.), canned (⅔ c.), juice,	150	35	2	trace	7	14	0.8	1,350	0.10	0.06	1.0	29
Tomato catsup (2 tbsp.)	35	30	1	trace	8	10	0.2	480	0.04	0.02	0.6	6
Other, cooked (beets, mushrooms, onions, turnips) (½ c.)	95	25	1	..	5	20	0.5	15	0.02	0.10	0.7	7
Others commonly served raw: cabbage (½ c., 50 Gm.), celery (3 sm. stalks, 40 Gm.), cucumber (¼ med., 50 Gm.), green pepper (½, 30 Gm.), radishes (5, 40 Gm.)	..	10	trace	trace	2	15	0.3	100	0.03	0.03	0.2	20
Carrots, raw (½ carrot)	25	10	trace	trace	2	10	0.2	2,750	0.02	0.02	0.2	2
Lettuce leaves (2 lg.)	50	10	1	trace	2	34	0.7	950	0.03	0.04	0.2	9
Fruits and Fruit Products												
Cantaloupe (½ med.)	385	60	1	trace	14	25	0.8	6,540	0.08	0.06	1.2	63
Citrus and strawberries: orange (1), grapefruit (½), juice (½ c.), strawberries (½ c.), lemon (1), tangerine (1)	..	50	1	..	13	25	0.4	165	0.08	0.03	0.3	55
Yellow, fresh: apricots (3), peach (2 med.); canned fruit and juice (½ c.) or dried, cooked, unsweetened: apricot, peaches (½ c.)	..	85	..	..	22	10	1.1	1,005	0.01	0.05	1.0	5
Other, dried: dates, pitted (4), figs (2), raisins (¼ c.)	40	120	1	..	31	35	1.4	20	0.04	0.04	0.5	..
Other, fresh: apple (1), banana (1), figs (3), pear (1)	..	80	..	..	21	15	0.5	140	0.04	0.03	0.2	6
Fruit pie: to 1 serving fruit add 1 tbsp. flour, 2 tbsp. sugar, 1 tbsp. fat	..	..	..	..	..	..	..	..	..	..	..	..
Grain Products												
Enriched and whole grain: bread (1 sl. 23 Gm.), biscuit (½), cooked cereals (½ c.), prepared cereals (1 oz.), Graham crackers (2 lg.), macaroni, noodles, spaghetti (½ c. cooked), pancake (1, 27 Gm.), roll (½), waffle (½, 38 Gm.)	..	65	2	1	16	20	0.6	10	0.09	0.05	0.7	..
Unenriched: bread (1 sl. 23 Gm.), cooked cereal (½ c.), macaroni, noodles, spaghetti (½ c.), popcorn (½ c.), pretzel sticks, small (15), roll (½)	..	65	2	1	16	10	0.3	5	0.02	0.02	0.3	..
Desserts												
Cake, plain (1 pc.), doughnut (1). For iced cake or doughnut add value for sugar (1 tbsp.). For chocolate cake add chocolate (30 Gm.)	45	145	2	5	24	30	0.4	65	0.02	0.05	0.2	..
Cookies, plain (1)	25	120	1	5	18	10	0.2	20	0.01	0.01	0.1	..
Piecrust, single crust (1/7 shell)	20	95	1	6	8	3	0.3	0	0.04	0.03	0.3	..
Flour, white, enriched (1 tbsp.)	7	25	1	trace	5	1	0.2	0	0.03	0.02	0.2	0

* From Wilson, Fisher and Fuqua: Principles of Nutrition. New York, Wiley, 1966.

TABLE 2.   Food Composition Table for Short Method of Dietary Analysis (3rd Revision) * (Continued)

Food and Approximate Measure	Weight Gm.	Food Energy Cal.	Protein Gm.	Fat Gm.	Carbo-hydrate Gm.	Calcium mg.	Iron mg.	Vitamin A IU	Thiamine mg.	Riboflavin mg.	Niacin mg.	Ascorbic Acid mg.
Fats and Oils												
Butter, margarine (1 pat, ½ tbsp.)	7	50	trace	6	trace	1	0	230	..	..	..	..
Fats and oils, cooking (1 tbsp.), French dressing (2 tbsp.)	14	125	0	14	0	0	0	0	0	0	0	0
Salad dressing, mayonnaise type (1 tbsp.)	15	80	trace	9	1	2	0.1	45	trace	trace	trace	0
Sugars, Sweets												
Candy, plain (½ oz.), jam and jelly (1 tbsp.), syrup (1 tbsp.), gelatin dessert, plain (½ c.), beverages, carbonated (1 c.)	..	60	0	0	14	3	0.1	trace	trace	trace	trace	trace
Chocolate fudge (1 oz.), chocolate syrup (3 tbsp.)	..	125	1	2	30	15	0.6	10	trace	0.02	0.1	trace
Molasses (1 tbsp.), caramel (⅓ oz.)	..	40	trace	trace	8	20	0.3	trace	trace	trace	trace	trace
Sugar (1 tbsp.)	12	45	0	0	12	0	trace	0	0	0	0	0
Miscellaneous												
Chocolate, bitter (1 oz.)	30	145	3	15	8	20	1.9	20	0.01	0.07	0.4	0
Sherbet (½ c.)	96	130	1	1	30	15	trace	55	0.01	0.03	trace	2
Soups: bean, pea (green) (1 c.)	..	150	7	4	22	50	1.6	495	0.09	0.06	1.0	4
Noodle, beef, chicken (1 c.)	..	65	4	2	7	10	0.7	50	0.03	0.04	0.9	trace
Clam chowder, minestrone, tomato, vegetable (1 c.)	..	90	3	2	14	25	0.9	1,880	0.05	0.04	1.1	3

From Wilson, Fisher and Fuqua: Principles of Nutrition. New York, Wiley, 1966.

TABLE 3. Selected Fatty Acids and Cholesterol in Common Foods

	Amount in 100 Gm. Edible Portion				
			Unsaturated Fatty Acids		
Item and Description	Total Fat	Total Saturated Fat	Oleic	Linoleic	Cholesterol mg.
Almonds, shelled....................	54.2	4	36	11	..
Avocado, raw......................	16.4	3	7	2	..
Bacon, broiled or fried...............	52.0	17	25	5	100
Beef, edible, raw, chuck..............	31.4	15	14	1	70
Porterhouse steak.................	36.2	17	16	1	..
Round, entire.....................	12.3	6	5	Tr.	125
Round, separable lean..............	4.7	2	2	Tr.	..
Rump, total edible................	25.3	12	11	1	..
Hamburg, regular..................	21.2	10	9	Tr.	..
lean....................	10.0	5	4	Tr.	..
Beef, corned, canned................	12.0	6	5	Tr.	..
Brazil nuts, shelled..................	66.9	13	32	17	..
Bread, white, 3-4% milk solids........	3.2	1	2	Tr.	..
Butter............................	81.0	46	27	2	250
Cake, plain, from mix with milk, egg and vegetable shortening...........	12.0	3	7	1	45
Candy, made with chocolate nuts and vegetable shortening Chocolate-coated peanuts.........	41.3	11	22	7	..
Fudge with walnuts...............	17.4	6	5	6	..
Cashew nuts.......................	45.7	8	32	3	..
Cheese, cheddar, natural.............	32.2	18	11	1	100
cottage, creamed.............	4.2	2	1	Tr.	15
Chicken, raw, edible portion Fryer..........................	7.2	2	2	2	60–90
Roasting........................	12.6	4	6	2	60–90
Stewing.........................	25.0	6	11	6	60–90
Chocolate, bitter, cooking.............	53.0	30	20	1	..
Coconut, shredded, sweetened.........	39.1	34	3	Tr.	..
Cookies, sugar, with v. f.*............	16.8	4	10	1	50
Cornbread or muffins, v. f.*...........	8.4	3	4	1	46
Crackers, Graham, v. f.*	10.0	2	6	1	..
plain soda, v. f.*	10.2	2	6	1	..
Cream, light, coffee.................	20.6	11	7	1	67
heavy whipping..............	37.6	21	12	1	120
Custard, baked, milk and egg..........	5.5	3	2	Tr.	86

* v.f.—vegetable fat.

TABLE 3. Selected Fatty Acids and Cholesterol in Common Foods *(Continued)*

	Amount in 100 Gm. Edible Portion				
			Unsaturated Fatty Acids		
Item and Description	Total Fat	Total Saturated Fat	Oleic	Linoleic	Cholesterol mg.
Duck, raw, edible portion..............	28.6	7	11	7	..
Eggs, whole........................	11.5	6	5	1	468
yolks only.....................	30.6	10	13	2	1,500
Filberts, shelled.....................	62.4	3	34	10	..
Herring, raw.......................	11.3	2	Tr.	2	..
Ice cream, 12% fat..................	12.5	7	4	Tr.	45
Ice milk...........................	5.1	3	2	Tr.	..
Lamb, raw, leg, edible portion........	16.2	9	6	Tr.	70
shoulder, edible portion..........	23.9	13	9	1	70
Lard..............................	100	38	46	10	106
Liver, pork, raw....................	3.7	1	1	Tr.	300
Luncheon meat.....................	24.2	9	10	2	..
Margarine, hydrogenated.............	81.0	18	47	14	..
Milk, whole, cow's..................	3.7	2	1	Tr.	11–15
canned, evaporated.............	7.9	4	3	Tr.	..
dry, whole	27.5	15	9	1	85
Noodles, egg, dry form..............	4.6	1	2	Tr.	..
Oils: corn.........................	100	10	28	53	..
cottonseed.....................	100	25	21	50	..
olive.........................	100	11	76	7	..
peanut........................	100	18	47	29	..
safflower seed..................	100	8	15	72	..
soybean.......................	100	15	20	52	..
Olives, ripe, Mission type.............	20.1	2	15	1	..
Oysters, raw or canned..............	2.0	..	..	..	200
Peanuts, roasted, shelled.............	48.7	11	21	14	..
Peanut butter, oil added.............	50.6	9	25	14	..
Pecans, shelled.....................	71.2	5	45	14	..
Pistachio nuts, shelled................	53.7	5	35	10	..
Popcorn, popped, plain..............	5.0	1	1	3	..
Pork, fresh, raw ham, edible portion..............	26.6	10	11	2	70–105
loin, edible portion..............	24.9	9	10	2	70–105

TABLE 3. Selected Fatty Acids and Cholesterol in Common Foods *(Continued)*

	Amount in 100 Gm. Edible Portion				
			Unsaturated Fatty Acids		
Item and Description	Total Fat	Total Saturated Fat	Oleic	Linoleic	Cholesterol mg.
Pork, cured, ham, edible portion........	23.0	8	10	2	70–105
canned......................	12.3	4	5	1	70–105
Potatoes, French-fried.................	13.2	3	3	7	..
mashed, milk and butter.......	4.3	2	1	Tr.	..
Potato chips.......................	39.8	10	8	20	..
Salad dressings: made with soybean, cottonseed or corn oil French, commercial...............	38.9	7	8	20	..
Italian, commercial...............	60.0	10	13	31	..
Mayonnaise with egg.............	79.9	14	17	40	..
Russian.......................	50.8	9	11	26	..
Salmon, canned, pink.................	5.9	2	1	Tr.	..
Salt pork..........................	85.0	32	39	5	..
Sausage, country style................	31.1	11	13	3	70–105
pork, link, cooked............	44.2	16	19	4	..
Shrimp, raw.......................	.8	..	..	..	125
Tuna fish, canned in oil, drained solids...	8.2	3	2	2	..
Turkey, dark meat...................	9.6	3	4	2	16–26
light meat...................	4.6	1	2	1	8–15
Veal, total edible, raw Chuck, medium fat................	10.0	5	4	Tr.	90
Rib, medium fat...................	14.0	7	6	Tr.	90
Walnuts, shelled, black...............	59.3	4	21	28	..
English type................	64.0	4	10	40	..
Wheat germ, commercial..............	11.5	2	3	6	..

Figures in this table are taken from Table 3, Handbook No. 8. Washington, U.S.D.A. 1963, and from Hardinge, M. G., and Crooks, H.: J. Am. Dietet. A., 34: 1065, 1958.

TABLE 4. Amino Acid Content of Foods per 100 Grams, Edible Portion*

Food Item	Nitrogen Conversion Factor	Protein Content Per Cent	Phenyl-alanine mg.	Iso-leucine mg.	Leucine mg.	Valine mg.	Sulfur Containing			Trypto-phan mg.	Threo-nine mg.	Lysine mg.	Tyrosine mg.	Arginine mg.	Histi-dine mg.
							Methio-nine mg.	Cystine mg.	Total mg.						
Milk, Milk Products															
Fluid, whole	6.38	3.5	170	223	344	240	86	31	117	49	161	272	178	128	92
Canned, evap. unsweetened	6.38	7.0	340	447	688	481	171	63	234	99	323	545	357	256	185
Dried, non-fat	6.38	35.6	1,724	2,271	3,493	2,444	870	318	1,188	502	1,641	2,768	1,814	1,300	937
Cheese, Cheddar, processed	6.38	23.2	1,244	1,563	2,262	1,665	604	131	735	316	862	1,702	1,109	847	756
Cottage	6.38	17.0	917	989	1,826	978	469	147	616	179	794	1,428	917	802	549
Eggs, whole															
fresh or stored	6.25	12.8	739	850	1,126	950	401	299	700	211	637	819	551	840	307
Meat, Poultry, Fish															
Beef, chuck, med. fat	6.25	18.6	765	973	1,524	1,033	461	235	696	217	821	1,625	631	1,199	646
Hamburg, reg.	6.25	16.0	658	837	1,311	888	397	202	599	187	707	1,398	543	1,032	556
Rib roast	6.25	17.4	715	910	1,425	590	432	220	652	203	768	1,520	590	1,122	604
Round	6.25	19.5	802	1,020	1,597	1,083	484	246	730	228	861	1,704	661	1,257	677
Rump	6.25	16.2	666	848	1,327	899	402	205	607	189	715	1,415	550	1,045	562
Lamb, med. fat	6.25														
leg	6.25	18.0	732	933	1,394	887	432	236	668	233	824	1,457	625	1,172	501
Rib	6.25	14.9	606	772	1,154	734	358	195	553	193	682	1,206	517	970	415
Pork, fresh, med. fat	6.25														
Ham	6.25	15.2	598	781	1,119	790	379	178	557	197	705	1,248	542	931	525
Loin	6.25	16.4	646	842	1,207	853	409	192	601	213	761	1,346	585	1,005	567
Pork, cured	6.25														
Bacon, med. fat	6.25	9.1	434	399	728	434	141	106	247	95	306	587	234	622	246
Ham	6.25	16.9	646	841	1,306	879	411	273	684	162	692	1,420	652	1,068	544
Luncheon meat, canned, spiced		14.9	570	741	1,151	775	362	241	603	143	610	1,252	879	942	479
Veal, med. fat	6.25														
Round	6.25	19.5	792	1,030	1,429	1,008	446	231	677	256	846	1,629	702	1,270	627
Poultry, flesh only	6.25														
Chicken, fryer	6.25	20.6	811	1,088	1,490	1,012	537	277	814	250	877	1,810	725	1,302	593
Turkey	6.25	24.0	960	1,260	1,836	1,187	664	330	994	..	1,014	2,173	..	1,513	649

TABLE 4. Amino Acid Content of Foods per 100 Grams, Edible Portion (Continued)

Food Item	Nitrogen Conversion Factor	Protein Content Per Cent	Phenyl-alanine mg.	Iso-leucine mg.	Leucine mg.	Valine mg.	Sulfur Containing			Trypto-phan mg.	Threo-nine mg.	Lysine mg.	Tyrosine mg.	Arginine mg.	Histidine mg.
							Methionine mg.	Cystine mg.	Total mg.						
Meat, Poultry, Fish (Continued)															
Fish	6.25														
Cod, fresh, raw	6.25	16.5	612	837	1,246	879	480	222	702	164	715	1,447	446	929	..
Haddock, raw	6.25	18.2	676	923	1,374	930	530	245	775	181	789	1,596	492	1,025	..
Halibut, raw	6.25	18.6	690	943	1,405	991	542	250	792	185	806	1,631	503	1,048	..
Salmon, Pacific, raw	6.25	17.4	646	883	1,314	927	507	234	741	173	754	1,526	470	980	..
Canned, sockeye or red	6.25	20.2	750	1,025	1,526	1,076	588	271	859	200	876	1,771	546	1,138	..
Meat Products	6.25														
Liver, calf	6.25	19.0	958	994	1,754	1,195	447	234	681	286	903	447	711	1,158	505
Bologna sausage	6.25	14.8	540	718	1,061	744	313	185	498	126	606	1,191	481	1,028	398
Frankfurters	6.25	14.2	518	688	1,018	713	300	177	477	120	582	1,143	461	986	382
Liverwurst	6.25	16.7	759	818	1,400	1,037	347	203	550	187	724	1,301	510	1,034	497
Legumes, dry and Nuts															
Bean, red kidney, canned	6.25	5.7	315	324	490	346	57	57	114	53	247	423	220	343	162
Peanuts	5.46	26.9	1,557	1,266	1,872	1,532	271	463	734	340	828	1,099	1,104	3,296	749
Peanut Butter	5.46	26.1	1,510	1,228	1,816	1,487	263	449	712	330	803	1,066	1,071	3,198	727
Pecans	5.30	9.4	564	553	773	525	153	216	369	138	389	435	316	1,185	273
Walnuts	5.30	15.0	767	767	1,228	974	306	320	626	175	589	441	583	2,287	405
Grains and Their Products															
Bread, white 4% milk solids	5.70	8.5	465	429	668	435	142	200	342	91	282	225	243	340	192
Cereal combinations Infant food, precooked mixed cereal & dry milk	6.25	19.4	543	..	..	..	310	137	447	118	..	273	447	447	233

*figures for the amino acid content of foods are taken from Orr, M. L., and Watt, B. K.: Amino Acid Content of Foods. Home Economics Research Report No. 4. Washington, U.S.D.A., 1957. Amino acid content is given in milligrams, using whole numbers, rather than in grams, using decimals. The order of listing the amino acids has been arranged for the convenience of dietitians dealing with inborn errors of metabolism. For further explanation of the nitrogen conversion factors see reference above.

TABLE 4. Amino Acid Content of Foods per 100 Grams, Edible Portion (Continued)

Food Item	Nitrogen Conversion Factor	Protein Content Per Cent	Phenyl-alanine mg.	Iso-leucine mg.	Leucine mg.	Valine mg.	Sulfur Containing			Trypto-phan mg.	Threo-nine mg.	Lysine mg.	Tyrosine mg.	Arginine mg.	Histi-dine mg.
							Methio-nine mg.	Cystine mg.	Total mg.						
Grains and Their Products (Continued)															
Oat-corn-rye, puffed	5.83	14.5	933	841	1,368	900	388	234	622	172	545	343	622	776	326
Corn Products															
Corn grits	6.25	8.7	395	402	1,128	444	161	113	274	53	347	251	532	306	180
Corn meal, degermed	6.25	7.9	359	365	1,024	403	147	102	249	48	315	228	483	278	163
Cornflakes	6.25	8.1	354	306	1,047	386	135	152	287	52	275	154	283	231	226
Hominy	6.25	8.7	333	349	810	398	99	..	..	84	316	358	331	444	203
Oatmeal, rolled oats	5.83	14.2	758	733	1,065	845	209	309	518	183	470	521	524	935	261
Rice, white or converted	5.95	7.6	382	356	655	531	137	103	240	82	298	300	347	438	128
Rice, products flakes or puffed	5.95	5.9	286	..	..	..	..	44	..	46	..	56	124	137	137
Wheat products Farina	5.70	10.9	579	..	..	..	143	184	327	124	..	199	447	424	268
Flakes	5.70	10.8	478	496	891	572	127	191	318	121	356	360	311	559	231
Macaroni or Spaghetti	5.70	12.8	669	642	849	728	193	243	436	150	499	413	422	582	303
Noodles, made with egg	5.70	12.6	610	621	834	745	212	245	457	133	533	411	312	621	301
Shredded wheat	5.83	12.8	755	..	..	..	..	246	..	136	..	466	481	742	371
Fruits															
Bananas, ripe	6.25	1.2	..	..	..	..	11	..	..	18	..	55	31	..	..
Grapefruit	6.25	0.5	..	..	..	..	10	..	..	1	..	30	..	..	..
Muskmelon	6.35	0.6	..	..	..	..	2	..	..	1	..	15	..	..	..
Oranges or orange juice	6.25	0.9	..	..	..	..	2	..	..	3	..	22	..	..	..
Pineapple	6.25	0.4	..	..	..	..	1	..	..	5	..	9	..	..	..

TABLE 4. Amino Acid Content of Foods per 100 Grams, Edible Portion (Continued)

| Food Item | Nitrogen Conversion Factor | Protein Content Per Cent | Phenyl-alanine mg. | Iso-leucine mg. | Leucine mg. | Valine mg. | Sulfur Containing | | | Trypto-phan mg. | Threo-nine mg. | Lysine mg. | Tyrosine mg. | Arginine mg. | Histi-dine mg. |
							Methio-nine mg.	Cystine mg.	Total mg.						
Vegetables															
Asparagus, canned	6.25	1.9	60	69	83	92	27	..	..	23	57	89	..	106	31
Beans, snap, canned	6.25	1.0	24	45	58	48	14	10	24	14	38	52	21	42	19
lima, canned	6.25	3.8	197	233	306	246	41	42	83	49	171	240	131	230	125
Beets, canned	6.25	0.9	15	29	31	28	3	..	..	8	19	48	..	16	12
Beet greens	6.25	2.0	116	84	129	101	34	..	..	24	76	108	..	83	26
Broccoli	6.25	3.3	119	126	163	170	50	..	..	37	122	147	..	192	63
Cabbage	6.25	1.4	30	40	57	43	13	28	41	11	39	66	30	105	25
Carrots, raw	6.25	1.2	42	46	65	56	10	29	39	10	43	52	20	41	17
Cauliflower	6.25	2.4	75	104	162	144	47	..	..	33	102	134	34	110	48
Celery	6.25	1.3	..	..	..	..	15	6	21	12	..	..	..	..	..
Corn, sweet, white or yellow, canned	6.25	2.0	112	74	220	125	39	33	72	12	82	74	67	94	52
Cucumber	6.25	0.7	..	..	..	..	8	..	..	14	..	..	..	..	..
Eggplant	6.25	1.1	48	56	68	65	6	..	..	10	38	30	..	37	19
Lettuce	6.25	1.2	..	..	..	..	4	..	..	..	..	70	..	..	..
Onions, mature	6.25	1.4	39	21	37	31	13	..	..	21	22	64	46	180	14
Peas, canned	6.25	3.4	131	156	212	139	27	37	64	28	125	160	83	302	55
Potatoes cooked or canned	6.25	1.7	75	75	85	91	21	16	37	18	67	91	30	84	24
Pumpkin	6.25	1.2	32	44	63	45	11	..	..	16	28	58	16	43	19
Radishes	6.25	1.2	..	..	..	30	2	..	..	5	59	34	..	..	..
Spinach	6.25	2.3	99	107	176	126	39	46	85	37	102	142	73	116	49
Squash, summer	6.25	0.6	16	19	27	22	8	..	..	5	14	23	..	27	9
Tomatoes, all types	6.25	1.0	28	29	41	28	7	..	..	9	33	42	14	29	15
Turnips	6.25	1.1	20	20	..	..	12	..	..	..	..	57	29	..	..

TABLE 5. Sodium, Potassium, and Magnesium Content of Foods

Food	Na	K	Mg
	Mg. per 100 Grams		
Acerola	8	83	..
Almonds, shelled	4	773	270
Apples:			
Raw, pared	1	110	5
Frozen slices, sweetened	14	68	4
Apple juice, canned	1	101	4
Applesauce, canned, sweetened	2	65	5
Apricots:			
Raw	1	281	12
Canned	1	246	7
Dried	26	979	62
Frozen	4	229	9
Nectar	Tr.	151	..
Asparagus:			
Fresh, cooked	1	183	20
Frozen, cooked	1	238	14
Avocados	4	604	45
Bacon:			
Broiled or fried	1,021	236	25
Canadian, broiled or fried	2,555	432	24
Baking powders*			
Bananas	1	370	33
Barley, pearled	3	160	37
Beans, baked canned, no pork	338	268	37
Beans:			
Snap, canned	236	95	14
Canned, low-sodium	2	95	14
Frozen, cooked	1	152	21
Lima, cooked, frozen	101	426	48
Beef:			
Lean, cooked	60	370	29
Heart, raw	86	193	18
Liver, cooked	184	380	18
Tongue, raw	73	197	16
Beets:			
Canned, solids	236	167	15
Cooked, unsalted	46	167	15
Beet greens, raw	130	570	106
Beverages, carbonated†			
Blackberries	1	170	30
Blueberries, raw or frozen	1	81	6
Boysenberries, frozen	1	153	18
Brazil nuts	1	715	225
Breads:			
Boston, brown	251	292	..
Cracked, wheat	529	134	35
Rye, regular	557	145	42
unsalted	30	115	42
White, enriched	507	105	22
unsalted	30	180	22

Food	Na	K	Mg
	Mg. per 100 Grams		
Whole wheat, regular	527	273	78
unsalted	30	230	78
Raisin	365	233	24
Broccoli, frozen	13	244	21
Brussels sprouts, raw	14	390	29
Butter:			
Salted	987	23	2
Unsalted	10	23	2
Buttermilk, cultured	130	140	14
Cabbage:			
Common	20	233	13
Chinese	23	253	14
Candy:			
Butterscotch	66	2	..
Caramels	226	192	..
Chocolate, milk	94	384	..
Fudge	190	147	..
Hard candy	32	4	Tr.
Peanut brittle	31	151	..
Cantaloupe or honeydew	12	251	16
Carrots, raw	47	341	23
Cashew nuts	15	464	267
Cauliflower, raw	13	295	24
Celery, raw	126	341	22
Cereals:			
Corn flakes	1,005	120	16
Corn grits, cooked	..	11	3
Cornmeal, yellow or white	1	120	106
Farina, cooked	690	188	3
Oatmeal, cooked	218	61	21
Rice, puffed, unsalted	2	100	..
Wheat, shredded, unsalted	3	348	133
Wheat, puffed, unsalted	4	340	..
Chard, raw	147	550	65
Cheese:			
Cheddar	700	82	45
Cottage, creamed	229	85	..
Parmesan	734	149	48
Cherries, sweet or sour	2	191	8-14
Chestnuts, fresh	6	454	41
Chicken, cooked,			
white meat	64	441	19
dark meat	86	321	..
liver	61	151	16
Chicory greens, raw	..	420	13
Chives, raw	..	250	32
Chocolate, bitter	4	830	292
Chocolate syrup	52	282	63
Clams, meat only	120	181	..
Coconut, shredded	..	353	77
Coffee, instant dry powder	72	3,256	456
Collards, raw	43	401	57

*Baking powders vary greatly in sodium and potassium content. The label on the package tells the type. One tsp. or 5 Gm. of baking powder contains:

	Mg. Na	Mg.K.
Alum type	500	8
Phosphate type	450	9
Tartrate type	360	250
Low-sodium type	2	500

† The sodium content of carbonated beverages depends upon the sodium content of the water in the area where they are manufactured. See J.A.M.A., *195*:236, 1966.

TABLE 5. Sodium, Potassium, and Magnesium Content of Foods (Continued)

Food	Na	K	Mg	Food	Na	K	Mg
	Mg. per 100 Grams				Mg. per 100 Grams		
Corn: sweet, cooked.......	15	165	..	Marmalade, citrus.........	14	33	4
frozen, cooked..........	1	184	22	Milk:			
canned.................	236	97	19	Whole or skim..........	50	144	13
Cornbread, from mix.......	744	127	13	Evap., unsweetened......	118	303	25
Crab, cooked meat, canned.	1,000	110	34	Molasses, light............	15	917	46
Crackers:				Mushrooms:			
Graham...............	670	384	51	Canned...............	400	197	8
Soda.................	1,100	120	29	Fresh.................	15	414	13
Cranberries:				Mussels.................	289	315	24
Juice.................	1	10	2	Mustard greens, cooked....	18	220	25
Sauce.................	1	30	2	Nectarines..............	6	294	13
Cream, light, coffee........	43	122	11	Noodles, cooked..........	2	44	..
Cress, garden............	14	606	..	Okra, fresh or frozen......	2	168	47
Cucumbers...............	6	160	11	Olives:			
Currants, raw, red.........	2	257	15	Green.................	2,400	55	22
Dates, natural and dry.....	1	648	58	Ripe.................	750	27	..
Eggplant, cooked..........	1	150	16	Onions, mature, raw.......	10	157	12
Eggs:				Oranges or orange juice....	1	200	11
Whole................	122	129	11	Oysters, raw.............	73	121	32
Whites................	146	139	9	Pancakes, from mix........	451	156	..
Yolk..................	52	98	16	Papaya, raw.............	3	234	..
Endive or Escarole........	14	294	10	Parsley.................	45	727	41
Figs, dried..............	34	640	71	Parsnips, cooked..........	8	379	32
Filberts (hazelnuts)	2	704	184	Peaches:			
Fish:				Raw..................	1	202	10
Cod, broiled...........	110	407	28	Canned...............	2	130	6
Haddock, fried.........	177	348	24	Peanuts, roasted, unsalted...	5	701	175
Halibut, broiled.........	134	525	..	Peanut butter.............	606	652	173
Salmon, baked, broiled...	116	443	30	Pears:			
Sardines, canned in oil...	823	590	24	Raw..................	2	130	7
Tuna, canned, water.....	41	279	..	Canned...............	1	84	5
Gooseberries.............	1	155	9	Peas:			
Grapefruit:				Canned, regular........	236	96	20
Pulp..................	1	135	12	Frozen................	115	135	24
Juice.................	1	162	12	Low sodium, canned......	3	96	24
Grapes:				Pecans.................	Tr.	603	142
American type.........	3	158	13	Peppers, raw............	13	213	18
European type..........	3	173	6	Persimmons..............	6	174	8
Grape juice, canned	2	116	12	Pickles:			
Guava, common, raw.......	4	289	13	Dill..................	1,428	200	12
Honey, strained...........	5	51	3	Sweet.................	527	..	1
Ice cream, regular.........	63	181	14	Pineapple:			
Ice milk.................	68	195	..	Raw..................	1	146	13
Jams, jellies, average......	15	81	12	Canned, heavy syrup.....	1	96	8
Lamb, any cut, broiled or				Juice, unsweetened......	1	149	12
roasted...............	70	290	19	Pistachio nuts.............	..	972	158
Leeks, raw..............	5	347	23	Plums:			
Lemon juice, fresh or frozen..	1	141	7	Raw..................	1	170	9
Lettuce, iceberg..........	9	175	11	Purple, canned, in syrup..	1	142	5
Lime juice...............	1	104	..	Pork:			
Lobster, cooked...........	210	180	22	All cuts, fresh cooked.....	65	390	23
Loganberries, raw.........	1	170	25	Ham, cured, cooked......	930	326	17
Macaroni, plain, cooked....	1	61	18	Sausage, pork, cooked...	958	269	16
Mangos, raw.............	7	189	18	Potatoes:			
Margarine:				Peeled, boiled, unsalted..	2	285	22
Regular...............	987	23	..	French fried, unsalted....	6	853	25
Unsalted..............	10 or less	10	..	Mashed, milk added.....	301	261	12
				Potato chips.............	1,000‡	1,130	..

‡Potato chips vary in sodium according to amount of salt added.

TABLE 5. Sodium, Potassium, and Magnesium Content of Foods *(Continued)*

Food	Na	K	Mg	Food	Na	K	Mg
	Mg. per 100 Grams				Mg. per 100 Grams		
Pretzels.................	1,680	130	..	Strawberries, raw.........	1	164	12
Prunes:				Sweet potato, baked......	12	300	31
Dried, uncooked.........	8	694	40	Tangerine, raw...........	1	126	..
Cooked..............	4	327	20	Tomatoes, raw...........	3	244	14
Pumpkin, canned, unsalted...	2	240	12	Tomato juice:			
Radishes, raw.............	18	322	15	Canned..............	200	227	10
Raisins, uncooked..........	27	763	35	Canned, low sodium.....	3	227	10
Raspberries:				Tomato catsup:			
Raw, red.............	1	168	20	Regular..............	1,338	370	21
Black.................	1	199	30	Low sodium...........	5-35	370	21
Rhubarb, cooked..........	2	203	13	Turkey, roasted..........	130	367	28
Rice:				Turnips:			
Cooked, regular, salted...	374	28	8	Raw.................	49	268	20
Cooked without salt......	2	28	8	Cooked, unsalted........	34	188	20
Rutabagas, cooked, unsalted	4	167	15	Turnip greens, frozen.......	17	149	26
Salad dressings:				Veal, all cuts, cooked......	80	500	18
French.................	1,370	79	10	Walnuts, English...........	2	450	131
Italian.................	2,092	15	..	Watercress..............	52	282	20
Mayonnaise...........	597	34	2	Watermelon..............	1	100	8
Russian................	868	157		Wheat:			
Scallops, cooked..........	265	476	..	Flour.................	2	95	25
Shrimp, cooked...........	186	229	51	Bran.................	9	1,121	490
Syrup, maple.............	10	176	11	Germ.................	3	827	336
Soybean curd (tofu)........	7	42	111	Yams.................	..	600	..
Spinach, cooked...........	50	324	63	Yoghurt.................	51	143	..
Squash:				Zweiback.................	250	150	..
Summer, cooked, unsalted.	1	141	16				
Winter, cooked, unsalted..	1	141	17				

Sodium, potassium and magnesium figures from Composition of Food, Raw, Processed Prepared. Agr. Handbook No. 8. U.S.D.A., Washington, D. C., 1963; or from Church, C. E., and Church, H. N.: Food Values of Portions Commonly Used. Ed. 10. Philadelphia, Lippincott, 1966.

Values for these minerals in canned and processed foods subject to variation because of methods of processing.

Additional References on Sodium, Potassium and Magnesium Content of Foods

Cancio, M., and Leon, J. M.: Sodium and potassium in Puerto Rican foods and waters. J. Am. Dietet. A., 35:1165, 1959.

Cancio, M.: Sodium and potassium in Puerto Rican meats and fish. J. Am. Dietet. A., 38:341, 1961.

Chan, S. L., and Kennedy, B. M.: Sodium in Chinese vegetables. J. Am. Dietet. A., 37:573, 1960.

Clifford, P. A.: Sodium content of food. J. Am. Dietet. A., 31:21, 1955.

Dahl, L. K.: Sodium in foods for a 100 Mg. diet. J. Am. Dietet. A., 34:717, 1958.

Davidson, C. S., et al.: Sodium-restricted diets. The rationale, complications, and practical aspects of their use. Nat. Research Council Pub. No. 325, 1954.

Holinger, B. W., et al.: Analyzed sodium values in foods ready to serve. J. Am. Dietet. A., 48:501, 1966.

Hopkins, H. T.: Minerals and proximate composition of organ meats. J. Am. Dietet. A., 38:344, 1961.

Hopkins, H. T., and Eisen, J.: Mineral elements in fresh vegetables from different geographical areas. J. Agr. Food Chem., 7:633, 1959.

Nelson, G. Y., and Gram, M. R.: Magnesium content of accessory foods. J. Am. Dietet. A., 38:437, 1961.

Oglesby, L. M., and Bannister, A. C.: Sodium and potassium in salt-water fish. J. Am. Dietet. A., 35:1163, 1959.

Thurston, C. E.: Sodium and potassium content of 34 species of fish. J. Am. Dietet. A., 34:396, 1958.

Thurston, C. E., and Osterhaug, K. L.: Sodium content of fish flesh. J. Am. Dietet. A., 36:212, 1960.

Copper Content of Foods

Tables giving the copper content of certain foods are too conflicting and incomplete to be included in the above table. For persons interested in the copper content of foods in dealing with Wilson's Disease the following references are listed:

Silverberg, M., and Gellis, S. S.: Wilson's Disease. Am. J. Dis. Child., 113:178, 1967 (Lists foods to be avoided).

————: Preventing Wilson's Disease Sequelae. J.A.M.A., 200:41, 1967.

Hook, L., and Brandt, I. K.: Copper content of some low copper foods. J. Am. Dietet. A., 49:202, 1966.

Review: Dietary copper in Wilson's Disease. Nutr. Rev., 23:301, 1965.

TABLE 6. Lesser Known Vitamins in Foods*: Vitamin B_6, pantothenic acid, biotin, folic acid, choline, and inositol content of foods, edible portion

Food	Amt.	Wt. Gm.	Vitamin B_6 Mcg./portion	Vitamin B_6 Mcg./100 Gm.	Pantothenic Acid Mg./portion	Pantothenic Acid Mg./100 Gm.	Biotin Mcg./portion	Biotin Mcg./100 Gm.	Folic Acid Mcg./portion	Folic Acid Mcg./100 Gm.	Choline Mg./portion	Choline Mg./100 Gm.	Inositol Mg./portion	Inositol Mg./100 Gm.
Cereals and Bread Products														
Cereals, cooked, whole														
Barley, whole	½ c.	30 (dry)	167.1	557	0.219	0.73	9.3	31.0	15.	50.0	41.7	139.0	117.6	392.0
Corn, yellow	½ c.	20 (dry)	93.4	467	0.128	0.64	4.2	21.0	5.3	26.5	12.2	61.0	10.0	50.0
Oats	½ c.	20 (dry)	41.0	205	0.300	1.50	4.8	24.0	6.6	33.0	31.2	156.0	53.8	269.0
Rice, brown	½ c.	30 (dry)	186.0	620	0.456	1.52	3.6	12.0	6.0	20.0	33.6	112.0	35.7	119.0
Wheat, whole	½ c.	30 (dry)	158.4	528	0.411	1.37	4.8	16.0	14.7	49.0	28.2	94.0	110.0	370.0
Cereals, refined, cooked														
Cornmeal														
White	½ c.	20 (dry)	(12.2)†	(61)	0.116	0.58	1.3	6.6	1.8	9.0	..	..	10.2	51
Yellow	½ c.	20 (dry)	..	..	0.138	0.69	..	..	1.8	9.0	2.0	10.0	..	..
Hominy grits	½ c.	20 (dry)	(1.2)	(6)	0.068	0.34	0.1	0.7	0.9	4.5	..	..	0.6	3
Rice														
Converted	½ c.	30 (dry)	20.4	68	0.393	1.31	2.4	8.0	6.0	20.0	26.7	89.0	6.0	20
Parboiled	½ c.	30 (dry)	30.0	100	0.411	1.37	3.0	10.0	5.7	19.0	29.4	98.0	7.5	25
White	½ c.	30 (dry)	11.1	37	0.225	0.75	1.5	5.0	4.8	16.0	17.7	59.0	3.0	10
Cereal concentrates, raw														
Rice														
Bran	1 oz.	30 (dry)	750.0	2500	0.831	2.77	18.0	60.0	43.8	146.0	51.0	170.0	138.9	463
Germ	1 oz.	30 (dry)	480.0	1600	0.900	3.00	17.4	58.0	129.0	430.0	90.0	300.0	111.6	372
Polishings	1 oz.	30 (dry)	600.0	2000	1.000	3.33	17.1	57.0	57.6	192.0	30.6	102.0	136.2	454
Wheat														
Bran	1 oz.	30 (dry)	414.0	1380	0.900	3.00	4.2	14.0	58.5	195.0	42.9	143.0	..	..
Germ	1 oz.	30 (dry)	275.4	918	0.660	2.20	..	..	91.5	305.0	121.8	406.0	231.0	770
Ready-to-eat, dark cereal														
Corn soya	1 c.	30	..	..	0.273	0.91	..	..	24.0	80.0	..	..	..	..
Oats	1 c.	25	..	..	0.230	0.92	..	..	5.6	22.4	..	..	..	..
Wheat														
Bran	1 c.	35	..	..	1.015	2.90	..	..	35.0	100.0	..	..	..	..
Flakes	1 c.	35	..	..	0.304	0.87	..	..	16.4	47.0	..	..	..	..
Shredded Wheat	1 bisc.	30	..	..	0.210	0.70	..	..	16.5	55.0	..	..	..	..
Ready-to-eat, white cereal														
Corn flakes	1 c.	25	(14.4)	(48)	0.047	0.19	0.4	1.3	1.4	5.5	..	..	..	..
Rice	1 c.	30	..	..	0.114	0.38	..	..	2.3	7.6	..	..	5.7	19
Bread														
White	1 sl.	23	23.0	100	0.101	0.44	0.3	1.1	3.4	15.0	..	..	11.7	51
Whole wheat	1 sl.	23	96.0	420	0.182	0.79	0.4	1.9	6.9	30.0	..	..	15.4	67

TABLE 6. Lesser Known Vitamins in Foods*: Vitamin B₆, pantothenic acid, biotin, folic acid, choline, and inositol content of foods, edible portion (Continued)

Food	Portion		Vitamin B$_6$		Pantothenic Acid		Biotin		Folic Acid		Choline		Inositol	
	Amt.	Wt. Gm.	Mcg./ portion	Mcg./ 100 Gm.	Mg./ portion	Mg./ 100 Gm.	Mcg./ portion	Mcg./ 100 Gm.	Mcg./ portion	Mcg./ 100 Gm.	Mg./ portion	Mg./ 100 Gm.	Mg./ portion	Mg./ 100 Gm.
Cereals and Bread Products (Continued)														
Flour														
White	1 c.	110	363.0	330	0.594	0.54	1.1	1.0	8.8	8.0	57.2	52	51.7	47
Whole wheat	1 c.	120	1116.0	930	1.296	1.08	10.8	9.0	45.6	38.0	...	...	132.0	110
Dairy Products														
Cheese														
Cheddar	1 oz.	30	(18.7)	(66)	0.114	0.40	1.0	3.6	4.5	16.0	13.6	48	7.0	7
Cottage	1 oz.	30	...	...	0.080	0.28	...	...	8.8	31.0	...	...	...	...
Processed	1 oz.	30	...	...	0.136	0.48	1.3	4.6	3.1	11.0	...	...	...	...
Egg														
Whole	1 med.	50	126.0	252	0.795	1.59	11.2	22.5	2.5	5.1	252.0	504	16.5	33
Yolk	1 med.	17	52.4	308	0.719	4.23	8.8	52.0	2.2	12.9	253.3	1490	...	...
White	1 med.	31	67.3	217	0.043	0.14	2.2	7.0	0.2	0.6	0.6	2	...	...
Milk														
Whole	1 c.	244	87.8	36	0.756	0.31	11.5	4.7	1.5	0.6	36.6	15	31.7	13
Evaporated reconstituted	1 c.	244	53.7	22	0.805	0.33	11.0	4.5	1.7	0.7	36.6	15	...	...
Nonfat dry reconstituted	1 c.	244	80.5	33	0.830	0.34	8.3	3.4	0.5	0.2	25.4	10.4	...	...
Fats, Oils, and Oily Foods														
Butter	1 tbsp.	14	...	...	...	...	...	...	...	...	0.7	5	...	...
Lard	1 tbsp.	14	...	...	...	...	...	...	...	...	0.7	5	...	...
Margarine	1 tbsp.	14	...	...	...	...	...	...	...	...	0.7	5	...	...
Vegetable oils	1 tbsp.	14	...	...	...	...	...	...	...	...	0.7	5	...	...
Fruits														
Fruits, fresh or frozen														
Apples, medium	1	130	39.0	30	0.130	0.10	1.2	0.9	2.6	2.0	...	...	31.2	24
Apricots	3 med.	100	71.0	71	0.290	0.29	...	...	3.3	3.3	...	...	...	...
Bananas	1 med.	100	320.0	320	0.310	0.31	4.4	4.4	9.7	9.7	...	...	34.0	34
Berries														
Blackberry	2/3 c.	100	...	...	0.260	0.26	...	...	13.7	13.7	...	...	...	...
Blueberry	2/3 c.	100	91.0	91	0.120	0.12	...	...	8.0	8.0	...	...	...	...
Raspberry, sweetened	3/4 c.	100	38.0	38	0.210	0.21	...	...	5.0	5.0	...	...	...	...
Strawberry, sweetened	2/3 c.	100	61.0	61	0.160	0.16	4.0	4.0	9.0	9.0	...	...	60.0	60
Cantaloupe, diced	2/3 c.	100	36.0	36	0.260	0.26	3.1	3.1	6.8	6.8	...	...	120.0	120
Cherries, sour, red, pitted	2/3 c.	100	85.0	85	0.070	0.07	...	...	6.0	6.0	...	...	...	...
Figs, small	3	114	148.2	130	0.388	0.34	...	...	16.0	14.0	...	...	...	...
Grapefruit, small	1/2	120	25.0	21	0.288	0.24	3.6	3.0	3.4	2.8	...	...	180.0	150
Grapes, 1 bunch	3 1/2 ozs.	100	85.0	85	0.050	0.05	1.6	1.6	5.2	5.2	...	...	...	...

Oranges, small	1	100	31.0	31	0.220	0.22	1.9	1.9	5.1	5.1			210.0	210
Peaches, sweetened	½ c.	100	20.0	20	0.120	0.12	1.7	1.7	4.0	4.0			96.0	96
Pineapple	3½ ozs.	100	75.0	75	0.170	0.17	..	..	6.0	6.0			..	..
Rhubarb, sweetened	3½ ozs.	100	29.0	29	0.070	0.07	..	..	4.0	4.0			..	..
Watermelon, diced	1 c.	150	49.5	33	0.450	0.30	5.4	3.6	0.9	0.6			96.0	64
Fruits, canned														
Apricots	½ c.	125	67.5	54	0.125	0.10	..	..	0.6	0.5			..	..
Blackberries	½ c.	125	30.0	24	0.100	0.08	..	..	17.5	14.0			..	..
Blueberries	½ c.	125	48.7	39	0.087	0.07	..	..	5.2	4.2			..	..
Cherries, sweet	½ c.	125	196.2	157	0.150	0.12	..	..	3.7	3.0			..	..
Peaches	½ c.	125	28.8	23	0.088	0.07	0.3	0.2	0.6	0.5			..	..
Pineapple	½ c.	125	88.7	71			..	..	1.0	0.8			..	..
Plums, purple	½ c.	125	33.7	27	0.100	0.08	..	..	1.2	1.0			..	..
Fruit, dried														
Apricots, small	6 halves	30	..	..	0.225	0.75	..	..	1.4	4.7			..	..
Dates, pitted	5	45	..	..	0.351	0.78	..	..	11.1	24.7			..	..
Figs, large	2	40	128.0	320	0.208	0.52	..	..	12.8	32.0			..	..
Prunes	5 med.	35	..	..	0.126	0.36	..	..	1.9	5.4			..	..
Raisins, seedless	3 tbsp.	30	98.0	327	0.030	0.10	1.4	4.5	3.0	10.0			36.0	120
Fruit Juices														
Canned fruit juice														
Apple	½ c.	120	42.0	35	..		1.0	0.8	0.2	0.2			..	..
Grapefruit	½ c.	120	15.6	13	0.204	0.17	..	..	2.3	1.9			..	..
Lemon	½ c.	120	61.2	51	0.156	0.13	1.0	0.8	0.2	0.2			120.0	100
Orange	½ c.	120	28.8	24	0.120	0.10	..	..	2.8	2.3			169.0	141
Pineapple	½ c.	120	115.2	96			..	..	1.1	0.9			..	..
Frozen or fresh														
Apple	½ c.	120	36.0	30	0.024	0.02	0.5	0.4	1.8	1.5	0.7	0.6	28.8	24
Grape	½ c.	120	25.2	21	0.048	0.04	0.4	0.3	3.6	3.0			..	..
Grapefruit	½ c.	120	16.8	14	0.192	0.16	0.8	0.7	1.6	1.3			120.0	100
Lemon, single	½ c.	120	46.8	39	0.108	0.09	..	..	1.2	1.0			..	..
Orange, fresh	½ c.	120	31.2	26	0.168	0.14	0.4	0.3	2.6	2.2	14.4	12	141.6	118
Orange, frozen	½ c.	120	26.4	22	0.168	0.14	0.4	0.3	2.6	2.2	14.4	12	110.4	92
Pineapple	½ c.	120	88.8	74	0.144	0.12	..	..	1.2	1.0			..	..
Legumes, cooked														
Mung bean	½ c.	32 (dry)	182.4	570	0.800	2.50	2.4	7.5	46.4	145	66.9	209	22.4	70
Cowpeas	½ c.	32 (dry)	(67.2)	(210)	0.397	1.24	6.7	21.0	140.5	439	82.2	257	76.9	240
Garbanzos	½ c.	32 (dry)	172.8	540	0.400	1.25	3.2	10.0	40.0	125	78.4	245	76.8	240
Lentils	½ c.	32 (dry)	156.8	490	0.480	1.50	4.2	13.2	34.2	107	71.4	223	41.6	130
Lima beans	½ c.	32 (dry)	176.0	550	0.416	1.30	3.1	9.8	41.0	128	..	..	54.4	130
Navy beans	½ c.	32 (dry)	..	..	0.387	1.21	..	..	40.0	125	..	..	160.0	500
Kidney beans	½ c.	32 (dry)	..	..	0.208	0.65	..	..	57.6	180	..	..	..	..
Split peas	½ c.	32 (dry)	105.0	328	0.700	2.18	5.9	18.4	16.3	51	64.3	201	48.0	150
Soy beans	½ c.	32 (dry)	204.8	640	0.538	1.68	19.5	61.0	71.7	224	108.8	340	64.0	200
Soy flour	1 c.	90 (dry)	590.4	656	1.512	1.68	63.0	70.0	383.4	426	202.5	225	184.5	205

TABLE 6. Lesser Known Vitamins in Foods*: Vitamin B₆, pantothenic acid, biotin, folic acid, choline, and inositol content of foods, edible portion (Continued)

Food	Portion		Vitamin B$_6$		Pantothenic Acid		Biotin		Folic Acid		Choline		Inositol	
	Amt.	Wt. Gm.	Mcg./portion	Mcg./100 Gm.	Mg./portion	Mg./100 Gm.	Mcg./portion	Mcg./100 Gm.	Mcg./portion	Mcg./100 Gm.	Mg./portion	Mg./100 Gm.	Mg./portion	Mg./100 Gm.
Meat and Poultry†														
Beef														
Ground	3½ ozs.	100	460.0‡	460	0.440‡	0.44	..	..	6.9	6.9	290.7	510	..	..
Liver	2 ozs.	57	378.5	664	5.324	9.34	54.7	96.0	167.6	294.0	82.0	82	29.1	51
Rib roast, lean	3 ozs.	100	480.0‡	480	0.600‡	0.60	3.4	3.4	..	..	68.0	68	..	..
Round	3 ozs.	100	495.0‡	495	0.520‡	0.52	2.6	2.6	10.5	10.5	..	..	11.5	11.5
Lamb														
Leg	3 ozs.	100	320.0‡	320	0.620‡	0.62	5.9	5.9	3.3	3.3	84.0	84	58.0	58
Liver	2 ozs.	57	..	..	4.047	7.10	72.4	127.0	157.3	276.0	..	76	..	..
Loin chop	3 ozs.	100	330.0‡	330	0.590‡	0.59	..	..	..	..	76.0	..	..	..
Veal														
Chop	3½ ozs.	100	430.0‡	430	0.550‡	0.50	2.0	2.0	..	..	96.0	96	33.0	33
Leg	3½ ozs.	100	200.0	200	0.914	0.914	..	..	..	..	132.0	132	..	..
Shoulder	3½ ozs.	100	300.0	300	..	..	..	..	..	..	93.0	93	..	..
Stew meat	3½ ozs.	100	330.0	330	0.852	0.852	..	..	4.6	4.6	96.0	96	..	..
Pork														
Bacon	2 sl.	16	88.0‡	550	0.070‡	0.440	1.2	7.6	..	..	12.8	80	6.9	43
Ham	3½ ozs.	100	440.0‡	440	0.640‡	0.640	5.0	5.0	10.6	10.6	122.0	122	31.0	31
Liver	2 ozs.	57	..	..	3.994	7.008	57.0	100.0	126.0	221.0	314.6	552	..	..
Loin	3½ ozs.	100	480.0‡	480	0.400‡	0.440	5.2	5.2	2.4	2.4	77.0	77	45.0	45
Poultry														
Chicken														
Dark meat	3½ ozs.	100	(25.0)	(25)	0.692	0.692	10.0	10.0	2.8	2.8	..	..	47.0	47
White meat	3½ ozs.	100	(130.0)	(130)	0.804	0.804	11.3	11.3	3.0	3.0	..	..	48.0	48
Turkey	3½ ozs.	100	..	..	0.748	0.748	..	..	7.5	7.5	..	60	..	..
Bologna, A. & P.	2 ozs.	57	65.0	130	..	..	..	..	..	..	34.2	57	..	..
Frankfurter, A. & P.	1	50	108.3	190	0.212	0.425	..	..	..	..	28.5	48	..	..
Sausage, pork, A. & P.	2 ozs.	57	..	..	0.321	0.563	..	..	6.5	11.5	27.4	..	..	..
Fish and Shellfish														
Fish														
Halibut, canned	3½ ozs.	100	(110.0)	(110)	0.150	0.150	8.0	8.0	..	..	..	..	17.0	17
Mackerel, Pacific, canned	3½ ozs.	100	270.0	270	0.470	0.470	18.0	18.0	0.6	0.6	..	..	..	..
Salmon, canned	3½ ozs.	100	450.0	450	0.580	0.580	15.0	15.0	0.5	0.5	..	..	17.0	17
Tuna, canned	3½ ozs.	100	670.0	670	0.420	0.420	3.0	3.0	1.8	1.8	..	..	..	..
Sardines, Pacific, canned	3½ ozs.	100	280.0	280	0.600	0.600	24.0	24.0	0.5	0.5	..	..	..	..
Shellfish, canned														
Clams	3½ ozs.	100	83.0	83	0.590	0.590	..	..	2.0	2.0	..	..	..	..
Crabs	3½ ozs.	100	364.0	364	..	..	..	..	0.4	0.4	..	..	..	..

Food	Measure													
Oysters	3½ ozs.	100	37.0	37	0.490	0.490	8.7	8.7	11.3	11.3	..	..	44.0	44
Shrimp	3½ ozs.	100	111.0	111	0.210	0.210	..	..	1.8	1.8	..	..	..	..
Nuts and Oily Fruits														
Almonds	12–15	15	15.0	100	0.087	0.578	2.7	18.0	6.7	45.0	..	..	..	..
Brazil nuts	2 med.	15	..	..	0.035	0.231	..	..	0.7	4.5	..	..	..	..
Cashews	6–8	15	..	..	0.174	1.62	..	..	4.1	27.6	..	..	..	..
Coconut, fresh	½ oz.	15	..	..	0.049	0.330	..	..	10.0	66.6	..	..	..	..
Filbert	10–12	15	..	..	0.172	1.146	5.1	34.0	8.5	56.5	..	..	27.0	180
Peanuts, roasted	15–17	15	45.0	300	0.320	2.137	4.0	27.0	4.0	27.0	24.3	162	..	..
Pecan halves	12	15	..	..	0.256	1.707	5.5	37.0	11.5	77.0	7.5	50	..	..
Walnut halves	8–15	15	144.0	960	0.146	0.970	6.2	39.0	8.5	56.5	..	..	28.8	180
Peanut butter	1 tbsp.	16	48.0	300	0.400	2.500	..	..	8.5	56.5	23.2	145	..	..
Fruits, oily														
Avocado, Fuerte (cubed)	½ c.	75	457.5	610	0.675	0.90	4.1	5.5	22.5	30.0	..	..	10.0	10.0
Olive, ripe, mammoth	6	40	6.4	16	0.008	0.02	..	..	0.3	0.7	..	..	..	..
Vegetables														
Fresh or frozen														
Asparagus	3½ ozs.	100	136.0	136	0.620	0.62	..	..	109.0	109.0	10.0	10.0	10.0	10.0
Beans, Lima	3½ ozs.	100	170.0	170	0.450	0.45	..	..	34.0	34.0	..	..	..	..
Beans, snap, green	3½ ozs.	100	63.0	63	0.200	0.20	1.9	1.9	27.5	27.5	42.0	42.0	42.0	42
Beets (diced)	⅔ c.	100	(37.0)	(37)	0.170	0.17	..	..	13.5	13.5	..	..	21.0	21
Broccoli	⅔ c.	100	171.0	171	1.290	1.29	..	..	53.5	53.5	..	..	..	..
Brussels sprouts	3½ ozs.	100	162.0	162	0.720	0.72	2.4	2.4	49.0	49.0	23.0	23.0	95.0	95
Cabbage (fine shreds)	1 c.	100	120.0	120	0.260	0.26	1.4	2.5	32.3	32.3	13.4	13.4	26.4	48
Carrots (grated)	½ c.	55	66.0	120	0.150	0.27	..	..	4.4	8.0	7.0	13.4	..	..
Cauliflower (buds)	1 c.	100	177.0	177	1.010	1.01	17.0	17.0	22.2	22.2	..	..	95.0	95
Celery (diced)	1 c.	100	..	..	0.430	0.43	6.0	6.0	7.0	7.0	..	..	..	..
Corn	3½ ozs.	100	222.0	222	0.890	0.89	3.1	3.1	28.0	28.0	..	..	..	..
Lettuce	¼ hd.	100	(71.0)	(71)	0.360	0.36	..	..	21.0	21.0	..	..	55.0	55
Mixed vegetables	3½ ozs.	100	122.0	122	0.310	0.31	3.8	3.5	16.0	16.0	..	..	..	..
Onion (2½ in.)	1	110	(69.3)	(63)	0.187	0.17	21.0	21.0	11.0	10.0	..	..	..	..
Peas, cow	3½ ozs.	100	118.0	118	0.400	0.40	9.4	9.4	41.0	41.0	..	..	96.8	88
Peas, green	3½ ozs.	100	150.0	150	0.820	0.82	..	..	25.0	25.0	97.0	97.0	240.0	240
Potatoes, peeled	1 med.	100	220.0	220	0.400	0.40	4.3	4.3	6.8	6.8	75.0	75.0	162.0	162
Potatoes, sweet	3½ ozs.	100	320.0	320	0.930	0.93	..	..	12.0	12.0	29.0	29.0	29.0	29
Squash, winter	3½ ozs.	100	91.0	91	0.490	0.49	..	..	12.0	12.0	11.5	11.5	66.0	66
Squash, yellow	3½ ozs.	100	63.0	63	0.390	0.39	4.4	4.0	17.0	17.0	..	..	..	..
Tomato	1 small	110	..	..	0.341	0.31	9.6	16.0	8.8	8.0	..	..	50.6	46
Mushrooms, fresh	2 ozs.	60	(27.0)	(45)	1.626	2.71	..	..	14.4	24.0	..	..	10.2	17
Greens														
Beet	3½ ozs.	100	..	..	0.260	0.26	2.7	2.7	60.0	60.0	..	..	21.0	21
Kale	3½ ozs.	100	185.0	185	1.290	1.29	..	..	70.0	70.0	..	..	..	..
Mustard	3½ ozs.	100	133.0	133	0.250	0.25	..	..	60.0	60.0	22.0	22.0	22.0	22
Spinach	3½ ozs.	100	198.0	198	0.310	0.31	6.9	6.9	75.0	75.0	22.0	22.0	27.0	27
Turnip	3½ ozs.	100	98.0	98	0.380	0.38	..	..	42.0	42.0	27.0	27.0	46.0	46

TABLE 6. Lesser Known Vitamins in Foods*: Vitamin B_6, pantothenic acid, biotin, folic acid, choline, and inositol content of foods, edible portion (Continued)

Food	Portion Amt.	Wt. Gm.	Vitamin B_6 Mcg./portion	Mcg./100 Gm.	Pantothenic Acid Mg./portion	Mg./100 Gm.	Biotin Mcg./portion	Mcg./100 Gm.	Folic Acid Mcg./portion	Mcg./100 Gm.	Choline Mg./portion	Mg./100 Gm.	Inositol Mg./portion	Mg./100 Gm.
Vegetables (Continued)														
Canned with liquid														
Asparagus, green	½ c.	120	90.0	75	0.240	0.20	2.0	1.7	32.4	27.0	..	..	..	..
Beans														
Lima	½ c.	120	97.2	81	0.132	0.11	..	..	15.6	13.0	..	..	..	..
Green string	½ c.	120	51.6	43	0.084	0.07	1.5	1.3	14.4	12.0	..	..	..	..
Beets (diced)	½ c.	125	67.5	54	0.125	0.10	..	..	3.5	2.8	..	..	..	..
Carrots (diced)	½ c.	125	51.2	41	0.137	0.11	1.9	1.5	4.1	3.3	..	..	..	..
Corn	½ c.	125	270.0	216	0.275	0.22	2.7	2.2	9.6	7.7	..	..	..	..
Mushrooms	½ c.	120	75.6	63	1.128	0.94	8.7	7.3	4.7	3.9	..	..	20.4	17
Peas														
Cow	½ c.	125	66.2	53	..	..	2.6	2.1	32.5	26.0	..	..	..	..
Green	½ c.	125	55.0	44	0.212	0.17	2.8	2.3	12.9	10.3	..	..	..	..
Spinach	½ c.	120	114.0	95	0.071	0.059	2.2	1.8	58.8	49.0	..	..	..	..
Tomatoes	½ c.	120	181.2	151	0.276	0.23	..	..	4.4	3.7	..	..	..	..
Tomato juice	½ c.	120	230.4	192	0.360	0.30	..	..	8.0	6.7	..	..	..	..
Miscellaneous														
Chocolate	1 oz.	28.4	(6.5)	(23)	0.054	0.19	9.0	32.0	28.1	99.0	..	..	24.1	85
Molasses	1 tbsp.	20	(54.0)	(270)	0.092	0.46	1.8	9.0	1.9	9.5	17.2	86	30.0	150
Yeast, brewer's	1 tbsp.	8	193.5	2419	0.880	11.0	16.0	200.0	161.8	2022.0	19.2	240	..	..
Food yeast, torula	1 tbsp.	8	280.0	3500	0.800	10.0	8.0	100.0	240.0	3000.0	20.0	250	21.6	270
Honey	1 tbsp.	20	2.0	10	0.012	0.06	..	..	0.6	3.0	..	..	..	..

Dots indicate that no representative value was found in the literature for particular constituent.

*Table adapted from Hardinge, M. G. and Crooks, H., J. Am. Dietet. A. 38:240, 1961, by permission of the authors and the Journal.

†Raw values, except where indicated.

‡Cooked values.

Supplementary References

Bunnell, R. H., et al.: Alpha-tocopherol content of foods. Am. J. Clin. Nutr., 17:1, 1965.

Dicks-Bushnell, M. W., and Davis, K. C.: Vitamin E content of infant formulas and cereals. Am. J. Clin. Nutr., 20:262, 1967.

Polansky, M. M., and Murphy, E. W.: Vitamin B_6 components in fruits and nuts. J. Am. Dietet. A., 48:109, 1966.

Roels, O. A.: Present knowledge of vitamin E. Nutr. Rev., 25:33, 1967.

TABLE 7. Alcoholic and Carbonated Beverages

Beverage	Average Portion	Weight Gm.	Calories	Carbo-hydrate Gm.	Alcohol* Gm.
Alcoholic Beverages:					
Ale, mild...................	8 oz. glass	230	98	8	9
Beer, average...............	8 oz. glass	240	114	11	9
Benedictine.................	cordial glass	20	69	7	7
Brandy, California..........	brandy glass	30	73	..	11
Cider, fermented............	6 oz. glass	180	71	2	9
Cordial, anisette............	cordial glass	20	74	7	7
Creme de menthe...........	cordial glass	20	67	6	7
Curacao...................	cordial glass	20	54	6	6
Daiquiri...................	cocktail glass	100	122	5	15
Eggnog, Christmas..........	4 oz. punch cup	123	335	18	15
Gin Rickey.................	4 oz. glass	120	150	1	21
Gin, dry...................	1 jigger, 1½ oz.	43	105	..	15
Highball, average..........	8 oz. glass	240	166	..	24
Manhattan.................	cocktail glass, 3½ oz.	100	164	8	19
Old Fashioned..............	4 oz. glass	100	179	4	24
Planter's punch.............	3½ oz. glass	100	175	8	22
Rum......................	1 jigger, 1½ oz.	43	105	..	15
Tom Collins.................	10 oz. glass	300	180	9	22
Whiskey, rye...............	1 jigger, 1½ oz.	43	119	..	17
Scotch.............	1 jigger, 1½ oz.	43	105	..	15
Wines:					
Champagne................	4 oz. glass	120	84	3	11
Muscatel or port............	3½ oz. glass	100	158	14	15
Sauterne...................	3½ oz. glass	100	84	4	10
Sherry, domestic.............	2 oz. glass	60	84	5	9
Table type................	3½ oz. glass	100	85	..	10
Vermouth, French...........	3½ oz. glass	100	105	1	15
Vermouth, Italian............	3½ oz. glass	100	167	12	18
Carbonated Beverages:					
Coca-cola..................	6 oz. bottle	170	78	20	..
Ginger ale.................	6 oz. bottle	230	80	21	..
Pepsi-cola.................	8 oz. bottle	230	106	28	..
Soda, fruit flavor...........	8 oz. bottle	230	94	24	..
Root beer.................	8 oz. bottle	230	106	28	..

Values taken from Church, C. F., and Church, H. N.: Food Values of Portions Commonly Used. 10th ed. Philadelphia, Lippincott, 1966.

* Alcohol yields 7 calories per gram.

TABLE 8. Acid-Base Reaction of Foods

Potentially Acid or Acid Ash Foods	Potentially Basic or Alkaline Ash Foods
Breads, all types	Fruits, all types (except cranberries, plums and prunes*)
Cakes and cookies, plain	Jams and jellies, honey
Cereals and crackers	Milk, cream and buttermilk†
Cheese, all types	Molasses
Eggs	Nuts: almonds, coconut, chestnuts
Fish and shellfish	Vegetables, all types (except corn and lentils)
Fruits: cranberries, plums and prunes	
Macaroni, spaghetti, noodles	
Meats and poultry	
Nuts: Brazil, filberts, peanuts, walnuts	
Vegetables: corn and lentils	

Neutral Foods

Butter or margarine	Syrups
Candy, plain	Starches, corn and arrowroot
Cooking fats and oils	Sugars

* Ash alkaline in vitro, partly acid in vivo, because organic acids are not completely utilized.

† Calcium largely excreted into intestinal tract. Therefore, effect upon pH of serum and urine tends to be acid because of high phosphate content.

TABLE 9. Blood and Urine Components

BLOOD		Deviations in Disease	
	Normal Range	Decreased	Increased

Hematology

Red blood cells

(erythrocytes).......	4.5–5 million per cu. mm.	Anemia Hemorrhage Chronic infectious diseases	Polycythemia Dehydration
White blood cells (leukocytes).........	5–10 thousand per cu. mm.	Leukopenia	Acute infections Leukemias
Hemoglobin, men......	14–16 Gm./100 ml.	Anemias Prolonged dietary deficiency of iron	Polycythemia Dehydration
women....	13.5–15 Gm./100 ml.		
Hematocrit...........	$\frac{\text{Red cells}}{\text{Serum}} = 42\text{–}50\%$ cells	Anemias Prolonged dietary deficiency of iron	Polycythemia

Chemistry

Cholesterol...........	150–250 mg./100 ml.	Pernicious anemia Malnutrition Hyperthyroidism	Atherosclerosis Biliary obstruction Myxedema Uncontrolled diabetes Renal disease
Glucose (true)........	65–110 mg./100 ml.	Hyperinsulinism Addison's disease	Diabetes mellitus Cushing's syndrome
Nonprotein nitrogen....	15–35 mg./100 ml.		Dehydration Renal disease
Uric acid...........	2.5–5 mg./100 ml.		Gout Nephrosis
Urea nitrogen.......	10–20 mg./100 ml.		Renal disease
Creatinine.........	0.7–1.5 mg./100 ml.		Renal disease
Ammonia (in blood)....	40–70 mcg./100 ml.		Liver disease
Protein, total...........	6–8 Gm./100 ml.	Nephrosis	Multiple myeloma (Bence-Jones protein)
Albumin...........	3.5–5.5 Gm./100 ml.	Nephritis with edema Liver disease	
Globulin...........	1.5–3 Gm./100 ml.		Liver disease

Minerals

Calcium...........	9–11 mg./100 ml.	Renal disease Hypoparathyroidism Chronic rickets Steatorrhea	Hyperparathyroidism Multiple myeloma
Chlorides..........	100–106 mEq./liter	Renal disease Addison's disease Vomiting	Dehydration Renal disease

TABLE 9. Blood and Urine Components (Continued)

BLOOD

	Normal Range	Deviations in Disease	
		Decreased	Increased
Chemistry (Continued)			
Magnesium.........	1.8–3 mg./100 ml.	Severe malnutrition Vomiting Diarrhea	
Phosphorus.........	3.0–4.5 mg./100 ml.	Rickets Renal disease Hyperparathyroidism	Hypoparathyroidism Renal disease Diabetic coma
Potassium..........	3.5–5.0 mEq./liter	Periodic paralysis	Addison's disease Renal disease
Sodium............	139–144 mEq./liter	Diabetic acidosis Addison's disease Diarrhea Dehydration	Dehydration
Other			
Bilirubin, total.......	0.3–1.1 mg./100 ml.		Jaundice
Carbon dioxide combining power...	24–29 mEq./liter or 53–64 Vol. %	Metabolic acidosis Hypoventilation	Metabolic alkalosis Hyperventilation
Phosphatase (alkaline)	2–4.5 units/100 ml. (Bodansky)		Certain bone diseases
Vitamin A..........	30–50 I.U./100 ml.	Cirrhosis Infectious hepatitis Myxedema Malnutrition	
Vitamin C (in blood)..	0.4–1.5 mg./100 ml.	Infection Dietary deficiency Leukemia	

COMPOSITION OF URINE

	Normal Range/24 Hrs.		Normal Range/24 Hrs.
Volume...............	1,000–1,500 ml.	Mineral salts:	
Specific gravity....1.003–1.030		Calcium....................	<250 mg.
pH........ 4.6–8		Chlorides (as NaCl)..........	10–15 Gm./L.
Total solids..............	30–70 Gm.	Magnesium.................	50–200 mg./L.
Nitrogenous constituents:		Oxalate....................	15–30 mg./L.
Total nitrogen.........	10–17 Gm./L.		
Urea.................	20–35 Gm./L.	Phosphate.................	1–1.2 Gm./L.
Uric acid.............	0.2–2.0 Gm./L.	Potassium..................	1.5–2.5 Gm./L.
Creatinine............	15–25 mg./Kg.		
Ammonia.............	0.5–1.0 Gm./L.	Sodium....................	4–5 Gm./L.
Amino acids..........	0.4–1.0 Gm./L.	Sulfates (total)..............	1–2 Gm./L.

TABLE 10. Equivalent Weights and Measures

Weight Equivalents

	Milligram	Gram	Kilo-gram	Grain	Ounce	Pound
1 microgram (mcg.).......	0.001	0.000001				
1 milligram (mg.).........	1.	0.001		0.0154		
1 gram (Gm.)............	1,000.	1.	0.001	15.4	0.035	0.0022
1 kilogram (Kg.)..........	1,000,000.	1,000.	1.	15,400.	35.2	2.2
1 grain (gr.).............	64.8	0.065		1.		
1 ounce (oz.).............		28.3		437.5	1.	0.063
1 pound (lb.)............		453.6	0.454		16.0	1.

Volume Equivalents

	Cubic Millimeter	Cubic Centimeter	Liter	Fluid Ounce	Pint	Quart
1 cubic millimeter (cu. mm.).......	1.	0.001				
1 cubic centimeter (cc.)..........	1,000.		0.001			
1 liter (L.)....................	1,000,000.	1,000.	1.	33.8	2.1	1.05
1 fluid ounce.................		30.(29.57)	0.03	1.		
1 pint (pt.)..................		473.	0.473	16.	1.	
1 quart (qt.).................		946.	0.946	32.	2.	1.

Linear Equivalents

	Millimeter	Centimeter	Meter	Inch	Foot	Yard
1 millimeter (mm.)............	1.	0.1	0.001	0.039	0.00325	0.0011
1 centimeter (cm.)............	10.	1.		0.39	0.0325	0.011
1 meter (M.).................	1,000.	100.	1.	39.37	3.25	1.08
1 inch (in.)..................	25.4	2.54	0.025	1.	0.083	0.028
1 foot (ft.).................	304.8	30.48	0.305	1.12	1.	0.33
1 yard (yd.).................	914.4	91.44	0.914	36.0	3.	1.

Comparative Values of Weight and Volume of Water

1 liter	=	1 kilo.	=	2.2 lbs.
1 fluid ounce	=	30 Gm.	=	1.04 ozs.
1 pint	=	473 Gm.	=	1.04 lbs.
1 quart	=	.946 kilo.	=	2.1 lbs.

Table of Common Measures and Metric Equivalents

1 tsp.	=	5 cc.
1 tbsp.	=	14 cc. (approx. 15 Gm.)
1 cup	=	225 cc. (approx. 240 Gm.)

Comparative Temperatures

	Centigrade	Fahrenheit
Boiling water, sea level........	100	212
Body temperature............	37	98.6
Tropical temperature..........	30	89
Room temperature, average.....	20	70
Freezing....................	0	32

Table of Measures and Approximate Weights

3 teaspoons......................	1 tbsp.	*1 tablespoon liquid....................	½ oz.
16 tablespoons......................	1 cup	1 tablespoon flour....................	¼ oz.
½ cup............................	1 gill	1 tablespoon sugar...................	⅗ oz.
2 cups............................	1 pt.	*1 cup liquid.......................	8 ozs.
4 cups............................	1 qt.	1 cup flour........................	4½ ozs.
2 pints............................	1 qt.	1 cup butter.......................	8 ozs.
4 quarts............................	1 gal.	1 cup sugar.......................	10 ozs.
1 tablespoon butter...................	½ oz.		

*Water or milk.

TABLE 11. Height and Weight for Age Percentile Standards, Boyd 1952

AGE YEARS	HEIGHT PERCENTILES					WEIGHT PERCENTILES				
	10	25	50	75	90	10	25	50	75	90
					BOYS					
	Ins.	Ins.	Ins.	Ins.	Ins.	Lbs.	Lbs.	Lbs.	Lbs.	Lbs.
2.............	32.7	33.2	33.8	34.3	34.6	24.2	25.8	27.3	28.7	30.6
3.............	36.0	36.6	37.2	37.6	38.1	28.9	30.4	31.7	33.5	35.5
4.............	39.0	39.7	40.2	40.8	41.4	30.0	33.1	34.8	35.9	37.9
5.............	41.7	42.4	43.0	43.6	44.3	37.3	38.8	40.6	42.8	45.4
6.............	44.1	44.9	45.7	46.3	47.0	41.7	43.2	45.4	48.3	51.6
7.............	46.3	47.2	48.1	48.9	49.9	46.1	47.8	50.9	54.7	58.6
8.............	48.5	49.4	50.5	51.4	52.6	50.5	52.9	57.4	61.9	66.6
9.............	50.6	51.7	52.8	53.8	54.8	55.1	58.6	64.4	70.1	75.2
10.............	52.5	53.7	54.9	56.1	57.0	60.4	64.8	71.4	78.0	84.2
11.............	54.3	55.4	56.7	58.2	59.1	65.7	71.2	78.9	86.4	93.5
12.............	56.0	57.1	58.7	60.3	61.5	71.0	77.8	86.0	94.8	102.7
13.............	58.1	59.3	61.2	62.6	64.3	76.9	85.3	95.7	105.8	114.6
14.............	60.4	62.1	64.1	65.5	67.2	88.0	98.5	111.1	119.5	128.7
15.............	63.0	65.0	66.9	68.3	69.8	101.6	112.2	124.3	134.5	143.3
16.............	65.6	67.3	68.9	70.4	71.7	112.4	122.6	133.8	146.4	157.4
17.............	66.5	68.2	69.8	71.2	72.4	120.4	130.1	139.8	153.9	169.3
18.............	67.1	68.6	70.2	71.5	72.7	127.0	134.3	142.4	158.7	173.3
					GIRLS					
2.............	31.8	32.7	33.5	34.3	34.9	21.6	23.6	25.8	27.6	29.1
3.............	34.9	35.8	37.0	38.0	38.7	25.6	27.3	30.6	32.4	34.4
4.............	37.8	38.9	40.4	41.3	42.0	29.3	31.3	35.5	37.5	40.1
5.............	40.5	41.6	43.3	44.3	45.0	33.1	35.9	40.3	43.4	45.9
6.............	43.1	44.0	45.9	47.2	47.7	37.0	40.6	45.4	49.6	51.6
7.............	45.4	46.2	48.5	49.8	50.3	41.4	45.2	51.1	55.8	60.0
8.............	47.7	48.4	51.0	52.2	52.8	46.2	50.0	58.0	61.9	70.5
9.............	49.8	50.7	53.5	54.6	55.2	51.1	56.0	65.7	70.5	82.5
10.............	51.9	53.1	55.6	56.9	58.0	56.0	62.2	74.3	81.8	93.9
11.............	53.7	55.7	58.1	59.7	60.9	60.8	69.4	83.8	94.6	104.7
12.............	55.5	59.0	61.3	62.6	63.6	70.5	80.9	96.1	106.5	115.1
13.............	58.3	61.0	63.9	65.1	65.9	79.4	91.5	108.9	114.9	124.8
14.............	60.5	62.2	65.0	66.1	67.2	85.5	98.3	116.6	121.7	133.6
15.............	61.8	63.2	65.6	66.5	67.7	89.1	102.7	121.0	127.0	140.7
16.............	62.4	63.8	65.9	66.8	68.0	91.5	106.0	123.9	131.0	144.2
17.............	62.6	64.1	66.1	67.0	68.3	93.0	108.5	125.7	133.8	145.9
18.............	62.7	64.3	66.2	67.6	68.9	93.7	110.0	126.1	135.4	146.8

From Hathaway, M. L.: Heights and Weights of Children and Youth in the United States. Home Economics Res. Bulletin No. 2, U.S.D.A., Washington, D. C., 1957.

TABLE 12. Height-Weight Table for Men and Women

Weight for height classifications based on measurements of young college men and women.*
(Measurements made without shoes or clothing)

Height in Inches	WEIGHT IN POUNDS					
	Underweight	Slender	Normal	Stocky	Overweight	Obese
YOUNG MEN						
63..................	111	121	131	141	151	170
64..................	114	124	134	144	155	175
65..................	117	128	138	148	159	179
66..................	120	131	141	152	163	184
67..................	123	134	145	156	167	188
68..................	126	138	149	160	171	193
69..................	130	141	152	164	175	198
70..................	133	145	156	168	180	203
71..................	136	148	160	172	184	209
72..................	140	152	165	177	189	214
73..................	143	156	169	181	194	219
74..................	147	160	173	186	199	225
75..................	151	164	178	191	204	231
76..................	155	168	182	196	209	237
77..................	159	173	187	201	215	243
78..................	163	177	192	206	220	249
YOUNG WOMEN						
58..................	88	95	103	111	119	134
59..................	90	98	106	114	122	138
60..................	93	101	109	117	125	142
61..................	95	104	112	120	129	146
62..................	98	106	115	124	132	150
63..................	101	109	118	127	136	154
64..................	103	112	122	131	140	158
65..................	106	116	125	134	144	162
66..................	109	119	128	138	148	167
67..................	112	122	132	142	152	172
68..................	115	126	136	146	156	176
69..................	119	129	140	150	160	181
70..................	122	133	143	154	165	186
71..................	125	136	147	158	170	192
72..................	129	140	152	163	174	197
73..................	132	144	156	167	179	202
74..................	136	148	160	172	184	208

* Underweight = 15 per cent or more below average weight.
Slender = 7.5–15 per cent below average weight.
Normal = Average weight for college men, 21–29 years of age and for college women, 17–29 years of age.
Stocky = 7.5–15 per cent above average weight.
Overweight = 15–30 per cent above average weight.
Obese = More than 30 per cent above average weight.

From Sargent, D. W.: Weight-Height Relationship of Young Men and Women. Am. J. Clin. Nutr., 13:318, 1963.

Bibliography

PART ONE

PRINCIPLES OF NUTRITION

GENERAL REFERENCES

Books:

Aykroyd, W. R.: Food for Man. Long Island City, Pergamon Press, 1964.

Anderson, L., and Browe, J. H.: Nutrition and Family Health Services. Philadelphia, Saunders, 1960.

Beaton, G. H., and McHenry, E. W.: Nutrition. A Comprehensive Treatise. Vol. III. Nutritional Status, Assessment and Application. New York, Academic Press, 1966.

Bogert, L. J., Briggs, G. M., and Calloway, D. H.: Nutrition and Physical Fitness. Ed. 8. Philadelphia, Saunders, 1966.

Brock, J. F.: Recent Advances in Human Nutrition. Boston, Little Brown & Co., 1961.

Chaney, M. S., and Ross, M. L.: Nutrition. Ed. 7. Boston, Houghton, 1966.

Davidson, S., and Passmore, R.: Human Nutrition and Dietetics. Ed. 3. Baltimore, Williams and Wilkins, 1966.

Eppright, E., Pattison, M., and Barbour, H.: Teaching Nutrition. Ames, Iowa. Iowa State College Press, 1963.

Fleck, H. C., and Munves, E. D.: Introduction to Nutrition. New York, Macmillan, 1962.

Goodhart, R. S., and Wohl, M. G.: Manual of Clinical Nutrition. Philadelphia, Lea and Febiger, 1964.

Guthrie, H. A.: Introductory Nutrition. St. Louis, Mosby, 1967.

Heinz Handbook of Nutrition. Ed. 3. New York, McGraw-Hill, 1967.

Krause, M. V.: Food, Nutrition and Diet Therapy. Ed. 4. Philadelphia, Saunders, 1966.

Lowenberg, M., Todhunter, E. N., and Wilson, E. D.: Food and Man. New York, John Wiley & Sons, 1968.

Martin, E. A.: Nutrition in Action. Ed. 2. New York, Holt, 1965.

McHenry, E. W.: Basic Nutrition. rev. ed. Philadelphia, J. B. Lippincott, 1963.

Mowry, L.: Basic Nutrition and Diet Therapy for Nurses. Ed. 3. St. Louis, Mosby, 1966.

Pike, R. L., and Brown, M. L.: Nutrition: An Integrated Approach. New York, John Wiley and Sons, 1967.

Robinson, C. H.: Normal and Therapeutic Nutrition. New York, Macmillan, 1967.

Taylor, C. M., and Pye, O. F.: Foundations of Nutrition. Ed. 6. New York, Macmillan, 1966.

Wayler, T. J., and Klein, R. S.: Applied Nutrition. New York, Macmillan, 1965.

Wilson, E. D., Fisher, K. H., and Fuqua, M. E.: Principles of Nutrition. Ed. 2. New York, John Wiley and Sons, 1966.

Wohl, M. G., and Goodhart, R. S.: Modern Nutrition in Health and Disease. Philadelphia, Lea and Febiger, 1964.

Journals and Annuals:

American Journal of Nursing
American Journal of Public Health
American Journal of Clinical Nutrition
Borden's Review of Nutrition Research
Food Research
Journal of the American Dietetic Association
Journal of Home Economics
Journal of Nutrition
Metabolism
Nutrition Abstracts and Reviews
Nutrition Reviews
Nutrition Today (Florida Citrus Com.)
World Review of Nutrition and Dietetics

Journal Articles:

Dietary adequacy and nutritional status in the United States. Dairy Coun. Digest, 38:31, 1967 (Nov.-Dec.).

Harris, R. S. (Ed.): Symposium on recent advances in the appraisal of the nutrient intake and the nutritional status of man. Am. J. Clin. Nutr., 11:331, 1962.

Hunscher, H. A., Leverton, R. M., and Cederquist, D.: The life cycle and its diet: symposium and bibliography. J. Home Econ., 49:101, 1957.

King, C. G.: Latest advances in nutrition. J. Am. Dietet. A., *38*:223, 1961.

————: Research and educational progress in nutrition. J. Am. Dietet. A., *42*:199, 1963.

Morris, E.: How does a nurse teach nutrition to patients? Am. J. Nursing, *60*:67, 1960.

Stiebling, H. K.: Food and nutrient consumption trends and consumer problems. Fed. Proc., *17*:770, 1958.

Todhunter, E. N.: Role of the home economist and dietitian. Fed. Proc., *17*:746, 1958.

Wellin, E.: In-patient dietary instruction and the hospital setting. J. Am. Dietet. A., *34*: 1179, 1958.

Books for Lay Readers:

Bieler, H. G.: Food is Your Best Medicine. New York, Random House, 1965.

Carter, R.: Your Food and Your Health. New York, Harper and Row, 1964.

Gerard, R. W.: Food for Life. Chicago, University of Chicago Press, 1965.

Graham, M. F.: Prescription for Life. New York, David McKay, 1966.

Howe, P. S.: Nutrition for Practical Nurses. Ed. 4. Philadelphia, Saunders, 1967.

Leverton, R. M.: Food Becomes You. Ames, Iowa, Iowa State Univ. Press. Garden City, Doubleday (paperback), 1965.

Mickelson, O.: Nutrition Science and You. Englewood Cliffs, N. J., Scholastic Books, 1964.

McHenry, E. W.: Food Without Fads. Philadelphia, J. B. Lippincott, 1960.

Peyton, A. B.: Practical Nutrition. Ed. 2. Philadelphia, J. B. Lippincott, 1962.

Shackelton, A. Dent: Practical Nurse Nutrition Education. Ed. 2. Philadelphia, Saunders, 1966.

Stare, F. J.: Eating for Good Health. Garden City, Doubleday, 1964.

Stefferud, A. (ed.): Food, The Yearbook of Agriculture 1959. U.S.D.A., Washington, D. C., 1959.

White, P. L.: Let's Talk About Food. Chicago, Am. Med. Ass., 1967.

Journal Articles in

Nutrition Today
Science Digest
Science News Letter
Today's Health

BIOCHEMISTRY AND PHYSIOLOGY

Books:

Albanese, A. A.: Newer Methods of Nutritional Biochemistry with Applications and Interpretations. New York, Academic Press, 1963.

Best, C. H., and Taylor, N. B.: The Human Body, Its Anatomy and Physiology. New York, Holt, Rinehart and Winston, 1963.

Best, C. H., and Taylor, N. B.: The Physiological Basis of Medical Practice. A Textbook of Applied Physiology. Ed. 8. Baltimore, Williams and Wilkins, 1966.

Cantarow, A., and Schepartz, B.: Biochemistry. Ed. 4. Philadelphia, Saunders, 1967.

Cantarow, A., and Trumper, M.: Clinical Biochemistry. Ed. 6. Philadelphia, Saunders, 1962.

Carlson, A. J., and Johnson, V. E.: The Machinery of the Body. Ed. 5. Chicago, Univ. Chicago Press, 1961.

Conn, E. E., and Stumpf, P. K.: Outlines of Biochemistry, New York, John Wiley and Sons, 1965.

Greisheimer, E. M., and Trayer, J. R.: Physiology and Anatomy. Ed. 8. Philadelphia, Lippincott, 1963.

Harper, H. A.: Review of Physiological Chemistry. Ed. 10. Los Altos, Cal., Lange Medical Pub., 1965.

Harrow, B., and Mazur, A.: Textbook of Biochemistry. Ed. 9. Philadelphia, Saunders, 1966.

Jevons, F. R.: The Biochemical Approach to Life. New York, Basic Books, 1964.

Kleiner, I. S., and Orten, J. M.: Biochemistry. Ed. 7. St. Louis, C. V. Mosby, 1966.

McDowall, R. J. S.: Handbook of Physiology. Ed. 43. Philadelphia, J. B. Lippincott, 1960.

Oser, B. L. (ed.): Hawk's Physiological Chemistry. Ed. 14, New York, Blakiston Div. McGraw-Hill, 1965.

West, E. S., *et al.*: Textbook of Biochemistry. Ed. 4. New York, Macmillan, 1966.

Journals:

American Journal of Physiology
Annual Review of Biochemistry
Annual Review of Physiology
Biochemical Journal
Journal of Biological Chemistry
Proceedings of Experimental Biology and Medicine
Physiological Reviews

HISTORY OF NUTRITION

Books:

Barber, M. I.: History of the American Dietetics Association. Philadelphia, J. B. Lippincott, 1959.

Beeuwkes, A. M., Todhunter, E. N., and Weigley, E. S.: Essays on History of Nutrition and Dietetics. Chicago, Am. Dietet. Ass., 1967.

Cummings, R. O.: The American and His Food. Chicago, Univ. Chicago Press, 1941.

Goldblith, S. A., and Joslyn, M. A.: Milestones in Nutrition. AVI Pub., Westport, Connecticut, 1964.

McCollum, E. V.: A History of Nutrition. Boston, Houghton Mifflin, 1957.

Orr, Lord Boyd: As I Recall. London, MacGibbon, 1966.

Todhunter, E. N.: The Story of Nutrition. *in* Food. The Yearbook of Agriculture, U.S.D.A., Washington, D. C., 1959.

Journal Articles:

Arrington, L. R.: Foods of the Bible. J. Am. Dietet. A., 35:816, 1959.

Carpenter, T. M.: The historical development of metabolism studies. J. Am. Dietet. A., 25:837, 1949.

Cooper, L. F.: Florence Nightingale's contribution to dietetics. J. Am. Dietet. A., 30:121, 1954.

Elvehjem, C. A.: A forty year look at nutrition research. J. Am. Dietet. A., 38:236, 1961.

McCollum, E. V.: An adventure in nutrition investigation. J. Am. Dietet. A., 35:806, 1959.

McCollum, E. V.: History of nutrition. World Rev. Nutr. Dietet., 1:1, 1959.

Rosen, G.: Metabolism: evolution of a concept. J. Am. Dietet. A., 31:861, 1955.

Sipple, H. L.: The Nutrition Foundation— First twenty-five years. Nutr. Rev., 24:353, 1966.

Stitt, K.: Nutritive value of diets today and fifty years ago. J. Am. Dietet. A., 36:433, 1960.

Todhunter, E. N.: Biographical sketches. J. Am. Dietet. A. (One or more sketches monthly of famous scientists in nutrition or related fields.)

GROWTH OF THE SCIENCE OF NUTRITION AND ITS APPLICATION

Books:

Barber, M. I.: History of the American Dietetics Association. Philadelphia, J. B. Lippincott, 1959.

Bourne, G. H. (ed.): World Review of Nutrition and Dietetics. Annual. New York, Hafner.

Hambidge, G.: The Story of FAO. New York, Van Nostrand, 1955.

Nat. Res. Council: Role of Nutrition in International Programs. Nat. Acad. Science, Washington, D. C., 1961.

Third World Food Survey. Rome, FAO, 1963.

World Food: World Health, 15: 1962 (Special issue on food).

Journal Articles:

Arrington, L. R.: Foods of the Bible. J. Am. Dietet. A., 35:816, 1959.

Berg, A. D.: Food for Peace—The U. S. effort in meeting world nutrition needs. J. Am. Dietet. A., 48:512, 1966.

Burney, L. E.: World health—A road to peace. J. Am. Dietet. A., 40:199, 1962.

Darby, W. J.: Basic contributions to medicine by research in nutrition. J.A.M.A., 180:816, 1962.

Davis, H. P.: Meeting foods needs with our agricultural abundance. J. Am. Dietet. A., 41:100, 1962.

Gortner, W. A.: International facets of U.S.D.A. nutrition research. J. Am. Dietet. A., 50:279, 1967.

György, P.: Education and training in nutrition. Am. J. Clin. Nutr., 10:1, 1962.

Holt, E. M., Jr.: Nutrition in a changing world. Am. J. Clin. Nutr., 11:543, 1962.

Johnson, O. C.: Nutrition education—what is the goal? Nutr. Rev., 23:353, 1966.

Leverton, R. M.: Nutrition programs in U.S.D.A. Am. J. Pub. Health, 56:812, 1966.

Pollack, H.: Nutritional problems as part of the total economy. Am. J. Clin. Nutr., 19:285, 1967.

Review: Planning and evaluation of applied nutrition programs. Nutr. Rev., 25:132, 1967.

Stiebeling, H. K.: Our share in better world nutrition. J. Am. Dietet. A., 45:315, 1964.

———: Improved use of nutrition knowledge—Progress and problems. J. Am. Dietet. A., 45:321, 1964.

Thompson, W. S.: World population and food supply. Council on Foods and Nutrition Report. J.A.M.A., 172:1647, 1960.

Todhunter, E. N.: Development of knowledge in nutrition. J. Am. Dietet. A., 41:328, 335, 1962.

———: Some classics of nutrition and dietetics. J. Am. Dietet. A., 44:100, 1964.

———: The evolution of nutrition concepts—perspectives and new horizons. J. Am. Dietet. A., 46:120, 1965.

Voris, L.: Activities of the Food and Nutrition Board. Nutr. Rev., 19:97, 1961.

WHO: The work of WHO in 1965. WHO Chronicle, 20:155, 1966.

TABLES OF FOOD COMPOSITION

Church, C. F., and Church, H. N.: Food Values of Portions Commonly Used. Ed. 10. Philadelphia, J. B. Lippincott, 1966.

FAO: Review of Food Composition Tables. Rome, Food Consumption and Planning Branch, FAO. 1965. (Food Composition tables from around the world.)

Hardinge, M. G., and Crooks, H.: Fatty acid composition of food fats. J. Am. Dietet. A., *34*:1065, 1958.

McCance, R. A., and Widdowson, E. M.: The Composition of Foods. Medical Research Council Special Report. Ser. No. 297. London, Her Majesty's Stationery Office, 1960.

Orr, M. L., and Watt, B. K.: Amino Acid Content of Foods. U.S.D.A. Washington, U. S. Gov't. Print. Off., 1957.

U.S.D.A.: Fatty Acids in Food Fats. Home Ec. Report No. 7. Washington, U. S. Gov't. Print. Off., 1959.

————: Nutritive Value of Foods. Home and Garden Bull. No. 72. Washington, U. S. Gov't. Print. Off., 1963.

Watt, B. K., and Merrill, A. L.: Composition of Foods—Raw, Processed, Prepared. U.S.D.A. Handbook No. 8. Washington, U. S. Gov't. Print. Off., 1963.

Widdowson, E. M.: British Food Composition Tables. J. Am. Dietet. A., *50*:363, 1967.

Wu Leung, Woot Tsuen: Food Composition Table for Use in Latin America. I.C.N.N.D. Nat. Inst. Health, Bethesda, Md., 1961.

————: A Selected Bibliography on African Foods and Nutrition and African Botanical Nomenclature. Office of International Research, Nutrition Sect., Bethesda, Md., 1966.

Szanton, J. G.: Food Values and Calorie Charts. New York, Fell, 1965.

RELIABLE SOURCES FROM WHICH TO OBTAIN NUTRITION INFORMATION

American Dietetic Ass., 620 N. Michigan Ave., Chicago, Ill. 60611.

American Home Economics Ass., 1600 Twentieth St., Washington, D. C., 20009.

The Borden Company, 350 Madison Ave., New York, N. Y. 10017.

Council on Foods and Nutrition, or Bureau of Investigation, American Medical Ass., 535 N. Dearborn St., Chicago, Ill. 60610.

Dept. of Health, Education and Welfare, Washington, D. C.

Food and Nutrition Board, National Research Council, 2101 Constitution Ave., Washington, D. C. 20418.

Food and Nutrition Section, American Public Health Ass., 1740 Broadway, New York, N. Y. 10019.

Food and Drug Administration, U. S. Dept. H.E.W., Washington, D. C. 20204.

Federal Trade Commission, Bureau of Investigation, Washington, D. C.

Money Management Institute, Household Finance Corp., Prudential Plaza, Chicago, Ill. 60601.

The Nutrition Foundation, Inc., 99 Park Ave., New York, N. Y. 10016.

Better Business Bureaus

State Health Departments

Food and Nutrition Dept. of State University

CARBOHYDRATES (*See also* references under Digestion, Absorption and Metabolism and Diabetes)

Books:

Beaton, G. H., and McHenry, E. W.: Nutrition. A Comprehensive Treatise. Vol. I. Macronutrients and Nutrient Elements, Chap. 2. New York, Academic Press, 1964.

Soskin, S., and Levine, R.: Carbohydrate Metabolism. Chicago, Univ. Chicago Press, 1952.

Journal Articles:

Anderson, J. T.: Dietary carbohydrate and serum triglycerides. Am. J. Clin. Nutr., *20*: 168, 1967.

Anderson, J. T., *et al.*: Glucose, sucrose and lactose in the diet and blood lipids in man. J. Nutr., 79:349, 1963.

Antar, M. A., *et al.*: Changes in retail market food supplies in the U. S. in the last seventy years in relation to the incidence of coronary heart disease, with special reference to dietary carbohydrates and essential fatty acids. Am. J. Clin. Nutr., *14*:169, 1964.

Bloom, W. L.: Carbohydrates and water balance. Am. J. Clin. Nutr., *20*:157, 1967.

Duncan, D. L.: The physiological effect of lactose. Nutr. Abstr. Rev., *25*:309, 1955.

Groen, J. J.: Effect of bread in the diet on serum cholesterol. Am. J. Clin. Nutr., *20*: 191, 1967.

Gryboski, J. D.: Diarrhea from dietetic candies (sorbitol). New Eng. J. Med., *275*:718, 1966.

Hardinge, M. G., *et al.*: Carbohydrates in foods. J. Am. Dietet. A., *46*:197, 1965.

Hartles, R. L.: Carbohydrate consumption and dental caries. Am. J. Clin. Nutr., *20*:152, 1967.

Heard, C. R. C.: Carbohydrates and protein. Proc. Nutr. Soc., *23*:109, 1964.

Hodges, R. E.: Present knowledge of carbohydrates. Nutr. Rev., *24*:65, 1966.

Hodges, R. E., and Krehl, W. A.: The role of carbohydrates in lipid metabolism. Am. J. Clin. Nutr., *17*:334, 1965.

Hollingsworth, D. F., and Greaves, J. P.: Consumption of carbohydrates in the United Kingdom. Am. J. Clin. Nutr., 20:65, 1967.

Keys, A., et al.: Fiber and pectin in the diet and serum cholesterol concentration in man. Proc. Soc. Exp. Biol. Med., 106:555, 1961.

Krehl, W. A., et al.: Some metabolic changes induced by low carbohydrate diets. Am. J. Clin. Nutr., 20:139, 1967.

Lopez, A., et al.: Some interesting relationships between dietary carbohydrates and serum cholesterol. Am. J. Clin. Nutr., 18:149, 1966.

MacDonald, I.: Dietary carbohydrates in normolipemia. Am. J. Clin. Nutr., 20:185, 1967.

McGandy, R. B., et al.: Dietary carbohydrate and serum cholesterol levels in man. Am. J. Clin. Nutr., 18:237, 1966.

Palmer, G. H., and Dixon, D.: Effect of pectin dose on serum cholesterol levels. Am. J. Clin. Nutr., 18:437, 1966.

Passmore, R., and Swindell, Y. E.: Observation on the respiratory quotients and weight gain of man after eating large quantities of carbohydrate. Brit. J. Nutr., 17:331, 1963.

Prather, E.: Effect of cellulose on serum lipids in young women. J. Am. Dietet. A., 45:230, 1964.

Review: Alcohol and the excretion of galactose in man. Nutr. Rev., 20:205, 1962.

———: Blood lipids and various dietary carbohydrates. Nutr. Rev., 24:35, 1966.

———: Carbohydrate and cataracts. Nutr. Rev., 20:245, 1962.

———: Carbohydrate intake and respiratory quotient. Nutr. Rev., 22:104, 1964.

———: Evaluation of cereal carbohydrates. Nutr. Rev., 17:24, 1959.

———: The role of carbohydrates in the diet. Nutr. Rev., 22:102, 1964.

Shamma'a, M., and Al-Khalidi, U.: Dietary carbohydrates and serum cholesterol. Am. J. Clin. Nutr., 13:194, 1963.

Speirs, R. L.: The systemic influence of carbohydrates on teeth. Proc. Nutr. Soc., 23:129, 1964.

Stevens, H. A., and Ohlson, M. A.: Estimated intake of simple and complex carbohydrates. J. Am. Dietet. A., 48:294, 1966.

Yudkin, J.: Evolutionary and historical changes in dietary carbohydrates. Am. J. Clin. Nutr., 20:108, 1967.

FATS AND LIPIDS (*See also* references under Digestion, Absorption and Metabolism and Atherosclerosis)

Books and Pamphlets:

Beaton, G. H., and McHenry, E. W.: Nutrition—A Comprehensive Treatise. Vol. I. Macronutrients and Nutrient Elements. Chap. 2. New York, Academic Press, 1964.

Food and Nutrition Board: Dietary Fat and Human Health. National Research Council Pub. No. 1147, 1966.

Home Economics Research Report, No. 7: Fatty Acids in Food Fats. Agr. Research Service, Washington, D. C., 1959.

Household Use of Fats and Oils in the U. S. Agr. Marketing Service, Washington, D. C., 1958.

Institute of Shortening and Edible Oils: Food Fats and Oils. Washington, D. C., 1963.

Journal Articles:

Aaes-Jorgensen, E.: Essential fatty acids. Physiol. Rev., 41:1, 1961.

Albrink, M. J.: The significance of serum triglycerides. J. Am. Dietet. A., 42:29, 1963.

Bernfeld, P., et al.: Fatty acid contents of margarines and other table fats. Am. J. Clin. Nutr., 11:554, 1962.

Casdorph, H. R.: Fats in the diet. Geriatrics, 20:168, 1965.

Council of Foods and Nutrition, A.M.A.: Regulation of dietary fat. J.A.M.A., 181:441, 1962.

Eastwood, G., et al.: Fatty acids and other lipids in mayonnaise. J. Am. Dietet. A., 42:518, 1963.

Groen, J. J., et al.: Influence of the nature of the fats in diets high in carbohydrate (mainly derived from bread) on the serum cholesterol. Am. J. Clin. Nutr., 17:296, 1965.

Gwinup, G., et al.: Effect of nibbling versus gorging on serum lipids in man. Am. J. Clin. Nutr., 13:209, 1963.

Hansen, A. E., et al.: Role of linoleic acid in infant nutrition. Pediatrics, 31:171, 1963.

Hegsted, D. M., et al.: Quantitative effects of dietary fats on serum cholesterol in man. Am. J. Clin. Nutr., 17:281, 1965.

Holman, R. T., et al.: The essential fatty acid requirement of infants and the assessment of their dietary intake of linoleate by serum fatty acid analysis. Am. J. Clin. Nutr., 14:70, 1964.

Hughes, A. A., et al.: Linoleic acid—an essential nutrient: its content in infant formulas and precooked cereals. Clin. Pediat., 2:555, 1963.

Imaichi, K., et al.: Studies with the use of fish oil fractions in human subjects. Am. J. Clin. Nutr., 13:158, 1963.

Kritchevsky, D., and Tepper, S. A.: Free and ester sterol content of various foodstuffs. J. Nutr., 74:441, 1961.

Kritchevsky, D., et al.: Influence of short term heating on composition of edible fats. J. Nutr., 77:127, 1962.

McLaren, D. S., *et al.*: Composition of human adipose tissue, with special reference to site and age differences. Am. J. Clin. Nutr., *17*: 171, 1965.

Mead, J. F.: Present knowledge of fat. Nutr. Rev. *24*:33, 1966.

Morse, E. H., *et al.*: Effect of two fats on blood lipids in young men. J. Am. Dietet. A., *46*: 193, 1965.

————: Relation of fats to blood lipids in young men. J. Am. Dietet. A., *41*:323, 1962.

Review: Body fat and adipose tissue. Nutr. Rev., *22*:99, 1964.

————: Dietary cholesterol and regulation of liver cholesterol synthesis. Nutr. Rev., *24*: 218, 1966.

————: Dietary fat in essential hyperlipemia. Nutr. Rev., *24*:103, 1966.

————: Effect of chain length of fatty acids upon serum lipids. Nutr. Rev., *20*:347, 1962.

————: Fat and cholesterol in the diet. Nutr. Rev., *23*:3, 1965.

————: Fatty acid composition of fish oils. Nutr. Rev., *23*:51, 1963.

————: Nutritional evaluation of inter-esterified fats. Nutr. Rev., *24*:201, 1966.

————: The intracellular free fatty acid pool in adipose tissue. Nutr. Rev., *20*:154, 1962.

————: Triton and fat balance. Nutr. Rev., *24*:338, 1966.

————: Unsaturated fatty acid isomers in nutrition. Nutr. Rev., *24*:1, 1966.

Rice, E. E.: Composition of modern margarines. J. Am. Dietet. A., *41*:319, 1962.

Roels, O. A., *et al.*: Serum lipids and diet: A comparison between three population groups with low, medium and high fat intake. J. Nutr., *79*:211, 1963.

Scott, R. R., *et al.*: Fatty acids of serum and adipose tissue in six groups eating natural diets. Am. J. Clin. Nutr., *14*:280, 1964.

Steiner, A., *et al.*: Importance of dietary cholesterol in man. J.A.M.A., *181*:186, 1962.

Symposium: Intravenous fat emulsions. Am. J. Clin. Nutr., *16*:1, 1965.

Tove, S. B.: Toxicity of saturated fats. J. Nutr., *84*:237, 1964.

Wiese, H., *et al.*: Essential fatty acids and human nutrition. J. Nutr., *52*:355, 1954.

————: Essential fatty acids in infant nutrition. J. Nutr., *66*:345, 1958.

PROTEIN (*See also* references under Digestion, Absorption and Metabolism)

Books and Pamphlets:

Albanese, A. A.: Protein and Amino Acid in Nutrition. New York, Academic Press, 1959.

Allison, J. B., and Fitzpatrick, W. H.: Dietary Proteins in Health and Disease. Springfield, Ill., Charles C Thomas, 1960.

Block, R. J., and Weiss, K. W.: Amino Acid Handbook. Springfield, Ill., Charles C Thomas, 1956.

FAO: Protein—At the Heart of the World Food Problem. Rome, FAO, 1967.

FAO/WHO Joint Expert Group: Protein Requirements. Rome, FAO, 1965.

Food and Nutrition Board: Evaluation of Protein Nutrition. Washington, D. C., National Research Council Pub. No. 711, 1959.

————: Evaluation of Protein Quality. National Research Council Pub. No. 1100, Washington, D. C., 1963.

————: Progress in Meeting Protein Needs of Infants and Children. National Research Council Pub. No. 843, 1961.

Orr, M. L., and Watt, B. K.: Amino Acid Content of Food. Home Econ. Res. Report No. 4, U.S.D.A., Washington, D. C., 1957.

Stare, F. J. (ed.): Protein Nutrition—A Monograph. Ann. N. Y. Acad. Sci., *69*:855, 1958.

Journal Articles:

Allison, J. B.: The ideal aminogram. Fed. Proc., *20*:66, 1961.

Allison, J. B., and Wannemacher, R. W.: The concept and significance of labile and overall protein reserves of the body. Am. J. Clin. Nutr., *16*:445, 1965.

Beveridge, J. M. R., *et al.*: Effect of the level of dietary protein with and without added cholesterol on plasma cholesterol levels in man. J. Nutr., *79*:289, 1963.

Coltman, C. A., *et al.*: The amino acid content of sweat in normal adults. Am. J. Clin. Nutr., *18*:373, 1966.

Consolazio, C. F., *et al.*: Nitrogen excretion in sweat and its relation to nitrogen balance requirements. J. Nutr., *79*:399, 1963.

György, P.: Protein-rich foods in calorie-protein malnutrition. Problems of evaluation. Am. J. Clin. Nutr., *14*:7, 1964.

Halac, E., Jr.: Studies of the relation between protein intake and resistance to protein deprivation. Am. J. Clin. Nutr., *11*:514, 1962.

Harper, A. E.: Some implications of amino acid supplementation. Am. J. Clin. Nutr., *9*: 533, 1961.

Holt, L. E., *et al.*: The concept of protein stores and its implication in diet. J.A.M.A., *181*: 699, 1962.

Holt, L. E., and Snyderman, S. E.: Protein and amino acid requirements of infants and children. Nutr. Abstr. & Rev., *35*:1, 1965.

Leverton, R. M., *et al.*: The quantitative amino acid requirements of young women. J. Nutr., *58*:83, 219, 341, 355, 1956.

Miller, G. T., *et al.:* Phenylalanine content of fruit. J. Am. Dietet. A., *46*:43, 1965.

Mitchell, H. S.: Protein limitation and human growth. J. Am. Dietet. A., *44*:165, 1966.

Oldham, H. G., and Dickinson, F. N.: Evaluation of nitrogen balance of young women fed amino acids proportioned as in the FAO provisional pattern and as in eggs, oats, milk and peanuts. Am. J. Clin. Nutr., *17*:360, 1965.

Review: Evaluation of a peanut-soybean mixture. Nutr. Rev., *23*:75, 1965.

————: Evaluation of the FAO amino acid reference pattern. Nutr. Rev., *21*:101, 1963.

————: Histidine requirements in infancy. Nutr. Rev., *22*:114, 1964.

————: Protein and amino acid requirements. Nutr. Rev., *20*:235, 1962.

————: The concept of protein stores. Nutr. Rev., *21*:45, 1963.

Rose, W. C.: Amino acid requirement of adult man. Nutr. Abstr. & Rev., *27*:631, 1957.

Scrimshaw, N. S., *et al.:* Protein metabolism of young men during university examinations. Am. J. Clin. Nutr., *18*:321, 1966.

Standal, B. R.: Nutritional value of proteins of oriental soybean foods. J. Nutr., *81*:279, 1963.

Swenseid, M. E., *et al.:* An evaluation of the FAO amino acid reference pattern in human nutrition. I. Studies with young men. J. Nutr., *75*:295, 1961.

————: An evaluation of the FAO amino acid reference pattern in human nutrition. II. Studies with youg women. J. Nutr., *77*:391, 1962.

————: Nitrogen balance studies with subjects fed the essential amino acids in plasma pattern proportions. J. Nutr., *79*:276, 1963.

Tolbert, B., and Watts, J. H.: Phenylalanine requirements of women consuming a minimal tyrosine diet and the sparing effect of tyrosine on the phenylalanine requirement. J. Nutr., *80*:111, 1963.

Tuttle, S. G., *et al.:* Study of the essential amino acid requirements of men over fifty. Metabolism, *6*:564, 1957.

————: Further observations on the amino acid requirements of older men. I. Effects of nonessential nitrogen supplements fed with different amounts of essential amino acids. Am. J. Clin. Nutr., *16*:225, 1965. II. Methionine and lysine. Am. J. Clin. Nutr., *16*:229, 1965.

Watts, J. H.: Evaluation of protein in selected American diets. J. Am. Dietet. A., *46*:116, 1965.

Wiener, R. P., *et al.:* Influence of various carbohydrates on the utilization of low protein rations by the white rat. V. Relationship among protein intake, calorie intake, growth and liver fat content. J. Nutr., *80*:279, 1963.

ENERGY METABOLISM

Books and Pamphlets:

Beaton, G. H., and McHenry, E. W.: Nutrition. A Comprehensive Treatise. Vol. I. Macronutrients and Nutrient Elements. Chap. 4. New York, Academic Press, 1964.

Bratton, E. C.: Some Factors of Cost to the Body in Standing to Work and Sitting to Work Under Different Postural Conditions. N. Y. State Agric. Experiment Station Memoir 365, 1959.

Consolazio, C. F., *et al.:* Physiological Measurements of Metabolic Functions in Man. New York, McGraw-Hill, 1963.

FAO Committee on Calorie Requirements: Calorie Requirements. FAO. FAO Nutrition Studies No. 15, Rome, 1957.

National Academy of Sciences: Techniques for Measuring Body Composition. Nat. Research Council, Washington, D. C., 1961.

Richardson, M., and McCracken, E. C.: Energy Expenditures of Women Performing Selected Activities. Agr. Research Service, Home Econ. Res. Report No. 11. Washington, D. C., 1960.

Sargent, D. W.: An Evaluation of Basal Metabolic Data for Children and Youth in the United States. Agr. Research Service, Home Econ. Res. Report No. 14, Washington, D. C., 1961.

————: An Evaluation of Basal Metabolic Data for Infants in the United States. Agr. Research Service, Home Econ. Res. Report No. 18. Washington, D. C., 1962.

Journal Articles:

Buskirk, E. R., *et al.:* Variations in resting metabolism with changes in food, exercise and climate. Metabolism, *6*:144, 1957.

————: Human energy expenditure studies in the National Institute of Arthritis and Metabolic Diseases. I. Interaction of cold environment and special dynamic effect. II. Sleep. Am. J. Clin. Nutr., *8*:602, 1960.

Call, D. L.: An examination of calorie availability and consumption in the United States, 1909-1963. Am. J. Clin. Nutr., *16*:374, 1965.

Consolazio, C. F., *et al.:* Environmental temperature and energy expenditure. J. Appl. Physiol., *18*:65, 1963.

Durnin, J. V. G. A.: The use of surface and of body weight as standards of reference in studies of human energy expenditure. Brit. J. Nutr., *13*:68, 1959.

Durnin, J. V. G. A., and Brockway, J. M.: Determination of total daily energy expenditure in man by indirect calorimetry: Assessment of the accuracy of a modern technique. Brit. J. Nutr., *13*:41, 1959.

Hampton, M. C., *et al.:* A longitudinal study of gross body composition and body conformation and their association with food and activity in a teen-age population: Anthropometric evaluation of body build. Am. J. Clin. Nutr., *19*:422, 1966.

Hunscher, H. A.: Pertinent factors in interpreting metabolic data. J. Am. Dietet. A., *39*: 209, 1961.

Issekutz, B., Jr., *et al.:* Effect of diet on work metabolism. J. Nutr., *79*:109, 1963.

Johnson, O. C.: Present knowledge of calories. Nutr. Rev., *25*:257, 1967.

Johnson, R. E.: Caloric requirements under adverse environmental conditions. Fed. Proc., *22*:1431, 1963.

Mason, E. D., *et al.:* Age differences in basal metabolism and body composition of Indian women in Bombay with prediction standards for the basal metabolic rate. Ind. J. Med. Res., *53*:309, 1965.

————: Racial group differences in basal metabolism and body composition of Indian and European women in Bombay. Human Biol., *36*:374, 1964.

Mayer, J.: Why people get hungry. Nutrition Today, *1*:2, 1966.

Review: Body fat in adolescent boys, Nutr. Rev., *22*:72, 1964.

————: Climate and caloric intake. Nutr. Rev., *16*:237, 1958.

————: Determination of human caloric requirements. Nutr. Rev., *12*:196, 1954.

————: Diet and work metabolism. Nutr. Rev., *21*:211, 1963.

————: Eating at various times before exercise. Nutr. Rev., *21*:40, 1963.

————: Energy metabolism in malnourished infants. Nutr. Rev., *18*:75, 1960.

————: Physical activity and the level of fats in the serum. Nutr. Rev., *20*:331, 1962.

Sasaki, T.: Relation of basal metabolism to changes in food composition and body composition. Fed. Proc., *25*(2):1165, 1966.

Symposium: Energy balance. Am. J. Clin. Nutr., *8*:527-774, 1960.

Weaver, E. I., and Elliot, D. E.: Factors affecting energy expended in home-making tasks. J. Am. Dietet. A., *39*:205, 1961.

Wheadon, G. D.: New research on human energy metabolism. Am. J. Dietet. A., *35*: 682, 1959.

Wilder, R. M.: Calorimetry: The basis of the science of nutrition. Arch. Int. Med., *103*: 146, 1959.

Yoshimura, M., *et al.:* Climatic adaptation of basal metabolism. Fed. Proc., *25*(2):1169, 1966.

Young, C. M.: Body composition studies of young women. Food Nutr. News, *34*:1, 1962.

WATER AND MINERALS

Books and Pamphlets:

Beaton, G. H., and McHenry, E. W.: Nutrition. A Comprehensive Treatise. Vol. I. Macronutrients and Nutrient Elements. Chaps. 5, 6, 7, 8, 9. New York, Academic Press, 1964.

Bothwell, T. H., and Finch, C. A.: Iron Metabolism. Boston, Little, Brown & Co., 1962.

FAO/WHO Expert Committee on Calcium Requirements: Calcium Requirements. FAO, Rome, 1962.

Hathaway, M. L.: Magnesium in Human Nutrition. Home Econ. Res. Report No. 19. U.S.D.A., Washington, D. C., 1962.

Snively, W. D., Jr.: Sea Within—The Story of Our Body Fluid. Philadelphia, J. B. Lippincott, 1960.

Swanson, P. P.: Calcium in Nutrition. Pamphlet. Chicago, National Dairy Council, 1963.

Underwood, E. J.: Trace Elements in Human and Animal Nutrition. New York, Academic Press, 1962.

Journal Articles:

A.M.A. Council on Food and Nutrition: Symposium on human calcium requirements. J.A.M.A., *185*:588, 1963.

Baker, E. M., *et al.:* Water requirements of men as related to salt intake. Am. J. Clin. Nutr., *12*:394, 1963.

Bothwell, T. H., *et al.:* Iron overload in Bantu subjects—Studies on the availability of iron in Bantu beer. Am. J. Clin. Nutr., *14*:47, 1964.

Briscoe, A., and Ragan, C.: Bile and endogenous calcium in man. Am. J. Clin. Nutr., *16*:281, 1965.

————: Effect of magnesium on calcium metabolism in man. Am. J. Clin. Nutr., *19*:296, 1966.

Brown, E. B.: The absorption of iron. Am. J. Clin. Nutr., *12*:205, 1963.

————: The utilization of iron in erythropoiesis. Am. J. Clin. Nutr., *12*:77, 1963.

Bunce, G. E., *et al.:* Influence of the dietary protein level on the magnesium requirement. J. Nutr., 79:220, 1963.

Callender, S. T.: Iron absorption. Proc. Nutr. Soc., 26:59, 1967.

Calloway, D. H., and McMullen, J.: Fecal excretion of iron and tin by men fed stored canned foods. Am. J. Clin. Nutr., 18:1, 1966.

Cartwright, G. E., and Wintrobe, M. M.: Copper metabolism in normal subjects. Am. J. Clin. Nutr., 14:224, 1964.

————: The question of copper deficiency in man. Am. J. Clin. Nutr., 15:94, 1964.

Chareton, R. W., *et al.:* The role of the intestinal mucosa in iron absorption. J. Clin. Invest., 44:543, 1965.

Coltman, C., and Rowe, N.: The iron content of sweat in normal adults. Am. J. Clin. Nutr., 18:270, 1966.

Consolazio, C. F., *et al.:* Excretion of sodium, potassium, magnesium and iron in human sweat and the relation of each to balance requirements. J. Nutr., 79:407, 1963.

Conway, E. J.: New light on the active transport of sodium ions. Fed. Proc., 23:680, 1964.

Cooper, G. R., and Heap, B.: Sodium ion in drinking water. II. Importance, problems, and potential applications of sodium-ion restricted therapy. J. Am. Dietet. A., 50:37, 1967.

Dunn, M. M., and Walser, M.: Magnesium depletion in normal man. Metabolism, 15:884, 1966.

Finch, C. A.: Iron balance in man. Nutr. Rev., 23:129, 1965.

Freiman, H. D., *et al.:* Iron absorption in the healthy aged. Geriatrics, 18:716, 1963.

Fujino, M., *et al.:* Interrelationships between estrogenic activity, serum iron and ascorbic acid levels during the menstural cycle. Am. J. Clin. Nutr., 18:256, 1966.

Githens, J. H., *et al.:* Iron deficiency anemia of infancy: Pathogenesis, diagnosis and management. Clin. Pediat., 2:477, 1963.

Glinsman, W. H., *et al.:* Plasma chromium after glucose administration. Science, 152:1243, 1966.

Greenwald, E., *et al.:* Effect of lactose on calcium metabolism in man. J. Nutr., 79:531, 1963.

Gundersen, K., and Shen, G.: Total body water in obesity. Am. J. Clin. Nutr., 19:77, 1966.

Harrison, M. T., *et al.:* Nature and availability of iodine in fish. Am. J. Clin. Nutr., 17:73, 1965.

Hodge, H. C.: Metabolism of fluorides. J.A.M.A., 177:313, 1961.

Hook, L., and Brandt, K.: Copper content of some low-copper foods. J. Am. Dietet. A., 49:202, 1966.

Hopkins, L. L., Jr., and Majaj, A. S.: Normalization of impaired glucose utilization and hypoglycemia by Cr(III) in malnourished infants. Fed. Proc., 25:303, 1966.

Hussain, R., *et al.:* Nutritive value of food iron. Am. J. Clin. Nutr., 16:464, 1965.

Krehl, W. A.: The potassium depletion syndrome. Nutrition Today, 1:20, 1966 (June).

————: Magnesium. Nutrition Today, 2:16, 1967 (Sept.).

Luecke, R. W.: The significance of zinc in nutrition. Borden's Rev. Nutr. Res., 26:45, 1965.

Lutwak, L., *et al.:* Effects of high dietary calcium and phosphorus on calcium, phosphorus, nitrogen and fat metabolism in children. Am. J. Clin. Nutr., 14:76, 1964.

Mayer, J.: Zinc deficiency: a cause of growth retardation. Postgrad. Med., 35:206, 1964.

McCallister, P. J., *et al.:* Urinary excretion of magnesium in man following the ingestion of ethanol. Am. J. Clin. Nutr., 12:415, 1963.

Mertz, W., *et al.:* Some aspects of glucose metabolism of chromium deficient rats raised in a strictly controlled environment. J. Nutr., 86:107, 1965.

Morgan, A. F., *et al.:* Bone density of an aging population. Am. J. Clin. Nutr., 10:337, 1962.

Morrey, L. W., *et al.:* Fluoridation of water and dental caries. J. Am. Dent. A., 65:587, 1962.

Naiman, J. L., *et al.:* The gastrointestinal effects of iron-deficiency anemia. Pediatrics, 33:83, 1964.

Nelson, G. Y., and Gram, M. R.: Magnesium content of accessory foods. J. Am. Dietet. A., 38:437, 1961.

Norden, B. E. C.: Calcium intake and calcium requirement of man. Proc. Nutr. Soc., 24:49, 1965.

North, B. B., *et al.:* Manganese metabolism in college women. J. Nutr., 72:217, 1960.

Parsons, D. S.: Sodium chloride absorption by the small intestine and the relationship between salt transport and the absorption of water and some organic molecules. Proc. Nutr. Soc., 26:46, 1967.

Prasad, A. S., *et al.:* Zinc and iron deficiencies in male subjects with dwarfism and hypogonadism. Am. J. Clin. Nutr., 12:437, 1963.

Reinhold, J. G., *et al.:* Zinc and copper concentrations in hair of Iranian villagers. Am. J. Clin. Nutr., 18:294, 1966.

Review: Calcium in sweat. Nutr. Rev., 21:13, 1963.

Review: Copper deficiency in malnourished infants. Nutr. Rev., 23:164, 1965.

———: Dietary sodium and experimental dental caries. Nutr. Rev., 23:117, 1965.

———: Effect of altitude on intestinal absorption of iron. Nutr. Rev., 20:8, 1962.

———: Enhancement of calcium absorption by carbohydrate. Nutr. Rev., 18:316, 1960.

———: Exercise and calcium utilization. Nutr. Rev., 19:42, 1961.

———: Fluoride bone crystal structure, and calcium balance. Nutr. Rev., 21:165, 1963.

———: Gastric function and structure in iron deficiency. Nutr. Rev., 24:326, 1966.

———: Gastrointestinal tract and iron deficiency anemia. Nutr. Rev., 22:323, 1964.

———: Hepatic iron stores and iron absorption. Nutr. Rev., 22:214, 1964.

———: Human renal calculus formation and magnesium. Nutr. Rev., 24:43, 1966.

———: Hypertension and salt aversion. Nutr. Rev., 19:57, 1961.

———: Influence of homogenization, copper, and ascorbic acid on flavor of milk. Nutr. Rev., 21:240, 1963.

———: Intestinal absorption of calcium. Nutr. Rev., 20:45, 1962.

———: Intestinal absorption of chromium. Nutr. Rev., 25:76, 1967.

———: Intestinal calcium and bone formation. Nutr. Rev., 23:6, 1965.

———: Iron absorption. Nutr. Rev., 24:247, 1967.

———: Iron absorption and diet. Nutr. Rev., 22:306, 1964.

———: Iron deficiency anemia. Nutr. Rev., 20:164, 1962.

———: Iron storage in bone marrow. Nutr. Rev., 21:329, 1963.

———: Loss of nutrients through the skin. Nutr. Rev., 21:266, 1963.

———: Magnesium deficiency. Nutr. Rev., 20:335, 1962.

———: Magnesium metabolism. Nutr. Rev., 20:250, 1962.

———: Manganese balance in children. Nutr. Rev., 23:236, 1965.

———: Mineral elements in wheat, flour and bread. Nutr. Rev., 22:223, 1964.

———: Phosphate influence on experimental dental caries. Nutr. Rev., 22:311, 1964.

———: Phytase and bone calcification. Nutr. Rev., 20:208, 1962.

———: Potential toxicity of fluorides. Nutr. Rev., 21:291, 1963.

———: Relation of zinc metabolism to a syndrome characterized by anemia, dwarfism, and hypogonadism. Nutr. Rev., 21:264, 1963.

Review: Salt supplementation during fasting in the cold. Nutr. Rev., 23:45, 1965.

———: Symptoms of iron deficiency anemia. Nutr. Rev., 25:86, 1967.

———: The therapeutic effectiveness of various compounds containing iron. Nutr. Rev., 24:232, 1966.

———: Trivalent chromium in human nutrition. Nutr. Rev., 25:50, 1967.

Roe, D.: Nutrient toxicity with excessive intake. II. Mineral overload. N. Y. State J. Med., 66:1233, 1966.

Rush, B., et al.: Effect of a low iron diet on iron absorption. Am. J. Clin. Nutr., 19:132, 1966.

Schroeder, H. A.: Renal cadmium and essential hypertension. J.A.M.A., 187:358, 1964.

———: Cadmium as a factor in hypertension. J. Chron. Dis., 18:647, 1965.

Schroeder, H. A., et al.: Abnormal trace metals in man: Chromium. J. Chron. Dis., 15:941, 1962.

———: Essential trace metals in man: Copper. J. Chron. Dis., 19:1007, 1966.

Seelig, M. S.: The requirement of magnesium by the normal adult. Summary and analysis of published data. Am. J. Clin. Nutr., 14:342, 1964.

Segar, W. E.: Multiple episodes of potassium deficiency. Am. J. Dis. Child, 109:295, 1965.

Seltzer, C. C., et al.: Serum iron and iron-binding capacity in adolescents. I. Standard values. Am. J. Clin. Nutr., 13:343, 1963.

Shils, M. E.: Experimental human magnesium depletion. Am. J. Clin Nutr., 15:133, 1965.

Smith, F. W.: Safety of water fluoridation. J. Am. Dent. A., 65:598, 1962.

Sullivan, J. F., and Lankford, H. G.: Zinc metabolism and alcoholism. Am. J. Clin. Nutr., 17:57, 1965.

Sullivan, J. F., et al.: Magnesium metabolism in alcoholism. Am. J. Clin. Nutr., 13:297, 1963.

Swanson, P. P., et al.: Patterns of calcium metabolism in women 50 years of age and older. Fed. Proc., 21:308, 1962.

Tal, E., and Guggenheim, K.: Effect of manganese on calcification of bone. Biochem. J., 95:94, 1965.

Vought, R. L., and London, W. T.: Dietary sources of iodine. Am. J. Clin. Nutr., 14:186, 1964.

Wacker, W. E. C.: Magnesium metabolism. J. Am. Dietet. A., 44:362, 1964.

Waldbott, G. L.: Fluoride in food. Am. J. Clin. Nutr., 12:455, 1963.

Walker, A. R. P.: Uncertainties in the interpretation and validity of long-term balance studies. Am. J. Clin. Nutr., 10:95, 1962.

White, J. M., *et al.*: Sodium ion in drinking water. I. Properties, analysis, and occurrence. J. Am. Dietet. A., *50*:32, 1967.

VITAMINS
General

(See also references under Malnutrition—A World-Wide Problem.)

Books and Pamphlets:

American Medical Association: Vitamin Supplements and Their Correct Use. Chicago, Ill. American Medical Association, 1964.

Beaton, G. H., and McHenry, E. W.: Nutrition. A Comprehensive Treatise. Vol. II. Chaps. 1, 2, 3, and 4. New York, Academic Press, 1964.

DeReuck, A. V. S., and O'Connor, M. (eds.): The Mechanism of Action of Water-soluble vitamins. Ciba Foundation Symposium. Boston, Little, Brown & Co., 1962.

Heinz, H. J., Co.: Nutritional Data. Pittsburgh, H. J. Heinz Co., 1965.

Report of a Joint FAO/WHO Expert Group: Requirements of Vitamin A, Thiamine, Riboflavin and Niacin. Rome, Italy, FAO, 1967.

U. S. Department of Agriculture: Conserving the Nutritive Values in Foods. Home and Garden Bulletin No. 90, Washington, D. C., U. S. Government Printing Office, 1963.

Vitamin Manual. Upjohn Co., Kalamazoo, Mich., 1963.

Wagner, A. F., and Folkers, K.: Vitamins and Coenzymes. Interscience Publishers, New York, 1964.

Journal Articles:

Campbell, J. A.: Dietary factors affecting vitamin requirements. Proc. Nutr. Soc., *23*:31, 1964.

Campbell, J. A., and Morrison, A. B.: Some factors affecting the absorption of vitamins. Am. J. Clin. Nutr., *12*:162, 1963.

Council on Foods and Nutrition: General Policy on addition of specific nutrients to foods. J.A.M.A., *178*:1024, 1961.

Daniel, L. J.: Inhibitors of the B complex vitamins. Nutr. Rev., *31*:1, 1961.

Gershoff, S. N.: Effects of dietary levels of macronutrients on vitamin requirements. Fed. Proc., *23*:1077, 1964.

Hardinge, M. G., and Crooks, H.: Lesser known vitamins in foods. J. Am. Dietet. A., *38*:240, 1961.

Maddox, G.: Vitamin pills are not a food substitute. Today's Health, Nov., p. 38, 1961.

Pearson, W. N.: Biochemical appraisal of the vitamin nutritional status in man. Council on Foods and Nutrition, J.A.M.A., *180*:49, 1962.

Review: Lipids and fat-soluble vitamins in cellular metabolism. Nutr. Rev., *24*:272, 1966.

Roe, D. A.: Nutrient toxicity with excessive intake. I. Vitamins. N. Y. J. Med., *66*:869, 1966.

Symposium: Advances in the detection of nutrition deficiencies in man. Am. J. Clin. Nutr., *20*: June 1967.

Vilter, R. W.: Vitamins, minerals, and anemia. J.A.M.A., *175*:152, 1961.

Vitamin A

Journal Articles:

Arroyave, G., *et al.*: Serum and liver vitamin A and lipids in children with severe protein malnutrition. Am. J. Clin. Nutr., 9:180, 1961.

Council on Foods and Nutrition: Fortification of nonfat milk solids with vitamins A and D. J.A.M.A., *198*:1107, 1966.

Di Benedetto, R. J.: Chronic hypervitaminosis A in an adult. J.A.M.A., *201*:130, 1967.

Fell, H. B.: Effect of vitamin A on tissue structure. Proc. Nutr. Soc., *19*:50, 1960.

Ganguly, J.: Absorption, transportation, and storage of vitamin A. Vitam. Horm., *18*:387, 1960.

Gopalan, C., *et al.*: Studies of vitamin A deficiency in children. Am. J. Clin. Nutr., *8*: 833, 1960.

Morrice, G., Jr., and Havener, W. H.: Vitamin A intoxication as a cause of pseudo-tumor cerebri. J.A.M.A., *173*:1802, 1960.

Olson, J. A.: The absorption of beta-carotene and its conversion into vitamin A. Am. J. Clin. Nutr., *9*:1, 1961.

Owen, E. C.: Some aspects of the metabolism of vitamin A and carotene. World Rev. Nutr. Dietet., *5*:132, 1965.

Pallotta, M. A., and Krause, R. F.: Effect of vitamin A on certain blood constituents of geriatric subjects. Am. J. Clin. Nutr., *13*: 201, 1963.

Pease, C. N.: Focal retardation and arrestment of growth of bones due to vitamin A intoxication. J.A.M.A., *182*:980, 1962.

Reddy, V., and Srikantia, S. G.: Serum vitamin A in kwaskiorkor. Am. J. Clin. Nutr., *18*: 105, 1966.

Review: An active metabolite of retinoic acid. Nutr. Rev., *24*:113, 1966.

Review: A comparison of the biological activity of vitamin A acid (retinoic acid) and vitamin A ester in rats. Nutr. Rev., *21*:341, 1963.

——: The conversion of retinene to vitamin A acid by liver enzymes. Nutr. Rev., *21*: 215, 1963.

——: The effect of an excess of vitamin A on membranes *in vitro*. Nutr. Rev., *22*:146, 1964.

——: The influence of vitamin A on sulfate and hexosamine metabolism. Nutr. Rev., *24*: 204, 1966.

——: Interrelationships between vitamins A and E. Nutr. Rev., *23*:82, 1965.

——: Intestinal absorption of vitamin A. Nutr. Rev., *22*:86, 1964.

——: Levels of vitamin A and E in human blood. Nutr. Rev., *19*:101, 1961.

——: Toxic reactions of vitamin A. Nutr. Rev., *22*:109, 1964.

——: Transport of vitamin A in the lymphatic system. Nutr. Rev., *24*:16, 1966.

——: Vitamin A acid and the function of vitamin A. Nutr. Rev., *18*:349, 1960.

——: Vitamin A intoxication in infancy. Nutr. Rev., *23*:263, 1965.

——: Vitamin A in human livers. Nutr. Rev., *21*:71, 1963.

——: Vitamin A and proteins in blood and liver. Nutr. Rev., *19*:344, 1961.

——: Vitamin A transport in man. Nutr. Rev., *25*:199, 1967.

——: Vitamin A and vascularization. Nutr. Rev., *23*:248, 1965.

Roderuck, C., *et al.:* Studies of serum carotenoids and vitamin A in Iowa school children. Am. J. Clin. Nutr., *13*:186, 1963.

Rodger, F. C., *et al.:* A reappraisal of the ocular lesion known as Bitot's spot. Brit. J. Nutr., *17*:475, 1963.

Roels, O. A.: The effect of protein and fat supplements on vitamin A-deficient Indonesian children. Am. J. Clin. Nutr., *12*:380, 1963.

——: Present knowledge of vitamin A. Nutr. Rev., *24*:129, 1966.

——: Vitamin A and protein metabolism. N. Y. J. Med., *64*:288, 1964.

Symposium. Vitamin A. Proc. Nutr. Soc., *24*: 127, 1965.

Venkatachalam, P. S., *et al.:* Studies on vitamin A nutritional status of mothers and infants in poor communities of India. J. Am. Dietet. A., *41*:476, 1962.

Wolfe, G.: Some thoughts on metabolic role of vitamin A. Nutr. Rev., *20*:161, 1962.

Vitamin D

Journal Articles:

Aboul-Dahab, Y. W., and Zaki, K.: Studies on rickets and malnutrition in the undernourished child. Am. J. Clin. Nutr., *13*:98, 1963.

Barnsby, E. R., *et al.:* Study of the vitamin D intake of infants in 1960. Brit. M. J., *1*:1661, 1964.

Broadfoot, B. V. R., *et al.:* Vitamin D intakes of Canadian children. Canad. M. A. J., *94*: 332, 1966.

Committee on Nutrition: The prophylactic requirement and toxicity of vitamin D. Pediatrics, *31*:512, 1963.

——: Vitamin D intake and the hypercalcemic syndrome. Pediatrics, *35*:1022, 1965.

Cuthbertson, W. F. J.: The vitamin D activity of plasma of children with idiopathic hypercalcemia. Brit. J. Nutr., *17*:627, 1963.

Dale, A. E., and Lowenberg, M. E.: Consumption of vitamin D in fortified and natural foods and in vitamin preparations. J. Pediat., *70*:952, 1967.

Dent, C. E.: Dangers of vitamin D intoxication. Brit. M. J., *5386*:834, 1964.

Fomon, S. J., *et al.:* Vitamin D and growth of infants. J. Nutr., *88*:345, 1965.

Forbes, G. B.: Present knowledge of vitamin D. Nutr. Rev., *25*:225, 1967.

Harrison, H. E., and Harrison, H. C.: Vitamin D and permeability of intestinal mucosa to calcium. Am. J. Physiol., *208*:370, 1965.

Harrison, H. E.: Vitamin D and calcium and phosphate transport. Pediatrics, *28*:53, 1961.

Norman, A. W.: Actinomycin D and the response to vitamin D. Science, *149*:184, 1965.

Review: Effect of vitamin A on vitamin D toxicity. Nutr. Rev., *20*:315, 1962.

——: Intestinal absorption of calcium. Nutr. Rev., *20*:45, 1962.

——: Nutritional rickets and parathyroid function. Nutr. Rev., *21*:271, 1963.

——: Safe levels of vitamin D intake for infants. Nutr. Rev., *24*:230, 1966.

——: Serum transport of vitamin D. Nutr. Rev., *24*:149, 1966.

——: Vitamin D and milk fever prevention. Nutr. Rev., *19*:141, 1961.

——: Vitamin D and protein synthesis. Nutr. Rev., *24*:18, 1966.

Wasserman, R. H.: Vitamin D and the intestinal absorption of calcium. N. Y. J. Med., *64*:1329, 1964.

Vitamin E

Journal Articles:

Alfin-Slater, R. B.: Relation of vitamin E to lipid metabolism. Am. J. Clin. Nutr., 8:445, 1960.

Bailey, P.: Cerebellar encephalomalacia produced by diets deficient in tocopherol. Am. J. Clin. Nutr., *12*:275, 1963.

Bieri, J. G., *et al.*: Serum vitamin E levels in a normal adult population in the Washington, D. C. area. Proc. Soc. Exp. Biol. Med., *117*:131, 1964.

Booth, V. H., and Bradford, M. P.: Tocopherol contents of vegetables and fruits. Brit. J. Nutr., *17*:575, 1963.

Bunnell, R. H., *et al.*: Alpha-tocopherol content of foods. Am. J. Clin. Nutr., *17*:1, 1965.

Century, B., and Horwitt, M. K.: Biological availability of various forms of vitamin E with respect to different indices of deficiency. Fed. Proc., *24*:906, 1965.

Committee on Nutrition: Vitamin E in human nutrition. Pediatrics, *31*:324, 1963.

Dinning, J. S.: Vitamin E responsive anemia in monkeys and man. Nutr. Rev., *21*:289, 1963.

Harris, R. D.: Influences of storage and processing on the retention of vitamin E in foods. Vitam. Horm., *20*:603, 1962.

Harris, P. L., and Embree, N. D.: Quantitative consideration of the effect of polyunsaturated fatty acid content of the diet upon the requirement for vitamin E. Am. J. Clin. Nutr., *13*:385, 1963.

Herting, D. C.: Perspective on Vitamin E. Am. J. Clin. Nutr., *19*:210, 1966.

Herting, D. C., and Drury, E. E.: Plasma tocopherol levels in man. Am. J. Clin. Nutr., *17*:351, 1965.

Horwitt, M. K.: Role of vitamin E, selenium, and polyunsaturated fatty acids in clinical and experimental muscle disease. Fed. Proc., *24*:68, 1964.

————: Vitamin E in human nutrition—an interpretive review. Borden's Rev., *22*:1, 1961.

————: Vitamin E and lipid metabolism in man. Am. J. Clin. Nutr., *8*:451, 1960.

Horwitt, M. K., *et al.*: Polyunsaturated lipids and tocopherol requirements. J. Am. Dietet. A., *38*:231, 1961.

Leonard, P. J.: Vitamin E deficiency in Uganda African subjects. Trans. Roy. Soc. Trop. Med. Hyg., *58*:517, 1964.

Majaj, A. S., *et al.*: Vitamin E responsive megaloblastic anemia in infants with protein-calorie malnutrition. Am. J. Clin. Nutr., *12*:374, 1963.

McMasters, V., *et al.*: Effect of supplementing the diet of man with tocopherol on the tocopherol levels of adipose tissue and plasma. Am. J. Clin. Nutr., *17*:357, 1965.

Moore, T.: The significance of selenium and vitamin E in nutrition. Proc. Nutr. Soc., *21*:179, 1962.

Nitowsky, H. M., *et al.*: Vitamin E requirements of human infants. Vitam. Horm., *20*:559, 1962.

Rahman, M. M., *et al.*: Serum vitamin E levels in the rural population of East Pakistan. Proc. Soc. Exp. Biol. Med., *117*:133, 1964.

Review: Antioxidant replacements for vitamin E. Nutr. Rev., *19*:217, 1961.

————: The determination of alpha-tocopherol in animal tissues. Nutr. Rev., *20*:111, 1962.

————: Erythrocyte hemolysis, lipid peroxidation, and vitamin E. Nutr. Rev., *20*:60, 1962.

————: Interrelationships between vitamins A and E. Nutr. Rev., *23*:82, 1965.

————: Metabolic role of vitamin E. Nutr. Rev., *23*:90, 1965.

————: "Therapy" with vitamin E. Nutr. Rev., *18*:227, 1960.

————: Tocopherol deficiency in infancy and childhood. Nutr. Rev., *19*:168, 1961.

————: Vitamin E and amino acid transport. Nutr. Rev., *24*:203, 1966.

————: Vitamin E and erythrocyte life span. Nutr. Rev., *19*:155, 1961.

————: Vitamin E responsive macrocytic anemia. Nutr. Rev., *21*:263, 1963.

————: Vitamin E status of adults on a vegetable oil diet. Nutr. Rev., *24*:41, 1966.

Roels, O. A.: Present knowledge of vitamin E. Nutr. Rev., *25*:33, 1967.

Schwartz, K.: Factor 3, selenium and vitamin E. Nutr. Rev., *18*:193, 1960.

Vitamin K

Journal Articles:

Aballi, A. J.: The action of vitamin K in the neonatal period. S. Med. J., *58*:1, 48, 1965.

Committee on Nutrition: Vitamin K compounds and the water soluble analogues. Pediatrics, *28*:501, 1961.

Dallam, R. D.: Possible function of vitamin K and related quinones in oxidative phosphorylation. Am. J. Clin. Nutr., *9*:104, 1961.

Johnson, B. C.: Dietary factors and vitamin K. Nutr. Rev., *22*:225, 1964.

Martius, C.: The metabolic relationships between the different K vitamins and the synthesis of the ubiquinones. Am. J. Clin. Nutr., *9*:97, 1961.

Paolucci, A. M., *et al.*: Vitamin K deficiency and oxidative phosphorylation. J. Nutr., *81*:17, 1963.

Review: The antagonistic effect of vitamin A on vitamin K in the germfree rat. Nutr. Rev., *24*:125, 1966.

Review: Hemolysis and bilirubinemia induced by vitamin K analog in the rat. Nutr. Rev., 22:78, 1964.

————: Irradiated beef and vitamin K. Nutr. Rev., *19*:14, 1961.

————: Sex differences in susceptibility to vitamin K deficiency. Nutr. Rev., *19*:110, 1961.

Shoshkes, M., *et al.:* Vitamin K_1 in neonatal hypoprothrombinemia. J. Am. Dietet. A., *38*: 380, 1961.

Smith, A. E., Jr., and Custer, R. P.: Vitamin K toxicity, induced hypoprothrombinemia and altered liver function. J.A.M.A., *173*:502, 1960.

Vietti, T. J.: Observations on the prophylactic use of vitamin K in the newborn infant. J. Pediat., *56*:343, 1960.

Wefring, K. W.: Hemorrhage in the newborn and vitamin K prophylaxis. J. Pediat., *63*: 663, 1963.

Thiamine

Journal Articles:

Baker, H., *et al.:* A method for assaying thiamine status in man and animals. Am. J. Clin. Nutr., *14*:197, 1964.

Bradley, W. B.: Thiamine enrichment in the United States. Ann. N. Y. Acad. Sci., *98*: 602, 1962.

Brin, M.: Erythrocyte as a biopsy tissue for functional evaluation of thiamine adequacy. J.A.M.A., *187*:762, 1964.

Dreyfus, R. M., and Victor, M.: Effects of thiamine deficiency on the central nervous system. Am. J. Clin. Nutr., *9*:414, 1961.

Jansen, B. C. P.: Early nutritional research on beriberi leading to the discovery of vitamin B_1. Nutr. Abstr. Rev., *26*:1, 1956.

Morrison, A. B., and Campbell, J. A.: Vitamin absorption studies. I. Factors influencing the excretion of oral test doses of thiamine and riboflavin by human subjects. J. Nutr., *72*: 435, 1960.

Noble, L. I.: Thiamine and riboflavin retention in braised meat. J. Am. Dietet. A., *47*:205, 1965.

Review: Availability of flora-synthesized thiamine. Nutr. Rev., *20*:124, 1962.

————: Carbohydrates and thiamine synthesis. Nutr. Rev., *20*:216, 1962.

————: Thiamine deficiency in an infant. Nutr. Rev., *20*:304, 1962.

Rogers, E. F.: Thiamine antagonists. Ann. N. Y. Acad. Sci., *98*:412, 1962.

Salcedo, J.: Experience in the etiology and prevention of thiamine deficiency in the Philippine Islands. Ann. N. Y. Acad. Sci., *98*: 568, 1962.

Sebrall, W. H.: A clinical evaluation of thiamine deficiency. Ann. N. Y. Acad. Sci., *98*: 563, 1962.

Wurst, H. M.: The history of thiamine. Ann. N. Y. Acad. Sci., *98*:385, 1962.

Ziporin, Z. Z., *et al.:* Excretion of thiamine and its metabolites in the urine of young adult males receiving restricted intakes of the vitamins. J. Nutr., *85*:287, 1965.

————: Thiamine requirement in the adult human as measured by urinary excretion of thiamine metabolites. J. Nutr., *85*:297, 1965.

Riboflavin

Journal Articles:

Belvady, B.: Riboflavin requirement of nursing mothers. Indian J. Med. Res., *50*:104, 1962.

Bro-Rasmussen, F.: The riboflavin requirement of animals and man and associated metabolic reactions. Nutr. Abstr. Rev., *28*:369, 1958.

Lane, M., *et al.:* The anemia of human riboflavin deficiency. Blood, *25*:632, 1965.

————: The rapid induction of human riboflavin deficiency with galactoflavin. J. Clin. Invest., *43*:357, 1964.

Review: Genetic differences in riboflavin utilization. Nutr. Rev., *22*:273, 1964.

————: Non-respiratory function of riboflavin. Nutr. Rev., *20*:95, 1962.

————: Riboflavin and adrenal cortical metabolism. Nutr. Rev., *18*:221, 1960.

————: Riboflavin coenzymes and congenital malformations. Nutr. Rev., *21*:24, 1963.

Tucker, R. G., *et al.:* The influence of sleep, work, diuresis, heat, acute starvation, thiamine intake, and bed rest on human riboflavin excretion. J. Nutr., *72*:251, 1960.

Windmueller, H. G., *et al.:* Elevated riboflavin levels in urine of fasting human subjects. Am. J. Clin. Nutr., *15*:73, 1964.

Niacin

Journal Articles:

Chick, H.: The causation of pellagra. Nutr. Abstr. Rev., *20*:523, 1950-51.

DeLange, D. J., and Joubert, C. P.: Assessment of nicotinic acid status of population groups. Am. J. Clin. Nutr., *15*:169, 1964.

Gabuzda, G. J., and Davidson, C. S.: Tryptophan and nicotinic acid metabolism in patients with cirrhosis of the liver. Am. J. Clin. Nutr., *11*:502, 1962.

Goldsmith, G.A.: Niacin-tryptophan relationships in man and niacin requirements. Am. J. Clin. Nutr., 6:479, 1958.

————: Niacin—antipellagra factor, hypercholesterolemic agent. J.A.M.A., 194:167, 1965.

Goldsmith, G. A., et al.: Efficiency of tryptophan as a niacin precursor in man. J. Nutr., 73:172, 1961.

Horwitt, M. K.: Niacin-tryptophan requirements of man, in terms of niacin equivalents. J. Am. Dietet. A., 34:914, 1958.

Moyer, E. Z., et al.: Metabolic patterns in preadolescent children. VII. Intake of niacin and tryptophan and excretion of niacin or tryptophan metabolites. J. Nutr., 79:423, 1963.

Review: Bound niacin. Nutr. Rev., 19:240, 1961.

————: Fetal death from nicotinamide deficiency. Nutr. Rev., 23:58, 1964.

————: Nicotinic acid and diabetes mellitus. Nutr. Rev., 22:166, 1964.

Rikans, L. L., et al.: Fatty livers produced in albino rats by excess niacin in high fat diets. I. Alterations in enzyme and coenzyme systems induced by supplementing 40 per cent fat diets with 0.1 per cent of niacin. J. Nutr., 82:83, 1964.

Vivian, V. M.: Relationship between tryptophan metabolism and changes in nitrogen balance. J. Nutr., 82:395, 1964.

Pyridoxine

Journal Articles:

Babcock, M. J., et al.: Evaluation of vitamin B_6 nutrition. J. Nutr., 70:369, 1960.

Baker, E. M., et al.: Vitamin B_6 requirement for adult man. Am. J. Clin. Nutr., 15:59, 1964.

Bunnell, R. H.: Vitamin B_6. Science, 146:674, 1964.

Cheslock, K. E., and McCully, M. T.: Response of human beings to a low-vitamin B_6 diet. J. Nutr., 70:507, 1960.

Coursin, D. B.: Present status of vitamin B_6 metabolism. Am. J. Clin. Nutr., 9:304, 1961.

————: Vitamin B_6 requirements. J.A.M.A., 189:27, 1964.

Everson, G. J., et al.: Aseptic canning of foods. III. Pyridoxine retention as influenced by processing method, storage, time, and temperature and type of container. Food Tech., 18:87, 1964.

Farogalla, F. F., and Gershoff, S. N.: Interrelationships among magnesium, vitamin B_6, sulfur and phosphorus in the formation of kidney stones in the rat. J. Nutr., 81:60, 1963.

Hines, J. D., and Harris, J. W.: Pyridoxine-responsive anemia. Description of three patients with megaloblastic erythropoiesis. Am. J. Clin. Nutr., 14:137, 1964.

————:Pyridoxine-responsive anemia. Am. J. Clin. Nutr., 15:59, 1964.

Hollister, L. E., et al.: Antipyridoxine effect of D-penicillamine in schizophrenic men. Am. J. Clin. Nutr., 19:307, 1966.

Johansson, S., et al.: Studies on the metabolism of labelled pyridoxine in man. Am. J. Clin. Nutr., 18:185, 1966.

Leitch, I., and Hepburn, A.: Pyridoxine metabolism and requirement. Nutr. Abstr. Rev., 31:389, 1961.

Linkswiler, H.: Biochemical and physiological changes in vitamin B_6 deficiency. Am. J. Clin. Nutr., 20:547, 1967.

Lushbough, C. H., et al.: The retention of vitamin B_6 in meat during cooking. J. Nutr., 67:451, 1959.

Mueller, J. F., and Tacono, J. M.: Effect of desoxypyridoxine-induced vitamin B_6 deficiency on polyunsaturated fatty acid metabolism in human beings. Am. J. Clin. Nutr., 12:358, 1963.

Nelson, E. M.: Association of vitamin B_6 deficiency with convulsions in infants. Pub. Health Rep., 71:445, 1956.

Polansky, M. M., et al.: Components of vitamin B_6 in grains and cereal products. J. A. Agr. Chem., 47:750, 1964.

Polansky, M. M., and Murphy, E. W.: Vitamin B_6 in fruits and nuts. J. Am. Dietet. A., 48:109, 1966.

Raica, N., Jr., and Sauberlich, H. E.: Blood cell transaminase activity in human vitamin B_6 deficiency. Am. J. Clin. Nutr., 15:67, 1964.

Review: Pyridoxine and dental caries; human studies. Nutr. Rev., 21:143, 1963.

————: Pyridoxine dependency. Nutr. Rev., 25:72, 1967.

————: Vitamin B_6 content of infant foods. Nutr. Rev., 19:223, 1961.

————: Vitamin B_6 deficiency and tryptophan metabolism. Nutr. Rev., 21:89, 1963.

————: Vitamin B_6 dependency state in infants. Nutr. Rev., 19:229, 1961.

————: Effects of insulin on carbohydrate and fat metabolism in vitamin B_6 deficiency. Nutr. Rev., 22:314, 1964.

Richardson, L. R., et al.: Comparative vitamin B_6 activity of frozen, irradiated and heat-processed foods. J. Nutr., 73:363, 1961.

Ritchey, S. J., and Feeley, R. M.: The excretion patterns of vitamin B_6 and B_{12} in preadolescent girls. J. Nutr., 89:411, 1966.

Sauberlich, H. E.: Human requirements for vitamin B_6. Vitam. Horm., 22:807, 1964.

Shriver, C. R., and Hutchison, J. H.: The vitamin B_6 deficiency syndrome in human infancy: biochemical and clinical observations. Pediatrics, 31:240, 1963.

Swendseid, M. E., *et al.*: Free amino acid in plasma and tissues of rats fed a vitamin B_6-deficient diet. J. Nutr., 82:206, 1964.

Folic Acid

Journal Articles:

Banerjee, D. K., and Chatterjea, J. B.: Folic activity of Indian dietary articles. Food Tech., 18:137, 1964.

Chung, A. S., *et al.*: Folic acid, vitamin B_6, pantothenic acid, and vitamin B_{12} in human dietaries. Am. J. Clin. Nutr., 9:573, 1961.

Ghitis, J.: The labile folate of milk. Am. J. Clin. Nutr., 18:452, 1966.

Herbert, V.: A palatable diet for producing experimental folate deficiency in man. Am. J. Clin. Nutr., 12:17, 1963.

Herbert, V.: Studies of folate deficiency in man. Proc. Roy. Soc. Med., 57:377, 1964.

————: Folic acid. Annual Rev. Med., 16:359, 1965.

Izak, G., *et al.*: The effect of small doses of folic acid in nutritional megaloblastic anemia. Am. J. Clin. Nutr., 13:369, 1963.

Klipstein, F. A., and Lindenbaum, J.: Folate deficiency in chronic liver disease. Blood, 25:443, 1965.

Review: Folacin activity in U. S. diets. Nutr. Rev., 22:142, 1964.

————: Folic acid restriction and cancer inhibition. Nutr. Rev., 21:82, 1963.

————: Folic acid in serum. Nutr. Rev., 20:83, 1962.

Santini, R., *et al.*: The distribution of folic acid active compounds in individual foods. Am. J. Clin. Nutr., 14:205, 1962.

————: Folic acid activity in Puerto Rican foods. J. Am. Dietet. A., 41:562, 1962.

Velez, H., *et al.*: Folic acid deficiency secondary to iron deficiency in man. Am. J. Clin. Nutr., 19:27, 1966.

Vilter, R. W., *et al.*: Interrelationships of vitamin B_{12}, folic acid and ascorbic acid in the megaloblastic anemias. Am. J. Clin. Nutr., 12:130, 1963.

Vitale, J. J.: Present knowledge of folacin. Nutr. Rev., 24:289, 1966.

Vitamin B_{12}

Journal Articles:

Chow, B. F.: Nutritional significance of vitamin B_{12}, World Rev. Nutr. Dietet., 1:127, 1960.

Cox, E. V., and White, A. M.: Methylmalonic acid excretion; An index of vitamin B_{12} deficiency. Lancet, 2:853, 1962.

Feeley, R. M., and Moyer, E. Z.: Metabolic patterns in preadolescent children. VI. Vitamin B_{12} intake and urinary excretion. J. Nutr., 75:447, 1961.

Hsu, J. M.: Effect of deficiencies of certain B vitamins and ascorbic acid on absorption of vitamin B_{12}. Am. J. Clin. Nutr., 12:170, 1963.

Jadhav, M., *et al.*: Vitamin B_{12} deficiency in Indian infants. Lancet, 2:903, 1962.

Morse, E. H., *et al.*: Vitamin B_{12} and ascorbic acid in protein utilization. J. Am. Dietet. A., 39:476, 1961.

Review: B_{12} transport in red cell membranes. Nutr. Rev., 25:248, 1967.

————: Intrinsic factor and absorption of vitamin B_{12}. Nutr. Rev., 19:177, 1961.

————: New antimetabolites of vitamin B_{12}. Nutr. Rev., 18:333, 1960.

————: Oral B_{12} therapy of pernicious anemia. Nutr. Rev., 22:10, 1964.

————: Relationship between thyroid hormone and vitamin B_{12}. Nutr. Rev., 19:274, 1961.

————: Vitamin B_{12} deficiency. Nutr. Rev., 18:121, 1960.

————: Vitamin B_6 and B_{12} relationships. Nutr. Rev., 19:122, 1961.

————: Vitamin B_{12} deficiency in vegetarians. Nutr. Rev., 14:73, 1956.

————: Vitamin B_{12} interrelationships. Nutr. Rev., 18:16, 1960.

Schweigert, B. S.: The role of vitamin B_{12} in nucleic acid synthesis. Borden Rev. Nutr. Res., 22:19, 1961.

Spray, G. H.: Absorption of vitamin B_{12} from the intestines. Proc. Nutr. Soc., 26:55, 1967.

Sullivan, L. W., and Herbert, V.: Studies on the minimum daily requirement for vitamin B_{12}. New Eng. J. Med., 272:340, 1965.

Symposium on vitamin B_{12}. Am. J. Clin. Nutr., 8:259, 1960.

U. S. Dept. of Agriculture: Vitamin B_{12} microbiological assay method and distribution in selected foods. Home Econ. Res. Report. No. 13. Washington, D. C., Gov't. Printing Office, 1961.

Weissbach, H., and Dickerman, H.: Biochemical role of vitamin B_{12}. Physiolog. Rev., 45:80, 1965.

Wilson, T. H.: Intrinsic factor and B_{12} absorption—a problem in cell physiology. Nutr. Rev., 23:33, 1965.

Biotin

Journal Articles:

Bridgers, W. F.: Present knowledge of biotin. Nutr. Rev., 25:65, 1967.

Ochoa, S., and Kaziro, Y.: Biotin enzymes, Fed. Proc., 20:982, 1961.

Review: Mechanism of action of biotin-enzymes. Nutr. Rev., 21:310, 1963.

————: The role of biotin in lipid metabolism. Nutr. Rev., 20:143, 1962.

Woodward, J. D.: Biotin. Sci. Am., 204:139, 1961.

Pantothenic Acid
Journal Articles:

Faber, S. R., *et al.*: The effects of an induced pyridoxine and pantothenic acid deficiency on excretions of oxalic and xanthurenic acids in the urine. Am. J. Clin. Nutr., 12:406, 1963.

Fox, H. M., and Linkswiler, H.: Pantothenic acid excretion on three levels of intake. J. Nutr., 75:451, 1961.

Hatano, M.: Blood and urinary pantothenic acid levels in the patients with liver diseases. J. Vitaminol., 8:161, 1962.

Ishiguro, K.: Studies on pantothenic acid and age. J. Am. Dietet. A., 40:450, 1962.

————: Studies on pantothenic acid intake. II. Pantothenic acid intake of farming and finishing villagers. J. Am. Dietet. A., 43:249, 1963.

Page, J. K., *et al.*: Metabolic patterns in preadolescent children. V. Intake and urinary excretion of pantothenic acid and of folic acid. J. Nutr., 74:345, 1961.

Review: Relation of pantothenic acid to adrenal cortical function. Nutr. Rev., 19:79, 1966.

Zook, E. G., *et al.*: Pantothenic acid in foods. Agr. Handbook No. 97. Washington, D. C., 1956.

Ascorbic Acid
Journal Articles:

Abt, A. F., von Schuching, S., and Enns, T.: Vitamin C requirement of man reexamined. Am. J. Clin. Nutr., 12:21, 1963.

Bring, S. V., and Raab, F. P.: Total ascorbic acid in potatoes. J. Am. Dietet. A., 45:149, 1964.

Demers, P., *et al.*: An epidemiological study of infantile scurvy in Canada, 1961-3. Canad. M. A. J., 93:573, 1965.

Grewar, D.: Infantile scurvy. Clin. Pediat., 4:82, 1965.

Livak, J. K., and Morse, E. H.: Ascorbic acid in vegetables purchased in Vermont. J. Am. Dietet. A., 41:111, 1962.

Lopez, A., *et al.*: Influence of time and temperature on ascorbic acid stability. J. Am. Dietet. A., 50:308, 1967.

McDonald, B. S.: Gingivitis-ascorbic acid deficiency in the Navajo. J. Am. Dietet. A., 43:331, 1963.

Merrill, A. L.: Facts behind the figures—citrus fruits values in "Handbook No. 8," revised. J. Am. Dietet. A., 44:264, 1964.

Noble, I.: Ascorbic acid and color of vegetables. Effect of length of cooking. J. Am. Dietet. A., 50:304, 1967.

Noel, G. L., and Robberstad, M. T.: Stability of vitamin C in canned apple juice and orange juice under refrigerated conditions. Food Tech., 17:127, 1963.

Pierce, H. B., *et al.*: Ascorbic acid supplementation. I. Response of gum tissue. II. Response of certain blood constituents. Am. J. Clin. Nutr., 8:353, 1960.

Review: Ascorbic acid and the common cold. Nutr. Rev., 25:228, 1967.

————: Endothelial changes in scorbutic guinea pigs. Nutr. Rev., 24:179, 1966.

————: Intake and tissue levels of ascorbic acids in surgical patients. Nutr. Rev., 20:328, 1962.

————: Respiratory catabolism of L-ascorbic acid. Nutr. Rev., 22:7, 1964.

————: Scurvy and blood coagulation. Nutr. Rev., 18:242, 1960.

Ritchey, S. J.: Metabolic patterns in preadolescent children. XV. Ascorbic acid intake, urinary excretion and serum concentration. A. J. Clin. Nutr., 17:78, 1965.

Rivers, J. M.: Ascorbic acid metabolism of connective tissue. N. Y. J. Med., 65:1235, 1965.

Stone, N., and Meister, A.: Function of ascorbic acid in the conversion of proline to collagen by hydroxyproline. Nature, 194:555, 1962.

Wang, M. M., *et al.*: Comparative metabolic response to erythorbic acid and ascorbic acid by the human. J. Nutr., 77:443, 1962.

Wells, C. E., *et al.*: Ascorbic acid in uncooked frozen green beans. J. Am. Dietet. A., 43:559, 1963.

DIGESTION, ABSORPTION AND METABOLISM

Books:

Davenport, H. W.: Physiology of the Digestive Tract. Chicago, Year Book Publishers, 1961.

Wilson, T. H.: Intestinal Absorption. Philadelphia, W. B. Saunders, 1962.

Wiseman, G.: Absorption from the Intestine. New York, Academic Press, 1964.

Journal Articles:

Barboriak, J. J., *et al.*: Changes in breakfast menu and blood lipids. J. Am. Dietet. A., 49:204, 1966.

Bergstrom, B.: Absorption of fats. Proc. Nutr. Soc., *26*:34, 1967.

Bowie, M. D., *et al.:* Carbohydrate absorption in malnourished children. Am. J. Clin. Nutr., *20*:89, 1967.

Brown, W. D.: Present knowledge of protein nutrition. Part 3. Postgraduate Medicine, *41*(A):119, 1967.

Christensen, H. N.: Transport of amino acids. Nutr. Rev., *21*:97, 1963.

Clifton, J. A.: Intestinal absorption and malabsorption. J. Am. Dietet. A., *39*:449, 1961.

Cohen, A. M.: Effect of dietary carbohydrate on the glucose tolerance curve in the normal and the carbohydrate-induced hyperlipemic subject. Am. J. Clin. Nutr., *20*:126, 1967.

Cornblath, M., *et al.* (eds.): Carbohydrate and energy metabolism in the newborn—an international exploration. Pediatrics, *39*:582, 1967.

Dahlqvist, A.: Disaccharide intolerance. J.A.M.A., *195*:38, 1966.

————: Localization of the small-intestinal disaccharidases. Am. J. Clin. Nutr., *20*:81, 1967.

Danielsson, H.: Influence of bile acids on digestion and absorption of lipids. Am. J. Clin. Nutr., *12*:214, 1963.

Dragstedt, L. R.: Why does not the stomach digest itself? J.A.M.A., *177*:758, 1961.

Efron, M. L.: Diet therapy for inborn errors in amino acid metabolism. J. Am. Dietet. A., *51*:40, 1967.

Fisher, R. B.: Absorption of proteins. Proc. Nutr. Soc., *26*:23, 1967.

Gardner, F. H.: Nutritional management of chronic diarrhea in adults. J.A.M.A., *179*: 69, 1962.

Gaylor, J. L.: Inhibition of cholesterol biosynthesis. N. Y. J. Med., *66*:1097, 1966.

Holt, L. E., *et al.:* The concept of protein stores and its implication in the diet. J.A.M.A., *181*:699, 1962.

Holter, H.: How things get into cells. Sci. Am., *205*:167, 1961.

Holzel, A.: Nutritional consequences of altered carbohydrate absorption in infancy and childhood. Proc. Nutr. Soc., *23*:123, 1964.

Isselbacher, K. J.: Metabolism and transport of lipids by intestinal mucosa. Fed. Proc., *24*:16, 1965.

Jacobs, F. A.: Dietary amino acid transport via lymph. Fed. Proc., *26*:302, 1967.

Joint Committee of American Dietetic Association and American Medical Association: Diet as related to gastrointestinal function. J. Am. Dietet. A., *38*:425, 1961.

Jukes, T. H.: Present status of the amino acid code. J. Am. Dietet. A., *45*:517, 1964.

Kenworthy, R.: Influence of bacteria on absorption from the small intestine. Proc. Nutr. Soc., *26*:18, 1967.

Laster, L., and Ingelfinger, F. J.: Intestinal absorption—aspects of structure, function and disease of the small-intestine mucosa. New Eng. J. Med., *264*:1192, 1246, 1961.

Lehninger, A. L.: Energy transformation in the cell. Sci. Am., *202*:102, 1960.

Lengemann, F. W., and Comar, C. L.: The presence of lactose in intestinal tissue. J. Nutr., *81*:95, 1963.

Levy, R. I., *et al.:* Studies in a patient with chyluria—Relationship of dietary lipid to urinary fat excretion. Am. J. Clin. Nutr., *18*:20, 1966.

Mansford, R. L.: Recent studies on carbohydrate absorption. Proc. Nutr. Soc., *26*:27, 1967.

McDonald, I.: Dietary carbohydrate and lipid metabolism. Proc. Nutr. Soc., *23*:119, 1964.

————: Dietary carbohydrates and lipid metabolism. Nutr. Rev., *22*:257, 1964.

Mead, J. F.: The metabolism of polyunsaturated fatty acids. Am. J. Clin. Nutr., *8*:55, 1960.

Miller, D., and Crane, R. K.: The digestion of carbohydrates in the small intestine. Am. J. Clin. Nutr., *12*:220, 1963.

Mayer, J.: Why people get hungry. Nutrition Today, *1*:2, 1966 (June).

Nasset, E. S.: Role of digestive system in protein metabolism. Fed. Proc., *24*:953, 1965.

Neurath, H.: Protein-digesting enzymes. Sci. Am., *211*:68, 1964.

Newey, H., and Smyth, D. H.: Assessment of absorptive capacity. Proc. Nutr. Soc., *26*:5, 1967.

Orton, A. A.: Intestinal phase of amino acid nutrition. Fed. Proc., *22*:1103, 1963.

Peraino, C., and Harper, A. E.: Observations on protein digestion in vivo. V. Free amino acids in blood plasma of rats force-fed zein, casein, or their respective hydrolysates. J. Nutr., *80*:270, 1963.

Portman, O. W.: Importance of diet, species and intestinal flora in bile acid metabolism. Fed. Proc., *21*:896, 1962.

Review: Amino acid transport and insulin release. Nutr. Rev., *25*:41, 1967.

————: The biosynthesis of fatty acids. Nutr. Rev., *21*:155, 1963.

————: Carbohydrate digestion and absorption. Nutr. Rev., *21*:279, 1963.

————: Citrate cleavage and lipogenesis. Nutr. Rev., *24*:153, 1966.

Review: Diarrhea caused by disaccharidase deficiency. Nutr. Rev., 22:43, 1964.

———: Digestibility of high-amylose corn starches. Nutr. Rev., 21:27, 1963.

———: Digestion and absorption of disaccharides in man. Nutr. Rev., 20:203, 1962.

———: Effects of cortisol on glucose metabolism. Nutr. Rev., 20:278, 1962.

———: Effect of dietary protein on proteolytic enzymes. Nutr. Rev., 22:317, 1964.

———: Factors affecting amino acid absorption. Nutr. Rev., 24:332, 1966.

———: Glucose metabolism in the red blood cell. Nutr. Rev., 18:206, 1960.

———: Medium chain triglycerides in tropical sprue. Nutr. Rev., 23:71, 1965.

———: Metabolic interrelationships of dietary carbohydrate and fat. Nutr. Rev., 22:216, 1964.

———: Mobilization of liver lipids by specific plasma proteins. Nutr. Rev., 24:87, 1966.

———: Nutritional state and hormonal regulation of liver enzymes. Nutr. Rev., 24:308, 1966.

———: Protein digestion and metabolism. Nutr. Rev., 20:67, 79, 139, 201, 1962.

———: Regulation of gluconeogenesis. Nutr. Rev., 24:347, 1966.

———: Sucrose intolerance: An enzymatic defect. Nutr. Rev., 23:101, 1965.

———: The effect of pectin on cholesterol absorption. Nutr. Rev., 24:209, 1966.

———: The site of intestinal absorption of neutral fat and fatty acids. Nutr. Rev., 20:90, 1962.

———: Transport of amino acids. Nutr. Rev., 21:97, 1963.

———: Utilization of fructose by the working muscle. Nutr. Rev., 18:296, 1960.

Sanford, P. A.: The inhibition and mechanism of intestinal absorption. Proc. Nutr. Soc., 26:12, 1967.

Shiner, M.: The structure of the small intestine and some interesting relations to its function. Proc. Nutr. Soc., 26:1, 1967.

Snook, J. T.: Effect of diet on enzymes of exocrine pancreas. N. Y. J. Med., 66:3171, 1966.

Snook, J. T., and Meyer, J. H.: Response of digestive enzymes to dietary protein. J. Nutr., 82:409, 1964.

Symposium on mechanisms of gastrointestinal absorption. Am. J. Clin. Nutr., 12:161, 1963.

Tower, D. B.: Interrelationship of oxidative and nitrogen metabolism with cellular nutrition and function in the central nervous system. Am. J. Clin. Nutr., 12:308, 1963.

Treadwell, C. R., *et al.*: Factors in sterol absorption. Fed. Proc., 21:903, 1962.

Udenfriend, S.: Factors in amino acid metabolism which can influence the central nervous system. Am. J. Clin. Nutr., 12:287, 1963.

MEAL PLANNING
TO MEET RECOMMENDED
DIETARY ALLOWANCES

(See also General References and under specific nutrients)

Books and Pamphlets:

Anderson, L., and Browe, J. H.: Nutrition and Family Health Service. Philadelphia, W. B. Saunders, 1960.

Journal Articles:

Leverton, R. M.: Basic nutrition concepts. J. Home Ec., 59:346, 1967.

Maynard, L. A.: An adequate diet. J.A.M.A., 170:457, 1959.

Ohlson, M. A., and Hart, B. P.: Influence of breakfast on total day's food intake. J. Am. Dietet. A., 47:282, 1965.

Rusoff, L. L.: The role of milk in modern nutrition. Borden's Rev., 25:17, 1964 (Apr.-Sept.).

Sebrell, W. H.: The role of the bread-cereal group in the well-balanced diet. Borden's Rev., 27:1, 1966. (Jan.-Mar., Apr.-June).

Seidler, A. J.: Nutritional contributions of the meat group to an adequate diet. Borden's Rev., 24:29, 1963 (July-Sept.).

Stiebeling, H. K.: Foods of the vegetable-fruit group—their contribution to nutritionally adequate diets. Borden's Rev., 25:51, 1964 (Oct.-Dec.).

Walker, A. R. P.: Optimal intake of nutrients. Nutr. Rev., 23:321, 1965.

REGIONAL, NATIONAL AND
RELIGIOUS FOOD PATTERNS

Journal Articles:

Adolph, W. H.: Nutrition in the Near East. J. Am. Dietet. A., 30:753, 1954.

Community Nutrition Section, American Dietetics A.: Selected List of References on National Food Patterns and Recipes. Am. Dietet. A., 1954.

Hardinge, M. G., Crooks, H., and Stare, F. J.: Nutritional studies of vegetarians. J. Am. Dietet. A., 48:25, 1966.

Horne, L.: The evolution of dietary habits in the West Indies. Nutr., 14:158, 1960.

Jelliffe, D. B.: Cultural variation and the practical pediatrician. J. Pediat., 49:661, 1957.

Johnson, O. C.: Conference on nutrition teaching in medical schools. Nutr. Rev., *21*:33, 1963.

Joseph, S., *et al.*: Composition of Israeli mixed dishes. J. Am. Dietet. A., *40*:125, 1962.

Judd, J. E.: Century-old dietary taboos in 20th century Japan. J. Am. Dietet. A., *33*:489, 1957.

Korff, S. I.: The Jewish Dietary Code. Food Technology, *20*:76, 1966.

Lee, D.: Cultural factors in dietary choice. Am. J. Clin. Nutr., 5:166, 1957.

Mayer, J.: The nutritional status of American Negroes. Nutr. Rev., *23*:161, 1965.

Mitchell, H. S., and Joffe, N. F.: Food patterns of some European countries: Background for study programs and guidance of relief workers. J. Am. Dietet. A., *20*:676, 1944.

Queen, G. S.: Culture, economics and food habits. J. Am. Dietet. A., *33*:1044, 1957.

Tepley, L. J.: Training of nutrition workers for developing countries. J. Am. Med. Women's A., *18*:389, 1963.

Young, C. M., and Lafortune, T. D.: Effect of food preferences on nutrient intake. J. Am. Dietet. A., *33*:98, 1957.

NUTRITION IN PREGNANCY AND LACTATION

Books and Pamphlets:

Beaton, G. H., and McHenry, E. W.: Nutrition. A Comprehensive Treatise. Vol. III. Chap. 3. New York, Academic Press, 1966.

Brewer, T. H.: Metabolic Toxemia of Late Pregnancy, A Disease of Malnutrition. Springfield, Ill., Charles C Thomas, 1966.

Hytten, F. E., and Leitch, I.: The Physiology of Human Pregnancy. Philadelphia, F. A. Davis, 1964.

Macy, I. G.: Physiological Adaptations and Nutritional Status During and After Pregnancy. Detroit, Children's Fund of Michigan, 1954.

Moyer, E. C., *et al.*: Nutritional Status of Mothers and Their Infants. Detroit, Children's Fund of Michigan, 1954.

Prenatal Care. Children's Bureau Publ. No. 4. U. S. Department of Health, Education and Welfare, Washington, D. C., 1962.

WHO: Nutrition in Pregnancy and Lactation. Tech. Report Series No. 302. Geneva, Switzerland, 1965.

Journal Articles:

Allen, C. E., *et al.*: Vigorous weight reduction during pregnancy—Nitrogen balance before and during normal gestation. J.A.M.A., *188*: 392, 1964.

Alperin, H. T., *et al.*: Studies of folic acid requirements in megaloblastic anemia of pregnancy. Arch. Int. Med., *117*:681, 1966.

Aznar, R., and Bennett, A. E.: Pregnancy in the adolescent girl. Am. J. Obstet. Gynec., *81*:935, 1961.

Bagchi, K., and Bose, A. K.: Effect of low nutrient intake during pregnancy on obstetrical performance and offspring. Am. J. Clin. Nutr., *11*:586, 1962.

Beaton, G. H.: Some physiological adjustments relating to nutrition in pregnancy, Canad. M. A. J., *95*:622, 1966.

Beaton, G. H.: Nutritional and physiological adaptations in pregnancy. Fed. Proc. *20* (No. 1, Part III):196, 1961.

Beck, J.: Guarding the unborn. Today's Health, *46*:38, 1968 (Jan.).

Bigwood, E. J.: Nitrogenous constituents and nutritive value of human and cow's milk. World Rev. Nutr. Dietet., *4*:95, 1963.

Burke, B. S., *et al.*: Nutritional studies during pregnancy. J. Nutr., *38*:453, 1949.

Cellier, K. M., and Hankin, M. E.: Studies of nutrition in pregnancy. I. Some considerations in collecting dietary information. Am. J. Clin. Nutr., *13*:55, 1963.

Clements, F. W.: Nutrition in maternal and infant feeding. Fed. Proc. *20* (Suppl. 7):165, 1961.

Coursin, D. B., and Brown, V. C.: Changes in vitamin B_6 during pregnancy. Am. J. Obstet. Gynec., *82*:1307, 1961.

Dawson, D. W., *et al.*: Prevention of megaloblastic anemia in pregnancy by folic acid. Lancet, *2*:1015, 1962.

Edwards, C. H., *et al.*: Clay- and cornstarch-eating women. J. Am. Dietet. A., *35*:810, 1959.

———: Effect of clay and cornstarch intake on women and their infants. J. Am. Dietet. A., *44*:109, 1964.

Egan, M. C.: Working together in community nutrition. J. Am. Dietet. A., *45*:355, 1964.

Emerson, R. G.: Obesity and its association with the complications in pregnancy. Brit. Med. J., *5303*:516, 1962.

Gopalan, C.: Maternal and infant nutrition in underdeveloped countries. J. Am. Dietet. A., *39*:129, 1961.

Gray, M. J., *et al.*: Regulation of sodium and total body water metabolism in pregnancy. Am. J. Obstet. Gynec., *89*:761, 1964.

Hansen, A. E., *et al.*: Influence of diet on blood serum lipids in pregnant women and newborn infants. Am. J. Clin. Nutr., *15*:11, 1964.

Hellman, R. W.: Nutrition in pregnancy and lactation. Med. Clin. N. Am., *48*:1141, 1964.

Hillman, R. W., *et al.*: Pyridoxine supplementation during pregnancy. Am. J. Clin. Nutr., *12*:427, 1963.

Holly, R. G.: Dynamics of iron metabolism in pregnancy. Am. J. Obstet. Gynec., *93*:370, 1965.

Jacobson, H. N., *et al.*: Effect of weight reduction in obese pregnant women on pregnancy, labor, and delivery and on the condition of the infant at birth. Am. J. Obstet. Gynec., *83*:1609, 1962.

Jeans, P. C., *et al.*: Dietary habits of pregnant women of low income in a rural state. J. Am. Dietet. A., *28*:27, 1952.

Landesman, R., and Knapp, R. C.: Diagnosis and treatment of toxemias of pregnancy; I and II. N. Y. J. Med., *60*:3830, 1960.

Larson, R. H.: Effect of prenatal nutrition on oral structures. J. Am. Dietet. A., *44*:368, 1964.

Little, B.: Current concepts: Treatment of pre-eclampsia. New Eng. J. Med., *270*:94, 1964.

Lowenstein, L., *et al.*: The incidence and prevention of folate deficiency in a pregnant clinic population. Canad. M. A. J., *95*:797, 1966.

————: Vitamin B_{12} in pregnancy and the puerperium. Am. J. Clin. Nutr., 8:265, 1960.

Lubchenco, L. O., *et al.*: Intrauterine growth as estimated from liveborn birth-weight data at 24 to 42 weeks of gestation. Pediatrics, *32*:793, 1963.

Luhby, A. L., *et al.*: Survey of folic acid deficiency in pregnancy. Am. J. Clin. Nutr., *12*:332, 1963.

Macy, I. G.: Metabolic and chemical changes in normal pregnancy. J.A.M.A., *168*:2265, 1958.

Matoth, Y., *et al.*: Studies on folic acid in infancy. III. Folates in breast-fed infants and their mothers. Am. J. Clin. Nutr., *16*:356, 1965.

Mayer, J.: Nutrition and lactation. Postgrad. Med., *33*:380, 1963.

McCollum, E. B.: Symposium on prenatal nutrition. J. Am. Dietet. A., *36*:236, 1960.

McGanity, W. J.: Obesity and the obstetrician. J.A.M.A., *186*:39, 1963.

McGanity, W. J., *et al.*: Vanderbilt cooperative study of maternal and infant nutrition. J.A.M.A., *168*:2138, 1958.

Mengert, W. F., and Tacchi, D. A.: Pregnancy, toxemia and sodium chloride. Am. J. Obstet. Gynec., *81*:601, 1961.

Metz, J., *et al.*: Effect of folic acid and vitamin B_{12} supplementation on tests of folate and vitamin B_{12} nutrition in pregnancy. Am. J. Clin. Nutr., *16*:472, 1965.

Mullick, S., *et al.*: Serum lipid studies in pregnancy. Am. J. Obst. Gynec., *89*:766, 1964.

Neff, M. E.: Helping low-income families use donated foods. J. Am. Dietet A., *45*:358, 1964.

Payton, E., *et al.*: Dietary habits of 571 pregnant southern Negro women. J. Am. Dietet. A., *37*:129, 1960.

Pike, R. L.: Sodium intake during pregnancy. J. Am. Dietet. A., *44*:176, 1964.

Questions and Answers—Nausea of pregnancy. J.A.M.A., *187*:165, 1964.

Review: Diet, detoxification, and toxemia of pregnancy. Nutr. Rev., *21*:269, 1963.

————: Intrauterine growth. Nutr. Rev., *22*:266, 1964.

————: Maternity Care: The world situation. WHO Chronicle, *21*:140, 1967.

————: Vigorous weight reduction during pregnancy. Nutr. Rev., *22*:237, 1964.

Rhodes, P.: Significance of weight gain in pregnancy. Lancet, *1*:663, 1962.

Rust, H.: Food habits of pregnant women. Am. J. Nursing, *60*:1636, 1960.

Seifert, E.: Changes in beliefs and food practices in pregnancy. J. Am. Dietet. A., *39*:455, 1961.

Semmens, J. P.: Implications of teen-age pregnancy. Obstet. Gynec., *26*:77, 1965.

Semmens, J. P., and McGlamory, J. C.: Teenage pregnancies. Obstet. Gynec., *16*:31, 1960.

Sodium intake in pregnancy: two views. J.A.M.A., *200*:42, 1967.

Stevens, H. A., and Ohlson, M. A.: Nutritive value of the diets of medically indigent pregnant women. J. Am. Dietet. A., *50*:290, 1967.

Streiff, R. R., and Little, A. B.: Folic acid deficiency in pregnancy. New Eng. J. Med., *276*:776, 1967.

Thomson, A. M., and Billewicz, W. Z.: Nutritional status, maternal physique and reproductive efficiency. Proc. Nutr. Soc., *22*:55, 1963.

Underwood, B. A.: Human milk lipids during prolonged lactation. Fed. Proc., *26*:304, 1967.

Warkany, J.: Production of congenital malformations by dietary measures. J.A.M.A., *168*:2020, 1958.

Willoughby, M. L. N., and Jewell, F. J.: Investigation of folic acid requirements in pregnancy. Brit. Med. J., *5529*:1568, 1966.

Woody, D. C., and Woody, H. B.: Management of breast feeding. J. Pediat., *68*:344, 1966.

NUTRITION OF INFANTS

(See also references under Protein, Minerals and Vitamins)

Books and Pamphlets:

Blake, F. G., and Wright, F. H.: Essentials of Pediatric Nursing. Ed. 7. Philadelphia, J. B. Lippincott, 1963.

Fomon, S. J.: Infant Nutrition. Philadelphia, W. B. Saunders, 1967.

Gerber Products Co.: Nutritive Values of Gerber Baby Foods. Fremont, Mich., Gerber Products Co., 1966.

Holt, L. E., Jr., *et al.:* Pediatrics. Ed. 13. New York, Appleton-Century-Crofts, 1961.

How to make a baby's formula; by terminal heat method, by aseptic method, by tap water method. Evaporated Milk Ass., Chicago, Ill.

Hunt, E. P.: Recent Demographic Trends and Their Effects on Maternal and Child Health Needs and Services. Children's Bureau, U.S.H.E.W., Washington, D. C., 1966.

Meyer, H. F.: Infant Foods and Feeding Practices. Springfield, Ill., Charles C Thomas, 1960.

Nelson, W. E.: Textbook of Pediatrics. Ed. 8. Philadelphia, W. B. Saunders, 1964.

Oski, F. A., and Naiman, J. L.: Hematologic Problems in the Newborn. Philadelphia, W. B. Saunders, 1966.

Silverman, W.: Dunham's Premature Infants. Ed. 3. New York, Hoeber-Harper, 1961.

Spock, B.: Baby and Child Care. New York, Pocket Books, 1957.

Spock, B., and Lowenberg, M. E.: Feeding Your Baby and Child. New York, Pocket Books, 1955.

Willis, N. H.: Basic Infant Nutrition. Philadelphia, J. B. Lippincott, 1964.

General

Journal Articles:

Cravioto, J.: Application of the newer knowledge of nutrition on physical and mental growth. Am. J. Pub. Health, 53:1803, 1963.

Filer, L. J., and Martinez, G. A.: Intake of selected nutrients by infants in the United States. Clin. Pediat., 3:633, 1964.

Guthrie, H. A.: Nutritional intake of infants. J. Am. Dietet. A., 43:120, 1963.

McLoughlin, P. T.: Investigational background of present-day infant nutrition. Arch. Pediat., 79:208, 1962.

Rueda-Williamson, Rose, H. E.: Growth and nutrition of infants. Pediatrics, 30:639, 1962.

Symposium VII: Infant Nutrition. Council on Foods and Nutrition. J.A.M.A., 175:100, 1961.

Breast Feeding

Aitken, F. C., and Hytten, F. E.: Infant feeding: Comparison of breast and artificial feeding. Nutr. Abstr. Rev., 30:341, 1960.

Robertson, W. O.: Breast feeding practices. Am. J. Pub. Health, 51:1035, 1961.

Prematures

Davidson, M.: Feeding prematurely born infants. J. Pediat., 57:604, 1960.

Gordon, H. H.: Protein allowances for premature infants. J.A.M.A., 175:107, 1961.

Hassan, H.: Syndrome in premature infants associated with low plasma vitamin E levels. Am. J. Clin. Nutr., 19:147, 1966.

Holt, E. J., Jr., *et al.:* A study of premature infants fed a cold formula. J. Pediat., 61:556, 1962.

Holt, L. E., Jr., and Snyderman, S. E.: The effect of high caloric feeding on premature infants. J. Pediat., 58:237, 1961.

Omans, W. B., *et al.:* Prolonged feeding studies in premature infants. J. Pediat., 59:951, 1961.

Milks

Comm. on Nutrition, Amer. Acad. Pediatrics: Appraisal of nutritional adequacy of infant formulas used as cow milk substitutes. Pediatrics, 31:329, 1963.

————: Composition of milks. Pediatrics, 26:1039, 1960.

Cow's milk versus human milk protein in infant feeding. Nutr. Rev., 20:67, 1962.

Fomon, S. J.: Comparative study of adequacy of protein from human and cow's milk in promoting nitrogen retention in normal full-term infants. Pediatrics, 29:51, 1960.

Jackson, R. L., *et al.:* Growth of "well-born" American infants fed human and cow's milk. Pediatrics, 33:642, 1964.

Smith, C. A.: Overuse of milk in the diets of infants. J.A.M.A., 172:567, 1960.

Protein Requirement

Editorial: The protein allowance controversy. J. Pediat., 54:545, 1959.

Effect of nitrogen intake on nitrogen balance in infants. Nutr. Rev., 20:105, 1962.

Gordon, H. H., and Ganzon, A. F.: On the protein allowance for young infants. J. Pediat., 54:503, 1959.

Holt, L. E., Jr.: The protein requirement of infants. J. Pediat., 54:496, 1959.

Holt, L. E., Jr., *et al.:* The concept of protein stores and its implication in diet. J.A.M.A., 181:699, 1962.

Iron and Trace Elements

Andelman, M. B., and Sered, B. R.: Utilization of dietary iron by term infants. Am. J. Dis. Child., *111*:45, 1966; *113*:403, 1967.

Beal, V. A., *et al.*: Iron intake, hemoglobin and physical growth during the first two years of life. Pediatrics, *30*:518, 1962.

Comm. on Nutrition, Amer. Acad. Pediatrics: Trace elements in infant nutrition. Pediatrics, *26*:715, 1960.

Editorial: Iron deficiency in infants. J.A.M.A., *195*:175, 1966.

Farquhar, J. D.: Iron supplementation during the first year of life. Am. J. Dis. Child., *106*:201, 1963.

Filer, L. J., and Martinez, G. A.: Calorie and iron intake by infants in the United States: an evaluation of 4000 representative six-month olds. Clin. Pediat., *2*:470, 1963.

Gorten, M. K., *et al.*: Iron metabolism in premature infants: I. Absorption and utilization of iron as measured by isotope studies.

———: II. Prevention if iron deficiency. J. Pediat., *63*:1063, 1963; *64*:509, 1964.

———: III. Utilization of iron as related to growth in infants with low birth weight. Am. J. Clin. Nutr., *17*:322, 1965.

Haughton, J. G.: Nutrition anemia of infancy and childhood. Am. J. Pub. Health, *53*:1121, 1963.

Ross, J. D.: Treatment and prevention of iron deficiency anemia of infancy. N. Eng. J. Med., *266*:1372, 1962.

Shaw, R., and Robertson, W. O.: Anemia among hospitalized infants. Ohio State Med. J., *60*:45, 1964.

Wilson, J. F., *et al.*: Studies on iron metabolism. IV. Milk-induced gastrointestinal bleeding in infants with hypochromic microcytic anemia. J.A.M.A., *189*:568, 1964.

Woodruff, C. W., and Goode, M. D.: Nutritional assessment of infants with hypochromic anemia. Am. J. Clin. Nutr., *7*:634, 1959.

Vitamins

Bakwin, M.: The overuse of vitamins in children. J. Pediat., *59*:154, 1961.

Comm. on Nutrition, Amer. Acad. Pediatrics: Infantile scurvy and nutritional rickets in the U. S. Pediatrics, *29*:646, 1962.

Council on Foods and Nutrition, A.M.A.: Vitamin preparations as dietary supplements and as therapeutic agents. J.A.M.A., *169*:41, 1959.

Fomon, S. J., *et al.*: Influence of vitamin D on linear growth of normal full-term infants. J. Nutr., *88*:345, 1966.

Ossofsky, H. J.: Infantile scurvy. Am. J. Dis. Child., *109*:173, 1965.

Addition of Solid Foods

Beal, V. A.: On the acceptance of solid foods and other food patterns of infants and children. Pediatrics, *20*:448, 1957.

Comm. on Nutrition, Amer. Acad. Pediatrics: On the feeding of solid foods to infants. Pediatrics, *21*:685, 1958.

Review: Solid foods in the nutrition of young infants. Nutr. Rev., *25*:233, 1967.

NUTRITION OF CHILDREN AND YOUTH

(See aslo references under Proteins, Minerals, Vitamins)

General

Books and Pamphlets:

David, L.: Slimming for Teenagers. New York, Pocket Books, 1966.

Gesell, A., Ilg, F., and Ames, L. B.: Youth: The Years from Ten to Sixteen. New York, Harper, 1955.

György, P., and Burgess, A.: Protecting the Pre-School Child. London, Tavistock, 1965.

Hill, M. M.: Food Choices of the Teen-age Girl. Nutrition Foundation, New York, 1966.

Martin, E. A.: Nutrition Education in Action. New York, Holt, 1963.

McWilliams, M.: Nutrition for the Growing Years. New York, John Wiley and Sons, 1967.

Morgan, A. F. (ed.): Nutritional Status, U.S.A.? Bull. 769, Cal. Agr. Exp. Station, Berkeley, Cal., 1959.

Salmon, M. B.: Food Facts for Teenagers. Springfield, Ill., Charles C Thomas, 1965.

Tanner, J. M.: Growth at Adolescence. Oxford, Eng., Blackwell, 1962.

U.S.D.A.: Food for the Family with Young Children. Bull. No. 5, 1960.

———: Food for the Family with School Children. Bull. No. 15, 1960.

WHO Expert Committee: Health Problems of Adolescence. WHO Pub. 308, Geneva, 1965.

General

Journal Articles:

Beal, V. A.: Nutrition in a longitudinal growth study. J. Am. Dietet. A., *46*:457, 1965.

Beeuwkes, A. M., and Wallin, B. D.: From this day forward. . . . J. Am. Dietet. A., *49*: 289, 1966.

Burke, B. S., *et al.*: Relationship between animal protein, total protein, and total caloric intakes in the diets of children one to eighteen years of age. Am. J. Clin. Nutr., *9*: 136, 1961.

Burke, B. S., *et al.*: A longitudinal study of animal protein intake of children from one to eighteen years of age. Am. J. Clin. Nutr., 9: 616, 1961.

————: A longitudinal study of the calcium intake of children from one to eighteen years of age. Am. J. Clin. Nutr., 10:79, 1962.

Getty, G., and Hollinsworth, M.: Through a child's eye seeing. Nutrition Today (Florida Citrus Com.), 2:17, 1967 (June).

Gutelius, M. F., *et al.*: Treatment of pica with vitamin and mineral supplement. Am. J. Clin. Nutr., 12:388, 1963.

Lourie, R. S., *et al.*: Why children eat things that are not food. Children, 10:143, 1963 (July-Aug.).

Pre-schoolers

Dierks, E. C., and Morse, L. M.: Food habits and nutrient intakes of pre-school children. J. Am. Dietet. A., 47:292, 1965.

Harrison, H. E.: The disappearance of rickets. Am. J. Pub. Health, 56:734, 1966.

Metheny, N. Y., *et al.*: The diets of preschool children. Am. J. Home Ec., 54:303, 1962.

Tepley, L. J.: Nutritional needs of the preschool child. Nutr. Rev., 22:65, 1964.

Adolescents

Cone, T. E., Jr.: Growth problems of the adolescent. Med. Clin. N. Am., 49:357, 1965.

Edwards, C. H., *et al.*: Nutrition survey of 6200 teen-age youth. J. Am. Dietet. A., 45: 543, 1964.

Gschneider, M. P., and Roderuck, C. E.: Nutriture of school girls of different physiques. J. Am. Dietet. A., 36:22, 1960.

Hampton, M. C., *et al.*: Caloric and nutrient intakes of teen-agers. J. Am. Dietet. A., 50: 385, 1967.

Hinton, M. A.: Eating behavior and dietary intakes of girls 12 to 14 years old. J. Am. Dietet. A., 43:223, 1963.

Huenemann, R. L.: A study of teenagers: body size and shape, dietary practices and physical activity. Food and Nutrition News, 37: Apr. 1966. (Nat. Live Stock and Meat Board.)

Johnson, J. A.: Nutritional aspects of adolescence. J. Pediat., 59:741, 1961.

Mitchell, H. S.: Nutrition in relation to stature. J. Am. Dietet. A., 40:521, 1962.

————: Protein limitation and human growth. J. Am. Dietet. A., 44:165, 1964.

Nutritional implications of some problems of adolescents. Dairy Council Digest, 38:25, 1967 (Sept.-Oct.).

Nutritional status of teenagers. Dairy Coun. Digest, 35:7, 1964 (Jan.-Feb.).

Young, C. M.: Eating problems in adolescence. N. Y. J. Med., 61:939, 1961.

Height and Weight Studies

Hathaway, M. L.: Heights and weights of children and youth in the United States. Home Econ. Res. Report No. 2. Institute of Home Economics, Agricultural Research Service, U.S.D.A., 1957.

————: Overweight in children. J. Am. Dietet. A., 40:511, 1962.

Review: Growth standards for infants and children. Nutr. Rev., 21:141, 1963.

School Feeding and Nutrition Education

Council on Foods and Nutrition, A.M.A.: Confections and carbonated beverages in schools. J.A.M.A., 180:92, 1962.

Cronan, M. L.: The School Lunch. Peoria, Ill., Bennett, 1962.

Daniels, A. M.: Training school nurses to work with groups of adolescents. Children, 13: 210, 1966 (Nov.-Dec.).

Eppright, E. S., and LeBaron, H. R.: Our responsibilities to children and youth. J. Am. Dietet. A., 38:354, 1961.

Lantis, M.: The child consumer; cultural factors influencing his food choices. J. Home Econ., 54:370, 1962.

Review: The effects of a balanced lunch program on the growth and nutritional status of school children. Nutr. Rev., 23:35, 1965.

Whitehead, F. E.: How nutrition education affects adolescent's food choices. J. Am. Dietet. A., 37:348, 1960.

GERIATRIC NUTRITION

Books and Pamphlets:

Newton, K.: Geriatric Nursing. Ed. 3. St. Louis, C. V. Mosby, 1960.

Journal Articles:

Bernstein, D. S.: Prevalence of osteoporosis in high- and low-fluoride areas in North Dakota. J.A.M.A., 198:499, 1966.

Caniggia, A.: Senile osteoporosis. J. Am. Dietet. A., 47:49, 1965.

Cashman, J. W., *et al.*: Nutritionists, dietitians and Medicare. J. Am. Dietet. A., 50:17, 1967.

Davidson, C. S., *et al.*: The nutrition of a group of apparently healthy aging persons. Am. J. Clin. Nutr., 10:181, 1962.

Dibble, M. V., *et al.*: Evaluation of the nutritional status of elderly subjects, with a comparison of Fall and Spring. J. Am. Geriat. Soc., 15:1031. 1967.

Eckerstrom, S.: Clinical aspects of metabolism in the elderly. Geriatrics, 21:161, 1966.

Gordon, B. M.: A feeding plan for geriatric patients. Hospitals, 39:92, 1965 (Apr. 16).

Guggenheim, K., and Margulee, I.: Factors in the nutrition of elderly people living alone or as couples and receiving community assistance. J. Am. Geriat. Soc., 13:561, 1965.

Hayes, O. B., *et al.*: Relation of dietary intake to bone fragility in the aged, J. Geront., 11: 154, 1956.

Hegsted, D. M.: Nutrition, bone and calcified tissue. J. Am. Dietet. A., 50:105, 1967.

Henry, C. E.: Feeding elderly people in their homes. J. Am. Dietet. A., 35:149, 1959.

Keller, M. D., and Smith, C. E.: Meals on wheels. Geriatrics, 16:237, 1961.

Phillips, E. C.: Meals a la car. Nursing Outlook, 8:76, 1960.

Review: On meeting certain recommended dietary allowances in the elderly and the indolent. Nutr. Rev., 24:319, 1966.

Ryder, C. F.: A decalogue of challenges: Chronic illness and disability. J. Am. Dietet. A., 39:193, 1961.

Sebrell, W. H.: It's not age that interferes with nutrition of the elderly. Nutrition Today, 1: 15, 1966 (June).

Settle, E.: Correction of malnutrition in the aged; comparative efficacy of an anabolic hormone and enzyme vitamin complex. Geriatrics, 21:173, 1966.

Swanson, P.: Adequacy in old age: I. Role of nutrition. II. Nutrition education program for the aging. J. Home Econ., 56:651, 728, 1964.

Walker, D. M.: New findings in nutrition of older people. Am. J. Pub. Health, 55:548, 1965.

Watkin, D. M.: Nutrition of older people. Am. J. Pub. Health, 55:548, 1965.

MALNUTRITION— A WORLD-WIDE PROBLEM

(See also references under Proteins, Minerals and Vitamins)

Books and Pamphlets:

Autret, M., and Behar, M.: Syndrome Policarencial Infantil (Kwashiorkor) and its Prevention in Central America. FAO Nutrition Study 13. Rome, Italy, 1954.

Brock, J. F., and Autret, M.: Kwashiorkor in Africa. FAO Nutrition Study 8. Rome, Italy, 1952.

Brock, J. F.: Recent Advances in Nutrition. Boston, Little, Brown & Co., 1961.

Burgess, A., and Dean. R. F. A.: Malnutrition and Food Habits. Report of an international and interprofessional conference on malnutrition held at Cuernavaca, Mexico, 1960. London, Tavistock, 1962.

FAO: Third World Food Survey. Rome, Italy, 1963.

———: Freedom from Hunger Campaign: Basic studies 1960-1963. Rome, Italy, FAO.

———: Protein—At the Heart of the World Food Problem. Rome, FAO, 1967.

Hambidge, G.: The Story of FAO. New York, Van Nostrand, 1955.

Latham, M.: Human Nutrition in Tropical Africa. Rome, Italy, FAO, 1965.

May, J. M., and Jarcho, I. S.: The Ecology of Malnutrition in the Far and Near East. Food Resources, Habits and Deficiencies. New York, Hafner, 1961.

May, J. M.: The Ecology of Malnutrition in Central and Southeastern Europe. Studies in Medical Geography. New York, Hafner, 1966.

Moomaw, I. W.: The Challenge of Hunger— A Program for More Effective Foreign Aid. New York, Praeger, 1966.

Nichols, L., Sinclair, H. M., and Jelliffe, D. B. (eds.): Tropical Nutrition and Dietetics. Baltimore, Williams and Wilkins, 1961.

Pre-School Child Malnutrition—Primary Deterrent to Human Progress. Washington, Nat. Acad. Science—Nat. Res. Council, 1966.

Riddle, K. P., and Gatewood, R. D.: Food with Dignity—A Survey Presentation of Major U. S. Protestant Efforts to Combat World Hunger. New York, Nat. Council of Churches of Christ in the U.S.A., 1966.

Stein, H. D. (ed.): Planning for the Needs of Children in Developing Countries. (Roundtable Conference in Bellagio, Italy.) New York, UNICEF, 1965.

UNICEF: Children of the Developing Countries. New York, World Pub., 1963.

WHO: Requirements of Vitamin A, Thiamine, Riboflavin and Niacin. WHO Report 362. FAO Report 41, Geneva, Switzerland, 1967.

Williams, R. R.: Toward the Conquest of Beriberi. Cambridge, Harvard University Press, 1961.

General Malnutrition

Journal References:

American University of Beirut: Papers from the Institute of Nutrition Sciences. Am. J. Clin. Nutr., 17:115, 1965.

Balcomb, J.: The World-wide problem of malnutrition. UNICEF News, No. 40, Dec., 1966.

Berg, A. D.: Malnutrition and national development. Foreign Affairs, *46*:126, 1967 (Oct.).

DeMaeyer, E. M.: International nutrition programs by the UN Agencies. Am. J. Pub. Health, *56*:619, 1966.

Howe, E. E., *et al.*: An approach toward the solution of the world food problem with special emphasis on protein supply. Am. J. Clin. Nutr., *20*:1134, 1967.

King, C. G.: Trends in international nutrition programs. J. Am. Dietet. A., *48*:297, 1966.

Odell, A. D.: Malnutrition in the mid-hemisphere, progress thru research, General Mills, Minneapolis, Minn. 21, No. 2, 1967.

Review: Long-term effects of severe infantile malnutrition. Nutr. Rev., *25*:261, 1967.

Sen, B. R.: Problems of food and nutrition—views and programs of FAO. Fed. Proc., *20*:384, 1961.

Stiebeling, H. K.: Our share in better world nutrition. J. Am. Dietet. A., *45*:315, 1964.

Swaminathan, M.: Nutrition and the world food problem. Borden's Rev. Nutr. Res., *28*:1, 1967 (Jan.-Mar.).

Symposium on detection of nutrition deficiencies in man. Proc. Scottsdale, Ariz. Conference. Am. J. Clin. Nutr., *20*:513, 1967.

Symposium, Nutrition Section; Relation of nutrition to central nervous system function. Fed. Am. Soc. Exp. Biol., *4*:13, 1966.

Tepley, L. J.: Complementary effects of local and imported foods in improvement of nutrition in developing countries. Am. J. Pub. Health, *55*:1194, 1965.

VanVeen, A. G.: U. S. food production and world food needs. J. Am. Dietet. A., *48*:473, 1966.

Williams, R. R.: Can we eradicate the classical deficiency diseases? J. Am. Dietet. A., *36*:31, 1960.

———: Classical deficiency diseases. Fed. Proc., *20*:323, 1961.

Woodruff, C.: Nutritional aspects of metabolism of growth and development. J.A.M.A., *196*:214, 1966.

WHO: The WHO Programme in Nutrition. WHO Chronicle, *19*:378, 429, 467, 1965.

———: Malnutrition in early childhood. WHO Chronicle, *20*:83, 1966.

Youmans, J. B.: The changing face of nutritional disease in America. J.A.M.A., *189*: 672, 1964.

Specific Deficiencies
Protein-Calorie Malnutrition

Barnes, R. H.: Influence of nutritional deprivation in early life on learning and behavior of rats as measured by performance in a water maze. J. Nutr., *89*:399, 1966.

Bowie, M. D., *et al.*: Diarrhoea in protein-calorie malnutrition. Lancet, *2*,550, 1963.

Cabak, V., *et al.*: (Yugoslavia Pediatric Clinic) Effect of undernutrition in early life on physical and mental development. Arch. Dis. Child., *40*:532, 1965.

Caddell, J. L., and Goddard, D. R.: Studies in protein-calorie malnutrition—chemical evidence of magnesium deficiency. New Eng. J. Med., *276*:533, 1967.

Caddell, J. L.: Studies in protein-calorie malnutrition; Two double blind clinical trials to assess magnesium therapy. New Eng. J. Med., *276*:535, 1967.

Chandra, R. K.: Nutrition and brain development. J. Trop. Pediat., *10*:37, 1964.

Coursin, D. B.: Undernutrition and brain function. Borden's Rev., *26*:1, 1965 (Jan.-Mar.).

Cravioto, J., and Robles, B.: Evolution of adaptive and motor behavior during rehabilitation from kwashiorkor. Am. J. Orthopsychology, *35*:449, 1965.

Cravioto, J., *et al.*: Nutrition, growth and neurointegrative development; an experimental ecology study. Pediatrics (Suppl.), *38*:319, 1966.

Douglas, J. W. B., *et al.*: The relation between height and measured educable ability in school children of the same social class, family size and stage of sexual development. Human Biol., *37*:178, 1965.

Downs, E. F.: Nutritional dwarfing: A syndrome of early protein-calorie malnutrition. Am. J. Clin. Nutr., *15*:275, 1965.

György, P.: Conference notes on pre-school malnutrition. Am. J. Clin. Nutr., *14*:65, 1964.

Hopwood, H. H.: Scholastic underachievement as related to subpar-physical growth. J. School Health, *35*:337, 1965.

Jansen, G. R., and Howie, E. E.: World problems in protein nutrition. Am. J. Clin. Nutr., *15*:262, 1964.

Jelliffe, D. B.: Incidence of protein-calorie malnutrition n early childhood. Am. J. Pub. Health, *53*:905, 1963.

Kugel, R. B., and Mohr, J.: Mental retardation and physical growth. Am. J. Mental Defic., *68*:41, 1963.

Mosier, H. D., Jr.: Physical growth in mental defectives. A study in an institutionalized population. Pediatrics, (Suppl.), *36*:465, 1965.

Pretorius, P. J., and Wehmeyer, A. S.: An assessment of nutritive value of fish flour in the treatment of convalescent kwashiorkor patients. Am. J. Clin. Nutr., *14*:147, 1964.

Review: Subsequent growth of children treated for malnutrition. Nutr. Rev., *24*:267, 1966.

Review: Diet, development and intelligence. Nutr. Rev., *22*:244, 1964.

Scrimshaw, N. S.: Contributions of biochemistry to understanding and solving the world problem of protein-calorie malnutrition. Am. J. Clin. Nutr., *11*:593, 1962.

Webb, J. K., *et al.*: Peanut protein and milk protein blends in the treatment of kwashiorkor. Am. J. Clin. Nutr., *14*:331, 1964.

Mineral Deficiencies

Bell, M. E.: Mineral deficiencies in New Zealand. J. Am. Dietet. A., *40*:204, 1962.

Cadell, J. L.: Mineral deficiency . . . in extremis. Nutrition Today, *2*:14, 1967 (Sept.).

Cartwright, G. E., and Wintrobe, M. M.: The question of calcium deficiency in man. Am. J. Clin. Nutr., *15*:94, 1964.

Krehl, W. A.: The potassium depletion syndrome. Nutrition Today, *1*:20, 1966 (June).

———: Magnesium. Nutrition Today, *2*:16, 1967 (Sept.).

Lowenstein, F. W.: Iodized salt in the prevention of endemic goiter: a world wide survey of present programs. Am. J. Pub. Health, *57*:1815, 1967.

Mayer, J.: Zinc deficiency: a cause of growth retardation. Postgrad. Med., *35*:206, 1964.

Prasad, A. S., *et al.*: Zinc and iron deficiencies in male subjects with dwarfism and hypogonadism. Am. J. Clin. Nutr., *12*:437, 1963.

Randall, R. E.: Magnesium depletion in man. Ann. Int. Med., *50*:257, 1960.

Review: Potassium deficiency and the kidney. Nutr. Rev., *19*:242, 1961.

———: Magnesium deficiency. Nutr. Rev., *20*: 335, 1962.

———: Relation of zinc metabolism to a syndrome characterized by a anemia, dwarfism and hypogonadism. Nutr. Rev., *21*:264, 1963.

———: Goiter and iodine deficiency. Nutr. Rev., *22*:169, 1964.

———: Calcium deficiency in malnourished infants. Nutr. Rev., *23*:164, 1965.

Segar, W. E.: Multiple episodes of potassium deficiency. Am. J. Dis. Child., *109*:295, 1965.

Shils, M. E.: Experimental human magnesium depletion. Am. J. Clin. Nutr., *15*:133, 1965.

Vallee, B. L., *et al.*: The magnesium-deficiency tetany syndrome in man. New Eng. J. Med., *262*:155, 1960.

Wacker, W. E. C., and Vallee, B. L.: The magnesium deficiency syndrome in man. Borden's Rev., *22*:51, 1961.

WHO: Endemic goitre. WHO Chronicle, *14*: 337, 1960.

Vitamin Deficiencies—Vitamin A

Friis-Hansen, B., and McCullough, F. S.: Vitamin A deficiency in African children in Northern Rhodesia. J. Pediat., *60*:114, 1962.

McLaren, D. S.: Nutritional Disease and the Eye. Borden's Rev., *25*:1, 1964.

———: Xerophthalmia. Am. J. Clin. Nutr., *11*:603, 1962.

———: Xerophthalmia: a neglected problem. Nutr. Rev., *22*:289, 1964.

———: Xerophthalmia in Jordan. Am. J. Clin. Nutr., *17*:117, 1965.

Review: Etiology of follicular hyperkeratosis. Nutr. Rev., *21*:106, 1963.

Thiamine

Chitre, R. G., *et al.*: Bombay. Some aspects of thiamine metabolism and its probable relationship with infantile beriberi. Nutr. Abstr. Rev., *32*:209, 1962.

Cochrane, W. A., *et al.*: Superior hemorrhagic polioencephalitis (Wernicke's disease) occurring in an infant. Pediatrics, *28*:771, 1961.

Cravioto, H., *et al.*: Wernicke's encephalopathy; a clinical and pathological study of 28 autopsy cases. Arch. Neurol., *4*:510, 1961.

Jansen, B. C. P.: Early nutritional researches on beriberi leading to the discovery of vitamin B_1. Nutr. Abstr. Rev., *26*:1, 1956.

Pitt, D. B., and Samson, P. E.: Congenital malformations and maternal diet. Nutr. Abstr. Rev., *32*:895, 1962.

Reid, D. H. S.: Acute infantile beriberi. J. Pediat., *58*:858, 1961.

Review: Thiamine deficiency in infants. Nutr. Rev., *16*:240, 1958.

Victor, M.: Alcohol and nutritional diseases of the nervous system. J.A.M.A., *167*:65, 1958.

Wolf, P. L., and Levin, M. B.: Shōshin beriberi. New Eng. J. Med., *261*:1302, 1960.

Niacin

Barrett-Connor, E.: The etiology of pellagra and its significance for modern medicine. Am. J. Med., *42*:859, 1967.

Sydenstricker, V. P.: History of pellagra; its recognition as a disorder of nutrition and its conquest. Am. J. Clin. Nutr., *6*:409, 1958.

Vitamin B_6

Linkswiler, H.: Biochemical and physiological changes in vitamin B_6 deficiency. Am. J. Clin. Nutr., *20*:547, 1967.

Vilter, R. W.: Vitamin B_6 in medical practice. J.A.M.A., *159*:1210, 1955.

Wachstein, M.: Evidence of abnormal vitamin B_6 metabolism in pregnancy and various disease states. Am. J. Clin. Nutr., 4:369, 1956.

Ascorbic Acid and Vitamin D

Committee on Nutrition, Am. Acad. Pediatrics: Infantile scurvy and nutritional rickets in the United States. Pediatrics, 29:646, 1962.

Demers, P., *et al.*: An epidemiological study of infantile scurvy in Canada, 1961-63. Can. M. A. J., 93:573, 1965.

Harrison, H. E.: The disappearance of rickets. Am. J. Pub. Health, 56:734, 1966.

Kuroda, K.: Gingival pigmentation. Nutr. Abstr. Rev., 32:220, 1962.

Lorenz, A. J.: The conquest of scurvy. J. Am. Dietet. A., 30:665, 1954.

Severs, D., *et al.*: Infantile scurvy—a public health problem. Can. J. Pub. Health, 52:214, 1961.

Wilcox, E. B.: Gingivitis—ascorbic acid deficiency in the Navajo. J. Nutr., 74:352, 1961.

SAFEGUARDING OUR FOOD SUPPLY
Books and Pamphlets:

FAO/WHO Joint Committee on Food Additives: General Principles Governing the Use of Food Additives. Rome, FAO, 1957.

Food Protection Committee, Food and Nutrition Board: Safety of Artificial Sweeteners for Use in Foods. Pub. 386, 1955.

————: New Developments in the Use of Pesticides. Pub. 1082, 1963.

————: An Evaluation of Public Health Hazards from Microbiological Contamination of Foods. Pub. 1195, 1964.

————: Chemicals Used in Food Processing. Pub. 1274, 1965.

————: Toxicants Occurring Naturally in Foods. Pub. 1354, 1966.

Manufacturing Chemists Ass.: Food Additives, Washington, M. C. A., 1961.

National Communicable Disease Center: Salmonella Surveillance. Report 58. U. S. Dept. H.E.W., Washington, D. C., 1967.

U.S.D.A.: Protecting Our Food. Yearbook of Agriculture 1967. Washington, D. C., 1967.

WHO: The Public Health Aspects of the Use of Antibiotics in Foods. Geneva, 1963.

Journal Articles:
Food Care and Preservation

Goldblith, S. A.: Possible applications to food of ionizing and non-ionizing radiations. J. Am. Dietet. A., 51:233, 1967.

Saleh, B. A., *et al.*: Microbial evaluation of commercial freeze-dried foods. Food Tech., 20:103, 1966.

Schultz, H. W., and Lee, J. S.: Food preservation by irradiation: present status. Food Tech., 20:38, 1966.

Staff, N., and Miyauchi, D.: Acceptability of irradiated fish and shellfish. J. Am. Dietet. A., 46:111, 1965.

Vaughn, R. H., and Stewart, G. F.: Antibiotics as food preservatives. J.A.M.A., 174:162, 1965.

Foodborne Diseases and Toxins

Adler, H. E.: Salmonella in eggs—an appraisal. Food Tech., 19:191, 1965.

Cheng, T. C.: Parasitology and food protection. J. Environ. Health, 28:208, 1965.

Cliver, D. O.: Implications of bood-borne infectious hepatitis. Pub. Health Rep., 81:185, 1966.

Despaul, J. E.: The gangrene organism—a food-poisoning agent. J. Am. Dietet. A., 49:185, 1966.

Eadie, G. A., *et al.*: Type E. botulism. J.A.M.A., 187:496, 1964.

Editorial: Salmonella control. J.A.M.A., 189:691, 1964.

————: The most deadly poison. J.A.M.A., 187:530, 1964.

————: Carcinogen in groundnuts. Brit. Med. J., 5043:204, 1964.

Feuell, A. J.: Toxic factors of mould origin. Can. M. A. J., 94:574, 1966.

Goddard, J. L.: Incident at Selby Junior High. Nutrition Today, 2:2, 1967 (Sept.).

Koff, R. S., *et al.*: Viral hepatitis from shellfish. New Eng. J. Med., 276:703, 1967.

LaChapelle, N. C., *et al.*: A gastroenteritis outbreak of Staphylococcus aureus, Type 29. Am. J. Pub. Health, 56:94, 1966.

Lipshitz, A.: Salmonella food poisoning. N. Y. J. Med., 64:1112, 1964.

Most, H.: Trichinellosis in the United States. J.A.M.A., 162:871, 1965.

Note: Limiting temperature and humidity for production of aflatoxin by Aspergillus flavus in peanuts. Nutr. Rev., 25:286, 1967.

Note: Thermostable Clostridium perfringens as the cause of a food poisoning outbreak. Nutr. Rev., 25:287, 1967.

Review: Contaminated peanut meal. Nutr. Rev., 20:174, 1962.

————: Foods and feeds as sources of carcinogenic factors. Nutr. Rev., 24:321, 1966.

Salmonella, the ubiquitous bug. FDA Papers, 1:13, 1967 (Feb.).

Strong, F. M.: Naturally occurring toxic factors in plants and animals used as food. Can. M. A. J., *94*:568, 1966.

Thatcher, F. S.: Food-borne bacterial toxins. Can. M. A. J., *94*:582, 1966.

Wogan, G. N.: Current research on toxic food contaminants. J. Am. Dietet. A., *49*:95, 1966.

Zimmerman, W. J.: Current status of trichiniasis in U. S. swine. Pub. Health Rep., *80*: 1061, 1965.

●

Food Additives, Intentional and Accidental

Additives in Our Foods. Food & Drug Adm., U.S.H.E.W., Washington, D. C., 1966.

Council on Foods and Nutrition, A.M.A.: Radioactivity in foods. J.A.M.A., *171*:119, 1959.

Council on Foods and Nutrition, A.M.A., and Food and Nutrition Board, N.R.C.: General policy on addition of specific nutrients to foods. J.A.M.A., *178*:1024, 1961; Pub. 8, Food and Nutr. Board, N.R.C.

Fitzhugh, O. G.: Problems related to the use of pesticides. Can. M. A. J., *94*:598, 1966.

Food Additives: Safety of food additives continually evaluated. Pub. Health Rep., *81*: 244, 1966.

Hodges, R. E.: The toxicity of pesticides and their residues in food. Nutr. Rev., *23*:230, 1965.

Johnson, P. E.: Health aspects of food additives. Am. J. Pub. Health, *56*:948, 1966.

Oser, B. L.: Problems related to the use of food additives. Can. M. A. J., *94*:604, 1966.

Review: Food additives. Nutr. Rev., *19*:227, 1961.

Smith, E. H.: Problems in the safe and effective use of pesticides in Agriculture, Nutr. Rev., *22*:193, 1964.

Regulations Protecting our Food Supply

Analysis of pesticide residues. FDA Papers, *1*: 17, 1967 (June).

Beacham, L. M.: Food standards. FDA Papers, *1*:5, 1967 (July-Aug.).

Day, P. L.: The F.D.A. faces new responsibilities. Nutr. Rev., *18*:1, 1960.

FAO/IAEA/WHO Committee on Technical Basis for Legislation on Irradiated Foods; The Irradiation of Food. WHO Chronicle, *20*:371, 1966.

Kingma, F. J.: Establishing and monitoring drug residue levels. FDA Papers, *1*:9, 1967 (July-Aug.).

Roe, R. S.: F.D.A. food additive requirements. FDA Papers, *1*:25, 1967 (May).

WHO: Technical basis for legislation on irradiated foods. Tech. Report Ser. 316, 1966.

————: Procedures for investigating intentional and unintentional food additives. Tech. Report Ser. 348, 1967.

PART TWO

DIET IN DISEASE

(It is suggested that the bibliography under Nutrition and the references and Supplementary Readings quoted in each chapter also be consulted.)

GENERAL REFERENCES

Books:

Anderson, L., and Browe, J. H.: Nutrition and Family Health Services, Philadelphia, W. B. Saunders, 1960.

Beeson, P. B., and McDermott, W.: Cecil-Loeb Textbook of Medicine. Ed. 12. Philadelphia, W. B. Saunders, 1967.

Best, C. H., and Taylor, N. B.: Physiological Basis of Medical Practice. Ed. 8. Baltimore, Williams & Wilkins, 1966.

Bruner, J. S.: The Process of Education. Cambridge, Harvard University Press, 1965.

Cantarow, A., and Trumper, M.: Clinical Biochemistry. Ed. 6. Philadelphia, W. B. Saunders, 1962.

Church, C. F., and Church, H. N.: Food Values of Portions Commonly Used, ed. 10, Philadelphia, J. B. Lippincott, 1966.

Davidson, S., and Passmore, R.: Human Nutrition and Dietetics, ed. 3, Baltimore, Williams & Wilkins, 1966.

Duncan, G. G.: Diseases of Metabolism. Ed. 5. Philadelphia, W. B. Saunders, 1964.

Goldsmith, G. A.: Nutritional Diagnosis. Springfield, Ill., Charles C Thomas, 1959.

Goodman, L., and Gilman, A.: Pharmacological Basis of Therapeutics. Ed. 3. New York, Macmillan, 1965.

Guyton, A. C.: Textbook of Medical Physiology. Ed. 3. Philadelphia, W. B. Saunders, 1966.

Jevons, F. R.: The Biochemical Approach to Life. New York, Basic Books, 1964.

Krause, M. V.: Food, Nutrition and Diet Therapy, ed. 4, Philadelphia, W. B. Saunders, 1966.

Lillienfeld, A. M., and Gifford, A. J.: Chronic Diseases and Public Health. Baltimore, The Johns Hopkins Press, 1966.

Peyton, A. B.: Practical Nutrition, ed. 2, Philadelphia, J. B. Lippincott, 1962.

Robinson, C. H.: Proudfit-Robinson's Normal and Therapeutic Nutrition. Ed. 13. New York, Macmillan, 1967.

Thompson, R. H. S., and King, E. J.: Biochemical Disorders in Human Disease. Ed. 2. New York, Academic Press, 1964.

Turner, D.: Handbook of Diet Therapy. Ed. 4. Chicago, University of Chicago Press, 1965.

Wayler, T. J., and Klein, R. S.: Applied Nutrition, New York, Macmillan, 1965.

Weiss, E., and English, O. S.: Psychosomatic Medicine, ed. 3, Philadelphia, W. B. Saunders, 1957.

Wohl, M. G., and Goodhart, R. S.: Modern Nutrition in Health and Disease, ed. 3, Lea and Febiger, 1964.

Diet Manuals:

Diet Manual. The Ohio State University—University Hospital. Ed. 3. Columbus, Ohio, 1963.

Diet Manual. West Virginia University Medical Center. Ed. 2. Morgantown, W. Va., 1965.

Handbook of Experimental and Therapeutic Diets. Margaret A. Ohlson (ed.): Burgess Publishing Co., Minneapolis, Minn., 1962.

Manual of Applied Nutrition. Ed. 5. The Johns Hopkins Hospital—Nutrition Department. Baltimore, Md., 1966.

Mayo Clinic Diet Manual. Ed. 3. Philadelphia, W. B. Saunders, 1961.

(See also Diet Manuals from state departments of health.)

Journals:

American Journal of Clinical Nutrition
American Journal of Digestive Diseases
American Journal of Diseases of Children
American Journal of Medicine
American Journal of Nursing
American Journal of Obstetrics and Gynecology
American Journal of Public Health
Archives of Internal Medicine
Bulletin New York Academy of Medicine
Diabetes
Gastroenterology
Journal of Clinical Investigation

Journal of Chronic Diseases
Journal of Home Economics
Journal of Pediatrics
Journal of the American Dietetic Association
Journal of the American Medical Association
Lancet
Metabolism
New England Journal of Medicine
Nursing Outlook
Nutrition Reviews
Pediatrics
Postgraduate Medicine
Public Health Reports
Today's Health

THE PATIENT AND HIS NUTRITIONAL PROBLEMS; ROUTINE HOSPITAL DIETS

Books:

Bermosk, L. S., and Mordan, M. J.: Interviewing in Nursing. New York, Macmillan, 1964.

Brown, E. L.: Newer Dimensions of Patient Care: Part 3. Patients as People. New York, Russell Sage Foundation, 1964.

Macgregor, F. C.: Social Science in Nursing. New York, Russell Sage Foundation, 1960; paper, John Wiley & Sons, 1965.

Mead, M.: Cultural Patterns and Technical Change. New York, Mentor, 1955.

———: Food Habits Research: Problems of the 1960's. Publ. No. 1225, National Academy of Sciences—National Research Council, Washington, D. C., 1964.

Skipper, J. K., and Leonard, R. C.: Social Interaction and Patient Care. Philadelphia, J. B. Lippincott, 1965.

Journal Articles:

General

Goode, M. A.: The patient with a cerebral vascular accident. Nursing Outlook, *14*:60, 1966 (Mar.).

Johnson, D.: Present concepts of diet therapy. World Review of Nutrition and Dietetics, *5*:79, 1965.

Patterson, M. I., and Marble, B. B.: Dietetic foods. Am. J. Clin. Nutr., *16*:440, 1965.

Rivers, J. M.: Dynamics of diet therapy. Am. J. Clin. Nutr., *19*:357, 1966.

Tarnower, W.: Psychological needs of the hospitalized patient. Nursing Outlook, *13*:28, 1965 (July).

Vaughn, M. E.: An agency nutritionist looks at home health care under Medicare. J. Am. Dietet. A., *51*:146, 1967.

———: Nutrition consultation for public health nurses. J. Am. Dietet. A., *49*:505, 1966.

Meaning of Food

Babcock, C. G.: Attitudes and the use of food. J. Am. Dietet. A., 38:546, 1961.

Cassel, J.: Social and cultural implications of food and food habits. Am. J. Publ. Health, 47:732, 1957.

Fathauer, G. H.: Food habits—an anthropologist's view. J. Am. Dietet. A., 37:335, 1960.

Manning, M. L.: The psychodynamics of dietetics. Nursing Outlook, 13:57, 1965 (April).

Pumpian-Mindlin, E.: The meanings of food. J. Am. Dietet. A., 30:576, 1954.

Teaching the Patient

Cornely, P. B., et al.: Nutritional beliefs among a low-income urban population. J. Am. Dietet. A., 42:131, 1963.

Hamburger, W. W.: The psychology of dietary change. Am. J. Publ. Health, 48:1342, 1958.

Johnson, D.: Effective diet counseling begins early in hospitalization. Hospitals, 41:94, 1967.

Matthews, L. I.: Principles of interviewing and patient counseling. J. Am. Dietet. A., 50:469, 1967.

Morris, E.: How does a nurse teach nutrition to patients? Am. J. Nursing, 60:67, 1960 (Jan.)

Paynich, M. L.: Cultural barriers to nurse communication. Am. J. Nursing, 64:87, 1964 (Feb.).

Wood, C. L.: How the chaplain and the dietitian can cooperate. J. Am. Dietet. A., 35:821, 1959.

Young, C. M.: Diet therapy—interviewing the patient. Am. J. Clin. Nutr., 8:523, 1960.

FEVERS AND INFECTIONS

Journal Articles:

Dubos, R. I., and Schaedler, R. W.: Nutrition and infection. J. Pediat., 55:1, 1959.

Goddard, J. L.: Incident at Selby Junior High. Nutrition Today, 2:2, 1967. (Florida Citrus Commission)

Kass, I., et al.: Isoniazid as a cause of optic neuritis and atrophy. J.A.M.A., 164:1740, 1957.

Novak, M. L.: Social and emotional problems of patients with tuberculosis. Nursing Outlook, 6:210, 1958.

Report: Tuberculosis control in Europe. WHO Chronicle, 21:155, 1967 (April).

Schwartz, W. S.: Developments in the treatment of tuberculosis and other pulmonary diseases. J.A.M.A., 178:43, 1961.

Simon, H. J., and Miller, R. C.: Ampicillin in the treatment of chronic typhoid carriers. New Eng. J. Med., 274:807, 1966.

Wilson, N. L., et al.: Nutrition in tuberculosis. J. Am. Dietet. A., 33:243, 1957.

WEIGHT CONTROL

Books:

Kain, I. J., and Gibson, M. B.: Stay Slim for Life. New York, Garden City, Doubleday, 1966.

Leverton, R. M.: Food Becomes You. Ed. 3. Ames, Iowa, Iowa State University Press, 1965.

Obesity and Health. Department of Health, Education and Welfare, Public Health Service, Division of Chronic Diseases, 1966.

Wyden, P.: The Overweight Society. New York, Morrow, 1965.

(See Chapter 37 for cookbooks for low-caloric diets.)

Journal Articles:

Overweight

Alexander, M. M.: Have formula diets helped? J. Am. Dietet. A., 40:538, 1962.

Barnes, R. H.: Weight control—a practical office approach. J.A.M.A., 166:898, 1958.

Bruch, H.: The emotional significance of the preferred weight. Am. J. Clin. Nutr., 5:192, 1957.

————: Psychological aspects of obesity in adolescents. Am. J. Publ. Health, 48:1349, 1958.

Bullen, B. A., et al.: Physical activity of obese and non-obese adolescent girls. Am. J. Clin. Nutr., 14:211, 1964.

Cederquist, D. C.: Comments on fad dieting, J. Am. Dietet. A., 40:535, 1962.

Council on Foods and Nutrition: Formula diets and weight control. J.A.M.A., 176:439, 1961.

Duncan, G. G., et al.: Correction and control of intractible obesity. J.A.M.A., 181:309, 1962.

Drenick, E. J., et al.: Prolonged starvation as treatment of severe obesity. J.A.M.A., 187:100, 1964.

Edit.: Fasting in the treatment of obesity. J.A.M.A., 197:363, 1966.

Goldblatt, P. B., et al.: Social factors in obesity. J.A.M.A., 192:1039, 1965.

Hamburger, W. W.: The psychology of weight reduction. J. Am. Dietet. A., 34:17, 1958.

Hashim, S. A., and van Itallie, T. B.: Clinical and physiologic aspects of obesity: a review. J. Am. Dietet. A., 46:15, 1965.

Hathaway, M. L., and Sargent, D. W.: Overweight in children. J. Am. Dietet. A., 40:511, 1962.

Heald, F. P., et al.: Measures of body fat and hydration in adolescent boys. Pediatrics, 31:226, 1963.

Mayer, J.: Some aspects of the problem of regulation of food intake and obesity. New Eng. J. Med., *274*:610, 662, 772, 1966.

————: Obesity control. Am. J. Nursing, *65*: 112, 1965 (June).

Monello, L. F., and Mayer, J.: Obese adolescent girls, an unrecognized "minority" group. Am. J. Clin. Nutr., *13*:35, 1963.

Moore, M. E., *et al.:* Obesity, social class and mental illness. J.A.M.A., *181*:962, 1962.

Read, M. S., and Heald, F. P.: Adolescent obesity—summary of a symposium. J. Am. Dietet. A., *47*:411, 1965.

Scheck, J., *et al.:* Mineral and protein losses during starvation. J. Am. Dietet. A., *49*:211, 1966.

Seltzer, C. C., *et al.:* The triceps skin fold as a predictive measure of body density and body fat in obese, adolescent boys. Pediatrics, *36*: 212, 1965.

Seltzer, C. C., and Mayer, J.: Body build and obesity: who are the obese. J.A.M.A., *189*: 677, 1964.

————: Greater reliability of triceps skin fold over the subscapular skin fold as an index of obesity. Am. J. Clin. Nutr., *20*:950, 1967.

Speckman, E. W., *et al.:* The effect of nutrition on body composition. Nutr. Rev., *25*:1, 1967.

Stunkard, A., and Mendelson, M.: Disturbances in body image of some obese persons. J. Am. Dietet. A., *38*:328, 1961.

Young, C. M.: Some comments on the obesities. J. Am. Dietet. A., *45*:134, 1964.

————: Management of the obese patient. J.A.M.A., *186*:903, 1963.

Anorexia Nervosa

Dally, P. J., and Sargent, W.: A new treatment of anorexia nervosa. Brit. Med. J., *5188*:1770, 1960 (June 11).

Farquharson, R. F., and Hyland, H. H.: Anorexia nervosa: the course of 15 patients treated from 20 to 30 years previously. Canad. M. A. J., *94*:411, 1966.

Nemiah, J. C.: Anorexia nervosa: fact and theory. Am. J. Digest. Dis., *3*:249, 1958.

DIABETES MELLITUS

Books:

Danowski, T. S. (ed.): Diabetes Mellitus: Diagnosis and Treatment. New York, American Diabetes Association, 1964.

Joslin, E. P.: Diabetic Manual. Ed. 10. Philadelphia, Lea & Febiger, 1959.

Joslin, E. P., *et al.:* The Treatment of Diabetes Mellitus. Ed. 11. Philadelphia, Lea & Febiger (in preparation).

Rosenthal, H., and Rosenthal, J.: Diabetic Care in Pictures. Ed. 4. Philadelphia, J. B. Lippincott (in preparation).

Tolstoi, E.: The Practical Management of Diabetes. Springfield, Ill., Charles C Thomas, 1954.

(See Chapter 37 for cookbooks for diabetic diets.)

Journal Articles:

General

Bergen, S. S., Jr., and van Itallie, T. B.: The glucagon problem. N. Y. J. Med., *61*:779, 1961.

Daughaday, W. H.: Present status of dietary treatment of diabetes. Nutr. Rev., *17*:289, 1959.

Edit.: Diabetes and blood insulin. New Eng. J. Med., *267*:990, 1962.

Entmacher, P. S., *et al.:* Longevity of diabetic patients in recent years. Diabetes, *13*:373, 1964.

Ernest, I., *et al.:* Carbohydrate rich, fat-poor diet in diabetes. Am. J. Med., *39*:594, 1965.

Glinsmann, W. H., and Mertz, W.: Effect of trivalent chromium on glucose tolerance. Metabolism, *15*:510, 1966.

Hamwi, G. J.: Treatment of diabetes. J.A.M.A., *181*:1064, 1962.

Hodges, R. E.: Present knowledge of nutrition in relation to diabetes mellitus. Nutr. Rev., *24*:257, 1966.

Katz, L. A., and Spiro, H. M.: Gastrointestinal manifestations of diabetes. New Eng. J. Med., *275*:1350, 1966.

Marble, A., *et al.:* Unstable diabetes. Diabetes, *5*:475, 1956.

Martin, M. M.: Diabetes mellitus: current concepts. Am. J. Nursing, *65*:510, 1965 (Dec.).

————: Insulin reactions. Am. J. Nursing, *67*: 328, 1967 (Feb.).

————: New trends in diabetes detection. Am. J. Nursing, *63*:101, 1963 (Aug.).

McDonald, G. W., and Fisher, G. F.: Diabetes prevalence in the U. S.: Implications for public health programming. Publ. Health Rep., *82*:334, 1967.

Sharkey, T. P.: Recent research developments in diabetes mellitus. J. Am. Dietet. A., *48*: 281, 288, 1966.

Somogyi, M., and Goldwasser, H. V.: Quantitative relationship between insulin dosage and amount of carbohydrate utilized in diabetic persons. Am. J. Med., *26*:165, 1959.

Stone, D. B.: A rational approach to diet and diabetes. J. Am. Dietet. A., *46*:30, 1965.

Stone, D. B., and Connor, W. E.: The prolonged effects of a low cholesterol, high carbohydrate diet upon the serum lipids in diabetic patients. Diabetes, *12*:127, 1963.

WHO Expert Committee on Diabetes Mellitus: Report, 1965. WHO Chronicle, *20*:39, 1966.

Williams, R. H., and Ensinck, J. W.: Secretion, fates and actions of insulin and related products. Diabetes, *15*:623, 1966.

Yanoff, M.: Diabetic retinopathy. New Eng. J. Med., *274*:1344, 1966.

Oral Hypoglycemic Agents

Beaser, S. B.: Oral treatment of diabetes mellitus. J.A.M.A., *187*:887, 1964.

Camarini-Dávalos, R. A., and Marble, A.: Incidence and causes of secondary failure in treatment with tolbutamide. J.A.M.A., *181*: 1, 1962.

DeLawter, DeW. E., and Moss, J. M.: A five-year study of tolbutamide in the treatment of diabetes. J.A.M.A., *181*:156, 1962.

Edit.: Oral hypoglycemic agents in diabetes. J.A.M.A., *181*:43, 1962.

Kaye, R., and Davidson, M. H.: Limitations in the use of oral hypoglycemic agents in juvenile patients with diabetes. J. Pediat., *66*: 844, 1965.

Singer, D. L., and Hurwitz, D.: Long-term experience with sulfonyl ureas and placebo. New Eng. J. Med., *277*:450, 1967.

Weller, C.: Oral hypoglycemic agents. Am. J. Nursing, *64*:90, 1964 (Mar.).

Diabetes and Pregnancy

McLendon, H., and Bottomy, J. R.: A critical analysis of the management of pregnancy in diabetic women. Am. J. Obstet. Gynec., *80*: 641, 1960.

Reis, R. A., *et al.*: Pregnancy in the diabetic woman. Am. J. Obstet. Gynec., *76*:1148, 1958.

White, P.: Pregnancy and diabetes. Diabetes, *7*:494, 1958.

Juvenile Diabetes

Collyer, R. T., and Hazlitt, B. E.: Retinopathy and neuropathy in one hundred growth-onset diabetic patients. Canad. M. A. J., *85*:1328, 1961.

Davis, D. M., *et al.*: Attitudes of diabetic boys and girls towards diabetes. Diabetes, *14*: 106, 1965.

Etzwiler, D. D.: Effect of glucagon hydrochloride on hypoglycemia of juvenile diabetics. J.A.M.A., *183*:795, 1963.

Etzwiler, D. D., and Sines, L. K.: Juvenile diabetes and its management. J.A.M.A., *181*: 304, 1962.

Etzwiler, D. D., *et al.*: Wilderness camping for the diabetic. Diabetes, *14*:676, 1965.

Knowles, H. C., *et al.*: The course of juvenile diabetes treated with unmeasured diet. Monograph. Diabetes, *14*:239, 1965.

Long, P. J.: The diabetic child at home. Nursing Outlook, *12*:55, 1964 (Dec.).

Loughlin, W. C.: Certain other aspects of juvenile diabetes. N. Y. J. Med., *65*:631, 1965.

Marble, A.: The future of the child with diabetes. J. Am. Dietet. A., *33*:569, 1957.

Moore, M. L.: Diabetes in children. Am. J. Nursing, *67*:104, 1967.

White, P.: Childhood diabetes: its course and influence on the second and third generations. Diabetes, *9*:345, 1960.

Teaching the Diabetic Patient

Allen, F. A.: Education of the diabetic patient. New Eng. J. Med., *268*:93, 1963.

Anderson, R. S., *et al.*: Evaluation of clinical, cultural and psychosomatic influences in the teaching and management of diabetic patients. Am. J. Med. Sci., *245*:682, 1963.

Edit.: Teaching diabetic self-care. New Eng. J. Med., *276*:182, 1967.

Etzwiler, D. D.: Who's teaching the diabetic? Diabetes, *16*:111, 1967.

FORECAST. Publ. monthly by the American Diabetes Assn., 18 East 48th Street, New York, 10017. $2.00 per year.

Johnson, D.: Planning a restricted sodium diet and bland, low fiber diet for the diabetic patient. Am. J. Clin. Nutr., 5:569, 1957.

Kaufman, M.: The many dimensions of diet counseling for diabetes. Am. J. Clin. Nutr., *15*:45, 1964.

————: Newer programs for patients with diabetes. J. Am. Dietet. A., *44*:277, 1964.

————: Programmed instruction materials on diabetes. J. Am. Dietet. A., *46*:36, 1965.

Krysan, G. S.: How do we teach four million diabetics? Am. J. Nursing, *65*:105, 1965 (Nov.).

McDonald, G. W., and Kaufman, M.: Teaching machines for patients with diabetes. J. Am. Dietet. A., *42*:209, 1963.

Skiff, A. W.: Programmed instruction and patient teaching. Am. J. Pub. Health, *55*:409, 1965.

Williams, T. F., *et al.*: The clinical picture of diabetic control, studied in four settings. Am. J. Publ. Health, *57*:441, 1967.

————: Dietary errors made at home by patients with diabetes. J. Am. Dietet. A., *51*: 19, 1967.

ATHEROSCLEROSIS

(See also references under Fats and Lipids.)

Books:

Blakeslee, A., and Stamler, J.: Your Heart Has Nine Lives. Englewood Cliffs, N. J., Prentice Hall, 1963.

Food and Nutrition Board: Dietary Fat and Human Health: National Research Council, Publ. No. 1147, 1966.

(See Chapter 38 for cookbooks for fat-restricted diets.)

Journal Articles:

Albrink, M.: Diet and cardiovascular disease. J. Am. Dietet. A., *46*:26, 1965.

Antar, M. A., and Ohlson, M. A.: Effects of simple and complex carbohydrates on total lipids, nonphospholipids and different fractions of phospholipids of serum in young men and women. J. Nutr., *85*:329, 1965.

Baker, B. M., *et al.:* The national diet–heart study, an initial report. J.A.M.A., *185*:105, 1963.

Bellet, S., *et al.:* The effect of caffeine on free fatty acids. Arch. Int. Med., *116*:750, 1965.

Bernfeld, P., *et al.:* Fatty acid contents of margarine and other table fats. Am. J. Clin. Nutr., *11*:554, 1962.

Bierenbaum, M. L., *et al.:* Fats and fatty acids in excess. J. Am. Dietet. A., *50*:368, 1967.

Browe, J. H., *et al.:* Diet and heart disease in the cardiovascular health center. J. Am. Dietet. A., *50*:376, 1967.

Brown, H. B., *et al.:* Design of practical fat-controlled diets. Foods, fat composition and cholesterol content. J.A.M.A., *196*:205, 1966.

Brown, H. B., and Page, I. H.: Critical balance between saturated and unsaturated dietary fat necessary to reduce serum cholesterol levels. Circulation, *24*:1085, 1961.

Brown, H. B., and Page, I. H.: Variable responses of hyperlipemic patients to altered food patterns. J.A.M.A., *173*:248, 1960.

Christakis, G., *et al.:* The Anti-Coronary Club: a dietary approach to the prevention of coronary heart disease. A seven year report. Am. J. Publ. Health, *56*:299, 1966.

Council on Foods and Nutrition: Diet and the possible prevention of coronary atheroma. J.A.M.A., *194*:1149, 1965.

———: Special shortenings. J.A.M.A., *187*: 766, 1964.

Cramer, K., *et al.:* Coronary angiographic findings in correlation with age, body weight, blood pressure, serum lipids and smoking habits. Circulation, *33*:888, 1966.

Dawber, T. R., and Kannel, W. B.: Coronary heart disease as an epidemiology entity. Am. J. Publ. Health, *53*:433, 1963.

Dayton, S., *et al.:* Can change in the American diet prevent coronary heart disease? Am. J. Dietet. A., *46*:20, 1965.

Edit.: Changing dietary habits. J.A.M.A., *196*: 281, 1966.

———: Environmental factors in ischemic heart disease. J.A.M.A., *188*:997, 1964.

Eisenberg, H., *et al.:* Epidemiology of coronary heart disease in Middlesex County, Conn. J. Am. Dietet. A., *47*:391, 1965.

Epstein, F. H.: The epidemiology of coronary heart disease. J. Chron. Dis., *18*:735, 1965.

Frederickson, D. S., *et al.:* Fat transport in lipoproteins—an integrated approach to mechanisms and disorders. New Eng. J. Med., *276*:34, 94, 148, 215, 273, 1967.

Galbraith, A., and Hatch, F. T.: A system of proportioned fat diets for clinical use. Am. J. Clin. Nutr., *16*:480, 1965.

Hamburger, W. W.: The psychology of dietary change. Am. J. Publ. Health, *48*:1342, 1958.

Hartroft, W. S.: Should the American diet be drastically modified? J. Am. Dietet. A., *41*: 13, 1962.

Hatch, F. T., *et al.:* A study of coronary heart disease in young men. Circulation, *33*:679, 1966.

Hegsted, D. M., *et al.:* Quantitative effects of dietary fat on serum cholesterol in man. Am. J. Clin. Nutr., *17*:281, 1965.

Hiscock, E., *et al.:* A palatable diet high in unsaturated fat. J. Am. Dietet. A., *40*:427, 1962.

Hodges, R. E., and Krehl, W. A.: The role of carbohydrates in lipid metabolism. Am. J. Clin. Nutr., *17*:334, 1965.

International Conference on Diet, Serum Lipids and Atherosclerosis. Fed. Proc. *21* (No. 4, Part II), 1962 (July-Aug.).

Kerschbaum, A., and Bellet, S.: Cigarette smoking and blood lipids. J.A.M.A., *187*:33, 1964.

Keys, A., and Parlin, R. W.: Serum cholesterol response to changes in dietary lipids. Am. J. Clin. Nutr., *19*:175, 1966.

Kinch, S. H., *et al.:* Risk factors in ischemic heart disease. Am. J. Publ. Health, *53*:438, 1963.

Kinsell, L. W., *et al.:* Dietary considerations with regard to type of fat. Am. J. Clin. Nutr., *15*:198, 1964.

Little, J. A., *et al.:* Studies of male survivors of myocardial infarction. Circulation, *31*:854, 1965.

Mann, G. V., *et al.:* Cardiovascular disease in the Masai. J. Atherosclerosis Res., *4*:289, 1964.

McGandy, R. B., *et al.:* Dietary carbohydrate and serum cholesterol levels in man. Am. J. Clin. Nutr., *18*:237, 1966.

————: Dietary fats, carbohydrates and atherosclerotic vascular disease. New Eng. J. Med., *277*:186, 242, 1967.

Montoye, H. J., *et al.:* Relationship between serum cholesterol and body fatness. Am. J. Clin. Nutr., *16*:397, 1966.

Olson, R. E.: Diet and coronary artery disease. Circulation, *22*:453, 1960.

Page, I.: Dietary fat and its relation to heart attacks and strokes. Circulation, *23*:133, 1961.

Phillips, J. A., and Vail, G. E.: Effect of heat on fatty acids. J. Am. Dietet. A., *50*:116, 1967.

Rosenman, R. H., *et al.:* Coronary heart disease in Western Collaborative Study. J.A.M.A., *195*:86, 1966.

Rosenman, R. H., and Friedman, M.: Association of specific behavior pattern in women with blood and cardio-vascular findings. Circulation, *24*:1173, 1961.

Schroeder, H. A.: Municipal drinking water and cardiovascular death rates. J.A.M.A., *195*:81, 1966.

Spain, D. M.: Atherosclerosis. Scientific American, *215*:48, 1966.

Stamler, J., *et al.:* Dietary changes and serum cholesterol responses in coronary-prone middle-aged men, participating in coronary prevention evaluation program. Circulation, *24*:1105, 1961.

————:Coronary risk factors. Med. Clin. N. Am., *50*:229, 1966.

Stare, F. J.: Nutritional suggestions for the primary prevention of coronary heart disease. J. Am. Dietet. A., *48*:88, 1966.

Wolf, S., *et al.:* Changes in serum lipids in relation to emotional stress during rigid control of diet and exercise. Circulation, *26*:379, 1962.

CARDIAC DISEASE; HYPERTENSION
Journal Articles:
Cardiac Disease

Berliner, R. W.: Recent advances in the knowledge of the causes of edema and in diuretic therapy. The regulation of water balance and plasma sodium concentration. Arch. Int. Med., *102*:986, 1958.

Cooper, G. R., and Heap, B.: Sodium ion in drinking water. J. Am. Dietet. A., *50*:37, 1967.

Council of Foods and Nutrition: Low sodium milk. J.A.M.A., *163*:739, 1957.

Danowski, T. S.: Low sodium diets—physiological adaptation and clinical usefulness. J.A.M.A., *168*:1886, 1958.

Dustan, H. P.: Diet and diuretics in the treatment of hypertensive cardiovascular disease. J.A.M.A., *172*:2052, 1960.

Elliott, G. B., and Alexander, E. A.: Sodium from drinking water as an unsuspected cause of cardiac decompensation. Circulation, *23*:562, 1961.

Farag, S. A., and Mozar, H. N.: Preventing recurrences of congestive heart failure. J. Am. Dietet. A., *51*:26, 1967.

Heap, B., and Robinson, C.: New booklets for patients on sodium restriction. J. Am. Dietet. A., *34*:277, 1958.

Johnson, D.: Planning a restricted sodium diet and bland–low fiber diet for the diabetic patient. Am. J. Clin. Nutr., *5*:569, 1957.

Newman, E. V.: Regulation of electrolytes in the management of heart disease. J.A.M.A., *172*:2045, 1960.

Schroeder, H. A.: Municipal drinking water and cardiovascular death rates. J.A.M.A., *195*:81, 1966.

Symposium—Council on Foods and Nutrition: Nutritional problems in medicine. J.A.M.A., *172*:2045, 1960.

White, J. M., *et al.:* Sodium ion in drinking water. J. Am. Dietet. A., *50*:32, 1967.

(See Chapter 39 for cookbooks for sodium-restricted diets.)

Hypertension

Arterial hypertension and ischaemic heart disease: comparison in epidemiological studies. WHO Chronicle, *17*:15, 1963.

Conn, J. W.: Hypertension, the potassium ion and impaired carbohydrate tolerance. New Eng. J. Med., *273*:1135, 1965.

Dahl, L. K.: Role of dietary sodium in essential hypertension. J. Am. Dietet. A., *34*:585, 1958.

————: Salt, fat and hypertension: the Japanese experience. Nutr. Rev., *18*:97, 1960.

————: Sodium intake of the American male: implications on the etiology of essential hypertension. Am. J. Clin. Nutr., *6*:1, 1958.

Dahl, L. K., and Love, R. A.: Etiological role of sodium chloride intake in essential hypertension in humans. J.A.M.A., *164*:397, 1957.

Fallis, N., and Ford, R. V.: Electrolyte excretion and hypotensive response. J.A.M.A., *176*:581, 1961.

Glazener, F. S., *et al.:* Pargyline, cheese and acute hypertension. J.A.M.A., *188*:754, 1964.

Hartroft, W. S.: The nutritional aspects of hypertension and its reversibility. Am. J. Publ. Health, 56:462, 1966.

Kimura, T., and Ota, M.: Epidemiologic study of hypertension. Am. J. Clin. Nutr., 17:381, 1965.

Lipman, D. C.: Stress and hypertension: use of anti-stress diet and antihistamine. J. Am. Geriat. Soc., 8:177, 1960.

Page, I. H.: The nature of arterial hypertension. Arch. Int. Med., 111:103, 1963.

Salzano, J. V., et al.: Effect of weight loss on blood pressure. J. Am. Dietet. A., 34:1309, 1958.

Shear, L.: Renal function and sodium metabolism in idiopathic, orthostatic hypotension. New Eng. J. Med., 268:347, 1963.

Weller, J. M., and Hoobler, S. W.: Salt metabolism in hypertension. Ann. Int. Med., 50:106, 1959.

DISEASES OF THE KIDNEY

Journal Articles:

Kidney Disease

Barnes, B. A.: Survival data on renal transplantations in patients. New Eng. J. Med., 272:776, 1965.

Berlyne, G. M., et al.: Dietary treatment of chronic renal failure. Nephron, 2:129, 1965.

———: Amino acid loss in peritoneal dialysis. Lancet, 7504:1339, 1967 (June 24).

Berlyne, G. M., and Shaw, A. B.: Giordano-Giovanetti diet in terminal renal failure. Lancet, 7401:7, 1965 (July 3).

Edit.: Cleverness of the kidney. New Eng. J. Med., 277:656, 1967.

Giordano, C.: Use of exogenous and endogenous urea for protein synthesis in normal and uremic subjects. J. Lab. Clin. Med., 62:231, 1963.

Giovanetti, S., and Maggiore, Q.: A low nitrogen diet with proteins of high biological value for severe uremia. Lancet, 7341:1000, 1964 (Vol. 1).

Johnson, W. J.: Fluid and electrolyte disorders in chronic renal disease. Geriatrics, 21:216, 1966.

Kolff, W. J.: Treatment of uremia with forced high caloric, low protein diet. Nutr. Rev., 11:193, 1953.

Levin, D. M., and Cade, R.: Metabolic effects of dietary protein in chronic renal failure. Ann. Int. Med., 63:642, 1965.

Levin, S., and Winkelstein, J. A.: Diet and infrequent peritoneal dialysis in chronic anuric uremia. New Eng. J. Med., 277:619, 1967.

Levinsky, N. G.: Acute renal failure. New Eng. J. Med., 274:1016, 1966.

———: Hyperkalemia. New Eng. J. Med., 274:1076, 1966.

Maher, J. F., and Schreiner, G. E.: Metabolic problems related to prolonged dialytic maintenance of life in oliguria. J.A.M.A., 176:399, 1961.

McCracken, B. H., et al.: Dietary protein and renal failure. New Eng. J. Med., 272:1050, 1965.

Merrill, A. J.: Nutrition in chronic renal failure. J.A.M.A., 173:905, 1960.

Silverberg, D. S., and Hunt, J. C.: Dietary considerations in treating chronic renal failure. J. Am. Dietet. A., 49:425, 1966.

Kidney Stones

Boyce, W. H.: Nutrition in the formation of urinary calculi. Borden's Rev., 21 (No. 4), 1960 (July-Aug.).

Crawhall, J. C., et al.: Further observations on the use of D-penicillamine in cystinuria. Brit. Med. J., 5395:1411, 1964 (May 30).

Dempsey, E. F., et al.: Urinary oxalate excretion. Metabolism, 9:52, 1960.

Edit.: A new look at cystinuria. New Eng. J. Med., 273:613, 1965.

Efron, M. L.: Aminoaciduria. New Eng. J. Med., 272:1058, 1965.

Henneman, P. H., et al.: Idiopathic hypercalcuria. New Eng. J. Med., 259:802, 1958.

Kahn, H. D.: Effect of cranberry juice on urine —implications for therapy of urinary tract infection and calculi. J. Am. Dietet. A., 51:251, 1967.

McDonald, J. E., and Henneman, P. H.: Stone dissolution in vivo and control of cystinuria with D-penicillamine. New Eng. J. Med., 273:578, 1965.

Rosenberg, L. E., et al.: Intestinal transport of cystine and cysteine in man. J. Clin. Invest., 46:30, 1967.

Rosenberg, L. E., and Hayslett, J. P.: Nephrotoxic effects of penicillamine in cystinuria. J.A.M.A., 201:128, 1967.

DISEASES OF THE ESOPHAGUS AND THE STOMACH

Journal Articles:

Cardiospasm

Weiss, E.: Cardiospasm. Am. J. Digest. Dis., 3:275, 1958.

Wolf, S., and Almy, T. P.: Experimental observations on cardiospasm in man. Gastroenterology, 13:401, 1949.

Peptic Ulcer

Cornwell, G. G., III, and Killenberg, P. G.: The effects of a low fat, low caloric synthetic nutrient (Metrecal) on gastric secretion and emptying in man. Am. J. Digest. Dis., *10*:22, 1965.

Dragstedt, L. R.: Why does not the stomach digest itself? J.A.M.A., *177*:758, 1961.

Hartroft, W. S.: The incidence of coronary artery disease in patients treated with the Sippy diet. Am. J. Clin. Nutr., *15*:205, 1964.

Joint Committee, American Dietetic Association and American Medical Association: Diet as related to gastrointestinal function. J. Am. Dietet. A., *38*:425, 1961.

Menguy, R.: Current concepts of the etiology of duodenal ulcer. Am. J. Digest. Dis., *9*: 199, 1964.

Monat, H. A.: Factors in the successful treatment of duodenal ulcer. Am. J. Gastroenterol., *38*:188, 1962.

Moore, I. B.: Treatment of peptic ulcer with a cholesterol lowering dietary supplement. J. Am. Geriat. Soc., *12*:1138, 1964.

Sandweiss, D. J.: The Sippy treatment for peptic ulcer. Am. J. Digest. Dis., *6*:929, 1961.

Symposium: Clinical management of peptic ulcer. Am. J. Clin. Nutr., *15*:191; Panel Discussion, *15*:235, 1964.

Symposium: Gastric, esophageal and pancreatic islet cell relationships related to gastric ulcer and HCl formation. J.A.M.A., *183*:998, 1963.

Weinstein, L., *et al.:* Diet as related to gastrointestinal function. J.A.M.A., *176*:935, 1961.

DISEASES OF THE INTESTINAL TRACT
Journal Articles:

Diarrhea

Gardner, F. H.: Nutritional management of chronic diarrhea in adults. J.A.M.A., *180*: 147, 1962.

Disaccharidase Deficiency and Glucose-Galactose Malabsorption

Chalfin, D., and Holt, P. R.: Lactase deficiency in ulcerative colitis, regional enteritis and viral hepatitis. Am. J. Digest. Dis., *12*:81, 1967.

Dahlqvist, A.: Disaccharide intolerance. J.A.M.A., *195*:225, 1966.

Edit.: Isolated lactase deficit in the adult: a present view. J.A.M.A., *195*:954, 1966.

Hardinge, M. G., *et al.:* Carbohydrates in foods. J. Am. Dietet. A., *46*:197, 1965.

Holzel, A., *et al.:* Severe lactose intolerance in infancy. Lancet, *2*:1346, 1962 (Dec. 29).

Huang, S. S., and Bayless, T. M.: Lactose intolerance in healthy children. New Eng. J. Med., *276*:1283, 1967.

Kern, F., Jr., and Struthers, J. E., Jr.: Intestinal lactase deficiency and lactose intolerance in adults. J.A.M.A., *195*:927, 1966.

Klotz, A. P., and Lubos, M. C.: Gastrointestinal symptoms and intestinal lactase deficiency—a word of caution. Am. J. Digest. Dis., *12*:421, 1967.

Lifshitz, F.: Congenital lactase deficiency. J. Pediat., *69*:229, 1966.

Marks, J. F., *et al.:* Glucose-galactose malabsorption. J. Pediat., *69*:225, 1966.

Prader, A., and Auricchio, S.: Defects of intestinal disaccharide absorption. Ann. Rev. Med., *16*:345, 1965.

Review: Sucrose intolerance: an enzymatic defect. Nutr. Rev., *23*:101, 1965.

Schneider, A. J., *et al.:* Glucose-galactose malabsorption. New Eng. J. Med., *274*:305, 1966.

Townley, R. R. W.: Disaccharidase deficiency in infancy and childhood. Pediatrics, *38*:127, 1966.

———: Disordered disaccharide digestion and absorption and its relation to other malabsorption disorders in childhood. Borden's Rev., *28* (No. 2), April-June, 1967.

Welsh, J. D., and Porter, M. G.: Reversible secondary disaccharidase deficiency. Am. J. Dis. Child., *113*:716, 1967.

Weser, E., *et al.:* Lactase deficiency in patients with the "irritable colon syndrome." New Eng. J. Med., *273*:1070, 1965.

Protein-losing Enteropathy

Etheridge, C. L.: Protein-losing enteropathy. Med. Clin. N. Am., *48*:75, 1964.

Celiac Disease

Baker, H., *et al.:* Mechanisms of folic acid deficiency in non-tropical sprue. J.A.M.A., *187*: 119, 1964.

Bayless, T. M., *et al.:* Adult celiac disease: Treatment with a gluten-free diet. Arch. Int. Med., *111*:83, 1963.

Benson, G. D., *et al.:* Adult celiac disease with emphasis upon response to gluten-free diet. Medicine, *43*:1, 1964 (Am. J. Med.).

Dicke, W. K., *et al.:* Coeliac disease. 2. The presence in wheat of a factor having a deleterious effect in cases of coeliac disease. Acta Paediat., *42*:34, 1953.

Friedman, M., and Hare, P. J.: Gluten-sensitive enteropathy and eczema. Lancet, *7384*: 521, 1965 (Mar. 6).

Herting, D. C.: Perspective on vitamin E. Am. J. Clin. Nutr., *19*:210, 1966.

Kowlesser, O. D., *et al.*: Abnormal tryptophan metabolism in patients with adult celiac disease, with evidence for deficiency of vitamin B_6. J. Clin. Invest., *43*:894, 1964.

Lifshitz, F., *et al.*: Intestinal disaccharidase deficiency in gluten-sensitive enteropathy. Am. J. Digest Dis., *10*:47, 1965.

Review: The celiac syndrome (malabsorption) in pediatrics. Nutr. Rev., *21*:195, 1963.

Ross, J. R., *et al.*: Gluten enteropathy and skeletal disease. J.A.M.A., *196*:270, 1966.

Ruffin, J. M., *et al.*: Gluten-free diet for nontropical sprue. J.A.M.A., *188*:42, 1964.

van de Kamer, J. H., *et al.*: Coeliac disease. 4. An investigation into the injurious constituents of wheat in connection with their action on patients with coeliac disease. Acta Paediat., *42*:223, 1953.

van de Kamer, J. H., and Weijers, H. A.: Coeliac disease. 5. Some experiments on the cause of the harmful effect of wheat gliadin. Acta Paediat., *44*:465, 1955.

Weser, E., and Sleisenger, M. H.: Lactosuria and lactase deficiency in adult celiac disease. Gastroenterology, *48*:571, 1965.

(See Chapter 40 for cookbooks for gluten-free diets.)

Tropical Sprue

Conference on intestinal malabsorption and allied hematologic problems. Am. J. Digest. Dis., *9*:769, 1964.

O'Brien, W., and England, N. W. J.: Folate deficiency in acute tropical sprue. Brit. Med. J., *5424*:1573, 1964 (Dec. 19).

Rivera, J. V., *et al.*: Anemia due to vitamin B_{12} deficiency after treatment with folic acid in tropical sprue. Am. J. Clin. Nutr., *18*:110, 1966.

Cystic Fibrosis

Matthews, L. W., *et al.*: A therapeutic regimen for patients with cystic fibrosis. J. Pediat., *65*:558, 1964.

Medium Chain Triglycerides

Hashim, S. A., *et al.*: Intestinal absorption and mode of transport in portal vein of medium chain fatty acids. J. Clin. Invest., *43*:1238, 1964.

Holt, P. R., *et al.*: Treatment of malabsorption syndrome and exudative enteropathy with synthetic medium chain triglycerides. Am. J. Gastroenterol., *43*:549, 1965.

Zurier, R. B., *et al.*: Use of medium chain triglycerides in management of patients with massive resection of the small intestine. New Eng. J. Med., *274*:490, 1966.

Regional Enteritis

Crohn, B. B.: Current status on therapy in regional enteritis. J.A.M.A., *166*:1479, 1958.

Meyers, S. G., *et al.*: The clinical course of regional enteritis. Am. J. Digest. Dis., *4*: 341, 1959.

Ulcerative Colitis

Chalfin, D., and Holt, P. R.: Lactase deficiency in ulcerative colitis, regional enteritis and viral hepatitis. Am. J. Digest. Dis., *12*:81, 1967.

Davidson, M., *et al.*: Chronic ulcerative colitis in childhood. J. Pediat., *67*:471, 1965.

Kirsner, J. B.: Current concept of the medical management of ulcerative colitis. J.A.M.A., *169*:433, 1959.

Rider, J. A., and Moeller, H. C.: Food hypersensitivity in ulcerative colitis. Am. J. Gastroenterol., *37*:487, 1962.

DISEASES OF THE LIVER, THE BILIARY TRACT AND THE PANCREAS

Journal Articles:

Infectious Hepatitis

Havens, W. P., Jr.: Viral hepatitis. Am. J. Med., *32*:665, 1962.

Krugman, S., and Giles, J. P.: Natural history of infectious hepatitis. Am. J. Med., *32*:717, 1962.

Nefzger, M. D., and Chalmers, T. G.: The treatment of acute infectious hepatitis: Ten year follow-up study on the effects of diet and rest. Am. J. Med., *35*:299, 1963.

Welch, G. E., *et al.*: Management of hepatitis in the female. Am. J. Digest. Dis., *9*:729, 1964.

Liver Cirrhosis

Davidson, C. S.: Diet in the treatment of liver disease. Am. J. Med., *25*:690, 1958.

Deller, D. J., *et al.*: Folic acid deficiency in cirrhosis of the liver. Am. J. Digest. Dis., *10*:35, 1965.

Feres, A., *et al.*: Intestinal fat absorption in cirrhosis of the liver. Am. J. Digest. Dis., *12*:65, 1967.

Garceau, A. J., *et al.*: The natural history of cirrhosis: I. Survival with esophageal varices. New Eng. J. Med., *268*:469, 1963.

Iber, F. L.: Protein loss into the gastrointestinal tract in cirrhosis of the liver. Am. J. Clin. Nutr., *19*:219, 1966.

Isselbacher, K. J., and Greenberger, N. J.: Metabolic effects of alcohol on the liver. New Eng. J. Med., *270*:351, 402, 1964.

LaLonde, J. B., et al.: Hepatic regulation of sodium and water in ascites. J.A.M.A., 187: 117, 1964.

Losowsky, M. S., and Davidson, C. S.: Current concepts in therapy: The treatment of cirrhosis of the liver. New Eng. J. Med., 267: 87, 1962.

MacDonald, R. A.: Pathogenesis of nutritional cirrhosis. Arch. Int. Med., 110:424, 1962.

Orloff, M. J.: Effect of side to side portacaval shunt on intractable ascites, sodium excretion and aldosterone metabolism in man. Am. J. Surg., 112:287, 1966.

Sullivan, J. F., et al.: Magnesium metabolism in alcoholism. Am. J. Clin. Nutr., 13:297, 1963.

Sullivan, J. F., and Lankford, H. G.: Zinc metabolism and chronic alcoholism. Am. J. Clin. Nutr., 17:57, 1965.

Victor, M., and Adams, R. D.: On the etiology of the alcoholic neurologic diseases. Am. J. Clin. Nutr., 9:379, 1961 (Part I).

Pancreatitis

Knight, W. A.: The basis of therapy in pancreatic disease. Am. J. Digest. Dis., 9:832, 1964.

McDonough, F. E., and Reaves, L. E., III: Chronic relapsing pancreatitis: recognition and management. Postgrad. Med., 40:593, 1966.

SURGICAL NUTRITION; BURNS

Books:

Cole, W. H., and Zollinger, R. M.: Textbook of Surgery. Ed. 8. New York, Appleton-Century-Crofts, 1963.

Pareira, M. D.: Therapeutic Nutrition with Tube Feeding. Springfield, Ill., Charles C Thomas, 1959.

Journal Articles:

Preoperative and Postoperative Nutrition

Brooke, C. E., and Anast, C. S.: Oral fluid and electrolytes. J.A.M.A., 179:792, 1962.

Holden, W. D., et al.: The effect of nutrition on nitrogen metabolism in the surgical patient. Ann. Surg., 146:563, 1957.

Leaf, A., and Santos, R. F.: Physiologic mechanisms in potassium deficiency. New Eng. J. Med., 264:335, 1961.

Mansberger, A. R.: Preoperative fluid electrolyte balance and blood volume. J.A.M.A., 174:1941, 1960.

Symposium: Fat emulsions for intravenous use. Am. J. Clin. Nutr., 16:1, 1965.

Gastric Surgery and the Dumping Syndrome

Biggar, B. L., et al.: Nutrition following gastric resection. J. Am. Dietet. A., 37:344, 1960.

Gryboski, J. D., et al.: A defect in disaccharide metabolism after gastrojejunostomy. New Eng. J. Med., 268:78, 1963.

Lieber, H.: The jejunal hyperosmolic syndrome (dumping), and its prophylaxis. J.A.M.A., 176:208, 1961.

Postlewait, R. W., et al.: Nutrition after resection for peptic ulcer. Gastroenterology, 40: 491, 1961.

Schlang, H. A., and McHenry, L. E.: Obstruction of the small bowel by orange in the post-gastrectomy patient. Ann. Surg., 159: 611, 1964.

Vanamee, P.: Nutrition after gastric resection. J.A.M.A., 172:2072, 1960.

Wilde, W. L.: Potato skin phytobezoars in edentulous gastrectomized patients. Am. J. Surg., 109:649, 1965.

Willis, M. T., and Postlewait, R. W.: Dietary problems after gastric resection. J. Am. Dietet. A., 40:111, 1962.

Other Surgery of the Intestinal Tract

Allcock, E.: Absorption of vitamin B_{12} in man following extensive resection of the jejunum, ileum. Gastroenterology, 40:81, 1961.

Cornell, G. N., et al.: The pattern of absorption following surgical shortening of the bowel. Bull. N. Y. Acad. Med. (second series), 37:675, 1961.

Machella, T. E., and Ravdin, R. G.: Jejunal feeding. Am. J. Clin. Nutr., 3:481, 1955.

Scheiner, E., et al.: Malabsorption following massive intestinal resection. Am. J. Clin. Nutr., 17:64, 1965.

Stahlgren, L. A., and Ferguson, L. K.: The results of surgical treatment of chronic regional enteritis. J.A.M.A., 175:986, 1961.

Winawer, S. J., et al.: Successful management of massive small-bowel resection based on assessment of absorption defects and nutritional needs. New Eng. J. Med., 274:72, 1966.

Nutrition in Burns

Artz, C. P.: Recent developments in burns. Am. J. Surg., 108:649, 1964.

Boles, E. T., and Terry, J. L.: Practical aspects of the management of severely burned children. Am. J. Surg., 101:668, 1961.

Chasmar, L. R.: Antibiotics, infection and immunological aspects of burns. Canad. M.A.J., 97:436, 1967.

Soroff, H. S., et al.: An estimation of the nitrogen requirements for equilibrium in burned patients. Surg., Gynec. Obstet., 112:159, 1961.

ALLERGY; DISEASES OF THE SKIN
Journal Articles:
Allergy

American Academy of Pediatrics, Committee on Nutrition: Appraisal of nutritional adequacy of infant formulas used as cow milk substitutes. Pediatrics, *31*:329, 1963.

Colldahl, H.: Allergy and certain diseases in relation to the digestive tract. Acta Allergologica, *20*:84, 1965.

Edit.: Gastrointestinal allergy resurgent. New Eng. J. Med., *276*:809, 1967.

Fitzelle, G. T.: Personality factors and certain attitudes toward child rearing among parents of asthmatic children. Psychosom. Med., *21*:208, 1959.

Friedman, M., and Hare, P. J.: Gluten-sensitive enteropathy and eczema. Lancet, *7384*: 521, 1965.

Fries, J. H., and Lightstone, A. C.: Pediatric allergy—a critical review of the literature. Ann. Allergy, *20*:351, 1962.

Johnstone, D. E., and Dutton, A. M.: Dietary prophylaxis of allergic disease in children. New Eng. J. Med., *274*:715, 1966.

Lahey, M. E., *et al.*: Milk-induced enteropathy. Am. J. Digest. Dis., *9*:809, 1964.

Miller, H., and Baruch, D. W.: Psychotherapy of parents of allergic children. Ann. Allergy, *18*:990, 1960.

Mitchell, J. H.: The emotional factors in eczema and urticaria. Ann. Allergy, *18*:170, 1960.

Mueller, H. L., *et al.*: The incidence of milk sensitivity and the development of allergy in infants. New Eng. J. Med., *268*:1220, 1963.

Waldmann, R. D., *et al.*: Allergic gastroenteropathy: a cause of excessive gastrointestinal protein loss. New Eng. J. Med., *276*:761, 1967.

Wilson, J. F., *et al.*: Milk-induced gastrointestinal bleeding in infants with hypochromic microcytic anemia. J.A.M.A., *189*: 568, 1964.

(See Chapter 41 for cookbooks for allergy diets.)

Diseases of the Skin

Baird, J. W.: Acne—a new approach to an old problem. J. Pediat., *52*:152, 1958.

Cornbleet, T., and Gigli, I.: Should we limit sugar in acne? Arch. Dermat., *83*:968, 1961.

Hartman, W. E.: Vegetarian protein foods. Food Technology, *20*:39, 1966.

Kingery, F. A. J.: Why psoriasis looks that way. J.A.M.A., *195*:953, 1966.

Mitchell, H. H., and Erdman, M.: Nutritional significance of the dermal losses of nutrients in man. Am. J. Clin. Nutr., *10*:163, 1962.

Roe, D. A., and Weston, M. O.: Potential significance of free taurine in the diet. Nature, *204*:287, 1965.

Roe, D. A.: Taurine intolerance in psoriasis. J. Invest. Dermat., *46*:420, 1966.

———: Current concepts of the low taurine diet in psoriasis. Cutis, *2*:1013, 1966.

DISEASES OF THE BLOOD
Journal Articles:

Ausman, D. C.: Cobalt-iron therapy for iron-deficiency anemia. J. Am. Geriat. Soc., *13*: 425, 1965.

Chung, A. S. M., *et al.*: Folic acid, vitamin B_6, pantothenic acid and vitamin B_{12} in human dietaries. Am. J. Clin. Nutr., *9*:573, 1961.

Conrad, M. E.: Iron balance and iron deficiency states. Borden's Rev., *28* (No. 3):49, 1967 (July-Sept.).

Conrad, M. E., *et al.*: The role of the intestine in iron kinetics. J. Clin. Invest., *43*:963, 1964.

Ellison, A. B. C.: Pernicious anemia masked by multivitamins containing folic acid. J.A.M.A., *173*:240, 1960.

Herbert, V.: Biochemical and hematologic lesions in folic acid deficiency. Am. J. Clin. Nutr., *20*:562, 1967.

Herbert, V., and Castle, W. B.: Intrinsic factor. New Eng. J. Med., *270*:1181, 1964.

Leevy, C. M., *et al.*: Incidence and significance of hypovitaminemia in a randomly selected municipal hospital population. Am. J. Clin. Nutr., *17*:259, 1965.

Miller, D. R., *et al.*: Juvenile "congenital" pernicious anemia. New Eng. J. Med., *275*: 978, 1966.

Review: Iron deficiency anemia. Nutr. Rev., *20*:164, 1962.

———: Gastrointestinal tract and iron deficiency anemia. Nutr. Rev., *22*:323, 1964.

———: Iron balance and iron deficiency states. Borden's Rev., *28*: No. 3 July-Sept. 1967.

Rivera, J. V., *et al.*: Anemia due to vitamin B_{12} deficiency after treatment with folic acid in tropical sprue. Am. J. Clin. Nutr., *18*:110, 1966.

Salvidio, E., *et al.*: Nature of hemolytic crises and the fate of G-6-PD deficient, drug-damaged erythrocytes in Sardinians. New Eng. J. Med., *276*:1339, 1967.

Sansone, G., and Signo, G.: Sensitivity to broad beans. Lancet, *2*:295, 1957.

Scott, D. E., and Pritchard, J. A.: Iron deficiency in healthy young college women. J.A.M.A., *199*:897, 1967.

Sheehy, T. W.: How much folic acid is safe in pernicious anemia? Am. J. Clin. Nutr., *9*:708, 1961.

Vilter, R. W., *et al.*: Interrelationships of vitamin B_{12}, folic acid and ascorbic acid in the megaloblastic anemias. Am. J. Clin. Nutr., *12*:130, 1963.

DISEASES OF
THE MUSCULOSKELETAL AND
THE NERVOUS SYSTEMS

Books:

Hollander, J. E.: Arthritis and Allied Conditions. Ed. 7. Philadelphia, Lea & Febiger, 1966.

Ingram, M. E.: Principles and Techniques of Psychiatric Nursing. Ed. 5. Philadelphia, W. B. Saunders, 1960.

May, E. E., *et al.*: Homemaking for the Handicapped. New York, Dodd, 1966.

Render, H. W., and Weiss, M. O.: Nurse-Patient Relationships in Psychiatry. Ed. 2. New York, McGraw-Hill, 1959.

Rusk, H. A.: Rehabilitation Medicine. Ed. 2. St. Louis, C. V. Mosby, 1964.

Journal Articles:
Arthritis

Herndon, B.: Diet in the treatment of rheumatic disease. Am. J. Clin. Nutr., *18*:68, 1966.

Lamont-Havers, R. W.: Arthritis quackery. Am. J. Nursing, *63*:92, 1963 (Mar.).

Lockie, L. M.: Steroid therapy in rheumatoid arthritis. J.A.M.A., *170*:1063, 1959.

Review: The diet of the patient with arthritis. Nutr. Rev., *21*:203, 1963.

Walike, B. C.: Personality factors in rheumatoid arthritis. Am. J. Nursing, *67*:1427, 1967.

Whedon, G. O., *et al.*: Corticosteroid osteoporosis in rheumatoid arthritis. Arth. Rheum., *4*:445, 1961.

Osteoporosis

Bernstein, D. S., *et al.*: Use of sodium fluoride in metabolic bone disease. J. Clin. Invest., *42*:916, 1963.

Birge, S. J., Jr., *et al.*: Osteoporosis, intestinal lactase deficiency and low dietary calcium intake. New Eng. J. Med., *276*:445, 1967.

Caniggia, A.: Medical problems in senile osteoporosis. Geriatrics, *20*:300, 1965.

Goggin, J. E., *et al.*: Incidence of femoral fractures in post-menopausal women before and after water fluoridation. Publ. Health Rep., *80*:1005, 1965.

Heaney, R. P.: A unified concept of osteoporosis. Am. J. Med., *39*:877, 1965.

High calcium diet for osteoporosis. Publ. Health Rep., *76*:974, 1961.

Lafferty, F. W., *et al.*: Effects of androgens, estrogens and high calcium intakes on bone formation and resorption in osteoporosis. Am. J. Med., *36*:514, 1964.

Lutwak, L.: Osteoporosis. J. Am. Dietet. A., *44*:173, 1964.

Schwartz, E., *et al.*: Metabolic balance studies of high calcium intake in osteoporosis. Am. J. Med., *36*:233, 1964.

Walker, A. R. P.: Osteoporosis and calcium deficiency. Am. J. Clin. Nutr., *16*:327, 1965.

Muscular Dystrophy

Blahd, W. H., *et al.*: Decreased body potassium in non-dystrophic relatives of patients with musclar dystrophy. New Eng. J. Med., *270*:197, 1964.

————: The significance of decreased body potassium concentrations in patients with muscular dystrophy and non-dystrophic relatives. New Eng. J. Med., *276*:1349, 1967.

Myasthenia Gravis

Magee, K. R.: Myasthenia gravis. Am. J. Nursing, *60*:336, 1960 (Mar.).

Ménière's Disease

Altmann, F.: Ménière's disease. J.A.M.A., *176*:215, 1961.

Rehabilitation

Blanchard, I.: Better feeding can mean better speaking. Am. J. Nursing, *63*:94, 1963 (Nov).

Hodgins, E.: Listen—The Patient. New Eng. J. Med., *274*:657, 1966.

Kahn, H. D.: Effect of cranberry juice on urine—implications for therapy of urinary tract infection and calculi. J. Am. Dietet. A., *51*:251, 1967.

Reams, A.: Nutrition in rehabilitation. J. Home Econ., *51*:207, 1959.

Spader, M.: When homemakers with physical handicaps return to their own kitchens—what then? J. Home Econ., *55*:770, 1963.

Mental Illness

Christakis, G., and Miridjanian, A.: Diet, drugs and their interrelationships. J. Am. Dietet. A., *52*:21, 1968.

Cuthill, J. M., *et al.*: Death associated with tranylcypromine and cheese. Lancet, *7342*:1076, 1964.

Donahue, H. H., and Fowler, P. A.: Some problems of feeding mental patients. Am. J. Clin. Nutr., *5*:180, 1957.

Gee, D. A.: Effect of psychiatric services on the hospital dietary department. J. Am. Dietet. A., *41*:345, 1962.

Ross, M.: Food in the mental hospital. J. Am. Dietet. A., *40*:318, 1962.

MISCELLANEOUS METABOLIC DISTURBANCES

Book:

Duncan, G. G.: Diseases of Metabolism. Ed. 5. Philadelphia, W. B. Saunders, 1964.

Journal Articles:

Hypoglycemia

Beeuwkes, A. M.: The dietary treatment of functional hyperinsulinism. J. Am. Dietet. A., *18*:731, 1942.

Conn, J. W., and Seltzer, H. S.: Spontaneous hypoglycemia. Am. J. Med., *19*:460, 1955.

(See also under Inborn Errors of Metabolism in Nutrition in Diseases of Infancy and Childhood.)

Gout

Berkowitz, D.: Blood lipids and uric acid inter-relationships. J.A.M.A., *190*:856, 1964.

Gutman, A. B., and Yu, T. F.: An abnormality of glutamine metabolism in primary gout. Am. J. Med., *35*:820, 1963.

Hall, A. P., *et al.*: Epidemiology of gout: A long term population study. Am. J. Med., *42*:27, 1967.

Lieber, C. S., *et al.*: Interrelation of uric acid and ethanol metabolism. J. Clin. Invest., *41*:1863, 1962.

Maclachlan, M. J., and Rodnan, G. P.: Effects of food, fast and alcohol on serum uric acid and acute attacks of gout. Am. J. Med., *42*:38, 1967.

Nugent, C. A., and Tyler, F. H.: The renal excretion of uric acid in patients with gout and in non-gouty subjects. J. Clin. Invest., *38*:1890, 1959.

Rakic, M. T., *et al.*: Observations on the natural history of hyperuricemia and gout. 1. An eighteen year follow-up of nineteen gouty families. Am. J. Med., *37*:862, 1964.

Spencer, H., *et al.*: Changes in metabolism in obese persons during starvation. Am. J. Med., *40*:27, 1966.

NUTRITION IN DISEASES OF INFANCY AND CHILDHOOD

(Also consult supplementary readings and bibliography for diseases discussed in other chapters.)

Books:

Chase, F.: A Visit to the Hospital. New York, Grosset and Dunlap, 1957.

Fomon, S. J.: Infant Nutrition. Philadelphia, W. B. Saunders, 1967.

French, E. L., and Scott, J. C.: Child in the Shadows: A Manual for Parents of Retarded Children. Philadelphia, J. B. Lippincott, 1960.

Gellis, S. S., and Kagan, B. M.: Current Pediatric Therapy. Philadelphia, W. B. Saunders, 1964; 1966.

Holt, L. E., Jr., *et al.*: Pediatrics. Ed. 13. New York, Appleton-Century-Crofts, 1962.

Lyman, F. L.: Phenylketonuria. Springfield, Ill., Charles C Thomas, 1963.

Nelson, W. E.: Textbook of Pediatrics. Ed. 8. Philadelphia, W. B. Saunders, 1964.

Patton, R. G., and Gardner, L. I.: Growth Failure in Maternal Deprivation. Springfield, Ill., Charles C Thomas, 1963.

Journal Articles:

Hospitalization of Children

Langford, W. S.: The child in the pediatric hospital: adaptation to illness and hospitalization. Am. J. Orthopsych., *31*:667, 1961.

Mason, E. A.: The hospitalized child: his emotional needs. New Eng. J. Med., *272*:406, 1965.

Stitt, P. G.: The family approach to feeding chronically ill children. Children, *5*:213, 1958.

Iron Deficiency Anemia

Elian, E., *et al.*: Intestinal blood loss: a factor in calculations of body iron in late infancy. J. Pediat., *69*:215, 1966.

Hoag, M. S., *et al.*: Occult blood loss in iron deficiency anemia of infancy. Pediatrics, *27*:199, 1961.

Lahey, M. E., and Wilson, J. F.: The etiology or iron deficiency anemia in infants—a reappraisal. J. Pediat., *69*:339, 1966.

Rasch, C. A., *et al.*: Blood loss as a contributing factor in the etiology of iron-lack anemia of infancy. Am. J. Dis. Child., *100*:627, 1960.

Scurvy; Rickets

Burnett, C. H., *et al.*: Vitamin D-resistant rickets. Am. J. Med., *36*:222, 1964.

Demers, P., *et al.*: An epidemiological study of infantile scurvy in Canada 1961-63. Canad. M. A. J., *93*:573, 1965.

Harrison, H. E.: The disappearance of rickets. Am. J. Publ. Health, *56*:734, 1966.

Johnston, C. C., Jr., *et al.*: Familial vitamin D resistant rickets in untreated adult. Arch. Int. Med., *117*:141, 1966.

Kahn, S. B., and Brodsky, I.: Vitamin B_{12}, ascorbic acid and iron metabolism in scurvy. Am. J. Med., *40*:119, 1966.

West, C. D., *et al.*: Use of phosphate salts as an adjunct of vitamin D in the treatment of hypophosphatemic vitamin D refractory rickets. J. Pediat., *64*:469, 1964.

Failure to Thrive; Emotional Deprivation

Gardner, L. I., *et al.*: Rumination and growth failure in male fraternal twin. Pediatrics, *36*:585, 1965.

Powell, G. F., *et al.*: Emotional deprivation and growth retardation simulating idiopathic hypopituitarism. New Eng. J. Med., *276*: 1271, 1279, 1967.

Vernon, D. T. A., *et al.*: Changes in children's behavior after hospitalization. Am. J. Dis. Child., *111*:581, 1966.

Obesity

Bruch, H.: Psychological aspects of obesity in adolescence. Am. J. Publ. Health, *48*:1349, 1958.

**Congenital Anomalies
of Gastrointestinal Tract and Nervous System**

Bryan, A. H., and Anderson, E. L.: Dietary and nutritional problems of crippled children in five rural counties of North Carolina. Am. J. Publ. Health, *55*:1545, 1965.

Kallaus, J., *et al.*: The child with cleft lip and palate. Am. J. Nursing, *65*:120, 1965 (April).

Karle, I. P., *et al.*: Nutritional status of cerebral palsied children. J. Am. Dietet. A., *38*:22, 1961.

Epilepsy

Edit.: Dietary control of childhood epilepsy. J.A.M.A., *197*:580, 1966.

Hughes, J. G., and Jabbour, J. T.: The treatment of the epileptic child. J. Pediat., *53*: 66, 1958.

Mental Retardation

Tarjan, G.: Research and clinical advances in mental retardation. J.A.M.A., *182*:617, 1962.

Nephrosis

Cornfield, D., and Schwartz, M. W.: Nephrosis: A long-term study of children treated with corticosteroids. J. Pediat., *68*:507, 1966.

Symposium: Nephrosis. J. Pediat., *58*:607, 1961.

Inborn Errors of Metabolism—Survey

Amer. Acad. Pediat.: Committee on Nutrition: Nutritional management in hereditary metabolic disease. Pediatrics, *40*:289, 1967.

Crouch, W. H., Jr., and Evanhoe, C. M.: Inborn errors of metabolism. Pediat. Clin. N. Am., Feb. 1967.

Efron, M. L.: Aminoaciduria. New Eng. J. Med., *272*:1058, 1965.

——: Diet therapy for inborn errors of amino acid metabolism. J. Am. Dietet. A., *51*:40, 1967.

Hsia, D. Y-Y. (ed.): Symposium: Treatment of amino acid disorders. Am. J. Dis. Child., *113*:1, 1967.

O'Brien, D.: Rare inborn errors of metabolism in children with mental retardation. Children's Bureau Publ. 429, Department of Health, Education and Welfare, 1965.

Phenylketonuria

Acosta, P. B., and Centerwall, W. R.: Phenylketonuria: Dietary management. J. Am. Dietet. A., *36*:206, 1960.

Acosta, P. B., and Chinnock, R. F.: Dietary management of phenylketonuria. Medical Arts and Sciences, *16*:24, 1962 (No. 1).

Berry, H. K., and Wright, S.: Conference on the treatment of phenylketonuria. J. Pediat., *70*:142, 1967.

Centerwall, W. R.: Phenylketonuria. J. Am. Dietet. A., *36*:201, 1960.

The Clinical Team Looks at Phenylketonuria. Children's Bureau, Dept. of Health, Education and Welfare, 1965.

Committee on Fetus and Newborn, Amer. Acad. Pediat.: Screening of newborn infants for metabolic disease. Pediatrics, *35*:499, 1965.

Committee on the Handicapped Child, Amer. Acad. Pediat.: Statement on treatment of phenylketonuria. Pediatrics, *35*:501, 1965.

Keleske, L., *et al.*: Parental reactions to phenylketonuria in the family. J. Pediat., *70*:793, 1967.

Mabry, C. C., *et al.*: Mental retardation in children of phenylketonuric mothers. New Eng. J. Med., *275*:1331, 1966.

Miller, G. T., *et al.*: Phenylalanine content of fruit. J. Am. Dietet. A., *46*:43, 1965.

Rouse, B. M.: Phenylalanine deficiency syndrome. J. Pediat., *69*:246, 1966.

Schild, S.: Parents of children with phenylketonuria. Children, *11*:92, 1964.

Solomons, G., *et al.*: Evaluation of the effects of terminating the diet in phenylketonuria. J. Pediat., *69*:596, 1966.

Stevenson, R. E., and Huntley, C. C.: Congenital malformations in offspring of phenylketonuric mothers. Pediatrics, *40*:33, 1967.

Sutherland, B. S., *et al.*: Treatment of phenylketonuria: A decade of results. Am. J. Dis. Child., *111*:505, 1966.

Umbarger, B.: Phenylketonuria—treating the disease and feeding the child. Am. J. Dis. Child., *100*:908, 1960.

Umbarger, B., *et al.*: Advances in the management of patients with phenylketonuria. J.A.M.A., *193*:784, 1965.

Galactosemia

Donnell, G. N., *et al.*: Galactose-1-phosphate in galactosemia. Pediatrics, *31*:802, 1963.

————: Growth and development of children with galactosemia. J. Pediat., *58*:836, 1961.

Guest, G. M.: Hereditary galactose disease. J.A.M.A., *168*:2015, 1958.

Hsia, D. Y-Y., *et al.*: Galactosemia. J.A.M.A., *178*:944, 1961.

Hsia, D. Y-Y., and Walker, F. A.: Variability in clinical manifestations of galactosemia. J. Pediat., *59*:872, 1961.

Koch, R., *et al.*: Nutritional therapy of galactosemia. Clin. Pediat., *4*:571, 1965.

Leucine-Induced Hypoglycemia

Roth, H., and Segal, H.: The dietary management of leucine-induced hypoglycemia with a report of a case. Pediatrics, *34*:831, 1964.

Snyder, R. D., and Robinson, A.: Leucine-induced hypoglycemia. Am. J. Dis. Child., *113*:566, 1967.

Maple Syrup Urine Disease

Snyderman, S. W., *et al.*: Maple syrup urine disease with particular reference to dietotherapy. Pediatrics, *34*:454, 1964.

Westall, R. G.: Dietary treatment of a child with maple syrup urine disease. Arch. Dis. Child., *38*:485, 1964.

Inborn Error of Fatty Acid Metabolism

Sidbury, J. B., *et al.*: An inborn error of short-chain fatty acid metabolism. J. Pediat., *70*:8, 1967.

Glossary

acetone bodies (as'e-tōn). Acetone, acetoacetic acid and beta-hydroxybutyric acid. Called also ketone bodies. (See *ketosis,* defined below.)

achlorhydria (ah'klor-hid're-ah). Absence of hydrochloric acid in the gastric secretions.

achylia gastrica (ah-ki'le-ah gas'tri-kah). A condition in which the secretion of gastric juice is diminished or absent.

acidosis (as'ĭ-do'sis). A condition in which the body's alkaline reserve is lowered, due to abnormal loss of alkaline salts or abnormal accumulation of acids.

acne (ak'ne). A chronic inflammatory disease of the sebaceous glands, occurring most frequently on the face, the back and the chest.

acrodynia (ak'ro-din'e-ah). An eruptive skin disease. In humans, it is marked by pain in the soles of the feet and the palms of the hands.

ACTH (a-c-t-h) adrenocorticotropic hormone. A hormone, liberated by the pituitary gland, which stimulates the cortex of the adrenal glands.

adrenalectomy (ad-re'nal-ek'to-me). Excision of the adrenal glands.

aflatoxins (a'flah-tok'sin). Several closely related toxic compounds produced by certain molds, which cause liver injury in poultry and may be carcinogenic.

agranulocytosis (a-gran'u-lo-si-to'sis). A condition in which there is total or nearly total absence of the granular leukocytes (granulocytes) from the blood and the bone marrow.

albuminuria (al'bu-mĭ-nu'ri-ah). The presence of albumin in the urine.

aldosterone (al-do-ster'ōn). Hormone produced by the adrenal cortex, which regulates sodium reabsorption.

alginate (ăl'jĭ-nāt). A compound made from marine kelp which forms a viscous solution or a gel.

alkaline reserve (al'kah-lin). The amount of alkaline or basic material available in the body to neutralize acids.

alkalosis (al'kah-lo'sis). A condition in which there is an excess of alkaline substances in the body.

allergen (al'er-jen). Any substance capable of inducing allergy.

alopecia (al'-o-pe'sh-ah). Baldness, deficiency of hair.

alpha-ketoglutaric acid (ke'to-gloo-tar'ik). Intermediary product in the Krebs cycle.

amblyopia (am'ble-o'pe-ah). Dimness of vision without detectable organic lesion of the eye.

amino acid (a-me'no as'id). A class of organic compounds known as the building blocks of the protein molecule.

amphetamine (am-fet'ah-min). A synthetic drug that stimulates the central nervous system, reduces appetite and reduces nasal congestion.

amylase (am'ĭ-lās). An enzyme that digests starch, as ptyalin in the saliva.

amylopectin (am'i-lo-pek'tin). The branched chain insoluble form of starch which stains violet red with iodine and forms a paste with hot water.

amylose (am'ĭ-lōs). The straight chain soluble form of starch which stains blue with iodine and does not form a paste with hot water.

anabolism (ah-nab'o-lizm). Term applied to that phase of metabolism which synthesizes new molecules, especially protoplasm.

anaphylaxis (an'a-fi-lak'sis). Unusual or exaggerated reaction or shock of the organism to foreign protein.

anastomosis (ah-nas'to-mo'sis). A communication between two vessels; surgical formation of a passage between two vessels.

androgenic hormone (an'dro-jen'ik hor'mōn). A hormone producing masculine characteristics.

angioneurosis (an'je-o-nu-ro'sis). A disorder due to disease or injury of the vasomotor nerves or center.

angioneurotic edema (an'je-o-nu-rot'ik e-de'mah). Patches of circumscribed swelling of the skin, mucous membranes and, sometimes, viscera. Giant hives.

anions (an'i-on). An ion carrying a negative charge. Since unlike forms of electricity attract each other, it is attracted by, and travels to, the anode or positive pole. The anions include all the non-metals, the acid radicals, and the hydroxyl ion.

anorexia (an'o-rek'se-ah). Lack or loss of appetite for food.

anorexigenic (an'o-rek'si-jen'ik). Producing anorexia or diminishing the appetite.

antibiotic (an'ti-bi-ot'ik). A substance which inhibits growth and multiplication of bacteria.

antihemorrhagic (an'ti-hem'o-raj'ik). Preventing hemorrhage. Often applied to vitamin K.

antineuritic (an'ti-nu-rit'ik). Counteracting neuritis. Often applied to thiamine.

antioxidant (an'ti-ok'se-dant). A substance that prevents or delays oxidation.

antirachitic (an'ti-rah-kit'ik). Preventive, curative or corrective of rickets. Often applied to vitamin D.

antiscorbutic (an'ti-skor-bu'tik). Preventing or curing scurvy. Often applied to ascorbic acid.

antivitamin (an'ti-vi'ta-min). A substance which may inactivate or destroy a vitamin.

anuria (ah-nu'ri-ah). Complete suppression of urinary secretion.

apoenzyme (ap'o-en'zīm). The protein portion of an enzyme to which the prosthetic group or coenzyme is attached.

arachidonic acid (ar'a-ki-don'ik as'id). A polyunsaturated fatty acid, essential for normal nutrition.

arteriosclerosis (ar-te're-o-skle-ro'sis). A thickening and a hardening of the walls of arteries and capillaries.

ascites (ah-si'tez). Accumulation of fluid in the abdominal cavity.

ascorbic acid (a-skor'bik). Vitamin C, deficiency of which is a causative factor in scurvy.

aspergillus flavus (as'per-jil'us fla-vus). A mold found on corn, peanuts and certain grains when improperly dried and stored; source of aflatoxin.

aspiration (as'pi-ra'shun). The act of breathing or drawing in.

assay (ah-sa'). Examination or analysis of a substance.

asthenia (as-the'ne-a). Without strength.

atherosclerosis (ath'er-o-skle-ro'sis). Fatty degeneration of the connective tissue of the arterial walls.

athetoid (ath'e-toid). Resembling athetosis; constant, recurring series of slow movements of hands and feet, usually due to a brain lesion.

atonic (a-ton'ik). Lack of normal tone or vigor of an organ or part.

atrophy (at'ro-fe). A wasting away of a cell, tissue, organ or part.

Aureomycin (aw're-o-mi'sin). A proprietary brand of chlortetracycline, an antibiotic.

autosomal (au'to-so'mal). Pertaining to an autosome, a paired chromosome, not a sex chromosome.

avidin (av'i-din). A proteinlike substance isolated from egg white; antagonist of biotin.

avitaminosis (a-vi'ta-min-o'sis). A condition due to the lack or the deficiency of a vitamin in the diet, or to lack of absorption or utilization of it.

azotemia (az'o-te'me-ah). An increased level of urea or other nitrogenous substances in the blood.

bactericidal (bak-ter'i-si'dal). Destructive to bacteria.

bacteriostatic (bak-te're-o-stat'ik). Inhibitive to growth of bacteria.

base (bās). A substance which combines with acids to form neutral compounds.

benign (be-nīn'). Mild, favorable for recovery.

bio-assay (bi'o-as-sa'). Examination or analysis of a substance by noting its effect on animals.

biotin (bi'o-tin). A member of the vitamin B complex.

botulism (bot'u-lizm). Poisoning from the toxin produced by the organism *Clostridium botulinum*. The toxin has a selective action on the nervous system.

bradycardia (brad'e-kar'de-ah). Abnormal slowness of the heartbeat.

calciferol (kal-sif'er-ol). Vitamin D_2, produced by irradiating ergosterol.

calcification (kal'si-fi-ka'shun). Process by which organic tissue becomes hardened by a deposit of calcium salts.

calculus, pl. **calculi** (kal'ku-lus). Commonly called stone.

calorimeter (kal'o-rim'e-ter). An instrument for measuring the heat change in any system (such as the types pictured in Chapter 5, one of which is used to measure the amount of heat produced by the body), and the bomb calorimeter used to measure the calorie (energy) value of foods.

carcinogenic (kar'sĭ-no-jen'ik). Cancer-producing.

carotene (kar'o-tēn). A yellow pigment which exists in several forms; alpha, beta and gamma carotene are provitamins which may be converted into vitamin A in the body.

carotenoid (kah-rot'e-noid). Pertaining to a number of compounds related to carotene. They are primarily yellow pigments.

carrageenin (kar'ah-gēn'in). From carrageen (Irish moss); the commercial colloid extract from the moss which forms a gel.

casein (ka'se-in). The principal protein of milk, the basis of cheese.

catabolism (kah-tab'o-lizm). That aspect of metabolism which converts nutrients or complex substances in living cells into simpler compounds, with the release of energy.

cataract (kat'ah-rakt). An opacity of the crystalline lens of the eye or its capsule.

cation (kat'i-on). An ion carrying a positive charge which is attracted to the negative pole or cathode. (See anion above.) Cations include all metals and hydrogen.

celiac disease (se'le-ak). A disease characterized by fatty diarrhea (steatorrhea) and caused by intolerance to gluten; similar to non-tropical sprue.

cephalin (sef'ah-lin). A phospholipid found in tissues, especially brain and nerve tissue.

cerebral hemorrhage (ser'e-bral hem'or-ij). Hemorrhage into the cerebrum, usually in the region of the internal capsule. Also known as cerebral vascular accident (CVA) or stroke.

ceruloplasmin (se'ru-lo-plaz'min). A copper-containing enzyme.

cheilosis (ki-lo'sis). A condition marked by lesions on the lips and cracks at the angles of the mouth.

chlorpropamide (klor-pro'pam-id). (Diabinese) Oral hypoglycemic agent used in the treatment of diabetes. A sulfonylurea.

cholecalciferol (ko'le-kal-sif'er-ol). Vitamin D_3 derived from dehydrocholesterol.

cholecystectomy (ko'le-sis-tek'to-me). Surgical removal of the gallbladder.

cholecystitis (kol'e-sis-ti'tis). Inflammation of the gallbladder.

cholecystokinin (ko'le-cyst'o-ki'nin). A hormone produced in the wall of the duodenum in the presence of fat, which stimulates the contraction of the gallbladder, with the emission of bile.

cholelithiasis (kol'e-li-thi'a-sis). The presence or formation of gallstones.

cholesterol (ko-les'ter-ol). The most common member of the sterol group, defined below. It is a precursor of Vitamin D and closely related to several hormones in the body. It constitutes a large part of the most frequently occurring type of gallstones, and occurs in atheroma of the arteries.

choline (ko'lēn). A component of lecithin. Necessary for fat transport in the body. Prevents the accumulation of fat in the liver.

chromatin (kro'mah-tin). The more stainable portion of the cell nucleus: contains the chromosomes.

chylomicrons (ki'lo-mi'kron). Particles of emulsified lipoproteins containing primarily triglycerides from dietary fat and very little protein.

chylothorax (ki'lo-tho'raks). Effusion of chyle (fat) from the thoracic duct into the thoracic cavity.

chyme (kīm). The thick, grayish, semiliquid mass into which food is converted by gastric digestion. In this form it passes into the small intestine.

chymotrypsin (ki'mo-trip'sin). One of the proteolytic enzymes of the pancreatic juice.

cirrhosis (si-ro'sis). Inflammation with hardening of the tissues of an organ, more especially the liver.

cis **form** (sis). The configuration of a fatty acid in which the molecule turns back on itself at the double bond.

citrovorum factor (sit'ro-vo'rum fak'ter). A biologically active form of folic acid (folinic acid).

clostridium (klos-trid'e-um). A genus of schizomycetes, an anaerobic spore-forming rod-shaped bacterium, *C. perfringens* (and other species); a cause of gangrene.

cobalamine (co-bal'a-min). The basic molecule of vitamin B_{12} several compounds of which have vitamin activity.

cobamide (ko-bam'id). Refers to vitamin B_{12}, containing coenzymes.

colchicine (kol'shi-sin). An alkaloid drug used in the treatment of gout. It interferes in the metabolic pathway of uric acid.

colitis (ko-li'tis). Inflammation of the colon.

collagen (kol'a-jen). The main organic constituent of connective tissue and of the organic substance of bones: changed into gelatin by boiling.

colloidal (ko-loi'dal). Pertaining to a colloid, which is a substance containing tiny, solid, evenly dispersed particles not dissolved in the medium, but which will not settle out.

colostomy (ko-los'to-me). The surgical formation of an artificial opening from the colon onto the abdominal wall.

configuration (kon-fig'u-ra'shun). In chemistry, the arrangement in space of the atoms of a molecule.

congenital (kon-jen'i-tal). Existing at or before birth.

conjunctiva (kon'junk-ti'va). The delicate membrane that lines the eyelids and covers the eyeball in front.

cortex (kor'teks). The outer layers of an organ as distinguished from its inner substance.

corticotrophin (kor'te-ko-tro'fin). A hormone of the anterior pituitary that specifically stimulates the adrenal cortex.

cortisone (cor'te-sōn). A synthetic, hormone-like substance, similar to the adrenal cortex hormones.

creatine (kre'a-tin). A nitrogenous end product of muscle metabolism.

creatinine (kre-at'i-nin). A basic substance creatine anhydride, derived from creatine.

Cushing's Syndrome. The term applied to the changes that take place in the body as a result of some tumors of the pituitary gland. The changes are obesity, hairiness, curvature of the spine, impotence and the appearance of red lines in the skin. Cushing, a famous American brain surgeon, died in 1939.

cyanocobalamin (si'ah-no-ko-bal'ah-men). Vitamin B$_{12}$, a dark red compound containing cobalt and a cyanide group.

cyclamate (si'kla-māt). Sodium or calcium cyclamate, known as Sucaryl, used as an artificial sweetener.

cystic fibrosis (sis'tik fi-bro'sis). Fibrosis of the pancreatic ducts resulting in diminished excretion of pancreatic digestive enzymes.

cystine (sis'tin). A nonessential amino acid containing sulfur.

cystinuria (sis'ti-nu're-ah). The occurrence of excessive cystine in the urine.

cystitis (sis-ti'tis). Inflammation of the urinary bladder.

deaminization (de-am'in-i-za'shun). The process of metabolism by which the nitrogen portion (amine group) is removed from amino acids.

decubitus ulcer (de-ku'bi-tus). A pressure sore caused by prolonged pressure in a patient confined to bed for a long time.

dehydration (de'hi-dra'shun). Removal of water from food or tissue; or the condition that results from undue loss of water.

dehydrogenase (de-hi'dro-jen-as). An enzyme which facilitates the transfer of hydrogen from one compound to another.

dermatitis (dur'ma-ti'tis). Inflammation of the skin.

dermatomyositis (der'mah-to-mi'o-si'tis). A non-suppurative inflammation of the skin, subcutaneous tissue, and underlying muscle.

desoxycorticosterone (des-ox'e-cort'e-co'ster-on). A hormone produced by the cortex of the adrenals.

detoxication (de-tok'si-ka'shun). Reduction of the toxic properties of a substance.

dicumarol (di-koo'mah-rol). Registered name of dicoumarin, a coumarin derivative isolated originally from spoiled sweet clover and later made synthetically. It is used clinically as an anticoagulant in thrombotic states, and acts by depressing the factors concerned with the formation of thrombin.

disaccharidase (di-sak'ah-ri-das). An enzyme which hydrolyzes disaccharides.

disaccharide (di-sak'a-rid). Any one of the sugars which yields two single sugars on hydrolysis.

diuresis (di'u-re'sis). Increased secretion of urine.

diverticulosis (di'ver-tik'u-lo'sis). The presence of small pouches or pockets leading off a main cavity or tube. Often occurs in the intestines.

DNA, deoxyribonucleic acid (de-ok'se-ri'bo-nu-kle'ik). Found in the nucleus of living cells; functions in the transfer of genetic characteristics.

dyscrasia (dis-kra'ze-ah). An old term; signifies an abnormal composition of the blood.

dysentery (dis'en-ter-e). Inflammation of intestinal mucous membrane, especially the colon. The causative agent may be bacteria or parasitic worms.

dyspnea (disp-ne'a). Difficult or labored breathing.

dyssebacea (dis'se-ba'shea). Disorder of the sebaceous follicles often seen in riboflavin deficiency.

dystrophy (dis'tro-fe). Progressive weakening of a muscle.

eclampsia (ek-lamp'si-a). A severe manifestation of toxemia of pregnancy accompanied by convulsions.

eczema (ek'ze-ma). A skin disease.

edema (e-de'ma). The presence of an abnormally large volume of fluid in the intertissue spaces

electrocorticoid hormone (e-lek'tro-kor'ti-coid). One of the hormones produced by the adrenal cortex; concerned with the retention of sodium and excretion of potassium in the urine.

electrolyte (e-lek'tro-līt). The ionized form of an element. Common electrolytes in the body are sodium, potassium and chloride.

emaciation (e-ma'se-a'shun). A wasted condition of the body.

emulsion (e-mul'shun). A finely divided mixture or suspension of two liquids not mutually soluble.

endemic (en-dem'ik). Pertaining to or prevalent in a particular district or region.

endocarditis (en'do-kar-di'tis). Inflammation of the endocardium (inner lining membrane of the heart).

endocrine (en'do-krin). Applied to organs whose function it is to secrete internally a hormone which plays an important role in metabolism.

endogenous (en-doj'e-nus). Originating within the organism.

endosperm (en′do-sperm). The nutritive substance within the embryo sac of plants.

enterocrinin (en-ter-o-kri′nin). Gastrointestinal hormone which stimulates secretion by glands in small intestines.

enterogastrone (en′ter-o-gas′tron). Hormone of the gastrointestinal tract, antagonist of gastrin, inhibits gastric secretion and motility.

enteropathy (en′ter-op′ah-the). Any disease of the intestine.

enterotoxin (en′ter-o-tok′sin). A toxin specific for the cells of the intestinal mucosa and arising in the intestine.

enzyme (en′zīm). A substance, usually protein in nature and formed in living cells, which brings about chemical changes.

epiphysis; epiphyseal (epif′i-sis; ep′i-fiz′e-al). In the long bones, a segment of bone at the ends of the shaft. It is separated from the long bone early in life by cartilage, but is part of the bone when longitudinal growth is complete.

epithelium (ep′i-the′le-um). The outer layers of the skin and the mucous membranes, consisting of cells of various forms and arrangement.

ergocalciferol (er′go-kal-cif′er-ol). Vitamin D_2 derived from ergosterol. (See calciferol.)

ergosterol (er-gos′ter-ol). A sterol found in plant and in animal tissues which, on exposure to ultraviolet light, is converted into vitamin D_2. (See *sterol.*)

ergot (er′got). A fungus found on cereal grains; used in medicine as a hemostatic.

erythema, erythematous (er′i-the′mah). A redness of the skin due to congestion of the capillaries.

erythrocyte (e-rith′ro-sīt). Red blood corpuscle.

estrogen (es′tro-jen). A generic term for any compound which produces estrus in the female.

etiology (e′te-ol′o-je). The study of the causation of a disease.

exocrine (ek-so′krin). Applied to a gland which secretes outwardly; the opposite of endocrine.

exogenous (eks-oj′e-nus). Originating outside the organism.

extrinsic (eks-trin′sik). Coming from, or originating from, outside.

exudation (eks′u-da′shun). The outpouring of an abnormal substance which becomes deposited in or on the tissues.

FAO. Food and Agriculture Organization of the United Nations, Headquarters in Rome, Italy.

fatty acids (fat′e as′ids). The organic acids which combine with glycerol to form fat.

favism (fa′vism). An acute hemolytic anemia due to contact with the fava or broad bean.

febrile (fe′bril). Pertaining to, or accompanied by, fever.

feces (fe′sez). Excrement; the discharge of the bowel.

ferritin (fer′i-tin). An iron-containing protein: the form in which iron is stored in the liver, spleen, intestinal mucosa and reticuloendothelial cells.

fetus (fe′tus). The product of conception after the fourth month of pregnancy.

fibrosis (fi-bro′sis). The formation of fibrous connective tissue.

fistula (fis′tu-la). An abnormal tubelike passage in the body.

flatulence (flat′u-lens). Distention of the intestinal tract with gas or air.

flavin-adenine dinucleotide (FAD) (fla′vin-ad′e-nin di-nu′kle-o-tide). A riboflavin-containing coenzyme which functions in cell respiration.

flavin mononucleotide (FMN) (fla′vin mon′o-nu′kle-o-tide). A compound containing riboflavin and a phosphate group; functions as an enzyme in the Krebs cycle. Also referred to as the "yellow enzyme."

flavoproteins (fla′vo-pro′te-in). Compounds containing riboflavin, certain nucleotides and proteins. They are important as enzymes in the Krebs cycle.

fluoridation (floo-or′i-da′shun). The addition of fluoride to a water supply as part of a public health program to reduce the incidence of dental caries.

folacin (fo′la-sin). Another term for folic acid.

folic acid (fo′lic as′id). A vitamin of the B complex group, known also as pteroylglutamic acid.

folinic acid (fo-lin′ik). A folic acid derivative closely related to the true enzyme, also called "citrovorum factor."

follicle (fol′i-kl). A very small excretory or secretory sac or gland such as a hair follicle.

formiminoglutamic acid (FIGLU) (form-im′i-no′glu-ta′mik). Intermediary product of histidine metabolism. Since folic acid is necessary for its breakdown, the urinary excretion of FIGLU may be measured to determine folic acid status.

friable (fri′a-bl). Easily broken or crumbled.

galactose (gah-lak′tos). A monosaccharide derived from lactose by hydrolysis.

galactose-1-phosphate (gas-lak′tos). An intermediate product of galactose metabolism.

galactosemia (gah-lak'to-se'me-ah). A hereditary condition characterized by excess galactose in the blood.

gastrectomy (gas-trek'to-me). Surgical removal of a part or all of the stomach.

gastrin (gas'trin). Hormone of the gastrointestinal tract which stimulates the secretion of HCl by the gastric glands.

gastrostomy (gas-tros'to-me). Surgical creation of an artificial gastric fistula.

gavage (ga'vazh'). Feeding by the stomach tube.

genes (jēns). Units of hereditary DNA, carried by chromosomes.

geriatrics (jer'e-at'riks). Study and treatment of the problems and the diseases of old age.

gerontology (jer'on-tol'o-je). The scientific study of old age.

gestation (jes-ta'shun). Period of fetal development. Pregnancy.

gingivitis (jin'ji-vi'tis). Inflammation involving the gums around the teeth.

gliadin (gli'a-din). One of the proteins found in wheat.

glossitis (glos-i'tis). Inflammation of the tongue.

glucagon (gloo'ka-gon). A hormone produced by the pancreas which breaks down liver glycogen to glucose.

glucocorticoid hormone (gloo'ko-kor'ti-koid). One of the hormones produced by the adrenal cortex; increases the rate of glucose formation, raising the concentration of liver glycogen and blood glucose.

glutathione (gloo'tah-thi'on). A tripeptide coenzyme involved in metabolism; isolated from plant and animal tissues.

gluten (gloo'ten; -t'n). A protein found in many cereal grains.

glyceride (glis'er-īd). A compound formed when glycerol and an acid are combined.

glycogen (gli'ko-jen). A carbohydrate, similar in composition to the amylopectin form of starch. In this form, carbohydrate is stored in the liver and the muscles.

glycosuria (gli'ko-su'ri-a). Presence of sugar in the urine.

goitrogen (goi'tro-jen). A goiter-producing substance.

hematocrit (he-mat'o-krit). The volume of erythrocytes in centrifuged oxalated blood, expressed as corpuscular volume per cent.

hematopoietic (hem'a-to-poi-et'ik). Affecting the formation of blood cells.

hematuria (hem'ah-tu're-ah). The presence of blood in the urine.

heme (hēm). The colored, insoluble component of hemoglobin, containing iron.

hemeralopia (hem'er-a-lo'pe-a). Day blindness; inability to see in a bright light.

hemicellulose (hem'e-sel'u-los). A complex carbohydrate similar to celluose found in the cell wall of plants; indigestible but absorbs water, thereby stimulating laxation.

hemiplegia (hem'e-ple'je-ah). Paralysis of one side of the body.

hemochromatosis (he'mo-kro-mah-to'sis). A metabolic disorder characterized by pigmentation of the skin and viscera with hemosiderin, producing interstitial fibrosis, severe diabetes, impotence and loss of axillary hair. It occurs especially in the male.

hemocyanin (he'mo-si'ah-nin). A copper-containing protein in the blood of certain invertebrates. It functions as an oxygen carrier similar to hemoglobin in vertebrates. Also called hematocyanin.

hemodialysis (he'mo-di-al'i-sis). Dialysis of the blood, as by circulation through an artificial kidney.

hemolytic (he'mo-lit'ik). Pertaining to the breaking down of red blood corpuscles.

hemorrhage (hem'o-rij). A copious escape of blood from the vessels; bleeding.

hemorrhoid(s) (hem'o-roid). Vascularlike tumors made up of infected varices of the rectal mucous membrane.

hemosiderin (he'mo-sid'er-in). A dark yellow pigment similar to ferritin but containing more iron. It is formed as a result of iron loading or excessive blood transfusions.

hepatic (he-pat'ik). Pertaining to the liver.

hexose (hek'sos). A single sugar containing six carbon atoms.

histamine (his'ta-min). A nitrogenous substance found in all animal and vegetable tissues. A stimulator of the autonomic nervous system and used to stimulate gastric secretion.

histidine (his'ti-din). An amino acid required by growing animals.

homeostasis (ho'me-o-sta'sis). A tendency to uniformity or stability in the normal body states of the organism.

homogenized (ho-moj'e-nizd). Made homogeneous. Usually applied to dispersing milk fat in such fine globules that cream will not rise to the top.

hormone (hor'mōn). A chemical substance which is secreted into body fluids and transported to another organ, where it produces a specific effect on metabolism.

hydrogenation (hi'dro-jen-a'shun). The process of introducing hydrogen into a compound, as when oils are hydrogenated to produce solid fats.

hydrolysate (hi-drol′i-sat). A product of hydrolysis. Often applied to protein hydrolysate.

hydrolysis (hi-drol′i-sis). A chemical reaction in which decomposition is due to the incorporation and splitting of water, resulting in the formation of two new compounds.

hydroxocobalamine (hi-drok′so-co′bal-ah-min). Vitamin B_{12} with a hydroxyl group.

hydroxyproline (hi-drok′se-pro′lin). An amino acid which occurs in structural proteins, primarily collagen.

hypercalcemia (hi′per-kal-se′me-ah). An excess of calcium in the blood.

hyperchlorhydria (hi′per-klor-hi′dre-a). Excessive secretion of hydrochloric acid in the stomach.

hypercholesteremia (hi′per-ko-les′ter-e′me-a). Excess of cholesterol in the blood.

hyperchromic (hi′per-kro′mik). Highly or excessively colored.

hyperemia (hi′per-e′me-a). Excess of blood in any part of the body.

hyperglycemia (hi′per-gli-se′me-a). An increase in the blood sugar level above normal.

hyperinsulinism (hi′per-in′su-lin-izm). Excessive secretion of insulin by the pancreas resulting in hypoglycemia.

hyperlipemia (hi′per-li-pe′me-a). Excess of fat or lipids in the blood.

hyperlipidemia (hi′per-lip-i-de′me-ah). An excess of lipids in the blood.

hyperphagia (hi′per-fa′je-ah). Ingestion of greater than optimal quantity of food; increased hunger.

hyperpituitarism (hi′per-pi-tu′i-tah-rizm). A condition due to pathologically increased activity of the pituitary gland.

hyperplasia (hi′per-pla′zhe-a; -ze-a). Abnormal multiplication of cells, with increase in size of the organ, but without formation of a tumor.

hyperthermia (hi′per-thur′me-a). Fever.

hypertrophic (hi′per-trof′ik). Pertaining to an enlargement or overgrowth of an organ, or part, due to a diseased condition.

hyperuricemia (hi′per-u′ri-se′me-ah). Excess of uric acid in the blood.

hypervitaminosis (hi′per-vi′ta-min-o′sis). A condition due to an excess of one or more vitamins.

hypoalbuminemia (hi′po-al-bu′min-e′me-a). Abnormally low albumin content of the blood.

hypocalcemia (hi′po-kal-se′me-a). Abnormally low blood calcium.

hypochlorhydria (hi′po-klor-hi′dre-a). Diminished secretion of hydrochloric acid in the stomach.

hypochromic (hi′po-kro′mik). Decrease in color; usually applied to decrease in hemoglobin content of the erythrocytes.

hypoglycemia (hi′po-gli-se′me-a). A decrease in the blood sugar level below normal.

hypophysectomy (hi′po-fiz-ek′to-me). Surgical removal of the hypophysis, or pituitary gland.

hypophysis (hi-pof′i-sis). Any outgrowth, especially referring to the pituitary gland.

hypoproteinemia (hi′po-pro′te-in-e′me-a). A decrease in the normal quantity of serum protein in the blood.

hypoprothrombinemia (hi′po-pro-throm′bin-e′me-ah). Deficiency of prothrombin in the blood.

hypothalamus (hi′po-thal′ah-mus). A portion of the mid-brain concerned with emotional expression, visceral responses, water balance, body temperature and sleep.

icterus (ik′ter-us). Jaundice.

idiopathic (id′i-o-path′ik). Self-originated; occurring without known cause.

ileitis (il′e-i′tis). Inflammation of the ileum.

ileostomy (il′e-os′to-me). Surgical creation of a permanent opening through the abdominal wall into the ileum.

ileum (il′e-um). Lower third portion of the small intestine.

incipient (in-sip′i-ent). Beginning to exist.

infarct (in′farkt). Death of tissue due to local anemia resulting from obstruction of circulation supplying the part. (myocardial infarct)

inositol (in-o′si-tol). A member of the vitamin B complex.

interstitial (in′ter-stish′al). In the spaces between the cells.

intracellular (in′trah-sel′u-lar). Situated or occurring within the cell.

intravenous (in′tra-ve′nus). Within or into a vein.

intrinsic (in-trin′sik). Situated entirely within; pertaining to itself.

iodopsin (i′o-dop′sin). A light-sensitive vitamin A protein complex necessary for vision in bright light.

isoleucine (i′so-lu′sin). An essential amino acid.

isoniazid (i′so-ni′a-zid). One of the isonicotinic acid derivatives used as an anti-infective agent especially in tuberculosis.

iso-osmotic (i′so-oz-mot′ik). Having the same osmotic pressure.

isotopes (i′so-tope). Two or more chemical elements which have the same atomic number and identical chemical properties, but which differ in atomic weight or in the structure of the nucleus.

jejunum (je-joo'num). Middle portion of the small intestine. About 8 feet long.

jejunostomy (je'joo-nos'to-me). Surgical creation of a permanent opening through the abdominal wall into the jejunum.

keratin (ker'ah-tin). A scleroprotein which is the principal constituent of epidermis, hair, nails, horny tissues and the organic matrix of the enamel of the teeth. It is a very insoluble protein, contains sulfur, and yields tyrosine and leucine on decomposition.

keratinize (ker'a-tin-iz). To become hornylike.

ketogenic (ke'to-jen'ik). Capable of being converted into ketone bodies. Ketogenic substances in metabolism are the fatty acids and certain amino acids.

ketone bodies (ke'tōn). Acetoacetic acid, β-hydroxybutyric acid and acetone.

ketosis (ke-to'sis). A condition in which there is an accumulation in the body of the ketone bodies as a result of incomplete oxidation of the fatty acids.

kwashiorkor (kwa-shi-or'ker). A severe protein-calorie deficiency disease occurring in small children. Endemic in many parts of the world.

labile (la'bil). Not fixed; unstable.

lacteal(s) (lak'te-al). Tiny vessels in the intestinal wall through which fat is absorbed; part of the lymphatic system.

lamina propria (lam'i-nah pro'pre-ah). The connective tissue coat of a mucous membrane.

lavage (lav-azh'). The washing out of an organ, such as the stomach.

lecithin (les'i-thin). A phospholipid containing glycerol, fatty acids, phosphoric acid and choline.

leucine (lu'sin). An essential amino acid.

leukemia (lu-ke'me-a). A disease of the blood-forming organs, characterized by a marked increase of the white corpuscles.

leukocyte (lu'ko-sīt). White blood corpuscle.

leukopenic (lu'ko-pen'ik). Pertaining to leukopenia (reduction of leukocytes in the blood).

linoleic acid (lin'o-le'ik as'id). A polyunsaturated fatty acid essential for nutrition.

linolenic acid (lin'o-le'nik as'id). A polyunsaturated fatty acid.

lipase (li'pās; lip'ās). An enzyme that digests fat.

lipid (lip'id), **lipoid** (lip'oid). Fat or fatlike substances.

lipoprotein (lip'o-pro'te-in). Combination of a protein with a fat, found in both animal and plant tissues.

lipotropic (lip'o-trop'ik). Applied to substances essential for fat metabolism.

lumen (lu'men). The space within an artery, vein, intestine or tube.

lysosomes (li'so-soms). Membranous structures in cytoplasm which contain hydrolytic enzymes.

macrocytic (mak'ro-sit-ik). Refers to the presence in the blood of abnormally large red blood corpuscles.

malabsorption syndrome (mal'ab-sorp'shun). A group of symptoms which result from the inability to digest or absorb food in the intestinal tract.

malignant (ma-lig'nant). Severe form of occurrence, tending to grow worse.

malocclusion (mal'o-kloo'shun). Failure of proper occlusion of the jaws which may interfere with the function of mastication.

malonyl coenzyme A (mal'o-nil). An intermediate compound in the biosynthesis of fatty acids.

marasmus (ma-raz'mus). Wasting and emaciation, especially in infants.

matrix (ma'triks). The intercellular framework of a tissue.

megaloblastic anemia (meg'ah-lo-blast'ik). Anemia marked by the presence of oversize nucleated red blood cells (megaloblasts).

melanin (mel'ah-nin). The dark amorphous pigment of the skin, hair and certain other tissues.

menadione (me-na-di'on). Synthetic vitamin K.

metabolism (me-tab'o-lizm). General term to designate all chemical changes which occur in food nutrients after they have been absorbed from the gastrointestinal tract and to the cellular activity involved in utilizing these nutrients.

methionine (meth-i'o-nin). An essential amino acid containing sulfur.

methyl-malonic acid (meth'il-ma-lo'nik). (MMA) Intermediary product in metabolism of certain fatty acids. Vitamin B_{12} is necessary for its breakdown to succinic acid; hence, its measurement in urine can be used to determine B_{12} status.

microcytic (mi'kro-sit-ik). Refers to the presence in the blood of undersized red blood corpuscles.

microsome (mi'kro-som). One of the finely granular elements of protoplasm.

miscible (mis'i-bl). Capable of being mixed.

mitochondria (mit'o-kron'dre-ah). Small granules or rod-shaped structures in the cell.

monosaccharide (mon'o-sak'a-rid). A simple sugar which cannot be decomposed by hydrolysis.

mono-unsaturated (mon'o-un-sat'u-rat-ed). An organic compound such as a fatty acid in which two carbon atoms are united by a double bond.

mucin (mu'sin). A mucopolysaccharide or glycoprotein; the chief constituent of mucus secreted by the digestive glands.

mucopolysaccharide (mu'ko-pol'e-sak'ah-rid). A group of polysaccharides which contains hexoseamine, which may or may not be combined with protein and which, dispersed in water, form many of the mucins.

mucoprotein (mu'ko-pro'te-in). Substance containing a polypeptide chain and disaccharides, found in mucous secretions of the digestive glands.

mucosa (mu-ko'sa). Mucous membrane lining passages and cavities, as in the gastrointestinal tract.

mucoviscidosis (mu'ko-vi-si-do'sis). The hereditary condition more often called cystic fibrosis or pancreatic fibrosis.

myasthenia gravis (mi'as-the'ne-ah). A syndrome of fatigue and exhaustion of the muscular system marked by progressive paralysis without sensory disturbance or atrophy.

myocarditis (mi'o-kar-di'tis). Inflammation of the myocardium (heart muscle).

myoglobin (mi'o-glo'bin). Compound similar to hemoglobin, found in muscles.

myosin (mi'o-sin). A protein of muscle fiber.

myxedema (mik'se-de'ma). Condition due to a deficiency of thyroid secretion.

naphthoquinone (naf'tho-kwin'on). A derivative of quinone; some of these derivatives have vitamin K activity.

nasogastric tube (na'zo-gas'trik) Tube inserted through the nose and passed by way of the esophagus into the stomach.

necrosis (ne-kro'sis). Death of a circumscribed area of tissue.

neoplasm (ne'o-plazm). Any new and abnormal growth such as a tumor.

nephropathy (ne-frop'ah-the). Disease of the kidneys.

nephrosis (ne-fro'sis). Any disease of the kidneys characterized by degenerative lesions of the renal tubules and marked edema, albuminuria and decrease serum albumin.

neurasthenia (nu'ras-the'ne-a). Nervous exhaustion characterized by abnormal fatigue.

neurogenic (nu'ro-jen'ik). Forming nerve tissue. Originating in the nervous tissue.

neuropathy (nu-rop'ah-the). A general term denoting functional disturbances and/or pathological changes in the peripheral nervous system.

niacin (ni'a-sin). A member of the vitamin B complex, formerly known as nicotinic acid. An antipellagra factor.

niacinamide (ni'ah-sin-am'id). Nicotinamide, the amide derivative of nicotinic acid (niacin).

nicotinamide adenine dinucleotide (NAD) (nik'o-tin'ah-mid ad'e-nin di-nu'kle-o-tid). Niacin, containing coenzyme which is necessary for tissue respiration.

nocturia (nok-tu're-ah). Excessive urination at night.

nucleoprotein (nu'kle-o-pro'tein). The conjugated protein found in the nuclei of cells.

nucleotide (nu'kle-o-tid). Compound containing a sugar-phosphate component and a purine or pyrimidine base.

nyctalopia (nik'ta-lo'pe-a). Night blindness; imperfection of vision at night or in a dim light.

nystagmus (nis-tag'mus). An involuntary rapid movement of the eyeball.

oleic acid (o-le'ik). A monounsaturated fatty acid.

oliguria (ol'i-gu're-ah). Diminished secretion of urine.

ophthalmia (of-thal'me-a). Severe inflammation of the eye.

ophthalmoplegia (of-thal'mople'je-ah). Paralysis of the eye muscles.

opsin (op'sin). Protein compound which combines with retinal, vitamin A aldehyde, to form rhodopsin, visual purple.

osmotic pressure (osmot'ik). The force that a dissolved substance exerts on a semipermeable membrane through which it cannot pass but which forces the solvent to pass through until the concentration of dissolved particles are approximately equal on both sides.

ossification (os'i-fi-ka'shun). Formation of bone or bony substance.

osteoarthritis (os'te-o-ar-thri'tis). Chronic joint disease occurring mostly in older people and marked by degeneration and hypertrophy of bone and cartilage and thickening of the synovial membranes.

osteomalacia (os'te-o-ma-la'she-a). Softening of the bone due to loss of calcium. Occurs chiefly in adults.

osteoporosis (os'te-o-po-ro'sis). Abnormal porousness or rarefaction of bone due to failure of the osteoblasts to lay down bone matrix, and occurring when resorption dominates over mineral deposition.

oxaluria (ok'sah-lu're-ah). The presence of an excess of oxalic acid or of oxalates in the urine.

oxidation (ok'si-da'shun). A chemical process by which a substance combines with oxygen. Chemically it is an increase of positive charges on an atom through the loss of electrons.

pancreozymin (pan'kre-o-zi'min). A hormone of the duodenal mucosa which stimulates the external secretory activity of the pancreas.

pantothenic acid (pan'to-then'ik). A member of the vitamin B complex.

parenchyma (pa-reng'ki-ma). The functional part of an organ as distinguished from its framework.

para-aminobenzoic acid (PABA) (par'a-a-men' no-ben-zo'ik as'id). A part of pteroylglutamic acid, one of the forms of folic acid.

paraplegia (par'ah-ple'je-ah). Paralysis of the legs and the lower part of the body, both motion and sensation being affected, caused by disease or injury to the spine.

parenteral (par-en'ter-al). Not through the alimentary canal; i.e., subcutaneously or intravenously.

parturition (par'tu-rish'un). The act or process of giving birth to a child.

pentose (pen'tos). A single sugar containing five carbon atoms. Ribose is a pentose.

peptide (pep'tid). An intermediary product of enzymatic hydrolysis of protein.

peptone(s) (pep'ton). An intermediary product of enzymatic hydrolysis of protein.

pericarditis (per'e-kar-di'tis). Inflammation of the pericardium (membrane surrounding the heart).

peristalsis (per'e-stal'sis). The wavelike movement by which the alimentary tract propels its contents.

pernicious (per-nish'us). Tending to be serious or fatal.

peroral (per-o'ral). Performed through or administered through the mouth.

pesticide (pes'ti-sid). A poison used to destroy pests of any sort. The term includes fungicides, insecticides and rodenticides.

phagocytosis (fag'o-si-to'sis). The engulfing of microorganisms and cells by phagocytes— usually white blood corpuscles or other related cells.

phenformin (fen-for'min). A biguanide; an oral hypoglycemic agent used in the treatment of diabetes.

phenylalanine (fen'il-al'a-nen; nin). An essential amino acid.

phenylketonuria (PKU) (fen'il-ke'ton-nu're-ah). An inborn error of the metabolism of phenylalanine; phenylpyruvic acid appears in the urine.

phenylpyruvic acid (fen'il-pi-ru'vik). An intermediate product in phenylalanine metabolism.

phospholipid (fos'fo-lip'id). A fat in which one fatty acid is replaced by phosphorus and a nitrogenous compound.

phosphorylation (fos'for-i-la'shun). The process of introducing the trivalent phosphate group into an organic molecule. The phosphate donor is usually ATP.

photopic (fo-top'ik). Pertaining to vision in bright light.

phylloquinone (fil'o-kwin'ōn). Compound used as a prothrombogenic agent.

physiologic saline (fiz'e-o-loj'ik sa'lin). A solution of sodium chloride isotonic with the blood.

pinocytosis (pi'no-si-to'sis). Ameba-like action of cells encompassing minute amounts of fluid, thus forming a fluid-like vacuole.

polioencephalitis (po'le-o-en-sef'ah-li'tis). Inflammatory disease of the gray substance of the brain.

polyarthritis (pol'e-ar-thri'tis). Inflammation of several joints at the same time.

polycythemia (pol'e-si-the'me-a). Excess of red corpuscles in the blood.

polydipsia (pol'e-dip'se-a). Excessive thirst.

polyneuritis (pol'e-nu-ri'tis). Inflammation of many nerves.

polyneuropathy (pol'e-nu-rop'ah-the). A disease which involves several nerves.

polyphagia (pol'e-fa'je-ah). Excessive hunger. Exessive or voracious eating.

polysaccharide (pol'e-sak'ah-rid). A complex carbohydrate which contains more than four molecules of monosaccharides combined with each other.

polyunsaturated (pol'e-un-sat'u-rat'ed). An organic compound such as a fatty acid in which there is more than one double bond.

polyuria (pol'i-u're-a). Excessive secretion and discharge of urine.

porphyrin (por'fi-rin). Any one of a group of iron-free, magnesium-free pyrrole derivatives which occur in protoplasm. They form the basis of respiratory pigments such as hemoglobin and chlorophyll.

precursor (pre-kur'ser). A substance which is converted into another.

premature infant (pre'ma-tur'). An infant born before term.

primaquine (pri'mah-kwin). An antimalarial drug.

proconvertin (pro'kon-ver'tin). One of the blood coagulation factors; Factor VII.

prognosis (prog-no'sis). Prospect as to recovery from a disease.

prophylaxis (pro'fi-lak'sis). The prevention of disease.

protease (pro'te-as). An enzyme that digests protein.

protein hydrolysate (pro'te-in hi-drol'i-zat). A solution containing the constituent amino acids of an artificially digested protein, usually milk or beef protein.

proteinuria (pro'te-i-nu're-a). Presence of protein in the urine.

proteolytic (pro'te-o-lit'ik). Effecting the digestion of proteins.

proteose(s) (pro'te-os). An intermediate product of enzymatic hydrolysis of protein between protein and peptone.

prothrombin (pro-throm'bin). A factor in blood plasma which is the precursor of thrombin, necessary for the clotting of blood.

protoplasm (pro'to-plazm). The essential living matter in a cell. The only known form of matter in which life is manifested.

protozoa (pro'to-zo'ah). The lowest division of the animal kingdom, including one-celled organisms.

provitamin (pro-vi'ta-min). The forerunner of a vitamin. Provitamin A is carotene.

pteroylglutamic acid (ter-ol-glu-tam'ic as'id). (See *folic acid*.)

ptyalin (ti'a-lin). The amylase of saliva.

purine(s) (pu'rēn). End products of nucleoprotein metabolism.

putrefaction (pu'tre-fak'shun). The decomposition of animal matter, especially protein, caused by certain kinds of bacteria.

pyelitis (pi'e-li'tis). Inflammation of the pelvis of the kidney.

pyelonephritis (pi'ĕ-lo-ne-fri'tis). Inflammation of the kidney and its pelvis.

pyridoxal phosphate (PALP). (pir'i-dok'sal). Vitamin B_6, containing coenzyme. The active group for catalyzing several different metabolic reactions.

pyridoxine (pi'ri-dok'sin). Vitamin B_6, a member of the vitamin B complex.

pyrophosphate (pi'ro-fos'fāt). Any salt of phosphoric acid containing two phosphate groups.

quadriplegia (kwod'ri-ple'je-ah). Paralysis of all four limbs, both motion and sensation being affected.

rachitogenic (rah-kit'o-jen'ik). Capable of causing rickets.

RAD. A unit of measurement of absorbed doses of ionizing radiation.

radiography (ra'de-og'ra-fe). Photography with roentgen rays. The making of x-ray pictures.

remission (re-mish'un). The period of abatement of symptoms, or the lessening of their severity.

renal (or **kidney**) **threshold** (re'nal thresh'old). That concentration of a given substance in the blood above which the excess will be eliminated in the urine. Usually applied to glucose.

rennin (ren'in). The milk-curdling enzyme of the gastric juice.

rep (Roentgen-equivalent-physical). A unit of the amount of radiation of any kind which yields an amount of energy in tissue equal to one Roentgen unit.

reticulocyte (re-tik'u-lo-sīt'). An immature red blood cell.

retina (ret'i-na). Innermost and the perceptive structure of the eye, formed by the expansion of the optic nerve. The rods and cones of the retina are specialized nerve cells sensitive to light and color.

retinal (ret'i-nal). The aldehyde form of vitamin A which is necessary for the synthesis of rhodopsin, visual purple.

retinoic acid (ret'i-no-ic). The acid form of vitamin A.

retinol (ret'i-nol). The chemical term for vitamin A alcohol.

retinopathy (ret'i-nop'ah-the). Any noninflammatory disease of the retina.

retinyl (ret'i-nel). Refers to the vitamin A portion of the ester form of the vitamin. Retinyl palmitate is hydrolyzed to vitamin A alcohol (retinol) and palmitic acid in the gastrointestinal trract.

rheumatoid arthritis (roo'mah-toid ar-thri'tis). A chronic disease of the joints, marked by inflammatory changes in the synovial membranes and the articular structures and by atrophy and rarefaction of the bones.

rhodopsin (ro-dop'sin). Visual purple, formed in the rods of the retina by combining the protein opsin and vitamin A aldehyde. It is necessary for scotopic vision.

riboflavin (ri'bo-fla'vin). Heat-stable factor of B complex, sometimes called vitamin B_2.

ribonucleic acid (RNA). (ri-bo-nu'kle-ik). A nucleic acid replicated from DNA and found in cytoplasm.

saccharine (sak'ah-rin). An intensely sweet, white crystalline compound used as a substitute for ordinary sugar. It has no food value.

safflower oil (saf'flou'er). An edible oil from the seeds of the safflower plant, *Carthamus tinctorius;* high in linoleic acid.

saponification (sa-pon'i-fi-ka'shun). The splitting of fat by an alkali, yielding glycerol and soap. This may occur during the digestion of fat.

satiety (sa-ti'e-te). Fullness or gratification of appetite.

scleroderma (skle'ro-der'mah). A disease of the skin in which thickened, hard, pigmented patches occur, the connective tissue of the corium and subcutaneous structures increase, producing a hidebound condition.

sclerosis (skle-ro'sis). Hardening; a chronic thickening of a part due to inflammation and disease.

scotopic (sko-top'ik). Pertaining to vision in dim light.

sebaceous glands (se-ba'shus). Glands in the skin which secrete a greasy substance.

secretin (se-kre'tin). A hormone secreted by the mucosa of the duodenum and jejunum when acid chyme enters the intestine. Carried by the blood, it stimulates the secretion of pancreatic juice and bile.

sodium benzoate (so'de-um ben'zo-āt). A salt of benzoic acid used as a preservative in foods.

spasmophilia (spaz'mo-fil'e-a). A tendency to spasm and convulsions.

spastic (spas'tik). Characterized by spasms or convulsions.

sphincter (sfingk'ter). A ringlike muscle which closes a natural opening.

sphingomyelin (sfing'go-mi'e-lin). A phospholipid found primarily in brain and lung tissue as a constituent of the myelin sheaths.

stachyose (stak'e-os). An indigestible tetrasaccharide containing galactose.

stasis (sta'sis). A stoppage of the flow of blood or other body fluid in any part.

stearic acid (ste'a-rik). A saturated fatty acid.

steatorrhea (ste'a-to-re'a). Presence of an excess of fat in the stools.

steroid (ste'roid). A group name for compounds that resemble cholesterol chemically. Some of the substances included in this group are sex hormones, adrenal cortex hormones; bile acids and some of the carcinogenic hydrocarbons.

sterol (ster'ol). Fat-soluble substance with a complex molecular structure.

stomatitis (sto'mat-i'tis). Inflammation of the mouth.

streptococcus (strep'to-kok'us). A spherical bacterium of the genus Streptococcus. It occurs predominantly in chains of cells. The species are differentiated on the bases of hemolysis, serology and certain physiologic reactions.

substrate (sub'strāt). A substance upon which an enzyme acts.

succinic acid (suk-sin'ik). Intermediary product in metabolism.

suet (su'et). Hard fat of beef or mutton.

syndrome (sin'drom). A set of symptoms which occur together.

synthesis (sin'the-sis). The process of building up a chemical compound.

synovium (si-no'vi-um). A synovial membrane, lubricated by synovial fluid or mucin.

Terramycin (ter'ah-mi'sin). A proprietary brand of oxytetracycline, an antibiotic and antiprotozoan.

tetany (tet'a-ne). A condition characterized by intermittent spasms, muscle twitchings and cramps usually involving the extremities. It is due to abnormal calcium metabolism and may occur in parathyroid hypofunction and in vitamin D deficiency.

thiamine (thi'am-in). Vitamin B_1. Antineuritic factor, member of the B complex.

thiochrome (thi'o-krom). The yellow coloring matter of yeast. It may be prepared by oxidizing thiamine.

thyrocalcitonin (thi'ro-cal'ci-to'nin). A thyroid hormone which prohibits release of calcium from bone.

thyroglobulin (thi'ro-glob'u-lin). The iodine-containing protein which is synthesized in the thyroid gland and can be broken down to thyroxin and small amounts of triiodothyronine.

thyrotoxicosis (thi'ro-tok'si-ko'sis). The disease produced by the excessive activity of the thyroid gland, with increased production of thyroxin.

thyroxin (thi-rok'sin). An iodine-containing compound possessing the physiologic properties of thyroid extract; prepared synthetically; used in cases of defective thyroid functioning.

tocopherol (to-kof'er-ol). An alcohol-like substance, several forms of which have vitamin E activity.

tolbutamide (tol-bu'ta-mide). (Orinase) An oral hypoglycemic agent used in the treatment of diabetes.

toxemia of pregnancy (toks-e'me-a; preg'nan-se). A toxic condition of unknown etiology which occurs only in pregnancy.

trans **form.** The configuration of a fatty acid in which the chain is stretched out.

transamination (trans'am-i-na'shun). The transferring of an amino group from an amino acid to another compound. By this process the body is able to synthesize the nonessential amino acids as well as form urea. A vitamin B_6-containing enzyme is necessary for this reaction.

transferrin (trans-fer'in). A protein compound found in the blood stream which transports iron to the bone marrow for hemoglobin synthesis, to the liver or spleen for storage or to the other tissues for their use.

transketolase (trans-ke'to-lās). Enzyme containing thiamine (thiamine pyrophosphate—TPP) as a coenzyme. It is found in blood, cells, liver, kidney and other tissues and is necessary for the synthesis of the five carbon sugars found in DNA and RNA.

trauma (tro'ma). An injury or a wound.

trehalose (tre-ha'los). A disaccharide found in yeast and some fungi; used to identify certain bacteria.

triceps skinfold measure. A measurement of fat-thickness by skin-fold calipers at a point midway at the back of the upper right arm flexed at 90°.

trichinosis (trik'i-no'sis). A disease due to infection with trichinae—parasites found in raw pork.

triiodothyronine (tri'i-o-do-thi'ro-nin). Thyroid hormone similar to thyroxin.

trypsin (trip'sin). An enzyme that digests protein.

tularemia (too'la-re'me-ah). A disease of rodents, resembling plague, which is transmitted by the bites of flies, fleas, ticks and lice and may be acquired by man through handling of infected animals.

tyrosine (ti-ro'sin). A nonessential amino acid.

ultraviolet light (ul'tra-vi'o-let). Rays of shorter wave length than visible light. Sunlight is the natural source, but it may be derived from various kinds of electrical devices.

UNESCO. United Nations Educational, Scientific and Cultural Organization. Headquarters, Paris, France.

urea (u-re'a). The chief nitrogenous end product of protein metabolism in the body.

uremia (u-re'me-a). The increase of urinary constituents in the blood and the toxic condition produced thereby. Also known as azotemia.

uric acid (u'rik). An acid found in urine, derived from the metabolism of purines.

uricosuric (u'ri-ko-su'rik). Promoting the urinary secretion of uric acid.

urobilinogen (u'ro-bi-lin'o-jen). An excretory product in the urine derived from one of the bile pigments. Bile pigments are derived from degenerated hemoglobin.

urticaria (ur'ti-ka're-a). Hives, nettle rash.

valine (val'in). An essential amino acid.

vascular (vas'ku-ler). Pertaining to, or full of, blood vessels.

viosterol (vi-o'ster-ol). A solution of irradiated ergosterol in oil; vitamin D_2.

virus (vi'rus). A submicroscopic agent of infectious disease which proliferates only in the presence of living healthy host cells in the animal body or in tissue culture. Viruses are characterized by lack of metabolism.

Wernicke-Korsakoff syndrome (ver'ni-ke–kor-sak'of). A psychosis which is usually based on chronic alcoholism, probably due to prolonged thiamine deficiency.

WHO. World Health Organization of the United Nations, Headquarters, Geneva, Switzerland.

xerophthalmia (ze'rof-thal'mi-a). A dry and lusterless conditon of the conjunctiva of the eyes resulting from a vitamin A deficiency.

xerosis (ze-ro'sis). Abnormal dryness of the eye or the skin.

zein (ze'in). A protein obtained from corn, a prolamine, insoluble in water.

Index

Page numbers in *italics* refer to illustrations and tabular material.